Think Inside the Box

A COURSE PLANNING KIT THAT SAVES YOU HOURS OF TIME

Media Manager

ABC News Video Clips

NEW! Health Support
Manual: First Time
Teaching Tips & Visual
Lecture Outlines

MyHealthLab
Instructor Access Kit

Take Charge of Your
Health! Worksheets

Transparencies

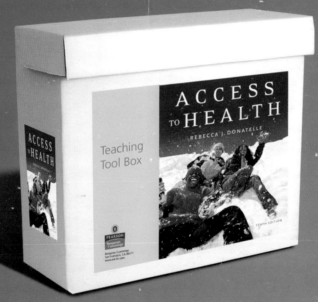

Clicker Questions for
Classroom Response Systems

NEW! Course-at-a-Glance

NEW! Game Show
Quiz Questions

Great Ideas: Active
Ways to Teach Health
and Wellness

Revised! Instructor
Resource Manual and
Printed/Computerized
Test Bank

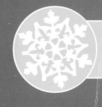

Teaching Tool Box

A COMPREHENSIVE INSTRUCTOR TEACHING TOOL BOX

MAKES CLASS PREP FAST AND EASY

Media Manager

This cross-platform CD-ROM includes all the PowerPoint® lecture outlines with embedded links to the ABC News video clips that can be customized for any lecture presentation. In addition, quiz show game and classroom "clicker" questions are included in PowerPoint® format. Additional resources include all figures and tables from the book, as well as Microsoft® Word® files of the Test Bank and Instructor Resource Manual.

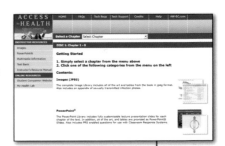

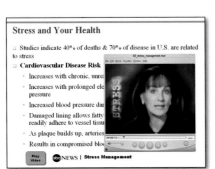

ABC News Video Clips

Created in partnership with ABC News, these 24 clips, each 8-12 minutes long, are a great way to start a lecture and spark interesting classroom discussions. And you'll find suggested discussion questions for each video on the Media Manager CD-ROM and in the Health Support Manual.

Think Inside the Box
A COURSE PLANNING KIT THAT SAVES YOU HOURS OF TIME

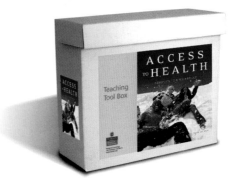

TEACHING TOOL BOX 0-321-49869-0

Save hours of valuable planning time with one comprehensive course planning kit. In one handy box, adjunct, part-time, and full-time faculty will find a wealth of supplements and resources that reinforce key learning from the text and suit virtually any teaching style.

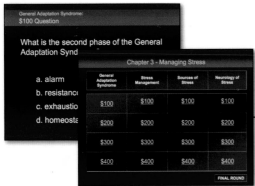

Game Show Quiz Questions

Students look forward to going to class when you make use of these questions styled after the popular TV game show Jeopardy. Provided in PowerPoint® format, you can use these questions in a variety of ways to reinforce key concepts.

COMPLETE CONTENTS OF TOOL BOX

- Media Manager
- Course-at-a-Glance
- Health Support Manual
- Printed Test Bank
- Computerized Test Bank
- Transparency Acetates
- Instructor Resource Manual and Media Guide
- Great Ideas: Active Ways to Teach Health and Wellness
- Game Show Quiz Questions
- MyHealthLab Instructor Access Kit
- Take Charge of Your Health! Worksheets
- Behavior Change Logbook and Wellness Journal

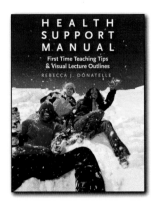

Health Support Manual: First Time Teaching Tips & Visual Lecture Outlines

Organized by chapter, this key manual provides a step-by-step visual walkthrough of all of the resources available to instructors. It includes information on available PowerPoint® lectures with the accompanying figures and art, integrated Lecture Launcher videos, suggested classroom discussion questions and in-class activities, tips and strategies for managing large classrooms, and the best ways to encourage active learning strategies.

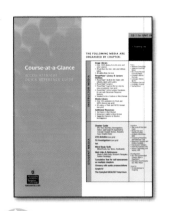

NEW! Course-at-a-Glance

This fold-out quick reference guide provides sample syllabi for both quarter and semester personal health courses. A great template for first-time instructors, or a rich resource of new ideas for established instructors, this concise guide presents an at-a-glance view of where the multiple course resources are located for both instructor and student support.

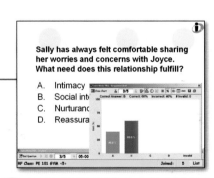

Clicker Questions for Classroom Response Systems

Now you can enhance interactivity in your classroom through clicker questions powered by the Classroom Response System (CRS) in PowerPoint® format. Use the questions provided—or import them into your own CRS—to start lively discussions and debates.

MyHealthLab

This online resource provides everything instructors need to teach the personal health course in one convenient place. MyHealthLab's course management system is loaded with valuable teaching resources that make giving assignments and tracking student progress easy.
www.myhealthlab.com

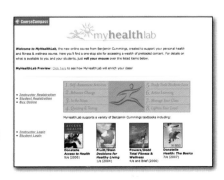

ENGAGE YOUR STUDENTS

Content updates

Today's students have many misperceptions about health. Through coverage of relevant issues, this updated text encourages students to be savvy and critical consumers of health information. And with the comprehensive supplements package and course planning tools, you can streamline pre-class preparation while teaching a course that students enjoy.

CONTENT UPDATES INCLUDE:

- Revised fitness chapter with more focus on daily physical activity
- Updated nutrition chapter featuring the 2005 dietary guidelines
- The latest information on coping with stress
- Hot topics such as fad diets, sleep, and the role of spirituality in a healthy life

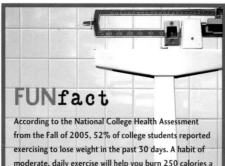

NEW! FUN FACTS ▶

Personalize health facts and statistics relevant to students and make learning even more enjoyable.

FUNfact

According to the National College Health Assessment from the Fall of 2005, 52% of college students reported exercising to lose weight in the past 30 days. A habit of moderate, daily exercise will help you burn 250 calories a day, or 91,250 calories per year, for a possible total weight loss of 26 pounds.

5

Healthy Relationships

COMMUNICATING EFFECTIVELY WITH FRIENDS, FAMILY, AND SIGNIFICANT OTHERS

NEW! CHAPTER OPENERS ▲

Introduce important health topics by grabbing attention with fascinating questions. The questions are repeated throughout each chapter, using a consistent design that shows students where to find the answers.

DOUBLE THE NUMBER OF PHOTOS ▶

Additional photos will visually engage students with more than 70 new ones appearing throughout the textbook.

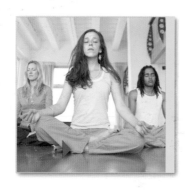

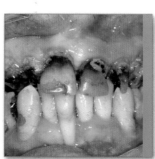

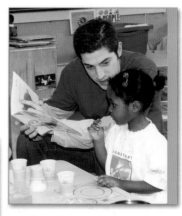

MOTIVATE STUDENTS

TO MAKE HEALTHY LIFE CHOICES

Does an **intimate** relationship have to be sexual?

How can I become a **better** communicator?

What can I do to cope with a **bad breakup**?

Is it good to **live** together before getting married?

How can I end a relationship without **hurting** my partner too much?

OBJECTIVES

- Discuss ways to improve communication skills and interpersonal interactions.
- Identify the characteristics of successful relationships, including how to maintain them and overcome common barriers.
- Explore similarities and differences between men and women in communication styles and decision making.
- Examine factors that are important in determining the success of an intimate relationship, and where to get help when a relationship has problems.
- Discuss actions that can improve interpersonal interactions.

Coping with Failed Relationships

What can I do to cope with a bad breakup?

No love relationship comes with a guarantee, no matter how many promises have been made by partners to be together forever. Losing a love is as much a part of life as falling in love. That being said, the uncoupling process can be very painful (see the Skills for Behavior Change box on ending a relationship). Whenever we risk getting close to another, we also risk being hurt if things don't work out. Remember that knowing, understanding, and feeling good about oneself before entering a relationship is very important. Consider these tips for coping with a failed relationship:[50]

1. *Recognize and acknowledge your feelings,* which may include grief, loneliness, rejection, anger, guilt, relief, or sadness. Seek professional help and support as needed.

2. ~~Find ways to express your~~

QUESTIONS

The questions that appear in the chapter opener are repeated within the chapter where the answers are found.

ASSESS YOURSELF! and MAKE IT HAPPEN! are combined

Assess Yourself! and **Make it Happen!** boxes are now combined in each chapter. The redesign of these features will further enhance students' assessment of their health behaviors, and strengthen the connection between assessment and action in making a positive behavior change. Students will be prompted to set a goal and make a plan right away, giving them a better chance of following through.

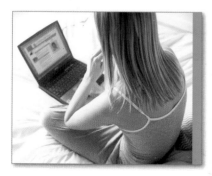

NEW! TRY IT NOW!

This feature motivates students to get an immediate start on a healthier life by highlighting the seemingly small, but highly significant, daily actions that can improve overall health.

try it NOW

Write it down! Journal writing is a great method to cleanse the mind, release emotions, and draft strategies for resolution. The next time you are feeling stressed, write down the event or situation that activated your stress response, identify the emotions that accompany it, and list several options to bring closure to the event. Writing these things down can be an effective means to cope with stressors.

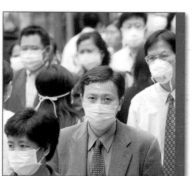

ADDITIONAL READING

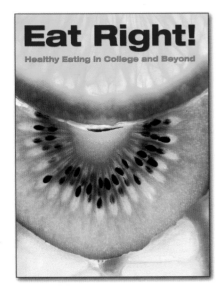

Eat Right! Healthy Eating in College and Beyond
by Janet Anderson, et al
0-8053-8288-7 • 978-0-8053-8288-4

This handy, full color 80-page booklet provides students with practical guidelines, tips, shopper's guides and recipes that turn healthy eating guidelines into blueprints for action. Topics include: healthy eating in the cafeteria, dorm room, and fast food restaurants; planning meals on a budget; weight management; vegetarian alternatives; and how alcohol impacts health.

Live Right! Beating Stress in College and Beyond
by Debra Atkinson
0-321-49149-1 • 978-0-321-49149-7

Live Right! gives students useful tips for coping with stressful life challenges both during college and for the rest of their lives. Topics include sleep, managing finances, time management, coping with academic pressure, and relationships. This book also presents an objective overview of some of the gimmicky health-oriented products now being advertised. Available packaged with a personal health text for no additional charge.

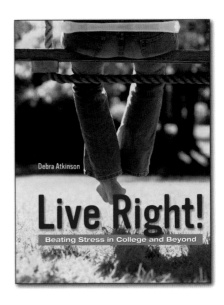

ADDITIONAL INSTRUCTOR SOLUTIONS FOR YOUR CLASSROOM

ABC NEWS LECTURE LAUNCHER VIDEO

0-8053-0438-X

DISCOVERY HEALTH CHANNEL LECTURE LAUNCHER VIDEOS

Vol. 1: 0-8053-5369-0 • Vol. 2: 0-8053-6001-8
Benjamin Cummings Lecture Launcher videos, created in partnership with the Discovery Health Channel, feature 24 video clips on health topics ranging from nutrition to stress management to substance abuse. Clips range from 5 to 12 minutes in length, and are available as a two-volume VHS set or on CD-ROM.

FILMS FOR THE HUMANITIES VIDEOS

Choose from more than 80 videos designed to supplement your lectures; available to qualified adopters.

CLICKERS IN THE CLASSROOM

0-8053-8728-5
Clickers (Classroom Response Systems) have quickly become one of the most popular and widely adopted new classroom teaching technologies in recent history. Whether you're a clicker novice or veteran, this is the book for learning how clickers can enhance your classroom lectures. In this handbook, experienced clicker educator Doug Duncan provides everything you need to know to successfully teach using clicker technology.

STUDENT SUPPLEMENTS

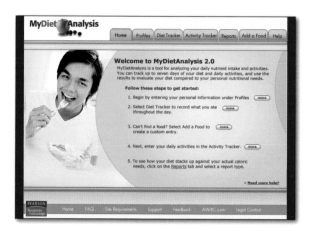

MyDietAnalysis 2.0 www.mydietanalysis.com
MyDietAnalysis 1.0 CD-ROM 0-3124-8799-0

MyDietAnalysis provides an accurate, reliable and easy-to-use program for students to analyze their diets effectively. This ESHA-based diet analysis software includes nearly 20,000 foods including ethnic foods, name brand fast foods, convenience foods, and supplements, and can be packaged with the text at a discount.

MyDiet Analysis

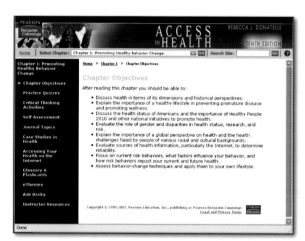

Companion Website www.aw-bc.com/donatelle

The companion website contains practice tests, activities, and web links to assist students in the study of personal health. The multiple choice and essay questions help students prepare for exams, while other activities may be completed as homework or extra credit assignments.

Take Charge of Your Health! Worksheets
0-321-49942-5

This collection of 50 self-assessment activities is available as a gummed pad and can be packaged at no additional charge with the main text.

MyHealthLab
www.myhealthlab.com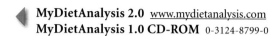
Turn the page to learn more about MyHealthLab.

Behavior Change Logbook and Wellness Journal
0-8053-7844-8

This assessment tool helps students track daily exercise and food intake and create a long-term nutritional and fitness plan. It also includes a Behavior Change Contract and topics for journal-based activities.

CLASSROOM RESPONSE SYSTEM

This wireless polling system enables you to pose questions, read results, and display those results instantly to your classroom. Whether you are considering a system for the first time or are interested in expanding a program department-wide, we can help you select the best system for your needs to accompany your Benjamin Cummings text.

COURSE MANAGEMENT OPTIONS

WebCT and **Blackboard** are available to make it easy to integrate online course materials into your course. All WebCT and Blackboard courses offer pre-loaded content including tests, quizzes, and more.

WebCT www.aw-bc.com/webct
Blackboard www.aw-bc.com/blackboard

EVERYTHING IN ONE CONVENIENT PLACE

ONLINE RESOURCES FOR BOTH INSTRUCTORS AND STUDENTS

MyHealthLab makes it easier than ever to organize your personal health class, personalize your students' educational experience, and push their learning to the next level. The site provides a one-stop spot for you and your students to access a wealth of preloaded content and tools for health and wellness.

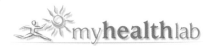

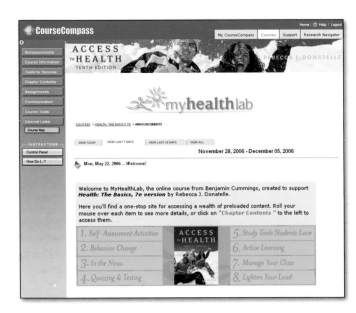

COURSE MANAGEMENT AND BEHAVIOR CHANGE TOOLS

MyHealthLab provides course management tools, including preloaded assignable quiz and test questions and a gradebook that automatically records student progress on assigned tests.

MyHealthLab also provides access to an interactive e-book and behavior change tools such as the "Behavior Change Log Book and Wellness Journal" with electronic journaling activities. Discussions of health issues in the news from a variety of resources, including the Link Library on Research Navigator™ are also included.

ELECTRONIC SELF-ASSESSMENTS

Students can access over 61 electronic self-assessments including in-text self-assessments and chapter-specific "Take Charge of Your Health! Worksheets."

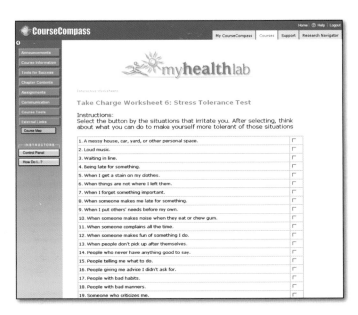

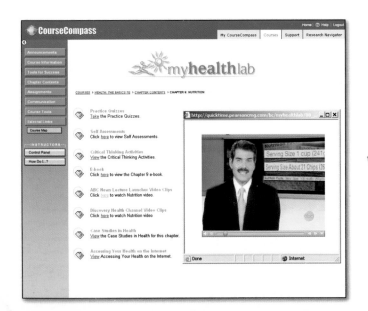

VIDEO CLIPS

Engage students and spark classroom discussion with ABC News Lecture Launcher video clips and Discovery Health Channel Health and Wellness video clips.

BEHAVIOR CHANGE CONTRACT

Complete the Assess Yourself questionnaire and read the Skills for Behavior Change box describing the stages of change. After reviewing your results and considering the various factors that influence your decisions, choose a health behavior that you would like to change, starting this quarter or semester. Sign the contract at the bottom to affirm your commitment to making a healthy change and ask a friend to witness it.

My behavior change will be:

_____

My long-term goal for this behavior change is:

_____

These are three obstacles to change (things that I am currently doing or situations that contribute to this behavior or make it harder to change):

1. _____
2. _____
3. _____

The strategies I will use to overcome these obstacles are:

1. _____
2. _____
3. _____

Resources I will use to help me change this behavior include:

a friend/partner/relative: _____
a school-based resource: _____
a community-based resource: _____
a book or reputable website: _____

In order to make my goal more attainable, I have devised these short-term goals

short-term goal	target date	reward
short-term goal	target date	reward
short-term goal	target date	reward

When I make the long-term behavior change described above, my reward will be:

_____ target date: _____

I intend to make the behavior change described above. I will use the strategies and rewards to achieve the goals that will contribute to a healthy behavior change.

Signed: _____   Witness: _____

Wondering how to eat a balanced diet?

Concerned about your drinking?

Looking for ways to reduce stress?

Hoping to quit smoking?

Here are all the tools you need to make it happen:

- Self-assessments to help you identify your strengths and your areas for improvement

- Behavior Change Contracts to help you put your goals for change into action

- Examples of students who made successful behavior changes

See the other side of this flap for a complete guide to the Assess Yourself self-assessments you will find in every chapter of *Access to Health*. Go to the "Make It Happen!" section at the end of each Assess Yourself for examples of behavior change plans. Some students' plans include:

BEHAVIOR CHANGE CONTRACT

Complete the Assess Yourself questionnaire and read the Skills for Behavior Change box describing the stages of change. After reviewing your results and considering the various factors that influence your decisions, choose a health behavior that you would like to change, starting this quarter or semester. Sign the contract at the bottom to affirm your commitment to making a healthy change and ask a friend to witness it.

My behavior change will be:

_____

My long-term goal for this behavior change is:

_____

These are three obstacles to change (things that I am currently doing or situations that contribute to this behavior or make it harder to change):

1. _____
2. _____
3. _____

The strategies I will use to overcome these obstacles are:

1. _____
2. _____
3. _____

Resources I will use to help me change this behavior include:

a friend/partner/relative: _____

a school-based resource: _____

a community-based resource: _____

a book or reputable website: _____

In order to make my goal more attainable, I have devised these short-term goals

short-term goal	target date	reward
short-term goal	target date	reward
short-term goal	target date	reward

When I make the long-term behavior change described above, my reward will be:

_____ target date: _____

I intend to make the behavior change described above. I will use the strategies and rewards to achieve the goals that will contribute to a healthy behavior change.

Signed: _____ Witness: _____

ACCESS
TO HEALTH

ACCESS

TO HEALTH

TENTH EDITION

REBECCA J. DONATELLE

Oregon State University

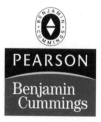

PEARSON

Benjamin Cummings

San Francisco   Boston   New York
Cape Town   Hong Kong   London   Madrid   Mexico City
Montreal   Munich   Paris   Singapore   Sydney   Tokyo   Toronto

Acquisitions Editor: Sandra Lindelof
Development Manager: Claire Alexander
Project Editor: Alison Rodal
Assistant Editor: Emily Portwood
Managing Editor: Deborah Cogan
Production Supervisor: Beth Masse
Production Management, Illustrator, and Compositor: The Left Coast Group, Inc.
Copy Editor: Anna Reynolds Trabucco
Photo Coordinator: Donna Kalal
Interior and Cover Designer: Yvo Riezebos Design
Photo Researcher: Kristin Piljay
Director, Image Resource Center: Melinda Patelli
Image Rights and Permissions Manager: Zina Arabia
Manufacturing Buyer: Stacy Wong
Marketing Manager: Neena Chandra
Text Printer: Courier, Kendalville
Cover Printer: Phoenix Color
Cover Photo Credit: Photodisc/Veer

Credits can be found on page C-1.

Library of Congress Cataloging-in-Publication Data

Donatelle, Rebecca J., 1950–
    Access to health / Rebecca J. Donatelle. — 10th ed.
        p.cm.
    Includes bibliographical references and index.
    ISBN-13: 978-0-8053-3249-0 (student ed.)
    ISBN-10: 0-8053-3249-9 (student ed.)
    ISBN-13: 978-0-321-46869-7 (professional)
    ISBN-10: 0-321-46869-4 (professional)
    1. Health. I. Title

RA776.D66 2008
613—dc22   2006100218

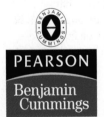

PEARSON

Benjamin
Cummings

www.aw-bc.com

1 2 3 4 5 6 7 8 9 10–CRK–11 10 09 08 07

PREFACE

It is difficult to imagine a time when concerns over health were not headline news. Fears over pandemic flu, new strains of infectious diseases, the safety of our drinking water, global warming and catastrophic environmental events such as hurricanes and winter storms, threats from sexually transmitted infections, and reports of epidemic increases in obesity and chronic disease seem to permeate our lives and cause concern for our future.

We are forced on a daily basis to make decisions that may impact our own health or the health of others based on a media blitz of information that is confusing to even the most savvy consumer. Will the foods we eat clog our arteries and cause cardiovascular disease? Is that person who sneezes two seats over in the airplane going to be responsible for our own illnesses? Should we eat more flaxseed to avoid risks from inflammatory diseases? Can changing our health behaviors really make a difference? In order to better understand the infinite health possibilities of our actions, it's necessary to look back and see how far we've advanced when it comes to health.

The challenges to our health that we face today could not have been imagined by our ancestors. Whereas pandemic disease has always been part of the human experience, modern-day issues were unthinkable just a generation or two ago. Disease and illness were seen as phenomena people had little power over and people who became sick from an infectious disease either weathered the illness and recovered or, in all too many cases, died. Few choices were available in foods, medicines, and services; consequently, health care decisions usually focused on cleanliness, avoiding known hazards, and staying away from others who were sick. Over the decades, our list of options for improved health has steadily grown. Improvements in vaccines and antibiotics, new treatments for a wide range of illnesses, and new scientific knowledge about risks and hazards have helped us sift through the information overload and begin to make some sense of things.

Juxtaposed against the threats to health are advances in medical research, recognition that we need to do more to remove barriers and reduce disparities for some groups when it comes to health, new attention to policies designed to preserve health and protect against harm, and improved strategies for promoting health and preventing premature disease and disability. Technologies continue to be developed, with concomitant improvements in diagnosis of disease and treatment. Daily, newspapers and scientific journals report evidence that

dietary choices, exercise behaviors, and improvements in interpersonal relationships really matter. At no time in history has it been more evident that by taking action, an individual can prevent illness and prolong a productive, fully functional life. Regardless of whether changes in public policy and community and corporate behavior are necessary to help improve health status, this much is true: the better individuals prepare themselves to make wise decisions, and the more community leaders and representatives of the health care system work together to help achieve and maintain excellent health status, the more likely that everyone's quality of life will improve.

Today's health-conscious individuals have an abundance of choice when making health decisions: pharmacies loaded with prescription and over-the-counter drugs, health food stores with thousands of products that claim to promote wellness and prevent illness, Yellow Pages filled with doctors and alternative practitioners to choose from, grocery stores and fast-food restaurants packed with every imaginable food, and transportation moving people to and from far-flung continents in a matter of hours. Books, television, the Internet, and other media-driven sources are constantly luring consumers into buying miracle products. Talk show hosts offer formulas for relationship success, sexual prowess, and a slew of other behaviors and products that promise happier and healthier living.

Each new class of college students represents a more savvy group of health consumers with its own unique perspectives on health. An astounding, often contradictory and confusing array of health information is available through the simple click of a mouse, the routine turning on of the television, cell phone, or other media device, or the casual perusal of a magazine. Because there is no one recipe for achieving health, it is important to consider the various opinions and options available to determine what information is the most scientifically defensible and which poses the least amount of risk to wellness.

After more than 30 years of teaching public health students from a wide range of health and other disciplines and after working on several editions of this book, I continue to be excited about the tremendous opportunities that students today have to make a difference to their health, the health of their loved ones, and the health of others. Part of my goal in writing this book is to help students be better "change agents" as they view the health controversies of today and those that will shape their future—not just in the arena of personal health behaviors, but also in the larger realm of policy changes and community behaviors, which ultimately can assist the global population in living smarter, longer, and better. In short, this book is designed not just to teach health facts but to present health as a much broader concept, something that everyone desires and deserves. By understanding the factors that contribute to health risk, exploring concepts provided in this text, contemplating action plans that might serve to reduce risk, and using the technological tools provided, students can take the first steps in accessing better health.

For health educators, preparing a new generation of students to be savvy consumers armed with accurate information for making wise health decisions is a formidable task. Writing an introductory health text for this population of students, in a field where information changes by the moment, can be extremely challenging. Clearly, no single text can answer all of a student's questions, give solid advice about all possible topics, or even attempt to cover the vast spectrum of hotly debated health issues.

Helping students select the best sources for information and teaching them how to ask the right questions is one of our primary goals. We want to teach students how to evaluate information and process it in a systematic, reasoned way as they endeavor to make informed decisions about health. We believe that by challenging students to think about and discuss controversial health topics, they will become the citizens that future generations can rely on to develop sound policies, programs, and key health services. This opportunity to assist a new generation of students to become future agents for change in the area of health is something we take seriously. Although issues of individual decision making and lifestyle are key features of *Access to Health,* we believe that individual health is also strongly influenced by public health actions and policy. Thus, we also focus on policies, programs, and services that promote health and prevent premature disease and disability. Each of us has positive assets and resources, as well as barriers and potential risks that make achieving health more difficult. Learning how to focus on our strengths and diminish our weaknesses is a key step in healthful living.

In addition, we are mindful of disparities in health and the underlying reasons for difference in risks based on race, ethnicity, age, gender, geographic region, and other factors. Recognizing that many of today's health problems know no national or international boundaries, we challenge students to think globally as they consider health risks and seek creative solutions to health problems. By reading, questioning, gaining greater understanding of the factors that contribute to individual and societal health, and contemplating possible actions that may reduce risk, *Access to Health* prepares students for their own development, as well as possible futures in the field.

As we prepared this text, we invited comments and suggestions on how to make this the best edition of *Access to Health* yet and the foremost personal health text on the market today. No text would be credible without scientific validation of information and inclusion of cutting-edge research on topics covered in each chapter. To this end, we have searched widely to insure that the information provided is accurate,

scientifically defensible, and representative of the latest and greatest scientific inquiries into human health.

We are pleased with the overwhelming success that *Access to Health* has enjoyed through its many revisions and changes, and we are gratified that many of you have continued to use this text. We hope that this edition once again meets the high standards we have previously established and that its rich foundation of scientifically valid and current citations, its wealth of technological tools and resources, and its thought-provoking exercises will continue to stimulate students to share our enthusiasm for health and to actively engage in health promotion and disease prevention.

New to This Edition

Each year as I face a new group of students, I am struck by the fact that these students will face a new set of health challenges surpassing anything that their parents or I could imagine at their age. These students must be able to find and assess accurate information about health, understand basic foundational material, and choose from a myriad of alternatives as they seek to maintain or improve their health. Each page of this text is designed to provide the latest information, engage students, guide them to reliable health information and services, and make health decisions based on the best science rather than pop mythology.

Though there are many well-written textbooks on the market, very few are written by actual health professionals who are trained in health promotion and disease prevention and who actually teach students, talk with them daily about their interests and concerns, and see their reactions to health knowledge in the classrooms of major universities. I believe that this helps make this text a "stand-out" in the introductory health market. I am committed to making this book an excellent tool for learning—and, with the help of an outstanding publishing team, I feel that it is the best edition to date.

As with previous editions of this text, I have ensured that this new edition provides students with the latest in research, discoveries, controversies, and realities that today's students face on a daily basis. This text maintains many features that it has become known for, while also focusing on exciting new health trends. The tenth edition has been updated, line by line; whether using classic references that helped set the stage for later discovery, current research from professional journals, or reputable national data sources, we have tried to provide students with not only the most current information, but also references for further exploration. This careful attention to detail ensures that students will be getting the latest information about health topics as this text goes to press. The most noteworthy changes include the following:

■ **Assess Yourself boxes now incorporate the Make It Happen! feature, previously located at the end of each chapter.** The Assess Yourself activity allows students to examine their health behaviors, and the Make It Happen! section provides students with a step-by-step guide to developing a behavior change plan, and includes one student's plan of action. The redesign of this feature will strengthen the connection between assessment and action in making a positive behavior change, giving students the tools they need to make real and lasting behavior changes, and something that can continue long after they have completed their health class. These assessments can also be completed online.

■ **New Chapter Opener questions touch on topics students are interested in** and help to capture students' attention and engage them in what they will be learning later in the chapter. Questions are repeated within the chapter, where answers can be found.

■ **The new Try It Now feature highlights simple actions a student can do immediately** to improve overall health and encourage positive lifestyle changes. These new activities, found in each chapter, further emphasize the overall course goal of behavior change, and the impact that small, daily changes have on overall wellness.

■ **New multiple-choice Chapter Review questions** appear in each chapter's Taking Charge end-of-chapter material, to help students immediately review what they have learned. Answers appear at the back of the text for easy chapter review.

■ **A brand-new design and enhanced photo program** includes a new chapter opener design, vibrant colors, redesigned boxes that key students into the importance of each type of box, and approximately five new photographs per chapter to enhance the visual appeal of the text. The redesign of the text provides the same pedagogical standards as in previous editions of *Access to Health*, with a modern and bold look aimed at engaging the student.

■ **New Fun Fact figures** highlight statistics and data that relate directly to the American college student population. These Fun Facts highlight the findings from the National College Health Association's National College Health Assessment, as well as numerous other studies that examine the health behaviors of college students. The graphic format allows students to visualize and personalize the information presented in each figure.

■ **The new Spotlight on Your Health box** replaces the Reality Check box from previous editions of *Access to Health*. This box highlights topics of particular interest and relevance to today's college student, such as common myths about marriage, the availability of emergency contraception, and the reality behind popular fad diets.

■ **References for numbered endnotes now appear at the end of each chapter.** This change will make it easier for professors and students to locate additional sources for i nformation and research. The references have also undergone a thorough review for currency.

■ **Updates on the status of our nation's health** include the concept of healthy life expectancy, improving overall quality of life, and health disparities that affect specific U.S. populations. We cover the latest trends and threats to health, including tobacco, emerging diseases, and obesity, and provide key information about risk reduction for major areas that are within individual control.

■ **Updated coverage of global health issues** acknowledges that in an era of constant travel and instant communication, we would be remiss in not addressing the interaction of individual, community, and global health. Textbooks that focus only on individual concerns leave out an important factor: we all live and work in a broader community and are increasingly affected by factors that evolve in our external world. Knowing how to cope and how to reduce risks at all levels is crucial to overall health.

■ **Updated information on the role our psychosocial health plays in overall wellness** covers the important role of adequate sleep in overall wellness, information on common sleep problems, the role of spirituality in enhancing psychosocial health, how certain personality traits may enhance our ability to cope with threats to psychosocial health, and how to evaluate your own level of happiness or satisfaction with life, and improve upon it.

■ **New information on how to evaluate stress levels,** the physical signs of stress, and techniques that can help students cope with stressful circumstances will give students valuable coping skills at a time when they are experiencing many changes, and new pressures associated with college life. This chapter also features revised references throughout, a new highlight box on the unique stressors international students face, and new coverage of common financial woes and how they can impact our stress level.

■ **New information on mental illness on campus** includes how to recognize depression, and ways campuses and universities are recognizing and addressing mental illness in college students. This coverage supplies students with the knowledge that they are not alone if they struggle with depression, and will help them to better understand how to recognize and cope with a deterioration in psychosocial health.

■ **Expanded and updated coverage on violence,** crime on campus, terrorism, and natural disaster preparedness is intended to increase student awareness of the tremendous toll that violence and disaster take. New facts and figures include trends in crime, the economic implications of crime, and the emotional and physical burden of violent crime among selected populations, particularly college students. Date rape, stranger rape, and marital rape are all discussed in terms of factors that contribute to these crimes, the impact on those affected by rape, and related societal issues. Precautions that students can take to stay safe, whether they walk home alone at night or live in an area at high risk for a disaster like an earthquake or hurricane, are discussed.

■ **Greatly updated nutrition information covers the USDA's new MyPyramid Plan.** It includes the key goals and features of the plan, detailed information on serving sizes and caloric needs, and the role of physical activity in the new plan. In addition, information on portion distortion, how to eat healthfully when dining out, and healthy eating tips for college students are discussed.

- **A revised fitness chapter** emphasizes the distinction between physical activity for overall health and wellness, and exercise for weight management or for the athlete. Examples of different types of activities to achieve different goals are provided. The chapter also explores the various contradictory activity guidelines prevalent in today's media, how to use interval training in your exercise routine, a new cardiorespiratory endurance assessment, eating disorders and obsessive exercise patterns in men, and strategies for starting and sticking to an exercise routine. We also cover a unique, often ignored, area: exercise programs for overweight, obese, and very out-of-shape individuals. Information on factors to consider when buying exercise equipment and fitness club memberships should be of interest to students of all ages.
- **A new figure looks at the rise in obesity rates throughout the last decade,** along with updated information on the global epidemic of obesity and the unique risks for people with weight problems. Risk factors for obesity, health problems related to obesity, new methods for assessing body composition, strategies for risk reduction, portion distortion, and the impact of advertising on the obesity epidemic are discussed.
- **Updated coverage of fad diets.** Coverage includes low-carb diets, low-fat diets, very low-calorie diets, and other weight management trends such as gastric bypass surgery, as well as information about the glycemic index and eating to control blood glucose and energy balance.
- **New and updated coverage of infectious diseases and chronic conditions** includes avian influenza, West Nile virus, meningitis, SARS, antibiotic resistance, hepatitis A, B, and C, tuberculosis, sleep apnea, and asthma.
- **Updated information is provided on the growing diabetes epidemic facing our nation,** including the relationship between diabetes and obesity, and information on evaluating your own risk for developing diabetes and actions you can take to prevent this chronic disease.
- **New coverage of widely publicized drugs** looks at drugs such as methamphetamine, GHB, Ecstasy, and other substances widely discussed in the media but whose risks are often misunderstood.
- **New information is included on recent steps the FDA has taken to ensure prescription drug safety** in light of health problems associated with the popular class of COX-2 inhibitor medications.
- **Expanded coverage of environmental issues and concerns** includes discussions of our roles and responsibilities for environmental health, conservation, and protection of the environment. We added updated information on overpopulation and the impact this has on our planet's resources, and new information on alternative energy resources, actions students can take to make their campus a "green" one, and the dangers from molds and other environmental health risks at home and outdoors. Comparisons

in consumption patterns between Americans and persons in other nations are designed to stimulate discussion and critical thinking.

- **Updated information on the newest contraceptive methods** available to students today, including their relative effectiveness, issues with use, and other key aspects of effective use, will be of interest. Lea's Shield, Ortho Evra, Seasonale, and Mirena are among the products described and assessed. Also included is information on ECPs, their safety, effectiveness, and controversy surrounding their availability.
- **The importance of creating a living will,** designating a health care proxy, and other difficult decisions brought to light by the Terry Schiavo case are discussed.
- **New coverage of topics of interest to college-aged populations,** whether the topic is gambling addiction, skin cancer and tanning booths, the connection between psychosocial health and sleep, or a vast array of other topics, we have tried to focus on areas of relevance to a new generation of health-savvy students. In many instances, we have updated facts and figures as we go to press and hope that you will find these data to be interesting and important.

If you have topics that you would like to see included or expanded upon, please feel free to e-mail the author at Becky.Donatelle@orst.edu.

Maintaining a Standard of Excellence

With every edition, the challenge has been to make the book better than before and to provide information and material that surpass the competition at every level. Thus, we have painstakingly considered our reviewer feedback from the previous edition and strengthened and improved pedagogical standards.

Chapter 1 establishes both the individual and social context of health and disease and promotes the importance of health to society as a whole, a dual approach used throughout the text. We believe that by using a dual approach, in which we acknowledge the many factors that may influence health decision making, students will have a more realistic approach to their own health. In order to assist students in their efforts to achieve health, we provide a foundation based on well-established theories of health behavior.

Decision making through critical thinking and awareness continues to form the cornerstone of each chapter. Pedagogical aids such as the What Do You Think? questions throughout the chapter encourage students to apply information acquired from the chapter to their own lives.

The roles of the community, health policies, and health services in disease prevention and health promotion are integrated throughout the text. The public health approach is often ignored in health texts in favor of individual action only. We believe that optimum health changes will occur only in environments that are conducive to change, in which individuals can maximize resources to make long-term behavior changes.

Within a strong pedagogical framework, the importance of building health skills is emphasized and integrated consistently throughout the text. Readers will learn specific applications in every chapter through the Assess Yourself, Skills for Behavior Change, and Spotlight on Your Health boxes, and Try It Now features throughout the text.

Special Features

Each chapter in *Access to Health* includes the following special feature boxes designed to help students think about healthy behavior skills, as well as how to apply the concepts in everyday life:

- **Assess Yourself** boxes provide quick, general indicators of personal health status in various areas, which students may consider when initiating behavior change. The Make It Happen! feature provides students with the opportunity to use the results of the self-assessment and create a plan for healthy behavior change.
- **Skills for Behavior Change** boxes focus on practical strategies that students can use to improve health or reduce their risks from negative health behaviors.
- **New Horizons in Health** boxes highlight new discoveries and research, as well as interesting trends in the health field.
- **Health Ethics: Conflict and Controversy** boxes highlight current controversial issues and allow students to explore their own opinions.
- **Spotlight on Your Health** boxes focus attention on specific health and wellness issues that relate to college-aged students. Statistical information and trends help students recognize risks as they relate to particular behaviors and outcomes.
- **Women's Health/Men's Health** boxes help students understand unique aspects of health for both genders.
- **Health in a Diverse World** boxes expand discussion of health topics to diverse groups within the United States and around the world.

Learning Aids

- Each chapter is introduced with **Chapter Objectives** to alert students to the key concepts to be covered in upcoming material.
- Groups of **What Do You Think?** questions that encourage students to think critically are highlighted and strategically placed throughout each chapter.
- To emphasize and support understanding of material, pertinent health terms are boldfaced in the text and defined in the **running glossary** appearing at the bottom of text pages.

- At the end of each chapter, the **Taking Charge** section wraps up the chapter content with a focus on application by the student. The Summary, multiple-choice Review Questions, Questions for Discussion and Reflection, Accessing Your Health on the Internet, and Further Reading sections offer more opportunities to explore areas of interest.
- **Health Resources** provides practical information in a convenient format at the end of the book. The Injury Prevention and Emergency Care section describes procedures that may prevent injury and save lives. Nutritive Value of Selected Foods and Fast Foods provides nutrient information for many common foods and can be used with the MyDiet-Analysis nutritional software described below. This section also includes a Behavior Change Contract and a sample filled-in contract.

Student Supplements

Available with *Access to Health*, Tenth Edition, is a comprehensive set of ancillary materials designed to enhance learning:

- **MyHealthLab** (www.aw-bc.com/myhealthlab). This online resource lets students access a wide range of print and media supplements that make studying convenient and fun. Contents include an interactive e-book, ABC News and Discovery Health Channel Lecture Launcher video clips, and over 70 electronic self-assessments. Contents also include selected logs and journaling activities from the Behavior Change Log Book and Wellness Journal, links to Research Navigator (three databases of credible and reliable source materials), and the text's Companion Website (described further below). The instructor resources on the site are described later in this preface.
- **Companion Website** (www.aw-bc.com/donatelle). This easy-to-navigate site offers 30 complete articles relevant to the text content from *The New York Times* and over 70 electronic self-assessments. The website also offers practice quizzes, open-ended critical-thinking questions, hypothetical case studies, and Web links for the Accessing Your Health on the Internet section found at the end of each chapter. The website includes the Flashcard program, with the entire list of terms and their definitions from the textbook available for study.
- **Take Charge of Your Health! Worksheets** (0-321-49942-5). This pad of 50 self-assessment activities allows students to further explore their health behaviors so as to make steps toward positive change.
- **Behavior Change Log Book and Wellness Journal** (0-8053-7844-8). This assessment tool helps students track daily exercise and nutritional intake and create a long-term nutrition and fitness prescription plan. It includes behavior change contracts and topics for journal-based activities.
- **MyDietAnalysis** (0-321-48797-4, access kit) (www.mydietanalysis.com). Powered by ESHA Research, Inc., MyDietAnalysis features a database of nearly 20,000 foods and multiple reports. This easy-to-use program allows

students to track their diet and activity using up to three profiles, and generate and submit reports electronically. It is available at a discount when packaged with Benjamin Cummings Nutrition, Personal Health, and Fitness & Wellness titles.

- **Stand-alone Access Code Tutor Center** (0-201-72170-8). Visit www.aw-bc.com/tutorcenter for 24/7 support from tutors who can help you get through some of the more difficult concepts you might encounter in your personal health course.
- **Live Right! Beating Stress in College and Beyond** (0-321-49149-1). New with this edition of *Access to Health*, *Live Right!* provides useful tips for coping with a variety of life's challenges, from sleep to finances, to managing time and academic pressures. Available at a discount when packaged with the text.

Instructor Supplements

A full resource package accompanies *Access to Health* to assist the instructor with classroom preparation and presentation:

- **MyHealthLab** (www.aw-bc.com/myhealthlab). This online resource provides everything instructors need to teach health in one convenient location. MyHealthLab's course management system is loaded with valuable free teaching resources that make giving assignments and tracking student progress easy. Powered by CourseCompass™, the preloaded content in MyHealthLab includes ABC News and Discovery Health Channel Lecture Launcher video clips, PowerPoint slides, Test Bank questions, Instructor's Manual material, and more.
- **ABC News Health and Wellness Lecture Launcher Videos** (0-8053-0438-X, VHS). Created in partnership with ABC News, these 24 clips, each 5 to 15 minutes in length, will enliven lectures, spark classroom discussion, and engage your students. They are also available on the Media Manager in the PowerPoint lectures, and on MyHealthLab.
- **Teaching Tool Box** (0-321-49869-0). Developed to support adjunct and part-time faculty teaching the personal health course, this kit will offer all the tools necessary to guide an instructor through the course. Requiring little to no preparation, this adjunct pack will provide detailed information on the resources available for each chapter, including

visual lecture outlines, class assignments, and discussion topics. The box includes the Instructor's Manual, Test Bank and Computerized Test Bank, Media Manager with ABC News Lecture Launcher videos, Course-at-a-Glance Grid, Health Support Manual, MyHealthLab Instructor Access Kit, Great Ideas: Active Ways to Teach Health and Wellness, the Behavior Change Logbook and Wellness Journal, Take Charge of Your Health worksheets, and transparencies.

- **Instructor's Resource Manual** (0-321-48948-9). This teaching tool provides student and classroom activities, chapter objectives, lecture outlines, and Companion Website resources to reinforce chapter concepts and develop effective student learning. It also includes ideas for incorporating the ABC News video clips into your course and discussion questions for the e-themes articles.
- **Printed Test Bank** (0-321-49107-6) and **Computerized Test Bank** (0-321-50018-0). The questions in the comprehensively revised test bank were reviewed by a panel of instructors for relevance and accuracy. The Test Bank includes approximately 2,500 multiple-choice, short-answer, true/false, matching, and essay questions, all with answers and page references. The cross-platform TestGen CD-ROM enables you to create tests, edit questions, and add your own material to existing exams.
- **Media Manager** (0-321-48949-7). This cross-platform CD-ROM includes figures and tables from the book and lecture outlines that may be customized for lecture presentation. In addition, links to media and appropriate questions for discussion have been added within each chapter lecture. It also includes the two-volume CD-ROM with ABC News video clips.
- **Transparency Acetates** (0-321-48761-3). The figures and tables from the text are also available as full-color transparencies.
- **Great Ideas: Active Ways to Teach Health and Wellness** (0-8053-2857-2). This publication provides effective, proactive strategies for teaching health topics in a variety of classroom settings, contributed by health educators from around the country.
- **Clickers in the Classroom** (0-8053-8728-5). This handbook provides detailed guidance in enhancing lectures using clicker (Classroom Response Systems) technology.
- **Course Management.** In addition to MyHealthLab, WebCT and Blackboard are also available. Contact your Benjamin Cummings sales representative for details.

ACKNOWLEDGMENTS

After writing ten editions of *Access to Health,* I can only marvel at the dedication and professionalism of the many fine publishing experts who have helped make such a text successful. With each subsequent edition of *Access,* their skills in dealing with the complexities and considerations of the publication process have become more apparent. Over the years, I have been extremely fortunate in having a steady stream of fine publishing teams to help me create the foundations of a text that was responsive to students, creative in approach, and reflective of the most important health trends of the times.

It is hard for me to believe that *Access to Health* is in its tenth edition! From my earliest teaching experiences at the University of Kansas to the present day, personal health books and the students who use them have undergone remarkable change. Formerly, college students didn't have Bluetooth phones and laptop computers, and their access to fast and high-quality information about health was limited to books and journals located on library shelves. Over the last editions, we've adapted to become more responsive to a new generation of students. Each step along the way in planning, developing, and marketing a high-quality textbook requires a tremendous amount of work by authors and the publishers that move the books from concept to reality. Since the acquisition of *Access to Health* and *Health: The Basics* by Benjamin Cummings, I have been extremely pleased by the professionalism, dedication, and attention to detail that this team has displayed as we've progressed through several editions of the text. They are truly outstanding and a pleasure to work with. From the highly skilled and enthusiastic Acquisitions Editor, Sandra Lindelof, to the outstanding editorial staff, I have been uniformly amazed at their consistent efforts to produce a great finished product. Although I wouldn't have thought it was possible to beat past publishing efforts, I must honestly say that my experiences with Benjamin Cummings have been the best of my publishing years, and, remarkably, they just keep getting better! The personnel personify key aspects of what it takes to be successful in the publishing world, from this author's perspective: (1) drive and motivation for hard work and efficient process, (2) commitment to excellence, (3) a vibrant, youthful, and enthusiastic approach that is in tune with college student needs, and (4) personalities that motivate an author to continually strive to produce market-leading texts. In previous editions of *Access to Health,* I was extremely impressed by the superb effort, expertise, level-headed perspective, and

guidance of Susan Malloy. With this edition, Alison Rodal has proved to be an outstanding addition to the writing team and provided the necessary skill, attention to detail, and creative flair that helped make this edition come alive. Like her predecessors, Alison is a wonderful project editor and it is largely through her efforts that this book was completed in a timely and efficient manner. She is very bright, creative, "gets it" when it comes to the needs of young adults, and is always thinking of innovative topics and cutting-edge research to stimulate college readers. I feel fortunate that Benjamin Cummings invests in its staff and picks outstanding professionals dedicated to producing high-quality texts. While authors provide the "bones" of the book, the editorial staff provides the flesh, life, and heart that entice students to step inside and enjoy the visual and pedagogical enhancements that make a book unique. Without her efforts, in particular, these texts would not have come to fruition or enjoyed the successes that they have achieved. Thank you, Alison!

In addition, I would like to acknowledge the wonderful editorial assistance provided by Developmental Editor Alice E. Fugate, who has been with this project for the last three editions. Her skill in helping merge text from *Health: The Basics* and *Access to Health* has been invaluable. In addition, she has made terrific suggestions on improving each edition of these texts based on reviewer comments and market demands. This was a huge and complicated task, and Alice did a remarkable job.

Although these women were key contributors to the finished work, there were many other people who worked on this revision of *Access to Health.* In particular, I would like to thank Beth Masse and The Left Coast Group for their invaluable assistance in final book development and refinement, and Emily Portwood, Assistant Editor, for overseeing the complete supplements package. I would also like to thank the Benjamin Cummings marketing and sales force, particularly Marketing Manager Neena Chandra, who does a superb job of making sure that *Access to Health* gets into instructors' hands and that adopters receive the service they deserve. This is an important, often overlooked, part of selling texts, and without Neena's direction and the superb work of a dedicated, professional sales force, *Access to Health* would not be as successful as it is. Part of the success of any book depends on those who work diligently to make sure that the strengths of the book are outlined and that instructors are able to make good decisions about what their students will be reading. In keeping with my overall experiences with Benjamin Cummings, the sales staff and editorial staff are among the best of the best. I am very lucky to have them working with me on this project and want to extend a special thanks to all of them!

Contributors to the Tenth Edition

Many colleagues, students, and staff members have provided the feedback, reviews, extra time and assistance, and encouragement that have helped me meet the demands of rigorous publishing deadlines over the years. With each edition of the book, your assistance has made the vision for *Access to Health* a reality. Rather than just creating an upscale version of a high school text, we have worked diligently to provide a text that is alive for readers. With each edition, we would not have developed a book like this one without the outstanding contributions of several key people. Whether acting as reviewers, generating new ideas, providing expert commentary, or writing chapters, each of these professionals has added his or her skills to our collective endeavor.

I would like to thank specific contributors to chapters in this edition: Dr. Christopher Eisenbarth (University of Idaho) did an outstanding job of updating and revising Chapter 3, Managing Stress, to reflect his many years of study and work in this area. Dr. Patricia Ketcham (Oregon State University), in Chapter 7, Reproductive Choices; Chapter 11, Addictions and Addictive Behavior; Chapter 12, Drinking Responsibly; Chapter 13, Tobacco and Caffeine; Chapter 14, Illicit Drugs; and Chapter 22, Consumerism, did a superb job of updating key chapters of concern to today's college students. In her position as Director of Health Promotion at OSU, she is in tune with the unique issues and concerns of students and is constantly developing strategies to help students achieve health and be successful in their college years and beyond. Dr. Peggy Pederson (Western Oregon State University), in Chapter 5, Healthy Relationships, and Chapter 6, Sexuality, provided both her expertise in this area and an engaging writing style that greatly enhanced the quality and presentation of updates to this chapter. Dr. Amy Eyler (St. Louis University) provided significant expertise and a wealth of teaching and research knowledge to update and expand Chapter 10, Personal Fitness. Several other individuals provided key information that helped insure an up-to-date published book. Graduate student Kelly

Droege provided invaluable background material and suggestions for enhancing Chapter 19, Healthy Aging, and Chapter 20, Dying and Death. John Kowalczyk (University of Minnesota, Duluth) created the review questions found at the end of each chapter.

Reviewers for the Tenth Edition

Clearly, *Access to Health* continues to be an evolving work. With each new edition, we have built on the combined expertise of many colleagues throughout the country who are dedicated to the education and behavioral changes of students. We thank the many reviewers of the past nine editions of *Access to Health* who have made such valuable contributions.

For the tenth edition, reviewers who have helped us continue this tradition of excellence include Leslie Hickcox, West Liberty State College; Denise Colaianni, Western Connecticut State University; Nick DiCicco, Camden County College; Molly Swick, Northern Illinois University; Benjamin Staupe, Rock Valley Community College; Shawn Houghton, Cabrillo College; Autumn Benner, Minnesota State University, Mankato; Gary McDowell, Tompkins-Cortland Community College; Jamie Rattray, Tompkins-Cortland Community College; Stephanie Perry, University of North Florida; John Kowalczyk, University of Minnesota, Duluth; James Maginel, Southeast Missouri State University; Marsha Greer, California State University, San Bernardino; Charlene Harkins, University of Minnesota, Duluth; Debra Atkinson, Iowa State University; Terry Silver-Davis, Tennessee State University; Brian Hickey, Florida AMU; Kim Clark, California State University, San Bernardino; Kathleen Malachowski, Ocean County College; Mary Iten, University of Nebraska, Kearny; Lana Zinger, Queensborough Community College; James Kahora, Middlesex County College; Cathy Hammond, Morehead State University; and Jennifer Howard, Morehead State University. Many thanks to all!

Rebecca J. Donatelle, Ph.D
Health & Kinesiology
Benjamin Cummings
1301 Sansome Street
San Francisco, California 94111

BRIEF CONTENTS

CONTENTS

FEATURE BOXES

ACCESS TO HEALTH

1

Promoting Healthy Behavior Change

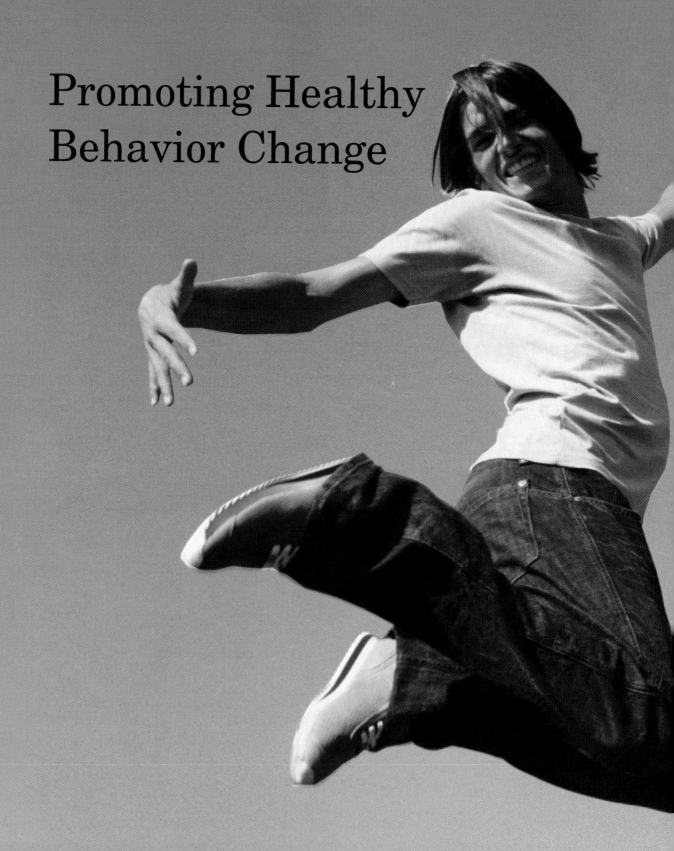

Are men and women different when it comes to their **health**?

Do my friends and family **influence** my health choices?

What can I do to **change** an unhealthy habit?

How can I **distinguish** between a bogus health claim and a real one?

How can I set a realistic health **goal**?

OBJECTIVES

- Discuss health in terms of its dimensions and historical perspectives.
- Explain the importance of a healthy lifestyle in preventing premature disease and promoting wellness.
- Discuss the health status of Americans and the importance of *Healthy People 2010* and other national initiatives to promote health.
- Evaluate the role of gender in disparities in health status, research, and risk.
- Explain the importance of a global perspective on health and the health challenges faced by people of various racial and cultural backgrounds.
- Evaluate sources of health information, particularly the Internet, to determine reliability.
- Focus on current risk behaviors, what factors influence your behavior, and how risk behaviors impact your current and future health.
- Assess behavior-change techniques and apply them to your own lifestyle.

Interested in improving your health? Concerned about the water you drink, the food you eat, or catching a new infectious disease like SARS or bird flu? If so, you are not alone. At no time in our nation's history have so many individuals, government agencies, community groups, policymakers, businesses, and health organizations focused so intently on a growing list of health-related issues. Epidemic rates of obesity and diabetes, a growing list of infectious and chronic diseases, a wide range of environmental threats, and other health problems are highlighted daily in the popular media. This widespread focus on health problems can make even the most healthy among us wonder what we can do to protect ourselves and our loved ones.

Juxtaposed against these very real threats to our health are the advertisements that offer pharmaceutical help for almost any problem. Drugs designed to help you get a full night of sleep, increase sexual responsiveness, reduce your levels of cholesterol, and eliminate stress, depression, or anxiety have exploded on the market. Books touting the newest "low-carb" fix for obesity and fitness regimens promising to give you that "six-pack stomach" fly from bookstore shelves. We are told that there are solutions to our health problems, and are led to believe that the fix is only a pill away.

For many of us, our health is a priority, and millions of us are working hard to try to change our lifestyles and improve our health. On a daily basis we are challenged to "Just do it, but don't overdo it"; "Be all you can be, but be yourself"; "Consider soy milk instead of regular dairy"; "Cut the bad carbs and bad fat, increase the good carbs and good fat"; and "Eat more fruits and vegetables, but make sure they are organic"—and "If you want to look and feel good, exercise, exercise, exercise!" Clearly, conflicting health claims abound, and we must learn to decipher health fads from truly reputable information. We often assume that the government, pharmaceutical industry, and medical profession will protect us or make everything better when we have a problem. Most of us are surprised when there isn't a drug to fix us or a treatment to make us better—or when we find out that the information we've received is, in fact, false.

Not only must we find reliable information, we must also be aware of how the media often exploits our weaknesses and businesses cater to our fears and desires through clever ad campaigns. Food advertisements encourage us to consume enormous portions of high-fat foods and influence us to eat when we aren't hungry, or are overstressed or feeling blue.

The struggle to make personal health choices is not just a matter of willpower and knowledge. Social and environmental conditions also play an important role in our options and health decisions. Positive lifestyle choices are even more difficult for people who lack the resources necessary to purchase healthy foods, have preventive screenings for diseases like diabetes and cancer, or join a gym to exercise indoors when the weather is too poor to get outside. Real disparities exist and not all have equal access to health opportunities. Many Americans, particularly students, have no health insurance or

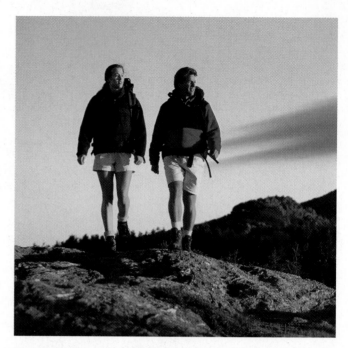

Today, health and wellness mean taking a positive, proactive attitude toward life, living it to its fullest.

are underinsured and only have coverage after paying large deductibles. These inequities in health care and information access can make our choices much more difficult.

In spite of the many challenges influencing our health, many people have made progress in reducing risks and making healthy lifestyle choices. Developing and maintaining healthy habits by becoming informed consumers takes work, determination, and time. Those who have achieved this goal ask more questions and learn to separate fact from fiction as they negotiate the various paths toward achieving health. Most importantly, these individuals have identified unique ways to make small changes to sustain long-term, positive behavior change. Learning to recognize unhealthy behaviors, identifying the factors that influence them, and planning the steps needed to reach personal health goals is a strategy that has worked for many.

This text cannot provide a foolproof recipe for achieving health or answer all of your questions. It is designed to provide fundamental knowledge about health topics, to help you use personal and community resources to create your own health profile, and to challenge you to think more carefully before making decisions that affect your health or the health of others. It shows how policies, programs, media, culture, ethnicity, gender, and socioeconomic status directly and indirectly influence health in the United States and around the world.

It is our hope that you will gain appreciation for the many achievements that we have made in health and the many challenges that lie ahead. In addition, we hope that you will begin to look at health not in an ethnocentric way, in which you are only able to appreciate those who look and talk like you and have habits and customs like yours, but rather in a more inclusive way.

NEW HORIZONS in health

Although the leading causes of death in the United States are usually described as selected diseases and conditions, the actual causes of these diseases have often been presented only as a footnote. These actual causes, also referred to as modifiable behavioral risk factors, help us understand the effects of recent trends and the implications of missed prevention opportunities. As shown in the figure, recent data from the Centers for Disease Control and Prevention (CDC) reveal that smoking is the leading cause of mortality in the United States, with poor diet and physical inactivity likely to overtake tobacco use as leading culprits in sharply rising death rates.

Note that many of these underlying causes are preventable. Their prevalence, along with sky-rocketing health care costs and an aging population, graphically point to the fact that we must work aggressively on more prevention and intervention programs. See the chapter for actions that you can take as an individual to reduce your own health risks.

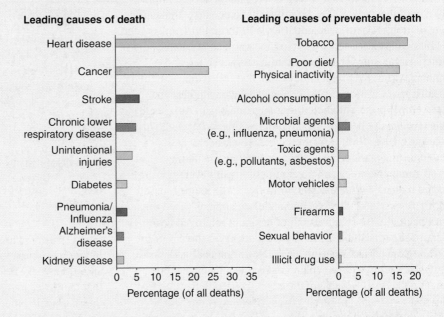

Leading Causes of Death and Leading Causes of Preventable Death in the United States, 2000

Sources: Leading causes of death data from A. M. Miniño, E. Arias, K. D. Kochanek, S. L. Murphy, and B. L. Smith, "Deaths: Final Data for 2000," *National Vital Statistics Reports* 50, no. 15 (Hyattsville, MD: National Center for Health Statistics, 2002), 1–120; leading causes of preventable death data from A. Mokdad, J. Marks, D. Stroup, and J. Geberding, "Actual Causes of Death in the United States, 2000," *Journal of the American Medical Association* 291, no. 10 (2004): 1238–1245.

Health decisions should be based on the best available research and should be consistent with who you are, your values and beliefs, and who you want to become. (See the Spotlight on Your Health box on page 18 for tips on using the Internet to gather valuable information.) Although health is not always totally within your control, certain behavior choices will affect you positively today and reduce future health risks. For risk factors beyond your control, you can learn to react, adapt, respond appropriately, and use a reasoned rather than purely emotional rationale for your choices. By making informed, rational decisions, you will improve the quality and the length of your own life and have a positive influence on those around you.

health simply means the antithesis of sickness. To others, it means being in good physical shape and able to resist illness. Still others use terms like **wellness**, or well-being, to include a wide array of factors that seem to lead to positive health status. Why all of these variations? In part, the differences are due to an increasingly enlightened way of viewing health that has taken shape over time. In addition, as our collective understanding of illness has improved, so has our ability to understand the many nuances of health. Our progress to current understandings about health has evolved over centuries, and we have a long way to go in achieving a truly comprehensive view of this complex subject.

Putting Your Health in Perspective

Although we use the term **health** almost unconsciously, few people understand the broad scope of the word. For some,

health   The ever-changing process of achieving individual potential in the physical, social, emotional, mental, spiritual, and environmental dimensions.

wellness   The achievement of the highest level of health possible in each of several dimensions.

Health: Yesterday and Today

Prior to the 1800s, if you weren't sick, you were regarded as lucky. When childhood diseases such as diphtheria were virtually unstoppable and deadly epidemics such as bubonic plague, influenza, and cholera killed millions of people, survivors were believed to be of hearty, healthy stock and congratulated themselves on their good fortune. Those in poor health often suffered from the stigma of being unsanitary and living in conditions that spread disease and harbored illness. Not until the early 1900s did researchers recognize that entire populations of poor people, particularly those living in certain locations, were victims of environmental factors (such as micro-organisms found in contaminated water, air, and human waste) over which they often had little control. Public health officials moved swiftly to clean water supplies and enact other policies to help those at greatest risk. As a result, the term *health* became synonymous with *good hygiene*. In the early 1900s, colleges offered courses in health and hygiene, the predecessors of the course you are taking today.

Throughout the years, perceptions of health were dominated by the **Medical Model**, in which health status focused primarily on the individual and a biological or diseased organ perspective. The surest way to bring about improved health was to cure disease in an individual, either via surgery or by treating the disease-causing agent. Restoring health via medicines or therapy was the main goal of this model, and government resources focused on initiatives that led to treatment of disease as a means of intervention. Even today, there are those who believe that it is cheaper to give someone a medicine to control a disease than it would be to prevent the disease from developing in the first place.

Around 1900, health professionals began to focus on an **Ecological or Public Health Model** of health. In this model, diseases and other negative health events are viewed more as a result of an individual's interaction with his or her social and physical environment. Thus, polluted air and water, hazardous work conditions, negative influences in the home and social environment, abuse of drugs and alcohol, stress, unsafe behavior, diet, a sedentary lifestyle, and cost, quality, and access to health care all are viewed as potent forces affecting one's health status. Because these external environmental factors affect health status, prevention must focus on both the individual and on improving policies and services that reduce risk. Under the Ecological Model, public health approaches work to improve individual health as well as the health of the population as a whole. The focus moves from treatment of

Medical Model   A model in which health status focuses primarily on the individual and a biological or diseased organ perspective.

Ecological or Public Health Model   A model in which diseases and other negative health events are viewed as a result of an individual's interaction with his or her social and physical environment.

TABLE 1.1	Ten Greatest Public Health Achievements of the Twentieth Century

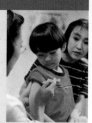

1. Vaccinations
2. Motor vehicle safety
3. Workplace safety
4. Control of infectious diseases
5. Reduction in cardiovascular disease (CVD) and stroke deaths
6. Safe and healthy foods
7. Maternal and infant care
8. Family planning
9. Fluoridated drinking water
10. Recognition of tobacco as a health hazard

Sources: Adapted from "Ten Great Public Health Achievements—United States, 1900–1999," *Morbidity and Mortality Weekly Report* 48, no. 12 (April 1999): 241–243; Centers for Disease Control and Prevention, "Poliomyelitis Prevention in the United States: Updated Recommendations of the Advisory Committee on Immunization Practices," *Morbidity and Mortality Weekly Report* (2000): 49 (RR-5).

individual illness to prevention of factors that cause illness and disease. By the 1940s, progressive thinkers began to note that there was more to health than hygiene or disease. At an international conference in 1947 focusing on global health issues, the World Health Organization (WHO) took the landmark step of clarifying what health truly meant: "Health is the state of complete physical, mental, and social well-being, not just the absence of disease or infirmity."[1]

Today, scientists recognize that health is much more than the absence of disease; in fact, today health includes multiple dimensions: the physical, social, and mental elements of life, as well as environmental, spiritual, emotional, and intellectual dimensions. To be truly healthy, a person must be capable of functioning at an optimal level in each of these areas, as well as interacting with others and the greater environment, in a productive and spiritually healthy manner. Rather than simply looking at how long we live, or the number of disease-free years we may have, public health researchers know that the quality of those years is equally important. Today, *quality of life* is considered as important as years of life.

Achievements in Public Health

To those of us in the field of public health, the saying "we've come a long way, baby" accurately reflects the health achievements of the past 100 years. Numerous policies, individual actions, and public services have worked to improve our health status. Table 1.1 lists the ten greatest public health achievements of the twentieth century.

Today, more people understand that it is often a broken "system" that causes major diseases to spread unchecked or for certain populations to be at higher risk for disease. As a classic example, consider life expectancy. In the early 1900s the average life expectancy in the United States was only 47 years, largely because of the vast numbers of individuals who died before age 5 from childhood diseases. Public health improvements in sanitation and the development of vaccines and antibiotics have added many years to the average life span since then.

Morbidity rates indicate that people less frequently contract common infectious diseases that devastated previous generations. Today, most childhood diseases are preventable or curable because of improvements in education, socioeconomic conditions, medical technology, vaccinations, and other public health measures. For these reasons, as of 2006 the average life expectancy at birth in the United States has risen to 77.85 years. According to **mortality** statistics, people are now living longer than at any time in our history.[2]

Will this trend continue? A recent study projects that today's newborns will be the first generation to have a lower life expectancy than that of their parents.[3] Largely attributable to the consequences of obesity, researchers report that life expectancy could decline by as much as 5 years over the next few decades.[4] It is also important to note that life expectancy predictions are just an average of the total population. Life expectancy can be affected by gender, race, and income. Though the average life expectancy of Americans as a whole has increased over the last 20 years, we rank 48th in the world, with countries such as Japan and Sweden leading the pack with life expectancies of 80 years and higher.

The Evolution toward Wellness

René Dubos, biologist and philosopher, aptly summarized the thinking of his contemporaries by defining health as "a quality of life, involving social, emotional, mental, spiritual, and biological fitness on the part of the individual, which results from adaptations to the environment."[5] The concept of adaptability, or the ability to successfully cope with life's ups and downs, became a key element of the overall health definition. Eventually the term *wellness* became popular and not only included the previously mentioned elements, but also implied that there were levels of health in each category. To achieve *high-level wellness,* a person would move progressively higher on a continuum of positive health indicators. Those who fail to achieve these levels may move to the illness side of the continuum. Today, the terms health and wellness are often used interchangeably to mean the dynamic, ever-changing process of trying to achieve one's potential in each of several interrelated dimensions. These dimensions typically include those presented in Figure 1.1.

- *Physical health.* This dimension includes characteristics such as body size and shape, sensory acuity and responsiveness, susceptibility to disease and disorders, body functioning, physical fitness, and recuperative abilities. Newer definitions of physical health also include our

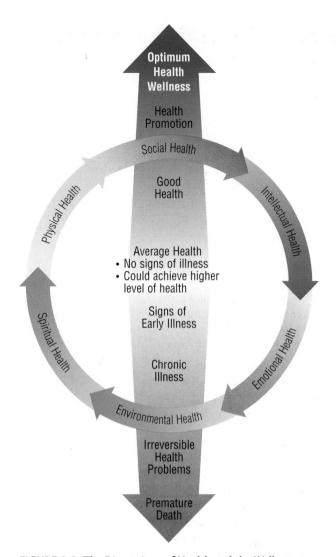

FIGURE 1.1 The Dimensions of Health and the Wellness Continuum

ability to perform normal **activities of daily living (ADLs)**, or those tasks that are necessary to normal existence in today's society. Being able to get out of bed in the morning, being able to bend over to tie your shoes, and other such tasks are examples of ADLs.

- *Social health.* This dimension consists of the ability to have satisfying interpersonal relationships: interactions with others, adaptations to various social situations, and daily behaviors.

- *Intellectual health.* The ability to think clearly, reason objectively, analyze critically, and use "brainpower" effectively to meet life's challenges are all part of this dimension. Intellectual health means learning from successes

morbidity   The relative incidence of disease.

mortality   The proportion of deaths to population.

activities of daily living (ADLs)   Performance of tasks of everyday living, such as bathing and walking up the stairs.

TABLE 1.2	How Many of These Healthy Behaviors Do *You* Practice?

- Get a good night's sleep (minimum of seven hours)
- Maintain healthy eating habits and manage your weight
- Participate in physical recreational activities
- Practice safer sex
- Limit your intake of alcohol and avoid tobacco products
- Schedule regular self-exams and medical checkups

Several other actions may not add years to your life, but they can add significant life to your years:

- Control real and imaginary stressors
- Maintain meaningful relationships with family and friends
- Make time for yourself and be kind to others
- Participate in at least one fun activity each day
- Respect the environment and the people in it
- Consider alternatives when making decisions; view mistakes as learning experiences
- Value each day and make the best of opportunities
- Understand the health care system and use it wisely

and mistakes and making sound, responsible decisions that take into consideration all aspects of a situation.

- *Emotional health.* This is the feeling component—being able to express emotions when appropriate, controlling them when not, and avoiding expressing them in an inappropriate manner. Self-esteem, self-confidence, self-efficacy, trust, love, and many other emotional reactions and responses are all part of emotional health.
- *Environmental health.* This dimension refers to an appreciation of the external environment and the role individuals play in preserving, protecting, and improving environmental conditions.
- *Spiritual health.* This dimension may involve a belief in a supreme being or a specified way of living prescribed by a particular religion. Spiritual health also includes the feeling of unity with the environment—a feeling of oneness with others and with nature—and a guiding sense of meaning or value in life. It also may include the ability to understand and express one's purpose in life; to feel a part of a greater spectrum of existence; to experience love, joy, pain, sorrow, peace, contentment, and wonder over life's experiences; and to care about and respect all living things.

Although typically not considered a dimension in most wellness continuums, **mental health** is an important concept.

mental health The thinking part of psychosocial health; includes your values, attitudes, and beliefs.

Often confused with emotional, social, spiritual, or intellectual health, it is a broader concept that encompasses all of these dimensions. According to the U.S. Surgeon General, this umbrella term refers to the "successful performance of mental function, resulting in productive activities, fulfilling relationships with others, and the ability to adapt to change and cope with adversity. From early childhood until late life, mental health is the springboard of thinking and communication skills, learning, emotional growth, resilience, and self-esteem."[6] Mental health is a critical public and community health priority. What are the characteristics a *well* individual might display? Table 1.2 lists some of these traits.

Many people believe that wellness can best be achieved by adopting a *holistic* approach, which emphasizes the integration of and balance among mind, body, and spirit. Achieving wellness means attaining the optimal level of wellness for a given person's unique limitations and strengths. A physically disabled person may function at his or her optimal level of performance; enjoy satisfying interpersonal relationships; work to maintain emotional, spiritual, and intellectual health; and have a strong interest in environmental concerns. In contrast, those who spend hours lifting weights to perfect the size and shape of each muscle but pay little attention to nutrition may look healthy but may not maintain a good balance in all areas of health. Although we often consider physical attractiveness and other external trappings in measuring the overall health of a person, appearance and physical performance indicators are actually only two signs of overall health, indicating little about the other dimensions.

How healthy are you? Complete the Assess Yourself box on page 10 to gain perspective on your own level of wellness in each dimension.

 what do you THINK?

René Dubos, a renowned bacteriologist who developed many key philosophies about health, is credited with saying, "Measure your health by your sympathy with morning and spring." What do you think Dubos meant by this statement? ■ Discuss how well your own health measures up when weighed against this criterion.

New Directions for Health

In 1990, the Surgeon General proposed a national plan for promoting health among individuals and groups. Known as *Healthy People 2000,* the plan outlined a series of long-term objectives. Many communities worked toward achieving these goals; nevertheless, as a nation we still had a long way to go by the new millennium.

TABLE 1.3   What Is *Healthy People 2010?*

OVERARCHING GOALS

1. Increase quality and years of healthy life
2. Eliminate health disparities

FOCUS AREAS

1. Access to quality health services
2. Arthritis, osteoporosis, and chronic back conditions
3. Cancer
4. Chronic kidney disease
5. Diabetes
6. Disability and secondary conditions
7. Educational and community-based programs
8. Environmental health
9. Family planning
10. Food safety
11. Health communication
12. Heart disease and stroke
13. Human immunodeficiency virus (HIV)
14. Immunization and infectious diseases
15. Injury and violence prevention
16. Maternal, infant, and child health
17. Medical product safety
18. Mental health and mental disorders
19. Nutrition and overweight
20. Occupational safety and health
21. Oral health
22. Physical activity and fitness
23. Public health infrastructure
24. Respiratory disease
25. Sexually transmitted disease
26. Substance abuse
27. Tobacco use
28. Vision and hearing

LEADING HEALTH INDICATORS

1. Physical activity
2. Overweight and obesity
3. Tobacco use
4. Substance abuse
5. Responsible sexual behavior
6. Mental health
7. Injury and violence
8. Environmental quality
9. Immunization
10. Access to health care

Source: Office of Disease Prevention and Health Promotion, U.S. Department of Health and Human Services, "Healthy People 2010," 2000, www.health.gov/healthypeople/About/hpfact.htm

Healthy People 2010 and Other Initiatives

A new plan, *Healthy People 2010,* takes the original initiative to the next level. *Healthy People 2010* is a nationwide program with two broad goals: (1) eliminate health disparities and (2) increase the life span and quality of life. The plan includes 28 focus areas, each representing a public health priority such as nutrition, tobacco use, substance abuse, access to quality health services, and common health conditions (for example, heart disease and diabetes). Under these focus areas is a list of Leading Health Indicators (LHIs) that spell out specific health issues (Table 1.3).

For each focus area, the plan presents specific objectives for the nation to achieve during the next decade. For instance, nutrition data show that only 42 percent of Americans aged 20 and older are at their healthy weight; the goal is to raise that number to 60 percent. In the focus area of physical activity and fitness, 40 percent of Americans aged 18 and older do not engage in any leisure-time physical activity. The objective is to reduce this number to 20 percent by 2010.[7]

Other programs and agencies also offer recommendations for improving overall health. In the public sector, the Agency for Health Care, Research, and Quality (AHRQ) offers additional direction for national health care efforts through its

AHRQ Guidelines, a set of objectives for health care providers to meet in specific areas of practice, such as treating pregnant women who smoke. The AHRQ also funds 13 Evidence-Based Practice Centers across the United States and Canada. These centers summarize key findings from the most current research, allowing consumers, policymakers, and health professionals to quickly make informed health decisions. The Institute of Medicine's *The Future of Public Health in the 21st Century* is another resource that recommends avenues of intervention for many critical public health issues.[8]

A New Focus on Health Promotion

The objectives of *Healthy People 2010* and other programs have prompted action to promote health and prevent premature disability through social, environmental, policy-related, and community-based programming. In addition, a new emphasis on assisting individuals in their pursuit of specific behavior changes is emerging. Changing behavior without help is not easy, however.

(Text continues on page 16)

ASSESS *yourself*

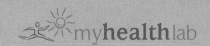

HOW HEALTHY ARE YOU?

Fill out this assessment online at
www.aw-bc.com/MyHealthLab or
www.aw-bc.com/donatelle.

Although we all recognize the importance of being healthy, it can be a challenge to sort out which behaviors are most likely to cause problems or which ones pose the greatest risk. Even when we recognize our unique risks and know what to do, it isn't always easy to stay motivated enough to maintain a specific set of health behaviors. Before you decide where to start, it is important to take a careful look at your health status right now. Think carefully about where you believe you are today in each of the dimensions of health. Circle the number in each category that you think best describes you. Rate your health status in each of the following dimensions by circling the number on the line that comes closest to describing the way you are most of the time.

	Poor Health		Average Health		Excellent Health
Physical health	1	2	3	4	5
Social health	1	2	3	4	5
Emotional health	1	2	3	4	5
Environmental health	1	2	3	4	5
Spiritual health	1	2	3	4	5
Intellectual health	1	2	3	4	5

After completing the above section, how would you rate your *overall* health?

_____

Which area(s), if any, do you think you should work on improving?

_____

If we were to ask your closest friends how healthy they think you are, which area(s) do you think they would say you need to work on and improve?

_____

By completing the following assessment, you will have a clearer picture of health areas in which you excel and those that could use varying degrees of work. Taking this assessment will also help you to reflect on various components of health that you may not have thought much about.

Use the results from this assessment as a guide and as a way to begin analyzing potential areas for improvement and/or maintenance. Answer each question, then total your score for each section and fill it in on the Personal Checklist at the end of the assessment for a general sense of your health profile. Think about the behaviors that influenced your score in each category. Would you like to change any of them? Choose the area that you'd like to improve, then complete the Behavior Change Contract at the front of your book. Use the contract to think through and implement a behavior change over the course of this class.

Each of the categories in this questionnaire is an important aspect of the total dimensions of health, but this is not a substitute for the advice of a qualified health care provider. Consider scheduling a thorough physical examination by a licensed physician or setting up an appointment with a mental health counselor at your school if you think you need help making a behavior change.

For each of the following, indicate how often you think the statements describe you.

	Never	Rarely	Some of the Time	Usually or Always
PHYSICAL HEALTH				
1. I am happy with my body size and weight.	1	2	3	4
2. I engage in vigorous exercises such as brisk walking, jogging, swimming, or running for at least 30 minutes per day, 3–4 times per week.	1	2	3	4
3. I do exercises designed to strengthen my muscles and increase endurance at least 2 times per week.	1	2	3	4

	Never	Rarely	Some of the Time	Usually or Always
4. I do stretching, limbering up, and balance exercises such as yoga, Pilates, or tai chi to increase my body awareness and control and increase my overall physical health.	1	2	3	4
5. I feel good about the condition of my body and would be able to respond to most demands placed upon it.	1	2	3	4
6. I get at least 7–8 hours of sleep each night.	1	2	3	4
7. I try to add moderate activity to each day, such as taking the stairs instead of the elevator and walking whenever I can instead of riding.	1	2	3	4
8. My immune system is strong, and my body heals itself quickly when I get sick or injured.	1	2	3	4
9. I have lots of energy and can get through the day without being overly tired.	1	2	3	4
10. I listen to my body; when there is something wrong, I try to make adjustments to heal it or seek professional advice.	1	2	3	4

Total score for this section: _____

SOCIAL HEALTH

	Never	Rarely	Some of the Time	Usually or Always
1. When I meet people, I feel good about the impression I make on them.	1	2	3	4
2. I am open, honest, and get along well with other people.	1	2	3	4
3. I participate in a wide variety of social activities and enjoy being with people who are different from me.	1	2	3	4
4. I try to be a "better person" and decrease behaviors that have caused problems in my interactions with others.	1	2	3	4
5. I get along well with the members of my family.	1	2	3	4
6. I am a good listener.	1	2	3	4
7. I am open and accessible to a loving and responsible relationship.	1	2	3	4
8. I have someone I can talk to about my private feelings.	1	2	3	4
9. I consider the feelings of others and do not act in hurtful or selfish ways.	1	2	3	4
10. I try to see the good in my friends and do whatever I can to support them and help them feel good about themselves.	1	2	3	4

Total score for this section: _____

EMOTIONAL HEALTH

	Never	Rarely	Some of the Time	Usually or Always
1. I find it easy to laugh, cry, and show emotions like love, fear, and anger and try to express these in positive, constructive ways.	1	2	3	4
2. I avoid using alcohol or other drugs as a means of helping me forget my problems.	1	2	3	4
3. When viewing a particularly challenging situation, I tend to view the glass as "half full" rather than "half empty" and perceive problems as opportunities for growth.	1	2	3	4
4. When I am angry, I try to let others know in nonconfrontational and nonhurtful ways and try to resolve issues rather than stewing about them.	1	2	3	4
5. I try not to worry unnecessarily and try to talk about my feelings, fears, and concerns rather than letting them become chronic issues.	1	2	3	4

(continued)

	Never	Rarely	Some of the Time	Usually or Always
6. I recognize when I am stressed and take steps to relax through exercise, quiet time, or other calming activities.	1	2	3	4
7. I feel good about myself and believe others like me for who I am.	1	2	3	4
8. I try not to be too critical and/or judgmental of others and to understand differences or quirks that I may note in others.	1	2	3	4
9. I am flexible and adapt or adjust to change in a positive way.	1	2	3	4
10. My friends regard me as a stable, emotionally well-adjusted person whom they trust and rely on for support.	1	2	3	4

Total score for this section: _____

ENVIRONMENTAL HEALTH

	Never	Rarely	Some of the Time	Usually or Always
1. I am concerned about environmental pollution and actively try to preserve and protect natural resources.	1	2	3	4
2. I buy recycled paper and purchase biodegradable detergents and cleaning agents whenever possible.	1	2	3	4
3. I recycle my garbage, purchase refillable containers when possible, and try to minimize the amount of paper and plastics that I use.	1	2	3	4
4. I try to wear my clothes for longer periods between washing to reduce water consumption and the amount of detergents in our water sources.	1	2	3	4
5. I vote for pro-environment candidates in elections.	1	2	3	4
6. I write to my elected leaders about environmental concerns.	1	2	3	4
7. I turn down the heat and wear warmer clothes at home in winter and use the air conditioner only when necessary or at higher temperatures in summer.	1	2	3	4
8. I am aware of lead pipes in my living area, chemicals in my carpet, and other potential hazards and try to reduce my exposure to them whenever possible.	1	2	3	4
9. I use both sides of the paper when taking class notes or doing assignments.	1	2	3	4
10. I try not to leave the faucet running too long when I brush my teeth, shave, or shower.	1	2	3	4

Total score for this section: _____

SPIRITUAL HEALTH

	Never	Rarely	Some of the Time	Usually or Always
1. I believe life is a precious gift that should be nurtured.	1	2	3	4
2. I take time to enjoy nature and the beauty around me.	1	2	3	4
3. I take time alone to think about what's important in life—who I am, what I value, where I fit in, and where I'm going.	1	2	3	4
4. I have faith in a greater power, be it a God-like force, nature, or the connectedness of all living things.	1	2	3	4
5. I engage in acts of caring and goodwill without expecting something in return.	1	2	3	4
6. I feel sorrow for those who are suffering and try to help them through difficult times.	1	2	3	4
7. I look forward to each day as an opportunity for further growth and challenge.	1	2	3	4

	Never	Rarely	Some of the Time	Usually or Always
8. I work for peace in my interpersonal relationships, in my community, and in the world at large.	1	2	3	4
9. I have a great love and respect for all living things, and regard animals, etc., as important links in a vital living chain.	1	2	3	4
10. I go for the gusto and experience life to the fullest.	1	2	3	4

Total score for this section: _____

INTELLECTUAL HEALTH

	Never	Rarely	Some of the Time	Usually or Always
1. I carefully consider my options and possible consequences as I make choices in life.	1	2	3	4
2. I learn from my mistakes and try to act differently the next time.	1	2	3	4
3. I follow directions or recommended guidelines, avoid risks, and act in ways likely to keep myself and others safe.	1	2	3	4
4. I consider myself a wise health consumer and check reliable information sources before making decisions.	1	2	3	4
5. I am alert and ready to respond to life's challenges in ways that reflect thought and sound judgment.	1	2	3	4
6. I have at least one hobby, learning activity, or personal growth activity that I make time for each week; something that improves me as a person.	1	2	3	4
7. I actively learn all I can about products and services before making decisions.	1	2	3	4
8. I manage my time well rather than let time manage me.	1	2	3	4
9. My friends and family trust my judgment.	1	2	3	4
10. I think about my self-talk (the things I tell myself) and then examine the evidence to see if my perceptions and feelings are sound.	1	2	3	4

Total score for this section: _____

Although each of these six dimensions of health is important, there are some factors that don't readily fit one dimension. As college students, you face some unique risks that others may not have. For this reason, we have added a section to this self-assessment that focuses on personal health promotion and disease prevention. Answer these questions and add your results to the Personal Checklist in the following section.

PERSONAL HEALTH PROMOTION/DISEASE PREVENTION

	Never	Rarely	Some of the Time	Usually or Always
1. I know the warning signs of common sexually transmitted infections, such as genital warts (HPV), chlamydia, and herpes, and read new information about these diseases as a way of protecting myself.	1	2	3	4
2. If I were to be sexually active, I would use protection such as latex condoms, dental dams, and other means of reducing my risk of sexually transmitted infections.	1	2	3	4
3. I find ways other than binge drinking when at parties or during happy hours to loosen up and have a good time.	1	2	3	4

(continued)

	Never	Rarely	Some of the Time	Usually or Always
4. When I have more than 1 or 2 drinks, I ask someone who is not drinking to drive me and my friends home.	1	2	3	4
5. I have eaten too much in the last month and have forced myself to vomit to avoid gaining weight.	4	3	2	1
6. I have several piercings and have found that I enjoy the rush that comes with each piercing event.	4	3	2	1
7. If I were to have a tattoo or piercing, I would go to a reputable person who follows strict standards of sterilization and precautions against bloodborne disease transmission.	1	2	3	4
8. I engage in extreme sports and find that I enjoy the highs that come with risking bodily harm through physical performance.	4	3	2	1
9. I am careful not to mix alcohol or other drugs with prescription and over-the-counter drugs.	1	2	3	4
10. I practice monthly breast/testicle self-examinations.	1	2	3	4

Total score for this section: _____

PERSONAL CHECKLIST

Now, total your scores in each of the health dimensions and compare them to what would be considered optimal scores. Which areas do you need to work on? How does your score compare with how you rated yourself in the first part of the questionnaire?

	Ideal Score	Your Score
Physical health	40	_____
Social health	40	_____
Emotional health	40	_____
Environmental health	40	_____
Spiritual health	40	_____
Intellectual health	40	_____
Personal health promotion/ disease prevention	40	_____

What Your Scores in Each Category Mean

Scores of 35–40: Outstanding! Your answers show that you are aware of the importance of these behaviors in your overall health. More important, you are putting your knowledge to work for you by practicing good health habits that should reduce your overall risks. Although you received a very high score on this part of the test, you may want to consider areas where your scores could be improved.

Scores of 30–34: Your health practices in these areas are very good, but there is room for improvement. Look again at the items you answered that scored one or two points. What changes could you make to improve your score? Even a small change in behavior can help you achieve better health.

Scores of 20–29: Your health risks are showing! Find information about the risks you are facing and why it is important to change these behaviors. Perhaps you need help in deciding how to make the changes you desire. Assistance is available from this book, your professor, and student health services at your school.

Scores below 20: You may be taking unnecessary risks with your health. Perhaps you are not aware of the risks and what to do about them. Identify each risk area and make a mental note as you read the associated chapter in the book. Whenever possible, seek additional resources, either on your campus or through your local community health resources, and make a serious commitment to behavior change. If any area is causing you to be less than functional in your class work or personal life, seek professional help. In this book you will find the information you need to help you improve your scores and your health. Remember that these scores are only indicators, not diagnostic tools.

MAKE it happen!

ASSESSMENT: The Assess Yourself activity gave you the chance to look at the status of your health in several dimensions. Now that you have considered these results, you can begin to take steps toward changing certain behaviors that may be detrimental to your health.

MAKING A CHANGE: In order to change your behavior, you need to develop a plan. Follow the steps below and complete your Behavior Change Contract to take action.

1. Evaluate your behavior and identify patterns and specific things you are doing. What can you change now? What can you change in the near future?

2. Select one pattern of behavior that you want to change.

3. Fill out the Behavior Change Contract found at the front of your book. It should include your long-term goal for change, your short-term goals, the rewards you'll give yourself for reaching these goals, potential obstacles along the way, and strategies for overcoming these obstacles. For each goal, list the small steps and specific actions that you will take.

4. Chart your progress in a journal. At the end of a week, consider how successful you were in following your plan. What helped you be successful? What made change more difficult? What will you do differently next week?

5. Revise your plan as needed: Are the short-term goals attainable? Are the rewards satisfying?

ONE STUDENT'S PLAN: Felipe assessed his health and discovered that his score in the personal health promotion section was low—25 points—because of some risky behaviors in which he was engaging. In particular, he realized that he had driven several times after drinking and that he was not performing monthly testicle self-examinations. Felipe decided to tackle one of these issues at a time. He completed a Behavior Change Contract to drive only when he had had fewer than two drinks. Steps in his contract included finding out about designated driver programs, moderating his drinking so that he was sober and competent to drive at the end of a night out with friends, and finding concerts and other events to attend that did not involve drinking. The rewards he chose for these steps included tickets to a concert and a new computer game. After a few months Felipe realized that he had been in several situations in which he might previously have driven under the influence. Instead, he had given himself alternatives such as designated drivers, budgeting for a taxi, and moderating his drinking, and thus had avoided unsafe situations.

Next month, Felipe will get a pamphlet from the health center on testicular self-exams and choose a day of the month to be his self-examination day. Every month that he does the exam, he'll sleep in an extra hour that weekend as a reward.

The term **health promotion** describes the educational, organizational, procedural, environmental, social, and financial supports that help individuals and groups reduce negative health behaviors and promote positive change. Health promotion programs identify healthy people who are engaging in **risk behaviors** (behaviors that increase susceptibility to negative health outcomes), motivate them to change their actions, and provide support that increases chances of success. Effective stop-smoking programs, for instance, don't simply say "Just do it." Instead, they provide information about risk behaviors and possible consequences to smokers and their secondhand smoke victims (educational supports); they encourage smokers to participate in smoking cessation classes and encourage employers to allow time off for worker attendance, or they set up buddy systems of social supports to help them (organizational supports); they establish rules governing smokers' behaviors and supporting their decisions to change, such as banning smoking in the workplace and removing cigarettes from vending machines (environmental supports); and they may provide monetary incentives to motivate people to participate (financial supports).

Health promotion programs also encourage those with sound health habits to maintain them. By attempting to modify behaviors, increase skills, change attitudes, increase knowledge, influence values, and improve health-related decision making, health promotion goes well beyond the simple information campaign. By basing programs and services in communities, organizations, schools, and other places where many people spend their time, health promotion increases the likelihood of long-term success in achieving health and wellness.

Whether we use the term *health* or *wellness,* we are talking about a person's overall responses to the challenges of living. Occasional dips into the ice cream bucket and other dietary slips, failures to exercise every day, flare-ups of anger, and other deviations from optimal behavior should not be viewed as major failures. Actually, the ability to recognize that each of us is an imperfect being, attempting to adapt in an imperfect world, signals individual well-being.

We must also remember to be tolerant of others. Rather than be warriors against pleasure in our zeal to change the health behaviors of others, we need to be supportive, understanding, and nonjudgmental in recognizing our unique differences. Health bashing—intolerance or negative feelings, words, or actions aimed at people who fail to meet our own expectations of health—may indicate our own deficiencies in the psychological, social, and/or spiritual dimensions of health.

Disease Prevention

Most health promotion initiatives include the term **disease prevention**. What does it really mean? Historically, the health literature describes three types of prevention: primary, secondary, and tertiary.

In a general sense, *prevention* means taking positive actions *now* to avoid becoming sick *later.* Getting immunized against diseases such as polio, deciding not to smoke cigarettes, and practicing safer sex constitute **primary prevention**—actions designed to reduce risk and avoid health problems before they start. **Secondary prevention** (also referred to as intervention) involves recognizing health risks or problems early and taking action (intervening) to stop the behavior before it leads to actual illness. Getting a young smoker to quit or reduce the number of cigarettes smoked is an example of secondary prevention. The third type of prevention, **tertiary prevention**, involves treatment and/or rehabilitation after the person is already ill. Typically, licensed health care professionals practice tertiary prevention.

Health Status Report: How Well Are We Doing?

In the United States, chronic diseases account for seven of the ten leading causes of death, and are linked to preventable lifestyle behaviors such as tobacco use, poor nutrition, and lack of physical activity leading to obesity, alcohol use, car crashes, risky sexual behavior, and drug use.[9] These preventable risk behaviors not only kill us, but they affect quality of life for nearly 100 million Americans and account for seventy percent of total medical expenditures.[10]

Primary and secondary prevention offer our best hope for reducing the **incidence** (number of new cases) and **prevalence** (number of existing cases) of disease and disability. Community intervention programs have proved effective and certain ones have become model programs for public health.[11]

A focus on prevention and early intervention rather than tertiary prevention can create a significant decrease in chronic diseases and the tolls they take on U.S. citizens. Health educators in our schools and communities offer an effective delivery mechanism for prevention and intervention programs.

---

health promotion   Combined educational, organizational, policy, financial, and environmental supports to help people reduce negative health behaviors and promote positive change.

risk behaviors   Behaviors that increase susceptibility to negative health outcomes.

disease prevention   Actions or behaviors designed to keep people from getting sick.

primary prevention   Actions designed to stop problems before they start.

secondary prevention (intervention)   Intervention early in the development of a health problem.

tertiary prevention   Treatment and/or rehabilitation efforts.

incidence   The number of new cases.

prevalence   The number of existing cases.

Certified Health Education Specialists (CHES) make up a trained cadre of public health educators with special credentials and competencies in planning, implementing, and evaluating prevention programs that offer scientific, valid, and behaviorally sound methods to help individuals and communities achieve optimal health. Trained exercise science and nutrition specialists can provide excellent advice on dietary and exercise behaviors that support specific aspects of health promotion activities. Together, these specialists have the skills and experience to greatly enhance the nation's health. A major shift in focus from treatment to prevention is necessary to achieve our national goals.

Improving Quality of Life

In the last decade, a shift in the way we look at health has been quietly emerging. This new view will have a profound impact on how we perceive our nation's health status. For decades we have looked at our steadily increasing life expectancy rates and proudly proclaimed that the health of Americans has never been better. However, recently health organizations and international groups have attempted to quantify the number of years a person lives with a disability or illness, compared with the number of healthy years. The World Health Organization summarizes this concept as **healthy life expectancy**. Simply stated, healthy life expectancy refers to the number of years a newborn can expect to live in full health, based on current rates of illness and mortality. For example, if we could delay the onset of diabetes so that a person didn't develop the disease until she was 60 years old, rather than developing it at 30, there would be a dramatic increase in this individual's healthy life expectancy. Several countries are currently working to develop policies that strive to increase healthy life expectancy.[12] A focus on disease prevention that improves quality of life could motivate individuals to change health risk behaviors earlier.

This concept of healthy life expectancy can have tremendous implications for your own health. Although you know that you should exercise, maintain a healthy weight, and not drink and drive, the threat of heart disease, cancer, or accident-related injuries seems decades away. Recognizing how your actions now will play a role in your future health can motivate you to make behavior changes to ensure the maximum number of happy, healthy years.

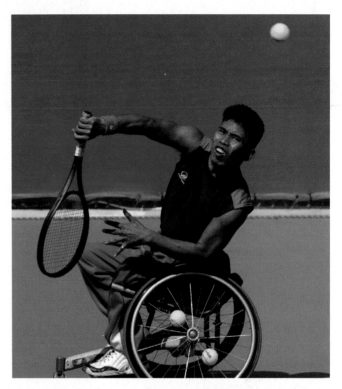

The motivation to improve quality of life within the framework of one's own unique capabilities is crucial to achieving health and wellness.

Reducing Health Disparities: New Challenges

The dramatic improvements in the health and life span of Americans in the twentieth century are largely the result of interactions between factors such as socioeconomic status, race, environment, education, cultural influences, and access to high-quality and affordable health care.[13] However, some populations are at a distinct disadvantage when it comes to getting healthy and staying healthy. For example, if you are a college student without health insurance and are on a limited budget, you may put off a visit to the doctor, or not go at all. If you have a serious illness, this can lower your chance of successful treatment. Factors such as language barriers can also impact an individual's health negatively. A recent study by the UCLA Center for Health Policy Research reported that

Certified Health Education Specialist (CHES) An academically trained health educator who has passed a national competency examination for prevention and intervention programming.

healthy life expectancy The equivalent number of years a newborn can expect to live, based on current rates of illness and mortality.

SPOTLIGHT on your health

FINDING RELIABLE HEALTH INFORMATION ON THE INTERNET

Seventy percent of college students obtain health information from the Internet. This makes the Internet second only to students' parents as a source of information.*

The Internet can be a wonderful resource for rapid answers. However, some of the answers you'll find are better than others. If you're not careful, you could end up feeling frazzled, confused, and—worst of all—misinformed.

How can I distinguish between a bogus health claim and a real one?

How can you maximize your chances of locating high-quality information? Follow these tips:

- Look for websites sponsored by an official government agency, a university or college, or a hospital/medical center. These typically offer accurate, up-to-date information about a wide range of health topics. Government sites are easily identified by their .gov extensions (for example, the National Institute of Mental Health is www.nimh.nih.gov); college and university sites typically have .edu extensions (Johns Hopkins University is www.jhu.edu). Hospitals often have a .org extension (Mayo Clinic: www.mayoclinic.org). Major philanthropic foundations, such as the Robert Wood Johnson Foundation, the Legacy Foundation, the Kellogg Foundation, and others, often provide information about selected health topics.
- Search for well-established, professionally peer-reviewed journals such as *The New England Journal of Medicine*

(www.nejm.org) or the *Journal of the American Medical Association (JAMA)* (http://jama.ama.org). Although some of these sites require a fee for access, often you can locate concise abstracts and information, such as a weekly table of contents, that can help you conduct a search. Other times, you can pay a basic fee for a certain number of hours of unlimited searching. You may also find that your college or university library receives an online subscription to a number of these journals.

- Consult the Centers for Disease Control and Prevention (www.cdc.gov) for consumer news and updates. The CDC also provides consumer alerts on topics such as buying antibiotics online and e-mail health hoaxes.
- For a global perspective on health issues, visit the World Health Organization (www.who.int/en).
- There are many government and education-based sites that are independently sponsored and reliable. The following is just a sample. We'll provide more in each chapter as we cover specific topics:
  1. Aetna Intelihealth: www.intelihealth.com
  2. Dr. Koop.com: www.drkoop.com
  3. Drug Infonet: www.druginfonet.com
  4. Health AtoZ.com: www.healthatoz.com
  5. WebMD health: http://my.webmd.com

The American Accreditation Healthcare Commission (www.urac.org), has devised over 50 criteria that health sites must satisfy to display its seal. Look for the "URAC Accredited Health Web Site"

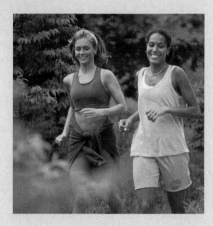

seal on websites you visit. In addition to policing the accuracy of health claims, URAC evaluates health information and provides a forum for reporting misinformation, privacy violations, and other complaints.

- And finally, don't believe everything you read. Cross-check information against reliable sources to see if facts and figures are consistent. Be especially wary of websites that try to sell you something. Just because a source claims to be a physician or an expert does not mean that this is true. When in doubt, check with your own physician, health education professor, or state health division website.

Sources: American College Health Association, "American College Health Association–National College Health Assessment (ACHA-NCHA) Web Summary," 2006, www.acha.org/projects _programs/ncha_sampledata.cfm. URAC, "Overview of URAC's Health Web Site Accreditation Review," 2006, www.urac.org/consumer_review .asp. *American College Health Association-National College Health Assessment, 2005.

---

health disparities   Differences in the incidence, prevalence, mortality, and burden of diseases and other health conditions among specific population groups.

people whose primary language is not English or who could not read prescription labels or follow written medical instructions had significant barriers to overall health.[14]

Recognizing the vast differences in health status, the *Healthy People 2010* plan included strong language about the importance of reducing **health disparities**, the differences in the incidence, prevalence, mortality, and burden of diseases and other adverse health conditions that exist among specific population groups in the United States and globally.[15]

Contributors to disparities include such factors as:

- *Race and ethnicity.* Research indicates dramatic health disparities among those with specific racial and ethnic backgrounds. These differences are not actually believed to be attributed to race or genetic susceptibility, but rather to socioeconomic differences, poor access to health care, cultural barriers, beliefs, discrimination, and limited education and employment opportunities.
- *Inadequate health insurance.* Large numbers of people are *uninsured* or *underinsured.* Those who do not have adequate insurance coverage may face high copayments, high deductibles, or limited care in their area (for more on health insurance, see Chapter 22).
- *Lifestyle behaviors.* Persistent poverty may make it difficult to buy healthy foods, get enough rest and exercise, cope with stress, and seek preventive medicine. Obesity, smoking, and lack of exercise are examples of health problems directly related to behavioral and cultural patterns we adopt from our families.
- *Transportation.* Whether you live in an urban or a rural area and have access to public transportation or your own vehicle can have a huge impact on what you choose to eat or your ability to visit the doctor or dentist. The elderly, the disabled, and those who lack the financial means to travel for preventive tests such as mammograms are clearly at a health disadvantage.

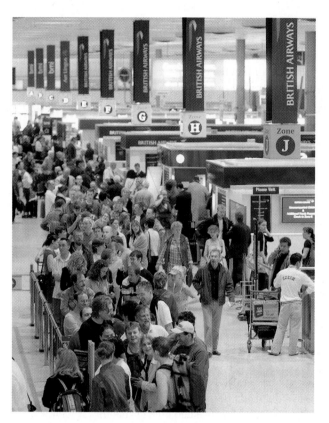

Modern travel has made health and the spread of disease a global issue. The deadly flu pandemic of 1918 took over one year to travel around the globe. Today, modern air travel could spread illness globally in a matter of weeks.

Preparing for Better Health in the Twenty-First Century

Although we've made dramatic improvements in many health areas, clearly there are challenges ahead. As we move through the twenty-first century, minority groups with different ethnic and racial backgrounds are expected to grow substantially in the United States. As these groups continue to make up a larger segment of the U.S. population, we will need to take action at the federal, state, local, and individual levels to reduce health disparities and achieve the goal of health for every person. Although it is important that each of us work to preserve and protect our own health, it is also important to become actively engaged in the health of our communities, our nation, and the global population. Central to this goal is the concept of **cultural competency**, defined as a set of congruent attitudes and policies that come together in a system or among individuals and enables effective work in cross-cultural situations.[16] The mark of a truly healthy person is whether the individual focuses beyond the "me" aspects of human existence and becomes equally concerned with the "we" aspects of health, as well as having a sense of

responsibility about the broader environment we live in. As a college student in the twenty-first century, it is important to understand the cultural differences among America's diverse population, examine our own health-related values and beliefs, and assist those who are different in navigating the health system and making healthy choices.

Focusing on Global Health Issues

Everyone's health is profoundly affected by economic, social, behavioral, scientific, and technological factors. The world economy has become increasingly interconnected and globalized; every day, millions of people worldwide move across national borders. Global commerce and communication have benefited people in virtually every country while creating a remarkable degree of mutual interdependence. In addition to the benefits of globalization, these changes also present

cultural competency A set of congruent attitudes and policies that come together in a system or among individuals and enables effective work in cross-cultural situations.

significant threats to our health, ranging from new diseases such as avian flu to contaminants in our food, air, and water supplies, natural disasters, and bioterrorism.[17]

Global health in the twenty-first century will require each of us to do our part to protect our own health and the health of others, whether at home or abroad.

what do you THINK?

What implications do developments in global health have for people living in the United States today? ■ What international programs, policies, and/or services might help control the world's health problems in the next decade? ■ Are there actions that individuals can take to help?

Gender Differences and Health Status

You don't have to be a health expert to know that there are physiological differences between men and women. Though much of the male and female anatomy is identical, researchers are discovering that the same diseases and treatments can affect men and women very differently. Many illnesses—for example osteoporosis, multiple sclerosis, diabetes, and Alzheimer's disease—are much more common in women, even though rates for these diseases seem to be increasing in men. Why these differences? Is it simply a matter of lifestyle? Clearly, it is much more complicated than that. Consider the following:[18]

Are men and women different when it comes to their health?

- The size, structure and function of the brain differs in women and men, particularly in areas that affect mood and behavior, and areas of the brain used to perform the same tasks. Reaction time is slower in women, but accuracy is higher.
- Bone mass in women reaches its maximum in the twenties; in men, it increases gradually until age 30. At menopause, women lose bone at an accelerated rate, and 80 percent of osteoporosis cases are women.
- Women's cardiovascular systems are different in size, shape, and nervous system impulses; women have faster heart rates.
- Women's immune systems are stronger than men's, but women are more prone to autoimmune diseases (disorders

Women's Health Initiative (WHI)   National study of postmenopausal women conducted in conjunction with the NIH mandate for equal research priorities for women's health issues.

in which the body attacks its own tissues, such as multiple sclerosis, lupus, and rheumatoid arthritis). Women experience pain in different ways than men and may react to pain medications differently.

Differences do not stop there; according to a report by the Society for Women's Health Research:[19]

- When consuming the same amount of alcohol, women have a higher blood alcohol content than men, even allowing for size differences.
- Women who smoke are 20 to 70 percent more likely to develop lung cancer than men who smoke the same number of cigarettes.
- Women are more likely than men to suffer a second heart attack within one year of their first heart attack.
- The same drug can cause different reactions and different side effects in women and men—even common drugs like antihistamines and antibiotics.
- Women are two times more likely than men to contract a sexually transmitted infection, and ten times more likely to contract HIV, when having unprotected intercourse.
- Depression is two to three times more common in women than in men.

Surprisingly, although these and countless other disparities in health have long been recognized, researchers largely ignored the unique aspects of women's health until the 1990s, when the National Institutes of Health (NIH) funded a highly publicized 15-year, $625 million study. Known as the **Women's Health Initiative (WHI),** this study was designed to focus research on the uniqueness of women when it came to drug trials, development of surgical instruments, and other health issues, rather than assuming that women were just like the males who had been studied. This research and follow-up studies are providing invaluable information about women's health risks and potential strategies for prevention, intervention, and treatment.

Improving Your Health

Table 1.4 summarizes the leading causes of death in the United States, by age. Note that Americans aged 15 to 24 are most likely to die from unintentional injuries, followed by homicide and suicide. Unintentional injuries are also the major killer in the next age group, aged 25 to 44, followed by malignant neoplasms and heart diseases. In 2005, for the first time in U.S. history, cancer replaced cardiovascular disease as the number-one cause of death for all persons under the age of 85.[20] It is important to note that when all age groups are included, cardiovascular disease remains the number-one cause of death in the United States as indicated in Table 1.4.

Individual behavior is a major determinant of good health. In fact, most experts believe that several key behaviors will help people live longer (Table 1.2). Heredity, access to health care, and the environment can also influence health status. (Figure 1.2, page 22). Though all of these factors are critical

TABLE 1.4 Leading Causes of Death in the United States by Age (Years), 2002

ALL AGES*		15–24	
Diseases of the heart	685,089	Unintentional injuries	15,412
Malignant neoplasms	556,902	Homicide	5,219
Cerebrovascular diseases	157,689	Suicide	4,010
Chronic lower respiratory diseases	126,382	Malignant neoplasms	1,730
Unintentional injuries	109,277	Diseases of the heart	1,022
UNDER 1 YEAR		**25–44**	
Congenital anomalies	5,621	Unintentional injuries	29,279
Short gestation or low birth weight	4,849	Malignant neoplasms	19,957
Sudden infant death syndrome	2,162	Diseases of the heart	16,853
Maternal complications	1,710	Suicide	11,897
Complications of placenta, cord, membranes	1,199	Homicide	7,728
1–4		**45–64**	
Unintentional injuries	1,641	Malignant neoplasms	143,028
Congenital anomalies	530	Diseases of the heart	101,804
Homicide	423	Unintentional injuries	23,020
Malignant neoplasms	402	Cerebrovascular diseases	15,952
Diseases of the heart	165	Diabetes mellitus	15,518
5–14		**65+**	
Unintentional injuries	2,718	Diseases of the heart	576,301
Malignant neoplasms	1,072	Malignant neoplasms	391,001
Congenital anomalies	417	Cerebrovascular diseases	143,293
Homicide	356	Chronic lower respiratory diseases	108,313
Suicide	260	Influenza and pneumonia	58,826

* *Note:* Data are age adjusted to take the aging population into account.

Source: R. N. Anderson and B. L. Smith, "Deaths: Leading Causes for 2002," in *National Vital Statistics Reports* 53 (Hyattsville, MD: National Center for Health Statistics, 2005).

to one's health status, our personal lifestyle decisions are one factor that most of us have complete control over, and can change for the better. Many public health recommendations emphasize that a healthy lifestyle has substantial health benefits, and we are bombarded with this message throughout our lives. In spite of the constant reminders to quit smoking, exercise for 30 to 60 minutes daily, and avoid *trans* fats, a recent study of the Behavioral Risk Factor Surveillance System data (see the Health in a Diverse World box on page 24) indicates that only 3 percent of the population adheres to the top four health recommendations.[21]

Clearly, change is not always easy. All of us, no matter where we are on the health and wellness continuum, have to start somewhere. All people have faced personal and external challenges to their attempts to change health behaviors— some have not done so well, some have been extremely successful, and some have made only small changes that add up to significant improvements in health over time. The key is to identify the behaviors you want to change, set goals and identify the necessary steps to achieve them, put the plan of ac-

tion in writing, and track your progress daily. Finally, don't say you'll start next week; start now! But first, let's take a look at factors that contribute to current patterns of behavior and assess how you can change things to make your goal easier to achieve (Figure 1.3, page 22).

Changing Your Health Behaviors

As Mark Twain said, "Habit is habit, and not to be flung out the window by anyone, but coaxed downstairs a step at a time." The chances of successfully changing negative habits improve when you identify a key behavior that you want to change and develop a plan for gradual change that allows you time to unlearn negative patterns and substitute positive ones. Many experts advocate dissecting a given health behavior into smaller parts and working on them one at a time in "baby steps" (see the Skills for Behavior Change box on page 26).

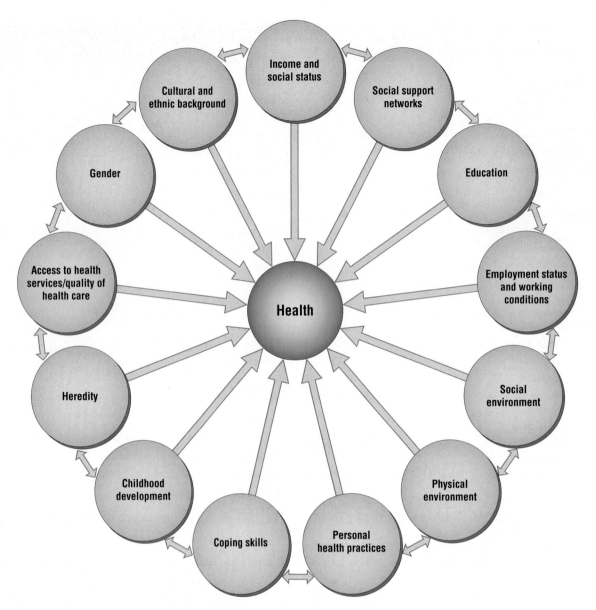

FIGURE 1.2 Key Determinants of Health

All of the factors shown influence your health. Can you think of others? How do these factors affect each other?

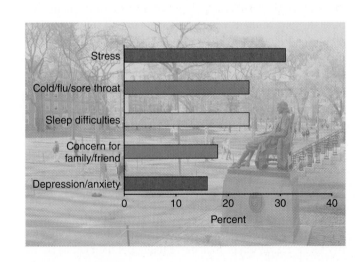

FIGURE 1.3 Top Five Reported Impediments to Academic Performance—Last 12 Months

Your personal health and wellness can affect your academic success. In a recent National College Health Association survey, students indicated specific health problems that prevented them from performing at their best.

Source: American College Health Association, "American College Health Association–National College Health Assessment (ACHA-NCHA) Web Summary," 2006, www.acha.org/projects_programs/ncha_sampledata.cfm.

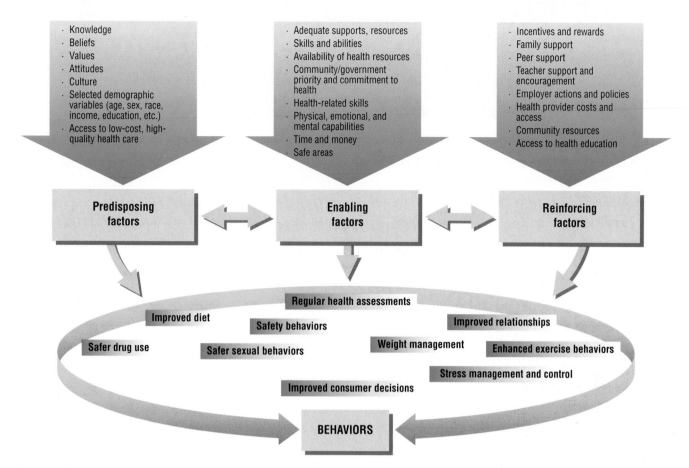

FIGURE 1.4 Factors That Influence Behavior-Change Decisions

First, identify what is most important to you or what causes you the greatest immediate and long-term risks. For example, if you are concerned about your weight, assess your eating patterns and decide where you can make changes that you can live with. Too many of us decide on New Year's Day that we are going to lose weight, exercise more, find more friends, and essentially reinvent ourselves overnight! Is it any wonder that we don't keep most of these resolutions?

Factors That Influence Behavior Change

Figure 1.4 identifies major factors that influence behavior and behavior-change decisions. They can be divided into three general categories: predisposing, enabling, and reinforcing.

Predisposing Factors Our life experiences, knowledge, cultural and ethnic inheritance, and current beliefs and values are all *predisposing factors* that influence behavior. Factors that may predispose us to certain conditions include age, sex, race, income, family background, educational background, and access to health care. For example, if your parents smoked, you are 90 percent more likely to start smoking than someone whose parents didn't. If your peers smoke, you

are 80 percent more likely to smoke than someone whose friends don't.

Enabling Factors Skills and abilities; physical, emotional, and mental capabilities; and resources and accessible facilities that make health decisions more convenient or difficult are *enabling factors*. Positive enablers encourage you to carry through on your intentions. Negative enablers work against your intentions to change. For example, if you would like to join a fitness center but discover that the closest one is four miles away and the membership fee is $500, those negative enablers may convince you to stay home. On the other hand, if your school's fitness center is two blocks away, stays open until midnight, and offers a special, low-priced student membership, those positive enablers will probably convince you to join. Identifying positive and negative enabling factors and devising alternative plans when the negative factors outweigh the positive are part of planning for behavior change.

Reinforcing Factors *Reinforcing factors* include the presence or absence of support, encouragement, or discouragement that significant people in your life bring to a situation. For example, if you decide to stop smoking and your family and friends continue smoking in your presence, you may be tempted to start smoking again. In other words, your smoking behavior is reinforced. If, however, you are

The amount of health advice you can find in newspaper headlines, on the evening news, or in popular magazines is enough to make your head spin. Consume at least 5 cups of vegetables daily, wash your hands for 30 seconds to avoid illness, a BMI greater than 25 puts you at risk for obesity-related illness, and other guidelines for a healthy life seem to come at us from every direction, and as if this isn't enough, they seem to change all the time! While trying to make sense of it all, you may be left wondering, "Who develops these recommendations?"

There are several key surveys and documents that guide health professionals as they create national guidelines for health. Health researchers, policymakers, and public health professionals administer a variety of surveys to random groups in the American population, and use the data they collect to examine trends and determine where we have the most room for improvement.

WHERE THE NUMBERS COME FROM

The following surveys aren't the only ones health professionals use, but they are a sampling of the most valuable sources of health data currently collected.

The Behavioral Risk Factor Surveillance System

The Behavioral Risk Factor Surveillance System (BRFSS) is a state-based system of health surveys. It collects information about health risk behaviors, clinical preventive practices, and health care access. State health departments conduct the survey by telephone using a standard questionnaire. BRFSS interviewers ask questions of adults, aged 18 and over, related to behaviors associated with preventable chronic diseases, injuries, and infectious diseases. Individual states can add their own questions to this survey. The states forward the responses to the Centers for Disease Control and Prevention, where monthly data are aggregated for each state, returned to the state, and then published on the BRFSS website. The data collected help

state and local health departments and national health organizations such as the American Cancer Society and the American Heart Association plan and target their health initiatives. The BRFSS may also be used to identify emerging health problems; establish and track health objectives; develop, implement, and evaluate a broad array of disease prevention activities; and support health-related legislative efforts. For more information about the BRFSS, visit www.cdc.gov/BRFSS.

The American College Health Association's National College Health Assessment

The American College Health Association's National College Health Assessment (ACHA-NCHA) is a national survey of college students organized by ACHA to assist college health service providers, health educators, counselors, and administrators in collecting data about their students' habits, behaviors, and perceptions on the most prevalent health topics:

- Alcohol, tobacco, and other drug use
- Sexual health

---

overweight, you lose a few pounds, and all your friends tell you how terrific you look, then your positive behavior will be reinforced and you will be more likely to continue your weight-loss plan.

The manner in which you reward or punish yourself also plays a role. Accepting small failures and concentrating on your successes can foster further achievements. Berating yourself because you binged on ice cream or argued with a friend may create an internal environment in which failure becomes almost inevitable. Telling yourself that you're worth the extra time and effort and giving yourself a pat on the back for small accomplishments are often overlooked factors in positive behavior change.

Motivation and Readiness to Change

Wanting to change is a prerequisite of the change process, but there is much more to the process than motivation. *Motiva-*

tion must be combined with common sense, commitment, and a realistic understanding of how best to move from point A to point B. Knowledge, attitudes, and skills are important components of being motivated to change. *Readiness* is the state of being that precedes behavior change, and those who are ready are likely to make the actual effort.[22] For someone to be ready for change, certain basic steps and adjustments in thinking must occur. The Skills for Behavior Change box on page 26 describes the Stages of Change model of health behavior change.

Some of us need a little boost before we are able to change our behavior. Rewards, or incentives for successfully reaching goals that we set, are effective ways to keep ourselves on track. Several studies have pointed out that those who set up a system of rewards for behavior change are often successful. For example, allow yourself something that you really enjoy after losing 5 pounds, rather than depriving yourself until you lose all 30 of the pounds that you want to lose.

- Weight, nutrition, and exercise
- Injury prevention, personal safety, and violence
- Mental health

While other health surveys of college students cover a single topic area, such as alcohol and drug use, the ACHA-NCHA offers the broadest range of health issues, as well as the ability to map the results over an extended time. To date, over 190,000 students at 324 colleges and universities have participated in the surveys, providing the college health and higher education fields with a vast spectrum of research on student health. Data from the ACHA-NCHA now spans from spring 2000 through fall 2004. The survey is administered by campus administration, then returned to the ACHA, which collates the data, then returns them in the form of reports and summaries to the university. The ACHA also maintains a national database, reflecting survey results from participating institutions. For more information about the survey, go to www.acha.org/projects_programs/assessment.cfm.

The National Health and Nutrition Examination Survey

The National Health and Nutrition Examination Survey (NHANES) is a population-based survey that was designed to collect information on the health and nutrition of those living in the United States. NHANES data have been used to influence policy and improve the health of the U.S. population in many ways, including getting lead removed from gasoline; creating and updating pediatric growth charts; and establishing national baseline estimates for cholesterol, blood pressure, and hepatitis C in the United States.

There are two parts to this survey: the home interview and the health examination. During the in-home interview, participants are asked questions about health status, disease history, and diet. The health examination is performed in a mobile exam center (MEC). The MEC is made up of four trailers, linked sideways, containing high-tech medical equipment. During the health examination many tests are performed; however, no internal exams or invasive procedures are done. Some of these tests (e.g., digital images of the retina) are not normally performed at a physician's office and could give the participant and his or her doctor additional information about the person's health. The examinations depend on that participant's age and gender. All participants receive a written *Report of Findings* approximately 12 weeks after the exam. If the survey program detects an abnormal value, the participant is notified immediately by letter. For more information about NHANES, visit www.cdc.gov/nchs/nhanes.htm.

Sources: National Center for Chronic Disease Prevention and Health Promotion, *About the Behavioral Risk Factor Surveillance System* (Atlanta: Centers for Disease Control and Prevention), www.cdc.gov/BRFSS/about.htm; The American College Health Association-National College Health Assessment, www.acha.org/projects_programs/assessment.cfm; The National Center for Health Statistics, *Introduction to the National Health and Nutrition Examination Survey, 2005–2006* (Atlanta: Centers for Disease Control and Prevention), www.cdc.gov/nchs/nhanes.htm.

Self-Efficacy

Why is self-efficacy among the most important of all factors that influence our health? Because it determines how we feel, think, motivate ourselves, and behave.[23] **Self-efficacy** is defined as an individual's belief that he or she is capable of achieving certain goals, or performing at a level that may influence events in life. In general, people who exhibit high self-efficacy are confident that they can succeed and approach challenges with a positive attitude. Prior success in academics, athletics, or social interactions will lead to expectations of success in the future. Self-efficacious people are more likely to feel a sense of **personal control** over situations, that their own internal resources allow them to control events. People who approach challenges, such as changing an unhealthy behavior, with confidence may be more motivated to change and achieve a greater level of success. On the other hand, someone with low self-efficacy may give up easily or never even try to change a behavior. Those with low self-efficacy tend to shy away from difficult challenges. These individuals may have failed before and when the going gets tough, are more likely to give up or revert to old patterns of behavior. How can one improve self-efficacy? Learning new skills and having successful experiences can help improve confidence and develop a "can-do" attitude.

External versus Internal Locus of Control

 The conviction that you have the ability to change is a powerful motivator. People who believe they lack control in a situation may become easily frustrated and give up. Those who feel they

self-efficacy Belief in one's ability to perform a task successfully.

personal control Belief that one's own internal resources allow one to control a situation.

SKILLS FOR behavior change

STAGING FOR CHANGE

On any given morning, many of us get out of bed and resolve to change a given behavior that day. Whether it be losing weight, drinking less, exercising more, being nicer to others, managing time better, or some other change, we start out with enthusiasm and high expectations. However, a vast majority of people return to doing whatever it was they thought they shouldn't be doing.

Why do so many good intentions fail? According to Dr. James Prochaska, University of Rhode Island, and Dr. Carlos DiClemente, University of Maryland, it's because we are going about things in the wrong way. According to Prochaska and DiClemente, fewer than 20 percent of us are really prepared to take action. After considerable research, they have concluded that behavior changes usually do not succeed if they start with the change itself. Instead, we must go through a series of stages to adequately prepare ourselves for that eventual change. Our chances of keeping those New Year's resolutions will be greatly enhanced if we have proper reinforcement and help during each of the following stages.

1. *Precontemplation.* People in the precontemplation stage have no current intention of changing. They may have tried to change a behavior before and given up, or they may be in denial and unaware of any problem.
   Strategies for Change: Sometimes a few frank yet kind words from friends may be enough to make precontemplators take a closer look at themselves. This is not to say that you should become a warrior against pleasure or tell people what to do when they haven't asked for advice. Recommending readings or making tactful suggestions, however, can be useful in helping precontemplators consider making a change.

2. *Contemplation.* In this phase, people recognize that they have a problem and begin to contemplate the need to change. Acknowledgment usually results from increased awareness, often due to feedback from family and friends or access to information. Despite this acknowledgment, people can languish in this stage for years, realizing that they have a problem but lacking the time or energy to make the change.
   Strategies for Change: Often, contemplators need a little push to get them started. This may come in the form of helping them set up a change plan (for example, an exercise routine), buying a helpful gift (such as a low-fat cookbook), sharing articles about a particular problem, or inviting them to go with you to hear a speaker on a related topic. People often need time to think about a course of action or to build a skill. Your assistance can help them move off the point of indecision.

3. *Preparation.* Most people at this point are close to taking action. They've thought about what they might do and may even have come up with a plan. Rather than thinking about why they can't begin, they have started to focus on what they can do.
   Strategies for Change: Follow a few standard guidelines: Set realistic goals (large and small), take small steps toward change, change only a couple of things at once, reward small milestones, and seek support from friends. Identify factors that have enabled or obstructed success in the past, and modify them where possible. Fill out the Behavior Change Contract in this book to help you commit to making these changes.

4. *Action.* In this stage, people begin to follow their action plans. Those who have prepared for change, thought about alternatives, engaged social support, and made a plan of action are more ready for action than those who have given it little thought. Unfortunately, too many people start behavior change here rather than going through the first three stages. Without a plan, without enlisting the help of others, or without a realistic goal, failure is likely.
   Strategies for Change: Publicly stating the desire to change helps ensure success. Encourage friends who are making a change to share their plans with you. Offer to help, and try to remove potential obstacles from the person's intended action plan. Social support and the buddy system can motivate even the most reluctant person.

5. *Maintenance.* Maintenance requires vigilance, attention to detail, and long-term commitment. Many people reach a goal, only to relax and slip back into the undesired behavior. In this stage, it is important to be aware of the potential for relapses and to develop strategies for dealing with such challenges. Common causes of relapse include overconfidence, daily temptations, stress or emotional distractions, and self-deprecation.
   Strategies for Change: During maintenance, continue taking the same actions that led to success in the first place. Find fun and creative ways to maintain positive behaviors. This is where a willing and caring support group can be vital. Knowing where on your campus to turn for help when you don't have a close support network is also helpful.

6. *Termination.* By this point, the behavior is so ingrained that the current level of vigilance may be unnecessary. The new behavior has become an essential part of daily living. Can you think of someone you know who has made a major behavior change that has now become an essential part of that person's life?

Source: J. O. Prochaska and C. C. DiClemente, "Stages and Processes of Self-Change of Smoking: Toward an Integrative Model of Change," *Journal of Consulting and Clinical Psychology* 51 (1983): 390–395.

have no personal control tend to have an *external locus of control* and lack confidence in their ability to succeed in a particular behavior. People who are confident that their behavior will influence the outcome tend to have an *internal locus of control*. Individuals who feel that they have limited control over their lives often find it more difficult to initiate positive changes.[24]

 what do you THINK?

If you were trying to adopt a healthy new behavior—for example, starting to exercise 30 minutes per day—who could you ask to support you? ■ What factors could make this change difficult? ■ What skills will you need to succeed? ■ How ready are you?

Beliefs and Attitudes

We often assume that when rational people realize there is a risk in what they are doing, they will act to reduce that risk. But this is not necessarily true. Consider the number of health professionals who smoke, consume junk food, and act in other unhealthful ways. They surely know better, but their "knowing" is disconnected from their "doing." Why is this so? Two strong influences on behavior are beliefs and attitudes.

A **belief** is an appraisal of the relationship between some object, action, or idea (for example, smoking) and some attribute of that object, action, or idea (for example, smoking is expensive, dirty, and causes cancer—or it is relaxing). Beliefs may develop from direct experience (perhaps you have trouble breathing after smoking for several years) or from secondhand experience or knowledge conveyed by other people (maybe you watched your grandfather, a longtime smoker, die of lung cancer). An **attitude** is a relatively stable set of beliefs, feelings, and behavioral tendencies in relation to something or someone.

Do Beliefs and Attitudes Influence Behavior?
It seems logical to conclude that your beliefs will affect your behavior. If you believe (make the appraisal) that taking drugs (an action) is harmful (attribute of that action), you will not use drugs. If you believe that drinking and driving are incompatible, you will never drink and drive. Or will you?

Psychologists studying the relationship between beliefs and health behaviors have determined that although beliefs may subtly influence behavior, they may not actually cause people to change behavior. As early as the 1950s, psychologists I. Rosenstock and G. Hochbaum developed a classic theory, the **Health Belief Model (HBM)**, to show when beliefs affect behavior change.[25]

Although many other models attempt to explain the influence of beliefs on behaviors, the HBM remains one of the most widely used. It holds that several factors must support a belief before change is likely:

- *Perceived seriousness of the health problem.* How severe would the medical and social consequences be if the health problem was to develop or be left untreated? The more serious the perceived effects, the more likely that action will be taken.
- *Perceived susceptibility to the health problem.* Next, what is the likelihood of developing the health problem? People who perceive themselves at high risk are more likely to take preventive action.
- *Cues to action.* Those who are reminded or alerted about a potential health problem are more likely to take action. If one believes she can prevent a negative outcome by a specific action that can be reasonably accomplished, she'll likely make that change.

Three other factors are linked to perceived risk for health problems: *demographic variables,* including age, gender, race, and ethnic background; *sociopsychological variables,* including personality traits, social class, and social pressure; and *structural variables,* including knowledge about or prior contact with the health problem.

People follow the Health Belief Model many times every day. Take, for example, smokers. Older smokers are likely to know other smokers who have developed serious heart or lung problems as a result of smoking. They are thus more likely to perceive tobacco as a threat to their health than does a teenager who has just begun smoking. The greater the perceived threat of health problems caused by smoking, the greater the chance a person will quit.

However, many chronic smokers know the risks yet continue to smoke. Why do they fail to take actions to avoid further harm? According to Rosenstock, some people do not believe that they will be affected by a severe problem—they act as if they believe they have some kind of immunity—and are unlikely to change their behavior. They also may feel that the immediate pleasure outweighs the long-range cost.

Intentions to Change

Our attitudes tend to reflect our emotional responses to situations and follow from our beliefs. According to the **Theory of Reasoned Action**, our behaviors result from our intentions to perform actions. An intention is a product of our attitude

belief   Appraisal of the relationship between some object, action, or idea and some attribute of that object, action, or idea.

attitude   Relatively stable set of beliefs, feelings, and behavioral tendencies in relation to something or someone.

Health Belief Model (HBM)   Model for explaining how beliefs may influence behaviors.

Theory of Reasoned Action   Model for explaining the importance of our intentions in determining behaviors.

toward an action and our beliefs about what others may want us to do.[26] A behavioral intention, then, is a written or stated commitment to perform an action.

In brief, the more consistent and powerful your attitudes about an action and the more you are influenced by others to take that action, the greater will be your stated intention to do so. The more you verbalize your commitment to change, the more likely you are to succeed.

Significant Others as Change Agents

Many of us are highly influenced by the approval or disapproval (real or imagined) of close friends, loved ones, and the social and cultural groups to which we belong. Such influences can support healthy behavior, or they can interfere with even the best intentions.

Your Family From the time of your birth, your parents and other family members have given you strong cues about which actions are socially acceptable and which are not.

Do my friends and family influence my health choices?

Brushing your teeth, bathing, and chewing food with your mouth closed are probably all behaviors that your family instilled in you long ago. Your family culture influenced your food choices, your religious beliefs, your political beliefs, and all your other values and actions. If you deviated from your family's norms, your mother or father probably let you know fairly quickly. Good family units share a dedication to the healthful development of all family members, unconditional trust, and a commitment to work out difficulties.

When the loving family unit does not exist, when it does not provide for basic human needs, or when irresponsible individuals try to build a family under the influence of drugs or alcohol, it becomes difficult for a child to learn positive health behaviors. Healthy behaviors get their start in healthy homes; unhealthy homes breed unhealthy habits. Healthy families provide the foundation for a clear and necessary understanding of what is right and wrong, what is positive and negative. Without this fundamental grounding, many young people have great difficulties.

Social Bonds and the Influence of Others

Just as your family influences your actions during your childhood, your friends and significant others influence your behaviors as you grow older. Most of us desire to fit the "norm." If you deviate from the actions expected in your hometown, or among your friends, you may suffer ostracism, strange looks, and other negative social consequences. If you couldn't care less what they think, you probably brush off their negative reactions or suggested changes. However, the lower your level of self-esteem and self-efficacy, the higher the chances that others will influence your actions.

The behavior choices we make can be explained by the *Theory of Planned Behavior.*[27] This theory outlines three reasons for how we choose to behave:

1. *Our attitudes toward the behavior,* for example, what we think about the positive or negative effects of our actions and the importance of each of those

2. *Our level of perceived behavioral control,* or our beliefs about the constraints and/or opportunities we might have concerning the behavior

3. *Our subjective norms,* or whether or not we think our actions will meet the approval or disapproval of people important to us

For example, if you want to lose weight because you believe it will make you more desirable, you'll have strong *intentions* to begin a weight-loss program (attitude toward the behavior). Intentions are powerful indicators of successful behavior change. If there is a convenient, affordable fitness center near you, you'll be motivated and believe you can make the change (control belief). Finally, the influence of others serves as a powerful *social support* for positive change. If friends offer encouragement (subjective norms), we are more likely to remain motivated to change our behavior. On the other hand, if we perceive that our friends will think we are "nerds" for going to the gym, we may quickly lose our motivation. The importance of cultivating and maintaining close *social bonds* with others is an important part of overall health. The key people in our lives play a powerful role in our motivation to change for the better, or for the worse.

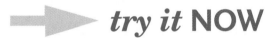

try it NOW

Stay connected. A broad base of social support is an important part of ensuring overall health. Make an effort to strengthen your social bonds. Call a friend right now and make a date for coffee, lunch, or "fun time" to catch up on each other's lives, and show you care. Make an effort to get to know your neighbors, too. The next time you pass someone in the dormitory hallway or bathroom, say hello. Neighbors can be an important social bond in times of need.

Choosing a Behavior-Change Technique

What can I do to change an unhealthy habit?

Once you have analyzed the factors that influence what you do, consider what actions you can take to change the negative ones. Behavior-change techniques include shaping, visualization, modeling, controlling the situation, reinforcement, changing self-talk, and problem solving. The options don't stop here, but these are the most common strategies.

Shaping

Regardless of how motivated you are, some behaviors are almost impossible to change immediately. To reach your goal, you may need to take a number of individual steps, each designed to change one small piece of the larger behavior. This process is known as **shaping**.

For example, suppose that you have not exercised for a while. You decide that you want to get into shape, and your goal is to be able to jog 3 to 4 miles every other day. You realize that you'd face a near-death experience if you tried to run even a few blocks in your current condition. So you decide to build up to your desired fitness level gradually. During week 1, you will walk for one hour every other day at a slow, relaxed pace. During week 2, you will walk for the same amount of time but will speed up your pace and cover slightly more ground. During week 3, you will speed up even more and will try to go even farther. You will continue taking such steps until you reach your goal.

Whatever the desired behavior change, all shaping involves the following actions:

- Start slowly, and try not to cause undue stress during the early stages of the program.
- Keep the steps small and achievable.
- Be flexible. If the original plan proves uncomfortable, or you deviate from it, don't give up! Start again and move forward.
- Don't skip steps or move to the next step until you have mastered the previous one.
- Reward yourself for meeting regular, pre-set goals.

Remember, behaviors don't develop overnight, so they won't change overnight.

Visualization

Mental practice and rehearsal can transform unhealthy behaviors into healthy ones. Athletes and others use a technique known as **imagined rehearsal** to reach their goals. By visualizing their planned action ahead of time, they will be prepared when they put themselves to the test.

For example, suppose you want to ask someone out on a date. Imagine the setting for the action (walking together to class). Then practice in your mind and out loud exactly what you're going to say. Mentally anticipate different responses and what you will say in reaction ("How about if I call you sometime this week?"). Careful mental and verbal rehearsal will greatly improve the likelihood of success.

Modeling

Modeling, or learning behaviors through careful observation of other people, is one of the most effective strategies for changing behavior. For example, suppose that you have trouble talking to people you don't know very well. One of the easiest ways to improve your communication skills is to select friends whose "gift of gab" you envy. Observe their social skills. Do they talk more or listen more? How do people

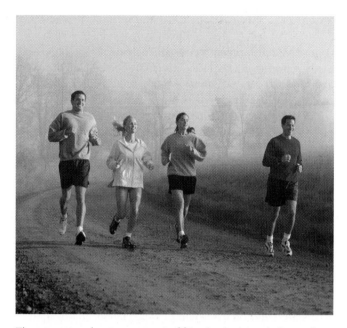

The support and encouragement of friends who have similar goals and interests will strengthen your commitment to develop and maintain positive health behaviors.

respond to them? Why are they such good communicators? If you carefully observe behaviors you admire and isolate their components, you can model the steps of your behavior-change strategy on a proven success.

Controlling the Situation

Sometimes, the right setting or the right group of people will positively influence your behaviors. Many situations and occasions trigger certain actions. The term **situational inducement** refers to an attempt to influence a behavior by using situations and occasions to control it.

For example, you may be more apt to stop smoking if you work in a smoke-free office, a positive situational inducement. But a smoke-filled bar, a negative situational inducement, may tempt you to resume. Careful consideration of which settings will help and which will hurt your effort to change, and your decision to seek the first and avoid the second, will improve your chances for change.

> **shaping** Using a series of small steps to gradually achieve a particular goal.
>
> **imagined rehearsal** Practicing, through mental imagery, to become better able to perform an event in actuality.
>
> **modeling** Learning specific behaviors by watching others perform them.
>
> **situational inducement** Attempt to influence a behavior through situations and occasions that are structured to exert control over that behavior.

Reinforcement

A **positive reinforcement** seeks to increase the likelihood that a behavior will occur by presenting something positive as a reward for it. Each of us is motivated by different reinforcers.

Most positive reinforcers can be classified under five headings: consumable, activity, manipulative, possessional, and social.

- *Consumable reinforcers* are delicious edibles such as candy, cookies, or gourmet meals.
- *Activity reinforcers* are opportunities to watch TV, go on a vacation, go swimming, or do something else enjoyable.
- *Manipulative reinforcers* are incentives such as lower rent in exchange for mowing the lawn or the promise of a better grade for doing an extra-credit project.
- *Possessional reinforcers* are tangible rewards such as a new TV or sports car.
- *Social reinforcers* are signs of appreciation, approval, or love, such as loving looks, affectionate hugs, and praise.

When choosing reinforcers, determine what would motivate you to act in a particular way. Research has shown that people can be motivated to change their behaviors, such as not smoking during pregnancy or abstaining from cocaine, if they set themselves up on a token economy system, whereby they earn tokens or points that can be exchanged for meaningful rewards such as money.[28] The difficulty often lies in determining which incentive will be most effective. Your reinforcers may initially come from others (extrinsic rewards); but as you see positive changes in yourself, you will begin to reward and reinforce yourself (intrinsic rewards). Keep in mind that reinforcers should immediately follow a behavior, but beware of overkill. If you reward yourself with a movie every time you go jogging, this reinforcer will soon lose its power. It would be better to give yourself this reward after, say, a full week of adherence to your jogging program.

❓ *what do you* THINK?

What consumable reinforcers would be a healthy reward for your new behavior? ▪ If you could choose one activity reinforcer to reward yourself after one day of success in your new behavior, what would it be? ▪ If you could obtain something (possessional reinforcer) after you reach your goal, what would it be? ▪ If you maintain your behavior for one week, what type of social reinforcer would you like to receive from your friends?

positive reinforcement Presenting something positive following a behavior that is being reinforced.

self-talk The customary manner of thinking and talking to yourself, which can impact your self-image.

Changing Self-Talk

Self-talk, or the way you think and talk to yourself, can also play a role in modifying health-related behaviors. Self-talk can reflect your feelings of *self-efficacy,* discussed earlier in this chapter on page 25. If you have had trouble with this activity in the past—for example, you have not enjoyed your previous experiences with speaking in public—you're not likely to feel self-efficacious about your ability to do it in the future.

When we don't feel self-efficacious, it's tempting to engage in negative self-talk, which can sabotage our best intentions. Here are some suggested strategies for changing self-talk.

Rational-Emotive Therapy
This form of cognitive therapy, or self-directed behavior change, is based on the premise that there is a close connection between what people say to themselves and how they feel. According to psychologist Albert Ellis, most everyday emotional problems and related behaviors stem from irrational statements that people make to themselves when events in their lives are different from what they would like them to be.[29]

For example, suppose that after doing poorly on an exam, you say to yourself, "I can't believe I flunked that easy exam. I'm so stupid." By changing this irrational, "catastrophic" self-talk into rational, positive statements about what is really going on, you can increase the likelihood that positive behaviors will occur. Positive self-talk might be phrased as follows: "I really didn't study enough for that exam, and I'm not surprised I didn't do very well. I'm certainly not stupid. I just need to prepare better for the next test." Such self-talk will help you to recover quickly from disappointment and take positive steps to correct the situation.

Blocking/Thought Stopping
By purposefully blocking or stopping negative thoughts, a person can concentrate on taking positive steps toward behavior change. For example, suppose you are preoccupied with your ex-partner, who has recently deserted you for someone else. You consciously stop thinking about the situation and force yourself to think about something more pleasant (perhaps dinner tomorrow with your best friend). By refusing to dwell on negative images and forcing yourself to focus elsewhere, you can avoid wasting energy, time, and emotional resources and move on to positive change.

Problem Solving: The Art of Self-Instruction

Some people seem to naturally take on challenges and deal with stressful life events in positive ways. However, most of us are not skilled at tackling and overcoming problems in our lives, but we can learn to do a better job. According to psychologist Donald Meichenbaum, we can learn to inoculate ourselves against stressful events or control our anger in certain situations. Before a stressful event (such as going to the doctor for sexually transmitted infection tests), Meichenbaum encourages his patients to practice coping skills, such as deep breathing or progressive muscle relaxation, or to practice self-instruction ("I'll feel better once I know what is going on here."). He provides a list of strategies that are designed to help each of us cope with stressors and modify anger reactions or other negative behaviors:[30]

- Define your stressor or stress reactions as problems to be solved.
- Set concrete, realistic goals and choose specific behaviors you can do to reach your goals.
- Try out the most acceptable and practical solution, and generate a wide range of possible alternative courses of action.
- Imagine and consider how others might respond if asked to deal with similar problems.
- Evaluate the pros and cons of each proposed solution and organize the solutions from least to most practical and desirable.
- Rehearse strategies and behaviors by means such as visualization or role-play the behavior in advance.
- Expect some failures, but reward yourself for having tried.
- Reconsider the original problem in light of your attempts at problem solving.

Changing Your Behavior

Many strategies have proved effective in making behavior changes. Before you begin this process, take stock of what has contributed to maintaining the behavior.

Self-Assessment: Antecedents and Consequences

Behaviors, thoughts, and feelings always occur in a context, that is, in a situation. Situations can be divided into two components: the events that come before and those that happen after. *Antecedents* are the setting events for a behavior; they cue or stimulate a person to act in certain ways. Antecedents can be physical events, thoughts, emotions, or the actions of other people. *Consequences*—the results of behavior—affect whether a person will repeat a behavior.[31] Consequences can also consist of physical events, thoughts, emotions, or the actions of other people.

Suppose you are shy and must give a speech in front of a large class. The antecedents include walking into the class, feeling frightened, wondering if you are capable of doing a good job, and being unable to remember a word of your speech. If the consequences are negative—if your classmates

OBSTACLE	STRATEGY
Stress (intrinsic and extrinsic)	Identify potential sources of stress. Find constructive ways to lower stress level.
Social pressures to repeat old habits	Enlist the support of friends. Identify specifics of these pressures.
Not accepting mistakes, being a perfectionist, hypercritical	Accept that slips are inevitable, but maintain control. Acknowledge that humans are imperfect beings.
Self-blame for poor coping or a weak personality	Blame pressures from the environment or lack of skills, rather than innate weakness.
Lack of effort, lack of motivation	Assess effort and make sure it is adequate. Provide rewards for successes.
Faulty beliefs, low self-efficacy	Develop new skills, focus on successes, and plan ahead for difficult situations. Change self-talk.

FIGURE 1.5 Overcoming Obstacles to Behavior Change
There are several types of obstacles that can make it difficult to succeed in making a behavior change. Each strategy can help overcome these obstacles.

Source: From *Self-Directed Behavior: Self-Modification for Personal Adjustment,* 9th ed. by D. L. Watson and R. G. Tharp. © 2006 Reprinted with permission of Wadsworth Publishing, a division of Thomson Learning. www.thomsonrights.com. Fax 800-730-2215.

make fun of you or you get a low grade—your terror about speaking in public will be reinforced, and you will continue to dread this kind of event. In contrast, if you receive positive feedback from the class and instructor, you may actually learn to like speaking in public.

Learning to recognize the antecedents of a behavior and acting to modify them is one method of changing behavior. A diary noting your undesirable behaviors and identifying the settings in which they occur can be a useful tool. Figure 1.5 on the previous page identifies several factors that can make behavior change more difficult.

Analyzing Personal Behavior

Successful behavior change requires determining what you want to change. All too often we berate ourselves by using generalities: "I'm lousy to my friends; I need to be a better person." Determining the specific behavior you would like to change—in contrast to the general problem—will allow you to set clear goals. What are you doing that makes you a lousy friend? Are you gossiping or lying about your friends? Have you been a taker rather than a giver? Or are you really a good friend most of the time?

Let's say the problem is gossiping. You can now analyze this behavior by examining the following components:

- *Frequency.* How often are you gossiping—all the time or only once in a while?
- *Duration.* How long have you been doing this?
- *Seriousness.* Is your gossiping just idle chatter, or are you really trying to injure the other person? What are the consequences for you? For your friend? For your friendship?
- *Basis for problem behavior.* Is your gossip based on facts, perceptions of facts, or deliberate embellishment of the truth?
- *Antecedents.* What kinds of situations trigger your gossiping? Do some settings or people bring out the gossip in you more than others? What triggers your feelings of dislike for or irritation toward your friends? Why are you talking behind their backs?

Once you assess your actions and determine what motivates you, consider what you can do to change your behavior.

Decision Making: Choices for Change

Now it is time to make a decision that will lead to positive health outcomes. Try to anticipate what might occur in a given setting and think through all possible safe alternatives.

For example, knowing that you are likely to be offered a drink when you go to a party, what kind of response could you make that would be okay in your social group? If someone is flirting with you and the situation takes on a distinct sexual overtone, what might you do to prevent the situation from turning bad? Advance preparation will help you stick to your behavior plan.

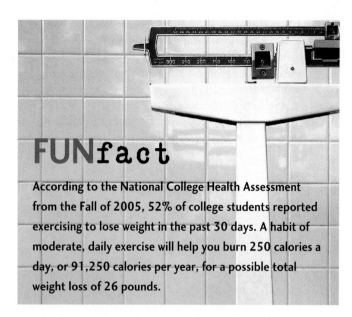

FUNfact

According to the National College Health Assessment from the Fall of 2005, 52% of college students reported exercising to lose weight in the past 30 days. A habit of moderate, daily exercise will help you burn 250 calories a day, or 91,250 calories per year, for a possible total weight loss of 26 pounds.

FIGURE 1.6 Do Your Peers Exercise?

Source: American College Health Association. National College Health Assessment, Reference Group Report, Fall 2005.

Fill out the Behavior Change Contract at the beginning of this book to help you set a goal, anticipate obstacles, and create strategies to overcome those obstacles. Remember that things typically don't "just happen." Making a commitment by completing a contract helps you stay alert to potential problems, be aware of your alternatives, maintain a good sense of your own values, and stick to your beliefs under pressure.

Setting Realistic Goals

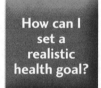

How can I set a realistic health goal?

Changing behavior is not easy, but sometimes we make it even harder by setting unrealistic and unattainable goals (Figure 1.6). To start making positive changes, ask yourself these questions.

- *What do I want?* What is your ultimate goal—to lose weight? Exercise more? Reduce stress? Have a lasting relationship? Whatever it is, you need a clear picture of your target outcome.
- *Which change is the greatest priority at this time?* Often people decide to change several things at once. Suppose that you are gaining unwanted weight. Rather than saying, "I need to eat less, start jogging, and really get in shape," you need to be specific about your current behavior. Are you eating too many sweets? Too many foods high in fat? Perhaps a realistic goal, therefore, would be, "I am going to try to eat less fat during dinner every day." Choose the behavior that constitutes your greatest problem, and tackle that first. You can always work on something else later.

Take small steps, experiment with alternatives, and find the best way to meet your goals.

- *Why is this important to me?* Think through why you want to change. Are you doing it because of your health? To look better? To win someone else's approval? Usually, doing something because it's right for you rather than to win others' approval is a sound strategy. If you are doing it for someone else, what happens when that other person isn't around?
- *What are the potential positive outcomes?* What do you hope to accomplish?
- *What health-promoting programs and services can help me get started?* Nearly all campuses and communities have programs and services designed to support positive behavior change. You might buy a self-help book at the campus bookstore, speak to a counselor, or enroll in an aerobics class at the local fitness center.

- *Are there family or friends whose help I can enlist?* Social support is one of your most powerful allies. Getting a friend to walk with you on a regular basis, asking your partner to help you stop smoking by quitting at the same time, and making a commitment with a friend to never let each other drive if you've had something to drink— these are all examples of how people can help each other make positive changes.

 what do you THINK?

Why is it sometimes hard to make decisions? ■ What factors influence your decision making? ■ Select one behavior that you want to change and refer to the Behavior Change Contract. ■ Using the goal-setting strategies discussed here, outline a plan for change.

TAKING charge

Summary

- Health encompasses the whole dynamic process of fulfilling one's individual potential in the physical, social, emotional, spiritual, intellectual, and environmental dimensions of life. Wellness means achieving the highest level of health possible along several dimensions.
- Although the average American life span has increased over the past century, we need to increase the span of quality life. Programs such as *Healthy People 2010* and the *AHRQ Guidelines* have established national objectives for achieving longer life and quality of life for all Americans through health promotion and disease prevention.
- Health disparities have become increasingly recognized as contributors to increased disease risks. Factors such as gender, race, and socioeconomic status continue to play a major role in health status and care. Women live longer but have more medical problems than do men. The recent inclusion of women in medical research and training and greater emphasis on minority populations are attempts to close gaps in health care.
- For the U.S. population as a whole, the leading causes of death are heart disease, cancer, and stroke. Cancer is the leading cause of death when looking at all those under age 85. But in the 15- to 24-year-old age group, the leading causes are unintentional injuries, homicide, and suicide. Many of the risks associated with cancer, heart disease, and stroke can be reduced through lifestyle changes. Many of

the risks associated with accidents, homicide, and suicide can be reduced through preventive measures.
- Worldwide commerce and travel are bringing dramatic changes in global health. In nonindustrialized countries, noncommunicable diseases such as depression and heart disease are replacing infectious disease and malnutrition as leading causes of disability and death.
- Several factors contribute to a person's health status, and a number of them are within our control. Beliefs and attitudes, self-efficacy, external and internal locus of control, intentions to change, support from significant others, and readiness to change are factors over which individuals have some degree of control. Access to health care, genetic predisposition, health policies that support positive choices, and other factors are all potential reinforcing, predisposing, and enabling factors that influence health decisions.
- Behavior-change techniques, such as shaping, visualization, modeling, controlling the situation, reinforcement, changing self-talk, and problem solving help people succeed in making behavior changes.
- Decision making has several key components. Each person must explore his or her own problems, the reasons for change, and the expected outcomes. The next step is to plan a course of action best suited to individual needs and fill out a Behavior Change Contract.

Chapter Review

1. The Public Health Model of health views disease and one's health status as a result of
   a. biological or diseased organ perspective.
   b. the individual's interaction with social and physical environments.
   c. curing the disease through surgery or treatment.
   d. restoring health with medicines and therapy.

2. Wellness can be defined as a
   a. choice one makes to move toward optimal health.
   b. lifestyle designed to achieve the highest potential for well-being.
   c. developing awareness that health and wellness go hand in hand.
   d. all of the above are true statements that define wellness

3. Which of the following wellness dimensions deals with the unity of one's surroundings to its environment?
   a. social health
   b. environmental health
   c. spiritual health
   d. emotional health

4. Which of the following is *not* an example of a risk behavior that a college student might unknowingly engage in?
   a. not practicing safer sex with a sexual partner
   b. eating a high-calorie and high-fat diet
   c. wearing a seat belt every time when driving in a vehicle
   d. using chewing tobacco

5. Which of the following is an example of *primary prevention*?
   a. attending a smoking cessation program
   b. using a condom during sexual intercourse
   c. receiving radiation therapy for cancer
   d. going to physical therapy for an injury resulting in a skiing accident

6. One of the main reasons for health disparities among poor people is due to
   a. inadequate health insurance.
   b. poor choices in lifestyle behaviors.
   c. not having transportation to get to the doctor's office or health clinic.
   d. socioeconomic differences in racial and ethnic backgrounds.

7. When Ashley began exercising and losing weight, her support group praised her efforts and encouraged her to continue her weight-loss plan. This process illustrates
   a. predisposing factors.
   b. reinforcing factors.
   c. locus of control.
   d. enabling factors.

8. Jake is exhibiting *self-efficacy* when he
   a. believes that he can and will be able to bench press from 75 pounds to 125 pounds in his specified time frame.
   b. is doubtful that his bad shoulder will heal enough to bench-press the desirable weights he is hoping for.
   c. beats up on himself that he is not good enough to do any physical exercise that will ever allow him to reach a 125-pound bench press.
   d. does not possess enough personal control over this situation.

9. An example of *shaping* when starting a new exercise program would be
   a. working on different sets of muscles each day to get the shape of the desired muscle tone.
   b. to gradually build up a running plan by walking, then jogging, and eventually being able to run the planned distance.
   c. to first lose weight in order to be in shape to do exercising.
   d. to practice modeling or learned behavior before starting the exercise program.

10. At Robert's place of employment, he participates in a smoking cessation program to quit his smoking habit. He obtains information, participates in a smoking cessation program during work hours and is provided monetary incentives to motivate his quitting smoking. This type of program is known as a
    a. primary prevention program.
    b. wellness program.
    c. employee brainwashing program.
    d. health promotion program.

Answers to these questions can be found on page A-1.

Questions for Discussion and Reflection

1. How are the terms *health* and *wellness* similar? What, if any, are important distinctions between these terms? What is health promotion? Disease prevention? What does it really mean to be healthy? Considering the various dimensions of health, describe someone whom you believe has many of these characteristics.

2. How healthy is the U.S. population today? Are we doing better or worse in health status than previously? Who is not doing better in an era when health is the "buzz" and everyone seems to be interested in improving health? What factors influence today's disparities in health?

3. What are some of the major global health problems today? Why is it increasingly important that we consider individual, community, U.S., and global health when we consider the health of populations?

4. What are some of the major differences in the way males and females are treated in the health care system? Why do you think these differences exist? Why are people treated differently based on race, sexual orientation, religion, marital status, and age?

5. What are the leading causes of death across different ages and races? What are the leading causes of death for people aged 15 to 24? Why are these statistics so different? Explain why it is important to look at these statistics by age

rather than just in total. What lifestyle changes can you make to lower your risks for contracting major diseases?

6. What major differences exist between the leading causes of death for Americans and those for people in other regions of the world?

7. What is the Health Belief Model? What is the Theory of Reasoned Action? How may each of these models be working when a young woman decides to smoke her first cigarette? Her last cigarette?

8. Explain the predisposing, reinforcing, and enabling factors that might influence a young mother who is dependent on welfare as she decides whether to sell drugs to support her children.

9. Using the Stages of Change model, discuss what you might do (in stages) to help a friend stop smoking. Why is it important that a person be ready to change before trying to change?

Accessing Your Health on the Internet

The following websites explore further topics and issues related to personal health. You'll also find links to each organization's website on the Companion Website for *Access to Health,* Tenth Edition, at www.aw-bc.com/donatelle.

1. *CDC Wonder.* Clearinghouse for comprehensive information from the Centers for Disease Control and Prevention (CDC), including special reports, guidelines, and access to national health data. http://wonder.cdc.gov

2. *Mayo Clinic.* Reputable resource for specific information about health topics, diseases, and treatment options. Easy to navigate and consumer friendly. www.mayo.edu

3. *National Center for Health Statistics.* Outstanding place to start for information about health status in the United States. Links to key documents such as Health United States (published annually), national survey information, and information on mortality by age, race, gender,

geographic location, and other important data. Includes comprehensive information provided by the CDC, as well as easy links to at least ten of the major health resources currently being utilized for policy and decision making about health in the United States. www.cdc.gov/nchs/default.htm

4. *National Health Information Center.* An excellent resource for consumer information about health. www.health.gov/nhic

5. *WebMD.* Reputable and comprehensive overview of various diseases and conditions. Written for the public in an easy-to-understand format with links to more in-depth information. www.webmd.com

Further Reading

Centers for Disease Control and Prevention, Health, United States, 2005 (Washington, DC: Government Printing Office, 2005).

Provides an up-to-date overview of U.S. health statistics, risk factors, and trends.

Institute of Medicine. *Who Will Keep the Public Healthy? Educating Public Health Professionals for the 21st Century.* Washington, DC: National Academies Press, 2003.

An edited text featuring experts from throughout the country discussing the role of health professionals in health change. It outlines an ecological approach to improving the nation's health and has served as a catalyst for initiatives focused on current health issues and future plans to improve health and prevent premature death and disability.

Institute of Medicine. *The Future of Public Health in the 21st Century.* Washington, DC: National Academies Press, 2003.

The summary of a national effort to examine the nation's health status describes how key individuals and organizations can work as a public health system to create conditions in which people can be healthy. This text also recommends the evidence-based actions necessary to make the U.S. health system work effectively.

Lee, P. and C. Estes. *The Nation's Health,* 7th ed. Sudbury, MA: Jones and Bartlett, 2003.

An overview of key writings on public health and issues affecting individuals and populations. Special emphasis is placed on health determinants, emerging threats to health, the health of diverse populations, and issues of health care quality, costs, and access.

U.S. Department of Health and Human Services. *Healthy People 2010: National Health Promotion and Disease Prevention Objectives for the Year 2010.* Washington, DC: Government Printing Office, 1998.

A plan containing the Surgeon General's long-range goals for improving the life span for all Americans by three years and improving access to health for all Americans, regardless of sex, race, socioeconomic status, and other variables.

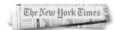

e-themes from *The New York Times*

For up-to-date articles about current health issues, visit www.aw-bc.com/donatelle, select *Access to Health,* Tenth Edition, Chapter 1, and click on "e-themes."

References

1. World Health Organization (WHO), "Constitution of the World Health Organization," *Chronicles of the World Health Organization* (Geneva, Switzerland: WHO, 1947).

2. Central Intelligence Agency, *Rank Order: Life Expectancy at Birth,* in The World Fact Book (Washington, DC: CIA, 2006); National Center for Health Statistics, *Health: United States, 2005,* with "Chartbook on Trends in the Health of Americans" and "Table 27" (Hyattsville, MD: National Center for Health Statistics, March 2006).

3. National Center for Health Statistics, Table 12 from "United States Life Tables, 2002," *National Vital Statistics Reports* 53, no. 6 (November 2004).

4. S. J. Olshansky et al., "A Potential Decline in Life Expectancy in the United States in the 21st Century," *New England Journal of Medicine* 352, no. 11 (March 2–5): 1138–1145.

5. R. Dubos, *So Human an Animal* (New York: Scribners, 1968), 15.

6. D. Satcher, *Keynote Address* (Washington, DC: National Association of School Psychologists, Government, and Professional Relations Committee, Public Policy Institute, February 2001), 10–12.

7. National Center for Health Statistics, "About *Healthy People 2010,*" www.cdc.gov/nchs.

8. Center for Outcomes and Evidence, "Evidence-Based Practice Centers: Synthesizing Scientific Evidence to Improve Quality and Effectiveness in Health Care" (Rockville, MD: Agency for Health Care, Research, and Quality, February 2006), www.ahrq.gov/clinic/epc; Centers for Disease Control and Prevention (CDC), *Best Practices for Comprehensive Tobacco Control Programs—August 1999* (Atlanta: U.S. Department of Health and Human Services, CDC, National Center for Chronic Disease Prevention and Health Promotion, Office on Smoking and Health, August 1999); Institute of Medicine, *The Future of Public Health in the 21st Century* (Washington, DC: National Academies Press, 2003).

9. Centers for Disease Control and Prevention, *Chronic Disease Prevention, 2004* (Atlanta: U.S. Department of Health and Human Services, 2004), www.cdc.gov/nccdphp.

10. Centers for Disease Control and Prevention, *The Burden of Chronic Diseases and Their Risk Factors: National and State Perspectives, 2004* (Atlanta: U.S. Department of Health and Human Services, 2004), www.cdc.gov/nccdphp/burdenbook2004.

11. Examples of organizations: American Cancer Society, Agency for Health Care, Research, and Quality, Centers for Disease Control and Prevention, National Cancer Institute, Substance Abuse and Mental Health Services Administration, 2005. See also Cancer Control Planet, which provides links to resources for comprehensive cancer control at http://cancercontrolplanet.cancer.gov.

12. World Health Organization (WHO), *The World Health Report 2002: Reducing Risks, Promoting Healthy Life* (Geneva, Switzerland: WHO, 2002), www.who.int/whr/2002/en; E. Khoman and M. Weale, "Incidence-Based Estimates of Healthy Life Expectancy for the United Kingdom: Coherence between Transition Probabilities and Aggregate Life Tables," National Institute Discussion Paper No. 270 (London: National Institute of Economic and Social Research, April 7, 2006).

13. Institute of Medicine, *Who Will Keep the Public Healthy? Educating Public Health Professionals for the 21st Century* (Washington, DC: National Academies Press, 2003).

14. UCLA Center for Health Policy Research, "Language Barrier Puts More than 1 Million Californians in HMOs at Risk for Health Problems," May 10, 2006, www.healthpolicy.ucla.edu/news_05102006 .html.

15. National Institutes of Health (NIH), *Strategic Research Plan and Budget to Reduce and Ultimately Eliminate Health Disparities: Volume 1, Fiscal Years 2002–2006* (Bethesda, MD: National Institutes of Health. Uploaded May 12, 2006).

16. National Institutes of Health, *What Is Cultural Competency?* (Bethesda, MD: National Institutes of Health 2006), www.omhrc .gov/templates/browse.aspx?lv1=1&1v1ID=3%20; A. Kleinman, L. Eisenberg, and B. Good. "Culture, Illness and Care: Clinical Lessons from Anthropologic and Cross-Cultural Research," *Focus: The Journal of Lifelong Learning in Psychiatry* 4, no. 140 (January 2006).

17. U.S. Department of Health and Human Services, The Fifty-Eighth World Health Assembly, Geneva, Switzerland, 2005, www.who.int/ mediacentre/events/2005/wha58/en/index.html.

18. C. Garnet, "What's Next for Women's Health Research?" The NIH Word on Health, April 2003, www.nih.gov/news/WordonHealth/ apr2003/womenshealth.htm.

19. Institute of Medicine, Committee on Understanding the Biology of Sex and Gender Differences, *Exploring the Biological Contributions to Human Health: Does Sex Matter?* (Washington, DC: National Academies Press, 2001).

20. A. Jemal et al., "Cancer Statistics," *A Cancer Journal for Clinicians* 55 (January/February 2005): 10–30; E. Ward, News Conference: American Cancer Society, ACS (January 19, 2005).

21. M. Reeves and A. Rafferty, "Healthy Lifestyle Characteristics Among Adults in the United States," *Archives of Internal Medicine* 165, no. 8 (2005): 854–857.

22. M. Hesse, "The Readiness Ruler as a Measure of Readiness to Change Polydrug Use in Drug Abusers," *Journal of Harm Reduction* 3, no. 3 (2006): 1477–1481; M. Cismaru, "Using Protection Motivation Theory to Increase the Persuasiveness of Public Service Communications," The Saskatchewan Institute of Public Policy, Public Policy Series paper no. 40 (February 2006); A. Fallon et al., "Health Care Provider Advice for African American Adults Not Meeting Health Behavior Recommendations," *Preventing Chronic Disease* 3,

no. 2 (2006); M. R. Chacko et al., "New Sexual Partners and Readiness to Seek Screening for Chlamydia and Gonorrhea: Predictors Among Minority Young Women," *Sexually Transmitted Infections* 82 (2006): 75–79.

23. A. Bandura, "Self-efficacy," in H. Friedman, ed., *Encyclopedia of Mental Health* (San Diego: Academic Press, 1998).

24. J. M. Twenge, Z. Liqing, and C. Im, "It's Beyond My Control: A Cross-Temporal Meta-Analysis of Increasing Externality in Locus of Control, 1960–2002," *Personality and Social Psychology Review* 8 (2004): 308–320.

25. I. Rosenstock, "Historical Origins of the Health Belief Model," *Health Education Monographs* 2, no. 4 (1974).

26. K. Glanz, F. Lewis, and B. Rimer, *Health Behavior and Health Education* (San Francisco: Jossey-Bass, 2003).

27. I. Ajzen, "The Theory of Planned Behavior," *Organizational Behavior and Human Decision Processes* 50 (1991): 179–211.

28. Hesse, "The Readiness Ruler as a Measure of Readiness"; Glanz et al., *Health Behavior and Health Education.*

29. A. Ellis and M. Benard, *Clinical Application of Rational Emotive Therapy* (New York: Plenum, 1985).

30. D. Meichenbaum, *Treatment of Patients with Anger Control Problems* (Toronto: Pergamon Press, 2003); D. Meichenbaum, *Stress Inoculation Training* (Toronto: Pergamon Press, 2004).

31. Glanz et al., *Health Behavior and Health Education.*

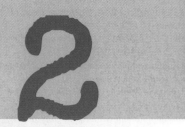

2

Psychosocial Health

BEING MENTALLY, EMOTIONALLY, SOCIALLY, AND SPIRITUALLY WELL

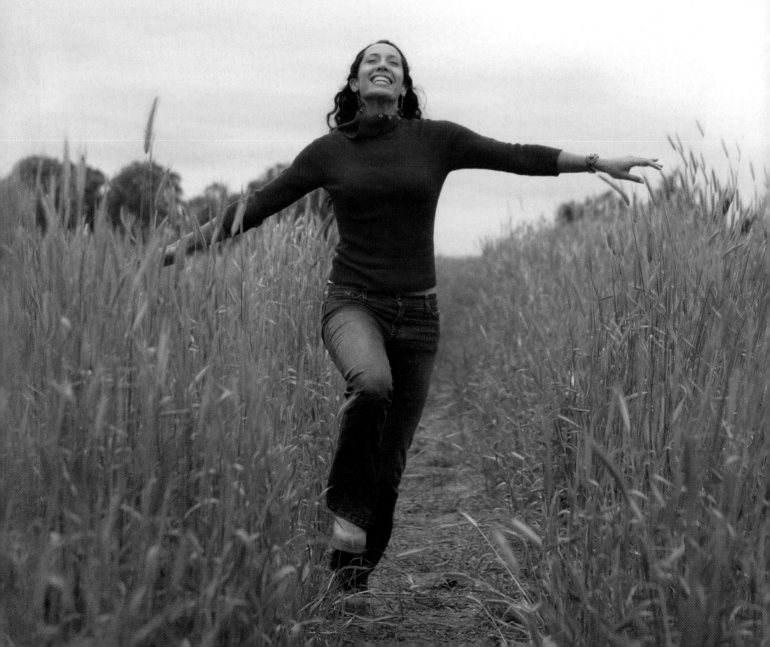

Do I have to be **religious** to be spiritual?

How do my **parents** influence my psychosocial health?

Can negative **emotions** make me sick?

How do I know if I've had a **panic attack**?

How can I choose the right **therapist** for me?

OBJECTIVES

- Define each of the four components of psychosocial health, and identify the basic traits shared by psychosocially healthy people.
- Learn how internal and external factors affect your psychosocial health; discuss the positive steps you can take to enhance psychosocial health.
- Discuss the dimension of spirituality and the role it plays in your health and wellness.
- Identify common psychosocial problems of adulthood, such as anxiety disorders and depression, and explain their causes and treatments.
- Discuss warning signs of suicide and actions that can be taken to help a suicidal individual.
- Explain the methods of different types of mental health professionals. Build a strategy for selecting a good therapist.

How often in the last month have you woken up feeling mentally and physically energized and alive, refreshed, and ready to go? When people smiled at you and you actually felt like smiling back? Perhaps you heard the birds singing outside your window and appreciated your surroundings, or had the drive to get through the day, accomplishing all of the things you wanted to do. In contrast, how many days in the last month have you groaned when the alarm went off, fought the urge to pull the covers over your head, and had to drag yourself out the door, only to feel listless and drained throughout the day? At the end of the day, did you wonder what happened and why you didn't accomplish one thing? Do these scenarios sound familiar? Daily fluctuations are not uncommon, and we all feel full of life one day, and maybe a little sluggish another.

Life can be challenging, painful, and frustrating; it can also be a source of great joy, fulfillment, and happiness. Regardless of what life throws at us, it is how we adapt to, cope with, and handle the day-to-day experiences that indicates our psychosocial and mental health.

Although the vast majority of college students describe their college years as among the best of their lives, many find the pressure of grades, financial concerns, relationship problems, and the struggle to find themselves to be extraordinarily difficult. Steven Hyman, provost of Harvard University and former director of the National Institute of Mental Health, states, "The mental state of many students is so precarious that it is interfering with the core mission of the university."[1] According to an annual survey of counseling center directors, the severity of the problems that students experience has been increasing since 1988.[2] Psychological distress caused by relationship issues, family issues, academic competition, and adjusting to life as a college student is rampant on college campuses today. Experts believe that the anxiety-inducing campus environment is a major contributor to poor health decisions such as high alcohol consumption and, in turn, health problems. "Much of collegiate social activity is centered on alcohol consumption because it's an anxiety reducer and demands no social skills. . . . It provides an instant identity; it lets people know that you are willing to belong."[3]

However, human beings possess a resiliency that enables us to cope, adapt, and thrive, regardless of life's challenges. How we feel and think about ourselves, those around us, and our environment can tell us a lot about our psychosocial health and whether we are healthy emotionally, spiritually, and mentally. Increasingly, health professionals recognize that having a solid social network, being emotionally and mentally healthy, and developing spiritual capacity don't just add years to life—they put life into years.

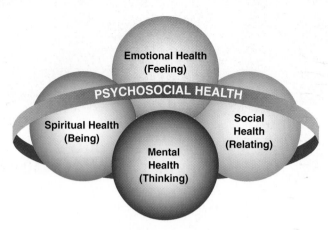

FIGURE 2.1 Psychosocial Health
Psychosocial health is a complex interaction of the mental, emotional, social, and spiritual dimensions of health.

Defining Psychosocial Health

Psychosocial health encompasses the mental, emotional, social, and spiritual dimensions of health (Figure 2.1). It is the result of a complex interaction between a person's history and conscious and unconscious thoughts and interpretations of the past. Psychosocially healthy people are emotionally, mentally, socially, intellectually, and spiritually resilient. They respond to challenges and frustrations in appropriate ways most of the time, despite occasional slips. Most authorities identify several basic elements shared by psychosocially healthy people:[4]

- *They feel good about themselves.* Healthy people are not typically overwhelmed by fear, love, anger, jealousy, guilt, or worry. They know who they are, have a realistic sense of their capabilities, and respect themselves even though they realize they aren't perfect.
- *They feel comfortable with other people.* Healthy people enjoy satisfying and lasting personal relationships and do not take advantage of others, nor do they allow others to take advantage of them. They can give love, consider others' interests, respect personal differences, and feel responsible for their fellow human beings.
- *They control tension and anxiety.* They recognize the underlying causes and symptoms of stress and anxiety in their lives and consciously work to avoid irrational thoughts, hostility, excessive excuse making, and blaming others for their problems.
- *They meet the demands of life.* They try to solve problems as they arise, accept responsibility, and plan ahead. Acknowledging that change is inevitable, they welcome new experiences.
- *They curb hate and guilt* by acknowledging and combating their tendencies to respond with anger, thoughtlessness, selfishness, vengeful acts, or feelings of inadequacy. Rather than knocking others aside to get ahead, they reach out to help others—even those they don't particularly like.

psychosocial health The mental, emotional, social, and spiritual dimensions of health.

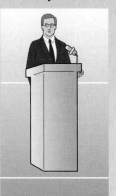

Psychosocially Healthy Person

— Zest for life, spiritually healthy and intellectually thriving
— High energy, resilient, enjoys challenges, focused
— Realistic sense of self and others, sound coping skills, open-minded
— Adapts to change easily, sensitive to others and environment

— Works to improve in all areas, recognizes strengths and weaknesses
— Healthy relationships with family and friends, capable of giving and receiving love and affection, accepts diversity
— Has strong social support, may need to work on improving social skills/interactions but usually no major problems
— Has occasional emotional "dips" but overall good mental/emotional adaptors

— Shows poorer coping than most, often overwhelmed by circumstances
— Has regular relationship problems, finds that others often disappoint
— Tends to be cynical/critical of others; has friends, but friends tend to be similarly negative/critical
— Lacks focus much of time, hard to keep intellectual acuity sharp
— Quick to anger, a bit volatile in interactions, sense of humor and fun evident less often
— Overly stressed, anxious and pessimistic attitude

— No zest for life; pessimistic/hopeless/cynical most of time; spiritually down
— Laughs, but usually at others, has little fun, no time for self
— Has serious bouts of depression, "down" and "tired" much of time; has suicidal, "life not worth living" thoughts
— A "challenge" to be around, socially isolated
— Developing neurosis/psychosis
— Experiences many illnesses, headaches, aches/pains, gets colds/infections easily

Psychosocially Unhealthy Person (Illness Likely)

FIGURE 2.2 Characteristics of Psychosocially Healthy and Unhealthy People
Where do you fall on this continuum?

■ *They maintain a positive outlook.* Psychosocially healthy people approach each day with a presumption that things will go well. They block out most negative and cynical thoughts and give star billing to the good things in life. They look to the future with enthusiasm rather than dread.
■ *They enrich the lives of others* because they recognize that there are people whose needs are greater than their own.
■ *They cherish the things that make them smile.* Reminders of good experiences brighten their day. Fun is an integral part of their lives. So is making time for themselves.
■ *They value diversity.* Healthy people do not feel threatened by those of a different race, gender, religion, sexual orientation, ethnicity, or political party. They appreciate creativity in others as well as in themselves.
■ *They respect nature.* They take time to enjoy their surroundings and are conscious of their place in the universe.

Of course, no one ever achieves perfection. Attaining psychosocial health and wellness involves many complex processes (Figure 2.2). This chapter will help you understand not only what it means to be psychosocially well, but also why we may run into problems. Learning how to assess your own health and take action to help yourself or others are important aspects of psychosocial health (see the Assess Yourself box).

 what do you THINK?

Which psychosocial qualities do you value the most in your friends? ■ Do you think that you are strong in these areas? ■ Explain your answer.

Mental Health: The Thinking You

The term **mental health** is often used to describe the "thinking" part of psychosocial health. It is defined as the

(Text continues on page 44)

mental health The thinking part of psychosocial health; includes your values, attitudes, and beliefs.

ASSESS *yourself*

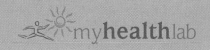

ASSESSING YOUR PSYCHOSOCIAL HEALTH

Fill out this assessment online at
www.aw-bc.com/MyHealthLab or
www.aw-bc.com/donatelle.

Being psychosocially healthy requires both introspection and the willingness to work on areas that need improvement. Begin by completing the following assessment scale. Use the scale to determine how much each statement describes you. When you've finished, ask someone who is very close to you to take the same test and respond with their perceptions of you. Carefully assess areas where your responses differ from those of your friend or family member. Which areas need some work? Which are in good shape?

	Never	Rarely	Fairly Frequently	Most of the Time	All of the Time
1. My actions and interactions indicate that I am confident in my abilities.	1	2	3	4	5
2. I am quick to blame others for things that go wrong in my life.	1	2	3	4	5
3. I am spontaneous and like to have fun with others.	1	2	3	4	5
4. I am able to give love and affection to others and show my feelings.	1	2	3	4	5
5. I am able to receive love and signs of affection from others without feeling uneasy.	1	2	3	4	5
6. I am generally positive and upbeat about things in my life.	1	2	3	4	5
7. I am cynical and tend to be critical of others.	1	2	3	4	5
8. I have a large group of people whom I consider to be good friends.	1	2	3	4	5
9. I make time for others in my life.	1	2	3	4	5
10. I take time each day for myself for quiet introspection, having fun, or just doing nothing.	1	2	3	4	5
11. I am compulsive and competitive in my actions.	1	2	3	4	5
12. I handle stress well and am seldom upset or stressed out by others.	1	2	3	4	5
13. I try to look for the good in everyone and every situation before finding fault.	1	2	3	4	5
14. I am comfortable meeting new people and interact well in social settings.	1	2	3	4	5
15. I would rather stay in and watch TV or read than go out with friends or interact with others.	1	2	3	4	5
16. I am flexible and can adapt to most situations, even if I don't like them.	1	2	3	4	5
17. Nature, the environment, and other living things are important aspects of my life.	1	2	3	4	5
18. I think before responding to my emotions.	1	2	3	4	5
19. I am selfish and tend to think of my own needs before those of others.	1	2	3	4	5
20. I am consciously trying to be a "better person."	1	2	3	4	5
21. I like to plan ahead and set realistic goals for myself and others.	1	2	3	4	5
22. I accept others for who they are.	1	2	3	4	5
23. I value diversity and respect others' rights, regardless of culture, race, sexual orientation, religion, or other differences.	1	2	3	4	5

	Never	Rarely	Fairly Frequently	Most of the Time	All of the Time
24. I try to live each day as if it might be my last.	1	2	3	4	5
25. I have a great deal of energy and appreciate the little things in life.	1	2	3	4	5
26. I cope with stress in appropriate ways.	1	2	3	4	5
27. I get enough sleep each day and seldom feel tired.	1	2	3	4	5
28. I have healthy relationships with my family.	1	2	3	4	5
29. I am confident that I can do most things if I put my mind to them.	1	2	3	4	5
30. I respect others' opinions and believe that others should be free to express their opinions, even when they differ from my own.	1	2	3	4	5

Interpreting Your Scores

Look at items 2, 7, 11, 15, and 19. Add up your score for these five items and divide by 5. Is your average for these items above or below 3? Did you score a 5 on any of these items? Do you need to work on any of these areas? Now look at your scores for the remaining items. (There should be 25 items.) Total these scores and divide by 25. Is your average above or below 3? On which items did you score a 5? Obviously you're doing well in these areas. Now remove these items from this grouping of 25 (scores of 5), and add up your scores for the remaining items. Then divide your total by the number of items included. Now what is your average?

Do the same for the scores completed by your friend or family member. How do your scores compare? Which ones, if any, are different, and how do they differ? Which areas do you need to work on? What actions can you take now to improve your ratings in these areas?

MAKE it happen!

ASSESSMENT: The Assess Yourself activity gave you the chance to look at various aspects of your psychosocial health and compare your self-assessment with a friend's perceptions. Now that you have considered these results, you can change certain behaviors that may be detrimental to your psychosocial health.

MAKING A CHANGE: In order to change your behavior, you need to develop a plan. Follow the steps below and complete your Behavior Change Contract to take action.

1. Evaluate your behavior and identify patterns and specific things you are doing. What can you change now? What can you change in the near future?

2. Select one pattern of behavior that you want to change.

3. Fill out the Behavior Change Contract found at the front of your book. It should include your long-term goal for change, your short-term goals, the rewards you'll give yourself for reaching these goals, potential obstacles along the way, and strategies for overcoming these obstacles. For each goal, list the small steps and specific actions that you will take.

4. Chart your progress in a journal. At the end of a week, consider how successful you were in following your plan. What helped you be successful? What made change more difficult? What will you do differently next week?

5. Revise your plan as needed: Are the short-term goals attainable? Are the rewards satisfying?

ONE STUDENT'S PLAN: John assessed himself as a positive and upbeat person, but the assessment his friend gave him rated him as impatient and cynical. John resolved to slow down and become more appreciative of the good things around him. Among his short-term goals: listening to his sister without interrupting her, and expressing a sincere compliment to a family member or friend every other day. John found that paying compliments made him stop to think about the qualities he appreciated in friends and family. While he struggled to listen without interrupting, John found that he was learning a lot about his sister that he had never known before. After several weeks, John's friends commented on his calmer and happier demeanor.

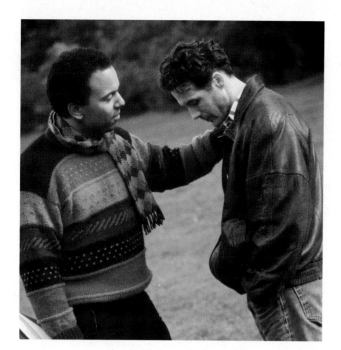

Support from family and friends is a vital component of your social health.

Emotional Health: The Feeling You

The term **emotional health** is often used interchangeably with mental health. Although the two are closely intertwined, emotional health more accurately refers to the "feeling," or subjective, side of psychosocial health. **Emotions** are intensified feelings or complex patterns of feelings that we experience on a minute-by-minute, day-to-day basis. Love, hate, frustration, anxiety, and joy are only a few of the many emotions we feel. Typically, emotions are described as the interplay of four components: physiological arousal, feelings, cognitive (thought) processes, and behavioral reactions. Each time you are placed in a stressful situation, you react physiologically while your mind tries to sort things out. You consciously or unconsciously react based on how rationally you interpret the situation.

Psychologist Richard Lazarus has indicated that there are four basic types of emotions: (1) emotions resulting from harm, loss, or threats; (2) emotions resulting from benefits; (3) borderline emotions, such as hope and compassion; and (4) more complex emotions, such as grief, disappointment, bewilderment, and curiosity.[6] Each of us may experience any of these feelings in any combination at any time. As rational beings, it is our responsibility to evaluate our individual emotional responses, the environment that is causing them, and the appropriateness of our actions.

Emotionally healthy people are usually able to respond in an appropriate manner to upsetting events. Emotionally unhealthy people are much more likely to let their feelings overpower them. They may be highly volatile and prone to unpredictable emotional responses. An ex-boyfriend who is so jealous of your new relationship that he hits you is showing an extremely unhealthy and dangerous emotional reaction.

Emotional health also affects *social health.* Someone feeling hostile, withdrawn, or moody may become socially isolated. Socially isolated people are not much fun to be around, so their friends may avoid them at the very time they are most in need of emotional support. For students, a more immediate concern is the impact of emotional trauma on academic performance. Have you ever tried to study for an exam after a fight with a close friend or family member? Emotional turmoil may seriously affect your ability to think, reason, and act rationally. Many otherwise rational, mentally healthy people do ridiculous things when they are going through a major emotional upset. Mental functioning and emotional responses are intricately connected.

successful performance of mental function, and results in productive activities, fulfilling relationships, and the ability to cope with life's challenges. Mental health plays a role in the way we think, communicate, express emotion, and feel about ourselves. A mentally healthy person has the intellectual ability to sort through information, messages, and life events, attach meaning, and respond appropriately. This is often referred to as *intellectual health,* a subset of mental health.[5]

A mentally healthy person is likely to respond to life's challenges constructively. For example, suppose you spend your spring break with friends on the beaches of Mexico, knowing that you have a major term paper due on the first day back from vacation. The night before the paper is due, you quickly throw it together. Rather than falling off the deep end and blaming the instructor if you get a "D" on the paper, a mentally healthy student would accept responsibility for the choices he or she made, learn from mistakes, and try to plan differently next time.

Learning to acknowledge that it is okay to be sad, unhappy, or frustrated and getting help through counseling or talking with trusted friends are all part of healthy adapting and coping. Unfortunately, far too many of us get caught up in our emotional upheavals and are unable to pull ourselves out of the deep "funks" we can find ourselves in.

emotional health   The feeling part of psychosocial health; includes your emotional reactions to life.

emotions   Intensified feelings or complex patterns of feelings we constantly experience.

 try it NOW

Get used to change. Change is an inevitable part of life, but it can also be a challenge to your psychosocial health. Develop skills to cope with change by creating it. Take a different route to class, study at the coffee shop instead of the library, or commit to trying a new food once a week.

Social Health: Interactions with Others

Social health, an important part of the broader concept of psychosocial health, includes your interactions with others on an individual and group basis, your ability to use social resources and support in times of need, and your ability to adapt to a variety of social situations.

Socially healthy individuals enjoy a wide range of interactions with family, friends, and acquaintances and are able to have healthy interactions with an intimate partner. They are able to listen, express themselves, form healthy relationships, act in socially acceptable and responsible ways, and find the best fit for themselves in society. Numerous studies have documented the importance of social health in promoting physical health, mental health, and enhanced longevity.[7]

As social animals, we grow stronger and learn valuable lessons in groups. From the moment we are born, we rely on parents for our care. We depend on others to learn new skills and develop much of our sense of self-worth as a result of our interactions with others. Our adult lives are spent working with others, developing relationships with family and friends, and participating in our community. Our value to society is measured by the number of connections we have and even by how many people attend our funerals. Few would disagree that social bonds are the very foundation of human life.

Social bonds reflect the level of closeness and attachment that we develop with individuals. They provide intimacy, feelings of belonging, opportunities for giving and receiving nurturance, reassurance of one's worth, assistance and guidance, and advice. Social bonds take multiple forms, the most common of which are social support and community engagements.

Social support consists of networks of people and services with whom you share ties. These ties can provide tangible support, such as babysitting services or money to help pay the bills, or intangible support, such as encouraging you to share intimate thoughts. Generally, the closer and the higher the quality of the social bond, the more likely a person is to ask for and receive social support. For example, if your car broke down on a dark country road in the middle of the night, who could you call for help and know that they would do everything possible to get there? People who are socially isolated, estranged from their families, and have few social connections will have difficulty thinking of someone to count on when they are in trouble. Psychosocially healthy people create and maintain a network of friends and family with whom they can give and receive support, and they work hard to maintain those relationships even in difficult times.

Social health also reflects the way we react to others. In its most extreme forms, a lack of social health may be represented by aggressive acts of prejudice toward other individuals or groups. In its most obvious manifestations, **prejudice** is reflected in acts of discrimination, hate, and bias, and in purposeful intent to harm individuals or groups.

Just as supportive ties promote health and longevity, the loss of such relationships threatens health. For example, on average, widows and widowers are at increased risk of mental and physical illness for up to two years after their spouse dies.

Spiritual Health: An Inner Quest for Well-Being

Although mental and emotional health are key factors in overall psychosocial functioning, it is possible to be mentally and emotionally healthy and still not achieve optimal well-being. What is missing? For many people, the difficult-to-describe element that gives zest to life is the spiritual dimension.

Most experts agree that **spirituality** refers to the personal quest for seeking answers to life's ultimate questions, finding meaning in one's life purpose, and seeking a sense of belonging to something greater than the purely physical or personal dimensions of existence.[8] For some, this unifying force is nature; for others, it is a feeling of connection to other people; for still others, the unifying force is a god or other spiritual symbol. Dr. N. Lee Smith, internist and associate professor of medicine at the University of Utah, defines spiritual health in the following ways:[9]

> **Do I have to be religious to be spiritual?**

- The quality of existence in which one is at peace with oneself and in good standing with the environment
- A sense of empowerment and personal control that includes feeling valued and in control over one's responses (but not necessarily in control of one's environment)
- A sense of connectedness to one's deepest self, to other people, and to all that is generally regarded as good
- A sense of meaning and purpose, which provides a sense of mission by finding meaning and wisdom in the here and now

On a day-to-day basis, many of us focus on acquiring material possessions and satisfying basic needs. But there comes a point when we discover that material possessions do not automatically bring happiness or a sense of self-worth. As we

---

social health Aspect of psychosocial health that includes interactions with others, ability to use social supports, and ability to adapt to various situations.

social bonds Degree and nature of interpersonal contacts.

social support Network of people and services with whom you share ties and get support.

prejudice A negative evaluation of an entire group of people that is typically based on unfavorable and often wrong ideas about the group.

spirituality A belief in a unifying force that gives meaning to life and transcends the purely physical or personal dimensions of existence.

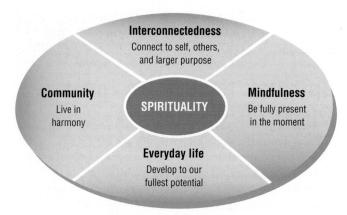

FIGURE 2.3 Four Major Themes of Spirituality

develop into spiritually healthy beings, we recognize our identity as unique individuals and gain a better appreciation of our strengths and shortcomings and our place in the universe.

In its purest sense, spirituality addresses four main themes: interconnectedness, the practice of mindfulness, spirituality as a part of everyday life, and living in harmony with the community (Figure 2.3).

- *Interconnectedness.* The term **interconnectedness** expresses a sense of harmony with oneself, with others, and with a larger meaning or purpose. Connecting with oneself involves exploring feelings, taking time to consider how you feel in a given situation, assessing your reactions to people and experiences, and taking mental notes when things or people cause you to lose equilibrium. It also involves considering your values and achieving congruence between your goals and what you can do to achieve them without compromising your values.
- *Practice of mindfulness.* **Mindfulness** refers to the ability to be fully present in the moment. Mindfulness has been described as a way of nurturing greater awareness, clarity, and acceptance of present-moment reality or a form of inner flow—a holistic sensation you feel when you are totally involved in the moment.[10] According to mindful-

interconnectedness A web of connections, including our relationship to ourselves, to others, and to a larger meaning or purpose in life.

mindfulness Awareness and acceptance of the reality of the present moment.

faith Belief that helps each person realize a unique purpose in life.

hope Belief that allows us to look confidently and courageously to the future.

love Acceptance, affirmation, and respect for the self and others.

ness experts, you can achieve this inner flow through an almost infinite range of opportunities for enjoyment and pleasure, either through the use of physical and sensory skills ranging from athletics to music to yoga or through the development of symbolic skills in areas such as poetry, philosophy, or mathematics. The psychologist Abraham Maslow referred to these moments as peak experiences, during which a person feels integrated, synergistic, and at one with the world.

- *Spirituality as a part of daily life.* Spirituality is embodied in the ability to discover and articulate our own basic purpose in life; to learn how to experience love, joy, peace, and fulfillment; and to help ourselves and others achieve their full potential.[11] This ongoing process of growth fosters three convictions: faith, hope, and love. **Faith** is the belief that helps us realize our purpose in life; **hope** is the belief that allows us to look confidently and courageously to the future; and **love** involves accepting, affirming, and respecting self and others, regardless of who they are.[12]
- *Living in harmony with our community.* Our values are an extension of our beliefs about the world and attitude toward life. They are formed over time through a series of life experiences, and they are reflected in our hopes, dreams, desires, goals, and ambitions.[13] Though most people have some idea of what is important to them, many spend life largely unaware of how their values impact themselves or those around them until a life-altering event shakes up their perspective on life.

Spirituality: A Key to Better Health

Although the specific impact of spirituality on health remains elusive, many experts affirm the importance of this dimension in achieving health and wellness. A recent study of spirituality among college students from 46 diverse universities and colleges indicates that spirituality may play a role in student health, grades, and other aspects of student life.[14] The study found a correlation between spirituality and health achievement, with more spiritually oriented students having better health, better grades, more involvement in charitable organizations or volunteerism, and more interest in helping others.

Other recent studies also indicate a correlation between certain elements of spirituality, such as "mindfulness," and positive health outcomes. Mindfulness therapies have been used effectively to treat depression, to reduce stress in outpatient therapy and in the nursing profession, with anxiety and heart disease treatments, and other problems.[15]

A Spiritual Resurgence Over recent decades, studies have shown that most Americans believe in God and consider spirituality to be important in their lives, although not necessarily in the form of religion. Many find spiritual fulfillment in music, poetry, literature, art, nature, and intimate relationships. Table 2.1 details some characteristics that distinguish religion from spirituality. Many religious groups have spawned new philosophies that are more inclusive and often influenced by "New Age" ideas, such as using positive thought to achieve your goals and striving to find your rightful place in the world.

For some, spirituality means a "quest for self and selflessness"—a form of therapy and respite from a sometimes challenging personal environment. This quest has received much scholarly and popular attention. Self-help books that focus on spirituality consistently top the bestseller lists. Television programs promote the virtues of a spiritual or natural existence. Writers and psychologists such as William James, Carl Jung, Gordon Allport, Erich Fromm, Viktor Frankl, Abraham Maslow, and Rollo May have made spirituality a major focus of their work.

Spiritual health courses have emerged in public health and medical school training. For example, the Harvard Medical School of Continuing Education offers a course called "Spirituality and Healing in Medicine," which brings together scholars and medical professionals from around the world to discuss the role of spirituality in treating illness and chronic pain. Self-help workshops focusing on spiritual elements of health are popular throughout the world.

Putting Spirituality into Practice

How can you enhance your spiritual dimension of psychosocial health? Some seek solace in religion and equate spirituality with religiosity. However, spirituality and religion are not the same thing. Enhancing your spiritual side takes just as much work as becoming physically fit, or improving your diet, or working on your mental health. The Skills for Behavior Change box on page 48 features some strategies you can implement to develop your spiritual side.

what do you THINK?

What do social, mental, emotional, and spiritual health mean to you? ▪ What are your strengths and weaknesses in these areas? ▪ What can you do to enhance your strengths? ▪ How can you improve areas that are not as strong?

Factors That Influence Psychosocial Health

Most of our mental, emotional, and social reactions to life are a direct outcome of our experiences and social and cultural expectations. Our psychosocial health is based, in part, on how we perceive life experiences.

TABLE 2.1	Characteristics Distinguishing Religion and Spirituality

Religion	Spirituality
Community focused	Individualistic
Observable, measurable, objective	Less visible and measurable, more subjective
Formal, orthodox, organized	Less formal, less orthodox, less systematic
Behavior oriented, outward practices	Emotionally oriented, inward directed
Authoritarian in terms of behaviors	Not authoritarian, little accountability
Doctrine separating good from evil	Unifying, not doctrine oriented

Source: National Institutes of Health, "Prayer and Spirituality in Health: Ancient Practices, Modern Science," *CAM at the NIH* 12, no. 1 (2005): 1–4.

External Factors

While some life experiences are under our control, others are not. External influences are those factors in life that we do not control, such as who raised us and where we lived in our youth.

The Family Families have a significant influence on psychosocial development. Children raised in healthy, nurturing, happy families are more likely to become well-adjusted, productive adults. Children raised in **dysfunctional families**— which show characteristics such as violence, distrust, anger,

How do my parents influence my psychosocial health?

dietary deprivation, drug abuse, parental discord, and sexual, physical, or emotional abuse—may have a harder time adapting to life. In dysfunctional families, love, security, and unconditional trust are so lacking that children often become confused and psychologically bruised. Yet not all people raised in dysfunctional families become psychosocially unhealthy, and not all people from healthy environments are well adjusted. Obviously, more factors are involved in our "process of becoming" than just our family.

The Broader Environment Although isolated negative events may do little damage to psychosocial health, persistent stressors, uncertainties, and threats can cause significant problems. Children raised in environments where

dysfunctional families Families in which there is violence; physical, emotional, or sexual abuse; parental discord; or other negative family interactions.

Spirituality involves connectedness to others and to the broader community, so it is important that we take time for meaningful interactions with our friends, family, and those within the community with whom we may not interact regularly. What types of actions foster connectedness?

VOLUNTEER

The ability to notice when others are in trouble and reaching out to help them through volunteering is an excellent way to feel connected with others, and enhance your own health. In the aftermath of Hurricane Katrina, thousands of people gave time, money, and effort to help an entire population that was suffering by volunteering or sending goods and providing services. Recognizing that we are all part of the greater system of humanity and that we have roles and responsibilities to help others in times of need is a key part of spirituality. Volunteering by helping your elderly neighbors clean their home,

working at the humane society, or participating in a beach or highway cleanup is all a part of being responsible and finding a place to help in the greater scheme of things. Volunteering can be a huge boost for you when you are feeling down or wondering how you fit in.

TAKE TIME TO REFLECT

Connecting with your self is another method of finding your spiritual side. Make a ritual out of taking a few moments each day to think about who you are, what you value, why you feel good, or what things are troubling you. Setting aside this special time to reflect will become a sacred time meant just for you, and can help to relieve tension, seek out answers to problems you are experiencing, or simply to empty your mind and enjoy this time to yourself.

GET INVOLVED IN SERVICE LEARNING

Service learning involves making meaningful and productive relationships with the greater community. Students have an opportunity to experience, learn new skills,

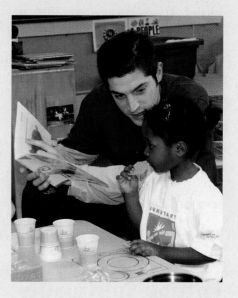

and grow. Community agencies and programs benefit from an enthusiastic, hardworking group of students. Students will learn to look at the greater community and world around them, rather than remaining absorbed in college life and thoughts of papers due, the party on Friday night, and basketball practice.

crime is rampant and daily safety is in question, for example, run an increased risk of psychosocial problems. Drugs, crime, violent acts, school failure, unemployment, and a host of other bad things can happen to good people. But it is believed that certain protective factors, such as having a positive role model in the midst of chaos, may help children from even the worst environments remain healthy and well adjusted.

Another important influence is access to health services and programs designed to enhance psychosocial health. Going to a support group or a trained therapist can be a crucial first step in prevention and intervention efforts. Individuals from poor socioeconomic environments who cannot afford such services often find it difficult to secure help in improving their psychosocial health.

Social Bonds Although often overlooked, a stable, loving support network of family and friends is key to psychosocial health. The social support of close relationships helps us get through even the most difficult times. Having those with

whom we can talk, share thoughts, and practice good and bad behaviors without fear of losing their love is an essential part of growth.

Internal Factors

Many internal factors also shape a person's development. These factors include hereditary traits, hormonal functioning, physical health status (including neurological functioning), physical fitness, and certain elements of mental and emotional health.

Self-Efficacy and Self-Esteem During our formative years, successes and failures in school, athletics, friendships, intimate relationships, our jobs, and every other aspect of life subtly shape our beliefs about our own personal worth and abilities. These beliefs in turn become internal influences on our psychosocial health.

Psychologist Albert Bandura used the term **self-efficacy** to describe a person's belief about whether he or she can successfully engage in and execute a specific behavior.

Self-esteem refers to one's sense of self-respect or self-worth. It can be defined as one's evaluation of oneself and one's own personal worth as an individual. People with high self-esteem tend to feel good about themselves and express a positive outlook on life. People with low self-esteem often do not like themselves, constantly demean themselves, and doubt their ability to succeed.

Our self-esteem is a result of the relationships we have with our parents and family during our formative years, with our friends as we grow older, with our significant others as we form intimate relationships, and with our teachers, coworkers, and others throughout our lives. If we felt loved and valued as children, our self-esteem allows us to believe that we are inherently lovable individuals. See the Skills for Behavior Change box on page 50 for some tips for increasing your self-esteem.

Learned Helplessness versus Learned Optimism
Psychologist Martin Seligman has proposed that people who continually experience failure may develop a pattern of responding known as **learned helplessness** in which they give up and fail to take any action to help themselves. Seligman ascribes this in part to society's tendency toward "victimology," blaming one's problems on other people and circumstances. Whereas viewing ourselves as victims may make us feel better temporarily, it does not address the underlying causes of a problem. Ultimately, it erodes self-efficacy and fosters learned helplessness by making us feel that we cannot do anything to improve the situation.[16]

Countering this is Seligman's principle of **learned optimism**: just as we learn to be helpless, so can we teach ourselves to be optimistic. His research provides growing evidence for the central place of mental health in overall positive development.[17]

In one study, university freshmen who had been identified as pessimistic on the basis of a questionnaire were randomly assigned to an experimental group or a control group. The experimental group attended a 16-hour workshop in which they practiced social and study skills and learned to dispute chronic negative thoughts. The control group did not participate. Eighteen months later, 15 percent of the control group members were experiencing severe anxiety and 32 percent were suffering from moderate to severe depression. In contrast, only 7 percent of workshop participants suffered from anxiety and 22 percent from depression. Seligman concluded that even relatively brief interventions, such as this workshop, can produce measurable improvements in coping skills.[18]

Personality
Your personality is the unique mix of characteristics that distinguish you from others. Hereditary, environmental, cultural, and experiential factors influence how each person develops. Personality determines how we react

to the challenges of life, interpret our feelings, and resolve conflicts.

Most of the recent psychosocial theories promote the idea that we have the power not only to understand our behavior, but also to actively change it and thus mold our own personalities. Yet although much has been written about the importance of a healthy personality, there is little consensus on what that concept really means. In general, people who possess the following traits often appear to be psychosocially healthy.[19]

- *Extroversion,* the ability to adapt to a social situation and demonstrate assertiveness, power, and/or interpersonal involvement
- *Agreeableness,* the ability to conform, be likable, and demonstrate friendly compliance as well as love
- *Openness to experience,* the willingness to demonstrate curiosity and independence (also referred to as inquiring intellect)
- *Emotional stability,* the ability to maintain social control
- *Conscientiousness,* the qualities of being dependable and demonstrating self-control, discipline, and a need to achieve

Life Span and Maturity
Our temperaments also change as we grow, as is illustrated by the extreme emotions experienced by many people in early adolescence. Most of us learn to control our emotions as we advance toward adulthood.

The college years mark a critical transition period for young adults as they move away from families and establish themselves as independent adults. For most, this step toward maturity entails changing the nature of the relationship to parents. Managing personal finances, career strategies, and interpersonal communication are among the developmental tasks college students must accomplish. Older students often have to balance the responsibilities of family, career, and school.

The transition to independence will be easier for those who have successfully accomplished earlier developmental tasks such as learning how to solve problems, make and evaluate decisions, define and adhere to personal values, and establish both casual and intimate relationships. People who have not fulfilled these earlier tasks may find their lives interrupted by recurrent crises left over from earlier stages. For example, if they did not learn to trust others in childhood, they may have difficulty establishing intimate relationships as adults.

self-efficacy   Belief in one's own ability to perform a task successfully.

self-esteem   Sense of self-respect or self-confidence.

learned helplessness   Pattern of responding to situations by giving up because of repeated failure in the past.

learned optimism   Teaching oneself to think optimistically.

How can you build self-esteem? Many things you can do daily can have a significant impact on the way you feel about yourself. Practice these tips regularly to bolster your self-esteem.

- *Pay attention to your own needs and wants.* Listen to what your body, your mind, and your heart are telling you.
- *Take good care of yourself.* Eat healthy foods, avoid junk foods, exercise, and plan fun activities for yourself.
- *Take time to do things you enjoy.* Make a list of things you enjoy doing. Then do something from that list every day.
- *Do something that you have been putting off.* Cleaning out your closet, going on a diet, or paying a bill that you've been putting off will make you feel like you've accomplished something.

- *Give yourself rewards.* Acknowledge that you are a great person by rewarding yourself occasionally.
- *Spend time with people.* People who make you feel better about yourself are great self-esteem boosters. Avoid people who treat you badly or make you feel bad about yourself.
- *Display items that you like.* You may have items that remind you of your achievements, your friends, or special times. Keep them close by.
- *Make your meals a special time.* Get rid of distractions like the television and really concentrate on enjoying your meal, whether by yourself or with others.
- *Learn something new every day.* Take advantage of any opportunity to learn something new every day—you'll feel

better about yourself and be more productive.
- *Do something nice for another person.* There is no greater way to feel better about yourself than to help someone in greater need. Check out local volunteer opportunities or make a special effort to be nice to those around you such as your parents or siblings.

Sources: A. L. Story, "Self-Esteem and Self-Certainty: A Meditational Analysis," *European Journal of Personality* 18, no. 2 (March 2004): 115; M. E. Copeland, "Building Self-Esteem: A Self-Help Guide," Center for Mental Health Services online booklet, May 10, 2004, www.mentalhealth.org/publications/allpubs/SMA-3715/default.asp.

Resiliency and Developmental Assets

Over the last decade, it has become well established that some people are much better prepared to meet the challenges of life than others. The combination of certain personality traits, coupled with a supportive environment, can equip one to deal effectively with life's many challenges. These individuals are able to cope and even thrive in times of great stress or pressure. **Resiliency** or **protective factors** are terms used to describe traits or characteristics that protect an individual

or community from threat or harm. In a sense, these traits may serve to inoculate one against potential ill health. People with **assets**, whether they be financial, emotional, spiritual, physical, intellectual, or mental, and other positive forces in their lives, are more likely to be resilient and able to recover when facing life's challenges.

Flourishing means living within an optimal range of human functioning—one that connotes goodness, productivity, growth, and resilience. For example, research shows that positive attitudes, such as interest and curiosity, produce more accurate subsequent knowledge than negative attitudes, like cynicism and boredom. It follows that if you start the first day in a class being "turned off" by the instructor and wondering what you are doing there, it is less likely that you will do well than if you strive for positiveness in your attitude and self-talk about the experience.[20]

resiliency (protective factors) An individual's capacity for adapting to change and stressful events in healthy and flexible ways.

assets Internal and external resources and community supports that help a person be more resilient in difficult times and more likely to make positive choices and respond in positive, healthful ways.

flourishing Living within an optimal range of human functioning—one that connotes goodness, productivity, growth, and resilience.

Strategies to Enhance Psychosocial Health

As we have seen, psychosocial health involves four dimensions. Attaining self-fulfillment is a lifelong, conscious process that involves enhancing each of these components. Strategies include building self-efficacy and self-esteem, understanding and controlling emotions, maintaining support networks, and learning to solve problems and make decisions. In addition to the advice in this chapter, see Chapter 3 for tips on effective stress reduction, relaxation techniques, and other tools for enhancing psychosocial health.

Developing and Maintaining Self-Esteem and Self-Efficacy

There are several ways to build self-esteem and self-efficacy. These include finding a support group, completing required tasks, forming realistic expectations, making time for yourself, maintaining your physical health, and examining your problems and seeking help.

Find a Support Group The best way to build self-esteem is through a support group—peers who share your values. The prime prerequisite for a support group is that it makes you feel good about yourself and forces you to take an honest look at your actions and choices. Although the idea of finding a support group seems to imply establishing a wholly new group, remember that old ties are often the strongest.

Keeping in contact with old friends and important family members can provide a foundation of unconditional love that will help you through the many life transitions ahead. Try to be a support for others, too. Join a discussion, political action, or recreational group. Write more postcards and "thinking of you" notes to people who matter. This will build both your own self-esteem and that of your friends.

Complete Required Tasks Develop a history of success by completing required tasks well. You are less likely to succeed in your studies if you leave term papers until the last minute or fail to ask about points that are confusing to you. Most college campuses provide study groups and learning centers that offer tips for managing time, understanding assignments, dealing with professors, and preparing for tests. Poor grades, or grades that do not meet expectations, are major contributors to emotional distress among college students.

Form Realistic Expectations Set realistic expectations for yourself. If you expect perfect grades, a steady stream of Saturday-night dates and soap-opera romances, and the perfect job, you may be setting yourself up for failure. Assess your current resources and the direction in which you are heading. Set small, incremental goals that are possible to meet.

Make Time for You Taking time to enjoy yourself is another way to boost self-esteem and psychosocial health. Trying to view each new activity as something to look forward to and an opportunity to have fun is an important part of keeping the excitement in your life. Wake up focusing on the fun things you have to look forward to each day, and try to make this anticipation a natural part of your day.

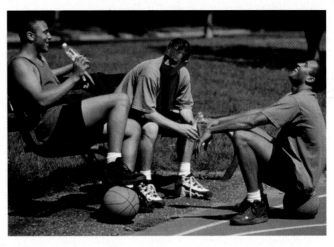

A solid support group can be as simple as spending time playing a team sport, like basketball, with friends.

Maintain Physical Health Regular exercise fosters a sense of well-being. Nourishing meals can help you avoid the weight gain experienced by many college students. Several studies support the role of exercise in improved mental health.[21] (See Chapter 8 for information on nutrition and Chapter 10 for more on the importance of exercise.)

Examine Problems and Seek Help When Necessary Knowing when to seek help from friends, support groups, family, or professionals is another important factor in boosting self-esteem. Sometimes you can handle life's problems alone; at other times, you need assistance.

Sleep: The Great Restorer

Sleep serves at least two biological purposes: (1) conservation of energy so that we are rested and ready to perform during high-performance daylight hours and (2) restoration so that neurotransmitters that have been depleted during waking hours can be replenished. This process clears the brain of daily minutiae to prepare for a new day. Getting enough sleep to feel ready to meet daily challenges is a key factor in physical and psychosocial health.

All of us can identify with that tired, listless feeling caused by sleep deprivation during periods of high stress. Either we can't find enough hours in the day for sleep, or once we get into bed, we can't fall asleep or stay asleep. Sleep, or lack of it, is especially common among college students; in a small survey of students at Notre Dame University, nearly 70 percent of students surveyed indicated they only receive 5 or 6 hours of sleep each weeknight. College students have a high workload, anxiety, and stress—all factors that may explain the collective lack of sleep among those aged 18 to 24.

How much sleep do we need? This depends on many factors. There is a genetically based need for sleep, and it differs

TABLE 2.2   Getting a Good Night's Sleep

- **Establish a consistent sleep schedule.** Go to bed and get up at about the same time every day.
- **Evaluate your sleep environment.** Is there something keeping you awake? If it's noise, wear earplugs or use a white-noise item such as running a fan. If it's light, try room-darkening shades.
- **Exercise regularly.** It's hard to feel drowsy if you have been sedentary all day. Don't exercise right before bedtime, because activity speeds up your metabolism and makes it harder to go to sleep.
- **Limit caffeine and alcohol.** Caffeine can linger in your body for up to 12 hours and cause insomnia. Although alcohol may make you drowsy at first, it interferes with the normal sleep–wake cycle.
- **Avoid eating a heavy meal or drinking large amounts of liquid before bed.**
- **Don't lie in bed, tossing and turning.** If you're unable to get to sleep in 30 minutes, get up and do something else. Read, play solitaire, or try other relaxing activities; return to bed when you feel drowsy.
- **Nap only in the afternoon.** This is when our circadian rhythms tend to make us sleepy. Don't let naps interfere with your normal sleep schedule.
- **Establish a relaxing nighttime ritual that puts you in the mood to sleep.** Take a warm shower, relax in a comfortable chair, don your favorite robe. Doing this consistently will cue your mind and body that it's time to wind down.

for each species. People may also alter sleep patterns by staying up late, drinking coffee, getting lots of physical exercise, eating a heavy meal, or using alarm clocks.

The most important period of sleep, known as the time of *rapid eye movement (REM)* sleep, is essential to feeling rested and refreshed. In REM sleep, heart rate increases, respiration speeds up, and dreaming tends to occur. If we miss REM sleep, we are left feeling groggy and sleep deprived.

Though many people turn to over-the-counter sleeping pills, barbiturates, or tranquilizers, look at Table 2.2 for more effective and less risky methods for conquering sleeplessness.

insomnia   Difficulty in falling asleep or staying asleep.

sleep apnea   Disorder in which a person has numerous episodes of breathing stoppage during a normal night's sleep.

psychoneuroimmunology   The science that exames the relationship between the brain and behavior and how this affects the body's immune system.

happiness   Feeling of contentment created when one's expectations and physical, psychological, and spiritual needs have been met and one enjoys life.

subjective well-being (SWB)   That uplifting feeling of inner peace and wonder that we call happiness.

Sleep Disorders   Today, nearly 70 million Americans suffer from sleep problems, and have difficulty getting a good night's rest due to a variety of sleep disorders. **Insomnia**—difficulty in falling asleep quickly, frequent arousals during sleep, or early morning awakening—is a common complaint among 20 to 40 percent of Americans. Insomnia is more common among women than men, and its prevalence is correlated with age and low socioeconomic status.

An increasingly common condition is **sleep apnea**, which is characterized by periodic episodes when the sleeper stops breathing completely or takes only shallow breaths for 10 seconds or longer at a time. In either case, the person does not get enough oxygen and may wake often. More than 12 million Americans suffer from sleep apnea, with the majority of sufferers being male.[22] (See the Women's Health/Men's Health box on page 56 for more on sleep problems that affect men and women.) Typically caused by upper respiratory tract problems in which weak muscle tone allows part of the airway to collapse, sleep apnea results in poor air exchange. This in turn raises blood pressure and lowers blood oxygen levels. Sleep apnea can pose a serious health risk.

The Mind–Body Connection

Can negative emotions make us physically ill? Can positive emotions and happiness help us stay well? Researchers are exploring the interaction between emotions and health, especially in conditions of uncontrolled, persistent stress. At the core of the mind–body connection is the study of **psychoneuroimmunology (PNI)**, or how the brain and behavior affect the body's immune system. The science of PNI focuses on the relationship between psychosocial factors, the central nervous system, the immune system, and disease and illness.[23] One area that appears to be particularly promising is the emotion of happiness.

Happiness and Physical Health

Happiness is defined as a kind of placeholder for a number of positive states in which individuals actively embrace the world around them.[24] As scientists have examined characteristics of happy people, they have found that this emotion can have a profound impact on the body. Researchers have discovered that happiness or related mental states like hopefulness, optimism, and contentment appear to reduce the risk or limit the severity of cardiovascular disease, pulmonary disease, diabetes, hypertension, colds, and other infections.

If happiness is good for your health, how does one "get happy"? **Subjective well-being (SWB)** refers to that uplifting feeling of inner peace or an overall "feel-good" state, which includes happiness. SWB is defined by three central components:[25]

1. *Satisfaction with present life.* People who are high in SWB tend to like their work and are satisfied with their current personal relationships. They are sociable, outgoing, and willing to open up to others. They also like themselves and enjoy good health and self-esteem.

2. *Relative presence of positive emotions.* People with high SWB more frequently feel pleasant emotions, mainly because they evaluate the world around them in a generally positive way. They have an optimistic outlook, and they expect success in what they undertake.

3. *Relative absence of negative emotions.* Individuals with a strong sense of subjective well-being experience fewer and less severe episodes of negative emotions, such as anxiety, depression, and anger.

You do not have to be happy all the time to achieve overall subjective well-being. Everyone experiences disappointments, unhappiness, and times when life seems unfair. However, people with SWB are typically resilient, able to look on the positive side, get themselves back on track fairly quickly, and less likely to fall into despair over setbacks. Most find some measure of happiness after the initial shock and pain of loss. Those who are otherwise healthy, in good physical condition, and part of a strong social support network can adapt and cope effectively. There are several myths about happiness: that it depends on age, gender, race, and socioeconomic status.

Scientists also suggest that people may be biologically predisposed to happiness. Psychologist Richard Davidson suggests that happiness may, in part, be related to actual differences in brain physiology—that *neurotransmitters,* the chemicals that transfer messages between neurons, may function more efficiently in happy people.[26] Other psychologists suggest that we can develop happiness by practicing positive psychological actions.[27]

How happy are you? Take the quiz in Figure 2.5 on the following page and see how you score.

Using Positive Psychology to Enhance Happiness

The emerging discipline of positive psychology focuses on helping us achieve the happiness we desire, find meaning in life, build our character strengths, and in general approach life from a more "positivistic" perspective. Currently, researchers are focusing efforts on developing methods that can be used to teach people how to focus on the positive.[28] Though this body of research is still in its early stages, several key aspects have emerged, and you can implement the following strategies to enhance happiness and employ a more positive outlook on life:[29]

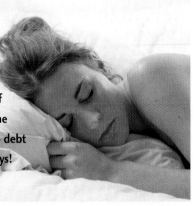

FUNfact

Every night you don't get 8 hours of sleep creates a "sleep debt." The average college student gets 5 hours of sleep a night. In just one semester, that's a sleep debt of 336 hours, or 28 days!

FIGURE 2.4 How Much Sleep Do You Get?

Source: W. Dement, "What All Undergraduates Should Know About How Their Sleeping Lives Affect Their Waking Lives," www.stanford.edu/~dement/index.html.

- *Develop gratitude.* **Gratitude** is a sense of thankfulness and appreciation for the good things in your life as well as for life's lessons.
- *Use capitalization.* **Capitalization** refers to the process by which we focus on the good things that happen to us and share those things with others. Research in this area indicates that telling others about a positive experience increases the positive emotion associated with the event and prolongs the good feelings.
- *Know when to say when.* Researchers have found that people who are always trying to do their absolute best may be more prone to depression, frustration, anxiety, and other problems. Researchers have coined the term "satisfice" to describe the ability to know when an outcome is good enough, rather than ideal. We should find a level of achievement that we will be satisfied with, make sure it is realistic, and stick to it.
- *Grow a signature strength.* Traits such as wisdom, courage, humanity, hope, vitality, curiosity, and love are all considered virtues one should work hard to grow. These strengths are believed to be the most important to one's overall health.

Does Laughter Enhance Health?

Remember the last time you laughed so hard that you cried? Remember how relaxed you felt afterward? Scientists are just

gratitude A sense of thankfulness and appreciation for the good things in your life as well as for life's lessons.

capitalization The process by which we focus on the good things that happen to us and share those things with others.

How Happy Are You?

Read the following statements, and then rate your level of agreement with each one using the 1–7 scale.

1	2	3	4	5	6	7
Strongly disagree	Disagree	Slightly disagree	Neither agree nor disagree	Slightly agree	Agree	Strongly agree

1. In most ways, my life is close to my ideal. _____
2. The conditions of my life are excellent. _____
3. I am satisfied with my life. _____
4. So far I have gotten the important things I want in life. _____
5. If I could live my life over, I would change almost nothing. _____

Total score: _____

Scoring:
31–35: You are very satisfied with your life 26–30: Satisfied 21–25: Slightly satisfied
20: You are neither satisfied nor dissatisfied 15–19: Slightly dissatisfied 10–14: Dissatisfied 5–9: Very dissatisfied

FIGURE 2.5 Satisfaction with Life Scale

Source: W. Pavot and E. Diener, "Review of the Satisfaction with Life Scale," *Psychological Assessment* 5 (1993): 164–172.

beginning to understand the role of humor in our lives and health:

■ Stressed-out people with a strong sense of humor become less depressed and anxious than those whose sense of humor is less well developed.
■ Students who use humor as a coping mechanism report that it predisposes them to a positive mood.
■ In a study of depressed and suicidal senior citizens, patients who recovered were the ones who demonstrated a sense of humor.
■ Telling a joke, particularly one that involves a shared experience, increases our sense of belonging and social cohesion.

Clearly, laughter enhances mental, emotional, and social health. Learning to laugh puts more joy into everyday experiences and increases the likelihood that fun-loving people will keep company with us.

Psychologist Barbara Fredrickson argues that positive emotions such as joy, interest, and contentment serve valuable life functions. These positive feelings empower us to cope effectively with life's challenges. Though the actual emotions may be transient, their effects can be permanent and provide lifelong enrichment.[30]

Laughter also seems to have positive physiological effects. A number of researchers, such as Lee Berk, MD, have noted that laughter and humor sharpens our immune system by activating natural killer cells, thus boosting our body's ability to stave off disease and infection. In one study, Dr. Berk looked at students who watched humorous videotapes, and those who didn't. Those who did watch the humorous videos had a significantly higher level of immune system activity than those who did not.[31] Other researchers have found that a fighting spirit, hope, and optimism are vital adjuncts to standard cancer therapy and successful treatment.[32]

While positive emotions appear to benefit physical health, evidence is accumulating that negative emotions can impair it. Studies of widowed and divorced people reveal below-normal immune system functioning and higher rates of illness and death than among married people. Other studies have shown unusually high rates of cancer among depressed people.[33]

Some researchers believe that certain psychosocial behaviors actually make people vulnerable to illness. Psychologist Lydia Temoshok studied people with malignant melanoma (a potentially deadly skin cancer) and found that 75 percent shared common traits. They tended to be unfailingly pleasant, repress their negative feelings and emotions, and make extraordinary attempts to accommodate others. She hypothesized that this "Type C" personality signals emotional repression, which may suppress the immune system.[34]

Do these studies provide conclusive evidence of a mind–body connection? Not necessarily, because they do not account for other factors known to be relevant to health. For example, some researchers suggest that people who are divorced, widowed, or depressed are more likely to drink and smoke, use drugs, eat and sleep poorly, and be sedentary—all of which may affect the immune system. We still have much to learn about this relationship. In the meantime, however, it appears that happiness and an optimistic mind-set don't just feel good—they are also good for you.

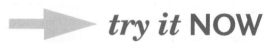 *try it* NOW

Find your flow! Flow is considered the contentment and happiness you experience when completely absorbed in an activity you enjoy. Scientists have discovered that flow induces a state of relaxed alertness, similar to meditation. To find your flow, paint a picture, write a story, or dance to your favorite music. Once you've found your flow, you'll be hooked!

When Psychosocial Health Deteriorates

Sometimes circumstances overwhelm us to such a degree that we need outside assistance to help us get back on track toward healthful living. Abusive relationships, stress, anxiety, loneliness, financial upheavals, and other traumatic events can sap our spirits, causing us to turn inward or to act in ways that are outside of what might be considered normal. Chemical imbalances, drug interactions, trauma, neurological disruptions, and other physical problems also may contribute to these behaviors. **Mental illnesses** are disorders that disrupt thinking, feeling, moods, and behaviors, and cause varying degrees of distress. They are believed to be caused by life events in some cases and by actual biochemical and/or brain dysfunction in other instances.[35] As with physical disease, mental illnesses can range from mild to severe and exact a heavy toll on the quality of life, both for those with the illnesses and those who come in contact with them.

Mental illness is universal, affecting all nationalities, ethnicities, and races around the globe. An estimated 26 percent of Americans aged 18 and older suffer from a diagnosed mental disorder in a given year. This is equal to one in every four people. Many individuals suffer from more than one mental disorder at a given time and there are huge disparities by age, culture, race, ethnicity and socioeconomic status in the recognition and treatment of mental disorders.[36]

Although there are many types of mental illnesses, we will focus here on those most likely to be experienced by large numbers of college students. For information about other disorders, consult the websites at the end of this chapter or ask your instructor for local resources.

Mood Disorders

Chronic mood disorders are disorders that affect how you feel, such as persistent sadness despair, or hopelessness. They include depression, dysthymic disorder, and bipolar disorder. In any given year, approximately 10 percent or 20.9 million Americans aged 18 or older suffer from one of the mood disorders.

Depression: The Full-Scale Tumble

According to a statement from the American Psychological Association, "Depression has been called the common cold of psychological disturbances, which underscores its prevalence, but trivializes its impact."[37] Just how serious is it? Depression affects approximately 14.8 million American adults, or about 7 percent of the U.S. population, each year.[38] Although depression can develop at any age, the median age at onset is 32. It is important to recognize that these numbers may reflect

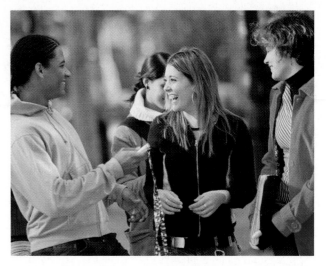

Sharing laughter and having fun with friends improves our social dimension of health and can put more joy into everyday life.

just the tip of the iceberg when it comes to true numbers of people with depression. Many more are misdiagnosed, underdiagnosed, not receiving treatment, or are not treated with the right combinations of therapy.[39]

College Students and Depression College students, particularly college freshmen, suddenly thrust into a new environment, without the support of family, friends, and their community, and confronted with high pressure to succeed, often are at high risk for depressive episodes. Over a four-year period, from 2000 to 2004, the number of students who reported "having been diagnosed with depression" increased by nearly 5 percent, from 10.3 percent in 2000 to 14.9 percent in 2004. Today, results from the same National College Health Assessment indicate that 21 percent of students rated depression among their top ten physical and mental problems in the last year. Another 14 percent reported that anxiety was a top ten problem.[40]

Depression can strike at any age, but the first episode usually occurs before age 40. (See Table 2.3 on page 58, which lists common symptoms.) Some people experience one bout of depression and never have problems again, but others suffer recurrences throughout their lives. Stressful life events are often catalysts for these recurrences.

Types of Depression

Sometimes life throws us down the proverbial stairs. We experience loss, pain, disappointment, or frustration and we can be left feeling beaten and bruised. How do we know if those

mental illnesses Disorders that disrupt thinking, feeling, moods, and behaviors, and impair daily functioning.

chronic mood disorder Experience of persistent sadness, despair, and hopelessness.

GENDER DIFFERENCES IN SLEEP PROBLEMS

Women and men face a unique set of issues that can affect sleep. In recent years, researchers have started to recognize that women are much more likely than men to suffer from sleep disorders. In a recent study conducted by the National Sleep Foundation, 70 percent of menstruating women of all age groups reported sleep disruptions during their period, and women were also more likely than men to suffer from insomnia in general. The table below explores the most common sources of sleep problems for women and men, and what can be done to treat them.

BIOLOGICAL REASONS FOR SLEEP DISORDER
Women

	Symptoms	Causes	Remedies
Menstruation	Bloating, soreness, cramps, and headaches disturb between two and three nights of sleep per month.	Hormonal fluctuation that affects the body and nervous system can disrupt normal sleep patterns.	Most symptoms get better with time. Otherwise, try over-the-counter painkillers and reduce caffeine.
Pregnancy	At first, frequent bathroom trips and daytime sleepiness. Later, restlessness, heartburn, and back pain.	Rising progesterone levels cause sleepiness. Other symptoms: pressure placed on the internal organs by the baby.	Short naps in the early afternoon, supportive pillows and lying on the side to sleep. Avoid spicy foods to prevent heartburn.
Menopause	Hot flashes, insomnia, and sleep apnea, in which the airway is briefly but repeatedly blocked during sleep.	Drops in progesterone and estrogen levels (the exact cause of hot flashes is still unclear) and weight gain.	Hormone therapy works for some but may increase the risk of blood clots or aggravate certain types of cancer.

feelings and emotions are really signs of a **major depressive disorder**? It's important to note that true depressive disorders are not the same as having a bad day or feeling down after a negative experience. It also isn't something that can be willed or wished away, or just a matter of learning to "grow a thicker skin." True major depressive disorders are characterized by a combination of symptoms that interfere with work, study, sleep, eating, relationships, and enjoyment of life. Symptoms can last for weeks, months, or years and vary in intensity.[41]

A less severe type of depression, known as **dysthymia**, is a milder, harder to recognize type of depression. Dysthymic individuals may appear to function okay, but they may lack energy or fatigue easily, be short-tempered, overly pessimistic, and ornery, or just not quite feel up to par without having any really overt symptoms. People with dysthymia may cycle into major depression over time. Without treatment, it won't go away.[42]

Still another type of depression is **bipolar disorder**, also called manic-depressive illness. People with bipolar disorder often have severe mood swings, ranging from extreme highs (mania) to lows (depression). Sometimes these swings are dramatic and rapid; other times they are slow and gradual. When in the manic phase, people may be overactive, talkative, and have tons of energy; in the depressed phase they may experience some or all of the typical major depressive symptoms.

major depressive disorder Severe depression that entails chronic mood disorder, physical effects such as sleep disturbance and exhaustion, and mental effects such as the inability to concentrate.

dysthymia A less severe type of depression that is milder, harder to recognize, and often characterized by fatigue, pessimism, or a short temper.

bipolar disorder Form of depression characterized by alternating mania and depression.

Men

	Symptoms	Causes	Remedies
Sleep apnea	Daytime exhaustion, snoring, gasping sounds	Overweight, fat around the neck, abnormal facial structure	Continuous positive airway pressure (CAP), weight loss, sleep on side
Prostatism	Frequent bathroom trips through the night	Enlarged prostate	Surgery to remove obstructing prostate tissue, medication

MENTAL AND PHYSICAL REASONS FOR SLEEP DISORDERS

Both Genders

	Symptoms	Causes	Remedies
Stress	Insomnia, a "racing" mind, restlessness, headaches, nightmares.	Tension brought on by stressful situations, like marital troubles or financial problems.	First, improve sleep, hygiene, and exercise early in the day; hypnotics are a short-term option.
Depression	Early-morning waking, fatigue, and excessive sleepiness during the day; insomnia at night.	Depression can change brain chemical levels and disrupt sleep.	Antidepressants (consult a doctor); psychotherapy.
Anxiety	Nighttime panic attacks that wake the sleeper; insomnia from chronic fear and worrying.	Anxiety triggers the release of chemicals that speed up breathing and heart rate; caffeine may also contribute.	Exercise regularly and avoid caffeine. If that isn't enough, anti-anxiety drugs like Xanax may help.

Source: M. Kryger, *A Woman's Guide to Sleep Disorders* (Boston: McGraw-Hill, 2004); National Sleep Foundation, "Sleep in America," 2002. www.sleepfoundation.org.

Although the exact cause of bipolar disorder is unknown, biological, genetic, and environmental factors seem to be involved in causing episodes of the illness. Factors that are believed to trigger episodes include drug abuse and stressful or psychologically traumatic events. Once diagnosed, persons with bipolar disorder have a number of counseling and pharmaceutical options, and most will be able to live a healthy, functional life while being treated.

Causes of Depression

Major depressive disorder is caused by the interaction between biology, learned behavioral responses, cognitive factors, environment, and situational triggers and stressors. Some types of depression, such as bipolar disorder, appear to run in families. People who have low self-esteem, who consistently view themselves and the world with pessimism, or who are readily overwhelmed by stress are prone to depression. Depression can also be triggered by a serious loss, diffi-cult relationship, financial problems, and pressure to get good grades or succeed in athletics. In recent years, researchers have shown that physical changes in the body can be accompanied by mental changes, particularly depression. Stroke, heart attack, cancer, Parkinson's disease, noninsulin-dependent diabetes, and hormonal disorders can cause depressive illness, making the sick person apathetic and unwilling to care for his or her physical needs, thus reducing chances of recovery.[43]

Depression in Diverse Populations

Depression and Women Women are almost twice as likely to experience depression as men. Hormonal changes related to the menstrual cycle, pregnancy, miscarriage, postpartum period, premenopause, and menopause may be factors in this increased rate.[44] Additionally, women face various

TABLE 2.3	Are You Depressed?

Sadness and despair are the main symptoms of depression. Other common signs include:

- Loss of motivation or interest in pleasurable activities
- Preoccupation with failures and inadequacies; concern over what others are thinking
- Difficulty concentrating; indecisiveness; memory lapses
- Loss of sex drive or interest in close interactions with others
- Fatigue and loss of energy; slow reactions
- Sleeping too much or too little; insomnia
- Feeling agitated, worthless, or hopeless
- Withdrawal from friends and family
- Diminished or increased appetite
- Recurring thoughts that life isn't worth living, thoughts of death or suicide
- Significant weight loss or weight gain

Some depressed people mask their symptoms with a forced, upbeat sense of humor or high energy levels. Communication may cease or seem frantic.

stressors in their lives related to dual responsibilities of work and child rearing, single parenthood, household work, and caring for elderly parents, at rates that are higher than those of men.

Although adolescent and adult females have been found to experience depression at twice the rate of males, the college population seems to represent a notable exception. Recent results from the National College Health Association survey indicate that rates of depression among college-aged women are only slightly higher than those of their male counterparts.[45] Why are women in a university setting no more prone to depression than men? Several theories have been suggested:[46]

- The social institutions of the college campus provide more egalitarian roles for men and women.
- College women experience fewer negative events than do high school females. Men in college report more negative events than they experienced in high school.
- College women report smaller and more supportive social networks.

Finally, researchers have observed gender differences in coping strategies (responses to certain events or stimuli) and have proposed that some women's strategies make them more vulnerable to depression. Presented with a list of things people do when depressed, college students were asked to indicate how likely they were to engage in each behavior. Men were more likely to assert that "I avoid thinking of reasons why I am depressed," "I do something physical," or "I play sports." Women were more likely to answer "I try to determine why I am depressed," "I talk to other people about my feelings," and "I cry to relieve the tension." In other words, the men tried to distract themselves from a depressed mood

whereas the women focused on it. If focusing obsessively on negative feelings intensifies these feelings, women who do this may predispose themselves to depression. This hypothesis has not been directly tested, but some supporting evidence suggests its validity.[47]

Depression and Men Six million men in the United States are currently in treatment for depression and countless others should be. Depression in men is often masked by alcohol or drug abuse, or by the socially acceptable habit of working excessively long hours. Typically, depressed men present not as hopeless and helpless, but as irritable, angry, and discouraged, often personifying a "tough guy" image. Men are less likely to admit they are depressed and doctors are less likely to suspect it, based on what men report during visits to a doctor.[48] Depression can also affect the physical health of men differently than women. Although depression is associated with an increased risk of coronary heart disease in both men and women, only men suffer a high death rate. Men are also more likely to act on suicidal feelings than are women, and are usually more successful at suicide as well; suicide rates among depressed men are four times those of women.[49] Encouragement and support from families and friends may help men to recognize symptoms and seek treatment.

Depression in the Elderly Contrary to popular thinking, it is not normal for older people to be depressed; in fact, most older people are satisfied with their lives. However, because the elderly are less likely to discuss feelings of sadness, loss, helplessness, or other symptoms, or to attribute their own depression to aging, they are likely to be undiagnosed or untreated. Additionally, because they often take multiple medications, many of which may result in depression symptoms, they may be at increased risk.

Depression Among Minority Populations
In a recent survey of U.S. citizens between the ages of 15 and 40, the prevalence of major depressive disorder was significantly higher in whites than in African Americans and Mexican Americans; the opposite was found for dysthymic disorder. Poverty was a significant risk factor for major depression among all racial groups.[50]

Depression in Children Today, depression in children is an increasingly reported phenomenon, with shocking cases of suicide and other outcomes in children as young as 4 and 5 years old. Depressed children may pretend to be sick, refuse to go to school, sleep incessantly, engage in self-mutilation, get into trouble with drugs or alcohol, feel misunderstood, and attempt suicide. Parents of children who are depressed may find it difficult to find therapists trained in working with kids who are depressed or physicians skilled in determining which adult antidepressants may be best for children. Why is depression increasing among the young? A recent report in the *American Journal of Psychiatry* indicates that offspring of a depressed parent are three times as likely to have anxiety disorders, major depression, or substance dependence and they are also at greater risk of social impairment on the job or in family life.[51]

Depression on Campus
The stressors of college life, such as anxiety over relationships, pressure to get good grades and win social acceptance, abuse of alcohol and other drugs, poor diet, and lack of sleep can create a toxic cocktail.[52] It is no surprise that depression on college campuses is a huge problem. According to a longitudinal study of students who sought help at Kansas State University over a 13-year period, sources of depression changed from relationship and money problems in the 1980s to more serious forms of stress-related anxiety in later years, paralleling trends in society as a whole.[53] International students are particularly vulnerable to mental health concerns. Being far from home without the security of family and friends can exacerbate problems and make coping difficult. Most campuses have cultural centers and other services available; however, many students do not utilize them. See the Spotlight on Your Health box on page 60 for more on campus mental health initiatives.

Treating Depression
The best treatment involves determining the person's type and degree of depression and its possible causes. Both psychotherapeutic and pharmacological modes of treatment are recommended for clinical (severe and prolonged) depression. Drugs often relieve the symptoms of depression, such as loss of sleep or appetite, while psychotherapy can be equally helpful by improving the ability to function. In some cases, psychotherapy alone may be the most successful treatment. The two most common psychotherapeutic treatments for depression are cognitive therapy and interpersonal therapy.

Cognitive Therapy
Cognitive therapy helps a patient look at life rationally and correct habitually pessimistic thought patterns. It focuses on the here and now rather than analyzing a patient's past. To pull a person out of depression, cognitive therapists usually need 6 to 18 months of weekly sessions comprising reasoning and behavioral exercises.

Interpersonal Therapy
Interpersonal therapy, sometimes combined with cognitive therapy, also addresses the present but focuses on correcting chronic relationship problems. Interpersonal therapists focus on patients' relationships with their families and other people.

Pharmacological Treatment
Antidepressant drugs offer several options for treating depressive disorders. See Table 2.4 on page 61 for a summary of the most common drug treatments. Generally, selective serotonin reuptake inhibitors (SSRIs) have fewer side effects than other options, but it is best to consult with a health care provider who is experienced in the treatment of depression with medication to determine the right one for you. The therapeutic effects of

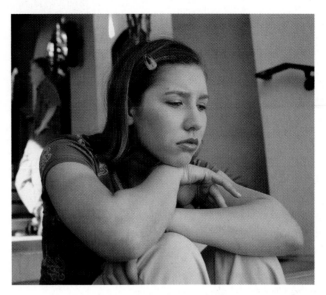

When experiencing problems such as depression, it is unwise to try to "go it alone." A qualified, caring therapist can help.

antidepressants may not be felt for several weeks, so patience is important. Medication should not be stopped all at once, but rather gradually, and its use should always be supervised by your doctor. However, countless emergency room visits occur when people misuse antidepressants, try to quit by going "cold turkey," or suffer reactions to the drugs.

The potency and dosage of each vary greatly. Antidepressants should be prescribed only after a thorough psychological and physiological examination. Recently, the U.S. Food and Drug Administration asked the makers of antidepressant drugs to add a warning to the labels advising that patients taking these drugs should be monitored for "worsening depression or the emergence of suicidality."[54]

If your doctor suggests an antidepressant, ask these questions first (beware of the health professional who gives you a five-minute exam, asks you if you are feeling down or blue, and prescribes an antidepressant to fix your problems):

- What biological indicators are you using to determine whether I really need this drug?
- What is the action of this drug? When will I start to feel the benefits? What are the side effects of using this drug? What happens if I stop taking it?
- What is your rationale for selecting this antidepressant over others?
- How long can I be on this medication without significant risk to my health?
- How will you follow up or monitor the levels of this drug in my body? How often will I need to be checked?

Electroconvulsive Therapy
Electroconvulsive therapy (ECT) is another treatment for depression. A patient given ECT is sedated under light general anesthesia, and an electric current is applied to the patient's temples for five seconds at a time for 15 or 20 minutes. However, because it

SPOTLIGHT on your health

MENTAL HEALTH PROBLEMS ON CAMPUS: UNIVERSITIES RESPOND

According to the results of the 2005 National College Health Assessment Survey, 41 percent of the respondents reported they have been diagnosed with depression in the last 12 months. Nineteen percent of respondents reported they felt too depressed to function 9 or more times in the last year.*

As students struggle to cope with the escalating pressures of college life, educational administrators are searching for a way to balance their needs with the responsibility of providing a safe learning environment for all. In a recent survey, more than 90 percent of college counseling centers reported seeing more students with more serious mental health problems. The increasing incidence of suicide is one major indicator, and schools are jumping to take action to combat the trend. For example, at the Massachusetts Institute of Technology, a series of suicides in the late 1990s and 2000 drove the university to completely overhaul its mental health program. Today, the school offers therapist support 24 hours a day, 7 days a week, in addition to seminars and informal gatherings in graduate and professional dorms, awareness training for faculty members, and a Web-based suicide prevention program that offers anonymous e-mail counseling.

Other universities have also responded to the dramatic increase in mental health problems among students. The option of "student leave" is a growing trend. New York University, Texas A&M, and Cornell are among the first that have enacted various forms of mandatory six-month or one-year student leave for those who seem to be at highest risk. In enacting these policies, colleges and universities are effectively saying that the mental health problems of

students are "family" matters better dealt with in the students' homes and communities than on campus. Because this is a relatively new policy, statistics on the success of student leave and the likelihood of a return to campus by students once their problems are resolved is unknown. Critics argue that such practices are not fair and violate the rights of students to have an education. For students who do not have health insurance, a six- to twelve-month mandated leave may not be well spent, because access to therapy becomes a serious challenge.

Universities are enacting a range of other policies as well, as overburdened counseling centers and student health centers struggle to figure out the best way to help their students cope with psychological problems.

- Some institutions, such as the University of Illinois at Urbana-Champaign, mandate counseling for students who are suicidal, requiring a minimum of four therapy sessions following a suicide attempt.
- Increasing numbers of institutions offer time management workshops; massage and de-stressing sessions during examinations; and workshops on relationships, coping with loss and grief, and other challenges through the academic year.
- Many schools have agreements with off-campus counseling centers, fitness centers, and other community-based resources to provide options for students.
- Classes on stress management, coping, relaxation, meditation, yoga, and other mental health strategies are increasingly common on campuses, either as elec-

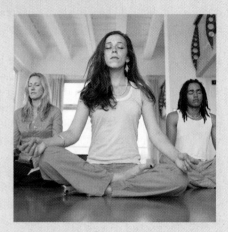

tives or as part of a professional curriculum.

- Most on-campus health services now include counseling centers with easy 24/7 access. Students are encouraged to use them and increased advertising in new-student orientations lets students know what kind of help is available.
- Many universities, such as Oregon State University, offer extensive orientations at the beginning of each academic year. Students engage in group activities, such as camping trips, outings, movies, and special seminars, to get to know each other in social settings. Professors, upper-class students, and others offer special assistance and lead discussion groups to help students cope with adjusting to life away from home.

Source: J. Feirman, "The New College Drop-Out," *Psychology Today* 38, no. 3 (2005): 38–39; *American College Health Association, National College Health Assessment, 2005, www.acha.org.

TABLE 2.4 | Drug Treatments for Depression

	SSRIs (Selective Serotonin Reuptake Inhibitors)	TCAs (Tricyclic Antidepressants)	MAOIs (Monoamine Oxidase Inhibitors)
How They Work	An SSRI works by stabilizing levels of serotonin, an important neurotransmitter. Low levels of serotonin have been linked to depression and other mood disorders.	An earlier family of anti-depressant drugs, TCAs increase the brain's levels of norepinephrine, a neurotransmitter.	MAOIs increase the levels of epinephrine, norepinephrine, and serotonin in the brain.
Commonly Prescribed Antidepressant Drugs	Zoloft, Prozac, Luvox, Paxil, Paxil CR, Celexa, Lexapro	Adapin, Endep, Norpramin, Pamelorf, Sinequan, Effexor	Nardil, Pamate, Remeron
Advantages	Relatively few side effects and no withdrawal symptoms. An SSRI is generally the first choice of most physicians.	Some patients respond better to TCA medication than they do to SSRIs.	May be used if other depression medications fail to treat the condition.
Disadvantages	Possible increase in suicidal tendencies under investigation. Can be transferred in breast milk; may cause weight gain, reduced sexual desire.	More side effects than SSRIs. May cause sensitivity to heat, which makes it harder for the body to adapt to temperature changes. Must be discontinued slowly or withdrawal symptoms may occur.	A strict dietary regime must be followed. Failure to do so can result in hypertensive crisis, which can be fatal. Many other medications react badly with MAOIs.

Source: "Selective Serotonin Reuptake Inhibitors," www.about-depression.com. Copyright © NCER, LLC, Oceanside, CA. Reprinted by permission.

carries a risk of permanent memory loss, some therapists do not recommend ECT under any circumstances.

Anxiety Disorders: Facing Your Fears

Anxiety disorders include panic disorders, obsessive-compulsive disorder, post-traumatic stress disorder, generalized anxiety disorder, and phobias. They are characterized by persistent feelings of threat and worry. Consider John Madden, former head coach of the Oakland Raiders and a true "man's man," who has outfitted his own bus and drives every weekend across the country to serve as commentator for NFL football games. What's the reason behind this exhausting driving schedule? Madden is terrified of getting on a plane.

Anxiety disorders are the number-one mental health problem in the United States, affecting over 40 million people aged 18 to 54 each year, or about 18 percent of all adults.[55] Anxiety is also a leading mental health problem among adolescents, affecting 13 million youngsters aged 9 to 17. Costs associated with an overly anxious populace are growing rapidly; conservative estimates cite nearly $50 billion a year spent in doctors' bills and workplace losses in America. These numbers don't begin to address the human costs incurred when a person is too fearful to leave the house or talk to anyone outside the immediate family.

Generalized Anxiety Disorder

One common form of anxiety disorder, **generalized anxiety disorder (GAD)**, is severe enough to interfere significantly with daily life. Generally, the person with GAD is a consummate worrier who develops a debilitating level of anxiety. Often multiple sources of worry exist, and it is hard to pinpoint the root cause of the anxiety. A diagnosis of GAD depends on showing at least three of the following symptoms for more days than not during a period of six months.[56]

1. Restlessness or feeling keyed up or on edge
2. Being easily fatigued
3. Difficulty concentrating or mind going blank
4. Irritability
5. Muscle tension
6. Sleep disturbances (difficulty falling or staying asleep or restless sleep)

anxiety disorders Disorders characterized by persistent feelings of threat and anxiousness in coping with everyday problems.

generalized anxiety disorder (GAD) A constant sense of worry that may cause restlessness, difficulty in concentrating, tension, and other symptoms.

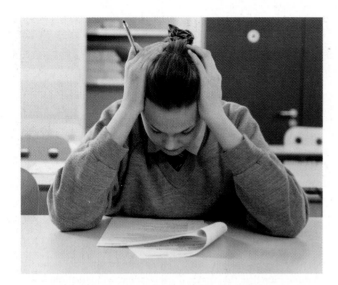

Panic attacks can occur without warning and be precipitated by a stressful or uncomfortable situation.

Often GAD runs in families and is readily treatable with benzodiazepines such as Librium, Valium, and Xanax, which calm the person for short periods. Individual therapy can be a more effective long-term treatment.

Panic Disorders

On a recent trip to a professional conference, Marilyn Erickson (not her real name) boarded a connecting flight at O'Hare International Airport, only to find that her husband John, a professor at a major university, was missing. Marilyn got off the plane and searched frantically throughout the airport for him. Finally, long after the plane had departed, she found John sitting on a bench outside the terminal; he was vomiting, dizzy, and distraught over the mere thought of boarding the plane. When Marilyn suggested catching another flight, he trembled violently and refused to move from the bench. They returned to their home on the West Coast on a bus and missed their scheduled conference appearance.

Professor Erickson suffered a **panic attack**, a form of acute anxiety reaction that brings on an intense physical reaction. Approximately 6 million Americans aged 18 and older experience panic attacks each year, usually in early adulthood. Although highly treatable, panic attacks and disorders are increasing in incidence, particularly among young women. Panic attacks may become debilitating and destructive, particularly if they happen often and cause the person to avoid going out in public or interacting with others.

panic attack   Severe anxiety reaction in which a particular situation, often for unknown reasons, causes terror.

phobia   A deep and persistent fear of a specific object, activity, or situation that results in a compelling desire to avoid the source of the fear.

A panic attack typically starts abruptly, peaks within 10 minutes, lasts about 30 minutes, and leaves the person tired and drained.[57] In addition to those just described, symptoms can include increased respiration rate, chills, hot flashes, shortness of breath, stomach cramps, chest pain, difficulty swallowing, and a sense of doom or impending death. This reaction may be so severe that you think you are going to have a heart attack and die. Or you may dismiss it as the "jitters" from too much stress.

Although researchers aren't sure of causation, heredity, stress, and certain biochemical factors may play a role. Your chances of having a panic attack increase if you have a close family member who has them. Some researchers believe that people who suffer panic attacks are experiencing an overreactive fight-or-flight physical response (see Chapter 3).

Obsessive-Compulsive Disorder

People who have to perform rituals over and over again, who are fearful of dirt or contamination, have an unnatural concern about order, symmetry, and exactness, or have persistent intrusive thoughts that they can't shake, may be suffering from *obsessive-compulsive disorder (OCD)*. Approximately 2 million Americans aged 18 or over have OCD.[58] Not to be confused with perfectionism, OCD individuals often know their behaviors are irrational and senseless, yet are powerless to stop them. According to the diagnostic manual of mental disorders, *DSM-IV-TR*, the obsessions must consume more than 1 hour per day and interfere with normal social and/or life activities. Although the exact cause is unknown, genetics, biological abnormalities, learned behaviors, and environmental factors have all been considered. OCD usually begins in adolescence or early adulthood and the median age when it starts is 19.

As with other anxiety-based disorders, medication and cognitive behavioral therapy are often the keys to treatment. Some individuals are given antidepressants, antianxiety drugs, or other drug combinations, which often prevent future attacks. Cognitive therapy can help sufferers recognize and avoid triggers or deal with triggers through meditation, deep breathing, and other relaxation techniques. Patients usually show improvement within eight to ten sessions.

Phobic Disorders

In contrast to anxiety disorders, **phobias**, or phobic disorders, involve a persistent and irrational fear of a specific object, activity, or situation, often out of proportion to the circumstances. Phobias result in a compelling desire to avoid the source of the fear. About 13 percent of Americans suffer from phobias, such as fear of spiders, snakes, public speaking, and so on. Social phobias are perhaps the most common phobic response.[59]

Social Phobias A **social phobia** is an anxiety disorder characterized by the persistent fear and avoidance of social situations. Essentially, the person dreads these situations for fear of being humiliated, embarrassed, or even looked at.[60] These disorders vary in scope. Some cause difficulty only in specific situations, such as getting up in front of the class to give a report. In more extreme cases, a person avoids all contact with others.

Sources of Anxiety and Phobic Disorders

Because anxiety and phobic disorders vary in complexity and degree, scientists have yet to find clear reasons why one person develops them and another doesn't. The following factors are often cited as possible causes.[61]

- *Biology.* Some scientists trace the origin of anxiety to the brain and brain functioning. Using sophisticated positron emission tomography scans (PET scans), scientists can analyze areas of the brain that react during anxiety-producing events. Families appear to display similar brain and physiological reactivity, so we may inherit our tendencies toward anxiety disorders.
- *Environment.* Anxiety may also be a learned response. Though genetic tendencies may exist, experiencing a repeated pattern of reaction to certain situations programs the brain to respond in a certain way. For example, monkeys separated from their mothers at an early age are more fearful and their stress hormones fire more readily than those that stayed with their mothers. If your mother (or father) screamed whenever a large spider crept into view or if other anxiety-raising events occurred frequently, you might be predisposed to react with anxiety to similar events later in your life. Interestingly, pets also experience such anxieties—perhaps from being around their edgy owners.
- *Social and cultural roles.* Because men and women are taught to assume different roles in society (such as man as protector, woman as victim), women may find it more acceptable to scream, shake, pass out, and otherwise express extreme anxiety. Men, on the other hand, have learned to repress such anxieties rather than act upon them. See the Spotlight on Your Health box on page 64 for information on another psychological disorder of growing concern—self-mutilation.

Other Mental Health Disorders

Seasonal Affective Disorder

An estimated 6 percent of Americans suffer from **seasonal affective disorder (SAD)**, a type of depression, and an additional 14 percent experience a milder form of the disorder known as the winter blues. SAD strikes during the winter

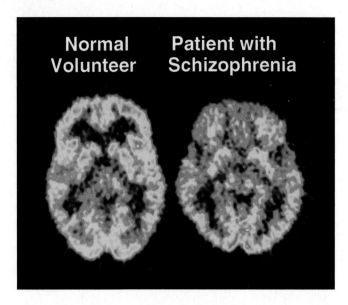

These brain images reveal significant differences between normal brain activity and that of a person with schizophrenia.

months and is associated with reduced exposure to sunlight. People with SAD suffer from irritability, apathy, carbohydrate craving and weight gain, increases in sleep time, and general sadness. Researchers believe that SAD is caused by a malfunction in the hypothalamus, the gland responsible for regulating responses to external stimuli. Stress may also play a role.

Therapies for SAD are simple but effective. The most beneficial is light therapy, which exposes patients to lamps that simulate sunlight. Eighty percent of patients experience relief from their symptoms within four days of treatment. Other treatments for SAD include diet change (eating more complex carbohydrates), increased exercise, stress management techniques, sleep restriction (limiting the number of hours slept in a 24-hour period), psychotherapy, and antidepressants.

Schizophrenia

Perhaps the most frightening of all mental disorders is **schizophrenia**, which affects about 1 percent of the U.S. population. Schizophrenia is characterized by alterations of the senses (including auditory and visual hallucinations); the inability to sort out incoming stimuli and to make appropriate responses; an altered sense of self; and radical changes in emotions, movements, and behaviors. Victims of this disease

social phobia A phobia characterized by fear and avoidance of social situations.

seasonal affective disorder (SAD) A type of depression that occurs in the winter months, when sunlight levels are low.

schizophrenia A mental illness with biological origins that is characterized by irrational behavior, severe alterations of the senses (hallucinations), and often an inability to function in society.

CUTTING THROUGH THE PAIN

Self-injury is an alarming phenomenon on the rise that especially affects bright, middle-class teens and young adults. Also called self-mutilation, self-hurt, self-abuse, or self-harm, this refers to deliberate harm inflicted on one's own body in an attempt to alter a mood state. Cutting (with razors, glass, knives, etc.) is the most common method, followed by burning, bruising, excessive nail biting, breaking bones, and pulling out hair. Those who self-injure don't feel the pain because they are in a state of dissociation, or mentally removed from reality.

Self-injury is a coping mechanism used to deal with stress and sadness. Some studies suggest that when people who self-injure feel emotionally overwhelmed, inflicting physical pain reduces stress almost immediately and calms them down.

The typical self-injurer is female, single, has average to high intelligence, low self-esteem, and comes from a middle- to upper-middle-class family. Self-injury usually starts during puberty (most self-injurers range in age from 11 to 17, although some are adults). An estimated 1 to 4 percent of the population in the United States (1,500 per 100,000 Americans) purposefully hurt themselves in some way. About half say they were physically or sexually abused in their childhoods, although some experts estimate that up to 90 percent have been abused.

Signs of self-injury include scars, current cuts or abrasions, and flimsy excuses for these wounds. A self-injurer may wear long sleeves and pants in warm weather to hide the wounds. Other symptoms can include difficulty handling anger, social withdrawal, sensitivity to rejection, or body alienation.

Treatments currently being explored range from psychotherapy to medications such as antidepressants and mood stabilizers. The goal is not just to stop the behavior, but to end the feelings that prompt the behavior in the first place.

Self-cutters who are currently in treatment offer the following tips:

- *Do something creative with your hands.* Keep your hands busy with painting, making a collage, or even cleaning.
- *Play with your pets.* Taking care of and playing with animals diverts your attention and your hands.
- *Communicate your feelings.* Confide in someone that you trust. You don't need to explain yourself, just let them know what you are going through.
- *Start a journal.* This is a place to write your thoughts and feelings down. Write in the journal as often as you need to.

For more information, try these sources:

National Self-Harm Network, www.nshn .co.uk; SAFE Alternatives, www.selfinjury .com; Secret Shame: Self-Injury Information and Support, www.crystal.palace.net/ ~llama/selfinjury.

Sources: S. Dobie, Oregon State University; Mayo Clinic Staff, "Cutting (Self-mutilation)," MayoClinic.com, May 13, 2004, www.mayoclinic .com/invoke.cfm?objectid=74946FF7-B41B- 456F-AF3E97F9BA898021; A. Derovin and T. Bravender, "Living on the Edge: The Current Phenomenon of Self-Mutilation in Adolescents," *MCN—The American Journal of Maternal Child Nursing* 29, no. 1 (Jan/Feb 2004): 12–18; "Student Self-Harm: Silent School Crisis," *Education Week,* December 2, 2003, vol. 23, no.14, 1; K. Goetz, "Cutting through the Pain," *The Cincinnati Enquirer,* July 28, 2002, www .enquirer.com/editions/2002/07/28/loc_cutting _through_pain.html; D. Martinson, "Self-Injury: A Quick Guide to the Basics," 1998, www.palace .net/~llama/psych/guide.html.

---

often cannot function in society. Contrary to popular belief, schizophrenia is not the same as split personality or multiple personality disorder.

For decades, scientists believed that schizophrenia was an environmentally provoked form of madness. They blamed abnormal family interactions or early childhood traumas. Since the mid-1980s, however, magnetic resonance imaging (MRI) and PET scans have allowed closer study of brain function, and scientists have recognized that schizophrenia is a biological disease of the brain. The brain damage occurs very early in life, possibly as early as the second trimester of fetal development. However, symptoms most commonly appear in late adolescence.

At present, schizophrenia is treatable but not curable. Treatments usually include some combination of hospitalization, medication, and supportive psychotherapy. Supportive psychotherapy, as opposed to psychoanalysis, can help the patient acquire skills for living in society.

Even though environmental theories of the causes of schizophrenia have been discarded in favor of biological theories, a stigma remains attached to the disease. Families of people with schizophrenia often experience anger and guilt associated with misunderstandings about the causes of the disease. They often need information, family counseling, and advice on how to meet the schizophrenic person's needs for shelter, medical care, vocational training, and social interaction.

Gender Issues in Psychosocial Health

Unfortunately, gender bias can hinder the correct diagnosis of psychosocial disorders. In one study, for instance, 175 mental health professionals of both genders were asked to diagnose a patient based upon a summarized case history. Some of the professionals were told that the patient was male, others that the patient was female. The gender of the patient made a substantial difference in the diagnosis (though the gender of the clinician did not). When subjects thought the patient was female, they were more likely to diagnose hysterical personality, which is often thought of as a women's disorder. When they believed the patient to be male, the more likely diagnosis was antisocial personality, frequently perceived as a male disorder.

PMS: Physical or Mental Disorder?

A major controversy is the inclusion of a provisional diagnosis for premenstrual syndrome (PMS) and premenstrual dysphoric disorder (PMDD) in the American Psychiatric Association's *Diagnostic and Statistical Manual of Mental Disorders*. Currently, PMDD, which is considered the more severe form of PMS, is included in the *DSM-IV-TR*. However, the ongoing controversy about its inclusion signals that PMS merits further study.

PMS is characterized by depression, irritability, and other symptoms of increased stress typically occurring just prior to menstruation and lasting for a day or two. Whereas PMS is somewhat disruptive and uncomfortable, it does not interfere with daily functions; PMDD does. To be diagnosed with PMDD, a woman must have at least five symptoms of PMS for a week to 10 days, with at least one symptom being serious enough to interfere with her ability to function at work or at home. In these more severe cases, antidepressants may be prescribed.

Suicide: Giving Up on Life

Each year there are over 35,000 reported suicides in the United States. Experts estimate that there may actually be closer to 100,000, due to the difficulty in determining the causes of many suspicious deaths. More lives are lost to suicide than to any other single cause except cardiovascular disease and cancer. Suicide often results from poor coping skills, lack of social support, lack of self-esteem, and the inability to see one's way out of a bad situation. Factors contributing to suicide are common risks in many regions of the world.

College students are more likely than the general population to attempt suicide; suicide is the second leading cause of death on college campuses. In fact, this age group accounts for nearly 20 percent of all suicides.[62] The pressures, joys, disappointments, challenges, and changes of the college environment are believed to be partially responsible. However, young adults who choose not to go to college but who are searching for direction in careers, relationships, and other life goals are also at risk.

Risk factors for suicide include a family history of suicide, previous suicide attempts, excessive drug and alcohol use, prolonged depression, financial difficulties, serious illness in the suicide contemplator or in his or her loved ones, and loss of a loved one through death or rejection. Societal pressures often serve as a catalyst.

In most cases, suicide does not occur unpredictably. In fact, 75 to 80 percent of people who commit suicide give a warning of their intentions.

Warning Signs of Suicide

Common signs of possible suicide include:[63]

- Recent loss and a seeming inability to let go of grief
- Change in personality—sadness, withdrawal, irritability, anxiety, tiredness, indecisiveness, apathy
- Change in behavior—inability to concentrate, loss of interest in classes, or work unexplained demonstration of happiness following a period of depression
- Diminished sexual interest—impotence, menstrual abnormalities
- Expressions of self-hatred and excessive risk taking, or an "I don't care what happens to me" attitude
- Change in sleep patterns and/or eating habits
- A direct statement about committing suicide, such as "I might as well end it all."
- An indirect statement, such as "You won't have to worry about me anymore."
- Final preparations such as writing a will, repairing poor relationships with family or friends, giving away prized possessions, or writing revealing letters
- A preoccupation with themes of death
- Marked changes in personal appearance

 what do you THINK?

If your roommate showed some of the warning signs of suicide, what action would you take? ■ Whom would you contact first? ■ Where on campus might your friend get help? ■ What if someone in class whom you hardly knew gave some of the warning signs? ■ What would you do then?

Taking Action to Prevent Suicide

Most people who attempt suicide really want to live but see death as the only way out of an intolerable situation. Crisis counselors and suicide hotlines may help temporarily, but the best way to prevent suicide is to get rid of conditions that may precipitate attempts, including alcoholism, drug abuse, loneliness, isolation, and access to guns.

If someone you know threatens suicide or displays any warning signs, take the following actions:

- *Monitor the warning signals.* Keep an eye on the person, or see that there is someone around the person as much as possible.
- *Take any threats seriously.* Don't brush them off.
- *Let the person know how much you care about him or her.* State that you are there to help.

- *Listen.* Empathize, sympathize, and keep the person talking. Try not to discredit or be shocked. Talk about stressors and listen to the responses.
- *Ask directly, "Are you thinking of hurting or killing yourself?"*
- *Do not belittle the person's feelings.* Don't say that he or she doesn't really mean it or couldn't succeed at suicide. To some people, these comments offer the challenge of proving you wrong.
- *Help the person think about alternatives.* Be ready to offer choices. Offer to go for help together. Call your local suicide hotline, and use all available community and campus resources. Recommend a counselor or other person to talk to.
- *Remember that your relationships with others involve responsibilities.* If you need to stay with the person, take the person to a health care facility, provide support, and give of yourself and your time.
- *Tell your friend's spouse, partner, parents, siblings, or counselor.* Do not keep your suspicions to yourself. Don't let a suicidal friend talk you into keeping your discussions confidential. If your friend succeeds in a suicide attempt, you may find that others will question your decision and you may blame yourself.

Seeking Professional Help

A physical ailment will readily send most of us to the nearest health professional, but many people view seeking professional help for psychosocial problems as an admission of personal failure. However, increasing numbers of Americans are turning to mental health professionals, and nearly one in five seeks such help. Researchers cite dysfunctional families, breakdowns in support systems, and high societal expectations of the individual as three major reasons why more people are asking for assistance than ever before.

Consider seeking help if:

- You think you need help
- You experience wild mood swings
- A problem is interfering with your daily life
- Your fears or feelings of guilt frequently distract your attention
- You begin to withdraw from others
- You have hallucinations
- You feel that life is not worth living
- You feel inadequate or worthless
- Your emotional responses are inappropriate to various situations
- Your daily life seems to be nothing but repeated crises
- You feel you can't "get your act together"
- You are considering suicide
- You turn to drugs or alcohol to escape from your problems
- You feel out of control

TABLE 2.5	How to Help Yourself if You Are Depressed

- Set realistic goals in light of the depression and assume a reasonable amount of responsibility.
- Break large tasks into small ones, set some priorities, and do what you can as you can.
- Try to be with other people and to confide in someone; it is usually better than being alone and secretive.
- Participate in activities that may make you feel better.
- Mild exercise, going to a movie, a ballgame, or participating in religious, social, or other activities may help.
- Expect your mood to improve gradually, not immediately. Feeling better takes time.
- It is advisable to postpone important decisions until the depression has lifted. Before deciding to make a significant transition, change jobs, or get married or divorced, discuss it with others who know you well and have a more objective view of your situation.
- People rarely "snap out of" a depression. But they can feel a little better day by day.
- *Remember,* positive thinking will replace the negative thinking that is part of the depression and will disappear as your depression responds to treatment.
- Let your family and friends help you.

There are also some measures you can take now to feel better, and pull yourself out of negative thoughts and feelings (Table 2.5).

Getting Evaluated for Treatment

If you are considering treatment for a psychosocial problem, schedule a complete evaluation first. Start with your campus health center. Consult a credentialed health professional for a thorough examination, which should include three parts:

- A physical checkup, which will rule out thyroid disorders, viral infections, and anemia—all of which can result in depression-like symptoms—and a neurological check of coordination, reflexes, and balance, to rule out brain disorders
- A psychiatric history, which will attempt to trace the course of the apparent disorder, genetic or family factors, and any past treatments
- A mental status examination, which will assess thoughts, speaking processes, and memory, as well as an in-depth interview with tests for other psychiatric symptoms[64]

Once physical factors have been ruled out, you may decide to consult a professional who specializes in psychosocial health.

Mental Health Professionals

How can I choose the right therapist for me?

Several types of mental health professionals are available to help you. The most important criterion is not how many degrees this person has, but whether you feel you can work together. Table 2.6 presents fundamental criteria to help you choose the best therapist for your needs.

Psychiatrist A **psychiatrist** is a medical doctor. After obtaining a medical doctor (MD) degree, a psychiatrist spends up to 12 years studying psychosocial health and disease. As a licensed MD, a psychiatrist can prescribe medications for various mental or emotional problems and may have admitting privileges at a local hospital. Some psychiatrists are affiliated with hospitals, while others are in private practice.

Psychologist A **psychologist** usually has a PhD degree in counseling or clinical psychology. In addition, many states require licensure. Psychologists are trained in various types of therapy, including behavior and insight therapy. Most can conduct both individual and group counseling sessions, and may also be trained in certain specialties, such as family counseling or sexual counseling.

Psychoanalyst A **psychoanalyst** is a psychiatrist or psychologist with special training in psychoanalysis. This is a type of therapy that helps patients remember early traumas that have blocked personal growth. Facing these traumas helps them resolve conflicts and lead more productive lives.

Clinical/Psychiatric Social Worker A **social worker** has at least a master's degree in social work (MSW) and two years of experience in a clinical setting. Many states require an examination for accreditation. Some social workers work in clinical settings, whereas others have private practices.

Counselor A **counselor** often has a master's degree in counseling, psychology, educational psychology, or related human service. Professional societies recommend at least two years of graduate coursework or supervised practice as a minimal requirement. Many counselors are trained to do individual and group therapy. They often specialize in one type of counseling, such as family, marital, relationship, child, drug, divorce, behavioral, or personal counseling.

Psychiatric Nurse Specialist Although all registered nurses can work in psychiatric settings, some continue their education and specialize in psychiatric practice. A **psychiatric nurse specialist** can be certified by the American Nursing Association in adult, child, or adolescent psychiatric nursing.

What to Expect in Therapy

Many different types of counseling exist, ranging from individual therapy, which involves one-on-one work between

TABLE 2.6	Questions to Ask When Choosing a Therapist

A qualified mental health professional should be willing to answer all your questions during an initial consultation. Questions to ask include the following:

- Can you interview the therapist before starting treatment? An initial meeting will help you determine whether this person will be a good fit for you.
- Do you like the therapist as a person? Can you talk to him or her comfortably?
- Is the therapist watching the clock or easily distracted? You should be the main focus of the session.
- Does the therapist demonstrate professionalism? Be concerned if your therapist is frequently late or breaks appointments, suggests social interactions outside your therapy sessions, talks inappropriately about himself or herself, has questionable billing practices, or resists releasing you from therapy.
- Will the therapist help you set your own goals? A good professional should evaluate your general situation and help you set small goals to work on between sessions. The therapist should not tell you how to help yourself but help you discover the steps.

Remember, in most states, the use of the title *therapist* or *counselor* is unregulated. Make your choice carefully.

therapist and client, to group therapy, in which two or more clients meet with a therapist to discuss problems.

The first trip to a therapist can be extremely difficult. Most of us have misconceptions about what therapy is and about what it can do. That first visit is a verbal and mental sizing up between you and the therapist. You may not accomplish much in that first hour. If you decide that this professional is not for you, you will at least have learned how to present your problem and what qualities you need in a therapist.

Before meeting, briefly explain your needs. Ask what the fee is. Arrive on time, wear comfortable clothing, and expect to spend about an hour during your first visit. The therapist will want to take down your history and details about the

psychiatrist A licensed physician who specializes in treating mental and emotional disorders.

psychologist A person with a PhD degree and training in psychology.

psychoanalyst A psychiatrist or psychologist with special training in psychoanalysis.

social worker A person with an MSW degree and clinical training.

counselor A person with a variety of academic and experiential training who deals with the treatment of emotional problems.

psychiatric nurse specialist A registered nurse specializing in psychiatric practice.

problems that have brought you to therapy. Answer as honestly as possible. Many will ask how you feel about aspects of your life. Do not be embarrassed to acknowledge your feelings. It is critical to the success of your treatment that you trust this person enough to be open and honest.

Do not expect the therapist to tell you what to do or how to behave. The responsibility for improved behavior lies with you. Ask if you can set your own therapeutic goals and timetables.

If after your first visit (or even after several visits), you feel you cannot work with this person, say so. You have the right to find a therapist with whom you feel comfortable.

? *what do you* THINK?

Have you ever thought about seeing a therapist? ■ What made you decide to go or not go? ■ If you were to consult a therapist, what factors would you take into consideration in choosing one who is right for you?

TAKING charge

Summary

- Psychosocial health is a complex phenomenon involving mental, emotional, social, and spiritual health.
- Many factors influence psychosocial health, including life experiences, family, the environment, other people, self-esteem, self-efficacy, and personality. Some of these are modifiable; others are not.
- Developing self-esteem and self-efficacy and getting enough sleep are key to enhancing psychosocial health.
- Many people believe spirituality is important to wellness. Though the exact reasons have not been established, many studies show a connection between the two.
- Happiness is a key factor in determining overall reaction to life's challenges. The mind–body connection is an important link in overall health and well-being.

- Depression is an indicator of deteriorating psychosocial health. Identifying depression is the first step in treating this disorder.
- Other common psychosocial problems include bipolar disorder, anxiety disorders, panic disorders, phobias, seasonal affective disorder, and schizophrenia.
- Suicide is a result of negative psychosocial reactions to life. Most people intending to commit suicide give warning signs of their intentions. They can often be helped.
- Mental health professionals include psychiatrists, psychoanalysts, psychologists, clinical/psychiatric social workers, counselors, and psychiatric nurse specialists. Many therapy methods exist, including group and individual therapy. It is wise to interview a therapist carefully before beginning treatment.

Chapter Review

1. Which of the following is *not* a characteristic of a mentally healthy individual?
   a. responds appropriately to life's challenges
   b. lives in a self centered environment
   c. carries out responsibilities
   d. accepts own limitations and possibilities

2. Emotional health is defined as
   a. feelings people have.
   b. moods one is experiencing.
   c. perceiving reality as it really is.
   d. answers A and B.

3. Which of the following is an example of a compulsive behavior?
   a. the killing of an animal
   b. catching a cold by shaking hands with other people

   c. the fear of dying from a plane crash
   d. washing one's hands 100 times in a day

4. The level of closeness and attachment to other people is referred to as
   a. sexual intimacy.
   b. social health.
   c. social bonds.
   d. spiritual health.

5. The leading reason college students seek psychological counseling is
   a. relationship issues.
   b. suicide thoughts.
   c. stress and anxiety.
   d. depression.

6. A major difference between *spirituality* and *religion* is that spirituality
   a. is not necessarily a component of religion.
   b. requires one to be a regular church-going individual.
   c. does not require living in harmony with the community.
   d. focuses on amassing large materialistic possessions.

7. Which of the following is *not* an example of possessing an internal locus of control?
   a. People who are autonomous in their decision making.
   b. Blaming other people for one's own failures.
   c. People who are in control of their circumstances.
   d. Having a positive attitude about a situation, even if the situation is negative.

8. A person with high *self-efficacy*
   a. possesses high self-respect and self-worth.
   b. believes he or she can successfully engage in a specific behavior.

   c. believes external influences shape one's psychosocial health.
   d. has a high altruistic capacity.

9. The following traits characterize psychosocially health people *except*
   a. agreeableness.
   b. openness to new experiences.
   c. conscientiousness.
   d. introversion in social settings.

10. The characteristic that describes a person's ability to bounce back in times of difficulty or threats in a healthy way is known as
    a. self-esteem.
    b. self-efficacy.
    c. resiliency.
    d. subjective well-being.

Answers to these questions can be found on page A-1.

Questions for Discussion and Reflection

1. What is psychosocial health? What indicates that you are or aren't psychosocially healthy? Why might the college environment provide a real challenge to psychosocial health?
2. Discuss the factors that influence your overall level of psychosocial health. Which factors can you change? Which ones may be more difficult to change?
3. What steps could you take today to improve your psychosocial health? Which steps require long-term effort?
4. What are four main themes of spirituality, and how are they expressed in daily life?
5. Why is laughter therapeutic? How can humor help you better achieve wellness?
6. What factors appear to contribute to psychosocial difficulties and illnesses? Which of the common psychosocial illnesses is likely to affect people in your age group?

7. What are the warning signs of suicide? Of depression? Why is depression so pervasive among young Americans today? Why are some groups more vulnerable to suicide and depression than others? What would you do if you heard a friend in the cafeteria say to no one in particular that he was going to "do the world a favor and end it all"?
8. Discuss the different types of health professionals and therapies. If you felt depressed about breaking off a long-term relationship, which professional and which therapy do you think would be most beneficial to you? Explain your answer. What services are provided by your student health center? What fees are charged to students?
9. What psychosocial areas do you need to work on? Which are most important to you, and why? What actions can you take today?

Accessing Your Health on the Internet

The following websites explore further topics and issues related to personal health. You'll also find links to each organization's website on the Companion Website for *Access to Health,* Tenth Edition, at www.aw-bc.com/donatelle.

1. *American Foundation for Suicide Prevention.* Resources for suicide prevention and support for family and friends of those who have committed suicide. www.afsp.org
2. *American Psychological Association Help Center.* Includes information on psychology at work, the mind–body connection, psychological responses to war, and other topics. http://helping.apa.org
3. *Anxiety Disorders Association of America.* Offers links to treatment resources, self-help tools, information on clinical trials, and other information. www.adaa.org

4. *National Alliance for the Mentally Ill.* A support and advocacy organization of families and friends of people with severe mental illnesses. Over 1,200 state and local affiliates; local branches can often help with finding treatment. www.nami.org
5. *National Institute of Mental Health (NIMH).* Overview of mental health information and new research relating to mental health. www.nimh.nih.gov
6. *National Mental Health Association.* Works to promote mental health through advocacy, education, research, and services. www.nmha.org

Further Reading

Dalai Lama and H. C. Cutler. *The Art of Happiness: A Handbook for Living.* New York: Riverhead, 1998.

> *Through a series of interviews, the authors explore questions of meaning, motives, and the interconnectedness of life, including the reasons why so many people are unhappy, and offer strategies for becoming happy.*

Norem, J. *The Positive Power of Negative Thinking.* New York: Basic Books, 2002.

> *Explores reasons for negative thinking and mechanisms for changing the way you think. Includes self-tests and analysis for helping you retrain your thinking processes.*

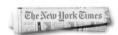

e-themes from *The New York Times*

For up-to-date articles about current health issues, visit www.aw-bc.com/donatelle, select *Access to Health,* Tenth Edition, Chapter 2, and click on "e-themes."

References

1. H. Marano, "A Nation of Wimps," *Psychology Today* 37, no. 6 (2004): 58–68.
2. S. Benton et al., "Changes in Counseling Center Client Problems across 13 Years," *Professional Psychology: Research and Practice* 34, no. 1 (2003): 66–72.
3. Marano, "A Nation of Wimps."
4. National Institute of Mental Health, National Survey of Counseling Center directors, 2005, www.nimh.nih.gov.
5. "Executive Summary of the Report of the Surgeon General on Mental Health," June 2006, www.surgeongeneral.gov/library/mentalhealth/summary.html.
6. R. Lazarus, *Stress and Emotion: A New Synthesis* (New York: Springer Publishing Company, 1999).
7. A. F. Jorm, "Social Networks and Health: It's Time for an Intervention Trial," *Journal of Epidemiology and Community Health* 59 (2005): 537–539; C. Huang, "Elderly Social Support System and Health Status in the Urban and Rural Areas," paper presented at the American Public Health Association Annual Meeting, New Orleans, 2005; C. Alarie, *The Impact of Social Support on Women's Health: A Literature Review,* Women's Center of Excellence, www.pwhce.ca/limpactDuSupport.htm.
8. Tufts University Program in Evidence-Based Complementary and Alternative Medicine, "Religion and Spirituality Overview," May 15, 2006, www.tufts.edu/med/ebcam/religion/index.html; H.G. Koenig et al., *Handbook of Religion and Health* (New York: Oxford University Press, 2001), 18.
9. S. R. Hawks et al., "Review of Spiritual Health: Definition, Role, and Intervention Strategies in Health Promotion," *American Journal of Health Promotion* 9, no. 5 (1995): 371–378; K. Karren et al., *Mind–Body Health* (San Francisco: Benjamin Cummings, 2006).
10. J. A. Astin and S. L. Shapiro et al., "Mind–Body Medicine: State of the Science, Implications for Practice," *Journal of the American Board of Family Practice* 16 (2003): 131–147; J. Bishop et al., "Mindfulness: A Proposed Operational Definition," *Clinical Psychology* 11 (2004): 230–241.
11. Ibid.
12. Ibid.
13. Ibid.
14. A. Astin et al., "Spirituality in Higher Education: A National Study of College Students' Search for Meaning and Purpose," 2004, www.spirituality.ucla.edu.
15. Z. Segal et al., *Mindfulness-Based Cognitive Therapy for Depression: A New Approach to Preventing Relapse* (New York: Guilford Publications, 2001); M. Weiss et al., "Mindfulness-Based Stress Reduction as an Adjunct to Outpatient Psychotherapy," *Psychotherapy and Psychosomatics* 74, no. 2 (2005): 108–112; J. Cohen-Katz et al., "The Effects of Mindfulness-Based Stress Reduction on Nurse Stress and Burnout, Part II: A Quantitative and Qualitative Study," *Holistic Nurse Practice* 1 (2005): 26–35; A Tacon et al., "Mindfulness Meditation, Anxiety Reduction, and Heart Disease: A Pilot Study," *Family and Community Health* 26, no. 1 (2003): 25–33.
16. M. Seligman and C. Peterson, "Learned Helplessness," in *International Encyclopedia for the Social and Behavioral Sciences,* vol. 13, ed. N. Smelser (New York: Elsevier, 2002), 8583–8586.
17. J. R. Grant, ed., "Positive Psychology," special issue, *Journal of Humanistic Psychology* 4, no. 1 (2001): 1–153.
18. S. Proffitt, "Pursuing Happiness with a Positive Outlook, Not a Pill," *Los Angeles Times,* January 24, 1999, www.apa.org/releases/pursuing.html; APA HelpCenter, "Mind/Body Connection: "Learned Optimism Yields Health Benefits," 1996, http://helping.apa.org; American Psychological Association, "Century of Research Confirms Impact of Psychosocial Factors on Health—Question Is How to Apply that Knowledge to Healthcare Systems," January 19, 2004, www.apa.org/releases/ mind.html.
19. M. Seligman, *Learned Optimism: How to Change Your Mind and Your Life* (New York: Free Press, 1998); J. H. Martin, "Motivation Processes and Performance: The Role of Global and Facet Personality," PhD diss., University of North Carolina at Chapel Hill, 2002.
20. B. Fredrickson and M. Losada, "Positive Affect and Complex Dynamics of Human Flourishing," *American Psychologist* 60, no. 7 (2005): 678–686.
21. D. Brown and C. Blanton, "Physical Activity, Sports Participation, and Suicidal Behavior Among College Students," *Medicine and Science in Sports and Exercise* 34, no. 7 (2002): 1087–1096.
22. National Heart, Lung and Blood Institute, "Sleep Apnea," February, 2006, www.nhlbi.nih.gov/health/dci/disease/sleepapnea/sleepapnea.html.
23. K. Goodkin and A. P. Vissar, *Psychoneuroimmunology: Stress, Mental Disorders, and Health* (Washington, D.C: American Psychiatric Press, Inc., 2000).
24. P. Herschberger, "Prescribing Happiness: Positive Psychology and Family Medicine," *Family Medicine* 37, no. 9 (2005): 630–634.

25. J. Kluger, "The Funny Thing about Laughter," *Time Magazine,* vol. 165, no. 3 (January 17, 2005): A25–A29.

26. R. Davidson et al., "The Privileged Status of Emotion in the Brain," *Proceedings of the National Academy of Sciences of the United States of America* 101, no. 33 (2004).

27. E. Diener and M. E. P. Seligman, "Beyond Money: Toward an Economy of Well-Being," *Psychological Science in the Public Interest* 5 (2004): 1–31; C. Peterson and M. Seligman, *Character Strengths and Virtues* (London: Oxford University Press, 2004).

28. P. Herschberger, "Prescribing Happiness"; M. E. Seligman et al., "Positive Psychology Progress: Empirical Validation of Interventions," *American Psychologist* 60, no. 5 (2005): 410–421.

29. M. Seligman, "Positive Interventions: More Evidence of Effectiveness," *Authentic Happiness Newsletter,* September 2004, www.authentichappiness.org/news/news10.html; S. I. Gable et al., "What Do You Do When Things Go Right? The Intrapersonal and Interpersonal Benefits of Sharing Positive Events," *Journal of Personal and Social Psychology* 87, no. 2 (2004): 228–245; B. Swartz, *The Paradox of Choice: Why More Is Less* (New York: HarperCollins Publishers, 2004); M. E. Seligman, *Character Strengths and Virtues: A Handbook and Classification* (New York: Oxford University Press, 2004).

30. B. L. Fredrickson, "Cultivating Positive Emotions to Optimize Health and Well-Being," *Prevention & Treatment* 3, Article 0001a, March 7, 2000.

31. L. Berk et al., "Modulation of Immune Parameters During the Eustress of Humor-Associated Mirthful Laughter," *Alternative Therapies in Health and Medicine* 9, no. 2 (2001): 62–67.

32. H. Dreher, "Cancer and the Mind: Current Concepts in Psycho-Oncology," *Advances, Institute for the Advancement of Health* 4, no. 3: 27–43.

33. Grady, "Think Right, Stay Well," *American Health* 11 (1992): 50–54.

34. L. Temoshok, *The Type C Connection* (New York: Random House, 1995).

35. MayoClinic.com, "Mental Health Definitions," 2006, www.mayoclinic.com.

36. R. C. Kessler et al., "Prevalence, Severity, and Comorbidity of Twelve-Month *DSM-IV* Disorders in the National Comorbidity Survey Replication (NCS-R)," *Archives of General Psychiatry* 62, no. 6 (2005): 617–627; National Institute of Mental Health, "The Numbers Count: Mental Disorders in America," February 17, 2006, www.nimh.nih.gov/publicat/numbers.cfm; DHHS, "Executive Summary: Mental Health, Culture, Race and Ethnicity, a Supplement to Mental Health: A Report of the Surgeon General," June 6, 2006, www.surgeongeneral.gov/library/mentalhealth/cre/execsummary-1.html).

37. L. A. Lefton, *Psychology,* 8th ed. (Boston: Allyn & Bacon, 2002).

38. National Institute of Mental Health, "The Numbers Count."

39. R. C. Kessler et al., "Lifetime Prevalence and Age-of-Onset Distributions of *DSM-IV* Disorders in the National Comorbidity Survey Replication (NCS-R)," *Archives of General Psychiatry* 62, no. 6 (2005): 593–602.

40. American College Health Association, "American College Health Association-National College Health Assessment (ACHA-NCHA) Web Summary," April 2006, www.acha.org/projects_programs/ncha_sampledata.cfm.

41. National Institute of Mental Health, "Depression," May 11, 2006, www.nimh.nih.gov/publicat/depression.cfm.

42. Ibid.

43. Ibid.

44. National Institute of Mental Health, "Depression"; N. Gavin et al., "Perinatal Depression: A Systematic Review of Prevalence and Incidence," *Obstetrics and Gynecology* 106 (2005): 1071–1083.

45. American College Health Association, "American College Health Association-National College Health Assessment (ACHA-NCHA) Web Summary."

46. National Institute of Mental Health, "Real Men, Real Depression," 2005, www.menanddepression.nimh.nih.gov.

47. A. K. Ferketick et al., "Depression as an Antecedent to Heart Disease among Women and Men in the NHANES I Study," National Health and Nutrition Examination Survey," *Archives of Internal Medicine* 160, no. 9 (2002): 1261–1268.

48. National Institute of Mental Health, "Depression."

49. Ibid; E. M. Berters, "Mental Health in U.S. Adults: The Role of Positive Social Support and Social Negativity in Personal Relationships," *Journal of Social and Personal Relationships* 22, no. 1 (date): 33–48, 2005.

50. S. Riolo et al., "Prevalence of Depression by Race/Ethnicity: Findings from the National Health and Nutrition Examination Survey III," *American Journal of Public Health* 95, no. 6 (2005): 998–1000.

51. M. Weissman et al., "Offspring of Depressed Parents: 20 Years Later," *American Journal of Psychiatry* 163 (2006): 1001–1008; J. Kim-Cohen et al., "The Caregiving Environments Provided to Children by Depressed Mothers With or Without an Antisocial History," *American Journal of Psychiatry* 163 (2006): 1009–1018.

52. R. Voelker, "Stress, Sleep Loss and Substance Abuse Create Potent Recipe for College Depression," *Journal of the American Medical Association* 291, no. 18 (2004): 2172–2174.

53. S. Benton et al., "Changes in Counseling Center Client Problems across 13 Years."

54. U.S. Food and Drug Administration (FDA), "FDA Issues Public Health Advisory on Cautions for Use of Antidepressants in Adults and Children" (FDA Talk Paper, T04-08), March 22, 2004, www.fda.gov/bbs/topics/ANSWERS/2004/ANS01283.html; U.S. FDA, Center for Drug Evaluation and Research, "Antidepressant Use in Children, Adolescents, and Young Adults," March 22, 2004, www.fda.gov/cder/drug/antidepressants/default.htm.

55. National Institute of Mental Health, "The Numbers Count."

56. National Institute of Mental Health, "Generalized Anxiety Disorder, GAD," February 2005, www.nimh.nih.gov/healthinformation/gadmenu.cfm.

57. MayoClinic.com, "Panic Attacks," 2006, www.mayoclinic.com.

58. National Institute of Mental Health, "The Numbers Count."

59. National Institute of Mental Health, "Generalized Anxiety Disorder, GAD."

60. Ibid.

61. Ibid.

62. American College Health Association, "Campus Violence White Paper," February 5, 2005, www.acha.org/info_resources/campus_violence.pdf.

63. National Institute of Mental Health, "In Harm's Way: Suicide in America," February 17, 2006, www.nimh.nih.gov/publicat/harmaway.cfm.

64. L. A. Lefton, *Psychology,* 9th ed. (Boston: Allyn & Bacon, 2005).

3

Managing Stress

COPING WITH LIFE'S CHALLENGES

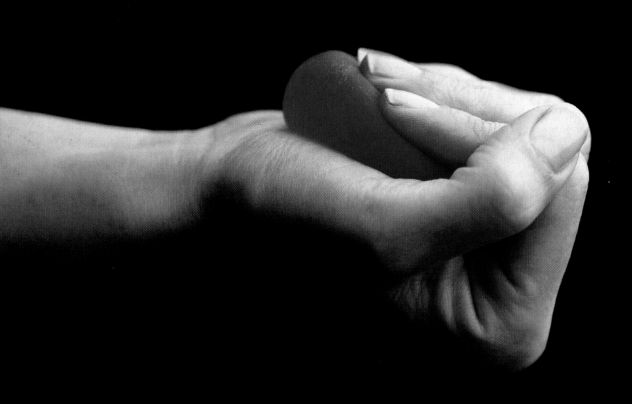

Why am I **physically** affected by stressful situations?

Why do I always catch a **cold** during finals week?

How can I **cope** with daily pressures and annoyances?

What actions can I take to deal with **anger** in a healthy way?

How can I **prioritize** everything I try to do in a day?

OBJECTIVES

- Define stress, and examine the potential impact of stress on health, relationships, and success in college.
- Explain the phases of the general adaptation syndrome and the physiological changes that occur.
- Discuss sources of stress and examine the special stressors that affect college students.
- Explore techniques for coping with or reducing exposure to stress and using positive stressors to enrich your life.
- Examine the role of spirituality in controlling or preventing the negative effects of stress.

Rising tuition, roommates who bug you, social-life drama, too much noise, no privacy, long lines at the bookstore, pressure to get good grades, never enough money, worries over war, terrorism, and natural disasters. STRESS! You can't run from it, you can't hide from it, and it invades our waking and sleeping hours.

Often, stress is insidious, and we don't even notice the things that affect us. As we sleep, it encroaches on our psyche through noise or incessant worries over things that need to be done. While we work at the computer, stress may interfere in the form of noise from next door, strain on our eyes, and tension in our backs. Even when we are out socializing with friends, we feel guilty about not enough time and so much left to do. The exact toll stress exacts from us during a lifetime of stress overload is unknown, but it is much more than an annoyance. Rather, it is a significant health hazard that can rob the body of needed nutrients, damage the cardiovascular system, raise blood pressure, and dampen the immune system's defenses, leaving us vulnerable to infections and disease. In addition, it can drain our emotional reserves, contribute to depression, anxiety, and irritability, and punctuate social interactions with hostility and anger. Although much has been written about stress, we are only beginning to understand the multifaceted nature of the stress response and its tremendous potential for harm or benefit.

What Is Stress?

Often, we think of stress as an externally imposed factor. But for most of us, stress results from an internal state of emotional tension that occurs in response to the various demands of living. Most current definitions state that **stress** is the mental and physical response of our bodies to the changes and challenges in our lives. Inherent in these definitions is the idea that we sometimes take ourselves too seriously; that we should loosen up, worry less, and gain greater control over our minds as well as our bodies. A **stressor** is any physical, social, or psychological event or condition that causes our bodies to adjust to a specific situation. Several factors influence one's response to stressors, including characteristics of the stressor (Can you control it? Is it predictable? Does it occur often?), biological factors (such as your age or gender), and past experiences.[1] Stressors may be tangible, such as an angry parent or a disgruntled roommate, or intangible, such as the mixed emotions associated with meeting your significant other's parents for the first time. **Strain** is the wear and tear the body and mind sustain during the stress process. **Coping** is the act of managing events or conditions to lessen the physical or psychological effects of excess stress.[2] Stress is literally in the eye of the beholder and each person's unique combination of heredity, life experiences, personality, and ability to cope influence how an event is perceived and the meaning attached to it.

Stress and strain are associated with most daily activities. Generally, positive stress, or stress that presents the opportunity for personal growth and satisfaction, is called **eustress**. Getting married, starting school, beginning a career, developing new friendships, and learning a new physical skill all give rise to eustress. **Distress**, or negative stress, is caused by events that result in debilitative stress and strain (such as financial problems, the death of a loved one, academic difficulties, and the breakup of a relationship).

We cannot get rid of distress entirely: like eustress, it is a part of life. However, we can train ourselves to recognize the events that cause distress and to anticipate our reactions to them. We can learn coping skills and strategies that will help us manage stress more effectively (see the Assess Yourself box on page 76).

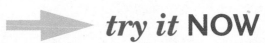 *try it* NOW

Write it down! Journal writing is a great method to cleanse the mind, release emotions, and draft strategies for resolution. The next time you are feeling stressed, write down the event or situation that activated your stress response, identify the emotions that accompany it, and list several options to bring closure to the event. Writing these things down can be an effective means to cope with stressors.

The Body's Response to Stress

The Fight-or-Flight Response

 Whenever we're surprised by a sudden stressor, such as someone swerving into our lane of traffic, the adrenal glands jump into action. Emotional reactions to a perceived threat trigger these two almond-sized glands sitting atop the kidneys to secrete adrenaline and other hormones into the bloodstream. As a result, the heart speeds up, breathing rate increases, blood pressure rises, and the flow of blood to the muscles increases with a rapid release of blood sugars into the bloodstream. This sudden burst of energy and strength is believed to provide the

---

stress Mental and physical responses to change.

stressor A physical, social, or psychological event or condition that requires our bodies to make an adjustment.

strain The wear and tear sustained by the body and mind in adjusting to or resisting a stressor.

coping The act of managing events or conditions to lessen the physical or psychological effects of excess stress.

eustress Stress that presents opportunities for personal growth.

distress Stress that can have a negative effect on health.

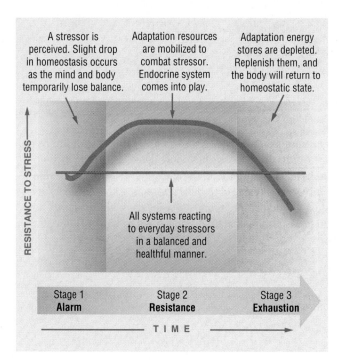

FIGURE 3.1 **The General Adaptation Syndrome**

A stressor is perceived. Slight drop in homeostasis occurs as the mind and body temporarily lose balance.

Adaptation resources are mobilized to combat stressor. Endocrine system comes into play.

Adaptation energy stores are depleted. Replenish them, and the body will return to homeostatic state.

All systems reacting to everyday stressors in a balanced and healthful manner.

RESISTANCE TO STRESS

Stage 1 **Alarm** Stage 2 **Resistance** Stage 3 **Exhaustion**

TIME

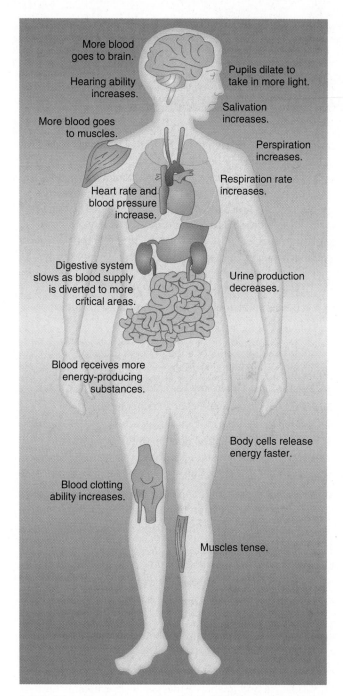

FIGURE 3.2 **The General Adaptation Syndrome: The Alarm Phase**

More blood goes to brain.

Pupils dilate to take in more light.

Hearing ability increases.

Salivation increases.

More blood goes to muscles.

Perspiration increases.

Respiration rate increases.

Heart rate and blood pressure increase.

Digestive system slows as blood supply is diverted to more critical areas.

Urine production decreases.

Blood receives more energy-producing substances.

Body cells release energy faster.

Blood clotting ability increases.

Muscles tense.

extra edge that has helped generations of humans survive during adversity. Known as the **fight-or-flight response**, this physiological reaction is believed to be one of our most basic, innate survival instincts.[3] It is a point at which our bodies go on the alert to either fight or escape.

The General Adaptation Syndrome

What we have just described in very general terms is a complicated physiological response to stress in which our bodies move from **homeostasis**, a level of functioning in which systems operate smoothly and maintain equilibrium, to one of crisis, in which the body attempts to return to homeostasis. This adjustment is referred to as an **adaptive response**. First characterized by Hans Selye in 1936, this internal fight to restore balance is known as the **general adaptation syndrome (GAS)** (Figure 3.1), which has three distinct phases: alarm, resistance, and exhaustion.[4]

Alarm Phase When the body is exposed to a stressor, whether real or perceived, the fight-or-flight response kicks into gear. Stress hormones flow into the body, and it prepares to do battle. The subconscious perceptions and appraisal of the stressor stimulate the areas in the brain responsible for emotions. Emotional stimulation, in turn, starts the physical reactions that we associate with stress (Figure 3.2). This entire process takes only a few seconds.

Suppose that you are walking to your car on a dimly lit campus after a late-night class. As you pass a particularly dark area, you hear someone cough behind you and sense that this person is fairly close. You walk faster, only to hear the

fight-or-flight response Physiological arousal response in which the body prepares to combat a real or perceived threat.

homeostasis A balanced physical state in which all the body's systems function smoothly.

adaptive response Form of adjustment in which the body attempts to restore homeostasis.

general adaptation syndrome (GAS) The pattern followed in the physiological response to stress, consisting of the alarm, resistance, and exhaustion phases.

ASSESS yourself

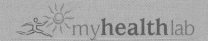

HOW STRESSED ARE YOU?

Fill out this assessment online at www.aw-bc.com/myhealthlab or www.aw-bc.com/donatelle.

Each of us reacts differently to life's little challenges. Faced with a long line at the bookstore, most of us will get anxious for a few seconds before we start grumbling or shrug and move on. For others—the one in five of us whom researchers call hot reactors—such incidents are part of a daily health assault. These individuals may get outwardly angry or appear calm and collected. It is what is going on under the surface that affects health. Surges in blood pressure, increases in heart rate, nausea, sweating, and other hot reactor indicators may occur. Completing the following assessment will help you think about the nature and extent of stress in your life and how you respond to daily stressors. Although this survey is just an indicator of what stress levels might be, it will help you focus on areas that you may need to work on to reduce stress.

PART ONE: WHAT IS STRESSING YOU OUT?

For each statement, indicate how often the following stressful situations or feelings are a part of your daily life.

	Never	Rarely	Sometimes	Often	Always
1. I find that there are not enough hours in the day to finish everything I have to do.	1	2	3	4	5
2. I am anxious about how I am performing in my classes.	1	2	3	4	5
3. People don't seem to notice whether or not I do a good job.	1	2	3	4	5
4. I am tired and feel like I don't have the energy to do everything that I need to get done.	1	2	3	4	5
5. I seem to be easily irritated by things that people do.	1	2	3	4	5
6. I worry about what is happening in my family (health of a loved one, financial problems, relationship problems, etc.).	1	2	3	4	5
7. I'm worried about my finances and having enough money to pay my bills.	1	2	3	4	5
8. I don't have enough time for fun.	1	2	3	4	5
9. I am unhappy with my body (weight, fitness level, etc.).	1	2	3	4	5
10. My family and friends count on me to help them with their problems.	1	2	3	4	5
11. I am concerned about my current relationship (or lack of a relationship).	1	2	3	4	5
12. I am impatient/intolerant of the weaknesses of others.	1	2	3	4	5
13. My house/apartment is a mess, and I'm embarrassed to have others see it.	1	2	3	4	5
14. I worry about whether I'll get a job and be able to support myself after graduation.	1	2	3	4	5
15. I worry that people don't like me.	1	2	3	4	5

Your Total Score: _____

Analyzing This Section

Scores of 60–75: Your stress level is probably quite high. Prioritize the areas where you scored 5s, and list two to three things for each area that you could do to reduce your stress level. Note any increase in headaches, backaches, or insomnia; your body is telling you to lighten your load. Plan at least one fun thing to do for yourself each day. Make yourself more of a daily priority.

Scores of 45–60: Your stress level is moderate. Look at those areas that are 5s and list two to three things that you would like to change now to help yourself reduce stress. Practice at least one stress management technique each day. Make more time for yourself.

Scores of 30–45: You seem to have a lower level of stress. This is good. However, there are still areas that you could work on. Think about what these are, and list things you could do now to reduce stress.

Scores below 30: You seem to be doing a great job. Whatever your problems, stress isn't one of them. Even when stressful events do occur—and they will—your health probably won't suffer.

Remember, each of us has "stress slips" along the way. Think about your reactions to situations like those above. Whenever possible, make conscious choices to reduce stress.

PART TWO: HOW DO YOU RESPOND TO STRESS?
Respond to each of the following statements with a rating of how likely you are to react to a given stressful event.

	Never	Rarely	Sometimes	Always

Scenario 1
You've been waiting 20 minutes for a table in a crowded restaurant, and the hostess seats a group that arrived after you.

	Never	Rarely	Sometimes	Always
1. You feel your anger rise as your face gets hot and your heart beats faster.	1	2	3	4
2. You yell "Hey! I was here first" in an irritated voice to the hostess.	1	2	3	4
3. You angrily confront the people who are being seated in front of you and tell them you were there first.	1	2	3	4
4. You say, "Excuse me" in a polite voice and inform the other group and/or the hostess that you were there first.	1	2	3	4
5. You note it, but don't react. It's no big deal, and the hostess obviously didn't notice the order of arrival.	1	2	3	4

Scenario 2
You get to a movie theater early so that you and a friend can get great seats. You strategically pick a seat that will give you a good view. Although the theater is nearly empty, a large, tall man plops himself in the seat directly in front of you. Try as you might, you cannot see the screen.

	Never	Rarely	Sometimes	Always
1. You say in a very loud voice: "There's a whole theater, and he has to sit right in front of us!"	1	2	3	4
2. You yell directly at the man, saying, "Can't you sit somewhere else? I can't see!"	1	2	3	4
3. You tap the man on the shoulder and say, "Excuse me, I wonder if you could slide down a seat. I can't see."	1	2	3	4
4. You calmly nudge your friend and decide to move.	1	2	3	4
5. You aren't bothered by the person in front of you. This is just part of going to the movies, and it is no big deal.	1	2	3	4

Other Scenarios
How would you respond to the following?

	Never	Rarely	Sometimes	Always
1. Your sister calls out of the blue and starts to tell you how much you mean to her. Uncomfortable, you change the subject without expressing what you feel.	1	2	3	4
2. You come home to find the kitchen looking like a disaster area and your spouse/roommate lounging in front of the TV. You tense up and can't seem to shake your anger, but you decide not to bring it up.	1	2	3	4

(continued)

	Never	Rarely	Sometimes	Always
3. Faced with a public speaking event, you get keyed up and lose sleep for a day or more, worrying about how you'll do.	1	2	3	4
4. Your boyfriend/girlfriend/partner is seen out with another person and appears to be acting quite close to the person. You are a trusting person and decide not to worry about it. If your significant other has anything to tell you, you know he/she will talk to you.	1	2	3	4
5. You aren't able to study as much as you'd like for an exam, yet you think that you really "nailed" the exam once you take it. When you get it back, you find that you did horribly. You make an appointment to talk with the professor and determine what you can do to improve on the next exam. You acknowledge that you are responsible for the low grade this time but vow to do better next time. You are disappointed, but you don't let it bother you.	1	2	3	4

Analyzing This Section

Look carefully at each of these scenarios. Obviously, none of us is perfect, and we sometimes react in ways that we later regret. The key here is to assess how you react the majority of the time.

If stressful events occur and you remain calm, do not experience increases in heart rate or blood pressure, or avoid excess anxiety, anger, or frustration, you are probably a cool reactor who tends to roll with the punches when a situation is out of your control. This usually indicates a good level of coping; overall, you will suffer fewer health consequences when stressed. The key here is that you really are not stressed, and you really are calm and unworried about the situation.

If you fret and stew about a stressor, can't sleep, or tend to react with hostility, anger, or other negative physiological overreactions, you probably are a hot reactor who responds to mildly stressful situations with a fight-or-flight adrenaline rush that drives up blood pressure and can lead to heart rhythm disturbances, accelerated clotting, and damaged blood vessel linings. Some hot reactors can seem cool on the outside, but inside their bodies are silently killing them. They may be on edge or jumpy or unable to sleep, even though most people would never suspect that they are in trouble. Before you honk or make obscene gestures at the guy who cuts you off in rush hour traffic, remember that getting angry can destroy thousands of heart muscle cells within minutes. Robert S. Eliot, author of *From Stress to Strength,* says hot

quickened footsteps of the other person. Your senses become increasingly alert, your breathing quickens, your heart races, and you begin to perspire. The stranger is getting closer and closer. In desperation you stop, clutching your book bag in your hands, determined to use force if necessary to protect yourself. You turn around quickly and let out a blood-curdling yell. To your surprise, the only person you see is your classmate Cindy, who has been trying to stay close to

you out of her own anxiety about walking alone in the dark. She screams and jumps back off the curb, only to trip and fall. You look at her in startled embarrassment, help her to her feet, and nervously laugh about your reaction. You have just experienced the alarm phase of GAS.

When the mind perceives a stressor (either real or imaginary), such as a potential attacker, the **cerebral cortex**, the region of the brain that interprets the nature of an event, is called to attention. If the cerebral cortex perceives a threat, it triggers an **autonomic nervous system (ANS)** response that prepares the body for action. The ANS is the portion of the central nervous system that regulates bodily functions that we do not normally consciously control, such as heart function, breathing, and glandular function. When we are stressed, the activity rate of all these bodily functions increases dramatically to give us the physical strength to protect ourselves or to mobilize internal forces to fight or flee.

The ANS has two branches: sympathetic and parasympathetic. The **sympathetic nervous system** energizes the body

cerebral cortex The region of the brain that interprets the nature of an event.

autonomic nervous system (ANS) The portion of the central nervous system that regulates bodily functions that a person does not normally consciously control.

sympathetic nervous system Branch of the autonomic nervous system responsible for stress arousal.

reactors have no choice but to calm themselves down with rational thought. Look at ways to change your perceptions and cope more effectively. Ponder the fact that the only thing you'll hasten by reacting is a decline in health. "You have to stop trying to change the world," Eliot advises, "and learn to change your response to it."

MAKE it happen!

ASSESSMENT: The Assess Yourself activity gave you the chance to look at your stress levels and identify situations in your life that particularly cause stress. Now that you are aware of these patterns, you can change a behavior that leads to increased stress.

MAKING A CHANGE: In order to change your behavior, you need to develop a plan. Follow the steps below and complete your Behavior Change Contract to take action.

1. Evaluate your behavior and identify patterns and specific things you are doing. What can you change now? What can you change in the near future?

2. Select one pattern of behavior that you want to change.

3. Fill out the Behavior Change Contract found at the front of your book. It should include your long-term goal for change, your short-term goals, the rewards you'll give yourself for reaching these goals, potential obstacles along the way, and strategies for overcoming these obstacles. For each goal, list the small steps and specific actions that you will take.

4. Chart your progress in a journal. At the end of a week, consider how successful you were in following your plan. What helped you be successful? What made change more difficult? What will you do differently next week?

5. Revise your plan as needed: Are the short-term goals attainable? Are the rewards satisfying?

ONE STUDENT'S PLAN: Kim discovered that much of her stress was caused by school deadlines. She wanted to learn how to manage her time more efficiently. Kim filled out a Behavior Change Contract, with a goal of finishing her history term paper five days before its due date to give herself enough time to study for her biology final. She broke the paper-writing process into manageable steps of research, writing, revising, and proofreading. Each time she finished a stage she rewarded herself with a movie or a trip to the local coffeehouse. She fell behind when her sister unexpectedly visited her for two days, but she got back on schedule when she worked on her paper instead of watching her afternoon soap opera. Kim completed her paper in plenty of time, was able to study efficiently for her biology exam, and didn't come down with her usual finals-period cold.

for fight or flight by signaling the release of several stress hormones that speed the heart rate, increase the breathing rate, and trigger many other stress responses. The **parasympathetic nervous system** functions to slow all the systems stimulated by the stress response. Thus, the parasympathetic branch of the ANS serves as a system of checks and balances on the sympathetic branch. In a healthy person, these two branches work together in a balance that controls the negative effects of stress. However, long-term stress can strain this balance, and chronic physical problems can occur as stress reactions become the dominant forces in a person's body.

The responses of the sympathetic nervous system to stress involve a complex series of biochemical exchanges between different parts of the body. The **hypothalamus**, a structure in the brain, functions as the control center of the sympathetic nervous system and determines the overall reaction to stressors. When the hypothalamus perceives that extra energy is needed to fight a stressor, it stimulates the adrenal glands, located near the top of the kidneys, to release the hormone **epinephrine**, also called adrenaline. Epinephrine causes more blood to be pumped with each beat of the heart, dilates the bronchioles (air sacs in the lungs) to increase oxygen intake, increases the breathing rate, enhances hearing,

Why am I physically affected by stressful situations?

parasympathetic nervous system Branch of the autonomic nervous system responsible for slowing systems stimulated by the stress response.

hypothalamus A section of the brain that controls the sympathetic nervous system and directs the stress response.

epinephrine Also called adrenaline, a hormone that stimulates body systems in response to stress.

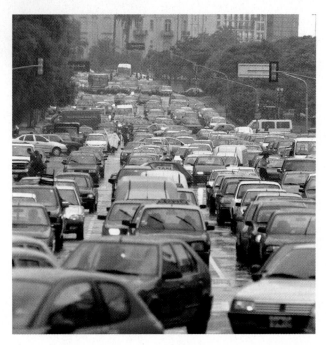

Traffic jams are a modern stressor and an example of the daily strains that can add up and jeopardize our health.

stimulates the liver to release more glucose (which fuels muscular exertion), and dilates the pupils to improve visual sensitivity. The body is then poised to act immediately.

As epinephrine secretion increases, blood is diverted away from the digestive system, possibly causing nausea and cramping if the distress occurs shortly after a meal, and drying of nasal and salivary tissues, producing dry mouth. The alarm phase also provides for longer-term reaction to stress. The hypothalamus triggers the pituitary gland, which in turn releases another powerful hormone, **adrenocorticotropic hormone (ACTH)**. ACTH signals the adrenal glands to release **cortisol**, a hormone that makes stored nutrients more readily available to meet energy demands. See the New Horizons in Health box on page 82 for more on the effect cortisol

adrenocorticotropic hormone (ACTH)   A pituitary hormone that stimulates the adrenal glands to secrete cortisol.

cortisol   Hormone released by the adrenal glands that makes stored nutrients more readily available to meet energy demands.

allostatic load   Wear and tear on the body caused by prolonged or excessive stress responses.

acute stress   Stress that is short in duration.

chronic stress   Stress that is not as intense as acute stress but that exists for prolonged periods of time.

adaptation energy stores   The physical and mental foundations of our ability to cope with stress.

immunocompetence   The ability of the immune system to respond to assaults.

can have on the body. Finally, other parts of the brain and body release endorphins, the body's naturally occurring opiates, which relieve pain that may be caused by a stressor.

Resistance Phase   The resistance phase of the GAS is similar to the alarm phase in that the same organs and systems are mobilized, but generally at a less intense level and for a longer period of time. The body tries to return to homeostasis but because some perceived stressor still exists, complete rest is never achieved. Instead, the body stays aroused at a level which causes a higher metabolic rate in some organ tissues. These organs and systems of resistance are in effect working overtime and after prolonged stress will become depleted to the point where they cannot function effectively.

Exhaustion Phase   Stress promotes adaptation but a prolonged response leads to **allostatic load** or exhaustive wear and tear on the body.[5] In the exhaustion phase of the GAS, the physical and emotional energy used to fight a stressor have been depleted. The toll it takes on the body depends on the type of stress or the period of time spent under stress. **Acute stress,** or short-term stress lasting for only a few minutes or hours, probably would not deplete all of a person's energy reserves, but **chronic stress** experienced over a period of time can create continuous states of alarm and resistance, resulting in total depletion of energy and susceptibility to illness. The key to warding off the effects of stress lies in what many researchers refer to as **adaptation energy stores**, the physical and mental foundations of our ability to cope with stress.

Two levels of adaptation energy stores exist: deep and superficial. We apparently have little control over deep stores, as their size appears to be preset by heredity. Superficial adaptation energy stores, however, are renewable and present the first line of defense against stress, as they are tapped into initially when the body fights stress. Only when superficial stores are exhausted does the body tap into the deep energy stores. As our adaptation energy stores are depleted, we tire more quickly and require more rest. Without this replenishing sleep, the alarm and resistance phases eventually will limit our ability to rebound properly.

As the body adjusts to chronic unresolved stress, the adrenal glands continue to release cortisol, which remains in the bloodstream for longer periods of time due to slower metabolic responsiveness. Over time, without relief, cortisol can reduce **immunocompetence**, or the ability of the immune system to respond to various onslaughts. Blood pressure can remain dangerously elevated, and our body systems become unable to respond with the same vigor they once did. The net effect? Greater chance of minor illnesses at one end of the continuum; greater risk of life-threatening disease at the other end.

Stress management, therefore, depends on the ability to replenish superficial stores and conserve deep stores. Besides getting adequate rest, adaptation energy stores can be replenished by aerobic exercise, finding a balance between work and relaxation, practicing good nutritional habits, setting realistic goals, and maintaining supportive relationships.

| TABLE 3.1 | What Stress Symptoms Do You Have? | 81 |

Circle the number that indicates the frequency of occurrence of each symptom.

	Never	At least once in the last 6 months	At least once in the last month	At least once in the last week
1. Tension headache	1	2	3	4
2. Migraine (vascular) headache	1	2	3	4
3. Stomachache	1	2	3	4
4. Cold hands	1	2	3	4
5. Acid stomach	1	2	3	4
6. Shallow, rapid breathing	1	2	3	4
7. Diarrhea	1	2	3	4
8. Muscle cramps	1	2	3	4
9. Burping	1	2	3	4
10. Gassiness	1	2	3	4
11. Increased urge to urinate	1	2	3	4
12. Sweaty hands/feet	1	2	3	4
13. Fatigue/exhausted feelings	1	2	3	4
14. Oily skin	1	2	3	4
15. Dry mouth	1	2	3	4
16. Hand tremor	1	2	3	4
17. Backache	1	2	3	4
18. Neck stiffness	1	2	3	4
19. Gum chewing	1	2	3	4
20. Constipation	1	2	3	4
21. Tightness in chest or heart	1	2	3	4
22. Dizziness	1	2	3	4
23. Nausea/vomiting	1	2	3	4
24. Butterflies in stomach	1	2	3	4
25. Skin blemishes	1	2	3	4
26. Heart pounding	1	2	3	4
27. Blushing	1	2	3	4
28. Palpitations	1	2	3	4
29. Indigestion	1	2	3	4
30. Hyperventilation	1	2	3	4
31. Skin rashes	1	2	3	4
32. Jaw pain	1	2	3	4
33. Grinding teeth	1	2	3	4

Evaluating Your Score

< 38 = low physiological symptoms
38–50 = moderate physiological symptoms
51–75 = high physiological symptoms
76–99 = excessive physiological symptoms

Source: R. Blonna, *Coping with Stress in a Changing World,* 4th ed. (Boston: McGraw-Hill, 2006), 126.

Stress and Your Health

Although much has been written about the negative effects of stress, researchers have only recently begun to untangle the complex web of physical and emotional interactions that can break down the body over time. Stress is often described as a "disease of prolonged arousal" that leads to other negative health effects. Nearly all body systems are potential targets, and the long-term effects may be devastating. Look at the stress symptom checklist in Table 3.1. Do you have any of these physical symptoms of stress?

Studies indicate that 40 percent of deaths and 70 percent of disease in the United States is related, in whole or part, to stress.[6] The list of ailments related to chronic stress includes heart disease, diabetes, cancer, headaches, ulcers, low back pain, depression, and the common cold. Alarming increases in rates of suicide, homicide, and domestic violence across

REDUCE STRESS TO REDUCE FAT?

Can chronic stress reshape your body? Research suggests that stress is linked to belly fat and, possibly, that you can keep the inches off your midsection by learning to manage stress.

The exact mechanisms still need clarification, but the hypothesis is that greater vulnerability to stress increases exposure to stress-induced cortisol, a powerful hormone that contributes to increased hunger (to replace fuel used during the fight-or-flight response) and to the deposit of fat in a particularly annoying spot—our waist.

When cortisol hits any cell, it activates fat-storing enzymes that cause the cell to enlarge. Fat cells in the belly have the largest number of receptors for cortisol so the hormone is particularly attracted to this area. The extra calories and the added abdominal fat are both unsightly and dangerous. Experts have identified excess weight around the middle (central fat) as a risk factor for several diseases, including hypertension, coronary heart disease, stroke, and diabetes.

Accumulating evidence from clinical to cellular to molecular studies tend to support the aforementioned hypothesis: for example, in animal studies, stress-induced cortisol secretion has been shown to increase central (or abdominal) fat. In human studies, women with central fat distribution have been shown to display heightened cortisol secretion in response to an acute laboratory stressor and an increase in food consumption following the stressful event. Only longitudinal and genetic studies will determine conclusively whether stress and central fat are causally related, but correlational data suggest that greater life stress and stress reactivity are linked to central fat.

If we want to win the battle of the bulge, we must focus on both stress management and weight-loss strategies. By learning to relax we can de-stress and prevent excess cortisol secretion. A simple stay-slim solution: engage in regular physical activity. Physical activity will reduce your stress hormones and minimize some of the appetite-triggering and fat-storage effects of cortisol.

Sources: M. F. Dallman et al., "Minireview: Glucocorticoids—Food Intake, Abdominal Obesity, and Wealthy Nations in 2004," *Endocrinology* 145, no. 6 (2004): 2633–2638; E. S. Epel et al., "Stress and Body Shape: Stress-Induced Cortisol Secretion Is Consistently Greater Among Women with Central Fat," *Psychosomatic Medicine* 62 (2000): 623–632; E. Epel et al., "Stress May Add Bite to Appetite in Women: A Laboratory Study of Stress-Induced Cortisol and Eating Behavior," *Psychoneuroendocrinology* 26 (2001): 37–49; J. Marniemi et al., "Visceral Fat and Psychosocial Stress in Identical Twins Discordant for Obesity," *Journal of Internal Medicine* 251 (2002): 35–43; M. Duclos et al., "Fat Distribution in Obese Women Is Associated with Subtle Alteration of the Hypothalamic-Pituitary-Adrenal Axis Activity and Sensitivity to Glucocorticoids," *Clinical Endocrinology* 55 (2001): 447–454.

the United States are additional symptoms of a nation under stress. While the battle over the legitimacy of these observations continues to be waged in research labs around the world, the theory that stress increases susceptibility to certain illnesses and infectious diseases has gained credibility and been substantiated by hundreds of studies.[7]

Stress and CVD

Perhaps the most studied and documented health consequence of unresolved stress is cardiovascular disease (CVD). The literature on this topic is quite expansive and many epidemiological and sociological observations have noted the impact of chronic stress on heart rate, blood pressure, heart attack, and stroke.[8] The largest epidemiological study to date, the INTERHEART Study with almost 30,000 participants in 52 countries, identified stress as one of the key modifiable risk factors for heart attack.[9] Similarly, the National Health Interview Study, conducted annually by the CDC's National Center for Health Statistics, has reported that stress accounts for approximately 30 percent of the attributable risk of myocardial infarction (heart attack).[10]

Historically, the increased risk of CVD from chronic stress has been linked to increased plaque buildup due to elevated cholesterol, hardening of the arteries, alterations in heart rhythm, increased and fluctuating blood pressures, and difficulties in cardiovascular responsiveness due to all of the above. Although these continue to be considered major risks, recent research also points to metabolic abnormalities, insulin resistance, and inflammation in blood vessels (perhaps due to lingering viral effects) as major contributors to heart disease.[11] (For more information about CVD, see Chapter 15.) In the past 15 to 20 years, research has grown exponentially and direct links have been identified between stressors such as job strain, care giving, bereavement, and natural disasters with the incidence and progression of CVD.[12] Whatever the mechanism, the evidence is clear that stress is a significant contributor to CVD morbidity and mortality.

Stress and Impaired Immunity

Why do I always catch a cold during finals week?

As discussed in Chapter 2, a burgeoning area of scientific investigation known as **psychoneuroimmunology (PNI)** analyzes the intricate relationship between the mind's response to stress and the ability of the immune system to function effectively. A review of more than 300 empirical studies linking stress to adverse health consequences suggests that too much stress, over a long period, can negatively regulate various aspects of the cellular immune response.[13] In particular, stress disrupts the communication networks between the nervous, endocrine, and immune systems. When these networks fail, messenger systems that regulate hormones, blood cell formation, and other health-regulating systems begin to falter or send faulty information. Whereas the acute stress response is essentially protecting, prolonged fight-or-flight readiness (alarm phase) exerts some immune system depression, particularly through the actions of cortisol.[14] During prolonged stress, elevated levels of cortisol and other adrenal hormones destroy or reduce the ability of certain white blood cells, known as killer T cells, to aid the immune response. When killer T cells are suppressed and other regulating systems aren't working correctly, illness may occur.

Loss of immune regulation can result in various disease states. The links between stress and the physiological features of cancer, arthritis, HIV/AIDS, asthma, and many other ailments have been studied through PNI.[15] Although each of these diseases has distinct clinical consequences, the change in the immune system from balanced and flexible to inflexible and unbalanced suggests increased vulnerability to stress-related immune impairment. (For more information about the immune system, see Chapter 17.)

How long does one have to be stressed to suffer from impaired immunity? A look at the research yields evidence of impaired immunity following acute stressors such as arguments, public speaking, and academic examinations; more prolonged stressors such as the loss of a spouse, exposure to a natural disaster, caregiving, living with a handicap, and unemployment also show declines in natural immune response among various populations.[16]

Other studies that link stress with infectious diseases include:

- More than 20 years of research examining psychosocial factors in susceptibility to upper respiratory infections has revealed a dose-response relationship between stress indexes and the rate of viral infection and clinical cold symptoms.[17]
- Psychological stress and loneliness correlate to poorer immune responses following influenza vaccinations in college students.[18]
- Exposure to academic stressors and self-reported stress are associated with increased upper-respiratory-tract infection among students.[19]

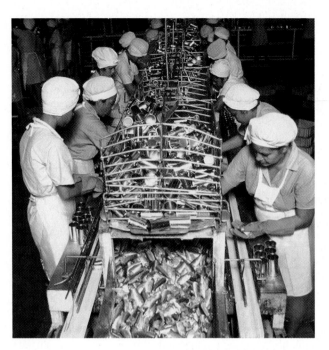

Studies indicate that those who have little control or decision-making powers in their employment are at increased risk for stress-related CVD.

Although strong indicators support the hypothesis of a relationship between high stress and increased risk for disease, we are only beginning to understand this link. Some research indicates that other factors, such as genetics and environmental stimuli, may be involved. However, in spite of questions, studies supporting this relationship outnumber those that don't and there is convincing evidence that susceptibility to disease is influenced by stress-induced alterations in immune functioning.[20]

Stress and Diabetes

Recent data from large epidemiological studies with humans has provided strong evidence of a link between psychological or physical stress and **diabetes**, a disease in which the pancreas fails to produce enough insulin or to use insulin effectively.[21] The activation of the sympathetic nervous system by the stress response can result in a combination of increased glucose (blood sugars) and inadequate production and release of *insulin,* a hormone that controls blood sugar levels.[22] While an occasional stress reaction might not harm you, high-stress jobs, unresolved problems with family, school, or finances, and other sources of chronic stress can contribute to the onset or progression of diabetes. Over time, high blood

psychoneuroimmunology (PNI) Science of the interaction between the mind and the immune system.

diabetes Disease in which the pancreas fails to produce enough insulin or to use insulin effectively.

sugar levels may begin to damage body organs such as the kidneys and blood vessels in the extremities and eyes.

Controlling stress levels is critical for successful short- and long-term diabetes management.[23] People under lots of stress often don't get enough sleep, don't eat well, and may drink or take other drugs to help them get through a stressful time. All of these behaviors can alter blood sugar levels further, on top of the increased blood sugars the body creates to fuel the fight-or-flight response. Exercise and relaxation techniques are particularly important. Even a short 15-minute walk can cause glucose levels to drop dramatically, as well as having other stress-reducing effects. Losing weight is also important. Being at a healthy weight contributes to overall glucose control and prevents the stress that people feel when they are overweight. For more information on diabetes, see Chapter 18.

Stress and the Mind

Stress may be one of the single greatest contributors to mental disability and emotional dysfunction in industrialized nations. Studies have shown that higher rates of mental disorders, particularly depression and anxiety, are associated with various environmental stressors, including divorce, marital conflict, economic hardship, and stressful life events.[24] In particular, young people aged 15 to 24 have higher prevalence rates of mental disorder than do other age groups. Based on this finding, researchers suggest that as individuals move from adolescence to adulthood, they face stressors of all kinds, from school to employment to relationships, that may challenge their mental health.[25]

Evidence suggests a strong relationship between stress and the potential for negative mental health reactions. Consider the following:[26]

- Stressful life events and inadequate sources of social support have been identified as predictors of psychiatric morbidity, including anxiety, insomnia, and depression.
- The high incidence of suicide among college students is assumed to be indicative of personal and societal stress in the lives of young people.
- Eighty-five percent of college counseling centers report an increase in the number of students they see with severe psychological problems—problems largely related to stress and adjustment difficulties.

Sources of Stress

Both eustress and distress have many sources. They include psychosocial factors, environmental stressors, and self-imposed stress.

Psychosocial Sources of Stress

Psychosocial stress refers to the factors in our daily lives that cause stress. Interactions with others, the subtle and not-so-subtle expectations we and others have of ourselves, and the social conditions we live in force us to readjust continually. Psychosocial stressors include change, hassles, pressure, inconsistent goals and behaviors, conflict, overload, burnout, and discrimination.

Change Any time change occurs in your normal routine, whether good or bad, you will experience stress. The more changes you experience and the more adjustments you must make, the greater the stress effects may be. Almost four decades ago, Drs. Thomas Holmes and Richard Rahe developed the Social Readjustment Rating Scale (SRRS) to identify if major life events preceded illness onsets.[27] They determined that certain events (both positive and negative) were predictive of increased risk for illness. Since then, the SRRS has served as the model for scales that measure stress levels of certain groups, including students, and research has documented that life events are related to a wide variety of physical and psychological problems. Table 3.2 shows the Student Stress Scale, one example of a scale based on the SRRS.

Hassles Whereas Holmes and Rahe focused on major stressors, psychologists such as Richard Lazarus and Susan Folkman pioneered research in the 1980s that focused on petty annoyances and frustrations, collectively referred to as *hassles*.[28] Minor hassles—losing your keys, slipping and falling in front of everyone as you walk to your seat in a new class, finding that you went through a whole afternoon with spinach stuck in your front teeth—seem unimportant. However, their cumulative effects have been shown to be harmful in the long run. In fact, hassles are related to subsequent illness and disease to a greater degree than are major life events.[29]

Pressure Pressure occurs when we feel forced to speed up, intensify, or shift the direction of our behavior to meet a higher standard of performance.[30] Pressures can be based on our personal goals and expectations, concern about what others think, or outside influences. Among the most significant outside influences are society's demands that we compete and be all that we can be. The forces that push us to compete for the best grades, nicest cars, most attractive significant others, and highest-paying jobs create significant pressure to be the personification of success.

Inconsistent Goals and Behaviors For many of us, negative stress effects are magnified when there is a disparity between our goals (what we value or hope to obtain in life) and our behaviors (actions that may or may not lead to these goals). For instance, you may want good grades, and your family may expect them. But if you party and procrastinate throughout the term, your behaviors are inconsistent with your goals, and significant stress in the form of guilt, last-minute frenzy before exams, and disappointing grades may result. On the other hand, if you dig in and work and remain committed to getting good grades, this may eliminate much of your negative stress. Thwarted goals can lead to

TABLE 3.2 | The Student Stress Scale

The Student Stress Scale represents an adaptation of Holmes and Rahe's Social Readjustment Rating Scale (SRRS). The SRRS has been modified to college-aged adults and provides a rough indication of stress levels and health consequences for instructional purposes.

In the Student Stress Scale, each event is given a score that represents the amount of readjustment a person has to make as a result of the life change. To determine your stress score, check each event that you have experienced in the last 12 months, and then sum the number of points corresponding to each event.

1. Death of a close family member	____	100
2. Death of a close friend	____	73
3. Divorce between parents	____	65
4. Jail term	____	63
5. Major personal injury or illness	____	63
6. Marriage	____	58
7. Firing from a job	____	50
8. Failure of an important course	____	47
9. Change in health of a family member	____	45
10. Pregnancy	____	45
11. Sex problems	____	44
12. Serious argument with close friend	____	40
13. Change in financial status	____	39
14. Change of major	____	39
15. Trouble with parents	____	39
16. New girlfriend or boyfriend	____	37
17. Increase in workload at school	____	37
18. Outstanding personal achievement	____	36
19. First quarter/semester in school	____	36
20. Change in living conditions	____	31
21. Serious argument with an instructor	____	30
22. Lower grades than expected	____	29
23. Change in sleeping habits	____	29
24. Change in social activities	____	29
25. Change in eating habits	____	28
26. Chronic car trouble	____	26
27. Change in number of family gatherings	____	26
28. Too many missed classes	____	25
29. Change of college	____	24
30. Dropping of more than one class	____	23
31. Minor traffic violations	____	20
	Total: ____	

Scoring: If your score is 300 or higher, you may be at high risk for developing a stress-related illness. If your score is between 150 and 300, you have approximately a 50:50 chance of experiencing a serious health problem within the next two years. If your score is below 150, you have a 1 in 3 chance of experiencing a serious health change in the next few years.

The following can help you to reduce your risk:

- Watch for early warning signs such as irritable bowels.
- Avoid negative thinking.
- Exercise regularly and eat nutritiously.
- Practice some form of relaxation regularly.
- Ask for help when necessary.

Source: Reproduced from R. Blonna, "The Social and Spiritual Basis of Stress," In: *Coping with Stress in a Changing World,* 4th edition, (Boston: McGraw-Hill, 2006). *Original source:* T. Holmes and R. H. Rahe, "The Social Readjustment Rating Scale," *Journal of Psychosomatic Research* 11 (1967): 213.

frustration, and frustration has been shown to be a significant disrupter of homeostasis.

Determining whether behaviors are consistent with goals is an essential component of maintaining balance in life. If we consciously strive to attain our goals in a direct manner, we greatly improve our chances of success.

Conflict

Conflict occurs when we are forced to make difficult decisions between competing motives, behaviors, or impulses, or when we are forced to face incompatible demands, opportunities, needs, or goals.[31] What if your best friends all choose to smoke marijuana and you don't want to smoke but fear rejection? Conflict often occurs as our values are tested. College students who are away from home for the first time often face conflict between parental values and their own set of developing beliefs.[32]

Overload

Excessive time pressure, too much responsibility, high expectations of yourself and those around you, and lack of support can lead to **overload**, a state of being overburdened. Have you ever felt you had so many responsibilities that you couldn't possibly begin to fulfill them all? Have you longed for a weekend when you could just take time out with friends and not feel guilty? These feelings are symptoms of overload. Students suffering from overload may experience anxiety about tests, poor self-concept, a desire to drop classes or drop out of school, and other problems. In severe cases, in which they are unable to see any solutions to their problems, students may suffer from depression or turn to substance abuse. Binge drinking (see Chapter 12) is one of the leading problems on college campuses today, and numerous studies have linked periods of academic overload with increased consumption of alcohol among college students.[33]

Burnout

People who regularly suffer from overload, frustration, and disappointment may eventually experience **burnout**, a state of physical and mental exhaustion caused by excessive stress. People involved in the "helping professions," such as teaching, social work, drug counseling,

overload A condition in which a person feels overly pressured by demands.

burnout Physical and mental exhaustion caused by excessive stress.

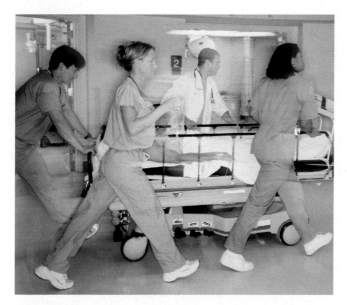

Individuals such as doctors and nurses face long work hours and a stressful work environment, making them especially prone to burnout.

nursing, and psychology, experience high levels of burnout, as do people such as police officers and air-traffic controllers who work in high-pressure, dangerous jobs. Accumulated evidence suggests that burnout resulting from prolonged exposure to stress is associated with increased risk of cardiovascular disease.[34]

Other Forms of Psychosocial Stress Other forms of psychosocial stress include problems with overcrowding, discrimination, and socioeconomic difficulties such as unemployment and poverty. People of different ages or ethnic backgrounds may face a disproportionately heavy impact from these sources of stress. In addition to all of these we face increasing threats from technological stressors. For more information see the Spotlight on Your Health box on page 88.

 what do you THINK?

Think about the changes that you have made during the past couple of years. Which of them would you regard as positive? As negative? ■ How did you react to these changes initially? ■ Did your reactions change later? ■ What are the biggest and most important changes that students must make as they enter colleges and universities, and what can they do to cope with unexpected changes?

background distressors Environmental stressors of which people are often unaware.

Stress and "-isms"

Today's racially and ethnically diverse group of students, faculty members, and staff enriches everyone's educational experience yet also challenges everyone to deal with differences. Students come to the campus from vastly different contexts and life experiences. Imagine what it would be like to come to campus and find yourself isolated, lacking friends, and ridiculed on the basis of who you are or how you look. Often, those who act, speak, dress, or appear different face additional pressures that do not affect students considered more typical. Students perceived as different may become victims of subtle and not-so-subtle forms of bigotry, insensitivity, harassment, or hostility. Race, ethnicity, religious affiliation, age, sexual orientation, or other "-*isms*"—different viewpoints and backgrounds—may hang like a dark cloud over these students.[35]

Evidence of the health effects of excessive stress in minority groups abounds. For example, African Americans suffer higher rates of hypertension, CVD, and most cancers than their white counterparts do. Although poverty and socioeconomic status have been blamed for much of the spike in hypertension rates for African Americans and other marginalized groups, this chronic, physically debilitating stress may reflect real and perceived status in society more than it reflects actual poverty. Feeling that you occupy a position of low status due to living conditions, financial security, or job status can be a source of stress. The problem is exacerbated for those who are socially disadvantaged early in life and grow up without a nurturing environment.[36] See the Health in a Diverse World box for more on stress and international students.

Environmental Stress

Environmental stress results from events occurring in the physical environment as opposed to social surroundings. Environmental stressors include natural disasters, such as floods and hurricanes, and industrial disasters, such as chemical spills and explosions. Often as damaging as one-time disasters are **background distressors**, such as noise, air, and water pollution, although we may be unaware of them and their effects may not become apparent for decades. As with other distressors, our bodies respond to environmental distressors with the general adaptation syndrome. People who cannot escape background distressors may exist in a constant resistance phase, which can contribute to the development of stress-related disorders.

Self-Imposed Stress

Appraisal and Stress We encounter many different types of life demands and potential stressors—some biological, some psychological, and others sociological. In any case, it is our appraisal of these demands, not the demands

HEALTH IN A *diverse world*

INTERNATIONAL STUDENT STRESS

Academic stress may pose a particular problem for the more than 400,000 international students who have left support networks of family and friends in their native countries to study in the United States. Accumulating evidence suggests that seeking and receiving emotional support from others is among the most effective ways to cope with stressful and upsetting situations. Unfortunately, many international students refrain from seeking emotional support due to cultural norms, shameful feelings, and the belief that support seeking is a sign of weakness that calls inappropriate attention to both the individual and his or her ethnic or cultural group. This reluctance to seek support, coupled with the language barriers, culture conflicts, racial prejudices, and other stressors, is theorized by researchers to explain why international students suffer significantly

more stress-related illnesses than do their American counterparts. There are no easy solutions to the myriad of stressors encountered by international students, yet there are things we can do to make one person's life (or maybe two or three persons' lives) a little less stressful: share companionship, communication, and assistance with others. To paraphrase a popular Hindu proverb: "Help thy neighbor's boat across and thine own boat will also reach the shore."

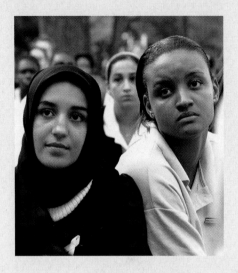

Sources: Institute of International Education, *Open Doors on the Web,* 2005, http://www. opendoorswed.org; M. R. Cunningham and A. P. Barbee, "Social Support," in *Close Relationships: A Sourcebook,* ed. C. Hendrick and S. S. Hendrick (Thousand Oaks, CA: Sage, 2000): 172–185; K. J. Edwards et al., "Stress, Negative Social Exchange, and Health Symptoms in University Students," *Journal of American College Health* 50 (2001): 75–79; S. T. Mortenson, "Cultural Differences and Similarities in Seeking Social Support as a Response to Academic Failure: A Comparison of American and Chinese College Students," *Communication Education* 55 no. 2 (2006): 127–146.

themselves, that results in the experience of stress. **Appraisal** is defined as the interpretation and evaluation of information provided to the brain by the senses. As new information becomes available, appraisal helps us recognize stressors, evaluate them on the basis of past experiences and emotions, and make decisions regarding how to cope with them. When an individual appraises his or her coping resources as sufficient to meet life demands, little or no stress is experienced. On the other hand, if an individual appraises life demands as exceeding his or her coping resources, strain and distress are likely to occur. Several coping resources that contribute to stressful appraisals, including self-esteem and self-efficacy, are discussed below.

Self-Esteem
As we learned in Chapter 2, self-esteem refers to a sense of positive self-regard or how you feel about yourself; it is a variable entity that can continually change. When we feel good about our self we are less likely to respond to or interpret an event as stressful. Conversely, if we place little or no value on our self and believe we have inadequate coping skills, we become susceptible to stress and strain.[37] Self-esteem appears to be related to coping behaviors and, in general, people with higher self-esteem tend to engage in more beneficial, problem-focused coping behaviors and seek advice and information more often than people with low self-esteem.[38]

Self-esteem is closely related to the emotions engendered by past experiences. Low self-esteem can lead to helpless anger. People suffering helpless anger usually have learned that they are wrong to feel anger, so instead of expressing it in healthy ways they turn it inward. They may swallow their rage in food, alcohol, or other drugs, or they may act in other self-destructive ways. Of particular concern, research with high school and college students has found that low self-esteem and stressful life events significantly predict **suicidal ideation,** a desire to die and thoughts about suicide. In Chapter 2 we discussed several methods to develop and maintain self-esteem, and it appears possible to increase an individual's ability to cope with stress by increasing his or her self-esteem.[39]

Self-Efficacy
Self-efficacy, also introduced in Chapter 2, is another important factor in the ability to cope with life's challenges. Self-efficacy refers to belief or confidence in

appraisal The interpretation and evaluation of information provided to the brain by the senses.

suicidal ideation A desire to die and thoughts about suicide.

TAMING TECHNOSTRESS

Cell phones that ring constantly; e-mail lists that grow on your Blackberry like an out-of-control fungus; laptop computers that somehow end up in your luggage when you go on vacation; voice message systems that don't allow you to talk to a live person. Can you feel your heart rate speeding up just thinking about these situations?

On college campuses across the country, students, faculty, and administrators are using electronic organizers, the Internet, and other forms of technology. E-mail, the World Wide Web, and personal digital assistant (PDA) devices are no longer flashy new tools but as commonplace as the backpack. Unfortunately, many people feel frustrated in their struggle to adapt to increasingly complex technology. As many as 85 percent of us feel at least some discomfort around technology.

If you are like millions of people today, you find that technology is often a daily terrorizer that raises your blood pressure, frustrates you, and prevents you from ever really getting away from it all. In short, you may be a victim of stressors that previous generations only dreamed (or had nightmares) about. Known as *technostress,* this problem is defined as "personal stress generated by reliance on technological devices . . . a panicky feeling when they fail, and a state of near-constant stimulation, or being perpetually 'plugged in.'" When technostress grabs you, it may interact with other forms of stress to create a synergistic, never-ending form of stimulation that keeps your stress response reverberating all day.

Part of the problem, ironically, is that technology enables us to be so productive. Because it encourages polyphasic activity, or "multitasking," people are forced to juggle multiple thoughts and actions at the same time, such as driving and talking on cell phones or checking handheld devices for appointments. People who multitask, however, are actually less efficient than those who focus on one project at a time. Moreover, there is clear evidence that multitasking contributes to auto accidents and other harmful consequences, including short-term memory loss. What is less clear is what happens to someone who is always plugged in.

What are the symptoms of technology overload? It evokes typical stress responses by increasing heart rate and blood pressure, and causing irritability and memory disturbances. Over time, many stressed-out people lose the ability to relax and find that they feel nervous and anxious when they are supposed to be having fun. Headaches, stomach and digestive problems, skin irritations, frequent colds, difficulty in wound healing, lack of sleep, ulcers, and other problems may result. Other red flags include gaps in your attentiveness and changes in your ability to concentrate. A study conducted by Yale University indicates that chronic stress may even thicken the waistline; increased secretions of cortisol caused even slender women to store added fat in the abdomen.

Authors Michelle Weil and Larry Rosen describe *technosis,* a syndrome in which people get so immersed in technology that they risk losing their own identity. If you answer "yes" to questions such as "Do you rely on preprogrammed systems to contact others?" and "Do you feel stressed if you haven't checked your e-mail within the last 12 hours?" you may be too dependent on technology.

---

one's skills and performance abilities.[40] Self-efficacy is considered one of the most important personality traits that influence psychological and physiological stress responses, and has been found to predict a number of health behaviors in college students.[41]

External versus Internal Locus of Control

Introduced in Chapter 1, and a concept very similar to self-efficacy, is that of perceived control. Individuals who feel they have no personal control tend to have an external locus of control, a low level of self-efficacy, and may become easily frustrated and give up in stressful circumstances. People with an internal locus of control are less likely to appraise a stressor as threatening, and more likely to believe that they possess the resources for coping with a stressful event. Studies have shown that high levels of internal control may reduce the impact of stressful events on psychological and physical health, whereas external control correlates with anxiety, depression, and other stress-related disorders.[42]

Type A Personality and Hostility Personality may contribute to the kind and degree of self-imposed stress we experience. In 1974, physicians Meyer Friedman and Ray Rosenman identified two stress-related personality types: Type A and Type B.[43] Type A personalities are hard-driving, competitive, anxious, time-driven, impatient, quick-tempered, and perfectionistic. Type B personalities are relaxed and noncompetitive. According to Rosenman and Friedman, people with Type A characteristics are more prone to heart attacks than are their Type B counterparts. Because some Type A behavior is learned, it can be modified. Some Type As are able to slow down and become more tolerant and patient. Unfortunately, many people do not decide to modify their Type A habits until after they become ill or suffer a heart attack.

TIPS FOR FIGHTING TECHNOSTRESS

- *Enjoy the natural environment.* Get away from any form of technology. Try to find a place that has few people and little noise—that usually means outdoors.
- *Become aware of what you are doing.* Log the time you spend on e-mail, voice mail, etc. Set up a schedule to limit your use of technology. For example, spend no more than a half-hour per day answering e-mails.
- *Give yourself more time for everything you do.* If you are surfing the Web for resources for a term paper, start early rather than the night before the paper is due.
- *Manage the telephone—don't let it manage you.* Rather than interrupting what you're doing to answer, screen calls with an answering machine or caller ID. Get rid of call waiting, which forces you to juggle multiple calls, and subscribe to a voice mail service that takes messages when you're on the phone.
- *Set "time out" periods when you don't answer the phone, listen to the stereo, use the computer, or watch TV.* Switch off e-mail notification systems so you aren't beeped during these periods.

- *Take regular breaks.* Even when working, get up, walk around, stretch, do deep breathing, or get a glass of water, every hour.
- *If you are working on the computer, look away from the screen and focus on something far away every 30 minutes.* Stretch your shoulders and neck periodically as you work. Playing soft background music can help you relax.
- *Resist the urge to buy the newest and fastest technology.* Such purchases not only cause financial stress, but also add to stress levels with the typical glitches that occur when installing and adjusting to new technology.
- *Do not take laptops, PDAs, or other technological gadgets on vacation.* If you must take a cell phone for emergencies, turn it and your voice messaging system off, and use the phone only in true emergencies.
- *Back up materials on your computer at regular intervals.* Writing a term paper only to lose it during a power outage will send you into hyperstress very quickly.
- *Expect technological change.* The only constant with technology is improvement and change. No matter how at

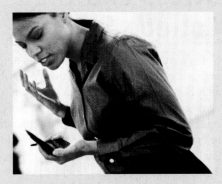

ease you are with your current computer, cell phone, PDA, etc., at some point you will need to move on to a new one.

Sources: D. Zielinski, "Techno-Stressed?" *Presentations* 18, no. 2 (2004): 28–34; L. D. Rosen and M. M. Weil, *TechnoStress: Coping with Technology @Work@Home@Play* (New York: John Wiley & Sons, 1997). Copyright © 1997. Material used by permission of John Wiley & Sons; M. Weil and L. Rosen, "Technostress: Are You a Victim of Technosis?" 2004, www.technostress.com/tstechnosis.htm; Yale University, "Stress May Cause Excess Abdominal Fat in Otherwise Slender Women, Study Conducted at Yale Shows," *ScienceDaily,* November 23, 2000; MayoClinic.com, "Are You a Slave to the Telephone?" November 1, 2000, www.mayoclinic.com.

Prevention of stress-related health problems requires recognizing and changing dangerous behaviors before damage is done.

Researchers today believe that more needs to be discovered about personality types. Most people are not one personality type all the time, and other unexplained variables must also be explored. For example, researchers at Duke University contend that the Type A personality may be more complex than previously described. They have identified a "toxic core" in some Type A personalities. People who have this toxic core are angry, distrustful of others, and cynical—a collection of characteristics commonly referred to as **hostility**.[44] It may be this toxic core rather than the hard-driving nature of the Type A personality that makes people more vulnerable to self-imposed stress. People who are hostile often have below-average levels of self-esteem and social support and other increased risks for ill health. A range of studies has identified hostility as an independent risk factor for coronary heart disease (CHD), hypertension, and premature mortality.[45]

Psychological Hardiness
According to psychologist Susanne Kobasa, **psychological hardiness** may negate self-imposed stress associated with Type A behavior. Psychologically hardy people are characterized by control, commitment, and challenge.[46] People with these three qualities are able to accept responsibility for their behaviors and change debilitating ones, have good self-esteem, understand their purpose in

---

hostility The cognitive, affective, and behavioral tendencies toward anger and cynicism.

psychological hardiness A personality trait characterized by control, commitment, and challenge.

life, and see change as a stimulating opportunity for personal growth. The concept of hardiness has been studied extensively and many researchers believe it is the foundation of an individual's ability to cope with stress and remain healthy.[47]

Stress and the College Student

College students thrive under a certain amount of pressure, but excessive stress can leave them overwhelmed and under-enthusiastic about their classes and social interactions. Students can experience numerous distressors, including changes related to being away from home for the first time, pressure to make friends in a new and sometimes intimidating setting, the feeling of anonymity imposed by large classes, and academic pressures and test-taking anxiety (Table 3.3).[48] Dealing with the tasks of transitioning to a new environment require that the college student develop new social roles and modify old ones. Such changes can result in role strain as a student attempts to form a new identity, and can lead to chronic stress responses.

Concerns about school are repeatedly the most frequently reported stressor among students and include the constant pressure of studying, too little time, writing papers, taking tests, and boring instructors.[49] Almost 32 percent of students surveyed for the National College Health Assessments reported that stress was the number-one factor affecting their individual academic performance, followed closely by stress-related problems such as cold/flu/sore throats (26.5 percent) and sleep difficulties (24.8 percent).[50]

A recent study by the Higher Education Research Institute at the University of California–Los Angeles reported that current college freshmen are more stressed than any class of freshmen before them. These researchers define **psychological stress** as the relationship between a person and the environment that the person judges to be beyond his or her resources and jeopardizes his or her well-being.[51] Freshmen seem to be the most vulnerable to the negative effects of psychological stress, with relationships, race relations, school events, physical assault (or being stalked), and feeling deviant from school norms being noted as particularly distressful. Not only did freshmen report more problems with these issues, but they also reported more emotional reactivity in the form of anger, hostility, frustration, and a greater sense of being out of control. Sophomores and juniors reported fewer problems with these issues, and seniors reported the fewest problems, which perhaps indicates progressive emotional growth through experience, maturity, increased awareness of support services, and more social connections.

psychological stress Stress caused by being in an environment perceived to be beyond one's control and endangering one's well-being.

TABLE 3.3	Overcoming Test-Taking Anxiety

Doing well on a test is an ability needed far beyond college. Here are some helpful hints to try on your next exam.

BEFORE THE EXAM

1. **Manage your time.** Plan to start studying a week before your test (longer if it's a professional exam required for your career). Being prepared will reduce anxiety. Do a limited review the night before, get a good night's sleep, and arrive for the exam early. This will ease your anxiety and increase your confidence.
2. **Build your test-taking self-esteem.** On a 3 × 5 inch card write down three reasons why you will pass the exam. Carry the card with you and look at it whenever you study. When you get the test, write your three reasons on the test or on a piece of scrap paper. Positive affirmations such as this will help you succeed.
3. **Eat a balanced meal before the exam.** Avoid sugar and rich or heavy foods, as well as foods that might upset your stomach. You want to feel your best.

DURING THE TEST

1. **Manage your time during the test.** Decide how much time you need to take the test, review your answers, and go back over questions you might be stuck on. Hold to this schedule. If you feel that you are a slow reader and need more time, talk to your teacher or test administrator before the exam.
2. **Slow down.** When you open your test book, always write RTFQ (Read the Full Question) at the top. Make sure you understand the question before answering.
3. **Stay on track.** If you begin to get anxious, reread your three reasons for success.

Male and female students also report different stressors. Women indicated that among their most frequent stressors were trying to diet, being overweight, and having an overload of school work. Men, in contrast, tended to list the following items as major stressors: being underweight, not having someone to date, not having enough sex, being behind in schoolwork, not having enough friends, and concerns about drug or alcohol use.

Differences in coping behaviors also have been identified: females report greater use of time management techniques to deal with stress, whereas males tend to engage in more leisure activities to lessen academic stress. Students generally report using health-enhancing methods to combat stress but research has found that students sometimes resort to health-compromising activities such as procrastination, avoidance, and substance use to escape the stress and anxiety of college.[52]

If you experience any of the stressors listed in Table 3.1, act promptly to reduce their impact. Most colleges offer stress management workshops through health centers or student counseling departments. Do not ignore the symptoms of stress overload, which include a vague sense of anxiety or nervousness; changes in sleep, diet, or exercise patterns; headaches; dizziness; short temper; increased negativism, cynicism, anger, or frustration; recurring colds and minor illnesses; persistent time pressures; increased difficulty in completing tasks; inability to concentrate; wanting to get away from others; and less tolerance of petty annoyances.

If stress is not dealt with, it can lead to long-lasting problems. Numerous researchers have recognized that stress among college students correlates to unhealthy behaviors such as substance abuse, lack of physical activity, poor psychological and physical health, lack of social problem solving, and low utilization of social support networks.[53] Many mental health problems may be traced to stress-related trauma that occurs at key periods of life, including the college years particularly.

Managing Your Stress

Recognizing stress is the first step toward making positive changes. Being on your own in college poses many challenges; however, it also lets you evaluate your unique situation and take steps that fit your own schedule and lifestyle in order to reduce negative stressors in your life.

One of the most effective ways to combat stressors is to build skills and coping strategies that will help inoculate you against them. Such efforts are known collectively as stress management techniques. They range from doing something as simple as taking 20 minutes each day to be alone to developing an elaborate time management plan for eating, socializing, and exercising.

Recall the process of shaping from Chapter 1 and how you may need to take a number of smaller steps to achieve a larger behavior change. Be careful not to change too many things at once, or your new stress management program could stress you out!

Building Skills to Reduce Stress

How can I cope with daily pressures and annoyances?

Dealing with stress involves assessing all aspects of a stressor, examining your response and how you can change it, and learning to cope. Often we cannot change the requirements at our college, assignments in class, or unexpected distressors. Although we cannot alter the facts, we can change our reactions to them.

Assess Your Stressors After recognizing a stressor, evaluate it. Can you alter the circumstances to reduce the amount of distress you are experiencing, or must you change your behavior and reactions to reduce stress levels? For example, if five term papers for five different courses are due during the semester, your professors are unlikely to drop such requirements. You can, however, change your behavior by beginning the papers early and spacing them over time to avoid last-minute stress.

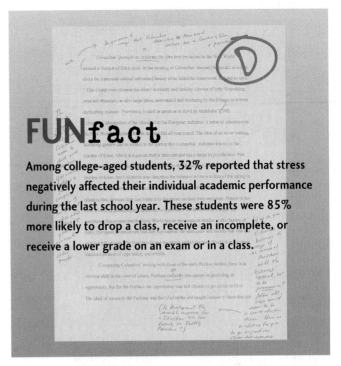

FIGURE 3.3 How Much Does Stress Affect Your School Work?

Source: American College Health Association, National College Health Assessment, 2005, www.acha.org.

Change Your Responses Changing your responses requires practice and emotional control. If your roommate is habitually messy and this causes you stress, you can choose among several responses. You can express your anger by yelling, you can pick up the mess and leave a nasty note, or you can defuse the situation with humor. The first reaction that comes to mind is not always the best. Stop before reacting to gain the time you need to find an appropriate response. Ask yourself, "What is to be gained from my response?"

Many people change their responses to potentially stressful events through cognitive coping strategies. These strategies help them prepare for stressors through gradual exposure to increasingly higher stress levels. The assumption is that by dealing with smaller stressors a person gathers resistance so that larger stressors do not seem so overwhelming.

Learn to Cope Everyone copes with stress in different ways. Some people drink or take drugs, others seek help from counselors, and still others try to forget about it or engage in positive activities such as exercise. **Stress inoculation** is a coping technique that helps people prepare for stressful events ahead of time. For example, suppose speaking in front of a class petrifies you. Practicing in front of friends or in front of a video camera are strategies that may inoculate you

stress inoculation Newer stress management technique in which a person consciously tries to prepare ahead of time for potential stressors.

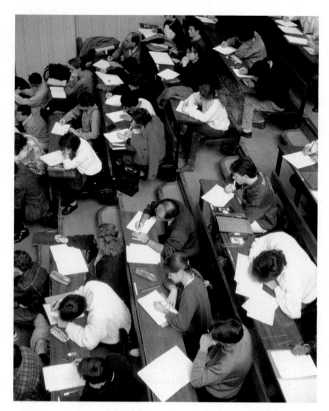

College can be a stressful time for students, whether they are young people choosing a career path or older adults returning to school to change directions later in life.

and prevent freezing up on the day of the presentation. Some health experts compare stress inoculation with a vaccine given to protect against a disease. Regardless of how you cope with a situation, your conscious effort to deal with it is an important step in stress management.

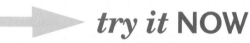

try it NOW

Think Triple A! Feeling overwhelmed? Experiencing overload? If the answer is yes, try the three A's of coping: Avoid, Alter, and Abolish.[54] If your school workload is causing distress, you may choose to *avoid* taking more than 15 credits, *alter* your schedule so that you attend classes in the morning when you are most alert, or *abolish* a few of your social events to devote more time to studying.

Consider Downshifting More and more people recognize that today's lifestyle is hectic and pressure-packed, and stress often comes from trying to keep up. Many people are questioning whether "having it all" is worth it, and they are taking a step back and simplifying their lives. This trend

---

downshifting Conscious attempt to simplify life in an effort to reduce the stresses and strains of modern living.

is known as **downshifting**. Moving from a large urban area to a smaller town, exchanging the expensive SUV for a modest sedan, and a host of other changes in lifestyle typify this move. Some dedicated downshifters have even given up television, phones, and computers.

Downshifting involves a fundamental shift in values and honest introspection about what is important in life. When considering any form of downshifting or perhaps even starting your career this way, it's important to move slowly and consider the following:

- *Determine your ultimate goal.* What is most important to you, and what will you need to reach that goal? What can you do without? Where do you want to live?
- *Make both short-term and long-term plans for simplifying your life.* Set up your plans in doable steps, and work slowly toward each step. Begin saying no to requests for your time, and determine those people with whom it is important for you to spend time.
- *Complete a financial inventory.* How much money will you need to do the things you want to do? Will you live alone or share costs with roommates? Do you need a car, or can you rely on public transportation? Pay off credit cards and eliminate current debt or consider debt consolidation. Get used to paying with cash. If you don't have the cash, don't buy. Remember, your lifestyle as a student will be different than living at home.
- *Plan for health care costs.* Make sure that you budget for health insurance and basic preventive health services if you're not covered under your parents' plan. This should be a top priority. Be sure you understand your coverage so you're not caught off guard.
- *Select the right career.* Look for work that you enjoy and that isn't necessarily driven by salary. Can you be happy in a lower-paying job that is less stressful and allows you the opportunity to have a life?
- *Consider options for saving money.* Downshifting doesn't mean you renounce money; it means you choose not to let money dictate your life. It's still important to save. If you're just getting started, you need to prepare for emergencies and for future plans.

Managing Social Interactions

As you plan a stress management program, don't underestimate the importance of social networks and social bonds. Consider the nature and extent of your friendships. Do you have someone with whom you can share intimate thoughts and feelings? Do you trust your friends to be supportive? Will your friends be honest with you if you are doing something risky or inappropriate? Friendships are an important aspect of inoculating yourself against harmful stressors. Studies have demonstrated the importance of social support in buffering individuals from the effects of stress.[55] It isn't necessary to have a large number of friends; however, different friends often serve different needs, so having more than one is usually beneficial. Particularly for those who lack close ties with family, friends often serve as a family away from home. As you work to develop and cultivate friendships, look for individuals who:

- Have values and interests that are similar to your own (as well as those with different interests who encourage you to grow and explore new ideas)
- Are good listeners, tolerant, give and share freely, and do not rush to judgment
- Are trustworthy and have your best interests at heart
- Are not unusually critical, negative, selfish, or bring you down. Avoid people who enjoy stirring things up and always seem to be in some crisis themselves. Such friends often precipitate, rather than reduce, stress responses.
- Are responsible, and value doing well in school, but also know when and how to have fun
- Are willing to be exercise and diet buddies or study partners and share an interest in a healthy lifestyle
- Know how to laugh, cry, engage in meaningful conversation, and listen to the silence

Just as it is important to find these characteristics in your friends, it is also important for you to bring these qualities to your friendships. Focusing on others may help you get your own problems into better focus and control.

Make the Most of Support Groups Support groups are an important part of stress management. Friends, family members, and coworkers can provide informational, emotional, and physical support.

If you do not have a close support group, find out where to turn when the pressures of life seem overwhelming. If friends or family are unavailable or unsupportive, most colleges and universities offer counseling services at no cost for short-term crises. Clergy, instructors, and dorm supervisors may also be excellent resources. If university services are unavailable or you are concerned about confidentiality, most communities offer low-cost counseling through mental health clinics.

Taking Mental Action

Stress management calls for mental action in two areas. First, positive self-esteem, which can help you cope with stressful situations, comes from learned habits and responses to people and events. Successful stress management involves mentally developing and practicing self-esteem skills, thinking positively about yourself, and examining self-talk to reduce irrational responses. Focus on the here and now rather than on past problems.

Second, because you can't always anticipate what the next stressor will be, develop the mental skills necessary to manage your reactions after it occurs. The ability to react productively and appropriately comes with time, practice, patience, and experience with a variety of stressful situations.

Change the Way You Think As noted earlier, our appraisals, thoughts, and ideas of people and situations are what make these things stressful, not the people or situations themselves. To combat negative self-talk we must first

become aware of it, then stop it, and finally replace the negative thoughts with positive ones—a process referred to as **cognitive restructuring**. Several types of negative self-talk exist but among the most common are pessimism, or focusing on the negative; perfectionism, or expecting super-human standards; "should-ing," or reprimanding yourself for items that you should have done; blaming, or condemning yourself or others for circumstances and events; and dichotomous thinking, in which everything is either black or white (good or bad) instead of in gradations.[56] Once you realize that some of your thoughts may be irrational or overreactive, interrupt this self-talk by saying "Stop" (under your breath or out loud) and make a conscious effort to adjust your thinking. Focus on more positive patterns. If we can learn to view potential stressors more positively we can reduce our stress levels without having to remove the stressors. Here are other actions you can take to develop these mental skills:

- *Reframe a distressing event from a positive perspective.* Reframing is a stress management technique that assists you to reconstruct or draft a "reframed" perspective on a situation from a positive vantage point.
- *Worry constructively.* Don't waste time and energy worrying about things you can't change or events that may never happen.
- *Look at life as being fluid.* If you accept that change is a natural part of living and growing, the jolt of changes will become less stressful.
- *Consider alternatives.* Remember, there is seldom only one appropriate action. Anticipating options will help you plan for change and adjust more rapidly.
- *Moderate your expectations.* Aim high, but be realistic about your circumstances and motivation.
- *Weed out trivia.* Cardiologist Robert Eliot offers two rules for coping with life's challenges: "Don't sweat the small stuff," and remember that "it's all small stuff."
- *Don't rush into action.* Think before you act.
- *Tolerate mistakes by yourself and others.* Rather than getting angry or frustrated by mishaps, evaluate what happened and learn from them.
- *Live simply.* Eliminate unnecessary things and obligations. Prioritize. Commitments should be to things you have to and want to do.

Once you have improved your mental outlook and gained a more positive perspective on life, you will find it easier to cope with stress.

Managing Emotional Responses

Have you ever gotten all worked up about something only to find that your perceptions were totally wrong? We often get

---

cognitive restructuring The modification of thoughts, ideas, and beliefs that contribute to stress.

POST-TRAUMATIC STRESS: DEALING WITH THE AFTERMATH

For many college students, war and other national threats were something studied in history classes—until the events of September 11, 2001, bombs on the London and Madrid underground systems, and the war in Iraq. For most, these were our first brushes with threats to a secure world, and reactions such as fear, anxiety, anger, and depression were not uncommon. These reactions were exacerbated in situations where individuals suffered personal losses or were separated from their loved ones due to impending threats. Even among college students with low exposure to the 9/11 attacks, terrorism-related stress was associated with greater depressive and illness symptoms. Significant trauma exposure has been documented in young, non-clinical samples with prevalence rates varying between 50 and 70 percent. According to the American Psychiatric Association, one-third to one-half of individuals exposed to a traumatic life event will go on to develop some form of psychopathology.

Each person, whether directly or indirectly affected by traumatic events, reacts differently. This range of responses is normal. Emotional responses can appear immediately or sometimes develop months later. According to the National Mental Health Association, common responses to trauma and disaster and their consequences include:

- Disbelief and shock
- Fear and anxiety about the future
- Disorientation, difficulty making decisions or concentrating
- Inability to focus on schoolwork and extracurricular activities
- Irritability and anger
- Extreme mood swings
- Feelings of powerlessness
- Changes in eating patterns; loss of appetite
- Crying for no apparent reason
- Headaches and stomach problems
- Difficulty sleeping
- Excessive use of drugs or alcohol

POST-TRAUMATIC STRESS DISORDER

In severe cases, an individual's response may be considered **post-traumatic stress disorder (PTSD)**. PTSD generally develops within the first hours or days after a traumatic event, but occasionally symptoms do not begin until months or years later. Typically, persons suffering from PTSD were soldiers returning from war, particularly those who saw friends killed or mangled or who experienced terrible pain themselves. Many of these soldiers continued to suffer from these experiences for decades afterward. Other extreme traumatic events include rape or other severe physical attacks, near-death experiences in accidents, witnessing a murder or death,

being caught in a natural disaster, or falling victim to terrorism such as the September 11 attack.

The development of PTSD is based on the hyperresponsive action of the "fight-or-flight" response, symptoms of which include:

- Dissociation, or perceived detachment of the mind from the emotional state or even the body. The person may have a sense of the world as a dreamlike or unreal place and have little memory of the events—a form of dissociative amnesia.
- Acute anxiety or nervousness, in which the person is hyperaroused; may cry easily or experience mood swings; and experience flashbacks, nightmares, and recurrent thoughts or visual images. Some people may sense vague uneasiness or feel like the event is happening again and again. Others may experience intense physiological reactions, such as shaking or nausea when something reminds them of the event. In some cases, they may have difficulty returning to areas that remind them of the trauma. For example, an individual who has been assaulted in a parking garage may have difficulty entering a garage again, be extremely fearful when walking in dark places when no one is around, or suffer from recurring nightmares.

---

upset not by reality, but by our faulty perceptions. For example, suppose you found out that everyone except you is invited to a party. You might easily begin to wonder why you were excluded. Does someone dislike you? Have you offended someone? Such thoughts are typical. However, the reality of the situation may have absolutely nothing to do with your being liked or disliked. Perhaps you were sent an invitation and it didn't reach you.

post-traumatic stress disorder (PTSD) An acute stress disorder caused by experiencing an extremely traumatic event, such as rape or combat.

In Chapter 1 the concept of self-talk was introduced. Stress management requires that you examine your self-talk and your emotional responses to interactions with others. With any emotional response to a distressor, you are responsible for the emotion and the behaviors elicited by the emotion. Learning to tell the difference between normal emotions and those based on irrational beliefs can help you either stop the emotion or express it in a healthy and appropriate way.

Learning to Laugh and Cry Have you noticed that you feel better after a good laugh or cry? It isn't your imagination. Laughter and crying stimulate the heart and temporarily rev up many body systems. Heart rate and blood pressure

PERSISTENT STRESS SYMPTOMS

Sufferers may have two or more of these symptoms:

- Difficulty falling or staying asleep
- Irritability or outbursts of anger or other emotions
- Difficulty concentrating
- Hypervigilance
- Exaggerated startle response

If these symptoms last more than one month, PTSD may be diagnosed, either as acute (less than three months' duration) or chronic (longer than three months). A delayed-onset form of PTSD may appear months after the event. In most people, symptoms disappear within six months.

TIPS FOR COPING

The National Institutes of Health indicates that as many as 5 to 8 percent of the American public may have chronic PTSD, with women having almost twice the prevalence of men. It is important to acknowledge the trauma and to address its effects. Ways to recover include:

- Talk about it and encourage others to share their perspectives.
- Take care of yourself. Get plenty of rest and exercise. Do things you find relaxing and soothing. Limit your exposure to media reports and images of the tragedy. As soon as possible, get back to normal routines.

- Stay connected to friends and family. Visit family or others who can offer reassurance and stability. If you can't travel or are nervous about it, use phone or e-mail contact.
- Do something positive that will help you gain a greater sense of control, such as giving blood, taking a first aid class, or donating food or clothing. Get involved with campus activities planned in response to a disaster, such as candlelight vigils, benefits, or discussion groups and speakers.
- Ask for help if you are feeling overwhelmed or out of control. It's not a sign of weakness. Talk with a trusted friend or faith leader. Use on-campus resources such as the counseling center or student health center. If you don't know where to go, talk with your health professor about options.
- Positive self-esteem, good problem-solving and communication skills, an internal locus of control, and a history of adaptive coping have been identified as protective factors against PTSD.

Therapies designed to help trauma victims recover are increasingly effective as our knowledge about this disorder grows. Schools, communities, and workplaces now routinely bring in crisis experts immediately after an event to help survivors talk

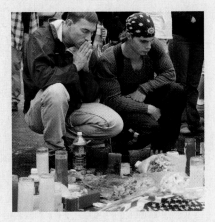

through their feelings and gain support from others. A supportive family, employer, and friends, and access to professional counseling, are important in the recovery process. New generations of antianxiety drugs can help individuals who have difficulties. Sleep aids and other options are available to ease short-term symptoms.

Sources: Posttraumatic Stress Disorder Society, "Posttraumatic Stress Disorder," 2003, www.mentalhealth.com/dis/p20-an06.html; National Center for Post Traumatic Stress, 2004, www.ncptsd.org; National Mental Health Association, "Coping with Disaster," 2001, www.nmha.org/reassurance/collegetips.cfm; Posttraumatic Stress Disorder Society, www.mentalhealth.com/dis/p20-an06.html; "Mental Health: A Report of the Surgeon General," www.surgeongeneral.gov/library/mentalhealth/.

---

then decrease significantly, allowing the body to relax. The positive psychological and physiological responses of laughter and crying have been demonstrated in a variety of settings, and outcomes include stress hormone reduction, improved mood, enhanced creativity, pain reduction, and improved immunity.[57]

Hostility: The Lethal Reaction
Earlier in this chapter we discussed personality type as a source of self-imposed stress. One characteristic in particular can have severe effects on cardiovascular health: the tendency toward hostility. Hostility has three components: (1) *cognitive*—negative beliefs about and attitudes toward others, including

cynicism and mistrust; (2) *affective*—anger, which can range from irritation to rage and be assessed with regard to frequency, intensity, and target; and (3) *behavioral*—actions intended to harm others, either verbally or physically, usually in an aggressive way. A wide range of studies has identified hostility as an independent risk factor for coronary heart disease (CHD), hypertension, and premature mortality. Hostility is thought to harm individuals by influencing health behaviors that themselves confer risk, such as smoking or fast driving, or by being associated with sociodemographic characteristics and physiological states that in turn increase the risk of heart disease.[58] White males and people with low socioeconomic status appear to be at highest risk for hostility, along with

TABLE 3.4	Strategies for Anger Control

1. **Calm yourself.** There are many relaxation techniques. Find one that works for you and bring yourself back to a level feeling.

2. **Change your thoughts about the situation.** When angry, many people act out in verbally abusive or other dramatic ways. Instead of screeching and yelling, tell yourself that you are justified in being angry and that you have a right to be upset, but don't act overtly. Remember that the "get it all out of your system" impulse is really not productive. It only makes you feel good for a bit, and then you realize that you have hurt others and said much more than you should have—and in the end, nothing is changed. Avoid thoughts or statements such as "never" or "always." Stay in the present.

3. **Improve your communication with the person who has made you angry or frustrated.** Talk with them when you are calm. Be direct and assertive. Let them know how you feel without being aggressive or attacking them. Social psychologist Carol Tavris, in her book *Anger: The Misunderstood Emotion,* says that anger should be expressed directly at the person or object that is perceived to have violated personal space, values, or identity, not randomly. If you can't express it immediately, try writing down your feelings and thoughts in a journal and describe what you'd like to see changed. Be clear when you talk with the person and try to keep your comments to "I"
rather than "you" statements (e.g., "I feel like I have been insulted in some way," rather than "You insulted me").

4. **Don't fight back.** It is natural to get upset if you feel attacked or criticized. Instead of reacting with anger, listen to what the person is saying, ask clarifying questions, and keep your cool. When the person has finished talking, acknowledge that you have heard and then express your own feelings.

5. **Use humor if possible.** Sometimes, the sheer volatility of a situation requires a bit of defusing, similar to the comic relief that accompanies a long dramatic passage in a movie or play. Try to defuse the situation if possible, and don't allow it to escalate. However, this doesn't mean sitting there with a smirk on your face or laughing at the other person or being sarcastic. Try to get the other person to laugh with you.

6. **Recognize that certain situations may cause little things to blow out of proportion.** Drinking, not enough sleep, responses to loss, and other situations may make people short fused. Avoid conflict when you are tired or too drained to respond appropriately, and respect these needs in others.

7. **Seek help.** If you feel about yourself or have others telling you that you are a chronically hostile or angry person, seek help. Your school has counselors who are able to help you. Talk with them or someone else you trust.

Source: C. Tavris, *Anger: The Misunderstood Emotion* (Carmichael, CA: Touchstone Books, 1989).

people who are overweight or obese, smokers, and people with excessive alcohol consumption, sedentary lifestyle, hypertension, or high total cholesterol.

Fighting the Anger Urge

Anger usually results when we feel we have lost control of a situation and/or are frustrated by a situation that we can do little about. The five main sources of anger are related to threats to (1) safety and well-being; (2) power; (3) perfectionism and pride; (4) self-sufficiency and autonomy; and (5) self-esteem and status.[59]

> **What actions can I take to deal with anger in a healthy way?**

Anger may vary in intensity from mild irritation to rage and may be expressed as cynicism, sarcasm, intimidation, frustration, impatience, quick flaring of temper, distrust, or anxiety. Not all anger is bad. Sometimes it can give us the energy we need to fight back if attacked or the resolve to work even harder to accomplish a goal. It is unresolved anger, the kind that festers and clouds our reasoning and our reactions, that we need to control.

Each of us has learned by this point in our lives that we have three main approaches to dealing with anger: expressing it, suppressing it, or calming it. You may be surprised to find out that *expressing* your anger is probably the healthiest thing to do in the long run, particularly if you express anger in an assertive, rather than aggressive, way. However, it's a natural reaction to want to respond aggressively and that is what we must learn to keep at bay. To accomplish this, there are several things you can do (see also Table 3.4):[60]

- Understand what anger is and how you tend to express it
- Develop an awareness and acceptance of your own tendency to anger
- Recognize your anger patterns: When do you get angry and how often? Who makes you angry?
- Learn and practice good communication
- Respect others and yourself

Taking Physical Action

Physical activities can complement the emotional and mental strategies of stress management.

Exercise All kinds of physical activity—walking, biking, bowling, and so on—are effective in reducing the stress response and also tend to improve our mood and self-esteem. This is because physical activity raises levels of endorphins—mood-elevating, painkilling hormones—in the bloodstream. So the next time you're feeling stressed, get moving, do something active, and subsequently you will feel much more relaxed!

Most of us have relieved stress by engaging in aggressive physical activity: for example, kicking a piece of furniture when we are angry. Exercise performed as an immediate response can help alleviate stress symptoms in a positive way. A regular exercise program yields substantial benefits. Try to engage in at least 25 minutes of aerobic exercise three or four times a week. Although it may not improve your aerobic capacity, even a quiet walk alone or with friends can refresh

Activity	Monday	Tuesday	Wednesday	Thursday	Friday	Saturday	Sunday	Total Hours
Getting ready								
On the road								
In class								
Working for pay								
Exercising								
Eating (meals & snacks)								
Studying								
Watching TV, videos								
Using computer (school-related)								
Using computer (recreational)								
Spending time with friends								
Leisure activities								
Other (specify)								
Total Hours								

FIGURE 3.4 How Do You Spend Your Time?

Fill in your daily activities for a week and assess how you spend your time. Are there any activities you can stop doing or that you would like to do more frequently?

your mind and calm your stress response. A short period of physical exercise may provide the break you really need. For more information on the beneficial effects of exercise, see Chapter 10.

Relax Like exercise, relaxation can help you cope with stressful feelings, preserve adaptation energy stores, dissipate excess hormones associated with the fight-or-flight response, and refocus your energies. Practice relaxation daily until it becomes a habit. You will probably find that you enjoy it.

Once you have learned simple relaxation techniques, you can use them at any time—during a difficult exam or stressful confrontation, for example. As your body relaxes, your heart rate slows, your blood pressure and metabolic rate decrease, and many other body-calming effects occur, all of which allow you to channel energy appropriately. See the Skills for Behavior Change box for more on relaxation techniques.

Eat Right Is food really a de-stressor? Whether foods can calm us and nourish our psyches is a controversial question. High-potency supplements that are supposed to boost resistance against stress-related ailments are nothing more than gimmicks. However, it is clear that eating a balanced, healthful diet will help provide the stamina you need to get through

problems and will stress-proof you in ways that are not fully understood. It is also known that poor eating habits may cause distress. In particular, avoid **sympathomimetics**, food substances that produce (or mimic) stresslike responses. The most common sympathomimetic is caffeine, commonly found in colas, coffee, tea, and chocolate. At high doses caffeine produces dose-related increases in anxiety, and excessive chronic caffeine consumption mimics generalized anxiety disorder.[61] For more information about the benefits of sound nutrition, see Chapter 8.

Managing Your Time

How can I prioritize everything I try to do in a day?

Time. Everybody needs more of it, especially students trying to balance the demands of classes, social life, earning money for school, and family obligations. Keep a journal for one week to become aware of your time patterns (Figure 3.4)

sympathomimetics Food substances that can produce stresslike responses.

SKILLS FOR behavior change

RELAXATION TECHNIQUES FOR STRESS MANAGEMENT

Relaxation techniques for stress reduction have been practiced for centuries, and there is a wide selection from which to choose. Take your time, experiment, and find the one that works best for you. In addition to those discussed in the chapter, four to consider are yoga, qigong, deep breathing, and progressive muscle relaxation.

YOGA

An estimated 20 million adults in America actively engage in yoga, an ancient tradition that combines meditation, stretching, and breathing exercises designed to relax, refresh, and rejuvenate. There are several popular versions.

Classical yoga is the ancestor of nearly all forms of yoga practiced today. Breathing, poses, and verbal mantras are often part of classical yoga.

Kripalu is a gentle, introspective practice in which much emphasis is placed on breathing techniques and releasing emotional blockages. Initially practitioners concentrate mainly on poses and deep breathing followed by emotional exercises.

In later stages, practitioners focus primarily on poses. Kripalu is particularly suited for those who want to go slowly and gently, or who have underlying injuries or problems.

Popularized by Madonna, *ashtanga yoga* is designed to improve sport performance with deep breathing and a progressive series of postures. Less well known than other forms, this type of yoga is growing in popularity.

Hot yoga, also known as *bikram yoga,* differs from traditional yoga in that classes are held in rooms where the temperatures are up to 105 degrees. After going through up to 26 poses, students emerge from these classes drained of energy, drenched in sweat, and feeling cleansed. Although bikram centers have sprung up across the country, there have been reports of heat exhaustion, dehydration, and other problems. This style of yoga is risky for those with hypertension, certain respiratory conditions, and other cardiovascular risks. If you feel weak, dizzy, nauseated, or have other ill effects, use caution. Before attending a class, speak with your doctor if you have questions or concerns, and make sure you go to a reputable facility with qualified staff.

QIGONG

Qigong (pronounced chee-kong) is one of the fastest-growing and most widely accepted forms of mind–body health exercises. Even some of the country's largest health care organizations, such as Kaiser Permanente, have incorporated this relaxation technique into their systems, particularly for those suffering from chronic pain or stress. Like acupuncture, qigong taps into a complex system of internal pathways called meridians, which are thought to run along the length of the body. According to Chinese medicine, meridians carry chi, or vital energy, throughout your body. If your chi becomes stagnant or blocked, you'll feel sluggish or powerless. Thus, a series of flowing movements, mental visualization exercises, and vocalizations of healing sounds such as "shhhuuu" are designed to integrate and refresh through easy-to-perform techniques.

DIAPHRAGMATIC OR DEEP BREATHING

Typically, we breathe using only the upper chest and thoracic region rather than involving the abdominal region. Simply

and use the following time management tips in your stress management program.

- *Take on only one thing at a time.* Don't try to pay bills, wash clothes, and write your term paper all at once. Stay focused.
- *Clean off your desk.* Go through the things on your desk, toss the unnecessary papers, and put into folders the papers for tasks that you must do. Read your mail, then file it or toss it.
- *Find a clean, comfortable place to work.* Go somewhere where you won't be distracted.
- *Prioritize your tasks.* Make a daily "to do" list and try to stick to it. Categorize the things you must do today, the things that you have to do but not immediately, and the things that it would be nice to do. Only consider the Nice to Do items if you finish the others or if the Nice to Do list includes something fun. Give yourself a reward as you finish each task.

- *Don't be afraid to say no.* All too often we do things out of fear of what someone may think about us. Set your school and personal priorities and live according to your own agenda, values, and goals.
- *Avoid interruptions.* When you have a project that requires total concentration, schedule uninterrupted time. Unplug the phone or let your answering machine get it. Close your door and post a *Do Not Disturb* sign. Go to a quiet room in the library or student union where no one will find you.
- *Reward yourself for being efficient.* Did you finish a task early? Take some time for yourself. See a movie or go for a walk. Differentiate between rest breaks and work breaks. Work breaks simply mean switching tasks for awhile. Rest breaks give you time to recharge and refresh your energy levels.
- *Use time to your advantage.* If you're a morning person, schedule activities to coincide with the time when you're at your best. Study and write papers in the morning, and

stated, diaphragmatic breathing is deep breathing that maximally expands the chest by involving the movement of the lower abdomen. This technique is commonly used in yoga exercises. The diaphragmatic breathing process occurs in three stages.

- Stage 1: Assume a comfortable position. Whether sitting or lying down on your back, find the most natural position to be in. Loosen or unfasten any tight or restrictive clothing (shirt, belt, pants) and close your eyes. Often it works best to fold your hands over your abdomen and get used to feeling the rise and fall of your stomach.
- Stage 2: Concentrate on the act of breathing. Shut out external noise. Focus on inhaling, exhaling, and the route the air is following. Try saying to yourself, "Feel the warm air coming into your nose, warming your windpipe, and flowing into your lungs. Feel your stomach rise and fall as you inhale slowly and exhale slowly, noting the air flowing out of your nose or mouth." Repeat this action several times.

- Stage 3: Visualize. The above stages seem to work best when combined with visualization. A common example is to visualize clean, fresh, invigorating air slowly entering the nose and being exhaled as gray, stale air that has accumulated in the body. Such processes, particularly when they involve the whole body, seem to help deep breathers become more refreshed from their experience.

PROGRESSIVE MUSCLE RELAXATION

Progressive muscle relaxation involves systematically contracting and relaxing each of several muscle groups; proper breathing and concentration are part of this process. Again, find a comfortable position similar to that discussed in the deep breathing section above, and begin a deep breathing cycle. The difference from diaphragmatic breathing is that, as you concentrate on inhaling, you also contract a particular muscle group (for example, the hand and fingers). Hold that position for a short period and then, as you exhale, slowly release the muscles that you have been contracting. Repeat and add

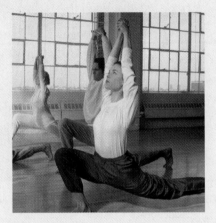

more muscle groups. You might start with a hand, then move to the forearm, the entire arm, the neck, to the shoulders, back, buttocks, thigh, and foot. You can add components of other relaxation techniques to this experience by saying, "My hands are getting warmer, my arm is getting warmer," and so on as you work to gain maximum control of blood flow and muscle tension in a region.

Source: Paragraph on qigong from C. Dold, "The New Yoga," *Health,* May 2004, 73–77.

take breaks when you start to slow down. Take a short nap when you need it.
- *Break overwhelming tasks into small pieces, and allocate a certain amount of time to each.* If you are floundering in a task, move on and come back to it when you're refreshed.
- *Remember that time is precious.* Many people learn to value their time only when they face a terminal illness. Try to value each day. Time spent not enjoying life is a tremendous waste of potential.

Managing Your Finances

Entering higher education in the twenty-first century involves a considerable financial burden for a growing number of students. Many students are working increasingly long hours to pay their way through school and others are incurring large consumer debt—both of which are related to decreased academic performance and psychological well-being.[62] The

pressure to succeed in college needs to be understood in the context of students' financial circumstances and the related implications for their health. Follow these tips for managing your money and reducing finance-related stress:

- *Develop a realistic budget.* What are your monthly expenses? What types of "luxuries" do you regularly splurge on?
- *When bills come in, take care of them immediately.* Write a check and hold it for mailing, or send it right away so you don't forget and then have to pay late fees.
- *Consider electronic banking.* This can make the process of paying bills faster and easier.
- *Become knowledgeable about how to manage your money.* Take advantage of campus workshops on financial aid, money management, and part-time jobs.
- *Avoid those tempting credit cards.* If you get tons of offers in the mail, just toss them. You need only one credit card, maybe two at most.

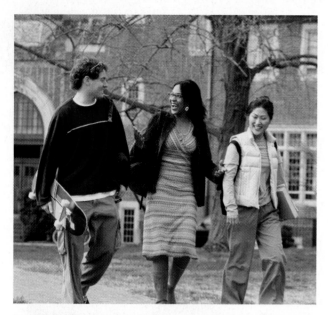

Communicating and socializing with friends is an important part of stress reduction.

■ *Don't get into debt.* If you don't have the money for an item now, don't buy it on credit and expect to pay for it later. If there is a pricey item you want, or a trip you want to take, create a savings plan.

Alternative Stress Management Techniques

Popular stress fighters include visualization, hypnosis, massage therapy, meditation, and biofeedback.

Visualization Often it is our own thoughts and imagination that provoke distress by conjuring up worst-case scenarios and exaggerating the significance of situations. Our imagination, however, can be an asset as well as a liability. **Visualization**, or the creation of mental scenes, works by engaging one's imagination of the physical senses of sight, sound, smell, taste, and feel to replace stressful stimuli with peaceful or pleasurable thoughts. The choice of mental images is unlimited but natural settings such as ocean beaches and mountain lakes are often used because they simulate

visualization The creation of mental images to promote relaxation.

hypnosis A process that allows people to become unusually responsive to suggestion.

meditation A relaxation technique that involves deep breathing and concentration.

biofeedback A technique involving using a machine to self-monitor physical responses to stress.

mindfulness The ability to be fully present in the moment.

vacation locations where people typically go to escape the stress of home, school, or work environments.[63] So the next time you feel stressed, close your eyes, imagine yourself at some tranquil location full of color, fresh air, soothing sounds, and other elements of nature, and take a mini mental vacation to allow your mind and body a chance to unwind.

Hypnosis **Hypnosis** is a process that requires a person to focus on one thought, object, or voice, thereby freeing the right hemisphere of the brain to become more active. The person then becomes unusually responsive to suggestion. Whether self-induced or induced by someone else, hypnosis can reduce certain types of stress.

Massage Therapy If you have ever had someone massage your stiff neck or aching feet, you know that massage is an excellent way to relax. Massage techniques vary from vigorous Swedish massage to the gentler acupressure and Esalen massage. Before selecting a massage therapist, check his or her credentials carefully. The therapist should have training from a reputable program that teaches scientific principles for anatomic manipulation and be certified through the American Massage Therapy Association (AMTA). Chapter 23 provides more information about the benefits of massage as well as other body-based methods such as acupressure and shiatsu.

Meditation There are many different forms of **meditation**. Most involve sitting quietly for 15 to 20 minutes, focusing on a particular word or symbol, controlling breathing, and getting in touch with the inner self. Practiced by Eastern religions for centuries, meditation is believed to be an important form of introspection and personal renewal. As a stress management tool, it can calm the body and quiet the mind, creating a sense of peace.

Biofeedback **Biofeedback** involves self-monitoring by machine of physical responses to stress and attempts to control these responses. The machine records perspiration, heart rate, respiration, blood pressure, surface body temperature, muscle tension, and other stress responses. Various relaxation techniques are employed while the person is hooked up to a biofeedback machine and, through trial and error and signals from the machine, the person learns to lower his or her stress response. Eventually, the person develops the ability to recognize and lower stress responses without using the machine.

Developing Your Spiritual Side: Mindfulness

A final piece of the stress puzzle is the role of spirituality in managing stress. As a meditative technique, **mindfulness**— the ability to be fully present in the moment—can aid relaxation, reduce emotional and physical pain, and help us connect more effectively with ourselves, with others, and with nature.[64] The practice of mindfulness focuses on the cultivation of awareness, openness, and a nonjudgmental attitude that includes strategies and activities that contribute to overall health and wellness. In fact, mindfulness and wellness are interconnected and can be developed concurrently, reinforcing each other. In addition to the themes of spirituality discussed in Chapter 2, we can think of spirituality as encompassing four dimensions: physical, emotional, social, and intellectual.

The Physical Dimension: Moving in Nature

A delightful way to strengthen the body, build endurance, and bring peace of mind is to interact with the natural environment. Activities such as walking, jogging, biking, and swimming foster this interaction, providing sensory experience (feeling, smelling, touching, seeing, and hearing) while strengthening muscles and the cardiovascular system. By focusing on the sounds of birdsong or the crunch of your shoes on freshly fallen snow, you can free yourself of worry or anxious thoughts. Appreciating and absorbing the beauty of nature allow us to unwind emotionally even as our bodies are at work.

The Emotional Dimension: Dealing with Negative Emotions

Each of us has positive and negative emotions that govern moods and behaviors throughout the day. We often take joy, happiness, and contentment for granted because we tend not to notice the *absence* of stress and distress. However, we typically are aware of negative emotions, such as jealousy, hatred, and anger because they deplete our energy reserves and cause us problems in interacting with others.

To improve our emotional health and access our spiritual side, we must take notice of the situations that trigger negative emotions, such as anger. (See "Fighting the Anger Urge" on page 96). By stopping in the midst of anger and concentrating on physical reactions, we begin to realize the full extent of the damage we inflict upon ourselves when we allow negativity to get the best of us. We might ask ourselves, "Is it worth it?"—and probably we will conclude: "I don't like allowing this kind of hit on my body. I've got to get a handle on this before I hurt myself or someone else." By practicing thought-stopping, blocking negative thoughts, and focusing on positive emotions via self-talk and other methods of diversion, we can help ourselves through a negative experience.

As important as the control of negative emotions is the development of spiritual wholeness characterized by faith, hope, and love, the beliefs mentioned in Chapter 2. These beliefs contribute to spiritual growth and lessen the negative effects of stress.

The Social Dimension: Interacting, Listening, and Communicating

Developing the spiritual side is not an individual internal process. It is also a social process that enhances relationships with others. The ability to give and take, speak and listen, and forgive and move on are all integral to spiritual development.

Today, life is busier than ever. While constantly juggling responsibilities, it is easy to get so caught up in the stresses of our own lives that we find it difficult to give to others. Here again, we need to stop and think about how being too self-enmeshed can affect relationships and the ability to communicate with others. Communication is a two-way process in which listening is every bit as important as speaking. The ability to *listen actively* is a potent asset. Active listeners take note of content, intent, and feelings being expressed. They listen to all levels of the communication. Sensitivity and honesty are also essential to the give and take of communication. Ask questions, rephrase the speaker's ideas, and focus genuine attention on the speaker. Through such active participation, we gain a greater insight into the other person, who in turn will be encouraged to share more. Sharing becomes more intimate and relationships more connected when people feel that others care for them and are genuinely interested in their well-being. Both parties benefit from such an interchange. For more on communication, see Chapter 5.

The Intellectual Dimension: Sharpening Intuition

Take the time to carefully assess events in life, their causes, and your own involvement in them. This often involves putting aside our emotional dimension for a moment to reflect, read, and ponder. Sometimes this process leads to startling new insights—"Ah-ha! Now I get it; this all makes sense!" Such moments mean so much, but few people include this mental activity in daily rituals. Examining the past, how we've gotten to where we are in the present, and what actions might have changed the course of events is a critical element of spiritual growth. By using our minds for objective reasoning, we develop the intellectual dimension of spiritual health.

TAKING charge

Summary

- Stress is an inevitable part of our lives. Eustress refers to stress associated with positive events, distress to negative events.

- The alarm, resistance, and exhaustion phases of the general adaptation syndrome (GAS) involve physiological responses to both real and imagined stressors and cause a complex cascade of hormones to rush through the body. Prolonged arousal may be detrimental to health.

- Undue stress for extended periods of time can compromise the immune system and result in serious health consequences. Psychoneuroimmunology is the science that analyzes the relationship between the mind's reaction to stress and the function of the immune system. Although increasing evidence links disease susceptibility to stress, much of this research remains controversial. However, stress has been linked to numerous health problems, including CVD, diabetes, cancer, and increased susceptibility to infectious diseases.

- Multiple factors contribute to stress and the stress response. Psychosocial factors include change, hassles, pressure, inconsistent goals and behaviors, conflict, overload, and

burnout. Other factors are environmental stressors and self-imposed stress. Persons subjected to discrimination or bias due to "-*isms*" may face unusually high levels of stress.

- College can be especially stressful. Recognizing the signs of stress is the first step toward better health. Learning to reduce test anxiety and cope with multiple stressors is also important.

- Managing stress begins with learning simple coping mechanisms: assessing stressors, changing responses, and learning to cope. Finding out what works best for you—probably some combination of managing emotional responses, taking mental or physical action, downshifting, learning time management, and using alternative stress management techniques—will help you cope with stress effectively.

- Developing the spiritual side involves practicing mindfulness and its many dimensions. These include the physical dimension (moving in nature); the emotional dimension (identifying and controlling negative feelings); the social dimension (interacting, listening, and communicating); and the intellectual dimension (sharpening intuition).

Chapter Review

1. An example of *eustress* is
   a. planning a wedding.
   b. having three exams in one day.
   c. breaking up with one's partner.
   d. a death in the family.

2. What is the "general adaptation syndrome"?
   a. the body's alarm to a stressor
   b. the body's mechanism to maintain homeostasis
   c. the stress that eventually causes the body to experience a state of exhaustion
   d. all of the above are true

3. Common effects of chronic stress on the human body include
   a. cold sores on the mouth.
   b. increased susceptibility to infections.
   c. elevated blood pressure ending in potential heart attack.
   d. all of the above are serious effects of chronic stress.

4. Which of the following test-taking techniques is not recommended to reduce test-taking stress?
   a. plan ahead and study over a period of time for the test
   b. take regular breaks to refresh the over-stimulated brain
   c. do all of the studying and preparation the night before the exam so it is fresh in your mind
   d. practice by testing yourself with other classmates' sample test questions

5. What are some techniques that can be used to reduce stress?
   a. deep breathing exercises
   b. refocusing to a positive image
   c. laughter
   d. all of the above

6. Which of the following is not an example of a time management technique?
   a. scheduling one's time with a calendar or day planner
   b. identifying time robbers
   c. practicing procrastination in completing homework assignments
   d. developing a game plan

7. Distress refers to the
   a. good stressors that occur in our life.
   b. negative effects of stress.
   c. finding creative solutions to our problems.
   d. building barriers to hide the stressors we don't want to deal with.

8. An example of a chronic stressor would be
   a. giving a talk in public.
   b. meeting a deadline for a big project.
   c. dealing with a permanent disability.
   d. death of a family member or close friend.

9. Which stage of the general adaptation syndrome (GAS) does the body mobilize its internal resources to maintain homeostasis?
   a. the exhaustion stage
   b. the alarm stage
   c. the resistance stage
   d. none of the above

10. In which stage does the 'fight-or-flight' response occur in the general adaptation syndrome?
   a. homeostasis
   b. alarm
   c. resistance
   d. exhaustion

Answers to these questions can be found on page A-1.

Questions for Discussion and Reflection

1. Compare and contrast distress and eustress. Are both types of stress potentially harmful?
2. Describe the alarm, resistance, and exhaustion phases of the general adaptation syndrome and the body's physiological response to stress. Does stress lead to more emotionality, or does emotionality lead to stress? Provide examples.
3. What are some of the health risks that result from chronic stress? How does the study of psychoneuroimmunology link stress and illness?
4. What major factors influence the nature and extent of a person's susceptibility to stress? Explain how social support, self-esteem, and personality can make a person more or less susceptible to stress.

5. Why are some students more susceptible to stress than others? What services are available on your campus to help you deal with excessive stress?
6. What can college students do to inoculate themselves against negative stress effects? What actions can you take to manage your stressors? How can you help others to manage their stressors more effectively?
7. How does anger affect the body? Discuss the steps you can take to fight your own anger urge and to help your friends control theirs.
8. What can you do to develop the dimensions of spirituality in your life? How can you apply the social dimension of spirituality to your current relationships?

Accessing Your Health on the Internet

The following websites explore further topics and issues related to personal health. You'll also find links to each organization's website on the Companion Website for *Access to Health,* Tenth Edition, at www.aw-bc.com/donatelle.

1. *American College Counseling Association.* The website of the professional organization for college counselors offers useful links and articles. www.collegecounseling.org
2. *American College Health Association.* This site provides information and data from the National College Health Assessment survey. www.acha.org

3. *Center for Anxiety and Stress Treatment.* Resources and services regarding a broad range of stress-related topics are offered. www.stressrelease.com
4. *Mind Tools.* This site focuses on all aspects of stress and stress management. www.psychwww.com/stsite/smpage.html
5. *National Institute of Mental Health.* This is a resource for information on all aspects of mental health, including the effects of stress. www.nimh.nih.gov

Further Reading

Greenberg, J. S. *Comprehensive Stress Management,* 9th ed. New York: McGraw-Hill, 2004.

  An overview of current perspectives on stress and the influence of personal control and behavior on health. Discusses stress management as a tool to control health problems.

Lovallo, W. R. *Stress and Health: Biological and Psychological Interactions,* 2nd ed. Thousand Oaks, CA: Sage, 2004.

  Latest scientific findings from psychology, neuroscience, and medicine on the relationship between stress and health.

Health and Stress: Newsletter of the American Institute of Stress. www.stress.org/news.htm.

  Monthly reports on developments in all areas of stress research. Each issue contains a listing of meetings of interest and a book review.

Romas, J. A. and M. Sharma. *Practical Stress Management,* 3rd ed. San Francisco: Benjamin Cummings, 2004.

  An accessible text that combines theory and principles with hands-on exercises to manage stress. Includes an audio CD with guided relaxation techniques.

Schindler, W. *Adults in College: A Survival Guide for Nontraditional Students.* Mt. Pleasant, TX: Dallas Publishing, 2002.

  Focuses on how older students cope with the stress of being an adult surrounded by recent high school graduates.

Seaward, B. *Managing Stress: Principles and Strategies for Health and Well-Being,* 4th ed. Sudbury, MA: Jones and Bartlett, 2004.

  A spirituality and stress expert provides a complete overview of stress and health effects, and strategies to reduce risk.

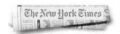

e-themes from *The New York Times*

For up-to-date articles about current health issues, visit
www.aw-bc.com/donatelle, select *Access to Health,* Tenth
Edition, Chapter 3, and click on "e-themes."

References

1. H. Anisman and Z. Merali, "Understanding Stress: Characteristics and Caveats," *Alcohol Research & Health* 23, no. 4 (1999): 241–249.
2. B. S McEwen, "Stress: Definitions and Concepts," in *Encyclopedia of Stress,* vol. 4, ed. G. Fink (London: Academic Press, 2000), 508–509.
3. W. B. Cannon, *The Wisdom of the Body* (New York: Norton, 1932).
4. H. Selye, *Stress Without Distress* (New York: Lippincott, 1974), 28–29.
5. B. S McEwen, "Mood Disorders and Allostatic Load," *Biological Psychiatry* 54 (2003): 200–207.
6. A. Mokdad et al., "Actual Causes of Death in the United States, 2000," *Journal of the American Medical Association* 291 (2004): 1238–1245.
7. S. C Segerstrom and G. E. Miller. "Psychological Stress and the Human Immune System: A Meta-Analytic Study of 30 Years of Inquiry," *Psychological Bulletin* 130, no. 4 (2004): 601–630.
8. S. Das and J. H. O'Keffe, "Behavioral Cardiology: Recognizing and Addressing the Profound Impact of Psychosocial Stress on Cardiovascular Health," *Current Atherosclerosis Reports* 8, no. 2 (2006): 111–118; A. K. Ferketich and P. F. Binkley, "Psychological Distress and Cardiovascular Disease: Results from the 2002 National Health Interview Study," *European Heart Journal* 26, no. 18 (2005): 1923–1929.
9. S. Yusef, S. Hawken et al., "Effect of Potentially Modifiable Risk Factors Associated with Myocardial Infarction in 52 Countries (The INTERHEART Study): Case-Control Study," *The Lancet* 364, no. 9438 (2004): 937–952.
10. A. K. Ferketich and P. F. Binkley, "Psychological Distress and Cardiovascular Disease," 1923–1929.
11. J. R. Hapuarachchi et al., "Changes in Clinically Relevant Metabolites with Psychological Stress Parameters," *Behavioral Medicine* 29 (2003): 52–60; C. N. Merz et al., "Psychosocial Stress and Cardiovascular Disease: Pathophysiological Links," *Behavioral Medicine* 27 (2002): 141–148; S. Das and J. H. O'Keffe, "Behavioral Cardiology," 111–118.
12. S. A. Everson-Rose and T. T. Lewis, "Psychosocial Risk Factors and Cardiovascular Disease," *Annual Review of Public Health* 26 (2005): 469–500.
13. S. C. Segerstrom and G. E. Miller, "Psychological Stress and the Human Immune System," 601–630.
14. M. E. Kemeny, "The Psychobiology of Stress," *Current Directions in Psychological Science* 12 (2003): 124–130; J. K. Kiecolt-Glaser et al., "Psychoneuroimmunology and Psychosomatic Medicine: Back to the Future," *Psychosomatic Medicine* 64 (2002): 15–28.
15. E. M. Reiche et al., "Stress, Depression, the Immune System, and Cancer," *The Lancet Oncology* 5, no. 10 (2004): 617–625; S. C. Segerstrom and G. E. Miller, "Psychological Stress and the Human Immune System," 601–630.
16. Ibid., Segerstrom and Miller.
17. S. Cohen, keynote presentation, Eighth International Congress of Behavioral Medicine: "The Pittsburgh Common Cold Studies: Psychosocial Predictors of Susceptibility to Respiratory Illness," *International Journal of Behavioral Medicine* 12, no. 3 (2005): 123–131; S. Cohen et al., "Reactivity and Vulnerability to Stress-Associated Risk for Upper Respiratory Illness," *Psychosomatic Medicine* 64 (2002): 302–310; B. Takkouche et al., "A Cohort Study of Stress and the Common Cold," *Epidemiology* 12, no. 3 (2001): 345–349.
18. S. D. Pressman et al., "Loneliness, Social Network Size, and Immune Responses to Influenza Vaccinations in College Freshmen," *Health Psychology* 24, no. 3 (2005): 297–306.
19. E. R. Volkman and N. Y. Weekes, "Basal SigA and Cortisol Levels Predict Stress-Related Health Outcomes," *Stress and Health* 22 (2006): 11–23.
20. E. V. Yang and R. Glaser, "Stress-Induced Immunomodulation and the Implications for Health," *International Immunopharmacology* 2 (2002): 315–324; R. Glaser, "Stress-Associated Immune Dysregulation and Its Importance for Human Health: A Personal History of Psychoneuroimmunology," *Brain, Behavior, and Immunity* 19 (2005): 3–11.
21. E. Shiloah and M. J. Rapoport, "Psychological Stress and New Onset Diabetes," *Pediatric Endocrinology Reviews* 3, no. 3 (2006): 272–275; American Diabetes Association, "Stress," 2004, www.diabetes.org/type-1-diabetes/stress.jsp.
22. R. Rosmond, "Role of Stress in the Pathogenesis of the Metabolic Syndrome," *Psychoneuroendocrinology* 30 (2005): 1–10.
23. M. Scollan-Koliopoulos, "Managing Stress Response to Control Hypertension in Type 2 Diabetes," *The Nurse Practitioner* 30, no. 2 (2005): 46–49.
24. D. A. Katerndahl and M. Parchman, "The Ability of the Stress Process Model to Explain Mental Health Outcomes," *Comprehensive Psychiatry* 43 (2002): 351–360; R. C. Kessler et al., "The Epidemiology of Major Depressive Disorder," *JAMA* 289 (2003): 3095–3105.
25. R. L. Turner and D. A. Lloyd, "Stress Burden and the Lifetime Incidence of Psychiatric Disorder in Young Adults: Racial and Ethnic Contrasts," *Archives of General Psychiatry* 61 (2004): 481–488.
26. V. R. Wilburn and D. E. Smith, "Stress, Self-Esteem, and Suicidal Ideation in Late Adolescence," *Adolescence* 40 (2005): 33–46. A. Väänänen et al., "Sources of Social Support as Determinants of Psychiatric Morbidity After Severe Life Events: Prospective Cohort Study of Female Employees," *Journal of Psychosomatic Research* 58 (2005): 459–467.
27. T. Holmes and R. Rahe, "The Social Readjustment Rating Scale," *Journal of Psychosocial Research* (1967): 213–217; B. P. Dohrenwend, "Inventorying Stressful Life Events as Risk Factors for Psychopathology: Toward Resolution of the Problem of Intracategory Variability," *Psychological Bulletin* 132, no. 3 (2006): 477–495.
28. R. Lazarus, "The Trivialization of Distress," in *Preventing Health Risk Behaviors and Promoting Coping with Illness,* ed. J. Rosen and L. Solomon (Hanover, NH: University Press of New England, 1985), 279–298.
29. D. J. Maybery and D. Graham, "Hassles and Uplifts: Including Interpersonal Events," *Stress and Health* 17 (2001): 91–104: R. Blonna, *Coping with Stress in a Changing World,* 3rd ed. (Boston: McGraw-Hill, 2005).
30. L. Lefton, *Psychology,* 9th ed. (Boston: Allyn & Bacon, 2005).
31. M. Kenny and K. Rice, "Attachment to Parents and Adjustment in College Students: Current Status, Applications, and Future Considerations," *Counseling Psychologist* 23 (1995): 433–456.
32. T. Bartlett, "Freshmen Pay Mentally and Physically as They Adjust to Life in College," *Chronicle of Higher Education,* February 1, 2002, 4.

33. C. L. Park, S. Armeli, and H. Tennen, "The Daily Stress and Coping Process and Alcohol Use Among College Students," *Journal of Studies on Alcohol* 65, no. 1 (2004): 126–130; B. E. Miller et al., "Alcohol Misuse Among College Athletes: Self-Medication for Psychiatric Symptoms?" *Journal of Drug Education* 32 (2002): 41–52.

34. J. M. Peiró et al., "Does Role Stress Predict Burnout Over Time Among Health Care Professionals?" *Psychology and Health* 16 (2001): 511–525; S. Melamed et al., "Burnout and Risk of Cardiovascular Disease: Evidence, Possible Causal Paths, and Promising Research Directions," *Psychological Bulletin* 132, no. 3 (2006): 327–353.

35. K. Nadal, "Ethnic Minority Students' Stressors: Their Impact on Campus Climate Perceptions and Academic Achievement," R. E. McNair Fellowship paper, http://members.tripod.com/~knall/minoritystress.html.

36. T. LaVeist, *Minority Populations and Health: An Introduction to Health Disparities* (San Francisco, CA: Jossey-Bass, 2006); T. Lewis, "Discrimination, Black Americans, and Health: Results of the SWAN Study," paper presented at the annual meeting of the American Heart Association, Washington, D.C., 2005.

37. K. Karren et al., *Mind/Body Health: The Effects of Attitudes, Emotions, and Relationships,* 3rd ed. (San Francisco: Benjamin Cummings, 2006); B. L. Seaward, *Managing Stress: Principles and Strategies for Health and Well-Being,* 4th ed. (Sudbury: Jones and Bartlett, 2004); V. R. Wilburn and D. E. Smith, "Stress, Self-Esteem, and Suicidal Ideation," 33–46.

38. M. C. Smith and M. C. Dust, "An Exploration of the Influence of Dispositional Traits and Appraisal on Coping Strategies in African American College Students," *Journal of Personality* 74, no. 1 (2006): 145–174.

39. V. R. Wilburn and D. E. Smith, "Stress, Self-Esteem, and Suicidal Ideation," 33–46; D. Robotham and C. Julian, "Stress and the Higher Education Student: A Critical Review of the Literature," *Journal of Further and Higher Education* 30, no. 2 (2006): 107–117.

40. K. Glanz, B. Rimer, and F. Levis, eds., *Health Behavior and Health Education: Theory, Research, and Practice,* 3rd ed. (San Francisco, CA: Jossey-Bass, 2002).

41. A. D. Von et al., "Predictors of Health Behaviors in College Students," *Journal of Advanced Nursing* 48, no. 5 (2004): 463–474.

42. W. R. Lovallo and W. Gerin, "Psychophysiological Reactivity: Mechanism and Pathways to Cardiovascular Disease," *Psychosomatic Medicine* 65 (2003): 36–45; S. E. Weinstein and K. S. Quigley, "Locus of Control Predicts Appraisals and Cardiovascular Reactivity to a Novel Active Coping Task," *Journal of Personality* 74, no. 3 (2006): 911–931; S. Catanzaro et al., "Coping Related to Expectancies and Dispositions as Prospective Predictors of Coping Responses and Symptoms," *Journal of Personality* 68 (2000): 757–788; A. Sanz et al., "Effects of Specific and Non-Specific Perceived Control on Blood Pressure in a Stressful Mental Task," *Biological Psychology* 71 (2006): 20–28; J. M. Twenge et al., "It's Beyond My Control: A Cross-Temporal Meta-Analysis of Increasing Externality in Locus of Control, 1960–2002," *Personality and Social Psychology Review* 8 (2004): 308–320.

43. M. Friedman and R. H. Rosenman, *Type A Behavior and Your Heart* (New York: Knopf, 1974).

44. K. Karren et al., *Mind/Body Health.*

45. R. Ragland and R. Brand, "Distrust, Rage May Be Toxic Cores That Put a Type A Person at Risk," *Journal of the American Medical Association* 261 (1989): 813, 814; J. C. Barefoot, W. G. Dahlstrom, and R. B. Williams, "Hostility, CHD Incidence, and Total Mortality: A 25-Year Follow-Up Study of 255 Physicians," *Psychosomatic Medicine* 51 (1983): 46–57; J. C. Barefoot et al., "Hostility Patterns and Health Implications: Correlates of Cook-Medley Hostility Scale Scores in a National Survey," *Health Psychology* 10 (1991): 18–24; K. Karren et al., *Mind/Body Health.*

46. S. Kobasa, "Stressful Life Events, Personality, and Health: An Inquiry into Hardiness," *Journal of Personality and Social Psychology* 37 (1979): 1–11.

47. B. J. Crowley, B. Hayslip, and J. Hobdy, "Psychological Hardiness and Adjustment to Life Events in Adulthood," *Journal of Adult Development* 10 (2003): 237–248; S. R. Maddi, "The Story of Hardiness: Twenty Years of Theorizing, Research, and Practice," *Consulting Psychology Journal: Practice and Research* 54 (2002): 173–186.

48. D. Robotham and C. Julian, "Stress and the Higher Education Student," 107–117.

49. L. Dusselier et al., "Personal, Health, Academic, and Environmental Predictors of Stress for Residence Hall Students," *Journal of American College Health* 54 (2005): 15–24; B. M. Hughes, "Study, Examinations, and Stress: Blood Pressure Assessments in College Students," *Educational Review* 57, no. 1 (2005): 21–36.

50. American College Health Association. "American College Health Association-National College Health Assessment: Reference Group Executive Summary, Spring 2005, Part C, Academic Impacts," Baltimore: American College Health Association, 2005, http://www.acha.org/projects_programs/NCHA_docs/ACHANCHA_Reference_Group_ExecutiveSummary_Spring2005.pdf.

51. J. H. Pryor et al., *The American Freshman: National Norms for Fall 2005* (Los Angeles: Higher Education Research Institute, 2006.

52. M. E. Pritchard and G. S. Wilson, "Do Coping Styles Change During the First Semester of College?" *Journal of Social Psychology* 146, no. 1 (2006): 125–127; C. L. Broman, "Stress, Race, and Substance Use in College," *College Student Journal* 39, no. 2 (2005): 340–352; D. Kariv and D. and T. Heilman, "Task-Oriented versus Emotion-Oriented Coping Strategies: The Case of College Students," *College Student Journal* 39, no. 1 (2005): 72–84; K. M. Kieffer et al., "Test and Study Worry and Emotionality in the Prediction of College Students' Reasons for Drinking: An Exploratory Investigation," *Journal of Alcohol and Drug Education* 50, no. 1 (2006): 57–81.

53. P. A. Bovier, E. Chamot, and T. V. Perneger, "Perceived Stress, Internal Resources, and Social Support as Determinants of Mental Health Among Young Adults," *Quality of Life Research* 13, no. 1 (2004): 161–170; E. Largo-Wright, P. M. Peterson, and W. W. Chen, "Perceived Problem Solving, Stress, and Health Among College Students," *American Journal of Health Behavior* 29, no. 4 C.L. Park et al., (2005): 360–370; "The Daily Stress and Coping Process and Alcohol Use Among College Students," 126–135.

54. Blonna, *Coping with Stress.*

55. P. A. Bovier et al., "Perceived Stress," 161–170; A. DeLongis and S. Holtzman, "Coping in Context: The Role of Stress, Social Support, and Personality in Coping," *Journal of Personality* 73, no. 6 (2005): 1633–1656.

56. Seaward, *Managing Stress.*

57. C. Hassed, "How Humor Keeps You Well," *Australian Family Physician* 30, no. 1 (2001): 25–28.

58. R. Niaura et al., "Hostility, Metabolic Syndrome, and Incident Coronary Heart Disease," *Health Psychology* 21, no. 6 (2002): 588–593.

59. P. Holmes, "Managing Anger: Understanding the Dynamics of Violence, Abuse and Control," SIUC Mental Health Web Site, 2004, www.siu.edu/offices/counsel/anger.htm.

60. Ibid.

61. M. Bonnet et al., "Effects of Caffeine on Heart Rate and QT Variability During Sleep," *Depression and Anxiety* 22, no. 3 (2005): 150–155.

62. B. Andrews and J. M. Wilding, "The Relations of Depression and Anxiety to Life-Stress and Achievement in Students," *British Journal of Psychology* 95 (2004): 509–521; J. M. Norvilitis et al., "Personality Factors, Money Attitudes, Financial Knowledge, and Credit-Card Debt in College Students," *Journal of Applied Social Psychology* 36 no. 6 (2006): 1395–1413.

63. R. Deckro et al., "The Evaluation of Mind/Body Intervention to Reduce Psychological Distress and Perceived Stress in College Students," *Journal of American College Health* 50, no. 6 (May 2002): 281–287.

64. N. B. Allen, R. Chambers, and W. Knight, "Mindfulness-Based Psychotherapies: A Review of Conceptual Foundations, Empirical Evidence, and Practical Considerations," *Australian and New Zealand Journal of Psychiatry* 40 (2006): 285–294.

4

Violence and Abuse

CREATING HEALTHY ENVIRONMENTS

Is **America** really more violent than other countries?

Is there anything I can do to **protect** myself from terrorism?

Are men ever **victims** of domestic violence?

What can I do if I think I am being **stalked**?

Can my university do anything to **help** me feel safer?

OBJECTIVES

- Differentiate between intentional and unintentional injuries, and discuss societal and personal factors that contribute to violence in American society.
- Examine factors that contribute to homicide, domestic violence, sexual victimization, and other intentional acts of violence.
- Explain how terrorism can affect individuals and populations, and summarize practical steps to lower your risk from terrorist attacks.
- Discuss strategies to prevent intentional injuries and reduce their risk of occurrence.
- Explain how the campus community, law enforcement officials, and individuals can prevent common campus crimes.
- Discuss the impact of unintentional injuries on American society, and identify actions that contribute to personal risk of injuries of all types.

Across the land, waves of violence seem to crest and break, terrorizing Americans in cities and suburbs, in prairie towns and mountain hollows.

To millions of Americans few things are more pervasive, more frightening, more real today than violent crime.... The fear of being victimized by criminal attack has touched us all in some way.

Among urban children ages 10–14, homicides are up 150 percent, robberies are up 192 percent, assaults are up 290 percent.

Do these sound like statements from today's newspapers or television news? They're not. The first quotation comes from President Herbert Hoover's 1929 inauguration speech, the second from the 1860 Senate report on crime, and the third from a 1967 report on children's violence.[1] Clearly, violence and our concern over its rising rates are not new concepts.

The term **violence** is used to indicate a set of behaviors that produce injuries, regardless of whether they are **intentional injuries** (committed with intent to harm) or **unintentional injuries** (committed without intent to harm, often accidentally), as well as the outcome of these behaviors. Any definition of violence implicitly includes the use of force, regardless of the intent, but as you'll see, some forms of violence are also extremely subtle.

In this chapter, we focus on the various types of intentional and unintentional violence, the underlying causes of or contributors to these problems, strategies to reduce risk of encountering violence, and possible methods for preventing violence. Although certain indicators of violence, such as the numbers of murders and deadly assaults, seem to be declining, other forms of violence, such as rape, hate crimes, and suicides, are on the increase.

Even more important is that for all we know about violence incidence and prevalence, a great deal remains unknown. Just how many people suffer in silence, failing to report violent acts due to fear of repercussions or accepting violence as "the way it is," remains unknown.

violence   A set of behaviors that produce injuries, as well as the outcomes of these behaviors (the injuries themselves).

intentional injuries   Injuries committed on purpose with intent to harm.

unintentional injuries   Injuries committed without intent to harm.

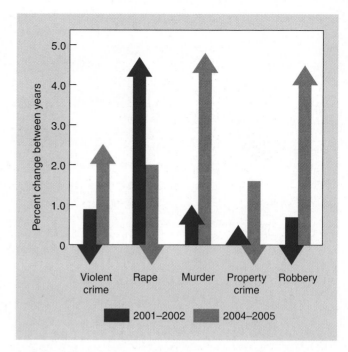

FIGURE 4.1   Changes in Violent Crime Rates, 2001–2002 and 2004–2005

Source: Federal Bureau of Investigation, Preliminary Annual Uniform Crime Report, 2005, Table 3: Percent Change for Consecutive Years, June 12, 2006, www.fbi.gov.ucr/2005preliminary.

Violence in the United States

Even though violence has long been a major concern in American society, not until 1985 did the U.S. Public Health Service formally identify violence as a leading public health problem that contributed significantly to death and disability. The Centers for Disease Control and Prevention (CDC) created the Division of Violence Prevention and considers violence a form of chronic disease that is pervasive at all levels of American society. Vulnerable populations, such as children, women, black males, and the elderly, were listed as being at high risk for certain types of crime, while older teens and young adults have the highest rates of both violent crime victimization and offending rates.[2]

Recent numbers indicate that we have made dramatic improvements in certain areas. Since 1973, statistics from the Federal Bureau of Investigation (FBI) had shown that overall crime and certain types of violent crime decreased each year. However, in 2005, overall rates of violent crime actually increased by 2.5 percent overall, with murder specifically increasing nearly 5 percent in 2005 over the previous year (see Figure 4.1).[3]

Is crime an issue on college and university campuses? Specific crime rates vary tremendously from region to region across the United States, and over the years, data indicate that college campuses are not immune. However, many question the accuracy of such campus crime reports, since petty theft, date rape, fighting, and other common campus incidents are

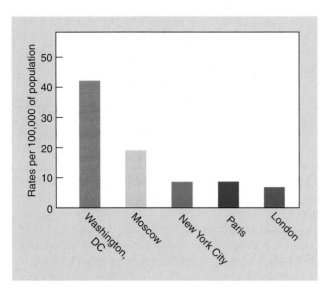

FIGURE 4.2 International Capital Murder Rates
Is it any wonder the international community views the United States as a violent place?

Source: Home Office of the United Kingdom, International Comparisons of Criminal Justice Statistics, 2001 (London: Home Office, 2003).

not always reported to police. Some also criticize campus administrators' reluctance to report incidents due to concern over reputation and other difficulties that could affect overall enrollment if a campus reports grim statistics. Most campuses are intensely aware of the potential for violent crime on campus, especially given the high-stress environment, where alcohol often plays a role. For this reason, universities and colleges do take steps to protect students. It is important to note that 70.8 percent of all deaths among persons aged 10 to 24 have violent elements and stem from just four causes: motor vehicle crashes (particularly when alcohol is involved), other unintentional injuries, homicide, and suicide.[4]

Is America really more violent than other countries?

Why should we be concerned about a violence-prone society? Violence affects everyone, directly or indirectly. Although the direct victims of violence and those close to them obviously suffer the most, others suffer in various ways because of the climate of fear that violence generates. Women are afraid to walk alone at night. The elderly are often afraid to go out even in the daytime. After terrorist episodes such as the 2001 World Trade Center attack and the Madrid and London subway attacks, some people are afraid to fly, use mass transit, work in tall buildings, or travel to popular international destinations. The cost of homeland security is staggering. You might be surprised to learn that international travelers often fear coming to the United States in much the same way that some Americans fear traveling to other regions of the world where attacks on U.S. citizens have taken place. Tourists from foreign countries are afraid of being brutalized in many of our nation's cities, and worry about being caught in the crosshairs of gang violence, or other forms of violent assault or robbery (see Figure 4.2). Many of these reports are carried in the international news media, depicting the United States as a violent

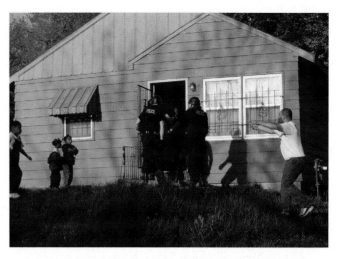

Violent acts do not just affect the victim and the perpetrator. Families and neighborhoods are also deeply affected by violent crime.

nation. Even people who live in supposedly safe areas can become victims of violence within their own homes or at the hands of family members.

Costs of Violence

Although the greatest costs of violence, those of human suffering and loss, are impossible to calculate, the direct and indirect economic toll is staggering, especially when we consider the cost of antiterrorism measures and war. According to a recent World Health Organization report, many nations spend more than 4 percent of their total gross domestic product dealing with violence-related injuries.[5] In the United States, traditional cost analysis of domestic violence alone among youth aged 10 to 24 indicates that our expenditures exceed $160 billion each year. Once we account for the costs associated with all other forms of violence, including terrorism, this easily amounts to trillions of dollars.[6] Societies face a monumental task in paying for these violence-related problems, funding prisons, and providing assistance to victims. At the very least, we all pay higher tax bills for law enforcement, homeland security, and surveillance intended to protect us from identity theft, terrorist acts, and other threats to ourselves and our property.

Societal Causes of Violence

Several social, cultural, and individual factors increase the likelihood of violent acts, including:

■ *Poverty.* Low socioeconomic status and poor living conditions can create an environment of hopelessness, leaving people feeling trapped and seeing violence as the only way to obtain what they want.

- *Unemployment.* It is a well-documented fact that when the economy goes sour, violent crime, suicide, assault, and other crimes increase.
- *Parental influence.* Violence is cyclical. Children raised in environments in which shouting, slapping, hitting, and other forms of violence are common are more apt to be violent as adults.
- *Cultural beliefs.* Cultures that objectify women and empower men to be tough and aggressive show increased rates of violence in the home.
- *The media.* Several studies indicate that violence on TV, the Internet, movies, and video games may increase the potential for violence among certain groups.
- *Discrimination/oppression.* Whenever one group is oppressed by another, for reasons ranging from religion to race to cultural difference, hate and bias crimes rise.
- *Breakdowns in the criminal justice system.* Overcrowded prisons, lenient sentences, early releases from prison, and errors in the justice and judicial system subtly encourage violence.
- *Stress.* People who are in crisis or under stress are more apt to be highly reactive, striking out at others or acting irrationally.
- *Heavy use of alcohol and other substances.* Alcohol and drug abuse are often catalysts for violence, and are risk factors for domestic violence, rape, child abuse, homicide, and other crimes. (Chapter 14 discusses the abuse of drugs. Chapter 12 goes into further detail about social and health problems related to alcohol abuse.)

Some say that the prevalence of guns in our society also contributes to the high death rate caused by violent acts. In addition to these broad, societally based factors, many personal factors also can lead to violence.[7]

 what do you THINK?

Why do you think rates of violence in the United States are so much higher than those of other nations, like Great Britain and Japan? ■ What actions can you take personally to prevent violence from occurring? ■ What could be done to reduce risk on your campus? ■ In your community?

Personal Precipitators of Violence

If you are like most people, you probably acted out your anger more readily as a child than you do today. However,

even the worst behaved children usually grow up. As we mature, we learn to control outbursts of anger and approach conflict rationally, because it is not socially acceptable to act out.

Yet, some go through life acting out their aggressive tendencies without regard for social norms, in much the same way as children. Why do two children from the same neighborhood, or even from the same family, go in different directions when it comes to violence? There are several predictors of future aggressive behavior.[8]

Anger *Anger* is a spontaneous, usually temporary, biological feeling or emotional state of displeasure that occurs most frequently during times of personal frustration. Because life is stressful, anger becomes a part of daily experience. Anger can range from slight irritation to *rage,* a violent and extreme form of anger. When it is acted out at home or on the road, the consequences can be deadly. (See the New Horizons in Health box.)

What makes some people flare up at the slightest provocation? Often, people who anger quickly have a low tolerance for frustration, believing that they should not have to put up with inconvenience or petty annoyances. The cause may be genetic or physiological; there is evidence that some people are born unstable, touchy, or easily angered. Another cause of anger is sociocultural. People who are taught not to express anger in public do not know how to handle it when it reaches a level that can no longer be hidden. Family background may be the most important factor. Typically, anger-prone people come from families that are disruptive, chaotic, and not skilled in emotional expression.[9]

Aggressive behavior is often a key aspect of violent interactions. **Primary aggression** is goal-directed, hostile self-assertion that is destructive in nature. **Reactive aggression** is more often part of an emotional reaction brought about by frustrating life experiences. Whether aggression is reactive or primary in nature, it is most likely to flare up in times of acute stress, during relationship difficulties or loss, or when a person is so frustrated that he or she feels the only recourse is to strike out at others.

 what do you THINK?

What are some examples of primary aggression? ■ Reactive aggression? ■ Can both result in the same degree of harm? ■ Do you think our laws are more lenient when violent acts result from reactive aggression? Why or why not?

Substance Abuse Although much has been written about a link between substance abuse and violence, we have yet to show that substance abuse actually causes violence. In fact, many violent episodes are carefully planned actions that involve no alcohol or drug abuse. In some situations, however, psychoactive substances appear to be a form of ignition for violence:[10]

(Text continues on page 112)

---

primary aggression Goal-directed, hostile self-assertion that is destructive in character.

reactive aggression Emotional reaction brought about by frustrating life experiences.

INTERMITTENT EXPLOSIVE DISORDER

Have you ever had someone scare you with a bout of road rage while you were in a car? Do you know someone who has exploded into a rage and punched a fist through a wall or door to show fury? If so, you are not alone. These very common, sometimes erratic and out-of-the-blue eruptions have recently received a scientific name: intermittent explosive disorder. We might commonly refer to this type of irrational anger as "road rage," or "explosive outbursts," but a study sponsored by the National Institute of Mental Health finds that these unwarranted reactions are so common and extreme that they deserve a name.

Intermittent explosive disorder (IED) is characterized by repeated episodes of aggressive, violent behavior that are grossly out of proportion to the situation. People with IED may attack others and their possessions, causing bodily injury and property damage. Typically beginning in the early teens, the disorder often precedes development of depression, bipolar disorder, anxiety, and substance abuse disorders.

HOW COMMON IS IT?

According to results from the NIMH study, IED affects over 7.3 percent of all adults—up to 16 million Americans—in their lifetimes. While over 82 percent of those affected suffer from depression, anxiety, or substance abuse, fewer than 28 percent ever get help for their angry outbursts. Experts suggest that treating anger early, particularly among youth, might help prevent later problems.

HOW IS IT DIFFERENT THAN JUST GETTING ANGRY ABOUT SOMETHING?

To be diagnosed with IED, a person must have had three episodes of impulsive aggression out of proportion to the situation at any time in his or her life. Effectively, the person must have "all of a sudden lost control and broke or smashed something worth more than a few dollars … hit or tried to hurt someone (including animals) …or threatened to hurt or hit someone." Often the person with IED may experience tingling, tremor, palpitations, chest tightness, head pressure, blood pressure increases, or redness in the face prior to the event.

ARE THERE VARIOUS FORMS OF IED?

Yes. If the person is driving a car, it may manifest itself as road rage, an IED episode that occurs while driving and is believed to be a leading cause of highway deaths. Several things may contribute to road rage and other forms of IED. Among them is a family history of violence in which a child learns that screaming, yelling, and other displays of power can get attention. Muscle cars, highway congestion, and traffic delays can increase stress and lead to IED. People with relationship or family problems, job stress, and other problems are also at risk for road rage and other forms of IED. Young women and men, particularly those under the influence of alcohol or other drugs, are often those most likely to engage in road rage. If the rage is acted out in the home, it is classified as domestic violence.

HOW TO AVOID BECOMING A VICTIM

- *Avoid becoming involved with "hotheads."* The best method of primary prevention is to not get involved with those who have a short fuse. If you start dating someone or hanging out with someone who flares easily and whose rage is unusual given the circumstances, keep your distance. We all get angry, but wild displays of anger are not a healthy reaction to life.
- *Avoid eye contact and engagement.* If you are driving or out in public and someone tries to get a reaction from you, avoid confrontation. Simply remove yourself from the situation.
- *Don't antagonize.* Slowing down in traffic to bug someone in an obvious hurry,

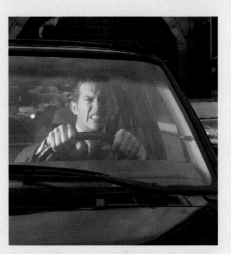

honking your horn, giving someone the bright lights, or other passive-aggressive gestures can get a rise out of even the mildest-mannered people.

- *If someone follows you after a nasty interaction, either in a car or on foot, do not immediately drive home or walk into your workplace.* Many shootings have occurred in workplaces when someone gunning for an individual goes on a shooting rampage. If you are driving, drive to a police station or area where there are lots of cars and traffic. Never isolate yourself.
- *Take names.* If you don't know the person, try to keep a mental description or get a license plate if driving. Report offenders, even if you are afraid of getting involved.
- *Stay calm.* Think before opening your mouth, and practice stress management whenever possible. Doing so, while avoiding alcohol and other substances that may cause you to lose your cool, are important strategies to avoid IED.

Sources: E. Coccaro et al., "National Comorbidity Survey Replication Study," National Institute of Mental Health, 2006, www.nimh.nih.gov/press/iedepi.cfm?Output=Print; J. Asher, "Intermittent Explosive Disorder Affects Up to 16 Million Americans," National Institute of Mental Health, Press Release, June 5, 2006, www.nimh.nih.gov.

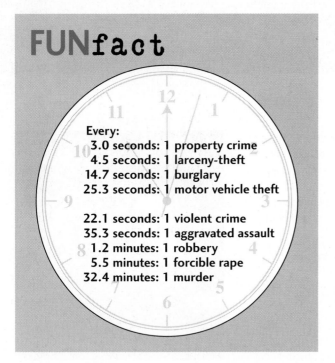

FUNfact

Every:
- **3.0 seconds:** 1 property crime
- **4.5 seconds:** 1 larceny-theft
- **14.7 seconds:** 1 burglary
- **25.3 seconds:** 1 motor vehicle theft

- **22.1 seconds:** 1 violent crime
- **35.3 seconds:** 1 aggravated assault
- **1.2 minutes:** 1 robbery
- **5.5 minutes:** 1 forcible rape
- **32.4 minutes:** 1 murder

FIGURE 4.3 Crime Clock: How Often Is a Crime Committed?
Are you surprised by the "Crime Clock"? Consider how long it takes you to brush your teeth, walk to class, or attend a class, then look at this data again. How does this information stack up against your own campus's crime?

Source: Federal Bureau of Investigation, "Crime in the United States," 2002, www.fbi.gov.

- Consumption of alcohol—by perpetrators of the crime, the victim, or both—immediately precedes over half of all violent crimes, including murder.
- Chronic drinkers are more likely than others to have histories of violent behavior.
- Criminals using illegal drugs commit robberies and assaults more frequently than nonusing criminals and do so especially during periods of heavy drug use.
- In domestic assault cases, more than 86 percent of the assailants and 42 percent of victims reported using alcohol at the time of the attack. Nearly 15 percent of victims and assailants reported using cocaine at the time of the attack.
- Ninety-two percent of assailants and 42 percent of victims reported using alcohol or other drugs on the day of the assault.
- Mentally ill patients who fail to adhere to prescription drug regimens and abuse alcohol and/or other drugs are significantly more likely to be involved in a serious violent act.

homicide Death that results from intent to injure or kill.

Intentional Injuries

Anytime someone sets out to harm other people or their property, the incident may be referred to as intentional violence. Such acts often result in intentional injuries, which come in many forms. Whether the situation entails a simple outburst of anger or a fatal attack with a weapon, the resulting intentional injuries cause pain and suffering at the very least and disability or death at the worst. Although nonviolent criminal acts are much more common, violent crimes occur all too frequently (Figure 4.3).

Gratuitous Violence

Violence can manifest itself in many ways. Often the most shocking or gratuitous crimes gain the greatest attention, such as stories of innocent victims of drive-by shootings or young students who turn their internal rage outward on family, classmates, and teachers.

Assault/Homicide
Homicide, defined as murder or nonnegligent manslaughter, was the fifteenth leading cause of death in 2004, but the second leading cause of death for persons aged 15 to 24.[11] It accounts for nearly 18,000 premature deaths in the United States annually.[12] Homicide is an area in which disparities among races are particularly clear. For an American, the average lifetime probability of being murdered is 1 in 153—but this average masks large differences for specific segments of the population. Asian/Pacific Islander, Hispanic or Latino, and African American groups all list homicide among the top ten causes of death, while homicide is not among the top ten killers of white Americans. Homicide rates for African American males are higher than for any other group.[13] For black men of any age, the risk of murder is 1 in 28; for a black man in the 20- to 22-year-old age group, the risk is 1 in 3.

The majority of homicides are not random acts of violence. Over half of all homicides occur among people who know one another. In two-thirds of these cases, the perpetrator and the victim are friends or acquaintances; in one-third, they belong to the same family.[14]

Bias and Hate Crimes

A hate or bias crime is a crime committed against a person, property, or group of people that is motivated by the offender's bias against a race, religion, disability, sexual orientation, or ethnicity.[15] In spite of national efforts in workplaces, schools, and communities to promote understanding and diversity-related appreciation, intolerance of differences continues to smolder in many parts of U.S. society. The 2002 murder of Gwen Araujo, a transgendered teen in California, and arson attacks on Alabama churches in 2006 remind Americans that violence based on sexuality, race, and other "-isms" still occurs. According to the FBI's most recent Hate Crime Statistics Report, 9,035 bias-motivated crimes were reported in 2004 (see Figure 4.4).

Since the 2001 terrorist attack in the United States and the conflicts in Iraq and Afghanistan, reports of hate-related incidents, beatings, and other physical and verbal assaults have escalated. In particular, persons of Muslim or Middle Eastern descent reported civil rights violations at work, in mass transit, and in communities throughout the United States. Many believe that the reported incidents are but the tip of the iceberg and actual numbers of bias- or hate-related crimes are much higher, but people do not report them for fear of possible retaliation.

Hate crimes vary along two dimensions: (1) the way they are carried out and (2) their effects on victims. Vicious gossip, nasty comments, and devilish pranks may not make headlines, but they can hurt nonetheless. Generally, about 30 percent of all hate crimes are against property, with the other 70 percent being against a person. Recent studies have identified three additional characteristics of hate crimes:[16]

- Excessively brutal
- Perpetrated at random on total strangers
- Perpetrated by multiple offenders

In addition, the perpetrators tend to be motivated by thrill, defensive feelings, or a hate-mongering mission.

Academic settings are not immune to hatred and bias. Campuses have responded to reports of hate crimes by offering courses that emphasize diversity, training faculty appropriately, and developing policies that strictly enforce punishment for hate crimes.[17] Sadly, many minor assaults do go unreported due to fear of retaliation or continued stigmatization for being different; this is a major impediment to reducing the rate of hate crimes on campus.

The tendency toward violent acts on campus might best be defined as campus **ethnoviolence,** a term that reflects relationships among groups in the larger society and is based on prejudice and discrimination. Although ethnoviolence often is directed randomly at persons affiliated with a particular group, the group itself is specifically targeted apart from other people, and that differentiation is usually ethnic in nature. Typically, the perpetrators agree that the group is an acceptable target, and amid fears of terrorism and war, this type of violence may increase.

Prejudice and discrimination are always at the base of ethnoviolence. **Prejudice** is a set of negative attitudes toward a group of people. To say that a person is prejudiced against some group is to say that the person holds a set of beliefs about the group, has an emotional reaction to the group, and is motivated to behave in a certain way toward the group. **Discrimination** constitutes actions that deny equal treatment or opportunities to a group of people, often based on prejudice.

Often intolerance stems from a fear of change and a desire to blame others when forces such as the economy and crime seem to be out of control. What can you do to be part of the solution rather than the problem?

- Support educational programs and campus groups that foster understanding and appreciation for differences in people. Many colleges now require diversity classes as part of their academic curriculum.

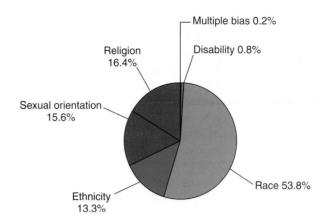

FIGURE 4.4 **Bias-Motivated Crimes, 2004**

Source: Federal Bureau of Investigation, "Hate Crime Statistics," 2004, www.fbi.gov/ucr/hc2004/openpage.htm.

- Examine your own values, attitudes, and behaviors. Are you intolerant of others? Do you engage in racist, sexist, or similar behaviors meant to demean a group of individuals? Do you judge people on appearances? If you have problems with a particular group, why?
- Do you discourage hurtful jokes and other forms of social or ethnic bigotry? Do not participate in such behaviors, and express your dissatisfaction with those who do.
- Educate yourself. Read, interact with, and attempt to understand people who appear to be different from you. Remember that you do not have to like everything about them, but respecting people's right to be different is a part of being a healthy, integrated individual.
- Encourage your legislators to support antihate and antibias legislation. Vote for those who support antidiscrimination policies and programs.

 what do you THINK?

Think about the bias or hate crimes that you have heard about in the past six months. Who were the victims? ■ Did you know any of them? ■ Why do you think people are motivated to initiate such crimes against people they don't know? ■ What can you do to reduce such crimes in your area? ■ What should be done nationally?

ethnoviolence Violence directed randomly at persons affiliated with a particular, usually ethnic, group.

prejudice A negative evaluation of an entire group of people that is typically based on unfavorable and often wrong ideas about the group.

discrimination Actions that deny equal treatment or opportunities to a group, often based on prejudice.

Gang Violence Why do young people join gangs? Although the reasons are complex, gangs seem to meet many of their needs. Gangs provide a sense of belonging to a "family" that gives them self-worth, companionship, security, and excitement. In other cases, gangs provide economic security through criminal activity, drug sales, or prostitution. Once young people become involved in the gang subculture, it is difficult to leave. Threats of violence or fear of not making it on their own discourage even those who are seriously trying to get out.

Who is at risk for gang membership? Membership varies considerably from region to region. The age range of gang members is typically 12 to 22 years. Risk factors include low self-esteem, academic problems, low socioeconomic status, alienation from family and society, a history of family violence, and living in gang-controlled neighborhoods.

The best way to prevent someone from joining a gang is to keep that person connected to positive influences and programs. From a child's early years, the focus should be on establishing bonds among friends, family, and school. Any student who has learning disabilities or other problems that make it hard to keep up should be involved in alternative activities that foster success and prevent a sense of alienation. Community-based programs that coordinate involvement of families, social service organizations, and law enforcement, school, and city officials have proved effective in keeping students out of gangs. Also, community members must begin to think of gang members not merely as trouble-making delinquents, but as people whose circumstances make them susceptible to the gang lifestyle.

In part because of growing gang and gang-related crime the U.S. Congress passed a crime bill in the early 1990s that included among other measures the establishment of "boot camps" for young nonviolent offenders. (Similar additions to our national policing and surveillance capabilities have been initiated post–September 11.) The boot camps were designed to keep offenders out of prison and instill discipline, self-esteem, and respect for the law. These "tough love" programs may not be as effective as many had hoped. Public health professionals have long advocated prevention rather than the current efforts spent on intervention. Examining the underlying causes of violence should provide evidence for supporting systemwide changes in the social environment.

Terrorism: Increased Risks from Multiple Sources

Not so long ago, Americans thought terrorism occurred only in distant cities, seldom amounting to more than a blip on the evening news. Since September 11, 2001, times have changed dramatically. Terrorist attacks on the World Trade Center and the Pentagon revealed the vulnerability of our nation to domestic and international threats. The terms *terrorist attack, bioterrorism,* and *biological weapons* catapulted us into the new millennium with an emotional reaction unlike any ever seen. America had lost its innocence and its illusion of invulnerability. An undercurrent of fear and anxiety about potential threats from faceless strangers shook many of us in ways that we had never even considered. Today, the specter of a terrorist attack looms ever present. Any time there is a national holiday or occasion where many Americans gather, we worry about a terrorist event.

What Is Terrorism? According to the FBI, **terrorism** is the use of unlawful force or violence against persons or property to intimidate or coerce a government, the civilian population, or any segment thereof in furtherance of political or social objectives. Typically, terrorism is of two major types:

- *Domestic terrorism* involves groups or individuals whose terrorist activities are directed at elements of our government or population, without foreign direction.
- *International terrorism* involves groups or individuals whose terrorist activities are foreign-based, transcend national boundaries, and are directed by countries or groups outside the United States.

Clearly, terrorist activities may have immediate impact in loss of lives and resources. However, the 2001 attacks also had far-reaching effects on the U.S. economy, airlines, and transportation systems. Perhaps most damaging in the aftermath of the attacks was the fear, anxiety, and altered behavior of countless Americans. How many people will fear working in skyscrapers for years to come? How many will fear climbing on a plane, crossing a bridge, or getting on the subway? Will worry about biological weapons and future terrorist attacks disrupt our lives and our interactions with others? (See the New Horizons in Health box on page 116.)

As the media spur our anxieties about germ, chemical, and nuclear warfare and the multitude of ways that terrorists can breach our defenses, is it any wonder that an already stressed American public is demonstrating increasing concern? What can we do to reduce our risk of terrorist attack?

Is there anything I can do to protect myself from terrorism?

The CDC has a wide range of ongoing programs and services to help Americans respond to terrorist threats and prepare for possible attacks. Information is available on the CDC website and is updated regularly. A new government entity, the Department of Homeland Security, has been established to prevent future attacks, and the FBI and other government agencies have also prepared a sweeping set of procedures and guidelines for ensuring citizen safety. Here are some things you can do to help reduce anxiety and harm related to terrorist attacks.

terrorism The use of unlawful force or violence against persons or property to intimidate or coerce a government, the civilian population, or any segment thereof in furtherance of political or social objectives.

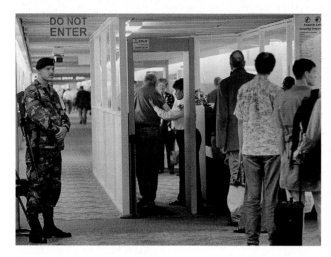

The threat of terrorism has affected many aspects of our daily lives.

- *Be aware of your own reactions to stress, anxiety, and fear.* Try to assess how much of your fear is justifiable in a given situation and how much is a product of media sensationalism. Practice stress reduction techniques, determine the source of your stressors, and react as prudently as possible. (See Chapter 3 for more information on post-traumatic stress disorder, which can be caused by exposure to events such as terrorist attacks.)
- *Be conscious of your surroundings.* If you notice suspicious activities or irregularities, report them to a person in authority. Being a passive observer and not speaking up when warranted may put you and others at risk.
- *Stay informed.* Try to stay on top of the news and understand the underlying roots of violent activity. Persistent poverty, pervasive religious or political fanaticism, and political situations in which there is an imbalance of power can provide fodder for violent acts. Consider when a self-righteous contempt for others may lead to persecution and violation of human rights. Be skeptical of acts perpetrated in the name of some cause, and intervene if possible to defuse violence.
- *Seek understanding.* Whenever two opposing groups stop engaging with each other mentally or communication breaks down, hatred, bigotry, and anger may result. Knowing about each other's customs, cultures, and beliefs and keeping the lines of communication open are good steps to avoid alienation.
- *Seek information.* When political parties fight for power in election years, know your candidates. What are their underlying beliefs regarding national defense, spending for consumer protection, policies on immigration, human rights violations, diversity issues, hate crimes, gun control, and so forth? Are they more aligned with one ideology than another? What is their stance on government interference and control, punishment of offenders, and other key issues?
- *Know what to do in an emergency.* Who would you call? How would you access local and regional assistance? Do

you have the necessary provisions for basic survival—food, water, prescription medications, first aid? What happens when your electricity is off, your phone and communication systems are down, and your access to health care is limited?

try it NOW

An emergency plan can make you feel more at ease, and eliminate anxiety. Get together with your family, friends, or roommates and make a plan for a natural disaster or terrorist attack. Keep an emergency kit on hand containing several days' worth of food and water, flashlights, batteries, and even a small battery-powered radio. Determine a meeting spot such as the quad, or the street corner on your block, in case there are no phones or other ways to get in touch with each other.

Domestic Violence

In the 1980s a popular country-western song crooned, "No one knows what goes on behind closed doors." Domestic violence shows us just how true that refrain can be. **Domestic violence** refers to the use of force to control and maintain power over another person in the home environment. It can occur between parent and child, spouses, or siblings and may involve emotional abuse, verbal abuse, threats of physical harm, and actual physical violence ranging from slapping and shoving to beatings, rape, and homicide. Today, domestic violence is at epidemic levels in America. It is the number-one cause of injury to women between the ages of 15 and 44, and each year 2–4 million women are battered, 2,000 of whom are beaten to death.[18]

Women as Victims While young men are more apt to become victims of violence from strangers, women are much more likely to become victims of violent acts perpetrated by spouses, lovers, ex-spouses, and ex-lovers. This aggression often includes pushing, slapping, and shoving, but it can take more severe forms. In reported assaults, only 31 percent of the men who attack women are in the "stranger" category. In fact, six of every ten women in the United States will be assaulted at some time in their lives by someone they know.[19] Every year, according to a national survey, approximately 12 percent of married women are the victims of physical aggression perpetrated by their husbands.[20]

On college campuses, relationship violence is a serious problem, and includes emotional, physical, and sexual abuse. In the American College Health Association's survey of Fall

domestic violence The use of force to control and maintain power over another person in the home environment, including both actual harm and the threat of harm.

BIOTERRORISM: PANDORA'S BOX

For many, the threat of a viable attack on the United States was incomprehensible until the World Trade Center and Pentagon attacks in 2001, and the train attacks in Madrid and London in 2004 and 2005. As shocking as those events were, they may pale in comparison to the opening of a Pandora's box of biological killers, which could threaten the global population. Before the 2001 attacks, many people had never heard of diseases such as anthrax, but within a few days Americans were watching endless newscasts that discussed the potential horrors of biological warfare.

As chilling as these threats might be, the actual potential for bioterrorism is more far-reaching than any of us might imagine, and includes a wide range of threats from both biological diseases and chemical agents, as indicated below. You can find a complete listing of potential agents and diseases, plus information on preparing for and dealing with emergencies, on the CDC website, www.bt.cdc.gov.

BIOLOGICAL AGENTS/DISEASES

Category A diseases are pathogens rarely seen in the United States and pose a risk to national security because they (1) can be easily disseminated or transmitted person to person; (2) cause high mortality, with potential for a major public health impact; (3) might cause widespread panic and social disruption; and (4) require special action for public health preparedness. The category A threats of greatest concern are highlighted below.

- *Bacillus anthracis* (**anthrax**): An acute infectious disease caused by a bacterium, anthrax typically occurs in host animals but can also infect humans. Three major forms of anthrax may occur: inhalation, cutaneous (skin), and intestinal, all with symptoms that usually appear within seven days after infection. Early symptoms of inhalation anthrax resemble a common cold, followed by respiratory symptoms and shock, which is often fatal. The intestinal form appears initially as nausea, vomiting, loss of appetite, and fever, followed by abdominal pain, bloody vomit, and severe diarrhea. It is believed that direct person-to-person spread of anthrax is very rare; thus, immunization and treatment of contacts are not recommended. Antibiotics are effective treatments in the early stages. Vaccination is effective if it occurs prior to contact.

- *Clostridium botulinum* toxin (**botulism**): Botulism is an acute muscle-paralyzing disease caused by a toxin produced by a bacterium. There are three major forms of botulism. Foodborne botulism, the most common strain, leads to illness within hours. Infant botulism affects babies who harbor the organism in their intestines. Wound botulism occurs when cuts are infected. Fortunately, botulism is not spread from person to person. Symptoms include double vision, blurred vision, slurred speech, difficulty swallowing, and muscle weakness that descends through

---

2005, 16 percent of women and 10 percent of men reported being emotionally abused in the last 12 months by a significant other. Nearly 5 percent of survey respondents reported physical abuse during this time period.[21]

The following U.S. statistics indicate the seriousness of this long-hidden problem.[22]

- African American women aged 25–29 are at 11 times the risk for being murdered while pregnant than their white equivalents.
- Homicide is the second leading cause of injury-related death among pregnant women and new mothers.
- Every 15 seconds, someone batters a woman; only 1 in every 250 such assaults is reported to the police.
- More than a third of female victims of domestic violence are severely abused on a regular basis.
- About five women are killed every day in domestic violence incidents; three-quarters of these women are killed by their husbands.

Although the ultimate result of these assaults can be murder, there are other devastating effects as well. Depression, panic attacks, disordered eating, chronic neck or back pain, migraine and other headaches, sexually transmitted infections, ulcers, and social isolation can all be results of domestic violence.

How many times have you heard of a woman who is repeatedly beaten by her partner and wondered, "Why doesn't she just leave him?" There are many reasons why some women find it difficult to break their ties with their abusers. Many women, particularly those with small children, are financially dependent on their partners. Others fear retaliation against themselves or their children. Some hope the situation will change with time (it rarely does), and others stay because cultural or religious beliefs forbid divorce. Finally, some women still love the abusive partner and are concerned about what will happen to him if they leave.

the body. It can eventually paralyze the ability to breathe and kill the person.

- *Yersinia pestis* (**plague**): An infectious disease of animals and humans that is found in many parts of the world, plague is caused by a bacterium carried by rodents and their fleas. The plague organism infects the lungs. Fever, headache, weakness, and a watery, blood-laden cough are frequent symptoms. Pneumonia follows quickly, and over 2 to 4 days may cause septic shock. Without treatment, plague can be fatal. Person-to-person contact with transfer of respiratory droplets spreads the disease. A vaccine has not been developed, but several antibiotics are effective if given early.

- *Variola major* (**smallpox**): Although smallpox was eliminated from the world in 1977, stockpiling of the virus that causes this disease has occurred in many regions of the world. Smallpox spreads from person to person by infected saliva droplets and is most contagious during the first week of illness. Initial symptoms include high fever, fatigue, and head- and backaches. In 2 or 3 days a characteristic rash develops, with flat red lesions that evolve into pustules most prominent on the face, arms, and legs. Lesions crust early in the second week. Scabs develop, separate, and fall off after about 3 to 4 weeks. Most people who get smallpox recover, but death occurs in up to 30 percent of cases. Most Americans were vaccinated prior to 1972, but it is uncertain whether these shots conferred lasting immunity. Although vaccines are effective, the current supply is limited. Treatment for smallpox focuses on relieving symptoms, but new antiviral agents are being tested.

Category B diseases are of concern but are less easily transmitted or have a lower mortality rate than those in category A. Examples include *Coxiella burnetii* (Q fever), *Brucella* species (brucellosis), *Burkholderia mallei* (glanders), ricin toxin from *Ricinus communis* (castor beans), epsilon toxin of *Clostridium perfringens,* and staphylococcal enterotoxin B.

Category C diseases are emerging pathogens that could be engineered for bioterrorism in the future because they have the potential for high morbidity and mortality rates and could be easily produced and disseminated. Examples include Nipah virus, hantavirus, tickborne hemorrhagic fever, tick-borne encephalitis viruses, yellow fever, and multidrug-resistant tuberculosis.

CHEMICAL AGENTS

These agents are classified by the body system they damage or the effects they produce. There are seven main categories of chemical agents, ranging from those that poison your blood, like hydrogen chloride, to those that inhibit nervous system function, like sarin. Chemical agents have been used in modern warfare, and images of those who live in countries such as Israel wearing gas masks are all too common.

Source: Centers for Disease Control and Prevention, "Emergency Preparedness and Response," 2004, www.bt.cdc.gov.

Psychologist Lenore Walker developed a theory known as the "cycle of violence" to explain how women can get caught in a downward spiral without realizing it.[23] The cycle has three phases:

1. *Tension building.* In this phase, minor battering occurs, and the woman may become more nurturant, more pleasing, and more intent on anticipating the spouse's needs to forestall further violence. She assumes guilt for doing something to provoke him and tries hard to avoid doing it again.

2. *Acute battering.* At this stage, pleasing her man doesn't help, and she can no longer control or predict the abuse. Usually, the spouse is trying to "teach her a lesson," and when he feels he has inflicted enough pain, he'll stop. When the acute attack is over, he may respond with shock and denial about his own behavior. Both batterer and victim may soft-pedal the seriousness of the attacks.

3. *Remorse/reconciliation.* During this "honeymoon" period, the batterer may be kind, loving, and apologetic, swearing he will never act violently again. He may "behave" for several weeks or months, and the woman may come to question whether she overreacted. However, when the tension that precipitated past abuse resurfaces, the man beats her again. Unless some form of intervention breaks this downward cycle of abuse—contrition, further abuse, denial, and contrition—it will repeat itself again and again, perhaps ending only in the woman's (or, rarely, the man's) death.

For most women who get caught in this cycle (which may include forced sexual relations and psychological and economic abuse as well as beatings), it is very hard to summon the resolution to extricate themselves. Most need effective outside intervention.

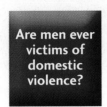

Men as Victims Are men also victims of domestic violence? Some women do abuse and even kill their partners. Approximately 12 percent of men reported that their wives had engaged in physically aggressive behaviors against them in the past year—nearly the same percentage of reported claims as for women.

However, there are two major differences between male and female batterers. First, although the frequency of physical aggression may be similar, the impact is drastically different: women are injured in domestic incidents two to three times more often than men.[24] These injuries tend to be more severe and have resulted in significantly more deaths. Women do engage in moderate aggression, such as pushing and shoving, at rates almost equal to those of men, but severe aggression that is likely to land the victim in the hospital is almost always male against female.

Second, a woman who is physically abused by a man is generally intimidated: she fears that he will use his power and control over her in some fashion. Men, however, generally report that they do not live in fear of their wives.

Causes of Domestic Violence
There is no single explanation for why people tend to be abusive in relationships. Although alcohol abuse is often associated with such violence, marital dissatisfaction is also a predictor.[25] Numerous studies also point to differences in the communication patterns between abusive and nonabusive relationships.[26] While some argue that the hormone testosterone causes male aggression, studies have failed to show a strong association between physical abuse in relationships and this hormone.[27] Many experts believe that men who engage in severe violence are more likely than other men to suffer from personality disorders.[28] Clearly, more research is needed to understand abusive relationships.

Regardless of the cause, it is the dynamics that both people bring to a relationship that result in violence and allow it to continue. Community support and counseling services can help determine underlying problems and allow the victim and batterer to break the cycle. The Assess Yourself box on page 120 may help you determine if you are involved in an abusive relationship.

Child Abuse and Neglect
Children raised in families in which domestic violence and/or sexual abuse occur are at great risk for damage to personal health and well-being. The effects of such violent acts are powerful and long lasting. **Child abuse** refers to the systematic harm of a child by a caregiver, generally a parent.[29] The abuse may be sexual,

child abuse The systematic harming of a child by a caregiver, typically a parent.

neglect Failure to provide for a child's basic needs such as food, shelter, medical care, and clothing.

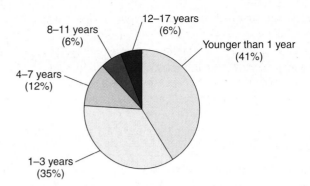

FIGURE 4.5 Child Abuse and Neglect Fatalities, by Age, 2002

Source: Bureau of Justice Statistics, "National Child Abuse and Neglect Data," 2002, http://nccanch.acf.hhf.gov/pubs/factsheets/fatality.cfm.

psychological, physical, or any combination of these. Although exact figures are lacking, many experts believe that nearly a million cases of child abuse and neglect occur every year in the United States, involving severe injury, permanent disability, or death.[30]

Neglect includes failure to provide for a child's basic needs for food, shelter, clothing, medical care, education, or proper supervision. How serious is the problem (Figure 4.5)? In 2004, 2.6 million reports concerning the welfare of approximately 4.5 million children were made to child protective services agencies in the United States.[31] In about two-thirds of these cases, sufficient abuse was detected to prompt investigation, resulting in over 896,000 cases, or 2,450 cases per day![32] Of these cases, 60 percent of victims experienced neglect.

There is no single profile of a perpetrator of fatal child abuse. Frequently, the perpetrator is a young adult in his or her midtwenties without a high school diploma, living at or below the poverty level, depressed, socially isolated, who has a poor self-image, and may have difficulty coping with stressful situations. In many instances, the perpetrator has experienced violence and is frustrated by life. Most fatalities from *physical abuse* are caused by fathers and other male caretakers. Mothers are most often held responsible for deaths resulting from *neglect*. However, in some cases this may be because women are the ones who spend the most time with the children and whom society deems responsible for their care. Though it is difficult to measure long-term consequences of abuse, an average of nearly 4 children die every day as a result of abuse or neglect.[33]

Child Sexual Abuse
Sexual abuse of children by adults or older children includes sexually suggestive conversations; inappropriate kissing; touching; petting; oral, anal, or vaginal intercourse; and other kinds of sexual interaction. The child may not understand these actions, and cannot give informed consent. The most frequent abusers are a child's parents or the companions or spouses of the child's parents. Next most frequent are grandfathers and siblings. Girls are more commonly abused than boys, although young boys are also frequent victims, usually of male family members. Between

20 and 30 percent of all adult women report having had an unwanted childhood sexual encounter with an adult male, usually a father, uncle, brother, or grandfather.[34] Perpetrators appear to be normal people, and are impossible to pick out by sight or behavior alone. There is much controversy surrounding sex offender databases that make offenders' identity known to neighbors, prospective employers, and other individuals.

Most sexual abuse occurs in the child's home. The following situations raise the risk:[35]

1. The child lives without one of his or her biological parents.
2. The mother is unavailable because she is disabled, ill, or working outside the home.
3. The parents' marriage is unhappy.
4. The child has a poor relationship with his or her parents or is subjected to extremely punitive discipline.
5. The child lives with a stepfather.

People who were abused as children bear spiritual, psychological, and/or physical scars. To appreciate the impact of child abuse on later life, studies have shown that children who experience maltreatment and abuse are at increased risk for risky adult behaviors such as smoking, alcoholism, drug abuse, eating disorders, mental health problems, and suicide.[36]

Parents and caretakers of children should be aware of behavioral changes that may signal sexual abuse:[37]

- Noticeable fear of a certain person or place
- Unusual or unexpected response when the child is asked if he or she has been touched by someone
- Unreasonable fear of a physical exam
- Drawings that show sexual acts
- Abrupt changes in behavior, such as bed-wetting
- Sudden or unusual awareness of genitals or sexual acts
- Attempts to get other children to perform sexual acts

Not all child violence is physical. Health can be severely affected by psychological violence—assaults on personality, character, competence, independence, or general dignity as a human being. The negative consequences of this kind of victimization can be harder to discern and therefore harder to combat. They include depression, low self-esteem, and a pervasive fear of offending the abuser.

Sexual Victimization

As with all forms of violence, men and women alike are susceptible to sexual victimization. However, sexual violence against women is of epidemic proportions, so we will focus on women. Physical battering and emotional abuse often leave psychological as well as physical scars. One-quarter to one-third of high school and college students report involve-

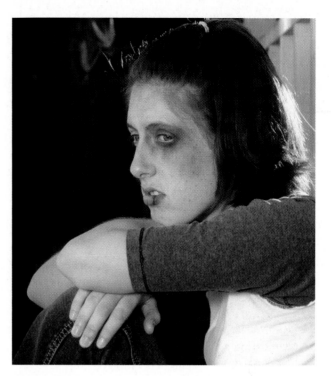

Despite obvious physical and psychological injury, it can be difficult for a person to leave an abusive partner.

ment in dating violence as perpetrators, victims, or both.[38]

Sexual Assault and Rape

Sexual assault is any act in which one person is sexually intimate with another person without that person's consent. This may range from simple touching to forceful penetration and may include such things as ignoring indications that intimacy is not wanted, threatening force or other negative consequences, and actually using force. Nearly six out of ten rapes and sexual assaults are reported by victims as occurring in their own or a friend's home.[39]

Rape **Rape**, the most extreme form of sexual assault, is defined as "penetration without the victim's consent."[40]

(Text continues on page 122)

sexual abuse of children Sexual interaction between a child and an adult or older child; includes, but is not limited to, sexually suggestive conversations, inappropriate kissing, touching, petting, and oral, anal, or vaginal intercourse.

sexual assault Any act in which one person is sexually intimate with another person without that person's consent.

rape Sexual penetration without the victim's consent.

ASSESS *yourself*

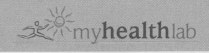

RELATIONSHIP VIOLENCE: ARE YOU AT RISK?

Fill out this assessment online at www.aw-bc.com/myhealthlab or www.aw-bc.com/donatelle.

Although we all want to have healthy relationships, many of us get caught in patterns of behavior that are a direct result of things we've learned or haven't learned in our past. Sometimes we don't even recognize that we are acting inappropriately; other times we know we should act in a particular way, but we get caught up in our own emotions and act out in ways that are physically or emotionally abusive to others. If you have been a victim of emotional or physical violence, you may have become so used to certain behaviors that you might not recognize them as inappropriate. To prevent violence, we have to be able to recognize it, deal with it in appropriate ways, and/or take action to avoid it. One place to start is to examine our intimate interpersonal relationships. Answer the following questions about your current or past relationships.

How often does your partner:

	Never	Sometimes	Often
1. Criticize you for your appearance (weight, dress, hair, etc.)?	❑	❑	❑
2. Embarrass you in front of others by putting you down?	❑	❑	❑
3. Blame you or others for his or her mistakes?	❑	❑	❑
4. Curse at you, say mean things, or mock you?	❑	❑	❑
5. Demonstrate uncontrollable anger?	❑	❑	❑
6. Criticize your friends, family, or others who are close to you?	❑	❑	❑
7. Threaten to leave you if you don't behave in a certain way?	❑	❑	❑
8. Manipulate you to prevent you from spending time with friends or family?	❑	❑	❑
9. Express jealousy, distrust, and anger when you spend time with other people?	❑	❑	❑
10. Tell you that you are crazy, irrational, or paranoid?	❑	❑	❑
11. Call you names to make you lose confidence in yourself?	❑	❑	❑
12. Make all the significant decisions in your relationship?	❑	❑	❑
13. Intimidate or threaten you, making you fearful or anxious?	❑	❑	❑
14. Make threats to harm others you care about?	❑	❑	❑
15. Prevent you from going out by taking your car keys?	❑	❑	❑
16. Control your telephone calls, listen in on your messages, or read your e-mail?	❑	❑	❑
17. Punch, hit, slap, or kick you?	❑	❑	❑
18. Gossip about you to turn others against you or make them think bad things about you?	❑	❑	❑
19. Make you feel guilty about something?	❑	❑	❑
20. Use money or possessions to control you?	❑	❑	❑
21. Force you to have sex or perform sexual acts that make you uncomfortable?	❑	❑	❑
22. Threaten to kill himself or herself if you leave?	❑	❑	❑
23. Control your money and make you ask for what you need?	❑	❑	❑
24. Set many rules that you must abide by?	❑	❑	❑
25. Follow you, call to check on you, or demonstrate a constant obsession with what you are doing?	❑	❑	❑

Interpreting Your Score

Now look at your responses to the above questions. If you answered "sometimes" to one or more of these questions, you may be at risk for emotional or physical abuse. If you answered "often" to any question, you may need to talk with someone about immediate threats to your emotional or physical health. Typically, such potentially abusive patterns only get worse over time as a person gains control and power in a relationship. If you are anxious about talking to your partner, seek counseling through your campus counseling center,

student health center, or community services. If you don't know where to go, ask your professor for possible options.

After you have completed the test about your partner's behavior, you should ask the same questions about your own behavior. If any of the questions describe your actions in a relationship, you should seek help to change these behavioral patterns. These actions are not conducive to healthy relationships and may result in harm to you or your loved ones. Seek help now to insure healthier relationships in the future.

MAKE it happen!

ASSESSMENT: The Assess Yourself activity gave you a chance to consider symptoms of abuse. If any of the symptoms describe a relationship experienced by you or someone you know, you should consider taking action.

MAKING A CHANGE: In order to change your behavior, you need to develop a plan. Follow the steps below and complete your Behavior Change Contract to take action.

1. Evaluate your behavior and identify patterns and specific things you are doing. What can you change now? What can you change in the near future?

2. Select one pattern of behavior that you want to change.

3. Fill out the Behavior Change Contract found at the front of your book. It should include your long-term goal for change, your short-term goals, the rewards you'll give yourself for reaching these goals, potential obstacles along the way, and strategies for overcoming these obstacles. For each goal, list the small steps and specific actions that you will take.

4. Chart your progress in a journal. At the end of a week, consider how successful you were in following your plan. What helped you be successful? What made change more difficult? What will you do differently next week?

5. Revise your plan as needed: Are the short-term goals attainable? Are the rewards satisfying?

ONE STUDENT'S PLAN Sondra thought that her roommate Jessie was experiencing several symptoms of abuse. Jessie's boyfriend Carl sometimes belittled her in front of her friends. He once broke her cell phone by throwing it against a wall toward Jessie and seemed resentful when she spent time with anyone but him. When Sondra talked to Jessie about her perceptions, Jessie was surprised and very defensive at first. The more she thought about it, though, she realized that sometimes she was afraid of Carl's actions. She started to consider what she could do about the situation. As a first step, Sondra helped Jessie make immediate appointments at the school counseling center, one for herself and one for her and Carl together.

Whether committed by an acquaintance, a date, or a stranger, rape is a criminal activity that usually has serious emotional, psychological, social, and physical consequences for the victim. Typically, victims are young females, with 29 percent under 11 years of age, 32 percent between the ages of 11 and 17, and 22 percent between the ages of 18 and 24.[41] Women aged 16 to 19 are four times as likely as the general population to be rape victims.[42]

One of the most startling aspects of sex crimes is how many go unreported, usually out of a belief that this is a private matter, fear of reprisal by the assailant, or unwarranted feelings of guilt and responsibility. It is thought that one out of every three women is the victim of an attempted or completed rape in her lifetime. Although as many as two-thirds of all rapes are never reported, there were over 683,000 reported cases of rape, attempted rape, or sexual assault in 2003.[43]

Incidents of rape generally fall into one of two types—aggravated or simple. An **aggravated rape** involves multiple attackers, strangers, weapons, or physical beatings. A **simple rape** is perpetrated by one person, whom the victim knows, and does not involve a physical beating or use of a weapon. Most incidents are classified as simple rapes, with one report suggesting that 82 percent of female rape victims have been victimized by acquaintances (53 percent), current or former boyfriends (16 percent), current or former spouses (10 percent), or other relatives (3 percent). With almost half of all rape charges dismissed before the cases reach trial and a perceived lack of male understanding of how rape affects women, it's easy to understand why experts feel that so-called "simple" rape is seriously underreported and ignored.

Acquaintance or Date Rape

Although the terms *date rape, friendship rape,* and *acquaintance rape* have become standard terminology, they are typically misused. Not all rapes occur on dates, not all the relationships are friendships, and sometimes the term *acquaintance* is used all too loosely. Many acquaintance rapes occur as the result of incidental contact at a party or when groups of people congregate at one person's house. These are crimes of opportunity, not necessarily a prearranged date. This is an important distinction because the term *date* suggests some type of reciprocal interaction arranged in advance. Whereas most date or acquaintance rapes happen to women aged 15 to 24 years, the 18-year-old new college student is the most likely victim. We'll talk more about dating violence later in this chapter.[44]

Consider the following:[45]

■ Eighty-four percent of rapes on college campuses are acquaintance rapes. Fifty-seven percent of these assaults occurred while on a date.

---

aggravated rape   Rape that involves multiple attackers, strangers, weapons, or physical beating.

simple rape   Rape by one person known to the victim that does not involve physical beating or use of a weapon.

■ Sexual coercion and aggression may occur at any stage of a relationship.
■ Acquaintance rape tends to occur on weekends, on the rapist's "turf," and may include verbal and physical force.
■ Alcohol and drugs are often involved.

Date rape is not simply miscommunication; it is an act of violence. Well-known expert on interpersonal relationships Susan Jacoby puts it this way:

Some women (especially the young) initially resist sex not out of real conviction, but as part of the elaborate persuasion and seduction rituals accompanying what was once called courtship. And it is true that many men (again, especially the young) take pride in their ability to coax a woman further than she intended to go. But these mating rituals do not justify or even explain date rape. Even the most callow youth is capable of understanding the difference between resistance and genuine fear; between a halfhearted "no, we shouldn't" and tears or screams.[46]

Marital Rape

Although the legal definition of marital rape varies within the United States, marital rape can be defined as any unwanted intercourse or penetration (vaginal, anal, or oral) obtained by force, threat of force, or when the wife is unable to consent.[47] Some researchers estimate that marital rape may account for 25 percent of all rapes; rape in marriage may be an extremely prevalent form of sexual violence.

Although this problem has undoubtedly existed since the origin of marriage as a social institution, it is noteworthy that marital rape did not become a crime in all 50 states until 1993. Even more noteworthy is the fact that in 33 states there are still exemptions from rape prosecution, meaning that the judicial system may treat it as a lesser crime.

Who is most vulnerable to marital rape? In general, women under the age of 25 and those from lower socioeconomic groups are at highest risk. Women from homes where other forms of domestic violence are common and where there is a high rate of alcoholism and/or substance abuse also tend to be victimized at greater rates. Women who are subjected to marital rape often report multiple offenses over a period of time; these events are likely to be forced anal and oral experiences.[48]

Again, abuse of power and a need to control and dominate seem to be key factors in the husband-rapist profile. Marital rape can have devastating short- and long-term consequences for women, including injuries to the vaginal and anal areas, lacerations, soreness, bruising, torn muscles, fatigue, panic attacks, sexually transmitted diseases, broken bones, wounds, and other emotional and physical scars.

Social Contributors to Sexual Assault

According to many experts, certain common assumptions in our society prevent recognition by both the perpetrator and the wider public of the true nature of sexual assault.[49] These assumptions include the following:

- *Minimization.* It is often assumed that sexual assault of women is rare because official crime statistics, including the Uniform Crime Reports of the FBI, show very few rapes per thousand population. However, rape is the most underreported of all serious crimes. Researchers have found that nearly 25 percent of women in the United States have been raped.
- *Trivialization.* Incredibly enough, sexual assault of women is still often viewed as a jocular matter. During a gubernatorial election in Texas a few years back, one of the candidates reportedly compared a bad patch of weather to rape: "If there's nothing you can do about it, just lie back and enjoy it." (He lost the election—to a woman.)
- *Blaming the victim.* Many discussions of sexual violence against women display a sometimes unconscious assumption that the woman did something to provoke the attack—that she flirted or dressed revealingly, for example.
- *"Boys will be boys."* According to this assumption, men just can't control themselves once they become aroused.

Over the years, psychologists and others have proposed several theories to explain why many males sexually victimize women. In one of the first major studies to explore this issue, almost two-thirds of the male respondents had engaged in intercourse unwanted by the woman, primarily because of male peer pressure.[50] By all indicators, these trends continue today. Peer pressure is certainly a strong factor, but a growing body of research suggests that sexual assault is encouraged by the socialization processes that males experience daily.

- *Male socialization.* Throughout our lives, we are exposed to social norms that objectify women—make them appear as objects that can be used. Media portrayals of half-dressed and undressed women in seductive poses promoting products, for instance, contribute to sex-role stereotyping. These portrayals often show males as aggressors and females as targets. In addition, men are exposed from an early age to antifemale jokes and vulgar and obscene terms for women. These reinforce the idea that females are lesser beings who may be pushed around with impunity. Males are also discouraged from acting in ways that society views as feminine. They are told to act tough and unemotional; strive for power, status, and control; be aggressive and take risks. Violence against women is not a phenomenon that is unique to America. See the Women's Health/Men's Health box on page 124.
- *Male attitudes.* Several studies have confirmed a greater tolerance of rape among men who accept the myth that rape is something women secretly desire, who believe in adversarial relationships between men and women, who condone violence against women, or who hold traditional attitudes toward sex roles. Such men are apt to blame the victim and more likely to commit rape themselves if they think they can get away with it.
- *Male sexual history and hostility.* Most rapists do not appear abnormal or psychologically disturbed. They

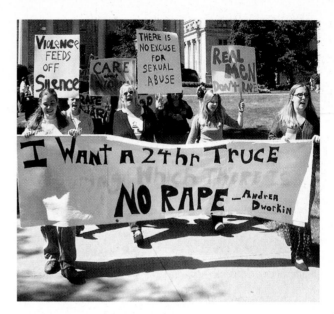

College students can organize vigils, marches, and educational programs to raise awareness about violence against women.

typically are employed, often married with families, and have a history of multiple sexual experiences (both forced and voluntary) during childhood. Many feel hostility toward women.

- *Male misperceptions.* Men who are convinced that women really want sex even if they say they don't are more likely to perpetrate sexual assaults. They more readily misinterpret a woman's words and behavior and act on their misperceptions—only to be surprised later when the woman says that she has been assaulted.
- *Situational factors.* Several factors increase the likelihood of sexual assault. Dates in which the male makes all the decisions, pays, drives, and in general controls what happens are more likely to end in aggression. Alcohol and drug use increase the risk and severity of assault. Length of relationship is another important situational factor: the more long-standing the relationship, the greater the chance of aggression. Finally, males who belong to a close-knit social group involving intense interaction are more prone to engage in a peer-pleasing assault.

Crime on Campus

It is not unusual for parents to send their sons and daughters away to colleges and universities with some trepidation. Parents worry that their children will have trouble adjusting to college life, drink too much and party too hard, and not eat right or sleep enough. Few parents realize that the 16 million students enrolled in some 4,200 colleges and universities in the United States also face risks from campus violence that can cause significant physical and mental problems for their children. The term *campus violence* include acts of physical violence such as homicide, suicide, rape, assault, dating violence, harassment and stalking, hazing, and hate crimes.[51]

GENDER VIOLENCE: A GLOBAL PHENOMENON

Over the last decade, the issue of gender violence, or violence against women, has increasingly captured the world's attention. Sexual, physical, and psychological violence are believed to cause as much ill health and death among women aged 15 to 44 as cancer and more than malaria and traffic accidents combined. Although men and women are both affected by violence, women bear a disproportionate burden. Consider the following facts:

- Globally, the World Health Organization believes that at least one woman in five has been physically or sexually abused by a man at some time in her life, usually by a husband, father, or neighbor rather than a stranger.
- Forty-eight surveys on intimate partner violence around the world asked respondents whether a partner had ever hit them with his fist or other object that could hurt them; 10 to 69 percent of women answered "yes."
- Studies in Mexico and the United States indicate that 40 to 52 percent of women who have been physically abused have also been sexually assaulted.
- Many large studies indicated that the victims had never told anyone about the violence they experienced. In Canada, 22 percent of women had remained silent before being queried for a study; in Chile, 30 percent; in Nicaragua, 37 percent; in the United Kingdom, 38 percent; in Egypt, 47 percent; and in Bangladesh, 68 percent.
- In many countries, women whose husbands beat them feel it is justified; in Egypt, as many as 81 percent felt this way.
- Recent research in the United Kingdom found that 50 percent of boys and 33 percent of girls thought it was OK to hit a woman or force her to have sex in certain circumstances, and 36 percent of boys thought they might personally hit a woman or force her to have sex.
- According to several researchers, physical and sexual abuse lie behind some of the most intractable reproductive health issues of our times: unwanted pregnancies, HIV and other sexually transmitted infections, and complications from pregnancy.

What do you think about each of these statistics? What factors contribute to them? How do societal values and beliefs contribute to global violence against women? Who are the most likely victims? What actions can be taken to reduce the rate of violence?

Source: World Health Organization, "The WHO Multi-Country Study on Women's Health and Domestic Violence Against Women," 2004, www.who.int/gender/violence/multicountry/en.

Consider the following facts on campus violence:[52]

- Approximately one out of every 14 men in the United States have been physically assaulted or raped by an intimate partner.
- Simple assault accounted for about two-thirds of college student violent crimes (63 percent), while rape or sexual assault accounted for 6 percent.
- Only about 5 percent of completed and attempted rapes committed against students are ever reported to the police.
- Nearly 80 percent of all rapes on campus are by persons the victim knows.
- Alcohol and other drugs are implicated in 55–74 percent of sexual assaults on campus.
- Approximately 93 percent of crimes against students occurred at off-campus locations.
- More than 36 percent of lesbian, gay, bisexual, and transgender (LGBT) students have experienced harassment within the last year.
- Non-Hispanic whites were more likely than any other races to be victims of overall violence or simple assault.

Black students were somewhat more likely than white students to suffer a simple assault.

However, these statistics represent only the tip of the iceberg. The sad fact is that fewer than 25 percent of campus crimes are reported to *any* authority.[53] Why would students fail to report such crimes? Typical reasons include concerns over privacy, embarrassment or shame, lack of support, perception that the crime was too minor, or uncertainty that it was a crime.

In 1992, Congress passed the Campus Sexual Assault Victim's Bill of Rights, known as the Ramstad Act. The act gives victims the right to call in off-campus authorities to investigate serious campus crimes. In addition, universities must set up educational programs and notify students of available counseling. More recent provisions of the act specify received notification procedures and options for victims, rights of victims and the accused perpetrators, and consequences if schools do not comply. It also requires the Department of Education to publish campus crime statistics annually.

Sexual Violence on Campus

Sexual Harassment **Sexual harassment** is defined as unwelcome sexual conduct that is related to any condition of employment or evaluation of student performance. It includes unwarranted sex-related comments, sexually explicit comments or graphics, unwelcome touching, and so forth.[54] Although often not thought of as harassment by many, making derogatory jokes based on sex or appearance, speaking in crude or offensive language, spreading rumors about a person's sexuality, placing compromising photos on the Web, or ogling are common forms of sexual harassment. Commonly, people only think of harassment as involving faculty members or persons in power, where sex is used to exhibit control of a situation. However, peers can harass one another too. Harassment can occur at many levels and can be extremely detrimental to those who are involved. Although exact numbers of cases of sexual harassment are difficult to determine, it is widely perceived to be a major problem on college campuses, forcing administrators to enact strict guidelines about interpersonal relationships between students and instructors or coworkers.

It's always important to watch what you say and how you say it. Learning now what constitutes sexual harassment may save you embarrassment or worse in the future. A simple compliment on someone's appearance can be offensive if stated without sensitivity, regardless of the intent. "You look very nice today" can become offensive if stated as, "That dress looks great on your body." Even if the person enjoys your comment, remember that others may overhear.

Most schools and companies have sexual harassment policies in place, as well as procedures for dealing with it. If you feel you are being harassed, the most important thing you can do is be assertive. Immediately after the incident occurs, follow the guidelines in Table 4.1.

what do you THINK?

What policies does your school have regarding consensual relationships between faculty members and students? ■ Should consenting adults have the right to interact, regardless of their positions within a system or workplace? ■ What are the potential dangers of such interactions?

Sexual Assault Earlier in this chapter, you learned about rape and sexual assault. Rape, acquaintance rape, sodomy, unwanted touching, and other forms of sexual assault occur daily on campuses throughout the United States and, like other forms of violence, these crimes have particularly high rates of nonreporting.[55] Sexual assault often involves force sufficient to cause serious injury, and psychological trauma may be substantial. A recent survey of college students found that the incidence of rape and attempted rape within the last academic year was 5.2 percent among women. The majority of sexual assaults occurred in living quarters.[56] Results of sexual assaults vary considerably between studies;

TABLE 4.1	Strategies for Preventing or Stopping Harassment
Tell the harasser to stop	Be clear and direct about what is bothering you and why you are upset.
Document the harassment	Make a record of the incident. If the harassment becomes intolerable, a record of exactly what occurred (and when and where) will help make your case.
Complain to a higher authority	Talk to your instructor, adviser, or counseling center about what happened. If they don't take you seriously, investigate your school's internal grievance procedures.
Remember that you have not done anything wrong	You will likely feel awful after being harassed (especially if you have to complain to superiors). However, feel proud that you are not keeping silent. The person who is harassing you is wrong, not you.

however, over the years, college men have consistently acknowledged forced intercourse at a rate of 5–15 percent and college sexual aggression at a rate of 15–25 percent.[57]

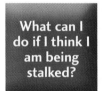

What can I do if I think I am being stalked?

Stalking The conduct directed at a specific person that involves repeated visual or physical proximity, nonconsensual communication that is written or verbal, and may imply threats is known as **stalking**.[58] Victims of stalking tend to be undergraduate students who are the same age as the stalker, know the stalker, and live alone. The most common form of stalking and that which poses the greatest risk of violence occurs following the termination of romantic relationships.[59] However, stalking may be more subtle, particularly with the use of modern technology. For example, cell-phone stalkers can keep track of a victim's actions by calling repeatedly to ask about the victim's current location and companions, and other seemingly harmless checks on activity. If this persists, the person experiencing it should let the caller know it's not appropriate behavior and ask him or her to stop calling. Although stalking occurs in virtually all populations, research suggests that stalking victimization rates may be higher among female college students than in the general population.[60]

sexual harassment Any form of unwanted sexual attention.

stalking The willful, repeated, and malicious following, harassing, or threatening of another person.

TABLE 4.2	Reducing Your Risk of Dating Violence

Remember that if a potential romantic partner truly cares for you and respects you, that person will respect your wishes and feelings. Here are some tips for dealing with sexual pressure or unwanted advances when dating:

- Before you go out on your date, think about your values, and set personal boundaries before you go out the door.
- Watch your alcohol consumption. Drinking might get you into situations you'd otherwise avoid.
- Practice communicating what you will say to your date if things are going in a direction you are uncomfortable with. You have the right to express your feelings and it is okay to be assertive.
- Do not be swayed by arguments such as, "What about my feelings?", "You were leading me on" and "If you really cared about me, you would."

Researchers suggest several reasons for stalking: (1) stalkers may have deficits in social skills; (2) they are young and have not yet learned how to deal with complex social relationships and situations; (3) they may not realize that their behavior is considered stalking; (4) they have a flexible schedule and free time; and (5) they are not accountable to authority figures for their daily activities.[61] How prevalent is stalking on campus? As with other violent acts, stalking behaviors are believed to be widely underreported; however, estimates are that between 25 and 30 percent of college women and between 11 and 17 percent of college men have been stalked.[62]

Campus Dating Violence

Actual or threatened physical or sexual violence or psychological and emotional abuse directed toward a current or former dating partner is known as campus dating violence. Table 4.2 details tips for safe dating. Intimate partners may be heterosexual, bisexual, or homosexual.[63] Often with intimate partner violence, it is repetitive and victims do not readily seek help. Studies of campus dating violence indicate that 15 percent of women and 9.2 percent of men reported being in emotionally abusive relationships during the last year, and 2.4 percent of women and 1.3 percent of men reported physically abusive relationships. Sexually abusive relationships were reported by 1.7 percent of women and 1.0 percent of men.[64] Like many forms of campus violence, alcohol use is frequently involved. (See the Spotlight on Your Health box.)

Reducing Your Risk

After a violent act is committed against someone we know, we acknowledge the horror of the event, express sympathy, and go on with our lives—but the person who has been brutalized may take months or years to recover. It is far better to prevent a violent act than to recover from it.

Self-Defense against Rape

Rape can occur no matter what preventive actions you take, but commonsense tactics can lower the risk. Self-defense is a process that includes increased awareness of your surroundings, learning self-defense techniques, taking reasonable precautions, and having the self-confidence and judgment needed to determine appropriate responses to different situations.

Taking Control Most rapes by unknown assailants are planned in advance. They are frequently preceded by a casual, friendly conversation. Although many women have said that they started to feel uneasy during this conversation, they denied the possibility of an attack to themselves until it was too late. Listen to your feelings and trust your intuition. Be assertive and direct to someone who is getting out of line or threatening—this may convince the would-be rapist to back off. Stifle your tendency to be "nice," and don't fear making a scene. Let him know that you mean what you say and are prepared to defend yourself. Consider the following:

- *Speak in a strong voice.* Use statements such as "Leave me alone" rather than questions like "Will you please leave me alone?" Sound like you mean it. Avoid apologies and excuses.
- *Maintain eye contact with the would-be attacker.*
- *Stand up straight, act confident, and remain alert.* Walk as if you own the sidewalk.

Many rapists use certain ploys to initiate their attacks. Among the most common are:

- *Request for help.* This allows him to get close—to enter your house to use the phone, for instance.
- *Offer of help.* This can also help him gain entrance to your home: "Let me help you carry that package."
- *Guilt trip.* "Gee, no one is friendly nowadays. I can't believe you won't talk with me for just a little while."
- *Deliberate accident.* He may bump into the back of your car, and then assault you when you get out to see the damage. Don't stop unless you have to in these situations, and if you do stop, stay in your car with the doors locked.
- *Authority.* Many women fall for the old "policeman at the door" ruse. If anyone comes to your door or vehicle dressed in uniform, ask him or her to show an ID before you unlock the door. You can also call the police department to confirm the ID.

If you are attacked, act immediately. Don't worry about causing a scene. You want to draw attention to yourself and your assailant. Scream "Fire!" loudly. Research has shown that passersby are much more likely to help if they hear the word fire rather than just a scream or calls using the word help. Your attacker may also be caught off balance by the action.

SPOTLIGHT on your health

DRUG-FACILITATED RAPES: ROHYPNOL AND OTHER DANGERS

Approximately 20–25 percent of women in colleges and universities across the United States have either been raped or endured an attempted rape, according to reported incidents alone.*

Of the over 600,000 sexual assaults and rapes that occur each year in the United States, many involve drugs or alcohol. In the late 1990s rape crisis centers became alarmed over reports of drugs being used to immobilize victims and make them unable to defend themselves from sexual attacks. These "date rape" drugs are typically slipped into the drinks of unsuspecting women, who wake up after being raped and can remember few details of the assault. Two of the most common drugs used are Rohypnol and GHB. Although these drugs are often called "date rape" drugs, their use is often unrelated to a date. Many times, they are slipped into the drinks of women whose only interface with the male perpetrator is to be bought a drink at a bar or handed a drink at a party. There is no date involved—just an opportunity to gain control and remove any chance of resistance.

Although not approved for sale in the United States, Rohypnol (flunitrazepam) is widely available in other countries as a sleep aid. Street names for it include Roaches, LaRocha, rope, Rib Roche, Roches, roofies, Ruffies, Mexican Valium, and roach-2. When dissolved in a drink, Rohypnol produces a sedative-hypnotic effect that includes muscle relaxation and amnesia. Generally, sedative effects occur within 20 to 30 minutes and incapacitation within 1 to 2 hours, often lasting for hours. People who take it may appear drunk or sleepy, dizzy, or confused. Tablets are white and contain the name "Roche" and an encircled "1" or "2" on one side indicating dosage. The manufacturer has now released a new, lower dose blue tablet designed to be impossible to slip into a drink without detection. Tests to determine if Rohypnol has been administered are available at rape crisis centers and emergency rooms, and through law enforcement agencies.

GHB (gamma-hydroxybutyrate) is known as Liquid E, Liquid Ecstasy, Liquid X, Grievous Bodily Harm, and Easy First. Illicitly used for its euphoric, sedative, and anabolic (bodybuilding) effects, today GHB is more commonly used than Rohypnol in sexual assaults. GHB is usually a colorless, odorless liquid that may taste salty. Used as a surgical anesthetic in Europe, it is not legal in the United States and can induce short-term coma, slowed heart rate, decreased breathing, seizures, and death.

Another drug that has recently appeared and that causes similar reactions is Burundanga, a light yellow powder that has no taste and takes effect immediately. Burundanga affects the central nervous system and can be highly dangerous.

Each year, there are several deaths from these rape-facilitating drugs. Survivors must cope with the fact that they have been violated without a chance to defend themselves. To reduce your risk, follow these guidelines:

- Do not accept drinks from strangers. In fact, do not take any beverages or open-container drinks from anyone you do not know well and trust.
- Never leave a drink unattended. If you get up to dance, have someone watch your drink or take it with you.
- At a bar or club, accept drinks only from the bartender or wait staff. Watch the bartender pour the drink and keep the drink in sight until it's in your hand.
- Be alert to the behavior of friends. If they seem disproportionately "out of it" in relation to what they've had to drink, stay with them and watch them carefully.
- Go out with friends and leave with friends. Make a rule never to leave a bar or party with someone you don't know well.
- If you think you may have been slipped something in a drink, tell a friend and have him or her get you to an emergency room. Call 911 if anyone appears to be unusually "out of it" or experiences seizures, difficulty breathing, or other complications.

Sources: National Institute of Drug Abuse, "NIDA Info Facts: Rohypnol and GHB," July 15, 2005, www.nida.nih.gov/infofax/RohypnolGHB.html; *B. S. Fisher, F. T. Cullen, and M. G. Turner, *The Sexual Victimization of College Women*, National Institute of Justice Publication No. NCJ 182369 (Washington, DC: Department of Justice (US), 2000).

To prevent an attack, remember the following points:

- *Always be vigilant.* Rapes occur in even the safest cities and towns, day or night. Don't be fooled by a sleepy-little-town atmosphere.
- *Use campus escort services whenever possible.*
- *Be assertive in demanding a well-lit campus.*
- *Don't use the same routes all the time.* Vary your movement patterns.
- *Don't leave a bar alone with a friendly stranger.* Stay with your friends, and look out for each other. Invite the stranger to hang out with your group of friends. Don't give your address to anyone you don't know.
- *Let friends and family know where you are going, what route you'll take, and when to expect your return.*
- *Stay close to others.* Avoid shortcuts through dark or unlit paths. Don't be the last one to leave the lab or library late at night. Be alert in parking lots and garages.
- *Keep your windows and doors locked.* Don't open the door to strangers.

What to Do if a Rape Occurs

If you are a rape victim, report the attack. This gives you a sense of control, and increases the chance the perpetrator will be caught. Follow these steps:

- Call 911 (if a phone is available).
- Do not bathe, shower, douche, clean up, or touch anything the attacker may have touched.
- Save the clothes you were wearing, and do not launder them. They will be needed as evidence.
- Bring a clean change of clothes to the clinic or hospital.
- Contact the rape assistance hotline in your area, and ask for advice on therapists or counseling if you need additional help or advice.

If a friend is raped, here's how you can help:

- Believe her. Don't ask questions that may appear to implicate her in the assault.
- Recognize that rape is a violent act and the victim was not looking for this to happen.
- Encourage her to see a doctor immediately. She may have medical needs but feel too embarrassed to seek help on her own. Offer to go with her.
- Encourage her to report the crime.
- Be understanding, and let her know you will be there for her.
- Recognize that this is an emotional recovery, and it may take six months to a year for her to bounce back.
- Encourage her to seek counseling.

A Campuswide Response to Violence

Can my university do anything to help me feel safer?

Increasingly, college campuses have become microcosms of the greater society, complete with the risks, hazards, and dangers people face in the world. Many college administrators have been proactive in establishing violence prevention policies, programs, and services. College administrators have also begun to examine the culture that promotes violent acts and tolerance for it.[65]

Changing Roles

To increase student protection, campus law enforcement has changed over the years in both numbers and authority to prosecute student offenders. Campus police are responsible for emergency responses to situations that threaten overall safety, human resources, the general campus environment, traffic and bicycle safety, and other dangers. They have the power to enforce laws with students in the same way they are handled in the general community. In fact, many campuses now hire state troopers or local law enforcement officers to deal with campus issues rather than maintain a separate police staff.

Many of these law enforcement groups follow a *community policing* model in which officers have specific responsibilities for certain areas of campus, departments, or events. By narrowing the scope of each officer's territory, officers get to know people in the area and are better able to anticipate and prevent risks. This differs from earlier policies, in which campus security typically swooped down only in times of trouble.

Prevention Efforts

Many universities now hire crime prevention and safety specialists. They commonly recommend the following activities:

- A rape awareness and education program for members of the campus community.
- A crime prevention orientation program for new faculty and staff, as well as students.
- Specialized safety workshops for particular groups, such as commuters, international students, athletes, and students with disabilities.
- Printed and electronic educational messages about personal safety.
- A notification process to distribute information about special hazards.
- Alcohol and drug programs dealing with policy, awareness, education, and enforcement.
- A "grounds safety" program, including measures such as installing good lighting and removing shrubs from dark areas.
- Emergency call boxes or telephones across campus.
- Escort services for students who must be out after dark.
- Motorist assistance programs for people with car trouble.
- Antitheft programs, including regular patrols of parking lots and other areas.
- Victim advocacy programs, such as rape and abuse counseling.

The Role of Student Affairs

Although there may be some overlap with law enforcement activities, student affairs offices need to play a vital role in all on-campus programs, both to prevent trouble and to resolve problems that do occur. Student groups should monitor progress, identify potential threats, and advocate for improvements in any areas found to be deficient. A student affairs office can play a key role in making sure that mental health services, student assistance programs, and other services are high quality and easily accessible, and that they meet student needs. A human services or student affairs office should seek to involve the entire student body and ensure that all are aware of its services. Any programs that are not visible or proactive in ensuring campus safety should be evaluated carefully. Student leaders can play a major role in shaping such services and advocating for the campus population.

Community Strategies for Preventing Violence

Because the causes of homicide and assaultive violence are complex, community strategies for prevention must be multi-dimensional. Successful strategies include the following:

- Developing and implementing educational programs to teach people communication, conflict resolution, and coping skills.
- Working with individuals to help them develop self-esteem and respect for others.
- Rewarding youngsters for good behavior, and never spanking a child when angry. (Children need to know that anger is sometimes acceptable, but violence never is. Use family meetings to resolve conflicts.)
- Establishing and enforcing policies that forbid discrimination on the basis of gender, religious affiliation, race, sexual orientation, marital status, and age.
- Increasing and enriching educational programs for family planning.
- Increasing efforts by health care and social service programs to identify victims of violence.
- Improving treatment and support for victims.
- Treating the psychological as well as the physical consequences of violence.

See the Skills for Behavior Change box on page 130 for personal steps you can take to stay safe.

Unintentional Injuries

As stated at the beginning of the chapter, unintentional injuries occur without planning or intention to harm. Examples of unintentional injuries include car accidents, falls, water accidents, accidental gunshots, recreational accidents, and workplace accidents. None of these injuries happen on purpose, yet they may result in pain, suffering, and possibly even death. Most efforts to prevent unintentional injuries focus on changing something about the person, the environment, or the circumstances (policies, procedures) that put people in harm's way.

Residential Safety

Injuries within the home typically take the form of falls, burns, or intrusions by others. Some populations, such as the elderly, are particularly vulnerable. However, the elderly are not the only victims; each year, hundreds of children suffer severe burns or die from accidental fires, falls, and other home-based injuries. To reduce the risk of accidents, consider the following.

Fall-Proof Your Home Falls are a common source of home injury. Eliminate objects you may stumble over,

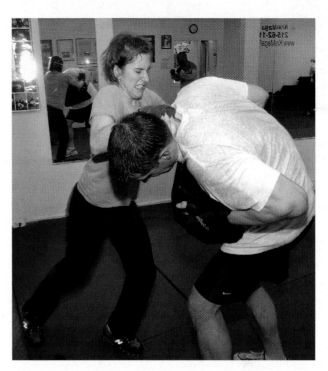

College campuses are increasingly offering safety workshops to equip students with skills to protect themselves from violent acts.

especially in the dark. Take the following measures to prevent falls:

- Eliminate clutter, and don't leave anything lying around on the floor or stairs.
- Fasten all rugs securely to the floor so they don't wrinkle or slide when stepped on. Inexpensive rubberized mats or strips will hold rugs in place.
- Train your pets to stay away from your feet. Many an unsuspecting person has ended up on the floor while trying to avoid a pet.
- Make sure handrails are secure and within easy reach. All stairs should have slip-proof treads.
- Install slip-proof mats or decals in showers and tubs. Add handrails and places to grab for stability in bathtubs and showers.

Avoid Burns Prevent injury from fires, such as burns, and take precautions to prevent fires from starting in the first place. Tips to prevent the risk of fires and related injury include:

- Extinguish all cigarettes in ashtrays before you go to bed.
- Don't smoke and drink before bed. In fact, don't smoke in bed at any time! Sparks can smolder in mattresses or upholstered furniture, and then flare into flames.
- Don't throw spent matches in the trash with combustibles. Soak matches in water before discarding.
- Set lamps away from drapes, linens, and paper, particularly halogen lights or specialty lamps that can get extremely hot.

SKILLS FOR behavior change

TIPS FOR PROTECTING YOURSELF

There are many steps you can take to protect yourself from personal assaults, whether you are home alone or on a date. Implement these steps to increase your awareness and reduce your risk of a violent attack.

WHEN DATING

- Set limits. If the situation feels like it is getting out of control, stop and talk, say no directly, and don't be coy or worry about hurting feelings. Be firm.
- Most rapes are committed by someone you know; if you feel uncomfortable, protect yourself or get away.
- Go out in couples or groups when dating someone new.
- Pay attention to your date's actions. If there is too much teasing and all of the decisions are made for you, it may mean trouble.
- Trust your intuition. Talk and try to get a sense of the person's history with others, what they say were issues with their past relationships, etc.
- Stick with your friends. Agree to keep an eye out for one another at parties, and have a plan for leaving together and checking in with each other.

- Avoid drinking too much. Never accept drinks from strangers and don't leave drinks unattended.

WHEN YOU'RE OUTSIDE ALONE

- Be aware of what is happening around you. Look, listen, and notice what is happening and how close people are to you. Avoid areas where people can lurk in bushes, etc.
- Carry a cell phone, but stay off it. Many people are attacked as they get in their cars or are out walking and on their cells and not paying attention.
- If you are being followed, don't go home. Head for a location where there are other people or if you decide to run, run fast and scream loudly to attract attention.
- Vary your routes; walk or jog with others at a steady pace.
- Park near lights; avoid dark areas where people could hide.
- Carry pepper spray or other deterrents.
- Tell others where you are going and when you expect to be back.

WHILE IN YOUR CAR

- Lock your doors.
- Purchase cars with alarm systems and remote entry with a light that goes on.

- If someone hits your car, stay in your car until help comes. Do not open your doors or windows to strangers.
- Call for help from police or road service.
- Never leave your keys in your vehicle. Have keys ready as you approach your car.
- Never leave a purse, backpack, or packages out in plain view in your car, even if it is locked.
- Be alert to cars that appear to be following you. Do not drive home. Drive to the nearest police station.

WHILE AT HOME

- Check doors and windows. Make sure the locks work.
- Lock doors when at home during the day. Home invasions while residents are home are becoming more common.
- Keep your garage door locked and closed.
- Don't leave a spare key outside or in the garage.
- When you move into a new residence, pay a locksmith to change the keys/locks.
- If your residence is broken into when you aren't home, don't enter—call the police.

- Keep hot pads and kitchen cloths away from stove burners. When not using a cloth, set it on a counter far from the stove.
- Keep candles under control and away from combustibles. Although it may seem romantic to go to sleep by candlelight, it is highly risky. Don't do it.
- Use caution when lighting barbecue grills and other home-based fires. Never spray combustible fluids such as lighter fluid directly onto the fire.
- Check chimneys and fireplaces regularly for buildup of flammable soot.
- Service furnaces annually, and be sure to change the filters.
- Avoid overloading electrical circuits with appliances and cords. Older buildings are at particular risk for fire from such overloads.

- Program phones with emergency numbers for speed dialing, and keep these numbers in clear sight near phones as well.
- Replace batteries in smoke alarms periodically, and test them regularly to make sure the batteries are working.
- Have the proper fire extinguishers ready in case of fire (Figure 4.6).

? *what do you* THINK?

Do a "spot check" of your home. What areas might pose a risk for home accidents or forced entry? ■ Do you know the numbers of your local fire and police departments? ■ Do you have a fire extinguisher in your house? Do you know how to use it? ■ What would you do if the house caught on fire and you needed to escape immediately?

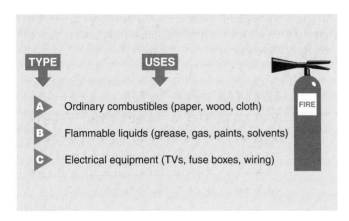

FIGURE 4.6 Do You Have the Right Fire Extinguisher?

Prevent Intruders Take precautions such as the following to ensure your safety at home:

- Close blinds and drapes whenever you are away and in the evening when you are home. Remove large bushes and obstructions from around your windows and doors so that anyone lurking outside will be visible.
- Install dead-bolt locks on all doors and locks on windows. Put a peephole in the main entryway to your home, and do not let anyone in without checking.
- If you have a screen door, lock it. If an unfamiliar visitor comes to the door, this door can serve as a barrier.
- Install a home alarm system.
- Rent apartments that require a security code or clearance to gain entry, and do not distribute that code to friends or delivery people.
- Avoid apartments that are easily accessible, such as first-floor units with large patio doors.
- Don't give information about your home or schedule to telephone solicitors. Try to vary the times of day that you come home for lunch or run errands.
- Don't let repairmen in without identification. Preferably, landlords should inform you about such visits well in advance. Have someone else with you when repairmen are there working. Just because a person is licensed to fix refrigerators does not mean he or she can be trusted.
- Avoid dark parking structures, laundry rooms, and the like. Try to use these areas only when others are around.
- Use initials for first names on mailboxes and in phone listings. Keep your address out of phone books.
- Keep a cell phone near your bed, and program it to 911. Unlike what you see on TV, many intruders do not cut phone lines. More often, they simply pick up the receiver in another room as they walk through, thereby disabling a bedroom phone.
- Get to know your neighbors. Organize a neighborhood watch.
- Be careful of "doggy doors." Some thieves have their smallest associate crawl through and unlock the door.
- Be careful of skylights and other areas that open from the outside. Keep them locked and bolted.

- When away, put the lights in different rooms on timers set to come on and go off at different times. Stop your mail and newspaper deliveries, or ask a neighbor to collect your mail.

Although no amount of security will prevent all threats of intrusion, following these precautions, as well as actively searching for well-maintained housing in low-crime areas, are good steps toward preventing break-ins. Usually intruders are searching for items to sell and enter with theft in mind. If you encounter an intruder, it is far better to give up your money than to fight.

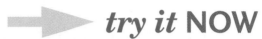
try it NOW

Take safety precautions in your home or dorm to prevent injuries. Using the information above, check your living space tomorrow. Identify places where a thief could break in, and write down a list of emergency phone numbers to keep by the phone. Get your roommates in on the plan, and spend a day ensuring home safety.

Workplace Safety

American adults spend most of their waking hours on the job. While most job situations are pleasant and productive, others pose physical and emotional hazards. Stress, burnout, hostile or abusive interactions with others, discrimination, power struggles, sexual harassment, and a host of other threats are possible whenever people are cloistered together for prolonged periods of time. The nature of the job itself, the corporate culture, and the policies and procedures that characterize certain professions can add to workplace stress.

Fatal Injuries Certain industries are inherently more hazardous than others; outdoor occupations show the highest fatality and injury rates. Although workplaces have instituted programs and services to reduce risks, the following statistics indicate a continuing problem:[66]

- In 2003, 5,534 people lost their lives at work. Rates had decreased slightly until 2002, but rose again in 2003, surpassing most previous fatality reports. There were 1.4 million injuries that required time off of work.
- Highway crashes were the leading cause of on-the-job fatalities and accounted for over 25 percent of fatal work injury totals in 2003. Most involved truck drivers.
- Sixteen percent of worker fatalities resulted from other types of transportation-related incidents, such as tractors and forklifts overturning in fields or warehouses, workers being struck by vehicles, aircraft and railway crashes, and water vehicles crashing or capsizing.
- Workplace homicides were higher in 2003 and continue to be a major cause of workplace danger, accounting for 631 murders at work in 2003. Workplace suicides are also on the rise.

Nonfatal Work Injuries Although deaths capture media attention, other workers may be seriously injured or disabled. Chronic, debilitating pain and other injuries can cause great economic strain on organizations due to workers' compensation claims and days lost from work. Injuries that cause the greatest number of lost-work days include carpal tunnel syndrome, hernia, amputation of a limb, fractures, sprains and strains (often of the back), cuts or lacerations, and chemical burns.[67] For example, nearly half of all workers with carpal tunnel syndrome miss 30 days or more of work each year. Because so many work injuries are due to repetitive motion, overexertion, or inappropriate motion, they are largely preventable through training and techniques designed to reduce employees' risks.

 what do you THINK?

What can be done to prevent injuries? ■ Are students on your campus at risk from any of the problems discussed? ■ Does your school have programs in place to prevent injuries? ■ Do you think more can be done, and if so, what?

TAKING charge

Summary

- Intentional injuries result from actions committed with intent to harm. Unintentional injuries are the result of actions involving no intent to harm. Violence is at epidemic levels in the United States. Many factors lead people to be violent. Among them are anger, substance abuse, and root causes of oppression, poor mental health, and economics.
- Acts of terrorism are becoming more common in the United States. In addition to their immediate impact on society, terrorist activities can exert damaging long-term effects by fostering an atmosphere of fear and anxiety.
- Violence affects everyone in society—from the direct victims, to those who live in fear, to those who pay higher taxes and insurance premiums. Over half of homicides are committed by people who know their victims. Bias and hate crimes divide people, but teaching tolerance can reduce risks. Gang violence continues to grow but can be combated

by programs that reduce the problems that lead to gang membership. Violence on campus may be increasing, but victims' rights have also increased as a result of major legislation.
- Prevention of violent acts begins with avoiding potentially dangerous situations. There are several avenues available for reducing risks, including community, school, workplace, and individual strategies. Many crimes of general society are now commonplace at universities and colleges, including personal assaults, harassment, hate crimes, and even murder.
- Unintentional injuries frequently occur in homes and worksites and can produce serious consequences, including death. By following commonsense guidelines, you can significantly reduce your risk of falls, burns, and other injuries.

Chapter Review

1. An example of an *unintentional injury* is
   a. a car accident.
   b. murder.
   c. domestic violence.
   d. drowning.

2. Hate crimes are motivated by the bias or hatred of which groups of people?
   a. gay people
   b. racial or ethnic groups
   c. religious groups
   d. All of the above.

3. An example of sexual harassment is
   a. displaying pornographic pictures.
   b. making sexual comments to the opposite sex.
   c. inappropriately touching another person.
   d. All of the above.

4. Which of the following is *not* an example of sexual coercion?
   a. Exerting peer pressure to get one's way with a person.
   b. Threatening to end a relationship if the partner doesn't do what the other wants to do.
   c. Getting someone intoxicated to take advantage of that person.
   d. Consensual sex between two adults.

5. What is considered to be the strongest predictor of acquaintance date rape?
   a. women who are known to be easy targets for sex
   b. consumption of alcohol
   c. how well the man knows the woman
   d. using a date rape drug on the woman

6. Which of the following is *not* a cause of violence?
   a. cultural beliefs
   b. poverty
   c. lack of education
   d. unemployment

7. An example of *primary aggression* is
   a. a planned attempted assault on a victim.
   b. hitting someone after being frustrated.
   c. road rage.
   d. flirting with the opposite sex.

8. Simple rape is
   a. a rape committed by multiple attackers.
   b. carrying out a sex act without the other's consent.
   c. a violent act committed by one person whom the victim may know.
   d. penetration by physical force on a person.

9. An example of *stalking* is
   a. making intimate and personal sexually-implied comments to another person.
   b. repeated visual or physical seeking out of another person.
   c. unwelcome sexual conduct by the perpetrator.
   d. sexual abuse of a child.

10. To help someone cope with a traumatic experience with violence, one should
    a. not pressure the victim to talk or not to talk, unless the victim chooses to do so.
    b. not deny that the incident ever happened.
    c. not blame the victim or make the victim feel that it was their fault for the violence.
    d. All of the above.

Answers to these questions can be found on page A-1.

Questions for Discussion and Reflection

1. What major types of crimes are committed in the United States? What is the difference between primary and reactive aggression?
2. What major factors lead to violent acts?
3. Who tends to be susceptible to the appeal of gang membership? What actions can be taken to keep kids out of gangs?
4. What is terrorism, and why does it occur? What can you do to protect yourself against terrorist attacks?
5. Compare domestic violence against men and against women: What are the differences and similarities? What causes domestic violence?
6. What conditions put a child at risk for abuse? What can be done to prevent or decrease child abuse?
7. What is sexual harassment, and what factors contribute to it in the workplace? On campus?
8. What factors increase risk for sexual assault?
9. What are the most effective violence prevention strategies on your campus?
10. What steps can you take to lower your risk of accidental injuries?

Accessing Your Health on the Internet

The following websites explore further topics and issues related to personal health. You'll also find links to each organization's website on the Companion Website for *Access to Health,* Tenth Edition, at www.aw-bc.com/donatelle.

1. *American College Counseling Association.* Provides useful information on a variety of violence issues facing college students. www.collegecounseling.org/content.html
2. *Communities Against Violence Network.* An extensive, searchable database for information about violence against women, with articles about everything from domestic violence to legal information and statistics. www.cavnet2.org
3. *Office of Post-Secondary Education, Campus Security.* Comprehensive source of information and statistics on campus safety across America. Includes tips for staying safe or reporting a crime. www.ed.gov/admins/lead/safety/campus.html

4. *National Center for Injury Prevention and Control.* The WISQARS database of this CDC section provides statistics and information on fatal and nonfatal injuries, both intentional and unintentional. www.cdc.gov/ncipc
5. *National Center for Victims of Crime.* Provides information and resources for victims of crimes ranging from hate crimes to sexual assault. Its "Get Help" series provides information on a wide range of crime victim topics, from bullying and harassment to identity theft. www.ncvc.org
6. *National Institute for Occupational Safety and Health (NIOSH).* Excellent reference for national statistics on injury and violence, in both the community and the workplace. www.cdc.gov/niosh

Further Reading

Hines, D. and K. Malley-Morrison. *Family Violence in the United States: Defining, Understanding, and Combating Abuse.* Thousand Oaks, CA: Sage Publications, Inc., 2005.

Overview of violence statistics, risk factors for various types of violence, and strategies for control and prevention.

Karjane, H., B. Fisher, and F. Cullen. *Sexual Assault on Campus: What Colleges and Universities Are Doing About It.* Washington, DC: National Institute of Justice, NCJ pub. no. 205521.

Overview of trends, causes, and contributors to violence on campus, as well as policies and programs designed to prevent violence.

Kruttschnitt, C., B. McLauglin, and C. Petrie. *Advancing the Federal Research Agenda on Violence Against Women.* Washington, DC: National Research Council, 2004.

Provides key statistics on the epidemic of violence against women, suspected contributors, and topics on which more research is needed.

Tjaden, P. and N. Thoenness. "Extent, Nature and Consequences of Rape Victimization: Findings from the National Violence Against Women Study." National Institute of Justice Special Report, 2006.

An excellent review of key findings from this survey and insights into the consequences of rape for victims, their families, and society.

Wellford, C. J. Pepper, and C. Petrie. *Firearms and Violence: A Critical Review.* Washington, DC: National Academies Press, 2004.

Overview of firearm violence and exploration of key issues relating to violence.

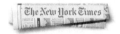

e-themes from *The New York Times*

For up-to-date articles about current health issues, visit www.aw-bc.com/donatelle, select *Access to Health,* Tenth Edition, Chapter 4, and click on "e-themes."

References

1. D. Zucchio, "Today's Violent Crime Is an Old Story with a New Twist," *San Jose Mercury News,* November 21, 1994.
2. Bureau of Justice Statistics, "Homicide Trends in the U.S.," September 2004, www.ojp.usdoj.gov/bjs.
3. Federal Bureau of Investigation, "Preliminary Uniform Crime Report, 2005, Table 3: Percent Change for Consecutive Years," June 12, 2006, www.fbi.gov.ucr/2005preliminary.
4. Centers for Disease Control, "Youth Risk Behavioral Surveillance U.S.," vol. 53/SS-2: 3, 2003, www.cdc.gov/mmwr/PDF.
5. World Health Organization, Seventh World Conference on Injury Prevention and Safety Promotion, Vienna, Austria, June 6–9, 2004, www.who.int/mediacentre/releases/2004/pr40/en/print.html.
6. National Center for Injury Prevention and Control, "Youth Violence Fact Sheet," 2006, www.cdc.gov/ncipc/factsheets/yvfacts.htm.
7. Federal Bureau of Investigation, "National and Regional Crime Statistics from 1970–2003: Summary Findings," 2005, www.fbi.gov.
8. M. Teicher et al., "Sticks, Stones and Hurtful Words: Relative Effects of Various Forms of Childhood Maltreatment," *American Journal of Psychiatry* 163 (2006): 993–1000.
9. Ibid.
10. M. Leeds, "Risk Factors for Violence," Guest Seminar at the Violence Prevention Summer Institute (2006), Oregon State University, Corvallis, OR; H. Foley et al., "Adolescent Sexual Victimization, Use of Alcohol and Other Substances, and Other Health Risk Behaviors," *Journal of Adolescent Health* 4 (2004): 321–328.
11. Centers for Disease Control and Prevention, "Leading Causes of Death by Age, Sex, and Race," Health—United States, 2005, www.cdc.gov/nchs/data/hus/hus05.pdf.
12. National Center for Health Statistics, "Deaths, Final Data," *National Vital Statistics Report* 54, no. 13 (2006), www.cdc.gov/nchs/data/nvsr/nvsr54/nvsr54_13.pdf.
13. Ibid.
14. Federal Bureau of Investigation, "Preliminary Uniform Crime Report," 2005, Geographic Trends in Crime, June 12, 2006, www.fbi.gove.ucr/2005preliminary.
15. Federal Bureau of Investigation, "Hate Crime Statistics—2004, Report Summary," 2005, www.fbi.gov/ucr/hc2004/openpage.htm.
16. C. Berlet, "Hate, Repression and the Apocalyptic Style: Facing Complex Questions and Challenges," *Journal of Hate Studies* 3 (2004): 145–158.
17. J. Carr, *American College Health Association Campus Violence White Paper* (Baltimore: American College Health Association, 2005).
18. American College of Emergency Physicians, "American College of Emergency Physicians Report on Domestic Violence," 2005, www.acep.org/violence/factsheet/domesticviolence.htm.
19. L. Rosen and J. Foutaine, *Compendium of Research on Violence Against Women, 1993–2005* (Washington, DC: National Institute of Justice, 2006).
20. National Coalition Against Domestic Violence, "Domestic Violence Facts 2006," www.ncadv.org.
21. American College Health Association, "Abusive Relationships—Last 12 Months," National College Health Assessment, Fall 2005, www.acha.org.
22. National Center for Injury Prevention and Control, "Domestic Violence Fact Sheet," 2005, www.cdc.gov/ncdv/factsheets.htm; J. Chang et al., "Homicide: A Leading Cause of Injury Deaths Among Pregnant

and Postpartum Women in the United States, 1991–1999," *American Journal of Public Health* 95, no. 3 (2005): 471–477.

23. N. West, "Crimes Against Women," *Community Safety Quarterly* 5 (1992): 3.

24. National Coalition Against Domestic Violence, "2005 Domestic Violence Facts," 2006, www.ncadv.org/resources/statistics_170.htm.

25. Rosen, *Compendium of Research on Violence Against Women.*

26. Ibid.

27. Ibid.

28. Ibid.

29. National Center for Injury Prevention and Control, "Child Maltreatment: Fact Sheet," 2006, www.cdc.gov/ncipc/factsheets/cmfacts.htm.

30. Ibid.

31. Administration for Children and Families, "An Issue Facing All Communities: The National Scope of the Problem," 2005, http://nccanch.acf.hhs.gov/topics/prevention/childabuse_neglect/scope.cfm.

32. Ibid.

33. Ibid.

34. World Health Organization, "Injuries and Violence Prevention: Child Abuse and Neglect," 2006, www.who.int/violence_injury _prevention/violence/neglect/en.

35. National Center for Injury Prevention and Control, "Sexual Violence Fact Sheet," 2006, www.cdc.gov/ncipc/factsheets/cmfacts.htm.

36. National Center for Injury Prevention and Control, "Sexual Violence Fact Sheet," D. Rungan et al., "Child Abuse and Neglect by Parents and Caregivers," in *World Health Report on Violence and Health,* ed. E. Krug et al. Geneva, Switzerland: World Health Organization, 2002, 59–86.

37. American Academy of Pediatrics Medical Library, "Child Abuse and Neglect," www.aap.org.

38. American College of Emergency Physicians, "American College of Emergency Physicians Report on Domestic Violence."

39. National Women's Health Information Center, "Sexual Assault," 2004, www.4woman.gov/fag/sexualassault.htm.

40. National Center for Injury Prevention and Control, "Sexual Violence Fact Sheet."

41. D. Elliot et al., "Adult Sexual Assault: Prevalence, Symptomology, and Sex Differences in the General Population," *Journal of Traumatic Stress* 17, no. 3 (2004): 203–211.

42. Ibid.

43. National Women's Health Information Center, "Sexual Assault."

44. Carr, *American College Health Association Campus Violence White Paper.*

45. University of Chicago, "Sexual Violence," 2006, http://sexual violence.uchicago.edu/resources.shtml.

46. Butcher et al., *Abnormal Psychology* (Boston: Allyn & Bacon, 2003).

47. R. K. Bergen, "Violence Against Women—Online Resources," University of Minnesota, 2002, www.vaw.umn.edu/Vawnet/mrape.htm.

48. Ibid.

49. P. Benson et al., "Acquaintance Rape on Campus," *Journal of American College Health* 40, (1992): 157–165.

50. A. Berkowitz, "College Men as Perpetrators of Aquaintance Rape and Sexual Assault," *Journal of American College Health* 40, (1992) 175–181.

51. U.S. Department of Education, "Summary of Campus Crime and Security Statistics: Criminal Offenses, 2004," 2005, www.ed.gov/admins/lead/safety/crime/criminaloffenses/index.html.

52. Carr, *American College Health Association Campus Violence White Paper.*

53. A. Hoffman et al., eds. *Violence on Campus: Defining the Problems, Strategies for Action* (Gaithersburg, MD: Aspen Publishers, 1998), 1–40.

54. Ibid.

55. J. Carr and K. Van Deusen, "Risk Factors for Male Sexual Aggression on College Campuses," *Journal of Family Violence* 19, no. 5 (2004): 279–289.

56. American College Health Association, "Sexual Abuse and Assault," National College Health Assessment, Fall 2005, www.acha.org.

57. Ibid.

58. National Center for Victims of Crime, "Stalking Resource Center," www.ncvc.org/srs/main.aspx?dbID=DB_onlineinternational251.

59. Carr, *American College Health Association Campus Violence White Paper.*

60. Ibid.

61. Ibid.

62. Ibid.

63. Ibid.

64. K. Baum and P. Klaus, *Violent Victimization of College Students, 1995–2002* (NCJ Publication No. 206836) (Washington, DC: U.S. Department of Justice, 2005).

65. Carr, *American College Health Association Campus Violence White Paper.*

66. Bureau of Labor Statistics, "2005 Census of Fatal Occupational Injuries Preliminary Data, 2005," 2006, www.bls.gov.

67. Ibid.

5

Healthy Relationships

COMMUNICATING EFFECTIVELY WITH FRIENDS, FAMILY, AND SIGNIFICANT OTHERS

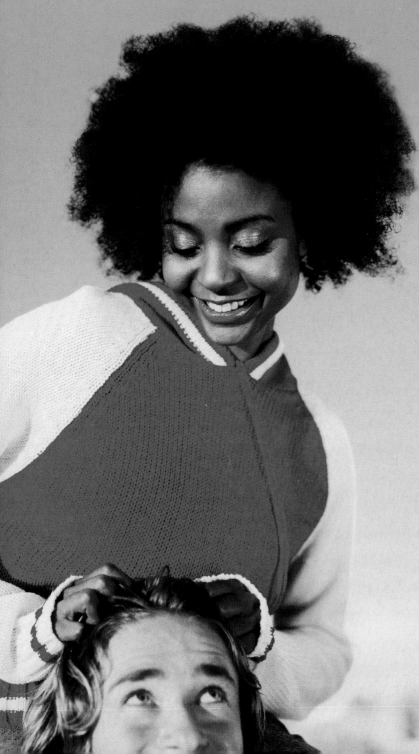

Does an **intimate** relationship have to be sexual?

How can I communicate **better**?

What can I do to cope with a **bad breakup**?

Is it good to **live** together before getting married?

How can I end a relationship without **hurting** my partner too much?

OBJECTIVES

- Discuss ways to improve communication skills and interpersonal interactions.
- Identify the characteristics of successful relationships, including how to maintain them and overcome common barriers.
- Explore similarities and differences between men and women in communication styles and decision making.
- Examine factors that are important in determining the success of an intimate relationship, and where to get help when a relationship has problems.
- Discuss actions that can improve interpersonal interactions.

Humans are social animals—we have a basic need to fit in to a human "pack," to feel loved and appreciated by others. We thrive in environments where we feel secure, needed, and respected, particularly if we are cared about by people who really matter to us. Although we can exist without these close interactions, our lives are enhanced and our days are more fulfilling when we can share our successes and failures with others. In fact, a study done by researchers at the Harvard School of Public Health shows that the ability to relate well with people throughout your life can have almost as much impact on your health as exercise and good nutrition.[1]

All relationships involve a degree of risk. Only by taking these risks, however, can we grow and truly experience all that life has to offer. In this chapter, we examine healthy relationships and the communication skills necessary to create and maintain them. Why is communication so important? For one thing, the way we communicate influences whether or not we are accepted by others. For another, most of us sincerely want to express ourselves clearly and honestly in our relationships. Clear communication can help us bridge our differences, and it can also affect health. Expressing ourselves well and knowing how to understand what others are saying are both vitally important to communication. These abilities lay the groundwork for healthy relationships, and satisfying relationships are significant factors in overall health.

Characterizing and Forming Intimate Relationships

> **Does an intimate relationship have to be sexual?**

Most people think of intimacy as two people having a loving, intense, often sexual, relationship in which there is a mutual desire for closeness, touching, and physical expression. However, in her book *The Dance of Intimacy*, Dr. Harriet Goldhor Lerner defines intimacy as "being who we are in a relationship and allowing the other person to be the same. An intimate relationship is one in which neither party silences or betrays the self and each party expresses strength and vulnerability, weakness and competence in a balanced way."[2] Thus, intimacy is less a physical state than it is a state of the mind, heart, and essence of those

intimate relationships Relationships with family members, friends, and romantic partners, characterized by closeness and understanding.

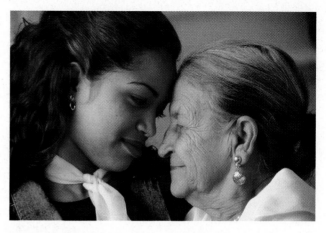

The emotional bonds that characterize intimate relationships often span the generations and help individuals gain insight and understanding into each other's worlds.

who share it. It may culminate in a physical way, but it is much more complex than the act of sexual intercourse or sexual expression. In fact, intimacy is sometimes described as an attitude; one that defines the quality of how two people relate to one another and their level of emotional and spiritual connectedness to each other in the times between lovemaking, as well as during lovemaking.

Experts in the field of interpersonal relationships define **intimate relationships** in terms of four characteristics: *behavioral interdependence*, *need fulfillment*, *emotional attachment*, and *emotional availability*. Each of these characteristics may be related to interactions with family, close friends, and romantic partners.[3]

Behavioral interdependence refers to the mutual impact that people have on each other as their lives and daily activities intertwine. What one person does influences what the other person wants to do and can do. Behavioral interdependence may become stronger over time to the point that each person would feel a great void if the other were gone.

Intimate relationships also fulfill psychological needs and so are a means of *need fulfillment*. Through relationships with others, we fulfill our needs for:

- *Intimacy,* someone with whom we can share our feelings freely
- *Social integration,* someone with whom we can share worries and concerns
- *Nurturance,* someone whom we can take care of and who will take care of us
- *Assistance,* someone to help us in times of need
- *Affirmation,* someone who will reassure us of our own worth and tell us that we matter

In rewarding, intimate relationships, partners and friends meet each other's needs. They disclose feelings, share confidences, and provide support and reassurance. Each person comes away feeling better for the interaction and validated by the other person.

In addition to behavioral interdependence and need fulfillment, intimate relationships involve strong bonds of *emotional attachment*, or feelings of love and attachment.

TABLE 5.1	Today's Changing Families

The United States is a melting pot of family types. The estimated percentages of school-aged children living in various family structures is listed below.

Family Structure	School-aged children living in identified family structure (%)
Nuclear family: husband and wife plus biological offspring	58
Stepparent family: one biological parent plus one stepparent	10
Blended family: parents plus children born to several families	5
Adoptive family: two parents	2
Single mother, never married	10
Single mother, divorced	10
Single father, divorced and never remarried	5

Source: Based on data from the U.S. Census Bureau, 2000.

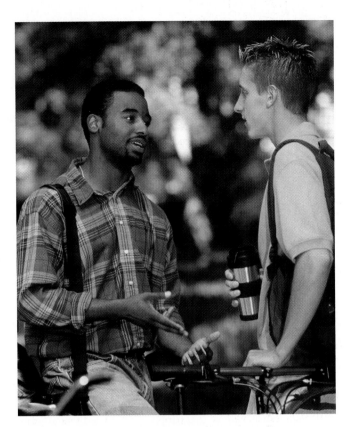

"The better part of one's life consists of his friendships."

—*Abraham Lincoln*

Emotional availability, the ability to give to and receive from others emotionally without fear of being hurt or rejected, is the fourth characteristic of intimate relationships. At times, all of us may limit our emotional availability—for example, after a painful breakup we may decide not to jump into another relationship immediately. Holding back can offer time for introspection and healing as well as considering the "lessons learned." However, because of intense trauma, some people find it difficult ever to be fully available emotionally. This limits their ability to experience and enjoy intimate relationships.

In the early years of life, families provide the most significant relationships. Gradually, the circle widens to include friends, coworkers, and acquaintances. Ultimately, most of us develop romantic relationships with a significant other. Each of these relationships plays a significant role in psychological, social, spiritual, and physical health.

Families: The Ties That Bind

A family is a recognizable group of people with roles, tasks, boundaries, and personalities whose central focus is to protect, care for, love, and socialize one another. Because the family is a dynamic institution that changes as society changes, the definition of family, and the individuals believed to constitute family membership, change over time as well. Who are members of today's families? Historically, most families have been made up of people related by blood, marriage, and long-term committed relationships or adoption.[4] Yet today, many other groups of people are being recognized and functioning as family units (see Table 5.1). Although there is no "best" family type, we do know the key roles and tasks a healthy family nurtures and supports. Healthy families

foster a sense of security and feelings of belonging that are central to growth and development. It is from our **family of origin**, the people present in our household during our first years of life, that we initially learn about feelings, problem solving, love, intimacy, and gender roles. We learn to negotiate relationships and have opportunities to communicate effectively, develop attitudes, beliefs, and values, and explore spiritual belief systems. It is not uncommon when we establish relationships outside of the family to rely on these initial experiences and skills modeled by our family of origin.

Establishing Friendships

A Friend is one who knows you as you are, understands where you've been, accepts who you've become, and still gently invites you to grow.

—*Author Unknown*

Good friends can make a boring day fun, a cold day warm, or a gut-wrenching worry disappear. They can make us feel that we matter and that we have the strength to get through just about anything. They can also make us angry, disappoint us, or seriously jolt our comfortable ideas about right and wrong.

family of origin People present in the household during a child's first years of life—usually parents and siblings.

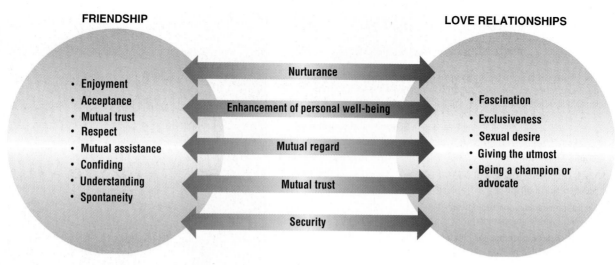

FRIENDSHIP

- Enjoyment
- Acceptance
- Mutual trust
- Respect
- Mutual assistance
- Confiding
- Understanding
- Spontaneity

Nurturance

Enhancement of personal well-being

Mutual regard

Mutual trust

Security

LOVE RELATIONSHIPS

- Fascination
- Exclusiveness
- Sexual desire
- Giving the utmost
- Being a champion or advocate

FIGURE 5.1 Common Bonds of Friends and Lovers

Friendships are relationships between two or more people that involve mutual respect, trust, support, and intimacy that may or may not include sexual intimacy. Like our family, our friends should have identified roles and boundaries. Persons in friendships should communicate their understandings, needs, expectations, limitations, and affections.[5]

Psychologists believe that people are attracted to and form relationships with people who give them positive reinforcement and that they dislike those who punish or overcriticize them. The basic idea is simple: you like people who like you. Another factor that affects the development of a friendship is a real or perceived similarity in attitudes, opinions, and background.[6] In addition, true friends have a sense of equity in which they share confidences, contribute fairly and equally to maintaining the friendship, and consistently try to give as much as they get back from the interactions.[7] See the Health in a Diverse World box for information on how the Internet is changing how we meet people and how to stay safe when socializing online.

Psychologists Jeffrey Turner and Laurna Rubinson summarized the consensus among experts on characteristics that make a good friendship:[8]

- *Enjoyment.* Although temporary states of anger, disappointment, or mutual annoyance may occur, friends enjoy each other's company most of the time.
- *Acceptance.* Friends accept each other as they are, without trying to change or make the other into a different person.
- *Mutual trust.* Each assumes that the other will act in his or her friend's best interest.
- *Respect.* Friends respect each other; each assumes that the other exercises good judgment in making life choices.
- *Mutual assistance.* Friends are inclined to assist and support one another. Specifically, they can count on each other in times of need, trouble, or personal distress.
- *Confiding.* Friends share experiences and feelings with each other that they don't share with other people.

- *Understanding.* Friends have a sense of what each person values. They are not puzzled or mystified by each other's actions.
- *Spontaneity.* Friends feel free to be themselves in the relationship, without being required to play a role or inhibit revelation of personal traits.

Take a few minutes to examine one of your current friendships. How many of these characteristics can you identify in that relationship?

Significant Others, Partners, and Couples

Most people choose at some point to enter into an intimate sexual relationship with another person. Numerous studies have analyzed the ways in which couples form significant partnering relationships. Most partners fit into one of four categories: married heterosexual couples, cohabiting heterosexual couples, lesbian couples, and gay male couples. These groups are discussed in greater detail later in this chapter.

Love relationships in each of these four groups typically include all the characteristics of friendship as well as other characteristics related to passion and caring:[9]

- *Fascination.* Lovers tend to pay attention to the other person even when they should be involved in other activities. They are preoccupied with the other and want to think about, look at, talk to, or merely be with that person.
- *Exclusiveness.* Lovers have a special relationship that usually precludes having the same bond with a third party. The love relationship takes priority over all others.
- *Sexual desire.* Lovers want physical intimacy with the partner, desiring to touch, hold, and engage in sexual activities with each other.
- *Giving the utmost.* Lovers care enough to give the utmost when the other is in need, sometimes to the point of extreme sacrifice.

MAKING CONNECTIONS THROUGH THE INTERNET WHILE STAYING SAFE

The Internet has revolutionized our access to information and the way we communicate, but it is not without potential dangers. Perhaps you recall recent newspaper headlines proclaiming, "Social networking site MySpace is hit with a $30 million lawsuit after a 14-year-old girl was allegedly raped by a 19-year-old man she met through the site." When you surf the Net looking for socializing opportunities or assistance with meeting people, do you know potential danger signs or what questions you should ask?

There are literally thousands of sites on the Web that specialize in helping people meet each other. Chat rooms and bulletin board systems are ways for people with similar interests to communicate about them. Sites like MySpace and Friendster allow people to network not only in their own community, but around the world, finding friends with similar interests in music and activities. Some sites specialize in providing dating services, like Match.com, which helps people find others who match particular profiles. These services may be free, while others may charge fees to participate. Dating service sites usually explicitly restrict participation to people over 18 years old, but most of them depend on possession of a credit card as their sole mechanism for authenticating age. How can these websites ensure that those under 18 are not signing on? There isn't much they can do if teenagers or younger children have access to credit card numbers.

Other social networking sites, such as MySpace, may have fewer restrictions and a younger audience, but also less policing. However, in light of recent crimes such as the one described at the beginning of this article, MySpace does try to educate users about safety and perform regular monitoring of users' pages. Site managers remove sexually explicit material and hate icons, and reserve the right to block some users. They also will kick off a user if they discover the individual is under the age of 14, in an effort to protect young teens from sexual predators.

In addition to creating casual friendships, matchmaking, or simply communicating with others, users of the Internet can also get involved in *cybersex*. People chatting online can describe themselves or each other in sexual situations or interactions that are age inappropriate and may be disturbing for some. Many divorces have resulted from cybersex when one spouse gets upset about the other's intimacy with a stranger, even via the Internet.

PRACTICAL GUIDELINES FOR CYBER-DATERS AND SOCIAL NETWORKERS OF ALL AGES

- As you are getting to know someone online, ask questions about lots of things you are interested in, such as hobbies, politics, religion, education, birthdate, family background, and marital history and status. Keep the answers you receive and beware of contradictions.
- Be suspicious of anyone who seems too good to be true, such as someone who agrees with your taste on every single preference or interest. Trying too hard to please may mark a manipulative and potentially dangerous personality.
- Be honest about yourself; state your own interests and characteristics fairly, including things you think might be less attractive than stereotypes and cultural norms dictate.
- If you get to the point of exchanging pictures, be sure that you see the person in a wide variety of situations and with other people, to make it harder to send pictures of someone else.
- Talk to your new friend by phone; be suspicious of resistance.
- Don't rush into face-to-face contact.
- Before you agree to meet, get the individual's full name, address, and telephone number. Be suspicious if the person refuses to give you a home number: could they have a spouse or a current live-in friend they are deceiving? Call the home number a couple of times to see if someone else answers.
- Be suspicious of anyone who tries to pressure you in any way, including demanding money or insisting on a meeting before you feel confident of their good intentions.
- Give your contact's name, address, and other identifying information and the exact details of where and when you are going to meet to friends and family. Do not meet anyone who wants to keep the location and time a secret. Meet in a well-lit, public place such as a coffee shop.
- If you like your new friend a lot, have a background check done using a professional service such as www.whoishe.com or www.whoisshe.com.

Source: Adapted from M. E. Kabay, "Cyber-Safety for Everyone, from Kids to Elders: Online Dating and Cyber-Sex," 2002, www2.norwich.edu/mkabay/cyberwatch/index.htm.

- *Being a champion or advocate.* Lovers actively champion each other's interests and attempt to ensure that the other succeeds.

For obvious reasons, the best love relationships share friendships, and the best friendships include several love components. Both relationships share common bonds of nurturance, enhancement of personal well-being, and a genuine sense of mutual regard, trust, and security. Healthy friendships and love relationships greatly enhance overall health and lead to sustained personal growth throughout life (see Figure 5.1).

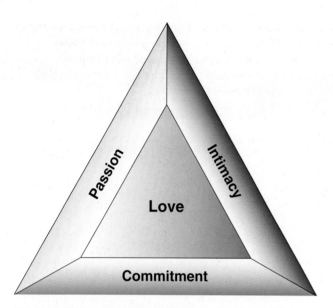

FIGURE 5.2 Sternberg's Triangular Theory of Love

- *Intimacy,* the emotional component, which involves feelings of closeness
- *Passion,* the motivational component, which reflects romantic, sexual attraction
- *Decision/commitment,* the cognitive component, which includes the decisions you make about being in love and the degree of commitment to your partner

According to Sternberg's model, the higher the levels of intimacy, passion, and commitment, the more likely a person is to be involved in a healthy, positive love relationship.

Anthropologist Helen Fisher has developed a large body of research on love and attraction. According to Dr. Fisher's classic studies, attraction and falling in love follow a fairly predictable pattern based on (1) *imprinting,* in which our evolutionary patterns, genetic predispositions, and past experiences trigger a romantic reaction; (2) *attraction,* in which neurochemicals produce feelings of euphoria and elation; (3) *attachment,* in which endorphins—natural opiates—cause lovers to feel peaceful, secure, and calm; and (4) *production of a "cuddle chemical,"* in which the brain secretes the chemical oxytocin, thereby stimulating sensations during lovemaking and eliciting feelings of satisfaction and attachment.[12]

Lovers who claim that they are swept away by passion may not, therefore, be far from the truth.

> A meeting of the eyes, a touch of the hands, or a whiff of scent may set off a flood that starts in the brain and races along the nerves and through the blood. The familiar results—flushed skin, sweaty palms, heavy breathing—are identical to those experienced when under stress. Why? Because the love-smitten person is secreting chemical substances such as dopamine, norepinephrine, and phenylethylamine (PEA) that are chemical cousins of amphetamines.[13]

Although attraction may in fact be a "natural high," with PEA levels soaring, this hit of passion loses effectiveness over time as the body builds up a tolerance. Needing a continual fix of passion, some people may become attraction junkies, seeking the intoxication of love much as the drug user seeks a chemical high.[14]

Fisher speculates that PEA levels drop significantly over a three- to four-year period, leading to the "four-year itch" that shows up in the peaking fourth-year divorce rates present in over 60 cultures. Romances that last beyond the four-year decline of PEA are influenced by another set of chemicals, the endorphins.[15]

Other researchers describe the first stage as the *lust phase,* in which our biological and genetic histories converge to pique our interest and intensity of response. In the lust phase, if someone comes into our range of awareness, a chemical surge can trigger our enthusiastic response. Known as pheromones, these triggers, said to be as unique as our fingerprints, are scent-infused chemicals found in perspiration under the armpits. They trigger a unique sensory reaction in the nose and result in attraction if their producer is a match for you.[16]

This Thing Called Love

What is love? Defining it may be more difficult than listing the characteristics of a loving relationship. This four-letter word has been written about and engraved on walls; it has been the theme of countless novels, movies, and plays. There is no one definition of love, and the word may mean different things to people depending on cultural values, age, gender, and situation. Yet, we all know what it is when it strikes.

Many social scientists maintain that love may be of two kinds: *companionate* and *passionate.* Companionate love is a secure, trusting attachment, similar to what we may feel for family members or close friends. In companionate love, two people are attracted, have much in common, care about each other's well-being, and express reciprocal liking and respect. Passionate love, in contrast, is defined as a state of high arousal, filled with the ecstasy of being loved and the agony of being rejected.[10] The person experiencing passionate love tends to be preoccupied with his or her partner and to perceive the love object as perfect.

According to classic research conducted by Elaine Hatfield and G. William Walster, passionate love will not occur unless three conditions are met.[11] First, the person must live in a culture in which the concept of "falling in love" is idealized. Second, a "suitable" love object must be present. If someone has been taught by parents, movies, books, and peers to seek partners of a certain appearance, socioeconomic status, or racial background, and if no such partner is available, the person may find it difficult to become involved. Finally, for passionate love to occur, there must be some type of physiological arousal that occurs when a person is in the presence of the beloved. Often this arousal takes the form of sexual excitement.

In his article "The Triangular Theory of Love" researcher Robert Sternberg attempts to clarify love by isolating three key ingredients (see Figure 5.2):

Following these pheromone triggers comes the *attraction phase*, often labeled the falling in love phase, and then the *attachment phase*. The two hormones most important in this last phase are oxytocin and vasopressin. Oxytocin not only increases the bond between lovers, but is also one of the chemicals responsible for contractions during childbirth and milk expression when breast-feeding and is released by both sexes during orgasm. The theory goes, therefore, that the more sex a couple has, the greater the bond between them.[17]

Vasopressin has been described as the "monogamy chemical." Much of what we know about oxytocin and vasopressin's roles in the chemistry of love comes from observations of voles, tiny mouse-size mammals that mate over a 24-hour period and bond for life. They prefer to spend their days together, nest together, and show affection toward one another and their offspring. In laboratory settings, if these two chemicals are blocked, voles' relationships become more like one-night stands, and they actively seek out other mates. If the chemicals are injected into voles, their monogamous ways continue. Although there are many other factors involved and the science is relatively new and specific to one species, there are interesting implications for humans.

In addition to such possible chemical influences, past experiences significantly affect our attractions for others. Our parents' modeling of traits we believe are desirable or undesirable may play a role in drawing us to people with similar traits.

Communicating: A Key to Good Relationships

Many of us find it difficult to tell people what we really think or to express how we feel. We constantly worry about making people angry, hurting their feelings, being misinterpreted, saying too much, or not saying enough. You may have communication problems with friends, family members, lovers, coworkers, professors, or others, and this is nothing new. Humans have found communication to be difficult ever since people began living together and forming common bonds. Some of this difficulty stems from our individual communication styles. Some of it comes from technology that allows us to whip expletives over the Internet whenever we feel the need. And some of it stems from the fact that learning to communicate effectively is something that never comes easily, even to those who consciously work at it.

Much of our communication difficulty is inherent in the complexity of language itself. As our nation becomes more diverse, numerous languages, dialects, and vocal inflections make understanding each other more difficult. If you were raised in Wisconsin, you may not only have a different accent than individuals from Texas or Massachusetts; you may find that you express yourself in a different manner overall, have different gestures and facial expressions, have a different speed and manner of speaking, and that certain words may sound downright odd. Even a simple word or gesture can cause confusion, send mixed messages, and create misunderstanding. When there are no eyes to look into or body language to interpret, as with e-mail communication, it is no wonder that we can quickly take offense, get frustrated, or misinterpret what others are saying.

Problems arise when we assume that others mean the same thing that we mean when we say certain words. Your friend's definition of love may be very different from yours, and if the two of you are talking about it and meaning two different things, the result may be disastrous. To someone raised in a home where yelling and angry outbursts are common occurrences that are quickly forgotten, a small raising of the voice or cursing on the phone may mean very little. To someone raised in an environment where peace and even-tempered discussions prevail, loud outbursts may be difficult to comprehend or even offensive. Awareness of the subtleties of language and the ways in which we react to various life situations, both verbally or nonverbally, is an important aspect of the communication process.

Different cultures, too, not only have different languages and dialects, but also different ways of expressing themselves and using body language.[18] Some cultures gesture wildly; others maintain a rigid posture while speaking. Some cultures are offended by direct eye contact; others welcome a steady look in the eyes.

This doesn't mean that one sex, culture, or group is better at communicating or should be a model for the others. It does mean that we have to be willing to accept differences and work to keep communication lines open and fluid. Remaining interested, actively engaged in the interaction, and open and willing to exchange ideas is something that we typically learn with practice and hard work.

Symbolism in Communication

How often have you heard someone say "We just can't communicate" or "You're sending me mixed messages"? These exchanges occur regularly as people struggle to solve a problem, learn a new skill, start a relationship, or work through difficulties in an existing relationship.[19] Whereas people typically use the word **communication** to mean "talking and listening, sending messages with words or your body," communication experts tend to describe this act as "the symbolic process of shared meanings."[20] Symbols transmit messages and represent people, events, places, or objects. Words or verbal expressions, facial expressions, vocal tone, eye contact, gestures, movement, body posture, appearance, context, and spatial distance all reflect various communication symbols. Gifts, food, cards, e-mails, and other objects are also forms of symbolic communication. The multiplicity of symbolic gestures and ways of interpreting them can make communication a challenge. Sometimes we think we are saying something

communication The transmission of information and meaning from one individual to another.

quite clearly, but even an attentive listener may misunderstand the symbols we use and thus our meaning.

Because communication is a process, our every action, word, and other symbols become part of our history with others—part of the evolving impression we make. If we are nasty and hostile with someone, even for a short period of time, those messages form a permanent part of our shared history. Each time we interact and communicate, this history evolves, for better or for worse. This is complicated by the fact that each person brings emotional "baggage" (both good and bad) from the past into an interaction. For example, a person who has become cynical and distrustful may be critical and guarded during interactions with others. Our interpretations of communication also become part of shared history, and interpretation can be tricky. If someone says, "I love you," it may mean friendship, the love shared by family members, or the passion reserved for a deep and intimate relationship. Knowing how to seek clarification, ask for what you want, and interpret words in the context of the situation are critical skills.

How Perception Affects Communication

Perception is the process by which people filter and interpret information from the senses in order to create a meaningful picture of the world.[21] It is the lens through which we view the world. Gender, culture, educational level, family behaviors, and a host of other factors influence this view. Important factors that affect your perceptions, and therefore your communication effectiveness, include the way you define yourself (*self-concept*) and the way you evaluate yourself (*self-esteem*). Your self-concept is like a mental mirror that reflects how you view your physical features, emotional states, talents, likes and dislikes, values, and roles.[22] Are you a student, a mother, an honors student, a Democrat, a pianist? How you define yourself is your self-concept. How you feel about yourself or evaluate yourself constitutes your self-esteem. You might consider yourself an excellent student, a horrible singer, a great lover, or a "10" in terms of appearance—such judgments indicate your level of self-esteem or self-evaluation.

Self-perceptions influence communication choices. If you feel unattractive, uncomfortable, or inferior to others, you may choose not to interact with them or to avoid social events. If you feel self-conscious and ill at ease around people who seem different, you might avoid or feel suspicious of them. Conversely, if you feel secure about your unique characteristics and talents, that positive self-concept will make it easier to interact with a variety of people in a healthy, balanced way.

---

perception   The process of filtering and interpreting information gathered through the senses.

self-disclosure   The process of revealing one's inner thoughts, feelings, and beliefs to another person.

Improving Your Communication Skills

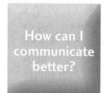

How can I communicate better?

All of us can learn to be better communicators. This lifelong process involves several challenges. We can start by learning how to share information through self-disclosure. This form of sharing will allow others to better understand us.

Likewise, we can work at becoming better listeners—a critical skill for starting or maintaining any relationship. A third skill involves understanding nonverbal communication—both how we convey nonverbal messages and how others use their bodies and facial expressions to convey information. Through understanding how to deliver and interpret information, we can enhance the relationships in our lives. In order to have healthy interactions with others and keep stress levels under control, it is important to deal with problems as early as possible. Learning communication skills that quickly resolve fights and misunderstandings can reduce unnecessary stress and lead to happier, more productive relationships.

Learning Appropriate Self-Disclosure

Self-disclosure is the sharing of personal information, ideas, and feelings with others. It is revealing something about yourself that is not obvious to others based on your external appearance.[23] If you are willing to share personal information with others, they will likely share personal information with you. In other words, if you want to learn more about someone, you have to be willing to share parts of your personal self with that person.

Self-disclosure can be a double-edged sword, for there is risk in divulging personal insights and feelings. If you sense that sharing feelings and personal thoughts will result in a closer relationship, you will likely take such a risk. On the other hand, if you believe that the disclosure may result in rejection or alienation, you may not open up so easily. If the confidentiality of previously shared information has been violated, you may hesitate to disclose yourself in the future.

However, the risk in not disclosing yourself to others is that you will lack intimacy in relationships. Psychologist Carl Rogers stressed the importance of understanding yourself and others through self-disclosure. Rogers believed that weak relationships were characterized by inhibited self-disclosure.[24]

If self-disclosure is a key element in creating healthy communication, but fear is a barrier to that process, what can we do? The following suggestions can help:

- *Get to know yourself.* Remember that your self includes your feelings, beliefs, thoughts, and concerns. The more you know about yourself, the more likely it is that you will be able to communicate with others about yourself. Think about who you are, what you are passionate about, and your strengths and limitations. Which of these do you feel good about? Which cause you concern?
- *Become more accepting of yourself.* No one is perfect or has to be. Even the people you look up to have their flaws. Only by accepting your imperfections can you expect others to accept them, too.
- *Be willing to discuss your sexual history.* In a culture that puts many taboos on discussions of sex in everyday conversation, it's no wonder we find it hard to disclose our sexual feelings to those with whom we are intimate. However, with the soaring rate of sexually transmitted infections and the ever-looming threat of AIDS, there has never been a more important time to disclose sexual feelings and history. The life-altering effects of an unwanted pregnancy or contracting the HIV virus underscore the need to communicate about sex before you become intimate.
- *Choose a safe context for self-disclosure.* Context refers to the setting in which the self-disclosure occurs. When and where you make such disclosures and to whom may greatly influence the response. Choose a setting in which you feel safe to let yourself be known.

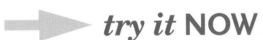 **try it NOW**

Create a "Johari Window." A Johari Window is a tool to help us understand the proportion of information about ourselves that we and others are aware of. Each quadrant of the window signifies the following. Open Self: Information about yourself known to you and others; Blind Self: Information about yourself others may recognize but you do not; Hidden Self: Information you are aware of, but do not share; Unknown Self: Information that is unknown to you or others, such as an addiction. Draw a window with four panes on a sheet of paper, and explore each portion of your "self." Try doing this with a trusted friend or partner and explore the reasons behind what you are and aren't willing to disclose to others.

Being a Better Listener

Listening is a vital part of interpersonal communication; it allows us to share feelings, express concerns, communicate wants and needs, and let our thoughts and opinions be known. We must do the necessary work to improve both our speaking and listening skills, which will enhance our relationships, improve our grasp of information, and allow us to interpret more effectively what others say. We listen best when (1) we believe that the message is somehow important and relevant to us, (2) the speaker holds our attention through humor, dramatic effect, use of the media, or other techniques, and (3) we are in the mood to listen (free of distractions and worries).

When we really listen effectively, we try to understand what people are thinking and feeling from their perspective. We not only hear the words, but we try to understand what is really being said. How many times have you been caught pretending to be listening when you were not? After several moments of nodding and saying "uh-huh" your friend finally asks you a question, and you haven't a clue about what she has been saying. Sometimes this tuned-out behavior is due to a lack of sleep, stress overload, being preoccupied, having too much to drink, or being under the influence of drugs. Other times it's because speakers are motormouths who talk for the sake of talking or because you find them or what they are talking about boring. Some of the most common listening difficulties are things that we can work to improve:[25]

- Being so interested in what you are going to say that you listen mainly to find an opening to get the floor
- Nodding your head vigorously or gesturing with every word that is said, displaying an obvious anxiousness to get "in" the conversation
- Mentally formulating a rebuttal to what is being said rather than really listening
- Evaluating or making judgments about the speaker or the message
- Not asking for clarification when there are things that you are unclear about
- Being frustrated because the other person is speaking in limited English or in another language
- Being so biased or emotional about your opinion that you are thinking of a counterargument the entire time the other person is speaking
- Engaging in side conversations with others while someone is speaking

Other external factors or things about the speaker that may make listening difficult and that could be improved include:

- Speaker speaks too fast or jumps from point to point
- Speaker speaks too loudly or too quietly
- External noise, commotion around you, or distractions
- Bad phone connections
- Lack of familiarity with a language or dialect

See the Skills for Behavior Change box on page 146 for more suggestions on improving your listening.

SKILLS FOR behavior change

LEARNING TO REALLY LISTEN

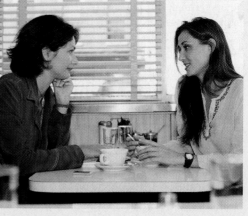

Most of us have lamented the fact that someone "never listens" and seems to monopolize the entire conversation. Although we are quick to recognize such flaws in others, we are often less likely to spot listening problems of our own. On a daily basis, we all have times when we just "tune out." When a professor drones on about a subject we don't relate to, we begin doodling or put on a fake interested facial expression, even though we are thinking about dinner or what to wear to the movies that night. When that boring friend tells the same story over and over again, we say "uh-huh," "yes," and worry that we'll be caught when he asks a question and we don't have a clue what he is talking about. We grimace at the thought of certain people calling but dash for the phone when the caller ID indicates that it is someone we love to talk with. Why do we tune out when some people speak and tune in for others?

We gravitate toward those who seem to understand us and with whom we have fun and interesting interactions. Truthfully, most of us are only mediocre listeners. What does it take to be an excellent listener? Practicing the following skills and consciously using them daily is an important part of improved communication.

- *Be present in the moment.* Contrary to what is often believed, good listeners don't just sit back with their mouths shut. They participate and acknowledge what the other person is saying. (Nodding, smiling, saying "yes" or "uh-huh," and asking questions at appropriate times are all part of this. Take care, however, not to numbly say "uh-huh" to every word, which is distracting and conveys insincerity.)
- *Use positive body language and voice tone.* Show that you are "with" the speaker by turning toward him or her

and staying focused (wandering eyeballs are a sure sign that your mind is elsewhere). Avoid barrier gestures such as shaking your head "no," making negative faces, or folding your arms; smile at appropriate times and maintain appropriate eye contact (deadpan stares can also be distracting). Voice tone, posture, and an attitude that conveys interest are all key.

- *Show empathy and sympathy.* Watch for verbal and nonverbal clues to the other person's feelings and try to relate. For example, saying, "That must have been really hard for you" can encourage the speaker to talk and feel more comfortable with you as an understanding listener.
- *Ask for clarification.* If you aren't sure what the speaker means, indicate that you're not sure you understand, or paraphrase what you think you heard. This kind of feedback is invaluable in avoiding misinterpretation and lapses in overall communication. As a speaker, you may ask," What did you think I was just saying?" but be sure to say this in a nonthreatening manner.
- *Control that deadly desire to interrupt.* Some people start nodding and gesturing before you ever get a word out of your mouth. If you are like that, squelch it, even if you have to put an inconspicuous hand over your mouth. Try taking a deep breath for two seconds, then hold your breath for another second and really listen to what is being said as you slowly exhale. Don't be so enthusiastically empathetic that you finish speakers' sentences or put words in people's mouths.
- *Avoid snap judgments based on what other people look like or are saying.* If you notice some strange mannerism,

try to focus on what is being said, not how it is being said. Avoid stereotyping or labeling.

- *Resist the temptation to "set the other person straight."* Control your urge to correct errors or react defensively. Listen and hear without reacting or trying to rationalize what the speaker is trying to say.
- *Try to focus on the speaker.* Sometimes it is very tough to listen to someone who is trying to talk about a painful situation, especially if we are experiencing or have recently experienced the same thing. Hold back the temptation to "tell all" and launch into your own rendition of a similar situation. Give the speaker the moment; later, after he or she is done talking, you may want to discuss your own experience as a way of validating the feelings expressed. Don't tell him how he is feeling or how he should feel.
- *Be tenacious.* Stick with the speaker and try to stay on the topic. If the person seems to wander, gently bring the topic back by saying, "You were just saying . . ." Offer your thoughts and suggestions, but remember that you should only advise up to a certain point. Clarify statements with "this is my opinion" as a reminder that it is only opinion, rather than fact.

The Three Basic Listening Modes There are three main ways in which we listen. Knowing when to use each of these will enhance the way in which you listen and improve the outcome.

1. *Competitive*, or *combative*, *listening* happens when we are more interested in promoting our own point of view than in understanding or exploring someone else's view. We listen either for openings to take the floor or for flaws and weak points that we can attack. Looking at your watch, sighing, nodding vigorously, staring into space, or other actions are meant to discourage speakers or cause them to relinquish the floor.

2. *Passive*, or *attentive*, *listening* occurs when we are genuinely interested in hearing and understanding the other person's point of view. By being attentive and passively listening, we encourage further discussion. We assume that we heard and understand correctly, but we stay passive and don't verify it.

3. *Active*, or *reflective*, *listening* is the single most useful and important listening skill. In active listening, we are also genuinely interested in understanding what the other person is thinking, feeling, and wanting in addition to what the message means, and we are active in confirming our understanding before we respond with our own new message. We restate or paraphrase our understanding of the other person's meaning and reflect it back to the sender for verification. This verification or feedback process is what distinguishes active listening and makes it effective.[26]

Benefits of Active Listening The most obvious benefit of active listening is that it reduces the risk of misunderstanding or, if a misunderstanding does occur, makes it immediately apparent. Other benefits include:[27]

- Sometimes people just need to be heard and acknowledged before they are willing to consider an alternative or soften their position.
- It is often easier for people to listen to and consider the other's position when they know the other person is listening to and considering theirs.
- It helps people spot the flaws in their reasoning when they hear it restated without criticism.
- Active listening helps identify areas of agreement so that the areas of disagreement are put into perspective and diminished rather than magnified.
- Reflecting back what we hear each other say makes each of us aware of the different levels of communication that are going on below the surface. This helps to bring issues into the open, where they can be resolved more readily.
- If we listen and try to understand other people's point of view, we can more effectively help them see the flaws in their position or discover the flaws in our own reasoning.

Using Nonverbal Communication

Understanding what someone is saying often involves much more than listening and speaking. Often, what is not actually said may speak louder than any words. Rolling the eyes, looking at the floor or ceiling rather than maintaining eye contact, making body movements and hand gestures—all these nonverbal clues influence the way we interpret messages. **Nonverbal communication** includes all unwritten and unspoken messages, both intentional and unintentional. Ideally, our nonverbal communication matches and supports our verbal communication. This is not always the case. Research shows that when verbal and nonverbal communications don't match, we are more likely to believe the nonverbal cues. This is one reason why it is important to be aware of all the nonverbal cues we use regularly and to understand how those cues might be interpreted by others.

Below are several styles of nonverbal communication. Read through this section and think about how and when you may have communicated using these nonverbal strategies.

- *Touch.* A handshake, a warm hug, a hand on the shoulder, a kiss on the cheek
- *Emblems.* Physical gestures that replace words such as a thumbs up or a wave hello or goodbye
- *Illustrators.* Movements that augment verbal communication such as fanning your face when you are hot or holding out your hands to show how big the fish was that got away
- *Affect displays.* Facial expressions of all kinds
- *Regulators.* Nonverbal cues used to regulate or manipulate a conversation such as glancing at one's watch, shifting weight from foot to foot, and eye movements. Sometimes regulators can be construed as rude.
- *Adaptors.* Body language such as folding your arms across your chest, crossing your legs, or leaning forward in your chair
- *Paralanguage.* Elements of speaking that color the use of words, such as pitch, volume, and speed[28]

In addition, territorial space and styles of clothing can also be elements of communication. To make your style of communication as effective as possible, it is important for you to recognize and utilize nonverbal cues that support and help clarify your verbal messages. Awareness and practice of your own verbal and nonverbal communication will also enhance your skills in interpreting the messages of others.

Expressing Difficult Feelings

How many times have you struggled to find just the right words in an emotionally charged situation? Imagine that Sarah has been dating Charles

> **nonverbal communication** All unwritten and unspoken messages, both intentional and unintentional.

and, though she feels he is a great person, he is not the one she wants to date exclusively. She wants to tell him that she likes him a lot, but she is not in love with him. Like most people, Sarah finds it difficult to express her feelings in a way that is not hurtful to another person. Professionals offer the following guidelines for expressing feelings:[29]

- *Try to be specific rather than general about how you feel.* Consistently using only one or two words to say how you are feeling, such as unhappy or upset, is too vague. Explain what you mean by upset: irritated, agitated, anxious, uncomfortable, angry, frightened, bothered?
- *Specify the degree of feelings, and you will reduce the chances of being misunderstood.* When you say angry, someone may think you are enraged when you are just a bit irritated.
- *When expressing anger or irritation, first describe the specific behavior you don't like, then your feelings.* The other person may become immediately defensive or intimidated when he or she first hears "I am angry with you" and could miss the test of the message.
- *If you have mixed feelings, say so; express each feeling, and explain what each feeling is about.* For example: "I really like your sense of humor and your values, but I don't feel comfortable around you 24–7." "I am thankful that I met you and we can be friends, but I don't have the depth of feeling that I think needs to be there for a relationship. We just are too different."

In general, the most tried and true techniques for expressing your feelings involve using **"I" messages** that include feelings like those stated above, rather than "you" statements that imply blame or something that the other person did wrong. "I" messages ("I like being with you"; "I'm sorry that I missed practice") are a direct, clear, and effective way to send information to others. When using "I" messages, the speaker takes responsibility for communicating his or her own feelings, thoughts, and beliefs. People who practice using "I" messages tend to have more positive interactions and generate less defensiveness from listeners.

The opposite of an "I" message is a "you" message. "You" messages are easy to distinguish because they begin with the communicator saying "you" ("You made me so mad"; "You never say you're sorry about anything"). "You" messages put the receiver of the information on the defensive and ready to attack. Consider this of "I" and "you" messages: Terry and Jim have been working together on a class project for most

of the term. Although they are both supposed to contribute 50 percent to the final product, Jim has done very little work thus far. Terry is very angry, but rather than saying, "Jim, you're really lazy, and you are not holding up your part of this assignment," she says, "Jim, I really am feeling overburdened by all of the work I've been putting into this project. I don't want to feel 'used' in this process, and I want both of us to get as much out of the effort as we can." Because Terry is putting this discussion in terms of how she is feeling (using "I" messages) rather than attacking Jim with "you" statements that make him want to defend himself, they are more likely to communicate constructively. Jim is apt to get the message and start contributing to the project.

To practice using "I" messages, follow these steps:

1. *"When you . . ."* Start by thinking about a problem behavior or situation that you want to discuss. Choose something specific—not a vague, sweeping complaint such as "My roommate is such a slob, and he needs to change." Concentrate on a particular ("When you leave your clothes all over the floor . . .").

2. *"I feel . . ."* Identify how the behavior or incident makes you feel, and state those feelings by starting your sentence with "I." Adding a feeling statement allows you to share your reaction honestly without placing blame or exerting power ("I feel frustrated and angry").

3. *"Because . . ."* Add a statement to explain, from your perspective, why the feeling occurred (". . . because I spend so much time trying to keep the place looking good").

Now put these steps together into one simple sentence: "When you leave your clothes all over the floor, I feel frustrated and angry because I spend so much time trying to keep the place looking good."

Communicating Assertively

Communicating assertively means using direct, honest communication that maintains and defends your rights in a positive manner. **Assertive communicators** are people who get their points across while at the same time respecting the rights of others. Assertiveness demands both verbal and nonverbal skills. Verbally, assertive communicators speak calmly, directly, and clearly to those around them. Nonverbally, they maintain direct eye contact, sit or stand facing the person they are speaking to, and sit or stand with an erect posture that indicates confidence and control.

Assertiveness is often distinguished from two other styles of communication that produce poor results: *nonassertiveness* and *aggressiveness*. **Nonassertive communicators** tend to be shy and inhibited. Verbally, nonassertive communicators may speak too rapidly, use a tone that is too low to be heard easily, or not say directly what's on their minds. Nonverbally, their body language frequently reveals timidity: their shoulders slump, they don't face the person they are talking to, or they avoid direct eye contact. Nonassertive people fear that if they really express how they feel, it will upset others. This fear

---

"I" messages Messages in which a person takes responsibility for communicating his or her own feelings, thoughts, and beliefs by using statements that begin with "I," not "you."

assertive communicators People who use direct, honest communication that maintains and defends their rights in a positive manner.

nonassertive communicators Individuals who tend to be shy and inhibited in their communication with others.

leaves them without positive ways of communicating their needs and concerns.

Aggressive communicators tend to employ an angry, confrontational, hostile manner in their interactions with others. Their communications are typically loud and verbally abusive, and they often blame others when things don't go their way. Someone who constantly uses "you" messages, causing the receiver of the information to feel on the defensive immediately, is usually an aggressive communicator.

What's your communication style? Complete the Assess Yourself activity on the next page to find out.

Establishing a Supportive Climate

An open climate for communication does not simply happen. Although selecting a safe place and a trustworthy confidant are important, carefully consider your own role in establishing a supportive climate for conversation. If you follow these steps when you speak, the other person is more likely to engage in an open, honest conversation.

- *Watch judgmental statements.* Words such as *stupid, ridiculous, great, crummy,* or *fantastic* show that an evaluation has already been made. Many of these judgmental statements leave no room for another opinion. Instead, use descriptive statements that reveal your feelings without labeling them as good, bad, right, or wrong. Say, "Your borrowing my car makes me very nervous," rather than, "You stupid jerk, you'll wreck my car and hurt yourself!"
- *Keep an open mind.* Because absolute statements tend to close off other opinions, thereby restricting communication, use qualifying statements to invite others to state their opinions. Say, "This may not always be true, depending on the circumstances," or, "I could be wrong, but it's what I think."
- *Avoid lecturing or projecting superiority.* If you really want someone's opinion, then respect it as having some value. As you learn to show respect for others' opinions, your own viewpoint will become more respected. Monitor your facial expressions, voice pitch and intonation, word choice, and actions to see whether they express true interest and respect.
- *Don't ask for feedback unless you want an honest answer.* How many times have you asked people what they thought, only to be hurt or angry when they told you? If you become visibly upset by honest feedback, people won't give it to you. Look at such feedback as an attempt to help. No one enjoys criticism, but you can't correct a negative action unless you are aware of it.
- *Avoid people who tend to give negative feedback.* Some people have such low self-esteem that they delight in criticizing others. Try to determine the underlying motives of such people, and then avoid them if possible.

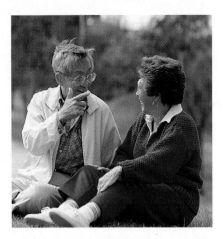

Positive communication means using positive body language. Laugh, smile, and gesture to assure your partner you are engaged.

Managing Conflict

A **conflict** is an emotional state that arises when the behavior of one person interferes with the behavior of another. Conflict is inevitable whenever people live or work together. Not all conflict is bad; in fact, airing feelings and coming to some form of resolution over differences can sometimes strengthen strained relationships. **Conflict resolution** and successful conflict management are a systematic approach to resolving differences fairly and constructively, rather than allowing them to fester. The goal of conflict resolution is to solve differences peacefully and creatively.

Most conflicts revolve around two message components: content and relationship. *Content* is usually easy to discern, as it is the subject of the sentences used by the participants. It deals with the issues on the surface. *Relationship* is more difficult to discern because it embodies the interactions between the people involved and usually involves issues that are much more deeply rooted. Because of the double-pronged nature of messages, many arguments arise out of seemingly innocuous situations. For instance, a housemate comes home from the library, walks into the kitchen, and asks, "What's for dinner?" The other responds, "Whatever you make! When are you going to take care of yourself for once?" On the surface, the conflict may be about dinner. From a relationship standpoint, however, one roommate feels used and underappreciated.

Prolonged conflict can destroy relationships unless the parties agree to resolve points of contention in a constructive manner. As two people learn to negotiate and compromise on

aggressive communicators People who use hostile, loud, and blaming communication styles.

conflict An emotional state that arises when the behavior of one person interferes with the behavior of another.

conflict resolution A concerted effort by all parties to resolve points in contention in a constructive manner.

ASSESS *yourself*

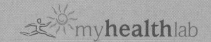

STANDING UP FOR YOURSELF

Fill out this assessment online at www.aw-bc.com/myhealthlab or www.aw-bc.com/donatelle.

You know that sinking feeling. Someone asks you to do something, and your stomach lurches. You don't want to go along, but you can't come up with a good excuse not to do so. It's hard to say no. How often are you caught in the "I can't say no" trap? Read the following situations and assess your response according to the following 5-point scale:

	Never	Seldom	Sometimes	Frequently	Always
1. Friends ask you to ride home with them after they've all been drinking. You know you shouldn't go, but you think one of them is cute and don't want to seem like a prude. You take the ride.	1	2	3	4	5
2. Your decisions can be easily swayed by a strong argument from someone else pushing you in the opposite direction.	1	2	3	4	5
3. You feel strongly about a political issue, but it is the opposite of the opinion your parents hold. You remain silent rather than getting into an argument.	1	2	3	4	5
4. You start out by saying no to something but get talked into doing it after a short time.	1	2	3	4	5
5. You're stressed out with too much to do and too little time, but you can't seem to say no when someone asks for a favor.	1	2	3	4	5
6. Someone says something really nasty about a person you like. You jump to the defense of the person being criticized, even though you are in the minority opinion.	1	2	3	4	5
7. You would describe yourself as assertive and tend to quickly let others know your thoughts about certain issues.	1	2	3	4	5
8. Someone is critical of something you do. You quickly defend your actions by explaining why you did what you did.	1	2	3	4	5

Interpreting Your Score

Think about your responses to each statement. Do your responses indicate an assertive communication style in which you stand up for your feelings or beliefs? What factors cause you to hold back when you should probably speak up? How can you work to improve your communication behaviors in this area? For statements 1 through 5, do you have several "5" responses? If yes, you should consider what skills you could develop to help you communicate more assertively.

---

their differences, the number and intensity of conflicts should diminish. Conflict resolution can therefore be a growth process as people learn to recognize problems and solutions based on past experience.

During a heated conflict, try to pause for a moment before responding, consider the possible impact of your comments or actions, and speak slowly and state your point positively and constructively. You can also dismiss yourself from the situation and walk away by saying something like "I can see we aren't going to resolve this right now. Let's save it for a time when we've both cooled off and can discuss this more calmly."

Rude or inconsiderate behavior usually develops in situations in which a person fails to recognize the feelings or rights of another. To avoid this type of behavior, try to see the other person's point of view, listen actively, avoid interrupting, and avoid making gestures, such as head-shaking or finger-pointing, that indicate disagreement. A key element of managing conflict successfully is to validate others' opinions and treat them as you would like to be treated. Maintain respect and concern for others' welfare at all times.

Here are some strategies for conflict resolution.[30]

1. *Focus on one topic at a time, and make other preoccupations clear,* such as in, "I may seem angry, but I had a

MAKE it happen!

ASSESSMENT: The Assess Yourself activity above gave you the chance to look at how you communicate in certain situations. It is important to be able to communicate assertively and to feel that you can stand up for yourself. Now that you have considered your responses to the statements, you may want to take steps toward becoming a more assertive communicator.

MAKING A CHANGE: In order to change your behavior, you need to develop a plan. Follow the steps below and complete your Behavior Change Contract to take action.

1. Evaluate your behavior and identify patterns and specific things you are doing. What can you change now? What can you change in the near future?

2. Select one pattern of behavior that you want to change.

3. Fill out the Behavior Change Contract found at the front of your book. It should include your long-term goal for change, your short-term goals, the rewards you'll give yourself for reaching these goals, potential obstacles along the way, and strategies for overcoming these obstacles. For each goal, list the small steps and specific actions that you will take.

4. Chart your progress in a journal. At the end of a week, consider how successful you were in following your plan.

What helped you be successful? What made change more difficult? What will you do differently next week?

5. Revise your plan as needed: Are the short-term goals attainable? Are the rewards satisfying?

ONE STUDENT'S PLAN: When Stacey assessed her responses to the statements about assertiveness, she realized that she tended to say yes when someone asked her for a favor, no matter how busy or stressed out she was. Stacey decided she wanted to learn to say no when necessary. She set a goal of imagining certain situations that she had faced recently and how she would handle them more assertively. The first week, she imagined her older sister asking her to babysit her son at the last minute and her roommates asking her for car rides while she was in the middle of studying. She planned what she would say and how she would explain her reasons for saying no. The second week, when her roommates asked for a ride to the movies, Stacey calmly stated that she was busy and needed two hours more for studying before she could take a break. Her roommates decided to walk to the video store instead and rented a movie they could all watch together when Stacey was ready for a break.

---

bad day at school today and I'm really worried about my grades." This takes the heat off the other person.

2. *Stop the action and cool down before things get out of control.* One sign of major distress in a couple is escalating hostility, often in the form of nagging that provokes angry responses. The escalation seems unstoppable once it gets started. Never send an e-mail to someone when you are upset. E-mails make it very easy to misinterpret what someone feels or intends. Talk in person: eye contact, gestures, and body language all speak louder than written words.

3. *Be specific in your criticisms or praises.* Prevent small complaints that you may stew over. You could say, "When I see your clothes on the floor, I feel that you are not doing your share of the work in the house and I feel taken advantage of," instead of, "You're a slob."

4. *Learn to "edit" what you say before you say it* to avoid remarks that would be needlessly hurtful. For example, don't dredge up past events and old grudges during a fight. Don't bring up additional issues before you've resolved the one at hand.

5. *Think about possible solutions that involve compromises for both parties.* Do some brainstorming to

discover options that work for both of you. Consider all the options first, then eliminate those that aren't acceptable to both of you. Be committed to change.

6. *Never think in terms of winning an argument.* Think instead of ways to prevent an argument from starting. By doing so, both parties win. Avoid becoming too invested in getting your way. Remember, your reality is not the only reality!

Gender Issues in Relationships

When it comes to relationships, are men really from Mars and women from Venus? If they are not planets apart, how far apart are they, and what are the implications of the disparities? In her landmark book *You Just Don't Understand: Women and Men in Conversation*, psychologist Deborah Tannen coined the term **genderlect** to characterize differences in word choices, interruption patterns, questioning patterns, language interpretations and misinterpretations, and vocal influences based on gender.[31] Tannen is not alone in her research. In fact, communication patterns between women and men have been studied for generations, with similar results. Recent research validates much of Tannen's work and indicates that women tend to be more expressive, relationship oriented, and concerned with creating and maintaining intimacy; men tend to be more instrumental, task oriented, and concerned with gathering information or establishing and maintaining social status or power.[32] Unlike women, men tend to believe that they are not supposed to show emotions and are brought up to believe that "being strong" is often more important than having close friendships. As a result, men are generally less likely to share their innermost thoughts. Figure 5.3 summarizes some of these characteristics found in each gender.

what do you THINK?

Who are the people with whom you feel most comfortable talking about personal issues? ■ Do you talk with both males and females about these issues, or do you tend to gravitate toward just one sex? ■ Why do you think you do this?

Picking Partners

For both males and females, the choice of partners is influenced by more than just chemical and psychological processes. One important factor is *proximity*, or being in the

same place at the same time. The more you see a person in your hometown, at social gatherings, or at work, the more likely that interaction will occur. Thus, if you live in New York, you'll probably end up with another New Yorker. If you live in Texas, you'll probably end up with another Texan. However, with the advent of the Internet, geographic proximity has become less important.

You also choose a partner based on *similarities* (in attitudes, values, intellect, and interests); the old adage that "opposites attract" usually isn't true. If your potential partner expresses interest or liking, you may react with mutual regard known as *reciprocity*. The more you express interest, the safer it is for someone else to return the regard, and the cycle spirals onward.

A final factor that apparently plays a significant role in selecting a partner is *physical attraction*. Whether such attraction is caused by chemical reactions or socially learned behavior, males and females appear to have different attraction criteria. Men tend to select their mates primarily on the basis of youth and physical attractiveness. Whereas women also value physical attractiveness, they tend to place higher emphasis on partners who are somewhat older, have good financial prospects, and are dependable and industrious.[33]

what do you THINK?

What factors do you consider most important in a potential partner? ■ Which are absolute musts? ■ Are there any differences between what you believe to be important in a relationship and the things your parents feel are important?

Sharing Feelings

Although men tend to talk about intimate issues with women more frequently than with men, women still complain that men do not communicate enough about what is really on their minds. This may reflect the powerfully different socialization processes experienced by women and men, which influence their communication styles. Throughout their lives, females are offered opportunities to practice sharing their thoughts and feelings with others. In contrast, males receive strong societal messages to withhold their feelings. The classic example of this training in very young males is the familiar saying, "Big boys don't cry." Men learn early that certain emotions are not to be shared, with the result that they are more information-focused and businesslike in their conversations. Understandably, such differences in communication styles contribute to misunderstandings and conflict. (See the Women's Health/Men's Health box on page 154.)

Although men are often perceived as being less emotional than women, do they really feel less or do they just have more difficulty expressing their emotions? In one study, when men and women were shown scenes of people in distress, the men exhibited little outward emotion, whereas the women

---

genderlect The "dialect," or individual speech pattern and conversational style, of each gender.

communicated feelings of concern and distress. However, physiological measures of emotional arousal (such as heart rate and blood pressure) indicated that the male subjects were actually as affected emotionally as the female subjects but inhibited the expression of their emotions, whereas the women openly expressed them. In other studies, men and women responded very differently to the same test.[34]

When men are angered, they tend to interpret the cause of their anger as something or someone in their environment and are likely to turn their anger outward in an aggressive manner. Women, on the other hand, tend to see themselves as the source of the problem and turn their anger inward, suppressing direct expression of it.[35]

We All Want to Be Understood

The bottom line is simple: both men and women want to be heard and understood. Understanding gender differences in communication patterns, rather than casting blame at each other, is the first step toward promoting effective communication. Tannen suggests that expecting persons of the other sex to change their style of communication is not an effective way to deal with the gender gap. Instead, learn to interpret messages while explaining your own unique way of communicating. Working to understand the different ways in which males and females use language will help us all achieve the goal of clear and honest communication.

 what do you THINK?

Do you believe that men and women really communicate in different styles? ■ What can you do to improve your communication with members of the other sex?

Overcoming Barriers to Intimacy

Obstacles to intimacy include lack of personal identity, emotional immaturity, and a poorly developed sense of responsibility. The fear of being hurt, low self-esteem, mishandled hostility, chronic "busyness" (and its attendant lack of emotional presence), a tendency to "parentify" loved ones, and a conflict of role expectations may be equally detrimental. In addition, individual insecurities and difficulties in recognizing and expressing emotional needs can lead to an intimacy barrier. These barriers to intimacy may have many causes, including miscommunication, a dysfunctional family background, and jealousy.

Barriers to Communication

In today's world of instant messages, cell phones, pagers, and technologically advanced information systems, communica-

Men

- Talk is primarily a means of preserving independence and negotiating and maintaining status.

- Men are more likely to give advice, tell a joke, change the subject, or remain silent when trouble arises.

- When women offer sympathy to men, men may feel that they are being placed in a lower-status position and find it condescending.

- Men are more likely to be avoidant.

Women

- Talk is primarily a means of rapport, a way of establishing connections and negotiating relationships. Emphasis is on displaying similarities and matching experiences.

- Women are more likely to share a similar problem or openly express sympathy, and to expect sympathy in return.

- When men give advice, women feel that their feelings are being invalidated, their problems are being minimized, or that the simple "fix" provided is condescending.

- Women are likely to be supportive.

FIGURE 5.3 Troubles Talk: How Men and Women Respond

Source: From S. L. Michaud and R. Warner, "Gender Differences in Self-Reported Responses in Troubles Talk," *Sex Roles: A Journal of Research* 37, no. 7–8 (1997): 527.

tion problems have grown exponentially. Our current means of communication differ greatly from those of our ancestors. In addition to physical changes in communication, people around the world must increasingly interact with others of vastly different backgrounds and values. Finding a means of communicating that accommodates everyone can be difficult. Barriers to communication take many forms.

Differences in Background
Age, education, social status, gender, culture, political beliefs, and many other variables can lead to differences between communicators. Your closest friends from high school, with whom you grew up, shared many similar experiences with you. Shared experiences contribute to shared meaning and understanding. At

HOW DIFFERENT ARE MEN AND WOMEN? RECOGNIZING UNIQUENESS

Although men and women may make decisions differently, act differently in terms of their sexual and partnering behaviors, and act in ways that are somewhat distinctive to their genders, these lines have begun to blur over time. Books such as *Men Are from Mars, Women Are from Venus* that focus on these differences capture media attention, but they also have their critics. According to Dr. Cynthia Burggraf Torppa at Ohio State University, differences in communication between men and women are really quite minor. What she says is most important is the way in which men and women interpret or process the same message. She indicates that studies support the idea that women, to a greater extent than men, are sensitive to the interpersonal meanings that lie between the lines in the messages they exchange with their mates. This is because societal expectations often make women responsible for regulating intimacy. Men, on the other hand, are more sensitive than women to subtle messages about status. For them, societal expectations dictate that they negotiate hierarchy, or who's the captain and who's the crew.

There are some gender-specific communication patterns and behaviors that are obvious to the casual observer, however. Recognizing these differences and how they make us unique is a good first step in avoiding unnecessary frustrations and irritations.

Men	Women
Body Language	
Occupy more space; gesture away from the body; lean back when listening; less feedback through body language; more forceful gestures (backslapping, stronger handshakes); overt fidgeting	Take up less space; movement is light and easy; gesture toward the body; lean forward when listening; provide feedback via body language; less likely to invade another's space; more gentle when touching others
Facial Expressions	
Often avoid eye contact; show less warmth in facial expression; frown more often	Maintain better eye contact; smile and nod more often
Speech Patterns	
More likely to interrupt, mumble, and use fewer speech tones (approximately three); voices are lower-pitched and usually louder; sound more abrupt; talk less personally about selves; make more direct statements than feeling statements; use fewer adjectives and descriptive statements; use fewer terms of endearment; tendency to lecture	Interrupt less often; articulate more clearly; use more speech tones (approximately five); may sound more emotional; voices are higher pitched and softer; more likely to discuss feelings and disclose more personal information; make more tentative statements ("kind of," "isn't it?")
Behavioral Differences	
More inclined to be analytical; give fewer compliments; use more sarcasm and teasing to show affection; cry less often; more argumentative; difficulty in expressing intimate feelings; hold fewer grudges; gossip less; less likely to ask for help; tend to take rejection less personally; apologize less often	More emotional approach to issues; give more compliments; show more expression; express feelings more readily; greater tendency to hold grudges; inclined to gossip more; more likely to ask for help; take rejection more personally; apologize more frequently

Sources: C. Burggraf Torppa, "Gender Issues: Communication Differences in Interpersonal Relationships," Family Life Packet, 2002, http://ohioline.osu.edu/flm02/FS04.html; J. Wood, *Gendered Lives: Communication, Gender, and Culture*, 7th ed. (Belmont, CA: Wadsworth, 2004); Kings Communications, "Men and Women Are Different!" 2002, www.KingsCommunications.com. Reprinted by permission; M. L. Knapp and A. L. Vangelisti, *Interpersonal Communication and Human Relationships*, 5th ed. (Boston: Allyn & Bacon, 2004).

college, however, you may suddenly find yourself among people having few shared experiences. Remember that the goal of good communication is not necessarily to have everyone agree with you; rather, it is to have others understand you.

Alcohol and Drugs Perhaps nothing stands in the way of effective communication more than alcohol and drugs. With an inhibited ability to encode messages, you may not be understood correctly. With an inhibited ability to decode messages, you may misinterpret someone else's message. Is it any wonder that 90 percent of campus rapes take place under the influence of alcohol? Avoiding date rape depends on a woman's ability to be clear in her own mind about what she wants and then to make herself clearly understood. It also depends on a man's ability to listen and hear what is being said, rather than what he thinks is being said. In most college campus sexual encounters that lead to date rape complaints, alcohol and drugs have played a role.

Dysfunctional Families As noted earlier, the ability to sustain genuine intimacy is largely developed in the family of origin. If you were to examine even the most pristine family under a microscope, you would likely find some problems. No group of people can interact perfectly all the time, but this does not necessarily make them dysfunctional. In a truly **dysfunctional family**, interaction between family members inhibits psychological growth, self-love, emotional expression, and individual development. Negative interactions are the norm rather than the exception.

Children raised in dysfunctional settings tend to face tremendous obstacles to growing up healthy. Coming to terms with past hurts may take years. However, with introspection, support from loved ones, and counseling when needed, children from even the worst homes have proved to be remarkably resilient. Many are able to move beyond the past and focus on the future, developing into healthy, well-adjusted adults. Some will have problems throughout their lives.

For example, many adult children of alcoholics (ACOAs) become involved in unhealthy relationships and have difficulty trusting others, communicating with partners, and defining a healthy relationship. Another tragically large group of people struggling with intimacy problems originating in the family of origin are survivors of childhood emotional, physical, or sexual abuse (see Chapter 4). It is important to note that dysfunctional families are found in every social, ethnic, religious, economic, and racial group.

Jealousy in Relationships

"Jealousy is like a San Andreas fault running beneath the smooth surface of an intimate relationship. Most of the time, its eruptive potential lies hidden. But when it begins to rumble, the destruction can be enormous."[36] **Jealousy** has been described as an aversive reaction evoked by a real or imagined relationship involving one's partner and a third person. Contrary to what many of us believe, jealousy is not a sign of intense devotion. Instead, jealousy often indicates underlying problems that may prove to be a significant barrier to a healthy intimate relationship. Causes of jealousy typically include:

- *Overdependence on the relationship*. People who have few social ties and who rely exclusively on their significant others tend to be fearful of losing them.
- *High value on sexual exclusivity*. People who believe that sexual exclusiveness is a crucial indicator of love are more likely to become jealous.

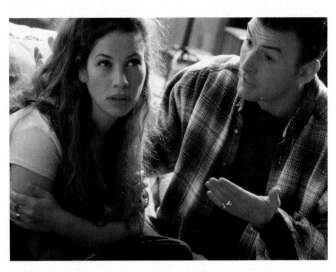

Open communication is key in addressing relationship problems. When one person shuts down, the argument can spin out of control.

- *Low self-esteem*. People who feel good about themselves are less likely to feel unworthy and fear that someone is going to snatch their partner away. The underlying question that torments people with low self-esteem is "Why would anyone want me?"
- *Fear of losing control*. Some people need to feel in control of any situation. Feeling that they may be losing the attachment of or control over a partner can cause jealousy.

In both sexes, jealousy is related to the expectation that it would be difficult to find another relationship if the current one should end. For men, jealousy is positively correlated with the degree to which the man's self-esteem is affected by his partner's judgments. Though a certain amount of jealousy can be expected in any loving relationship, it doesn't have to threaten a relationship as long as partners communicate openly about it.[37]

 what do you THINK?

"Jealousy is not a barometer by which the depth of love can be read. It merely records the depth of the lover's insecurity" (anthropologist Margaret Mead, 1901–1978). Do you agree or disagree with this statement? ■ What other factors may play a role in jealousy?

> **dysfunctional family** A family in which the interaction between family members inhibits rather than enhances psychological growth.
>
> **jealousy** An aversive reaction evoked by a real or imagined relationship involving a person's partner and a third person.

Committed Relationships

Commitment in a relationship means that there is an intent to act over time in a way that perpetuates the well-being of the other person, oneself, and the relationship. Polls show that the majority of Americans—as many as 96 percent—strive to develop a committed relationship. These relationships can take several forms, including marriage, cohabitation, and gay and lesbian partnerships.

Marriage

In many societies around the world, traditional committed relationships take the form of marriage. In the United States, marriage means entering into a legal agreement that includes shared financial plans, property, and responsibility for raising children. Many Americans also view marriage as a religious sacrament that emphasizes certain rights and obligations for each spouse.

Historically, close to 90 percent of Americans marry at least once during their lifetime, although in recent years Americans have become less likely to marry. From 1970 to 2004, there was a 50 percent decline in annual marriages of unmarried adult women.[38] This decrease may be due to several factors, including delay of first marriages, increase in cohabitation, and a small decrease in the number of divorced persons who remarry. In 1970, the median age for first marriage was 22.5 years for men and 20.6 years for women; in 2004, the median age of first marriage had risen to 27 for males and 26 for females.[39]

Many Americans believe that marriage involves **monogamy**, or exclusive sexual involvement with one partner. In fact, the lifetime pattern for many Americans appears to be **serial monogamy**, which means that a person has a monogamous sexual relationship with one partner before moving on to another monogamous relationship. However, some people prefer an **open relationship**, or open marriage, in which both partners agree that there may be sexual involvement for each person outside their relationship.

Humans are not naturally monogamous; most of us are capable of being sexually and/or emotionally involved with more than one person at a time. Sexual infidelity is an extremely common factor in divorces and breakups. So why do we continue to get married?

Certainly marriage is socially sanctioned and highly celebrated in our culture, so there are numerous incentives for couples to formalize their relationship with a wedding ceremony. A

monogamy Exclusive sexual involvement with one partner.

serial monogamy A series of monogamous sexual relationships.

open relationship A relationship in which partners agree that sexual involvement can occur outside the relationship.

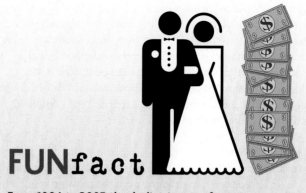

FUNfact

From 1984 to 2003 the decline in rate of marriage in men and women was 44% and 41%, respectively. In 2002, average college debt was $18,900, a 66% increase since 1997.

FIGURE 5.4 Recent research suggests a relationship between the decline in marriage rates among people aged 20–24 and student debt.

Source: A. C. Carlson, "Anti-Dowry? The Effects of Student Loan Debt on Marriage and Childbearing," *The Family in America* online edition 19, no. 12 (2005), www.profam.org.

healthy marriage provides emotional support by combining the benefits of friendship and a loving committed relationship. A happy marriage also provides stability for both the couple and for those involved in the couple's life. Considerable research indicates that married people live longer, feel happier, remain mentally alert longer, and suffer fewer physical and mental health problems.[40] Couples in healthy marriages have decreased stress, which in turn contributes to better overall health. Healthy marriage contributes to lower levels of stress in three important ways: financial stability, expanded support networks, and improved personal behaviors. Married adults are about half as likely to be smokers as single, divorced, or separated adults. They are also less likely to be heavy drinkers or to engage in risky sexual behavior. The one negative health indicator for married people is body weight. Married adults, particularly men, weigh more than do single adults.[41]

Although a successful marriage can bring much satisfaction, traditional marriage does not work for everyone and it is not the only path to a successful committed relationship. See the Spotlight on your Health box for some common misperceptions about marriage.

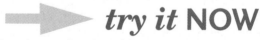 *try it* NOW

After class, make a list of factors you have used, or you think would be useful, in choosing a partner for a committed relationship. Then review the information on common myths associated with marriage and choosing a partner found in the Spotlight on Your Health box. Were you surprised when you compared the information on your list with current research findings?

MARRIAGE DEMYSTIFIED: HELPFUL FACTS AND COMMON MYTHS

For many young adults the idea of marriage conjures images of their parents, and other older adults they may know. What does marriage mean to you? Marriage is the great unknown for many young people, and it is possible that you wonder when Mr. or Ms. Right will come along, where you'll find your lifetime partner, or if there is such a thing as the "perfect" marriage.

The National Marriage Project, a research initiative at Rutgers University in New Jersey, is researching the attitudes of young adults toward marriage, and working to educate them on how to prepare for marriage in the future. The following facts and myths are from the National Marriage Project's current research findings:

Fact—*The most likely way to find a future marriage partner is through an introduction by family, friends, or acquaintances.* Despite the romantic notion that people meet and fall in love through chance or fate, the evidence suggests that social networks are important in bringing together individuals of similar interests and backgrounds, especially when it comes to selecting a marriage partner. According to a large-scale national survey of sexuality, almost 60 percent of married people were introduced by family, friends, coworkers, or other acquaintances.

Myth—*Marriage benefits men much more than women.*

Fact—*Contrary to earlier and widely publicized reports, recent research finds men and women benefit about equally from marriage, although in different ways.* Both men and women live longer, happier, healthier, and wealthier lives when they are married. Husbands typically gain greater health benefits while wives gain greater financial advantages.

Fact—*The more similar people are in their values, backgrounds, and life goals, the more likely they are to have a successful marriage.* Opposites may attract but they may not live together harmoniously as married couples. People who share common backgrounds and similar social networks are better suited as marriage partners than people who are very different in their backgrounds and networks.

Myth—*Couples who live together before marriage, and are thus able to test how well suited they are for each other, have more satisfying and longer-lasting marriages than couples who do not.*

Is it good to live together before getting married?

Fact—*Many studies have found that those who live together before marriage have less satisfying marriages and a considerably higher chance of eventually breaking up.* One reason is that people who cohabit may be more skittish of commitment and more likely to call it quits when problems arise. But in addition, the very act of living together may lead to attitudes that make happy marriages more difficult. The findings of one recent study, for example, suggest "there may be less motivation for cohabiting partners to develop their conflict resolution and support skills." (One important exception: cohabiting couples who are already planning to marry each other in the near future have just as good a chance of staying together as couples who don't live together before marriage.)

Fact—*For large segments of the population, the risk of divorce is far below 50 percent.* Although the overall divorce rate in America remains close to 50 percent of all marriages, it has been dropping gradually over the past two decades. Also, the risk of divorce is far below 50 percent for educated people going into their first marriage, and lower still for people who wait to marry until at least their mid-twenties, haven't lived with many different partners prior to marriage, or are strongly religious and marry someone of the same faith.

Myth—*Married people have less satisfying sex lives, and less sex, than single people.*

Fact—*According to a large-scale national study, married people have both more and better sex than do their unmarried counterparts.* Not only do they have sex more often but they enjoy it more, both physically and emotionally.

Sources: D. Popenoe, "The Top Ten Myths of Marriage," The National Marriage Project Ten Things to Know Series, 2005 http://marriage.rutgers.edu; D. Popenoe, "Ten Important Research Findings on Marriage and Choosing a Marriage Partner: Helpful Facts for Young Adults," 2005, The National Marriage Project, http://marriage.rutgers.edu.

Cohabitation

Cohabitation is defined as two people with an intimate connection who live together in the same household. For a variety of reasons, increasing numbers of Americans are choosing cohabitation. These relationships can be very stable and happy, with a high level of commitment between the partners. In some states, cohabitation that lasts a designated number of years (usually seven) legally allows for some of the same benefits as marriage. This constitutes a **common-law marriage**.

Cohabitation can offer many of the same benefits that marriage does: love, sex, companionship, and the ongoing opportunity to know a partner better over time. In addition to enjoying emotional and physical benefits, some people may cohabit for practical reasons such as the opportunity to share bills and housing costs. Though many cohabitants are young, some older adults choose this lifestyle because they would lose income, such as Social Security or a late spouse's pension, if they were to marry.

Between 1960 and 2004, the number of cohabiting adults in America increased by over 1,000 percent. In fact, today over half of all first marriages are preceded by living together.[42] Cohabitation can serve as a prelude to marriage, but for some, it is an alternative to marriage. Cohabitation is more common among those of lower socioeconomic status, those who are less religious, those who have been divorced, and those who have experienced high levels of parental conflict or parental divorce during childhood. Many people believe that living together before marriage is a good way to find out how compatible a potential partner is and possibly avoid a bad marriage. However, current data do not support this belief. The long-term outcomes or implications of living together may be related more to who chooses to cohabit rather than the experience of cohabitation itself.

Although cohabitation has its advantages, it also has some drawbacks. Perhaps the greatest disadvantage is the lack of societal validation for the relationship, especially if the couple then has children. Many cohabitants must deal with pressures from parents and friends, difficulties in obtaining insurance and tax benefits, and legal issues over property. In 1986, the U.S. Congress reaffirmed tax advantages for married couples and effectively blocked cohabiting heterosexual and homosexual couples from these benefits through the Defense of Marriage Act (DOMA). The purpose of DOMA was to normalize heterosexual marriage on a federal level and permit each state to decide for itself whether to recognize same-sex unions or not. Six states currently have established laws legalizing domestic partnerships that provide access to benefits previously reserved only for marriage partners. In addition, Massachusetts legally recognizes gay marriage. The discussion continues over the traditional religious or faith-based definition and value of marriage versus recognition and equal access to legal rights and privileges afforded persons in long-term committed relationships.

Gay and Lesbian Partnerships

Most adults want intimate, committed relationships, whether they are gay or straight, men or women. Lesbians and gay men seek the same things in primary relationships that heterosexual partners do: friendship, communication, validation, companionship, and a sense of stability.

The 2000 U.S. Census revealed a significant increase in the number of same-sex partner households across the country—more than three times the total reported in the 1990 Census. The states with the most reported same-sex households are California, New York, Florida, Illinois, and Georgia. According to Lee Badgett, research director of the Institute for Gay and Lesbian Strategic Studies, the actual number of households is probably much higher. Many gay and lesbian partners hesitate to report their relationship due to concerns about discrimination.[43]

Studies of lesbian couples indicate high levels of attachment and satisfaction and a tendency toward monogamous long-term relationships. Gay men, too, tend to form committed, long-term relationships, especially as they age, much like their heterosexual counterparts.

Challenges to successful lesbian and gay male relationships often stem from discrimination and difficulties dealing with social, legal, and religious doctrines. For lesbian and gay couples, obtaining the same level of "marriage benefits," such as tax deductions, power of attorney, child custody, and other rights, continues to be a challenge. However, commitment ceremonies and marriage ceremonies are becoming more frequent in some U.S. cities and in several countries. In 2004, courts in Massachusetts legalized marriages between same-sex partners. Worldwide, same sex marriages are legal in the Netherlands, Belgium, Spain, South Africa, and Canada.

Staying Single

Increasing numbers of adults of all ages are electing to marry later or to remain single altogether. Data from 2004 indicate that 75 percent of women aged 20 to 24 have never been married. Likewise, men in this age group postponed marriage in increasing numbers, with over 86 percent remaining unmarried in 2004.[44] According to the most recent figures from the Census Bureau and the National Center for Health Statistics, the number of unmarried women aged 15 and older will soon surpass the number of married women.[45] The number of unmarried men is also increasing. Other changes are reflected in the following facts:

- Over 10 percent of all people say they would never marry.
- People marrying today have about a 50 percent chance of divorcing.

---

cohabitation   Living together without being married.

common-law marriage   Cohabitation lasting a designated period of time (usually seven years) that is considered legally binding in some states.

- As more women enjoy financial independence, they are less likely to remarry after divorce.
- Increasing numbers of widows and widowers are opting not to remarry.

Today, large numbers of people prefer to remain single or to delay marriage. Singles clubs, social outings arranged by communities and religious groups, extended family environments, and a large number of social services support the single lifestyle. Many singles live rich, rewarding lives and maintain a large network of close friends and families. Although sexual intimacy may or may not be present, the intimacy achieved through other interactions with loved ones is a key aspect of the single lifestyle.

Some research indicates that single people live shorter lives, are more unhappy, and are more likely to experience financial and health problems than their married peers. However, other studies refute these conclusions. Few studies to date have controlled for other confounding variables, such as environmental conditions, past histories, and other factors that may carry more weight than the married or single state.

 what do you THINK?

What are the advantages to remaining single? ■ What are potential disadvantages? ■ What societal or organizational supports are available for the single lifestyle?

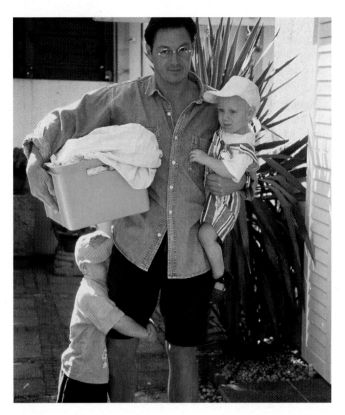

Single parents face additional challenges in juggling their work and family responsibilities. Many use community resources such as after-school day care centers.

Success in Relationships

 Our definition of success in a relationship tends to be based on whether a couple stays together over the years. Learning to communicate, respecting each other, and sharing a genuine fondness are crucial to relationship success. Many social scientists agree that the happiest committed relationships are flexible enough to allow the partners to grow throughout their lives.

Partnering Scripts

Parents often believe that their children will achieve happiness by living much as they have. Accordingly, most children are reared with a very strong script for what is expected of them as adults. Each group in society has its own partnering script that includes similarities of sex, age, social class, race, religion, physical attributes, and personality types. By adolescence, people generally know exactly what type of person they are expected to befriend or date. By which partnering script were you raised? Just picture whom you could or couldn't bring home to meet your family.

Society provides constant reinforcement for traditional couples, but it may withhold this reinforcement from couples of the same sex, mixed race, mixed religion, or mixed age.

People who have not chosen an "appropriate" partner are subject to a great deal of external stress. In addition to denying recognition to such couples, friends and family often blame the "inappropriateness" of the couple if the relationship fails. Recognizing that this stress is external to the relationship can help alleviate criticism and distancing between the partners.

Nonetheless, many nontraditional relationships survive and flourish. For example, the number of interracial marriages has quadrupled since the late 1960s, and the number of same-sex partner households has grown from 145,130 to almost half a million over the past ten years.[46]

 what do you THINK?

What characteristics are most important to you in a potential partner? ■ Which of these would be important to your parents or friends? ■ If your parents or friends didn't like a potential partner, how important would their opinion be to you? ■ What would you do in this situation?

Being Self-Nurturant

It is often stated that you must love yourself before you can love someone else. What does this mean? Learning how you function emotionally and how to nurture yourself through all life's situations is a lifelong task. You should certainly not postpone intimate connections with others until you have achieved this state. However, a certain level of individual maturity helps in maintaining a committed relationship. For example, divorce rates are much higher for couples under age 30 than for older couples.

Two concepts that are especially important to a good relationship are accountability and self-nurturance. **Accountability** means that both partners in a relationship see themselves as responsible for their own decisions and actions. They don't hold the other person responsible for positive or negative experiences.

Self-nurturance goes hand in hand with accountability. In order to make good choices in life, a person needs to maintain a balance of sleeping, eating, exercising, working, relaxing, and socializing. When the balance is disrupted, as it will inevitably be, self-nurturing people are patient with themselves and try to put things back on course. It is a lifelong process to learn to live in a balanced and healthy way. Two people who are on a path of accountability and self-nurturance together have a much better chance of maintaining a satisfying relationship.

Confronting Couple Issues

Couples seeking a long-term relationship have to confront a number of issues that can enhance or ruin their chances of success. Some of these issues involve gender roles and power sharing.

Changing Gender Roles Throughout history, women and men have taken on various roles in their relationships. In agricultural America, gender roles were determined by tradition, and each task within a family unit held equal importance. Our modern society has very few gender-specific roles. Women and men alike drive cars, care for children, operate computers, manage finances, and perform equally well in the tasks of daily living. Rather than taking on the traditional female and male roles, many couples find it makes more sense to divide tasks on the basis of schedule, convenience, and preference. However, while it may make sense to divide household chores, it rarely works out that the division is equal. Today's working woman, living in a dual-career family and coping with the responsibilities of being a partner, a mother, and a professional, is often stressed and frustrated. Men who may have expected a more traditional role for their partners may also experience difficulties. Even when women work full time, they tend to bear heavy family and household

responsibilities. Over time, if couples are unable to communicate about how they feel about performing certain tasks, the relationship may suffer.

Sharing Power **Power** can be defined as the ability to make and implement decisions. There are many ways to exercise power, but powerful people are those who know what they want and have the ability to attain it. In traditional relationships, men were the wage earners and consequently had decision-making power. Women exerted much influence, but in the final analysis they needed a man's income for survival. As women became wage earners in increasing numbers, the power dynamics between women and men changed. Within individual households, however, the dynamics have shifted considerably, with greater numbers of women working and enjoying their own financial resources. Part of the increase in the divorce rate undoubtedly reflects the recognition by working women that they can leave bad relationships in which they previously felt trapped. In general, successful couples have power relationships that reflect their unique needs rather than popular stereotypes.

Having Children . . . or Not?

When a couple decides to raise children, the relationship changes. Resources of time, energy, and money are split many ways, and the partners no longer have each other's undivided attention. Babies and young children do not time their requests for food, sleep, and care to the convenience of adults. Therefore, individuals or couples whose own basic needs for security, love, and purpose are already met make better parents. Any stresses that already exist in a relationship will be further accentuated when parenting is added to the responsibilities. Having a child does not save a bad relationship—in fact, it only seems to compound the problems that already exist. A child cannot and should not be expected to provide the parents with self-esteem and security.

Changing patterns in family life affect the way children are raised. In modern society, it is not always clear which partner will adjust his or her work schedule to provide the primary care of children. Nearly half a million children each year become part of a blended family when their parents remarry; remarriage creates a new family of stepparents and stepsiblings. In addition, an increasing number of individuals are choosing to have children in a family structure other than a heterosexual marriage (see Table 5.1). Single women or lesbian couples can choose adoption or alternative insemination as a way to create a family. Single men can choose to adopt or can obtain the services of a surrogate mother. According to the 2000 Census, over 25 percent of all school-aged children were living in families headed by a man or woman raising a child alone, reflecting a growing trend in America and in the international community.[47] Regardless of the structure of the family, certain factors remain important to

---

accountability   Accepting responsibility for personal decisions, choices, and actions.

self-nurturance   Developing individual potential through a balanced and realistic appreciation of self-worth and ability.

power   The ability to make and implement decisions.

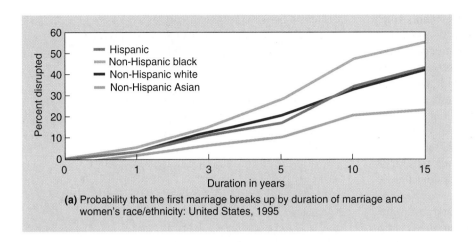

(a) Probability that the first marriage breaks up by duration of marriage and women's race/ethnicity: United States, 1995

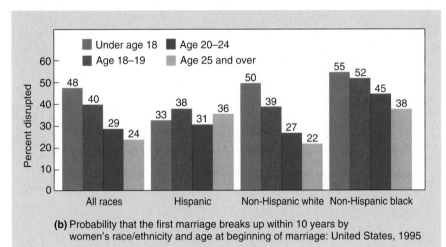

(b) Probability that the first marriage breaks up within 10 years by women's race/ethnicity and age at beginning of marriage: United States, 1995

FIGURE 5.5 Effects of Women's Age and Ethnicity on Marriage Success

Source: National Center for Health Statistics, "Cohabitation, Divorce, and Remarriage in the United States," *National Vital Statistics Report* 23, no. 22 (July 2002): 1–103.

the well-being of the unit: consistency, communication, affection, and mutual respect.

Some people become parents without a lot of forethought. Some children are born into a relationship that was supposed to last and didn't. This does not mean it is too late to do a good job of parenting. Children are amazingly resilient and forgiving if parents show respect and communicate about household activities that affect their lives. Even children who grew up in a household of conflict can feel loved and respected if the parents treat them fairly. This means that parents must take responsibility for their own emotions and make it clear to children that they are not the reason for the conflict.

Finally, consider the financial implications of deciding to have a child. Today, many families find that two incomes are needed just to make ends meet. It is estimated that a family that had a child in 2004 will spend close to $250,000 to raise the child over the next 17 years, and this does not take into account the costs of college.[48] Indeed, more than 80 percent of all mothers with children under the age of 5 work outside the home. Day care workers, family members, friends, grandparents, neighbors, and nannies "mind the kids." Some employers offer family leave arrangements that allow parents more latitude in taking time away from work.

 what do you THINK?

What characteristics of a healthy family environment are important to you? ■ Do you think that day care centers, extended families, and full-time babysitters can provide a positive environment for children? Why or why not?

When Relationships Falter

Breakdowns in relationships usually begin with a change in communication, however subtle. Either partner may stop listening, ceasing to be emotionally present for the other. In turn, the other feels ignored, unappreciated, or unwanted. Unresolved conflicts increase, and unresolved anger can cause problems in sexual relations, sometimes leading to infidelity. Over time, relationships with such difficulties may end in divorce. Age at first marriage, race, and socioeconomic status also affect the success of relationships (Figure 5.5).

When a couple who previously enjoyed spending time together find themselves continually in the company of others, spending time apart, or preferring to stay home alone, it may be a sign that the relationship is in trouble. Of course, seeing to the need for individual privacy and **autonomy** (the ability to care for oneself emotionally, socially, and physically) is not a cause for worry—it's essential to health. If, however, a partner decides to change the amount and quality of time spent together without the input or understanding of the other, it may be a sign of hidden problems.

College students, particularly those who are socially isolated and far from family and hometown friends, may be particularly vulnerable to staying in unhealthy relationships. They may become emotionally dependent on a partner for everything from eating meals to recreational and study time, and mutual obligations such as shared rental arrangements, transportation, and child care can make it tough to leave.

It's also easy to mistake sexual advances for physical attraction or love. Without a network of friends and supporters to talk with, to obtain validation for feelings, or to share concerns, a student may feel stuck in a relationship that is headed nowhere.

Honesty and verbal affection are usually positive aspects of a relationship. In a troubled relationship, however, they can be used to cover up irresponsible or hurtful behavior. "At least I was honest" is not an acceptable substitute for acting in a trustworthy way. The words "But I really do love you" should not be used as a license to be inconsiderate or rude.

Getting Help

The first place most people look for help for relationship problems is a trusted friend. However, although friends can offer support during trying times, few have the training and detachment necessary to resolve serious relationship problems.

Most communities have trained therapists who specialize in relationship difficulties. These practitioners may be psychiatrists, licensed psychologists, social workers, or counselors with advanced degrees. Most student health centers or on-campus counseling centers offer these services at low cost. If you don't know how to find such services, ask your instructor for suggestions.

If a couple's commitment to the relationship is strong, the chances of solving problems increase. The counselor typically interviews the partners separately and together, gradually helping them recognize and change the behaviors and attitudes that are detrimental to the relationship. Counseling may take a few weeks, several months, or even years as couples examine their values and reestablish their commitment.

Beware of the counselor who tells you during the first visit to drop the relationship or who tries to give advice without hearing the full story. Most good counselors will spend a

---

autonomy The ability to care for oneself emotionally, socially, and physically.

TABLE 5.2	World Divorce Rates

Divorce is legal in the countries shown in this list; the divorce rates are per 100 marriages.

Sweden	54.9
United States	54.8
Belarus	52.9
Finland	51.2
Luxembourg	47.4
Denmark	44.5
Belgium	44.0
Austria	43.4
Czech Republic	43.3
Russia	43.3
United Kingdom	42.6
Norway	40.4
Ukraine	40.0
Germany	39.4
France	38.3
Netherlands	38.3
Hungary	37.5
Canada	37.0
Moldova	28.1
Portugal	26.2
Switzerland	25.5
Bulgaria	21.1
Romania	19.1
Poland	17.3
Greece	15.7
Spain	15.2
Italy	10.0
Turkey	6.0

Sources: Americans for Divorce Reform, "World Divorce Rates," 2002, www.divorcereform.org; *Recent Demographic Developments in Europe, 2001* (Strasbourg, France: Council of Europe Publishing, 2001); Jean-Paul Sardon, "Recent Demographic Trends in the Developed Countries," *Population: English Edition* 57 (January–February 2002): 111–156.

good deal of time letting you tell them what you want and helping you work through your feelings rather than adopting theirs.

Trial Separations

Sometimes a relationship becomes so dysfunctional that even counseling cannot bring about significant change. Moving apart for a period of time may allow some preliminary healing and give both parties an opportunity to reassess themselves and their commitment. Trial separations do not guarantee that the situation will improve, nor do they mean the relationship is ending. If both people are involved in counseling or have other support systems and mutually agree on the need for a trial separation, it may be a way to regroup and save a failing relationship.

SKILLS FOR behavior change

ENDING A RELATIONSHIP

Relationship endings are just as important as relationship beginnings. Everyone wants to know why a relationship didn't work. Healthy closure affords both parties the opportunity to move on without wondering or worrying about what went wrong and whose fault it was. If you need to end a relationship, take the time to do so in a manner that preserves and respects the dignity of both partners. If you are the person "breaking up," you have probably had time to think about the process and may be at a different stage than the other party involved. Here are some tips for ending a relationship in a respectful and caring manner.

> **How can I end a relationship without hurting my partner too much?**

- Arrange a time and quiet place where you can talk without interruption.
- Say in advance that there is something important that you want to discuss.
- Accept that your partner may express strong feelings and be prepared to quietly listen.
- Consider in advance if you might also become upset and what support you might need.
- Communicate honestly using "I" messages and without personal attacks. Explain your reasons as much as you can without being cruel or insensitive.
- Don't let things escalate into a fight, even if you have very strong feelings.
- Provide another opportunity to talk about the end of the relationship when you both have had time to reflect.

Source: Adapted from "How to End a Relationship," www.professionalcounselling.co.uk/ending_relationship.html.

When and Why Relationships End

The lifetime probability of divorce or separation of a recently married couple in the United States is between 40 and 50 percent. Though this is still high, it does represent a small decline from previous decades. This small decrease may be related to an increase in the age at which persons first marry and also a higher level of education among those who are marrying. Increased age and education both contribute to marital stability.[49] Table 5.2 compares the American divorce rate with that of other countries.

While the divorce rate may seem alarming, the actual number of failed relationships is probably much higher. Many people never go through a legal divorce process and, as a result, are not counted in these statistics. Cohabitants and unmarried partners, who raise children, own homes together, and exhibit all the outward appearances of marriage without the license, are also not included.

Why do relationships end? There are many reasons, including illness, financial concerns, and career problems. Other breakups arise from unmet expectations. Many people enter a relationship with certain expectations about how they and their partner will behave. Failure to communicate these beliefs can lead to resentment and disappointment. Differences in sexual needs may also contribute to the demise of a relationship. Under stress, communication and cooperation between partners can break down. Conflict and negative interactions as well as a general lack of respect between partners can erode even the most loving relationship. One rather telling predictor of divorce appears to be husband dissatisfaction in the first five years of marriage.

 what do you THINK?

What factors do you think contribute to the high U.S. divorce rate? ■ How would you explain Americans' attitudes about marriage and divorce to a friend from another country?

Coping with Failed Relationships

> **What can I do to cope with a bad breakup?**

No love relationship comes with a guarantee, no matter how many promises have been made by partners to be together forever. Losing a love is as much a part of life as falling in love. That being said, the uncoupling process can be very painful (see the Skills for Behavior Change box on ending a relationship). Whenever we risk getting close to another, we also risk being hurt if things don't work out. Remember that knowing, understanding, and feeling good about oneself before entering a relationship is very important. Consider these tips for coping with a failed relationship:[50]

1. *Recognize and acknowledge your feelings,* which may include grief, loneliness, rejection, anger, guilt, relief, or sadness. Seek professional help and support as needed.

TABLE 5.3 Healthy versus Unhealthy Relationships

Being in a *healthy relationship* means . . .	If you are in an *unhealthy relationship* . . .
Loving and taking care of yourself before and while in a relationship.	You care for and focus on another person only and neglect yourself or you focus only on yourself and neglect the other person.
Respecting individuality, embracing differences, and allowing each person to "be themselves."	You feel pressure to change to meet the other person's standards, you are afraid to disagree, and your ideas are criticized. Or, you pressure the other person to meet your standards and criticize his/her ideas.
Doing things with friends and family and having activities independent of each other.	One of you has to justify what you do, where you go, and who you see.
Discussing things, allowing for differences of opinion, and compromising equally.	One of you makes all the decisions and controls everything without listening to the other's input.
Expressing and listening to each other's feelings, needs, and desires.	One of you feels unheard and is unable to communicate what you want.
Trusting and being honest with yourself and each other.	You lie to each other and find yourself making excuses for the other person.
Respecting each other's need for privacy.	You don't have any personal space and have to share everything with the other person.
Sharing sexual histories and sexual health status with a partner.	Your partner keeps his/her sexual history a secret or hides a sexually transmitted infection from you, or you do not disclose your history to your partner.
Practicing safer sex methods.	You feel scared of asking your partner to use protection or he or she has refused your requests for safer sex. Or, you refuse to use safer sex methods after your partner has requested, or you make your partner feel scared.
Respecting sexual boundaries and being able to say no to sex.	Your partner has forced you to have sex or you have had sex when you don't really want to. Or, you have forced or coerced your partner to have sex.
Resolving conflicts in a rational, peaceful, and mutually agreed upon way.	One of you yells and hits, shoves, or throws things at the other in an argument.
Having room for positive growth, and learning more about each other as you develop and mature.	You feel stifled, trapped, and stagnant. You are unable to escape the pressures of the relationship.

Source: Advocates for Youth, "Healthy versus Unhealthy Relationships," 2005, www.advocatesforyouth.org/youth/health/relationships/healthy.htm.

2. *Find healthful ways to express your emotions*, rather than turning them inward. Go for a walk, talk to friends, listen to music, work out at the gym, volunteer with a community organization, or write in a journal.

3. *Spend time with current friends or reconnecting with old friends.* Get reacquainted with yourself and what you enjoy doing.

4. *Don't rush into a "rebound" relationship.* You need time to resolve your past experience rather than escape from it. You can't be trusting and intimate in a new relationship if you are still working on getting over a past relationship.

psychoeducation The teaching of crucial psychological skills, giving people knowledge so they can help themselves.

Building Better Relationships

Most relationships start with great optimism and true love. So why do so many run into trouble? "We just don't know how to handle the negative feelings that are the unavoidable by-product of the differences between two people, the very differences that attract them to each other in the first place. Think of it as the friction any two bodies would generate rubbing against each other countless times each day," says Howard Markman, PhD, professor of psychology at the University of Denver.[51] According to Markman, most unhappy couples don't need therapy; they need education in how relationships work and the special skills that make them work well. Markman and others promote **psychoeducation**, the teaching of crucial psychological skills—giving people knowledge so they can help themselves. Psychoeducation courses aren't therapy per se, but they typically have a therapeutic effect on couples.

Elements of Healthy Relationships

Stable, satisfying relationships are characterized by good communication, intimacy, friendship, and other factors discussed in this chapter (Table 5.3). A key ingredient is **trust**, the degree of confidence felt in a relationship. Without trust, intimacy will not develop and the relationship could fail. Trust includes three fundamental elements:

- *Predictability* means that you can predict your partner's behavior, based on the knowledge that your partner acts in consistently positive ways.
- *Dependability* means that you can rely on your partner to give support in all situations, particularly those in which you feel threatened with hurt or rejection.
- *Faith* means that you feel absolutely certain about your partner's intentions and behavior.

Trust can develop even when it is initially lacking. This requires opening yourself to others, which carries the risk of hurt or rejection.

Other characteristics of happy relationships include the following items.

- Partners interpret each other's behavior in the context of their own relationship, without overreacting to behaviors that remind them of past relationships. For example, if a previous partner continually flirted with other people and cheated on you, the sight of your current partner dancing with someone else at a party could trigger unpleasant memories. However, don't assume that your current partner will behave the same way.
- Partners who like each other and find each other interesting are happier than those who don't. Many people describe their partners as their best friends. Although most relationships have their share of ups and downs, members of successful couples are able to talk, listen, and touch each other in an atmosphere of caring. They value a good sense of humor and exhibit clear communication, cooperation, and the ability to resolve conflicts constructively.
- Sexual intimacy is a major component of healthy relationships, but sex is not a major reason for the existence of the relationship. Some couples admit to sexual dissatisfaction but find the relationship itself more important than sexual pleasure. Many couples report that as communication and trust increase, the sexual relationship also improves.
- Another important quality is a shared and cherished history, including private jokes, special places where key events have occurred, nicknames, rituals, emotions, and significant shared time and activities.

After reading this chapter, it should be apparent that relationships—whether with partners, parents, friends, or others—involve complex interactions that don't always work the way you'd like them to. Occasionally, they'll lead to frustration and disappointment. However, they also will be a source of great joy and fulfillment. Developing skills that will protect you in a relationship and also help your relationship grow and flourish is an important step in achieving good relationship health. In addition, learning not to take yourself quite so seriously, to forgive others' slips, and to overcome your own fears and overreactions will help keep relationships on course.

> **trust** The degree of confidence felt in a relationship.

TAKING charge

Summary

- Intimate relationships have certain important characteristics, including behavioral interdependence, need fulfillment, emotional attachment, and emotional availability. These characteristics influence how we interact with others and the types of intimate relationships we form. Family, friends, and partners or lovers provide the most common opportunities for intimacy. Each relationship may include healthy and unhealthy characteristics that may affect daily functioning.
- Gender differences in communication can include different conversation styles as well as differences in sharing feelings and disclosing personal facts and fears. These differences explain why men and women may relate differently in intimate relationships. Understanding these differences and learning how to deal with them are important aspects of healthy relationships.
- Communication is a complex process that dictates how we interact with others. Understanding each other's words and symbols is an important part of communication. Our perceptions of these words and symbols, or our way of interpreting incoming information, is equally consequential as we forge relationships throughout our lives.

- To improve our ability to communicate with others, we need to address a number of factors. These include learning how to use self-disclosure, listen effectively, convey and interpret nonverbal communication, establish a proper climate for communicating, and manage and resolve conflicts.
- Barriers to intimacy often involve barriers in communication, which could result from a difference in background or the effects of alcohol and drugs. Other barriers may include the different emotional needs of the partners, jealousy, and emotional wounds that could result from being raised in a dysfunctional family.
- Commitment is an important ingredient in successful relationships for most people. The major types of committed relationships include marriage, cohabitation, and gay and lesbian partnerships.
- Success in committed relationships requires understanding the roles of partnering scripts, the importance of self-nurturance, the elements of a good relationship, and the ability to confront couple issues.

- Life decisions such as whether to marry or whether to have children require serious consideration. Remaining single is more common than ever before. Most single people lead healthy, happy, and well-adjusted lives. Those who decide to have or not to have children can also lead rewarding, productive lives as long as they have given this decision the utmost thought, weighing the pros and cons of each alternative in the context of their lifestyles. Today's family structure may look different from that of previous generations, but love, trust, and commitment to a child's welfare continue to be the cornerstones of successful childrearing.
- Before relationships fail, often many warning signs appear. By recognizing these signs and taking action to change behaviors, partners may save and enhance their relationship.
- There are many strategies for building better relationships. Examining one's own behaviors to determine what to change and how to change it is an important ingredient of success.

Chapter Review

1. Intense feelings of elation, sexual desire, and ecstasy being with a partner is characteristic of
   a. companionate love.
   b. mature love.
   c. passionate love.
   d. intimacy.

2. Cohabitation by unmarried couples is more likely to be a relationship among
   a. African American or Hispanic couples.
   b. Asian couples.
   c. white couples.
   d. higher income couples.

3. Half of first marriages end in divorce after an average of how many years?
   a. five
   b. seven to eight
   c. ten
   d. over 20

4. A common predictor of marital discord or unhappiness is
   a. defensive behavior.
   b. expressions of contempt about the other partner.
   c. stonewalling by showing no response to the partner's concerns or fears.
   d. All of the above.

5. *Perception* is a process that people use to
   a. select those individuals in which to carry on meaningful conversations.
   b. learn more about their own likes and dislikes in other people.
   c. filter and interpret information from all the senses to create a meaningful picture of the world.
   d. assume what the other person is trying to communicate.

6. Terms such as *behavioral interdependence, need fulfillment,* and *emotional availability* describe which type of relationship?
   a. dysfunctional relationship
   b. sexual relationship
   c. intimate relationship
   d. behavioral relationship

7. All of the following terms are used to describe what true love means *except*
   a. intimacy.
   b. passion.
   c. codependency.
   d. commitment.

8. Competitive listening refers to
   a. attentive listening to what the other person is saying.
   b. paraphrasing what the other person is communicating to you.
   c. arguing or debating without listening to what the other person is trying to express.
   d. promoting our own point of view.

9. One of the most important ways to express difficult feelings with another person is to
   a. be specific rather than general about how you feel.
   b. express anger and resentment so the other person feels your heartache.
   c. point your finger at the other person.
   d. blame the other person for the difficulty you are experiencing.

10. The communication style that conveys one's point of view while respecting the rights of others is known as
   a. aggressive communication.
   b. nonassertive communication.
   c. assertive communication.
   d. conflict resolution communication.

Answers to these questions can be found on page A-1.

Questions for Discussion and Reflection

1. Why are symbolism and individual perception so critical to the communication process?
2. How are self-esteem and stress directly related to physical well-being? How does communication improve self-esteem and reduce stress?
3. Why is self-disclosure so important to mental well-being? At what times is it better not to disclose personal information?
4. What is nonverbal communication, and why is it important to develop skills in this area? Give examples of some things that you do to communicate without words.
5. What are the characteristics of intimate relationships? What are behavioral interdependence, need fulfillment, emotional attachment, and emotional availability, and why is each important in relationship development?
6. Why are relationships with family important? Explain how your family unit was similar to or different from the traditional family unit in early America. Who made up your family of origin? your nuclear family?

7. How can you tell the difference between a love relationship and one that is based primarily on attraction? What characteristics do love relationships share?
8. What problems can form barriers to intimacy? What actions can you take to reduce or remove these barriers?
9. What are common elements of good relationships? Warning signs of trouble? What actions can you take to improve your own interpersonal relationships?
10. Name some common misconceptions about people who choose to remain single and about couples who choose not to have children. Do you want to have children? Why or why not? What characteristics show that a couple is ready to have children?
11. How have gender roles changed over the past twenty years? Do you view the changes as positive for women? For men?

Accessing Your Health on the Internet

The following websites explore further topics and issues related to personal health. You'll also find links to each organization's website on the Companion Website for *Access to Health,* Tenth Edition, at www.aw-bc.com/donatelle.

1. *Couples National Network.* Link into a network for same-sex couples and singles, with resources about gay and lesbian issues. http://couples-national.org
2. *Mental Health Notes.* User-friendly information about dysfunctional families from a licensed clinical psychologist. Includes links to related mental health articles. www.ontario.cmha.ca/content/readingroom/mhnotes.asp

3. *National Center for Health Statistics.* This division of the Centers for Disease Control and Prevention has up-to-date statistics on trends in marriage, divorce, and cohabitation. www.cdc.gov/nchs
4. *Relationship Growth Online.* Provides information, quizzes, games, advice, and links to more information on how to build better relationships. www.relationshipweb.com
5. *University of Missouri Counseling Center Self-Help Area.* Provides a bibliography of books and other resources dealing with intimacy issues. http://campus.umr.edu/counsel/selfhelp

Further Reading

Bailey, J. *Slowing Down to the Speed of Love*. New York: McGraw-Hill, 2005.

> *A faculty member at the Center for Spirituality and Healing at the University of Minnesota School of Medicine gives his advice on love and relationships.*

Busby, D. and V. Loyer-Carlson. *Pathways to Marriage with RELATE Online Relationship Inventory: Premarital and Early Marital Relationships*. Boston: Allyn & Bacon/Longman, 2003.

> *Step-by-step approach to building better relationships.*

Erber, R. and M. Wang-Erber. *Intimate Relationships: Issues, Theories, and Research*. Boston: Allyn & Bacon, 2001.

> *Overview of common issues in relationships, theories about why relationships succeed and fail, and discussions of relevant research.*

Fisher, H. *Why We Love: The Nature and Chemistry of Romantic Love*. New York: Henry Holt, 2004.

> *Overview of biological and chemical physiological reactions that stimulate love, lust, and romantic attachment.*

Galvin, K. and P. Cooper. *Making Connections*. Los Angeles: Roxbury Publishing, 2000.

> *Outstanding overview of the importance of interpersonal communication in everyday lives. Provides practical strategies to assist us at all stages of life.*

Sichel, M. *Healing from Family Rifts*. New York: McGraw-Hill, 2004.

> *The author, a therapist and clinical social worker, provides advice on dealing with family issues and problems that may seem insurmountable.*

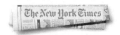

e-themes from *The New York Times*

For up-to-date articles about current health issues, visit www.aw-bc.com/donatelle, select *Access to Health,* Tenth Edition, Chapter 5, and click on "e-themes."

References

1. MayoClinic.com, "Nurture Relationships: A Healthy Investment," Mayo Foundation for Medical Education and Research (MFMER), 2002, www.mayohealth.org/home.
2. H. Lerner, *The Dance of Intimacy* (New York: Perennial, 1990).
3. S. Brehm et al., *Intimate Relationships*, 4th ed. (New York: McGraw-Hill, 2006), 6–7.
4. E. Weinstein and E. Rosen, *Teaching About Human Sexuality and Family: A Skills-Based Approach* (Belmont, CA: Thompson Higher Education, 2006)
5. Ibid.
6. L. Lefton and L. Brannon, *Psychology*, 9th ed. (Boston: Allyn & Bacon, 2005), 474.
7. Ibid.
8. J. Turner and L. Rubinson, *Contemporary Human Sexuality* (Englewood Cliffs, NJ: Prentice Hall, 1993), 457.
9. Ibid.
10. E. Hatfield, "Passionate and Compassionate Love," in *The Psychology of Love*, ed. R. J. Sternberg and M. Barnes (New Haven: Yale University Press, 1988), 191–217.
11. E. Hatfield and G. W. Walster, *A New Look at Love* (Reading, MA: Addison-Wesley, 1981).
12. H. Fisher, *Why We Love: The Nature and Chemistry of Romantic Love* (New York: Henry Holt, 2004).
13. A. Toufexis and P. Gray, "What Is Love? The Right Chemistry," *Time* 1993, 47–52.
14. Ibid.
15. Ibid.
16. C. McLoughlin, "Science of Love—Cupid's Chemistry," 2003, www.thenakedscientist.com/HTML/Columnists/clairemcloughlincolumn1.htm.
17. Ibid.
18. C. Snapp and M. Leary, "Hurt Feelings Among New Acquaintances: Moderating Effects of Interpersonal Familiarity," *Journal of Social and Personal Relationships* 18, no. 3 (June 2001): 1344–1350.
19. D. Busby and V. Loyer-Carlson, *Pathways to Marriage with RELATE Online Relationship Inventory: Premarital and Early Marital Relationships* (Boston: Allyn & Bacon/Longman, 2003).
20. K. Galvin and P. Cooper, *Making Connections* (Los Angeles: Roxbury Publishing, 2000), 4.
21. Ibid., 6.
22. R. Adler and G. Rodman, "Perceiving the Self," in *Making Connections*, ed. K. Galvin and P. Cooper (Los Angeles: Roxbury Press, 2000), 23.
23. B. L. Seaward, *Managing Stress: Principles and Practices for Health and Well-Being*, 4th ed. (Boston: Jones and Bartlett, 2004), 290.
24. Ibid., 100.
25. L. A. Nadig, "Effective Listening," 2004, www.drnadig.com/listening.htm.
26. Ibid.
27. Ibid.
28. Seaward, *Managing Stress: Principles and Practices for Health and Well-Being*.
29. L. A. Nadig, "How to Express Difficult Feelings," 2004, www.drnadig.com/feelings.htm.
30. L. A. Nadig, "Relationship Conflict: Healthy or Unhealthy," 2004, www.drnadig.com.conflict.htm.
31. D. Tannen, *You Just Don't Understand: Women and Men in Conversation* (New York: William Morrow, 1990).
32. S. Michaud and R. Warner, "Gender Differences," *Sex Roles* 37 (1997): 528–540; K. Pasley, J. Kerpelman, and D. Guilbert, "Gender

Conflict; Identity Disruption and Marital Instability. Expanding Gottman's Model," *Journal of Social and Personal Relationships* 18, no. 1 (2001): 1107–1114; L. C. Gallo and T. W. Smith, "Attachment Style in Marriage: Adjustments and Responses to Interaction," *Journal of Social and Personal Relationships* 18, no. 2 (2001): 263–289; J. Manusov and J. Harvey, eds., *Attribution, Communication Behavior, and Close Relationships* (New York: Cambridge University Press, 2001).

33. S. A. Rathus, J. Nevid, and L. Fichner-Rathus, *Human Sexuality in a World of Diversity*, 6th ed. (Boston: Allyn & Bacon, 2005).

34. C. Morris and A. Maisto, *Psychology: An Introduction*, 12th ed. (Upper Saddle River, NJ: Prentice Hall, 2005).

35. Ibid.

36. Brehm et al., *Intimate Relationships*.

37. G. F. Kelly, *Sexuality Today: The Human Perspective*, 8th ed. (Boston: McGraw-Hill, 2006), 270.

38. The National Marriage Project, Rutgers, the State University of New Jersey, "The State of Our Unions," 2005, http://marriage.rutgers.edu.

39. U.S. Census Bureau, "Estimated Median Age at First Marriage, by Sex: 1890 to Present," June 12, 2003, www.census.gov/population/www/socdemo/hh-fam.html history.

40. Mayo Clinic Staff, "Healthy Marriage: Why Love Is Good For You," Mayo Foundation for Medical Education and Research (MFMER), February 8, 2006, www.mayoclinic.com/print/healthy-marriage/MH00108.

41. C. A. Schoenborn, "Marital Status and Health: United States, 1999–2002," December 15, 2004, Advance Data from Vital and Health Statistics, CDC.

42. U.S. Census Bureau, "Estimated Median Age at First Marriage, by Sex: 1890 to Present."

43. Ibid.

44. U.S. Census Bureau, "Current Population Survey," March 2004, www.census.gov/population/www/socdemo/hh-fam.html.

45. U.S. Census Bureau, "Marital Status of People 15 Years and Older, March 2002," June 2003, www.census.gov/population/www.socdemo/hh-fam.html; Centers for Disease Control and Prevention, "Advance Data, First Marriage Dissolution, Divorce, and Remarriage: United States," 2001, www.cdc.gov/nchs/data/ad/ad323.pdf.

46. P. Alsop, "As Same-Sex Households Grow, More Mainstream Business takes Note, *The Wall Street Journal*, August 8, 2001.

47. National Center for Health Statistics, *National Vital Statistics Report* 49, no. 6 (August 2001).

48. U.S. Department of Labor Statistics, "Consumer Expenditure Survey," 2004, www.bls.gov/eex/csxover.htm.

49. The National Marriage Project, Rutgers, "The State of Our Unions," 2005.

50. Kelly, *Sexuality Today*.

51. H. Markman, "Love Lessons: Six New Moves to Improve your Relationship," *Psychology Today* (March/April 1997): 42–49.

6

Sexuality

CHOICES IN SEXUAL BEHAVIOR

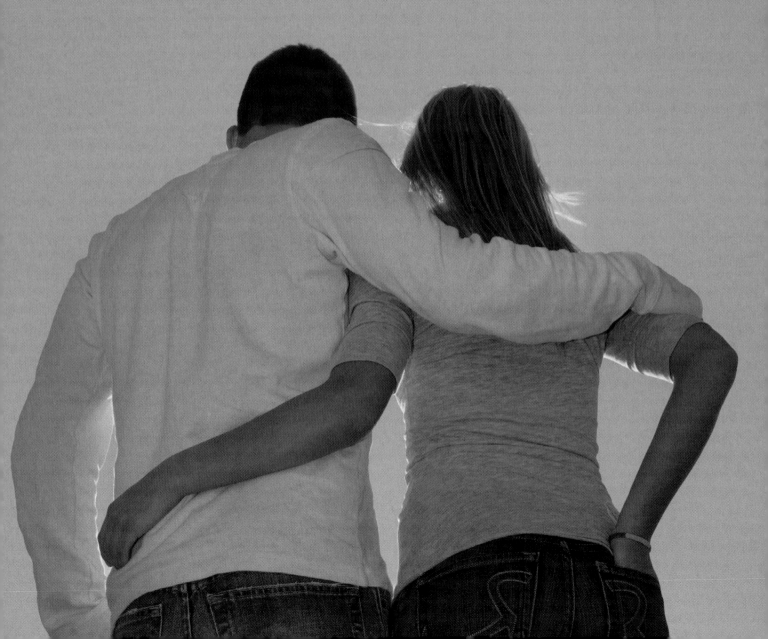

What else influences sexual **identity** besides biological gender?

Do men and women have the same sexual **response**?

What is **"normal"** sexual behavior?

How do **drugs** like Viagra work?

How much **sex** do my peers have?

OBJECTIVES

- Define sexual identity, and discuss its major components, including biology, gender identity, gender roles, and sexual orientation.
- Identify major features and functions of sexual anatomy and physiology.
- Discuss the options available for the expression of one's sexuality.
- Classify sexual dysfunctions, and describe major disorders.

Human sexuality can be fascinating, complex, contradictory, and sometimes frustrating. In reality, sexuality is interwoven into every aspect of being human. No single theory or perspective can explain all its subtleties. It presents challenges in the areas of personal values, interpersonal relationships, cultural traditions, social norms, new technologies, current research findings, and changing political agendas.

This interwoven nature of our sexuality is illustrated in Figure 6.1. Sexuality is much more than sexual feelings or sexual intercourse. Rather, it includes all the thoughts, feelings, and behaviors associated with being male or female, experiencing attraction, being in love, and being in relationships that include sexual intimacy and sexual activity. The five circles of sexuality include:[1]

- *Sensuality.* Awareness and feelings about your own body and other people's bodies, especially the body of your sexual partner. Sensuality enables us to feel good about how our bodies look and feel and to enjoy the pleasure our bodies can give us and others.
- *Intimacy.* Sexual intimacy is the ability to be emotionally close to another human being and to accept closeness in return.
- *Sexual identity.* A person's understanding of who she or he is sexually, including one's sense of maleness or femaleness.
- *Sexual health and reproduction.* A person's attitudes and behaviors related to producing children, care and maintenance of the sex and reproductive organs, and health consequences of sexual behavior.
- *Sexualization.* The use of sexuality to influence, control, or manipulate others, in either a harmful or harmless manner.

In this chapter, we will focus primarily on sexual identity, aspects of sexual health and reproduction, and sensuality. Because our sexuality is central to who we are, many of these topics are discussed throughout this text. In the end, having a comprehensive understanding of your sexuality will help prepare you to make healthful, responsible, and satisfying decisions about your life and your interpersonal relationships.

sexual identity   Recognition of oneself as a sexual being; a composite of biological sex characteristics, gender identity, gender roles, and sexual orientation.

intersexuality   Not exhibiting exclusively female or male primary and secondary sex characteristics.

gonads   The reproductive organs in a male (testes) or female (ovaries).

puberty   The period of sexual maturation.

secondary sex characteristics   Characteristics associated with gender but not directly related to reproduction, such as vocal pitch, degree of body hair, and location of fat deposits.

gender   The psychological condition of being feminine or masculine as defined by the society in which one lives.

Your Sexual Identity: More Than Biology

What else influences sexual identity besides biological gender?

Sexual identity, the recognition and acknowledgment of oneself as a sexual being, is determined by a complex interaction of genetic, physiological, environmental, and social factors. The beginning of sexual identity occurs at conception with the combining of chromosomes that determine sex. It is the biological father who determines whether a baby will be a boy or a girl. All eggs (ova) carry an X chromosome; sperm may carry either an X or a Y chromosome. If a sperm carrying an X chromosome fertilizes an egg, the resulting combination of sex chromosomes (XX) provides the blueprint to produce a female. If a sperm carrying a Y chromosome fertilizes an egg, the XY combination produces a male.

Not all people, however, have XX or XY chromosomes, nor do they all necessarily exhibit exclusively female or male primary and secondary sex characteristics. **Intersexuality** may occur as often as one in 100 live births (see the Health in a Diverse World box on page 174).

The genetic instructions included in the sex chromosomes lead to the differential development of male and female **gonads** (reproductive organs) at about the eighth week of fetal life. Once the male gonads (testes) and the female gonads (ovaries) are developed, they play a key role in all future sexual development because the gonads are responsible for the production of sex hormones. The primary sex hormones produced by females are estrogen and progesterone. In males, the sex hormone of primary importance is testosterone, which is converted from androgens, hormones secreted by the adrenal glands. The release of testosterone in a maturing fetus signals the development of a penis and other male genitals. If no testosterone is produced, female genitals form.

At the time of **puberty**, sex hormones again play major roles in development. Hormones released by the pituitary gland, called gonadotropins, stimulate the testes and ovaries to make appropriate sex hormones. The increase of estrogen production in females and testosterone production in males leads to the development of **secondary sex characteristics**. Male secondary sex characteristics include deepening of the voice, development of facial and body hair, and growth of the skeleton and musculature. Female secondary sex characteristics include growth of the breasts, widening of the hips, and the development of pubic and underarm hair.

Thus far, we have described sexual identity only in terms of a person's biology. While biology is an important facet of sexual identity, the relationship between biology and culture is much more complicated than the popular notion of sex as biology and gender as a social factor. Biological facts are themselves always understood and interpreted within the cultural framework that gives meaning to those facts. Sex simply refers to the biological condition of being male or female based on physiological and hormonal differences.

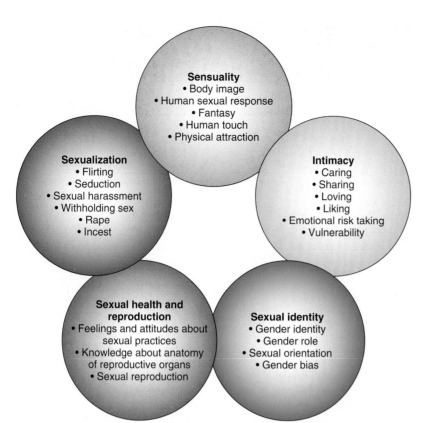

Sensuality
• Body image
• Human sexual response
• Fantasy
• Human touch
• Physical attraction

Sexualization
• Flirting
• Seduction
• Sexual harassment
• Withholding sex
• Rape
• Incest

Intimacy
• Caring
• Sharing
• Loving
• Liking
• Emotional risk taking
• Vulnerability

Sexual health and reproduction
• Feelings and attitudes about sexual practices
• Knowledge about anatomy of reproductive organs
• Sexual reproduction

Sexual identity
• Gender identity
• Gender role
• Sexual orientation
• Gender bias

FIGURE 6.1 Circles of Sexuality

Source: Advocates for Youth, *Life Planning Education: A Comprehensive Sex Education Curriculum* (Washington, DC: Advocates for Youth, in press)

Gender is the practice of behaving in masculine or feminine ways as defined by the society in which one lives and as a component of our identity, while sex is more related to physical form and function. In this sense, gender is a performance, something we do rather than something we have, and we learn gender through the process of **socialization**. Through interactions with family, peers, teachers, media, and other social organizations, we learn to act in ways that society deems appropriate. Think about the television shows you watch. Do the characters play out traditional gender roles?

Each of us expresses our maleness or femaleness to others on a daily basis by the **gender roles** we play. **Gender identity** refers to the

personal sense or awareness of being masculine or feminine, a male or a female. A person's gender identity does not always match his or her biological sex: this is called being **transgendered**. It may sometimes be difficult to express one's true sexual identity because of the bounds established by **gender-role stereotypes**, or bias about how males and females should express themselves and the characteristics each possesses. Our traditional sex roles are an example of gender-role stereotyping. Men are expected to be independent, aggressive, better in math and science, logical, and always in control of their emotions. Women, on the other hand, are traditionally expected to be passive, nurturing, intuitive, sensitive, and emotional.

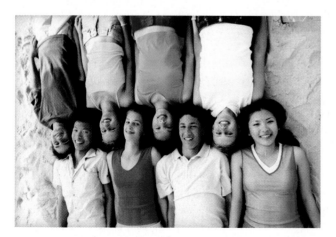

Signs of physical maturity are not always indicators of emotional adulthood.

socialization   Process by which a society communicates behavioral expectations to its individual members.

gender roles   Expression of maleness or femaleness in everyday life.

gender identity   Personal sense or awareness of being masculine or feminine, a male or a female.

transgendered   When one's gender identity does not match one's biological sex.

gender-role stereotypes   Generalizations concerning how males and females should express themselves and the characteristics each possesses.

INTERSEXUALITY

Intersexual people are born with various levels of male and female biological characteristics, ranging from different chromosomal arrangements to a variety of primary and secondary sex characteristics. Whereas most people are born with either XX or XY chromosomes, some are born with XXY or XO chromosomes (where O signifies a missing or damaged chromosome). In some people, gonads do not develop fully into ovaries or testicles, and in others external genitalia may be ambiguous. For example, a person may possess a phallus that could be a large clitoris or a small penis and a structure that resembles partially fused labia or a split scrotum.

Common forms of intersexuality include:

- *Androgen insensitivity syndrome (AIS).* Two forms of AIS exist: complete and partial. In complete AIS, people with XY chromosomes develop testes and produce androgens (hormones that produce male characteristics), but their bodies cannot respond to androgens and, therefore, their external genitalia are female. In adolescence, they experience breast development and sparse pubic hair growth but do not menstruate. In partial AIS, external genitalia are ambiguous.
- *Gonadal dysgenesis.* Like AIS, gonadal dysgenesis has two forms: complete and partial. In complete gonadal dysgenesis, people with XY chromosomes do not develop testes capable of producing androgen, and they have female external genitalia. People with partial gonadal dysgenesis develop ambiguous external genitalia.
- *Congenital adrenal hyperplasia (CAH).* In CAH, excess adrenal androgens lead to the development of ambiguous genitalia in people with XX chromosomes. People with CAH have masculine features such as facial hair, grow quickly but stop growing before they should, have difficulty fighting off infections, and may have difficulty retaining enough salt. People with mild CAH usually have irregular periods and may have trouble becoming pregnant.
- *Turner's syndrome.* People with Turner's syndrome have a single X chromosome and a missing or damaged X chromosome. Turner's occurs in about 1 out of 3,000 live births. Symptoms include short stature, webbed neck, absent or retarded development of secondary sex characteristics, absence of menstruation, and drooping eyelids.
- *Klinefelter's syndrome.* People with Klinefelter's syndrome have an extra sex chromosome—XXY instead of XY. This chromosome arrangement occurs in 1 in 500 to 1,000 male births. Not all XXY males will develop Klinefelter's syndrome, and many will never know they have an extra chromosome. Those who do develop the syndrome will have male external genitalia, although the penis may be smaller than in most males. They may develop breasts, lack facial and body hair, develop rounder bodies, and be overweight. They may also have some degree of language impairment.

Intersexuality has often been treated as a birth defect. Very often parents and physicians make determinations about the sex of a child born with ambiguous genitalia and have surgery performed to make the child's genitalia conform to expectations for the assigned sex. Many members of the intersex community have begun to protest this practice as a form of genital mutilation. They argue that conditions that are not life-threatening should not be surgically altered and society should become more accepting of the wide range of sexual differences.

Sources: Intersex Society of North America, "Intersexuality Basics," 2004, www.itpeople.org/ frameset.html; "Intersex Conditions," 2006, www.isna.org/faq/conditions; The Johns Hopkins Children's Center, "Syndromes of Abnormal Sex Differentiation," 2004, www .hopkinsmedicine.org/pediatricendocrinology/ intersex/index.html; National Institute of Child Health and Human Development, "A Guide for XXY Males and Their Families," 2004, http:// 156.40.88.3/publications/pubs/klinefelter.htm.

Androgyny is the expression of both masculine and feminine traits in a single person. Androgynous people do not always follow traditional sex roles but instead choose behaviors based on the given situation.

androgyny High levels of traditional masculine and feminine traits in a single person.

transsexuality Condition in which a person is psychologically of one sex but physically of the other.

Transsexuality, also known as *gender dysphoria*, refers to a condition in which a person is in a state of conflict between gender identity and physical sex. Simply stated, a transsexual is a mind physically trapped in the body of the opposite sex. The condition is not related to sexual orientation, nor should it be confused with transvestism, or cross-dressing.

By now you can see that defining sexual identity is not a simple matter. It is a lifelong process of growing and learning. Your sexual identity is made up of the unique combination of your biology, gender identity, chosen gender roles, sexual orientation, and personal experiences. It is up to you to take every opportunity to get to know and like yourself so that you may enjoy your life to the fullest.

 what do you THINK?

How often do you face gender-role stereotypes or gender bias? ▪ What is the outcome? ▪ Do you think men and women have the same degree of freedom in gender-role expression?

Sexual Orientation

Sexual orientation refers to a person's enduring emotional, romantic, sexual, or affectionate attraction to other persons. You may be primarily attracted to members of the other sex (**heterosexual**), your same sex (**homosexual**), or both sexes (**bisexual**).

Many homosexuals prefer the terms **gay** and **lesbian** to describe their sexual orientations, as these terms go beyond the exclusively sexual connotation of the term *homosexual*. The term *gay* can apply to both men and women, but *lesbian* refers specifically to women.

Irrational fear or hatred of homosexuality creates antigay prejudice and is expressed as **homophobia**. Homophobic behaviors range from avoiding hugging same-sex friends to name-calling and physical attacks. Recent data from the Department of Justice indicated that bias regarding sexual orientation was the motivation for over 15 percent of all hate crimes reported.[2]

Most researchers today agree that sexual orientation is best understood using a multifactorial model, which incorporates biological, psychological, and socioenvironmental factors. Biological explanations focus on research into genetics, hormones (perinatal and postpubertal), and differences in brain anatomy, while psychological and socioenvironmental explanations examine parent–child interactions, sex roles, and early sexual and interpersonal interactions. Collectively, this growing body of research suggests that the origins of homosexuality, like heterosexuality, are complex. To diminish the complexity of sexual orientation to "a choice" is a clear misrepresentation of current research. Homosexuals do not "choose" their sexual orientation any more than heterosexuals do.

There are other theories that try to understand sexual orientation and the factors that influence it. Though it is often viewed as a simple concept based entirely upon whom one has sex with, researcher F. Klein developed a questionnaire that explores not only who you are sexually attracted to, fantasize about, and actually have sex with, but considers factors such as who you feel closer to emotionally, like to socialize with, and in which "community" you feel most comfortable. Complete the worksheet in Table 6.1 on page 176. You may realize that there are not just two (homosexual, heterosexual) or three (homosexual, heterosexual, bisexual) orientations, but indeed a whole range of complex, interacting, and fluid factors influencing our sexuality over time.

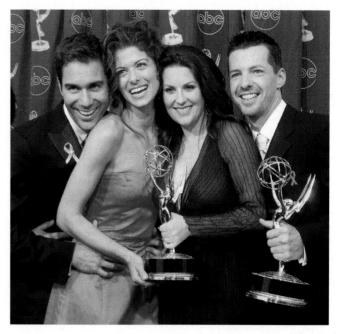

The presence of gay and lesbian characters and their friends, such as those portrayed by these actors on TV's *Will and Grace,* contributes to the increasing acceptance of gay relationships in everyday life.

 try it NOW

Analyze your own or a friend's feelings about heterosexuality. Go to http://advocatesforyouth.org/lessonplans/heterosexual2.htm and answer the questions, or complete this activity with a friend to take a closer look at what shapes our sexuality.

sexual orientation A person's enduring emotional, romantic, sexual, or affectionate attraction to other persons.

heterosexual Experiencing primary attraction to and preference for sexual activity with people of the other sex.

homosexual Experiencing primary attraction to and preference for sexual activity with people of the same sex.

bisexual Experiencing attraction to and preference for sexual activity with people of both sexes.

gay Sexual orientation involving primary attraction to people of the same sex; usually but not always applies to men attracted to men.

lesbian Sexual orientation involving attraction of women to other women.

homophobia Irrational hatred or fear of homosexuals or homosexuality.

TABLE 6.1 Analyzing Sexual Preferences

To complete this worksheet, use the scales provided below and choose a number for each of the three aspects of your life: your past, your present, and your ideal. Remember that there are no right or wrong answers.

Variable	Past (your entire life up until one year ago)	Present (the last 12 months)	Ideal (if you could order your life any way you wanted)
A. SEXUAL ATTRACTION: To whom are you sexually attracted?	_____	_____	_____
B. SEXUAL BEHAVIOR: With whom do you have sex?	_____	_____	_____
C. SEXUAL FANTASIES: Who do you fantasize about?	_____	_____	_____
D. EMOTIONAL PREFERENCE: Who do you feel more drawn to or close to emotionally?	_____	_____	_____
E. SOCIAL PREFERENCE: With whom do you spend most of your social life?	_____	_____	_____
F. LIFESTYLE PREFERENCE: In which community (gay, straight, mixed) do you prefer to spend your time or feel most comfortable?	_____	_____	_____
G. SELF-IDENTIFICATION: How do you label or identify yourself?	_____	_____	_____

SCALE FOR A–E

0 = other sex only
1 = other sex mostly
2 = other sex somewhat more
3 = both sexes equally
4 = same sex somewhat more
5 = same sex mostly
6 = same sex only

SCALE FOR F AND G

0 = heterosexual only
1 = heterosexual mostly
2 = heterosexual somewhat more
3 = equally heterosexual and homosexual
4 = homosexual somewhat more
5 = homosexual mostly
6 = homosexual only

Source: F. Klein, The Bisexual Option, copyright © 1978 The Haworth Press, Inc. Used with permission.

Sexual Anatomy and Physiology

An understanding of the functions of the male and female sexual systems will help you make responsible choices regarding your own sexual health, derive pleasure and satisfaction from your sexual relationships, and be sensitive to your partner's wants and needs.

external female genitals   The mons pubis, labia majora and minora, clitoris, urethral and vaginal openings, and the vestibule of the vagina and its glands.

vulva   Region that encloses the female's external genitalia.

mons pubis   Fatty tissue covering the pubic bone in females; in physically mature women, the mons is covered with coarse hair.

labia minora   "Inner lips," or folds of tissue just inside the labia majora.

labia majora   "Outer lips," or folds of tissue covering the female sexual organs.

Female Sexual Anatomy and Physiology

The female sexual system includes two major groups of structures, the external genitals (Figure 6.2) and the internal genitals (Figure 6.3, page 178). The **external female genitals** include all structures that are outwardly visible and are enclosed in a region known as the **vulva**. Specifically, the external genitalia include the mons pubis, the labia minora and majora, the clitoris, the urethral and vaginal openings, and the vestibule of the vagina. The **mons pubis** is a pad of fatty tissue covering the anterior part of the pubic bone. The mons serves to protect the bone, and after puberty it becomes covered with coarse hair. The **labia minora** are folds of thin skin, and the **labia majora** are folds of skin and tissue that enclose the urethral and vaginal openings. The labia minora are found just inside the labia majora.

The **clitoris** is the female sexual organ whose only known function is sexual pleasure. It is located at the upper end of the labia minora and beneath the mons pubis. Directly below the clitoris is the **urethral opening** through which urine leaves the body. Below the urethral opening is the vaginal opening. In some women, the vaginal opening is covered by a

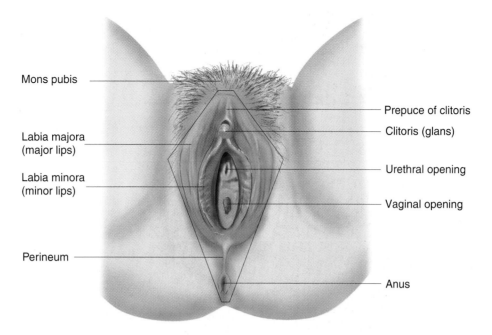

FIGURE 6.2 External Female Genital Structures

Source: From R. McAnulty and M. Burnette, *Exploring Human Sexuality: Making Healthy Decisions* 2nd ed (Boston: Allyn & Bacon, 2004). Copyright © 2004 by Pearson Education. Reprinted by permission of the publisher.

thin membrane called the **hymen**. It is a myth that an intact hymen is proof of virginity. The **perineum** is the "floor" that supports the endmost regions of the urogenital and gastrointestinal tracts (see Figure 6.2). Although not technically part of the external genitalia, the tissue in this area has many nerve endings and is sensitive to touch; it can play a part in sexual excitement.

The **internal female genitals** of the reproductive system include the vagina, uterus, uterine tubes, and ovaries. The **vagina** is a tubular organ that serves as a passageway from the uterus to the outside of a female's body. This passageway allows menstrual flow to exit from the uterus during a female's monthly cycle and serves as the birth canal during childbirth. The vagina also receives the penis during intercourse. The **uterus**, also known as the **womb**, is a hollow, muscular, pear-shaped organ. Hormones acting on the inner lining of the uterus, called the **endometrium**, either prepare the uterus for implantation and development of a fertilized egg or signal that no fertilization has taken place, in which case the endometrium deteriorates and its tissue and blood become menstrual flow.

The lower end of the uterus, the **cervix**, extends down into the vagina. The **ovaries** are almond-size structures suspended on either side of the uterus. The ovaries produce the hormones estrogen and progesterone and are also the reservoir for immature eggs. All the eggs a female will ever have are present in the ovaries at birth. Eggs mature and are released from the ovaries in response to hormone levels. Extending from the upper end of the uterus are two thin, flexible tubes called the **uterine (fallopian) tubes**. The uterine tubes, which

clitoris   A pea-sized nodule of tissue located at the top of the labia minora; central to sexual arousal in women.

urethral opening   The opening through which urine is expelled.

hymen   Thin tissue covering the vaginal opening in some women.

perineum   Tissue that forms the "floor" of the pelvic region; it covers a kite-shaped region including the external genitalia and anus.

internal female genitals   The vagina, uterus, uterine (fallopian) tubes, and ovaries.

vagina   The passage in females leading from the vulva into the uterus.

uterus (womb)   Hollow, pear-shaped muscular organ whose function is to contain the developing fetus.

endometrium   Soft, spongy matter that makes up the uterine lining.

cervix   Lower end of the uterus that opens into the vagina.

ovaries   Almond-size organs that house developing eggs and produce hormones.

uterine (fallopian) tubes   Tubes that extend from near the ovaries to the uterus.

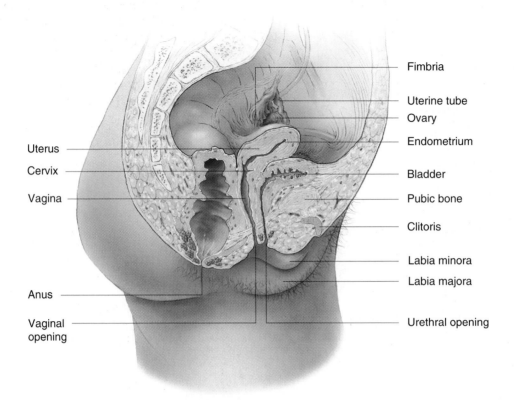

FIGURE 6.3 Side View of the Female Reproductive Organs

Labels on figure:
Fimbria
Uterine tube
Ovary
Endometrium
Bladder
Pubic bone
Clitoris
Labia minora
Labia majora
Urethral opening
Uterus
Cervix
Vagina
Anus
Vaginal opening

puberty   The maturation of the female or male reproduction system.

pituitary gland   The endocrine gland located deep within the brain; controls reproductive functions.

hypothalamus   An area of the brain located near the pituitary gland. The hypothalamus works in conjunction with the pituitary gland to control reproductive functions.

gonadotropin-releasing hormone (GnRH)   Hormone that signals the pituitary gland to release gonadotropins.

follicle-stimulating hormone (FSH)   Hormone that signals the ovaries to prepare to release eggs and to begin producing estrogens.

luteinizing hormone (LH)   Hormone that signals the ovaries to release an egg and to begin producing progesterone.

estrogens   Hormones secreted by the ovaries; control the menstrual cycle.

progesterone   Hormone secreted by the ovaries; helps keep the endometrium developing in order to nourish a fertilized egg; also helps maintain pregnancy.

do not actually touch the ovaries, capture eggs as they are released from the ovaries during ovulation, and they are where sperm and egg meet and fertilization takes place. Following fertilization, the uterine tubes serve as the passageway to the uterus, where the fertilized egg is implanted in the wall and development continues.

The Onset of Puberty and the Menstrual Cycle   With the onset of **puberty**, the female reproductive system matures, and the development of secondary sex characteristics transforms young girls into young women. The first sign of puberty is the beginning of breast development, which occurs around age 11. Under the direction of the endocrine system, the **pituitary gland**, the **hypothalamus**, and the ovaries all secrete hormones that act as chemical messengers among them. Working in a feedback system, hormonal levels in the bloodstream act as the trigger mechanism for release of more or different hormones.

At around age 9½ to 11½ in females, the hypothalamus receives the message to begin secreting **gonadotropin-releasing hormone (GnRH)**. The release of GnRH in turn signals the pituitary gland to release hormones called gonadotropins. Two gonadotropins, **follicle-stimulating hormone (FSH)** and **luteinizing hormone (LH)**, signal the ovaries to start producing **estrogens** and **progesterone**. Increased estrogen levels assist in the development of female secondary sex characteristics. In addition, estrogens regulate

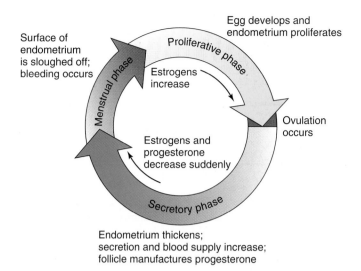

Surface of endometrium is sloughed off; bleeding occurs

Egg develops and endometrium proliferates

Proliferative phase

Menstrual phase

Estrogens increase

Ovulation occurs

Estrogens and progesterone decrease suddenly

Secretory phase

Endometrium thickens; secretion and blood supply increase; follicle manufactures progesterone

FIGURE 6.4 The Four Phases of the Menstrual Cycle

Source: S. Rathus, J. Nevid, and L. Rathus, *Human Sexuality in a World of Diversity* (Boston: Allyn & Bacon, 2005). Copyright © 2005 by Pearson Education. Reprinted by permission of the publisher.

the reproductive cycle. The normal age range for the onset of the first menstrual period, termed **menarche**, is 9 to 17 years, with the average age being 11½ to 13½ years. Body fat heavily influences the onset of puberty, and increasing rates of obesity in children may account for the fact that girls here and in other countries seem to be reaching puberty much earlier than they used to.[3] Very thin girls, such as young athletes, tend to start menstruating later.

The average menstrual cycle is 28 days long and consists of three phases: the proliferative phase, the secretory phase, and the menstrual phase (Figure 6.4). The first phase, the **proliferative phase,** begins with the end of menstruation. During this time, the endometrium develops, or "proliferates." How does this process work (Figure 6.5 on page 180)? By the end of menstruation, the hypothalamus senses very low levels of estrogen and progesterone in the blood. In response to these low levels, the hypothalamus increases its secretions of GnRH, which in turn triggers the pituitary gland to release FSH. When FSH reaches the ovaries, it signals several **ovarian follicles** (the part of the ovary where eggs develop) to begin to mature. Normally, only one of the follicles, called the **graafian follicle**, reaches full maturity in the days preceding ovulation. While the follicles mature, they begin to produce estrogen, which in turn signals the lining of the uterus, the endometrium, to grow and develop, or proliferate. If fertilization occurs, the endometrial tissue will become a nesting place for the developing embryo. High estrogen levels signal the pituitary to slow down FSH production and increase release of LH. Under the influence of LH, the graafian follicle ruptures and releases a mature ovum near a fallopian tube (around day 14). This is the process of **ovulation**. The other ripening follicles degenerate and are reabsorbed by the body. Occasionally, two ova mature and are released during ovulation. If both are fertilized, fraternal (nonidentical) twins develop. Identical twins develop when one fertilized ovum divides into two separate egg cells.

The phase following ovulation is called the **secretory phase**. The ruptured graafian follicle, which has remained in the ovary, is transformed into the corpus luteum and begins to secrete large amounts of estrogen and progesterone. These hormone secretions peak around the twentieth or twenty-first days of the average cycle and cause the endometrium to thicken and continue to prepare for a potential fertilized ovum. If fertilization and implantation take place, cells surrounding the developing embryo release a hormone called **human chorionic gonadotropin (HCG)**, increasing estrogen and progesterone secretions that maintain the endometrium and signal the pituitary not to start a new menstrual cycle. If no implantation occurs, the hypothalamus responds to peak levels of progesterone in the blood by signaling the pituitary to stop producing FSH and LH. As levels of FSH and LH quickly fall, the corpus luteum begins to decompose. The decomposition of the corpus luteum leads to rapid declines in estrogen and progesterone levels. These hormones are needed to sustain the lining of the uterus, the endometrium. Without them, the endometrium is sloughed off in the menstrual flow and this begins the **menstrual phase**. The low estrogen levels of the menstrual phase signal the hypothalamus to release GnRH, which acts on the pituitary to secrete FSH, and the cyclical process begins again.

Menstrual Problems Premenstrual syndrome **(PMS)** comprises the mood changes and physical symptoms that occur in some women during the one or two weeks prior to menstruation. Symptoms may include any or all of the

menarche The first menstrual period.

proliferative phase First phase of the menstrual cycle.

ovarian follicles (egg sacs) Areas within the ovary in which individual eggs develop.

graafian follicle Mature ovarian follicle that contains a fully developed ovum, or egg.

ovulation The point of the menstrual cycle at which a mature egg ruptures through the ovarian wall.

secretory phase Second phase of the menstrual cycle during which the endometrium continues to prepare for a fertilized egg.

human chorionic gonadotropin (HCG) Hormone that calls for increased levels of estrogen and progesterone secretion if fertilization has taken place.

menstrual phase Final phase of the menstrual cycle in which the endometrium sloughs off, and estrogen and progesterone levels decline in response to no fertilization taking place.

premenstrual syndrome (PMS) Comprises the mood changes and physical symptoms that occur in some women during the one or two weeks prior to menstruation.

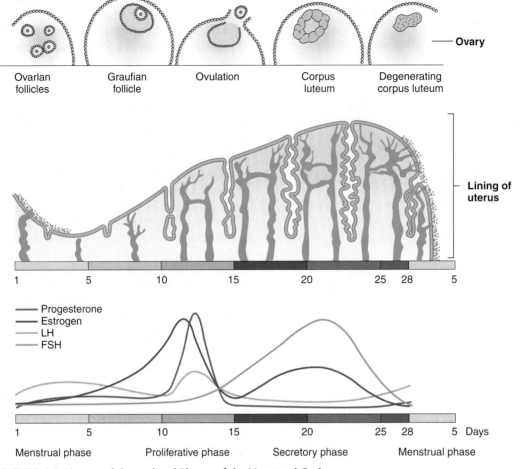

Ovary

| Ovarlan follicles | Graufian follicle | Ovulation | Corpus luteum | Degenerating corpus luteum |

Lining of uterus

1 5 10 15 20 25 28 5

— Progesterone
— Estrogen
— LH
— FSH

1 5 10 15 20 25 28 5 Days

Menstrual phase · Proliferative phase · Secretory phase · Menstrual phase

FIGURE 6.5 Hormonal Control and Phases of the Menstrual Cycle

following: breast swelling and tenderness, fatigue, trouble sleeping, upset stomach, bloating, constipation or diarrhea, headache, changes in appetite or food cravings, joint or muscle pain, weight gain, swelling of hands and feet, poor concentration, and feeling blue or irritable.

As many as 80 percent of women have some negative symptoms associated with the menstrual cycle. Of these, about 3 to 5 percent have symptoms that are similar to but more severe than PMS. Collectively, these symptoms are labeled **premenstrual dysphoric disorder**, or **PMDD**. Unlike PMS, PMDD symptoms are severe and difficult to manage. In addition to the physical symptoms described for PMS, PMDD is marked by severe mood disturbances including depressed mood, anxiety, irritability, angry outbursts, and/or

periods of sudden tearfulness or sadness. Many PMDD sufferers also experience insomnia and difficulty in concentrating. Women with PMDD experience significantly impaired lives for one to two weeks every month, and the quality of their social relationships is often affected. Only about 25 percent of women who seek medical attention for this disorder are actually diagnosed with this rare condition. Women usually do not develop PMDD until their late twenties or early thirties, and PMDD worsens until menopause.[4]

Many natural approaches to managing PMS can also help PMDD. These strategies include: (1) eating more carbohydrates (grains, fruits, and vegetables); (2) reducing caffeine and salt intake; (3) exercising regularly; and (4) taking measures to reduce stress. Recent investigation into methods of controlling the severe emotional swings has led to the use of antidepressant medications for treating PMDD. A particular type of antidepressant, selective serotonin reuptake inhibitors (SSRIs such as Prozac and Zoloft), has been shown to be beneficial in reducing the mood disturbances associated with PMDD. Overall, more than 60 percent of women with PMDD respond to SSRIs, even in low doses and when taking them only while premenstrual. Side effects are generally minimal.

Toxic shock syndrome (TSS), although rare today, is still something women should be aware of. It is caused by a

premenstrual dysphoric disorder (PMDD) Collective name for a group of negative symptoms similar to but more severe than PMS, including severe mood disturbances.

toxic shock syndrome (TSS) A potentially life-threatening disease that occurs when specific bacterial toxins are allowed to multiply unchecked in wounds or through improper use of tampons or diaphragms.

bacterial infection facilitated by tampon or diaphragm use (see Chapters 7 and 17). Since the early 1980s, the U.S. Food and Drug Administration (FDA) has mandated that manufacturers of tampons conduct a battery of tests for safety clearance, but regardless of the safeguards, all women who use tampons should be aware of the potential for TSS. Symptoms are sometimes hard to recognize because they mimic the flu and include sudden high fever, vomiting, diarrhea, dizziness, fainting, or a rash that looks like sunburn during one's period or a few days after. Proper treatment usually assures recovery in two to three weeks.

Dysmenorrhea is a condition that causes pain or discomfort in the lower abdomen just before or after menstruation. Primary dysmenorrhea usually begins one to two years after a woman's first period, while secondary dysmenorrhea is caused by a specific disease or disorder and may appear years after regular menstruation begins.

Many women find relief for painful menstrual periods through over-the-counter nonsteroidal anti-inflammatory drugs (NSAIDs) such as ibuprofen and aspirin. Applying a heating pad to the abdomen, taking a hot bath or shower, and massaging the abdomen may also provide relief.

Menopause Just as menarche signals the beginning of a female's potential reproductive years, **menopause**—the permanent cessation of menstruation—signals the end. Generally occurring between the ages of 40 and 60, and at age 51 on average, menopause results in decreased estrogen levels, which may produce troublesome symptoms in some women. Decreased vaginal lubrication, hot flashes, headaches, dizziness, and joint pain have been associated with the onset of menopause.

Hormones, such as estrogen and progesterone through **hormone replacement therapy (HRT)**, have long been prescribed to relieve menopausal symptoms and reduce the risk of heart disease and osteoporosis. (The National Institutes of Health prefers the term **menopausal hormone therapy** because hormone treatment is not a replacement and does not restore the physiology of youth.) However, recent studies, including results from the Women's Health Initiative (WHI), suggest that hormone therapy may actually do more harm than good. In fact, the WHI terminated this research ahead of schedule due to concerns about participants' increased risk of breast cancer, heart attack, stroke, blood clots, and other health problems.[5] All women need to discuss the risks and benefits of HRT with their health care provider and come to an informed decision. It is crucial to find a doctor who specializes in women's health and keeps up to date with the latest research findings. Certainly a healthy lifestyle, such as regular exercise, a balanced diet, and adequate calcium intake, can also help protect postmenopausal women from heart disease and osteoporosis.

Male Sexual Anatomy and Physiology

The structures of the male sexual system may be divided into external and internal genitals (Figure 6.6 on page 182). The penis and the scrotum make up the **external male genitals**. (See the Health Ethics box on page 183 for a discussion of the controversy surrounding circumcision, or removal of the foreskin of the penis.) The **internal male genitals** include the testes, epididymides, vasa deferentia, and the urethra and three other structures—the seminal vesicles, the prostate gland, and the Cowper's glands—that secrete components that, with sperm, make up semen. These three structures are sometimes referred to as the **accessory glands**.

The **penis** serves as the organ that deposits sperm in the vagina during intercourse. The urethra, which passes through the center of the penis, acts as the passageway for both semen and urine to exit the body. During sexual arousal, the spongy tissue in the penis becomes filled with blood, making the organ stiff, or erect. Further sexual excitement leads to **ejaculation**, a series of rapid, spasmodic contractions that propel semen out of the penis.

Situated behind the penis and also outside the body is a sac called the **scrotum**. The scrotum protects the testes and also helps control the temperature within the testes, which is vital to proper sperm production. The **testes** (singular: *testis*) are egg-shaped structures in which sperm are manufactured. The testes also contain cells that manufacture **testosterone**, the hormone responsible for the development of male secondary sex characteristics.

The development of sperm is referred to as **spermatogenesis**. Like the maturation of eggs in the female, this process is governed by the pituitary gland. FSH is secreted

---

dysmenorrhea   Condition that causes pain or discomfort in the lower abdomen just before or after menstruation.

menopause   The permanent cessation of menstruation, generally between the ages of 40 and 60.

hormone replacement therapy (HRT) or menopausal hormone therapy   Use of synthetic or animal estrogens and progesterone to compensate for decreases in estrogens in a woman's body.

external male genitals   The penis and scrotum.

internal male genitals   The testes, epididymides, vasa deferentia, ejaculatory ducts, urethra, and accessory glands.

accessory glands   The seminal vesicles, prostate gland, and Cowper's glands.

penis   Male sexual organ that releases sperm into the vagina.

ejaculation   The propulsion of semen from the penis.

scrotum   Sac of tissue that encloses the testes.

testes   Two organs, located in the scrotum, that manufacture sperm and produce hormones.

testosterone   The male sex hormone manufactured in the testes.

spermatogenesis   The development of sperm.

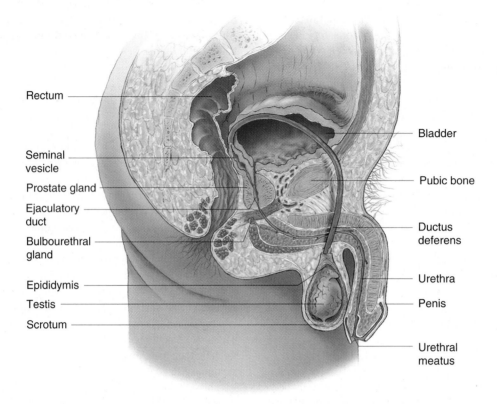

Labels on figure:
Rectum
Seminal vesicle
Prostate gland
Ejaculatory duct
Bulbourethral gland
Epididymis
Testis
Scrotum
Bladder
Pubic bone
Ductus deferens
Urethra
Penis
Urethral meatus

FIGURE 6.6 Side View of the Male Reproductive Organs

into the bloodstream to stimulate the testes to manufacture sperm. Immature sperm are released into a comma-shaped structure on the back of the testis called the **epididymis** (plural, *epididymides*), where they ripen and reach full maturity.

The epididymis contains coiled tubules that gradually "unwind" and straighten out to become the **vas deferens**. The

---

epididymis A comma-shaped structure atop the testis where sperm mature.

vas deferens A tube that stores and transports sperm toward the penis.

seminal vesicles Storage areas for sperm where nutrient fluids are added to them.

semen Fluid containing sperm and nutrient fluids that increase sperm viability and neutralize vaginal acid.

prostate gland Gland that secretes nutrients and neutralizing fluids into the semen.

Cowper's glands Glands that secrete a fluid that lubricates the urethra and neutralizes any acid remaining in the urethra after urination.

---

two vasa deferentia, as they are called in the plural, make up the tubular transportation system whose sole function is to store and move sperm. Along the way, the **seminal vesicles** provide sperm with nutrients and other fluids that compose **semen**.

The vasa deferentia eventually connect the epididymides to the ejaculatory ducts, which pass through the prostate gland and empty into the urethra. The **prostate gland** contributes more fluids to the semen, including chemicals that aid the sperm in fertilizing an ovum and neutralize the acidic environment of the vagina to make it more conducive to sperm motility (ability to move) and potency (potential for fertilizing an ovum).

Just below the prostate gland are two pea-shaped nodules called the **Cowper's glands**. The Cowper's glands secrete a fluid that lubricates the urethra and neutralizes any acid that may remain in the urethra after urination. Urine and semen do not come into contact with each other. During ejaculation of semen, a small valve closes off the tube to the urinary bladder.

Human Sexual Response

Psychological traits greatly influence sexual response and sexual desire. Thus, we may find relationships with one partner vastly different from those we might experience with others.

HEALTH ETHICS
conflict and controversy

CIRCUMCISION: RISK VERSUS BENEFIT

New parents must decide whether their infant son will be circumcised. Circumcision involves the surgical removal of the foreskin (prepuce), a fold of skin covering the end (glans) of the penis. Most circumcisions in the United States are performed for religious or cultural reasons or because of concerns about hygiene. (The foreskin is fully attached to the glans at birth and naturally separates from it anywhere from weeks to several years after birth.)

As with any surgical procedure, there are potential risks such as bleeding and infection. Circumcision is considered a permanent procedure and some insurance companies do not cover the costs of circumcision. If the procedure is done, it is important that proper anesthesia be used. The medical benefits of circumcision include decreased risk of urinary tract infections in the first year, decreased risk of penile cancer (although cancer of the penis is very rare), and decreased risk of sexually transmitted infections. Recently, the results of the first randomized controlled trials evaluating the impact of circumcision on HIV transmission were published. Results indicated that male circumcision does provide a degree of protection against HIV infection. This finding may have important implications in regions of the world where AIDS is epidemic.

Approximately 56 percent (1.1 million) of all newborn boys are circumcised in the United States each year. The procedure is much more common in the United States, Canada, and the Middle East than in Asia, South America, Central America, and most of Europe.

At present, the American Academy of Pediatrics does not consider circumcision medically necessary. Parents who choose to circumcise do so for religious, aesthetic, or other personal reasons. If it is performed, pain relief should be given to the infant.

What decision do you think you would make for your son? Give your reasons. If you are male, does your circumcised or uncircumcised status affect your opinion?

Sources: N. Siegfried et al., "HIV and Male Circumcision—A Systematic Review with Assessment of the Quality of Studies," *The Lancet Infectious Diseases* 5, no. 3 (2005): 165–173; A. Bertran et al., "Randomized, Controlled Intervention Trial of Male Circumcision for Reduction of HIV Infection Risk: The ANRS 1265 Trial," *PLoS Medicine* 2, no. 11 (2005): 1112–1122; B. G. Williams et al., "The Potential Impact of Male Circumcision on HIV in Sub-Saharan Africa," *PLoS Medicine* 3, no. 7 (2006): e262; B. P. Homeier, "Circumcision," KidsHealth for Parents, Nemours Foundation, January 2005, http://kidshealth.org/parent/system/surgical/circumcision.html; Mayo Clinic Staff, "Circumcision: Weighing the Pros and Cons," MayoClinic.com, March 2006, www.mayoclinic.com/health/circumcision/PR00040.

Do men and women have the same sexual response?

Sexual response is a physiological process that generally follows a pattern. Both males' and females' sexual responses are somewhat arbitrarily divided into four stages: excitement/arousal, plateau, orgasm, and resolution (Figure 6.7, page 184). Researchers agree that each individual has a personal response pattern that may or may not conform to these phases. Regardless of the type of sexual activity (stimulation by a partner or self-stimulation), the response stages are the same.

During the first stage, excitement/arousal, **vasocongestion**, or increased blood flow in the genital region, stimulates male and female genital responses. Increased blood flow to these organs causes them to swell. The vagina begins to lubricate in preparation for penile penetration, and the penis becomes partially erect. Both sexes may exhibit a "sex flush," or light blush all over their bodies. Excitement/arousal can be generated by touching other parts of the body, by kissing, through fantasy, by viewing films or videos, or by reading erotic literature.

During the plateau phase, the initial responses intensify. Voluntary and involuntary muscle tensions increase. The female's nipples and the male's penis become erect. The penis secretes a few drops of preejaculatory fluid, which may contain sperm.

During the orgasmic phase, vasocongestion and muscle tensions reach their peak, and rhythmic contractions occur through the genital regions. In females, these contractions are centered in the uterus, outer vagina, and anal sphincter. In males, the contractions occur in two stages. First, contractions within the prostate gland begin propelling semen through the urethra. In the second stage, the muscles of the pelvic floor, urethra, and anal sphincter contract. Semen usually, but not always, is ejaculated from the penis. In both sexes, spasms in other major muscle groups also occur, particularly in the buttocks and abdomen. Feet and hands may also contract, and facial features often contort.

Muscle tension and congested blood subside in the resolution phase, as the genital organs return to their pre-arousal states. Both sexes may experience feelings of well-being and profound relaxation. After orgasm and resolution, many

vasocongestion The engorgement of the genital organs with blood.

1. Excitement/Arousal Phase

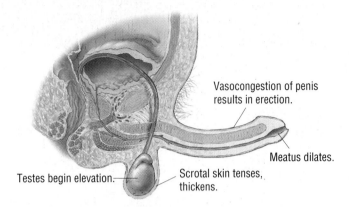

Vasocongestion of penis results in erection.

Meatus dilates.

Testes begin elevation.

Scrotal skin tenses, thickens.

1. Excitement/Arousal Phase

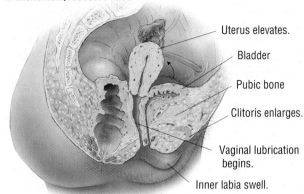

Uterus elevates.

Bladder

Pubic bone

Clitoris enlarges.

Vaginal lubrication begins.

Inner labia swell.

2. Plateau Phase

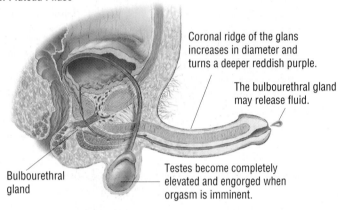

Coronal ridge of the glans increases in diameter and turns a deeper reddish purple.

The bulbourethral gland may release fluid.

Bulbourethral gland

Testes become completely elevated and engorged when orgasm is imminent.

2. Plateau Phase

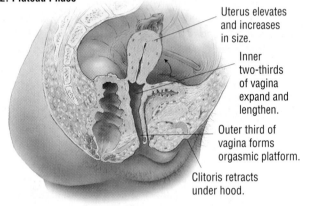

Uterus elevates and increases in size.

Inner two-thirds of vagina expand and lengthen.

Outer third of vagina forms orgasmic platform.

Clitoris retracts under hood.

3. Orgasmic Phase

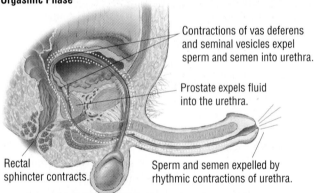

Contractions of vas deferens and seminal vesicles expel sperm and semen into urethra.

Prostate expels fluid into the urethra.

Rectal sphincter contracts.

Sperm and semen expelled by rhythmic contractions of urethra.

3. Orgasmic Phase

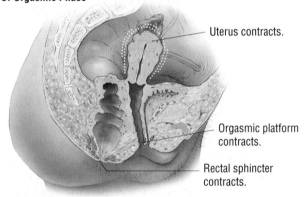

Uterus contracts.

Orgasmic platform contracts.

Rectal sphincter contracts.

4. Resolution Phase

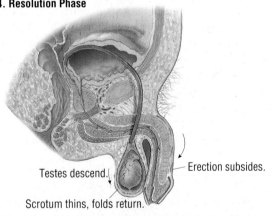

Erection subsides.

Testes descend.

Scrotum thins, folds return.

4. Resolution Phase

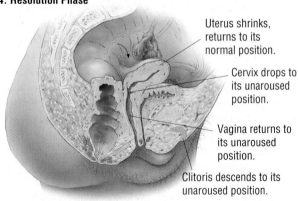

Uterus shrinks, returns to its normal position.

Cervix drops to its unaroused position.

Vagina returns to its unaroused position.

Clitoris descends to its unaroused position.

FIGURE 6.7 Comparison of Male and Female Sexual Response

females can become aroused again and experience additional orgasms. However, most men experience a refractory period, during which their systems are incapable of subsequent arousal. This refractory period may last from a few minutes to several hours, and tends to lengthen with age.

Although men and women experience the same stages in the sexual response cycle, the length of time spent in any one stage varies. Thus, one partner may be in the plateau phase while the other is in the excitement/arousal or orgasmic phase. Such variations in response rates are entirely normal. Some couples believe that simultaneous orgasm is desirable for sexual satisfaction. Although simultaneous orgasm is pleasant, it may be difficult to achieve because of differences in arousal and response.

Sexual pleasure and satisfaction are also possible without orgasm or even intercourse. Expressing sexual feelings for another person involves many pleasurable activities, of which intercourse and orgasm may be only a part.

 ## *what do you* THINK?

Why do we place so much importance on orgasm? ■ Can sexual pleasure and satisfaction be achieved without orgasm? ■ What is the role of desire in sexual response?

Sexual Responses among Older Adults

Older adults are commonly stereotyped as being incapable of or uninterested in sexual relations. The truth is, though we do experience some physical changes as we age, these changes generally do not cause us to stop enjoying sex.

In women, the most significant physical changes follow menopause. Skin becomes less elastic; most internal sexual organs, including the uterus and cervix, shrink somewhat; the vaginal walls become thinner; and vaginal lubrication during sexual arousal may decrease. The resulting increased friction during penetration can be painful. The use of artificial lubricants usually resolves the problem of insufficient lubrication. The typical physical change during orgasm is that the duration tends to be shorter. Women who remain sexually active as they age report fewer problems with age-related changes in sexual functioning.

Although men do not experience menopause, their bodies also change as a result of the aging process. They require more direct and prolonged stimulation to achieve an erection, and erections become less firm. They are slower to obtain a full erection and to reach orgasm, and their refractory periods are longer. Older men also experience a decrease in the intensity of ejaculation. Semen seeps out during ejaculation rather than being forcefully expelled as is typical in younger men. However, the majority of healthy older men, like healthy older women, enjoy a regular and satisfying sex life.

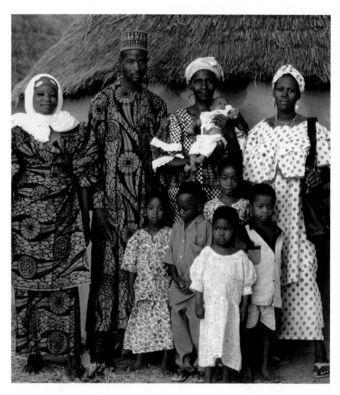

Our Western standard of monogamous heterosexual relationships may not be perceived as normal in other cultures. For example, this African family consists of one husband and several wives.

Expressing Your Sexuality

Finding healthy ways to express your sexuality is an important part of developing sexual maturity. Many avenues of sexual expression are available.

Sexual Behavior: What Is "Normal"?

What is "normal" sexual behavior?

Most of us want to fit in and be identified as normal, but how do we know which sexual behaviors are considered normal? What or whose criteria should we use? These are not easy questions.

Every society sets standards and attempts to regulate sexual behavior. Boundaries arise that distinguish good from bad, acceptable from unacceptable, and result in criteria used to establish what is viewed as normal or abnormal. Common sociocultural standards for sexual behavior in Western culture today include:[6]

■ *The heterosexual standard.* Sexual attraction should be limited to members of the other sex.
■ *The coital standard.* Penile–vaginal intercourse (coitus) is viewed as the ultimate sex act.

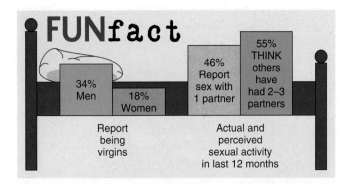

FIGURE 6.8 Sex on Campus: Perceptions and Reality Revealed

Sources: Smarter Sex Survey, "Sexual Attitudes and Behaviors of U.S. Students Aged 18–24," www.smartersex.org; American College Health Association-National College Health Assessment, *Reference Group Report, Fall 2005.*

- *The orgasmic standard.* All sexual interaction should lead to orgasm.
- *The two-person standard.* Sex is an activity to be experienced by two people.
- *The romantic standard.* Sex should be related to love.
- *The safer sex standard.* If we choose to be sexually active, we should act to prevent unintended pregnancy or disease transmission.

These are not laws or rules, but rather social scripts that have been adopted over time. Sexual standards often shift through the years, and many people choose not to follow them. Rather than making blanket judgments about normal versus abnormal, we might ask the following questions:[7]

- Is a sexual behavior healthy and fulfilling for a particular person?
- Is it safe?
- Does it involve the exploitation of others?
- Does it take place between responsible, consenting adults?

In this way, we can view behavior along a continuum that takes into account many individual factors. As you read about the options for sexual expression in the pages ahead, use these questions to explore your feelings about what is normal for you. See the Assess Yourself box on page 188 to examine your own feelings about sexual differences.

celibacy   State of not being involved in a sexual relationship.

autoerotic behaviors   Sexual self-stimulation.

sexual fantasies   Sexually arousing thoughts and dreams.

masturbation   Self-stimulation of genitals.

erogenous zones   Areas of the body of both males and females that, when touched, lead to sexual arousal.

Options for Sexual Expression

The range of human sexual expression is virtually infinite. What you find enjoyable may not be an option for someone else. The ways you choose to meet your sexual needs today may be very different from how you meet them two years from now. Accepting yourself as a sexual person with individual desires and preferences is the first step in achieving sexual satisfaction. Curious about your college peers' sexual behavior? See the Spotlight on Your Health box on page 190.

Celibacy
Celibacy is avoidance of or abstention from sexual activities with others. A completely celibate person also does not engage in masturbation (self-stimulation), whereas a partially celibate person avoids sexual activities with others but may enjoy autoerotic behaviors such as masturbation. Some people choose celibacy for religious or moral reasons. Others may be celibate for a period of time due to illness, the breakup of a long-term relationship, or lack of an acceptable partner. For some, celibacy is a lonely, agonizing state, but others find it an opportunity for introspection, values assessment, and personal growth.

Autoerotic Behaviors
Autoerotic behaviors involve sexual self-stimulation. The two most common are sexual fantasy and masturbation.

Sexual fantasies are sexually arousing thoughts and dreams. Fantasies may reflect real-life experiences, forbidden desires, or the opportunity to practice new or anticipated sexual experiences. The fact that you fantasize about a particular sexual experience does not necessarily mean that you want to, or have to, act that experience out. Sexual fantasies are just that—fantasy.

Masturbation is self-stimulation of the genitals. Although many people feel uncomfortable discussing masturbation, it is a common sexual practice across the life span. Masturbation is a natural, pleasure-seeking behavior in infants and children. It is a valuable and important means for adolescent males and females, as well as adults, to explore sexual feelings and responsiveness.

Kissing and Erotic Touching
Kissing and erotic touching are two very common forms of nonverbal sexual communication. Both males and females have **erogenous zones**, areas of the body that when touched lead to sexual arousal. Erogenous zones may include genital as well as nongenital areas, such as the earlobes, mouth, breasts, and inner thighs. Almost any area of the body can be conditioned to respond erotically to touch. Spending time with your partner to explore and learn about his or her erogenous areas is another pleasurable, safe, and satisfying means of sexual expression.

Manual Stimulation
Both men and women can be sexually aroused and achieve orgasm through manual stimulation of the genitals by a partner. For many women, orgasm is more likely to be achieved through manual stimulation than

through intercourse. *Sex toys* include a wide variety of objects that can be used for sexual stimulation alone or with a partner. Vibrators and dildos are two common types of toys and can be found in a variety of shapes, styles, and sizes. Sex toys can add zest to sexual experiences and, for women who may not reach orgasm by intercourse, may provide another option for satisfaction. Toys must be cleaned after each use.

Oral–Genital Stimulation

Cunnilingus refers to oral stimulation of a female's genitals, and **fellatio** to oral stimulation of a male's genitals. Many partners find oral–genital stimulation intensely pleasurable. Over 75 percent of college-aged men and women have had oral sex.[8] For some people, oral sex is not an option because of moral or religious beliefs.

Note that HIV and other sexually transmitted infections (STIs) can be transmitted via unprotected oral–genital sex just as through intercourse. Use of an appropriate barrier device is strongly recommended if either partner's health status is in question.

Vaginal Intercourse

The term *intercourse* generally refers to **vaginal intercourse** (*coitus*, or insertion of the penis into the vagina), which is the most frequently practiced form of sexual expression. Coitus can involve a variety of positions, including the missionary position (man on top facing the woman), woman on top, side by side, or man behind (rear entry). Many partners enjoy experimenting with different positions. Knowledge of yourself and your body, along with your ability to communicate effectively, will play a large part in determining the enjoyment and meaning of intercourse for you and your partner. Whatever your circumstances, you should practice safer sex to avoid disease and unwanted pregnancy.

Anal Intercourse

The anal area is highly sensitive to touch, and some couples find pleasure in the stimulation of this area. **Anal intercourse** is insertion of the penis into the anus. Over 26 percent of college-aged men and women have had anal sex.[9] Stimulation of the anus by mouth or with the fingers is also practiced. As with all forms of sexual expression, anal stimulation or intercourse is not for everyone. If you do enjoy this form of sexual expression, remember to use condoms to avoid transmitting disease. Also, anything inserted into the anus should not be directly inserted into the vagina, as bacteria commonly found in the anus can cause vaginal infections.

Variant Sexual Behavior

Although attitudes toward sexuality have changed radically since the Victorian era, some people still believe that any sexual behavior other than heterosexual intercourse is abnormal or perverted. People who study sexuality prefer to use the neutral term **variant sexual behavior** to describe sexual behaviors that are not engaged in by most people; for example:

- *Group sex.* Sexual activity involving more than two people. Participants in group sex run a higher risk of exposure to AIDS and other sexually transmitted infections.
- *Transvestism.* Wearing the clothing of the opposite sex. Most transvestites are male, heterosexual, and married.
- *Fetishism.* Sexual arousal achieved by looking at or touching inanimate objects, such as underclothing or shoes.

Some variant sexual behaviors can be harmful to the individual, to others, or to both. Many of the following activities are illegal in at least some states.

- *Exhibitionism.* Exposing one's genitals to strangers in public places. Most exhibitionists are seeking a reaction of shock or fear from their victims. Exhibitionism is a minor felony in most states.
- *Voyeurism.* Observing other people for sexual gratification. Most voyeurs are men who attempt to watch women undressing or bathing. Voyeurism is an invasion of privacy and illegal in most states.
- *Sadomasochism.* Sexual activities in which gratification is received by inflicting pain (verbal or physical) on a partner or by being the object of such infliction. A sadist is a person who receives gratification from inflicting pain, and a masochist receives gratification from experiencing pain.
- *Pedophilia.* Sexual activity or attraction between an adult and a child. Any sexual activity involving a minor, including possession of child pornography, is illegal.
- *Autoerotic asphyxiation.* The practice of reducing or eliminating oxygen to the brain, usually by tying a cord around one's neck while masturbating to orgasm. Tragically, asphyxiation is usually discovered when people accidentally hang themselves.

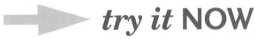

try it NOW

How do you communicate with your partner about sex? Sex can be a difficult subject to talk about, even with a trusted partner. Right now, take a moment to think about a sexual problem or desire you'd like to discuss with your partner, and brainstorm ways you can approach the subject.

(Text continues on page 190)

cunnilingus Oral stimulation of a female's genitals.

fellatio Oral stimulation of a male's genitals.

vaginal intercourse The insertion of the penis into the vagina.

anal intercourse The insertion of the penis into the anus.

variant sexual behavior A sexual behavior that is not engaged in by most people.

ASSESS yourself

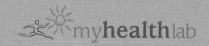

ATTITUDES TOWARD SEXUAL DIFFERENCES

Fill out this assessment online at
www.aw-bc.com/myhealthlab or
www.aw-bc.com/donatelle

How comfortable would you be in the following situations? Why?

	Completely Comfortable			Not at All Comfortable	
1. Your close same-sex friend reveals to you her/his preference for same-sex partners.	1	2	3	4	5
2. Your roommate tells you that she/he likes sexual encounters that involve three or more partners at one time.	1	2	3	4	5
3. Your sister tells you that she would like to have a sex-change operation.	1	2	3	4	5
4. You visit a friend's house, and she/he shows you her/his sexual fantasy room that includes vibrators, sexually explicit magazines, and erotic videos.	1	2	3	4	5
5. Your close friend of another sex reveals to you her/his preference for same-sex partners.	1	2	3	4	5
6. Your 85-year-old grandfather reveals that he is sexually active with his 85-year-old female partner.	1	2	3	4	5
7. A male friend reveals that, although he is primarily heterosexual, he occasionally has sex with other men.	1	2	3	4	5
8. Your lab partner, who looks and acts like a man, reveals that he is really a transgendered woman.	1	2	3	4	5
9. Your blind date tells you that she/he occasionally likes to engage in sadomasochistic sexual play.	1	2	3	4	5
10. Two women from your health class invite you to attend their commitment ceremony at the end of the term.	1	2	3	4	5
11. Your best friend reveals that she/he has made a personal commitment not to engage in sexual activity until marriage.	1	2	3	4	5
12. Your best male friend tells you that he enjoys phone sex.	1	2	3	4	5
13. The person with whom you are romantically involved asks you to tell her/him your sexual fantasies.	1	2	3	4	5
14. You meet someone in an Internet chat room who wants to engage in cybersex.	1	2	3	4	5
15. Your divorced mother reveals that she is dating a man who is your age.	1	2	3	4	5

MAKE it happen!

ASSESSMENT: The Assess Yourself activity gave you a chance to think about your comfort level with a variety of sexual situations and preferences. If you were surprised or unhappy with any of your responses, you may want to consider how to change the attitudes that disturb you.

MAKING A CHANGE: In order to change your behavior, you need to develop a plan. Follow the steps below and complete your Behavior Change Contract to take action.

1. Evaluate your behavior and identify patterns and specific things you are doing. What can you change now? What can you change in the near future?

2. Select one pattern of behavior that you want to change.

3. Fill out the Behavior Change Contract found at the front of your book. It should include your long-term goal for change, your short-term goals, the rewards you'll give yourself for reaching these goals, potential obstacles along the way, and strategies for overcoming these obstacles. For each goal, list the small steps and specific actions that you will take.

4. Chart your progress in a journal. At the end of a week, consider how successful you were in following your plan. What helped you be successful? What made change more difficult? What will you do differently next week?

5. Revise your plan as needed: Are the short-term goals attainable? Are the rewards satisfying?

ONE STUDENT'S PLAN: Jerome considered himself an open-minded and even experimental person. In fact, one of his goals in attending college was to meet people of all different types. Taking the self-assessment made him reevaluate some of his assumptions about his comfort level when it came to sexual differences. He found that most of the situations described made him very uncomfortable. Although he was comfortable with his personal decisions about sexuality, he was unhappy to feel judgmental about others' choices. Jerome knew that there was a student group dedicated to representing gay, lesbian, and bisexual students. Among other activities, they sponsored speakers and lectures. Jerome checked their schedule and attended a talk about gay students' experiences on his campus. Later in the month, he signed up for a lecture by a transgender activist. His goal was not necessarily to change his beliefs about sexuality but to learn as much about its variations as possible, then to accept his comfort level based on his increased understanding.

ANALYZING STUDENT MISPERCEPTIONS OF SEX ON CAMPUS

C ollege students often think everyone is having more sex than they are and with numerous partners. These perceptions may cause them to feel self-conscious about their own lack of sexual activity, or encourage increased promiscuity in order to "measure up." In reality, college students' opinions about sex, relationships, contraception, and attitudes toward sexual activity vary greatly. Results from a survey answered by college students nationwide might help you sort through some of these misperceptions.

How much sex do my peers have?

- Within the past school year approximately 72 percent of college students reported having had 0–1 sexual (oral, anal, or vaginal) partners. However, over 14 percent thought the typical student at their school had 0–1 sexual partners in the past school year.
- In the past 30 days, 48 percent of students reported having had oral sex 1 or more times, but 95 percent thought the typical student had oral sex 1 or more times in the past 30 days.
- In the past 30 days, 50 percent of students reported having vaginal intercourse 1 or more times, yet 96 percent thought the typical student had vaginal intercourse 1 or more times in the past 30 days.
- In the past 30 days, 5 percent of students reported having anal intercourse 1 or more times, whereas 59 percent thought the typical student had anal sex 1 or more times in the past 30 days.
- 1.5 percent of college students who had vaginal intercourse within the past school year reported experiencing an unintentional pregnancy within the last school year.
- Approximately 29 percent of students reported ever being tested for HIV.
- The most common methods of birth control used by sexually active students or their partners to prevent pregnancy the last time they had vaginal intercourse were:
  - Birth control pill, 40%
  - Condoms, 39%

Source: American College Health Association, *National College Health Assessment 2005,* in press.

Difficulties That Can Hinder Sexual Function

Research indicates that **sexual dysfunction**, the term used to describe problems that can hinder sexual functioning, is quite common. Don't feel embarrassed if you experience sexual dysfunction at some point in your life. The sexual part of you does not come with a lifetime warranty. You can have breakdowns involving your sexual function just as in any other body system. Sexual dysfunction can be divided into five major classes: disorders of sexual desire, sexual arousal, orgasm, and sexual performance, and sexual pain. All of them can be treated successfully.

sexual dysfunction　Problems associated with achieving sexual satisfaction.

inhibited sexual desire (ISD)　Lack of sexual appetite or simply a lack of interest and pleasure in sexual activity.

sexual aversion disorder　Type of desire dysfunction characterized by sexual phobias and anxiety about sexual contact.

erectile dysfunction (ED)　Difficulty in achieving or maintaining a penile erection sufficient for intercourse.

Sexual Desire Disorders

The most frequent reason why people seek out a sex therapist is **ISD**, or **inhibited sexual desire**.[10] ISD is the lack of a sexual appetite or simply a lack of interest and pleasure in sexual activity. In some instances, it can result from stress or boredom. **Sexual aversion disorder** is another type of desire dysfunction, characterized by sexual phobias (unreasonable fears) and anxiety about sexual contact. The psychological stress of a punitive upbringing, a rigid religious background, or a history of physical or sexual abuse may be sources of these desire disorders.

Sexual Arousal Disorders

The most common disorder in this category is **erectile dysfunction (ED)**—difficulty in achieving or maintaining a penile erection sufficient for intercourse. At some time in his life, every man experiences impotence. Causes are varied and include underlying diseases, such as diabetes or prostate problems; reactions to some medications (for example, drugs for high blood pressure); depression; fatigue; stress; alcohol; performance anxiety; and guilt over real or imaginary problems (such as when a man compares himself to his partner's past lovers). Some 30 million men in this country, half of them under age 65, suffer from ED. ED generally becomes more of a problem as men age, affecting one in four men over the age of 65.[11] In March 1998, the Food and Drug Administration (FDA) approved Viagra, the first pill to treat ED. Since that time, vardenafil hydrochloride (Levitra) and tadalafil (Cialis) have also been approved. Additional oral medicines are being tested for safety and effectiveness.

How do drugs like Viagra work? Viagra, Levitra, and Cialis all belong to a class of drugs called phosphodiesterase (PDE) inhibitors. Taken an hour before sexual activity, these drugs work by enhancing the effects of nitric oxide, a chemical that relaxes smooth muscles in the penis during sexual stimulation and allows increased blood flow.

These medications are not, however, without risk. The most commonly reported side effects include headache, flushing, stomachache, urinary tract infection, diarrhea, dizziness, rash, and visual changes. In addition, there have been several deaths in the United States among Viagra users, prompting more caution in prescribing it to patients with known cardiovascular disease and those taking commonly prescribed short- and long-acting nitrates, such as nitroglycerin.[12]

Orgasm Disorders

Premature ejaculation—ejaculation that occurs prior to or very soon after the insertion of the penis into the vagina—affects up to 50 percent of the male population at some time in their lives. Treatment for premature ejaculation first involves a physical examination to rule out organic causes. If the cause of the problem is not physiological, therapy is available to help a man learn how to control the timing of his ejaculation. Fatigue, stress, performance pressure, and alcohol use can all contribute to orgasmic disorders in men.

In a woman, the inability to achieve orgasm is termed **female orgasmic disorder**. A woman with this disorder often blames herself and learns to fake orgasm to avoid embarrassment or preserve her partner's ego. Contributing to this response are the messages women have historically been given about sex as a duty rather than a pleasurable act. As with men who experience orgasmic disorders, the first step in treatment is a physical exam to rule out organic causes. However, the problem is often solved by simple self-exploration to learn more about what forms of stimulation are arousing enough to produce orgasm. Through masturbation, a woman can learn how her body responds sexually to various types of touch. Once she has become orgasmic through masturbation, she learns to communicate her needs to her partner.

Sexual Performance Disorders

Both men and women can experience **sexual performance anxiety** when they anticipate some sort of problem in the sex act. A man may become anxious and unable to maintain an erection, or he may experience premature ejaculation. A woman may be unable to achieve orgasm or to allow penetration because of the involuntary contraction of vaginal muscles. Both can overcome performance anxiety by learning to focus on immediate sensations and pleasures rather than on orgasm.

Sexual Pain Disorders

Two common disorders in this category are dyspareunia and vaginismus. **Dyspareunia** is pain experienced by a female during intercourse. This pain may be caused by diseases such as endometriosis, uterine tumors, chlamydia, gonorrhea, or urinary tract infections. Damage to tissues during childbirth and insufficient lubrication during intercourse may also cause discomfort. Dyspareunia can also be psychological in origin. As with other sexual problems, dyspareunia can be treated, with good results.

Vaginismus is the involuntary contraction of vaginal muscles, making penile insertion painful or impossible. Most cases of vaginismus are related to fear of intercourse or to unresolved sexual conflicts. Treatment involves teaching a woman to achieve orgasm through nonvaginal stimulation.

Seeking Help for Sexual Dysfunction

Many theories and treatment models can help people with sexual dysfunction. A first important step is choosing a qualified sex therapist or counselor. A national organization, the American Association of Sex Educators, Counselors, and Therapists (AASECT), has been in the forefront of establishing criteria for certifying sex therapists. These criteria include appropriate degree(s) in the helping professions, specialized coursework in human sexuality, and sufficient hours of practical therapy work under the direct supervision of a certified sex therapist. Lists of certified counselors and sex therapists, as well as clinics that treat sexual dysfunctions, can be obtained by contacting AASECT or the Sexuality Information and Education Council of the United States (SIECUS).

---

premature ejaculation   Ejaculation that occurs prior to or almost immediately following penile penetration of the vagina.

female orgasmic disorder   The inability to achieve orgasm.

sexual performance anxiety   A condition of sexual difficulties caused by anticipating some sort of problem with the sex act.

dyspareunia   Pain experienced by women during intercourse.

vaginismus   A state in which the vaginal muscles contract so forcefully that penetration cannot be accomplished.

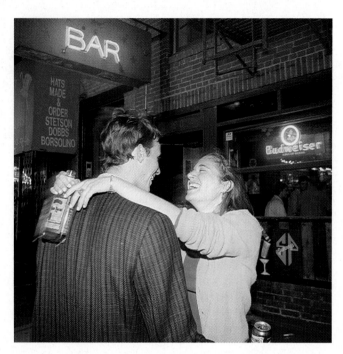
Alcohol and drug use can impair judgment and lead to sexual encounters that are later regretted.

Drugs and Sex

Because psychoactive drugs affect the entire physiology, it is only logical that they affect sexual behavior. Promises of increased pleasure make drugs very tempting to those seeking greater sexual satisfaction. Too often, however, drugs become central to sexual activities and damage the relationship. Drug use can also lead to undesired sexual activity.

Alcohol is notorious for reducing inhibitions and promoting feelings of well-being and desirability. At the same time, alcohol inhibits sexual response; thus, the mind may be willing, but not the body.

Perhaps the greatest danger associated with use of drugs during sex is the tendency to blame the drug for negative behavior. "I can't help what I did last night because I was drunk" is a statement that demonstrates sexual immaturity. A sexually mature person carefully examines risks and benefits and makes decisions accordingly. If drugs are necessary to increase erotic feelings, it is likely that the partners are being dishonest about their feelings for each other. Good sex should not depend on chemical substances.

"Date rape" drugs are becoming a greater concern. They are popular among college students and are often used in combination with alcohol. Rohypnol ("roofies," "rope," "forget pill"), GHB (gamma-hydroxybutyrate, or "liquid X," "Grievous Bodily Harm," "easy lay," "Mickey Finn"), and ketamine ("K," "Special K," "cat valium") have been used to facilitate rape. GHB and Rohypnol are difficult-to-detect drugs that depress the central nervous system. Ketamine can cause dreamlike states, hallucinations, delirium, amnesia, and impaired motor function. These drugs are often introduced to unsuspecting women through alcoholic drinks in order to render them unconscious and vulnerable to rape. This problem is so serious that the U.S. Congress passed the Drug-Induced Rape Prevention and Punishment Act of 1996 to provide increased federal penalties for using drugs to facilitate sexual assault. The dangers of these drugs are discussed in more detail in Chapter 4 (see the Spotlight on Your Health box) and Chapter 14 (see the Club Drugs section).

? *what do you* THINK?

Why do we find it so difficult to discuss sexual dysfunction in our society? ■ Do you think it is more difficult for men than for women to talk about dysfunction? ■ Have you ever used alcohol or some other drug to enhance your sexual performance? ■ Why are "roofies" of major concern on college campuses?

TAKING charge

Summary

- Sexual identity is determined by a complex interaction of genetic, physiological, and environmental factors. Biological sex, gender identity, gender roles, and sexual orientation are all blended into our sexual identity.
- The major components of the female sexual anatomy include the mons pubis, labia minora and majora, clitoris, urethral and vaginal openings, vagina, cervix, uterine tubes, and ovaries. The major components of the male sexual anatomy are the penis, scrotum, testes, epididymides, vasa deferentia, ejaculatory ducts, and urethra.
- Physiologically, males and females experience four phases of sexual response: excitement/arousal, plateau, orgasm, and resolution.

- Humans can express their sexual selves in a variety of ways, including celibacy, autoerotic behaviors, kissing and erotic touch, manual stimulation, oral–genital stimulation, vaginal intercourse, and anal intercourse. Sexual orientation refers to a person's enduring emotional, romantic, sexual, or affectionate attraction to other persons. Irrational hatred or fear of homosexuality or gay and lesbian persons is termed homophobia.
- Sexual dysfunctions can be classified into disorders of sexual desire, sexual arousal, orgasm, sexual performance, and sexual pain. Drug use can also lead to sexual dysfunction.

Chapter Review

1. Intense feelings of elation, sexual desire, and ecstasy about a partner are characteristic of
   a. companionate love.
   b. mature love.
   c. passionate love.
   d. intimacy.

2. Intimacy is what type of romantic feeling?
   a. romantic love
   b. sensual feelings
   c. empty commitment love
   d. mutual feelings of giving and receiving emotional closeness

3. The most sensitive or erotic spot in the female genital region is considered to be the
   a. mons pubis.
   b. vagina.
   c. clitoris.
   d. labia.

4. When a woman is in ovulation
   a. she has released an ovum egg cell.
   b. she is experiencing menstrual bleeding.
   c. an egg has been fertilized and she is pregnant.
   d. None of the above.

5. Which of the following is *not* true about a woman's menstrual cycle?
   a. All women will experience premenstrual syndrome (PMS).

   b. The estrogen levels drop during ovulation.
   c. The hypothalamus monitors the hormone levels in the blood.
   d. The endometrium becomes engorged with blood and causes bleeding if the ovum is not fertilized.

6. A condition in which women may stop menstruating is known as
   a. premenstrual syndrome.
   b. menstrual cramps.
   c. premenstrual dysphoric disorder.
   d. amenorrhea.

7. What is the role of testosterone in the male reproductive system?
   a. It is used to produce sperm for reproduction.
   b. It is the hormone that stimulates development of secondary male sex characteristics.
   c. It allows the penis to harden during sexual arousal.
   d. It secretes the seminal fluid preceding ejaculation.

8. The pre-ejaculate fluid that sometimes results before a man ejaculates comes from which gland in the male reproductive system?
   a. prostate gland
   b. Cowper's gland
   c. vas deferens
   d. testicles

9. Individuals who are sexually attracted to both sexes are identified as
   a. heterosexual.
   b. bisexual.
   c. homosexual.
   d. intersexed.

10. Fellatio is the oral stimulation of the
    a. male genitals.
    b. female genitals.
    c. anus region.
    d. mouth and tongue.

Answers to these questions can be found on page A-1.

Questions for Discussion and Reflection

1. How have gender roles changed over your lifetime? Do you view the changes as positive for both men and women?
2. Discuss the cycle of changes that occurs in our bodies in response to various hormones (for example, sexual differentiation while in the womb, secondary sex characteristics at puberty, menopause).
3. What is "normal" sexual behavior? What criteria should we use to determine healthful sexual practice?

4. If scientists finally establish the combination of factors that interact to produce homosexual, heterosexual, or bisexual orientation, will that put an end to antigay prejudice? Why or why not?
5. How can we remove the stigma that surrounds sexual dysfunction so that individuals feel more open to seeking help? Are men and women impacted differently by sexual dysfunction?

Accessing Your Health on the Internet

The following websites explore further topics and issues related to personal health. You'll also find links to each organization's website on the Companion Website for *Access to Health,* Tenth Edition, at www.aw-bc.com/donatelle.

1. *American Association of Sex Educators, Counselors, and Therapists (AASECT).* Professional organization providing standards of practice for treatment of sexual issues and disorders. www.aasect.org
2. *Bacchus and Gamma Peer Education Network.* Student-friendly source of information about sexual and other health issues. www.bacchusgamma.org
3. *Go Ask Alice.* An interactive question-and-answer resource from Columbia University Health Services. "Alice" is

available to answer questions each week about any health-related issues, including relationships, nutrition and diet, exercise, drugs, sex, alcohol, and stress. www.goaskalice.columbia.edu

4. *Sexuality Information and Education Council of the United States (SIECUS).* Information, guidelines, and materials for advancement of healthy and proper sex education. www.siecus.org
5. *Advocates for Youth.* Current news, policy updates, research, and other resources about the sexual health of and choices particular to high school and college-aged students. www.advocatesforyouth.org

Further Reading

Caron, S. L. *Sex Matters for College Students: Sex FAQs in Human Sexuality.* Englewood Cliffs, NJ: Prentice Hall, 2002.

This is a brief, easy-to-read, and affordable paperback designed specifically to answer the basic sexual questions of today's young adults in a friendly and age-appropriate way.

Caster, W. *The Lesbian Sex Book: A Guide for Women Who Love Women,* 2nd ed. New York: Alyson, 2003.

A handbook for lesbian sexual practices and health.

Goldstone, S. *The Ins and Outs of Gay Sex: A Medical Handbook for Men.* New York: Dell, 1999.

A comprehensive guide to the sexual and medical concerns of gay men.

Men's Health Books, ed. *The Complete Book of Men's Health: The Definitive, Illustrated Guide to Healthy Living, Exercise, and Sex.* Emmaus, PA: Rodale Press, 2000.

A comprehensive and lushly illustrated guide to information on healthy lifestyles for men.

Sexuality Information and Education Council of the United States (SIECUS) Report. 130 West 42nd Street, New York, NY 10036.

Highly acclaimed and readable bimonthly journal. Includes timely and thought-provoking articles on human sexuality, sexuality education, and AIDS.

Wingood, G. M. and R. DiClemente, eds. *Handbook of Women's Sexual and Reproductive Health.* Boston: Plenum Publishing, 2002.

Medical researchers, including those in behavioral sciences and health education, summarize in depth the epidemiology, social and behavioral factors, policies, and effective intervention and prevention strategies related to women's sexual and reproductive health.

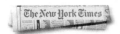

e-themes from *The New York Times*

For up-to-date articles about current health issues, visit www.aw-bc.com/donatelle, select *Access to Health,* Tenth Edition, Chapter 6, and click on "e-themes."

References

1. Advocates for Youth, *Life Planning Education: A Comprehensive Sex Education Curriculum* (Washington, DC: Advocates for Youth, in press).
2. Federal Bureau of Investigation, "Hate Crime Statistics, 2004," www.fbi.gov/ucr/hc2004/section1.htm.
3. S. E. Anderson, G. E. Dallal, and A. Must, "Relative Weight and Race Influence Average Age at Menarche: Results from Two Nationally Representative Surveys of U.S. Girls Studied 25 Years Apart," *Pediatrics* 111, no. 4 (2003): 844–850.
4. Madison Institute of Medicine, Inc., "Premenstrual Dysphoric Disorder," 2006, www.pmdd.factsforhealth.org/index.html.
5. National Institutes of Health, *Facts About Menopausal Hormone Therapy,* NIH Publication Number 05-5200, 2005.
6. G. F. Kelly, "Sexual Individuality and Sexual Values," in *Sexuality Today: The Human Perspective,* 8th ed. (New York: McGraw-Hill, 2006).
7. Ibid.
8. American College Health Association, "American College Health Association-National College Health Assessment (ACHA-NCHA) Web Summary," April 2006, www.acha.org/projects_programs/ncha _sampledata.cfm.
9. Ibid.
10. Kelly, "Sexual Individuality and Sexual Values."
11. National Kidney and Urological Diseases Information Clearinghouse, "Erectile Dysfunction," 2005, http://kidney.niddk.nih.gov/kudiseases/ pubs/impotence/index.htm.
12. U.S. Food and Drug Administration, "FDA Alert: Viagra (sildenafil citrate) Information," July 2005, www.fda.gov/cder/consumerinfo/ viagra/default.htm.

7

Reproductive Choices

MAKING RESPONSIBLE DECISIONS

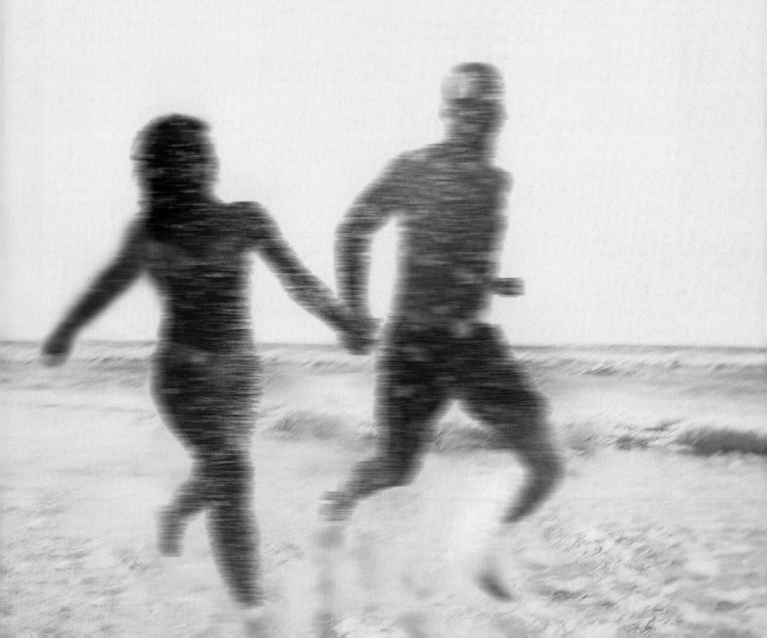

Which method of **birth control** is best for me?

Is emergency **contraception** the same as abortion?

How does the pill affect my physical **health**?

Are home **pregnancy** testing kits reliable?

What causes **infertility**?

OBJECTIVES

- Compare the different types of contraceptive methods and their effectiveness in preventing pregnancy and sexually transmitted infections.
- Summarize the legal decisions surrounding abortion and the various types of abortion procedures.
- Discuss key issues to consider when planning a pregnancy.
- Explain the importance of prenatal care and the physical and emotional aspects of pregnancy.
- Describe the basic stages of childbirth, and methods and complications that can arise during labor and delivery.
- Review primary causes of and possible solutions to infertility.

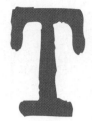

Today, we not only understand the intimate details of reproduction, but also possess technologies that can control or enhance our **fertility**. Along with information and technological advances comes choice, and choice goes hand in hand with responsibility. Choosing if and when to have children is one of our greatest responsibilities. A woman and her partner have much to consider before planning or risking a pregnancy. Children, whether planned or unplanned, change people's lives. They require a lifelong personal commitment of love and nurturing. Are you physically, emotionally, and financially prepared to care for another human being?

One measure of maturity is the ability to discuss reproduction and birth control with one's sexual partner before acting on sexual urges. Men often assume that their partners are taking care of birth control. Women often feel that bringing up the subject implies that they are promiscuous. Both may feel that this discussion interferes with romance and spontaneity. You will find embarrassment-free discussion a lot easier if you understand human reproduction and contraception and honestly consider your attitudes toward these matters before you find yourself in a compromising situation.

Methods of Fertility Management

Conception refers to the fertilization of an ovum by a sperm. The following conditions are necessary for conception:

1. A viable egg
2. A viable sperm
3. Access to the egg by the sperm

---

fertility   A person's ability to reproduce.

conception   The fertilization of an ovum by a sperm.

contraception (birth control)   Methods of preventing conception.

sexually transmitted infections (STIs)   A variety of infections that can be acquired through sexual contact.

barrier methods   Contraceptive methods that block the meeting of egg and sperm by means of a physical barrier (such as condom, diaphragm, or cervical cap), a chemical barrier (such as spermicide), or both.

hormonal methods   Contraceptive method that introduces synthetic hormones into the woman's system to prevent ovulation, thicken cervical mucus, or prevent a fertilized egg from implanting.

male condom   A single-use sheath of thin latex or other material designed to fit over an erect penis and to catch semen upon ejaculation.

The term **contraception** (also called **birth control**) refers to methods of preventing conception. These methods offer varying degrees of control over when and whether pregnancy occurs. However, since people first associated sexual activity with pregnancy, society has searched for a simple, infallible, and risk-free way to prevent pregnancy. We have not yet found one.

To evaluate the effectiveness of a particular contraceptive method, you must be familiar with two concepts: perfect use failure rate and typical use failure rate. *Perfect use failure rate* refers to the number of pregnancies that are likely to occur in the first year of use (per 100 uses of the method during sexual intercourse) if the method is used absolutely perfectly, that is, without any error. The *typical use failure rate* refers to the number of pregnancies that are likely to occur in the first year of use with typical use, that is, with the normal number of errors, memory lapses, and incorrect or incomplete use. This information is much more practical for making informed decisions about contraceptive methods. Table 7.1 details the effectiveness of various contraceptive methods, many of which we'll discuss in this chapter.

Many contraceptive methods can also protect, at least to some degree, against **sexually transmitted infections (STIs)**. This is an important factor to consider in choosing a contraceptive, and as we discuss various methods of contraception in this chapter, we'll also describe their effectiveness against STIs and HIV. See Chapter 17 for more about specific STIs.

Present methods of contraception fall into several categories. **Barrier methods** block the egg and sperm from joining. **Hormonal methods** introduce synthetic hormones into the woman's system that prevent ovulation, thicken cervical mucus, or prevent a fertilized egg from implanting. Surgical methods can permanently prevent pregnancy. Other methods of contraception involve temporary or permanent abstinence or planning intercourse in accordance with fertility patterns. See the Assess Yourself box on page 200 to determine what method is right for you and your partner.

> Which method of birth control is best for me?

Barrier Methods

The Male Condom
The **male condom** is a thin sheath designed to cover the erect penis and catch semen before it enters the vagina. The majority of male condoms are made of latex, although condoms made of polyurethane or lambskin are now available. The condom is the only temporary means of birth control available for men, and latex and polyurethane condoms are the only barriers that effectively prevent the spread of STIs and HIV. ("Skin" condoms, made from lamb intestines, are not effective against STIs.)

Condoms come in a wide variety of styles; all may be purchased with or without spermicide in pharmacies, in some supermarkets and public bathrooms, and in many health clinics. A new condom must be used for each act of vaginal, oral, or anal intercourse.

(Text continues on page 202)

TABLE 7.1 **Contraceptive Effectiveness and STI Prevention: Number of Unintended Pregnancies per 100 Women during First Year of Use**

Method	Typical Use	Perfect Use
Continuous Abstinence[*]	0.00	0.00
Outercourse[†]	N/A	N/A
Norplant Implant	0.05	0.05
Sterilization		
Men	0.15	0.1
Women	0.5	0.5
Depo-Provera Injection	0.3	0.3
IUD (Intrauterine Device)		
ParaGard (copper T380A)	0.8	0.6
Mirena	0.1	0.1
Oral Contraceptives (The Pill)	8.0	0.3
Male Condom[†]	15.0	2.0
Sponge		
Women who have not given birth	16.0	9.0
Women who have given birth	32.0	20.0
Ortho Evra (The Patch)	8.0	0.3
NuvaRing	8.0	0.3
Withdrawal	27.0	4.0
Diaphragm[†]	20.0	6.0
Cervical Cap[†]		
Women who have not given birth	16.0	9.0
Women who have given birth	32.0	26.0
Female Condom[†]	21.0	5.0
Periodic Abstinence	25.0	
Postovulation method		1.0
Symptothermal method		2.0
Cervical mucus (ovulation) method		3.0
Calendar method		9.0
Fertility Awareness Methods	N/A	N/A
Spermicide[†]	26.0	6.0
No Method	85.0	85.0
Emergency Contraception		

Emergency contraception pills: Treatment initiated within 72 hours after unprotected intercourse reduces the risk of pregnancy by 75–89% (with no protection against STIs). Emergency IUD insertion: Treatment initiated within seven days after unprotected intercourse reduces the risk of pregnancy by more than 99% (with no protection against STIs).

Note: "Typical Use" refers to failure rates for men and women whose use is not consistent or always correct. "Perfect Use" refers to failure rates for those whose use is consistent and always correct.

N/A means that effectiveness rates are not available.

[*]Indicates complete protection from STIs

[†]Indicates limited protection from STIs

Source: R. Hatcher et al., "Contraceptive Effectiveness Rates," *Contraceptive Technology,* 18th ed. (New York: Ardent Media, 2004). Reprinted by permission of Ardent Media.

ASSESS yourself

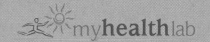

CONTRACEPTIVE COMFORT AND CONFIDENCE SCALE

Fill out this assessment online at www.aw-bc.com/MyHealthLab or www.aw-bc.com/donatelle.

These questions will help you assess whether the method of contraception you are using now or may consider using in the future will be effective for you. Answering yes to any of these questions predicts potential problems. Most individuals will have a few yes answers. If you have more than a few yes responses, however, you may want to talk to a health care provider, counselor, partner, or friend to decide whether to use this method or how to use it so that it will really be effective. In general, the more yes answers you have, the less likely you are to use this method consistently and correctly with every act of intercourse.

Method of contraception you use now or are considering: _____

Length of time you used this method in the past: _____

Answer yes or no to the following questions:

		Yes	No
1.	Have I ever had problems using this method?	❏	❏
2.	Have I ever become pregnant while using this method?	❏	❏
3.	Am I afraid of using this method?	❏	❏
4.	Would I really rather not use this method?	❏	❏
5.	Will I have trouble remembering to use this method?	❏	❏
6.	Will I have trouble using this method correctly?	❏	❏
7.	Do I still have unanswered questions about this method?	❏	❏
8.	Does this method make menstrual periods longer or more painful?	❏	❏
9.	Does this method cost more than I can afford?	❏	❏
10.	Could this method cause serious complications?	❏	❏
11.	Am I opposed to this method because of any religious or moral beliefs?	❏	❏
12.	Is my partner opposed to this method?	❏	❏
13.	Am I using this method without my partner's knowledge?	❏	❏
14.	Will using this method embarrass my partner?	❏	❏
15.	Will using this method embarrass me?	❏	❏
16.	Will I enjoy intercourse less because of this method?	❏	❏
17.	If this method interrupts lovemaking, will I avoid using it?	❏	❏
18.	Has a nurse or doctor ever told me not to use this method?	❏	❏
19.	Is there anything about my personality that could lead me to use this method incorrectly?	❏	❏
20.	Am I at risk of being exposed to HIV (the human immunodeficiency virus) or other sexually transmitted infections (STIs) if I use this method?	❏	❏

Total number of yes answers: _____

Source: From R. A. Hatcher et al., *Contraceptive Technology*, 18th ed. (New York: Ardent Media, 2004), 238. Reprinted by permission of Ardent Media.

MAKE it happen!

ASSESSMENT: The Assess Yourself activity gave you the chance to assess your comfort and confidence with a contraceptive method you are using now or may use in the future. Depending on the results of the assessment, you may consider making a change in your birth control method.

MAKING A CHANGE: In order to change your behavior, you need to develop a plan. Follow the steps below and complete your Behavior Change Contract to take action.

1. Evaluate your behavior and identify patterns and specific things you are doing. What can you change now? What can you change in the near future?

2. Select one pattern of behavior that you want to change.

3. Fill out the Behavior Change Contract found at the front of your book. It should include your long-term goal for change, your short-term goals, the rewards you'll give yourself for reaching these goals, potential obstacles along the way, and strategies for overcoming these obstacles. For each goal, list the small steps and specific actions that you will take.

4. Chart your progress in a journal. At the end of a week, consider how successful you were in following your plan. What helped you be successful? What made change more difficult? What will you do differently next week?

5. Revise your plan as needed: Are the short-term goals attainable? Are the rewards satisfying?

ONE STUDENT'S PLAN: Marissa had been using a diaphragm as her form of birth control. When she completed the self-assessment, she discovered that there were several aspects of it that made her uncomfortable. The questions to which she answered "yes" showed that she sometimes forgot to bring her diaphragm when she planned to see her boyfriend Ben, and she disliked using it because it interrupted her sexual activity. She also was embarrassed to use it because she didn't like inserting it in front of Ben. She decided she should investigate other birth control options and discuss them with her boyfriend. Her first step was to visit her student health center and, based on her likes and dislikes, to choose one or two alternatives to the diaphragm. Among the options suggested to her were the contraceptive patch (Ortho Evra) and the vaginal ring (NuvaRing), both of which she would not have to remember to use and would not interrupt sexual activity. Marissa's next step was to talk to her boyfriend about his likes and dislikes and then to make a final decision based on her confidence in the method, its convenience, and its cost.

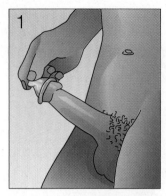
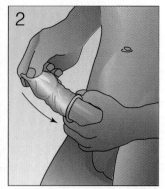
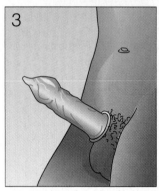
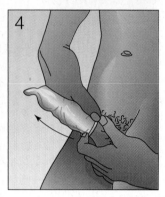

FIGURE 7.1 How to Use a Condom

The condom should be rolled over the erect penis before any penetration occurs. A small space (about ¹/₂ inch) should be left at the end of the condom to collect the semen after ejaculation. Hold the tip of the condom, and unroll it all the way to the base of the penis. Hold the base of the condom before withdrawal to avoid spilling any semen.

A condom must be rolled onto the penis before the penis touches the vagina, and held in place when removing the penis from the vagina after ejaculation (Figure 7.1). For greatest efficacy, the condom should be used with a spermicide. If necessary or desired, users can lubricate their own condoms with contraceptive foams, creams, and jellies or other water-based lubricants, such as K-Y jelly, ForPlay lubricants, Astroglide, or Wet or Aqua Lube, to name just a few. However, one should never use products such as baby oil, cold cream, petroleum jelly, vaginal yeast infection medications, or hand and body lotion with a condom. These products contain mineral oil and will make the latex begin to disintegrate within 60 seconds.

Condoms are less effective and more likely to break during intercourse if they are old or poorly stored. To maintain effectiveness, store them in a cool place (not in a wallet or hip pocket), and inspect them for small tears before use.

For some people, a condom ruins the spontaneity of sex. Stopping to put it on breaks the mood for them. Others report

spermicides Substances designed to kill sperm.

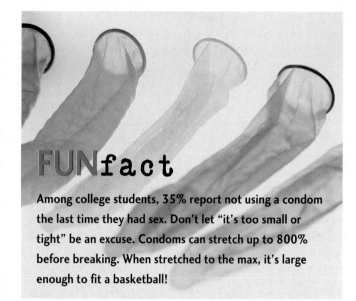

FIGURE 7.2 A Closer Look at College Students' Condom Use

that the condom decreases sensation. These inconveniences contribute to improper use of the device. Partners who incorporate putting a condom on during foreplay are generally more successful with this form of birth control.

Foams, Suppositories, Jellies, Creams, and Film

Like condoms, jellies, creams, suppositories, and foam do not require a prescription. Chemically, they are referred to as **spermicides**—substances designed to kill sperm. Recent studies indicate that spermicides containing nonoxynol 9 (N-9) are not effective in preventing certain STIs such as gonorrhea, chlamydia, and HIV. In fact, frequent use of N-9 spermicides has been shown to cause irritation and breaks in the mucous layer or skin of the genital tract, creating a point of entry for viruses and bacteria that cause disease.[1] Although they are not recommended as the primary form of contraception, spermicides are often recommended for use with other methods and are most effective when used in conjunction with a condom.

Jellies and creams are packaged in tubes, and foams are available in aerosol cans. All have tubes designed for insertion into the vagina. They must be inserted far enough to cover the cervix, providing both a chemical barrier that kills sperm and a physical barrier that stops sperm from continuing toward an egg (Figure 7.3).

Suppositories are waxy capsules that are inserted deep in the vagina, where they melt. They must be inserted 10 to 20 minutes before intercourse to have time to melt but no longer than one hour prior to intercourse or they lose their effectiveness. Additional spermicide must be applied for each subsequent act of intercourse.

Vaginal contraceptive film is another method of spermicide delivery. A thin film infused with spermicidal gel is inserted into the vagina, so that it covers the cervix. The film dissolves into a spermicidal gel that is effective for up to

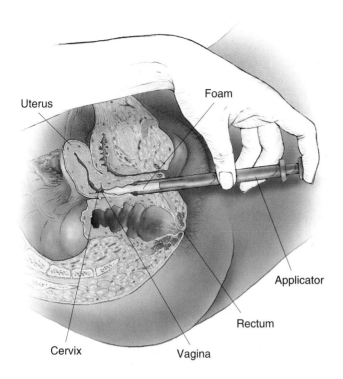

FIGURE 7.3 **The Proper Method of Applying Spermicide within the Vagina**

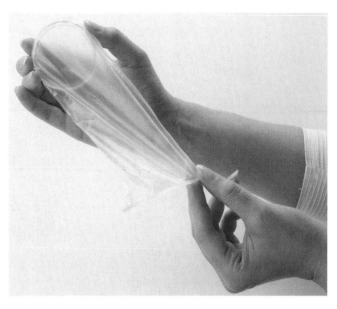

The Female Condom.

three hours. As with other spermicides, a new film must be inserted for each act of intercourse.

The Female Condom
The **female condom** is a single-use, soft, loose-fitting polyurethane sheath meant for internal use by women. It is designed as one unit with two diaphragm-like rings. One ring, which lies inside the sheath, serves as an insertion mechanism and internal anchor. The other ring, which remains outside the vagina once the device is inserted, protects the labia and the base of the penis from infection. Many women like the female condom because it gives them more control than does the male condom. When used correctly, the female condom provides protection against HIV and STIs comparable to that of a latex male condom. The female condom is not meant solely for women and can also be used for male anal sex.

The Diaphragm with Spermicidal Jelly or Cream
Invented in the mid-nineteenth century, the **diaphragm** was the first widely used birth control method for women. The device is a soft, shallow cup made of thin latex rubber. Its flexible, rubber-coated ring is designed to fit snugly behind the pubic bone in front of the cervix and over the back of the cervix on the other side. Diaphragms are manufactured in different sizes and must be fitted to the woman by a trained practitioner. The practitioner should also be certain that the user knows how to insert her diaphragm correctly before she leaves the practitioner's office.

Diaphragms must be used with spermicidal cream or jelly, which is applied to the inside of the diaphragm before it is inserted. The diaphragm holds the spermicide in place, creating a physical and chemical barrier against sperm. Additional spermicide must be applied before each subsequent act of intercourse, and the diaphragm must be left in place for six to eight hours after intercourse to allow the chemical to kill any sperm remaining in the vagina. When used with spermicidal jelly or cream, it offers significant protection against gonorrhea and possibly chlamydia and human papilloma virus (HPV) (Figure 7.4, on the next page).

Using a diaphragm during the menstrual period or leaving it in place longer than 24 hours slightly increases the user's risk of developing **toxic shock syndrome (TSS)**. This condition results from the multiplication of bacteria that spread to the bloodstream and cause sudden high fever, rash, nausea, vomiting, diarrhea, and a rapid drop in blood pressure. If not treated, TSS can be fatal. The diaphragm (as well as a tampon left too long in place) creates conditions conducive to the growth of these bacteria. To reduce the risk of TSS, women should wash their hands carefully with soap and water before inserting or removing the diaphragm.

female condom A single-use polyurethane sheath for internal use by women.

diaphragm A latex, cup-shaped device designed to cover the cervix and block access to the uterus; should always be used with spermicide.

toxic shock syndrome (TSS) A potentially life-threatening disease that occurs when specific bacterial toxins are allowed to multiply unchecked in wounds or through improper use of tampons or diaphragms.

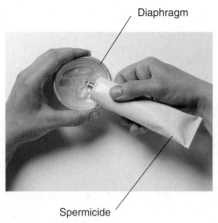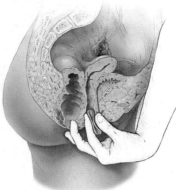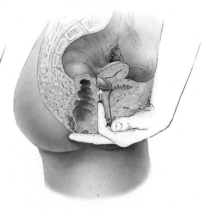

Diaphragm

Spermicide

a. Place spermicide inside and around the rim of the diaphragm.

b. Insertion: squeeze rim together; insert with spermicide-side up.

c. Check placement, making certain cervix is covered.

FIGURE 7.4 **The Proper Use and Placement of a Diaphragm**

Another problem with the diaphragm is that it can put undue pressure on the urethra, blocking urinary flow and predisposing the user to bladder infections. Inserting the device can be awkward, especially if the woman is rushed. When inserted incorrectly, diaphragms are much less effective.

The Cervical Cap with Spermicidal Jelly or Cream

One of the oldest methods used to prevent pregnancy, early cervical caps were made from beeswax, silver, or copper. Today's **cervical cap** is a small cup made of latex that fits snugly over the entire cervix. It must be fitted by a practitioner and is designed for use with contraceptive jelly or cream. It is somewhat more difficult to insert than a diaphragm because of its smaller size.

The cap works by blocking sperm from the uterus. It is held in place by suction created during application. Insertion may take place up to 6 hours prior to intercourse, and the device must be left in place for 6 to 8 hours after intercourse. The maximum length of time the cap can be left on the cervix is 48 hours. If removed and cleaned, it can be reinserted immediately. The cervical cap may offer protection against some STIs but not HIV.

Some women report unpleasant vaginal odors after use. Because the device can become dislodged during intercourse, placement must be checked frequently. It cannot be used during the menstrual period or for longer than 48 hours because of the risk of TSS.

Lea's Shield and FemCap

Lea's Shield is a one-size-fits-all silicon rubber device that covers the cervix. The device can be inserted any time prior to intercourse, but must remain in place for 8 hours after intercourse; it can remain in place for a maximum of 48 hours. The shield is outfitted with a small loop that aids in both insertion and removal. It must be used with spermicidal jelly or cream, similar to the diaphragm or cervical cap. Approved by the FDA in 2002, it is available by prescription. Because the shield is made of silicon rubber, not latex, it is a suitable alternative for those allergic to latex.

Like Lea's Shield, the *FemCap* is a latex-free barrier contraceptive that fits over the cervix, must be used with spermicide, and is available by prescription. FemCap comes in three sizes: the smallest size is meant for a woman who has never been pregnant, and the largest for a woman who has delivered a full-term baby. This allows for maximum fit and comfort. The device should remain in place for 6 hours after intercourse, and no more than 48 hours.

The Sponge

The original version of the **sponge**, the *Today Sponge,* was available in the United States from 1983 to 1995, at which time the manufacturer shut down production rather than bring its facility up to FDA standards. In 2005, the Today Sponge, produced by a different company, was again approved by the FDA, and is now available for purchase in retail stores.

The sponge is made of polyurethane foam and contains nonoxynol 9. It fits over the cervix and creates a barrier

cervical cap A small cup made of latex that is designed to fit snugly over the entire cervix.

Lea's Shield A one-size-fits-all silicon rubber device that covers the cervix and is available by prescription.

sponge A contraceptive device, made of polyurethane foam and containing nonoxynol 9, that fits over the cervix to create a barrier against sperm.

against sperm. A main advantage is convenience, as it does not require a trip to the doctor for fitting. It can be inserted in advance, and remain in place for 24 hours. Disadvantages of the sponge are limited protection from STIs and only moderate protection from pregnancy.

Hormonal Methods

Oral Contraceptives

Oral contraceptive pills were first marketed in the United States in 1960. Their convenience quickly made them the most widely used reversible method of fertility control. Today, oral contraceptives are the most commonly used contraceptive among college-aged women (Figure 7.5).

Most oral contraceptives work through the combined effects of synthetic estrogen and progesterone (*combination pills*). Because the levels of estrogen in the pill are higher than those produced by the body, the pituitary gland is never signaled to produce follicle-stimulating hormone (FSH), without which ova will not develop in the ovaries. Progesterone in the pill prevents proper growth of the uterine lining and thickens the cervical mucus, forming a barrier against sperm.

Combination pills are meant to be taken in a cycle. At the end of each three-week cycle, the user discontinues the drug or takes placebo pills for one week. The resultant drop in hormones causes the uterine lining to disintegrate, and the user will have a menstrual period, usually within 1 to 3 days. The same cycle is repeated every 28 days. Menstrual flow is generally lighter than it is for women who don't use the pill because the hormones in the pill prevent thick endometrial buildup.

Today's pill is different from the one introduced more than four decades ago. The original pill contained large amounts of estrogen, which caused certain risks, whereas the current pill contains the minimal amount of estrogen necessary to prevent pregnancy.

A new type of pill available since 2003 is **Seasonale**, a 91-day (extended-cycle) oral contraceptive. A woman using this type of regimen takes active pills for 12 weeks, followed by 1 week of placebos. Under this cycle, women can expect to have a menstrual period every 3 months. Early data indicate that women have an increased occurrence of spotting or bleeding in the first few cycles.[2] Side effects and risks are similar to 28-day-cycle pills.

> **How does the pill affect my physical health?**

Because the chemicals in oral contraceptives change the way the body metabolizes certain nutrients, women using the pill should check with their practitioners to see if dietary supplements are advisable, especially vitamins C, B_2 (riboflavin), B_6 (pyridoxine), and B_{12} (cobalamin). A nutritious diet that includes whole grains, fresh fruits and vegetables, lean meats, fish, and poultry, and nonfat dairy products is important.

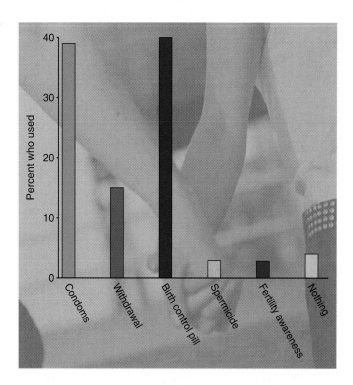

FIGURE 7.5 Type of Contraception Sexually Active College Students Have Used in the Past 30 Days

Source: American College Health Association (ACHA), "ACHA-National College Health Assessment," April 2006. Available at www.acha.org.

Oral contraceptives can also interact negatively with other drugs. For example, some antibiotics diminish the pill's effectiveness and may require an adjustment in dosage. Someone taking tetracycline, for example, should use a backup contraceptive for the entire duration of treatment or 14 days, whichever is shorter, plus 7 days.[3] Women in doubt should check with their practitioners or pharmacists.

Return of fertility may be delayed after discontinuing the pill, but the pill is not known to cause infertility. Women who had irregular menstrual cycles before going on the pill are more likely to have problems conceiving, regardless of pill use.

The pill is convenient and does not interfere with lovemaking, which can lead to enhanced sexual enjoyment. It may lessen menstrual difficulties, such as cramps and premenstrual syndrome (PMS). Oral contraceptives also lower the risk of several health conditions, including endometrial and ovarian cancers, fibrocystic breast disease, ectopic pregnancies, ovarian cysts, pelvic inflammatory disease, and iron-deficiency anemia.[4] Possible serious health problems

oral contraceptives Pills taken daily for three weeks of the menstrual cycle that prevent ovulation by regulating hormones.

Seasonale An extended-cycle oral contraceptive that causes a woman to menstruate only every three months.

A	Abdominal pain (severe)
C	Chest pain (severe, with cough, shortness of breath, or sharp pain on breathing in)
H	Headache (severe), dizziness, weakness, numbness, especially if it occurs on one side only
E	Eye problems (vision loss or blurring), speech problems
S	Severe leg pain (calf or thigh)

FIGURE 7.6 Early Warning Signs of Medical Complications for Pill Users

Source: R. A. Hatcher et al., *Contraceptive Technology*, 18th ed. (New York: Ardent Media, 2004).

associated with the pill include blood clots, which can lead to strokes or heart attacks, and an increased risk of high blood pressure. The risk is low for most healthy women under 35 who do not smoke; it increases with age and especially with cigarette smoking. (See Figure 7.6 for early warning signs of complications associated with oral contraceptives.)

Apart from these risk factors and certain side effects associated with the pill, its greatest disadvantage is that it must be taken every day. If a woman misses one pill, she should use an alternative form of contraception for the remainder of that cycle. Another drawback is that the pill does not protect against STIs. Some teenagers report that the requirement to have a complete gynecological examination in order to get a prescription for the pill is a huge obstacle. Educating young women about what goes on in a gynecological exam would certainly help ease their anxiety. Finally, cost may be a problem for some women.

Progestin-Only Pills Progestin-only pills (or mini-pills) contain small doses of progesterone. Women who feel uncertain about using estrogen pills, who suffer from side effects related to estrogen, or who are nursing may choose these medications rather than combination pills. There is still some question about how progestin-only pills work. Current thought is that they change the composition of the

Ortho Evra A patch that releases hormones similar to those in oral contraceptives; each patch is worn for one week.

NuvaRing A soft, flexible ring inserted into the vagina that releases hormones, preventing pregnancy.

Depo-Provera An injectable method of birth control that lasts for three months.

cervical mucus, thus impeding sperm travel. They may also inhibit ovulation in some women. The effectiveness rate of progestin-only pills is 96 percent, which is slightly lower than that of estrogen-containing pills. Also, their use usually leads to irregular menstrual bleeding. As with all oral contraceptives, the user has no protection against STIs.

Ortho Evra (The Patch) A hormonal contraceptive patch, **Ortho Evra**, became available by prescription in 2002. The patch is worn for one week and replaced on the same day of the week for three consecutive weeks, with the fourth week patch-free. Ortho Evra is 99 percent effective and works by delivering continuous levels of estrogen and progestin through the skin and into the bloodstream. It can be worn on one of four areas of the body: buttocks, abdomen, upper torso (front or back, excluding the breasts), or upper outer arm. The patch does not protect against HIV or other STIs.

In November 2005, amidst evidence that the patch may increase a woman's risk for life-threatening blood clots, the FDA mandated an additional warning label explaining that women who use the patch are exposed to about 60 percent more total estrogen than if they were taking a typical birth control pill. While studies on this health concern continue, the FDA will monitor the safety of Ortho Evra, and women should discuss these risks with their health care provider when determining if the patch is right for them.[5]

NuvaRing Introduced in 2002, this effective contraceptive offers protection for 4 weeks at a time when used as prescribed. **NuvaRing** is a soft, flexible, transparent ring about two inches in diameter. The user inserts it into her vagina, leaves it in place for three weeks, and removes it for one week for her menstrual period. Once the ring is inserted, it continuously releases a steady flow of estrogen and progestin.

Advantages of NuvaRing include protection against pregnancy for one month; no pill to take daily; no need to be fitted by a clinician; does not require spermicide; and the ability to become pregnant returns quickly when use is stopped. Some of the disadvantages that women might experience include increased vaginal discharge; vaginal irritation or infection; oil-based vaginal medicines to treat yeast infections cannot be used when the ring is in place; and a diaphragm or cervical cap cannot be used as a backup method for contraception.

Depo-Provera **Depo-Provera** is a long-acting synthetic progesterone that is injected intramuscularly every three months. Researchers believe that the drug prevents ovulation. There are fewer health problems associated with Depo-Provera than with estrogen-containing pills. The main disadvantage is irregular bleeding, which can be troublesome at first, but within a year, most women are amenorrheic (have no menstrual periods). Weight gain (an average of five pounds in the first year) is common. Other possible side effects include dizziness, nervousness, and headache. Some women feel Depo-Provera encourages sexual spontaneity because they do not have to remember to take a pill or insert a

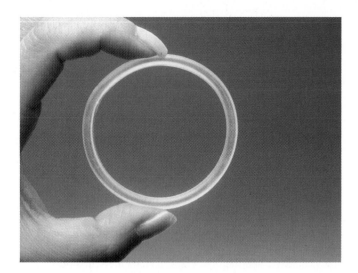

NuvaRing (actual size).

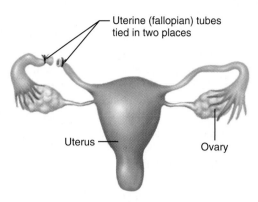

(a) Tubal ligation

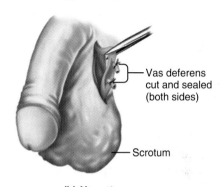

(b) Vasectomy

FIGURE 7.7 Sterilization

(a) In a tubal ligation, the uterine tubes are tied or sealed shut.
(b) In a vasectomy, the surgeon makes an incision in the scrotum, then locates the vas deferens, and either seals or ties both sides shut.

Source: M. Johnson, *Human Biology: Concepts and Current Issues,* 4th ed. (San Francisco: Benjamin Cummings, 2008).

device. However, unlike other methods of contraception, this method cannot be stopped immediately if problems arise. Also, women who wish to become pregnant may find that it takes up to a year after their last injection to succeed.

Norplant and Other Implants Norplant, an early contraceptive implant, was a set of six silicon capsules containing progestin that were surgically inserted under the skin of a woman's upper arm. The progestin worked in the same way as oral contraceptives to suppress ovulation. Norplant was withdrawn from the market due to legal issues. Two new types of implants, one with two rods (Jadelle) and one with a single rod (Implanon), slowly release progestin into the body. They are not on the market in the United States yet, but have been approved for sale.

 what do you THINK?

Who do you think is responsible for deciding which method of contraception should be used in a sexual relationship? ■ What are some examples of good opportunities for you and your partner to have a discussion about contraceptives? ■ What do you think are the biggest barriers in our society to the use of condoms?

Surgical Methods

Sterilization has become the second leading method of contraception for women of all ages in the United States, and the leading method of contraception among married women in the United States.[6] Because sterilization is permanent, those considering it should think through possibilities such as divorce and remarriage or a future improvement in financial status that might make a larger family realistic.

Female Sterilization **Tubal ligation** is one method of sterilization for females (see Figure 7.7a). The operation is usually done in a hospital on an outpatient basis. First, the abdomen is inflated with carbon dioxide gas through a small incision in the navel. The surgeon then inserts a *laparoscope* into another incision just above the pubic bone. This specially designed instrument has a fiber-optic light source that enables the physician to see the uterine tubes clearly.

A tubal ligation does not affect ovarian and uterine function. The woman's menstrual cycle continues, and released eggs simply disintegrate and are absorbed by the lymphatic system. As soon as her incision heals, the woman may resume sexual intercourse with no fear of pregnancy.

sterilization Permanent fertility control achieved through surgical procedures.

tubal ligation Sterilization of the female that involves the cutting and tying off or cauterizing of the uterine tubes.

As with any surgery, there are risks. Although rare, the possible complications of a tubal ligation include infection, pulmonary embolism, hemorrhage, anesthesia complication, and ectopic pregnancy. The procedure itself usually takes less than an hour, and the patient is generally allowed to return home within a short time. Women considering a tubal ligation should thoroughly discuss all the risks with their physician before the operation.

A new sterilization procedure, **Essure**, involves the placement of small microcoils into the fallopian tubes via the vagina by a physician. Once in place, the microcoils expand to the shape of the fallopian tubes. The coils promote the growth of scar tissue around the device and lead to the fallopian tubes becoming blocked. Like traditional forms of tubal ligation, Essure is permanent.

A potential advantage of the procedure is that it does not require an incision. The entire procedure takes only 35 minutes and can be performed in the doctor's office. It is recommended for women who definitely do not want more children and especially for those who cannot have a tubal ligation due to chronic health conditions such as obesity or heart disease. Essure is a relatively new technique, and as a result the long-term risks are unknown.

A **hysterectomy**, or removal of the uterus, is a method of sterilization requiring major surgery. It is usually done only when the patient's uterus is diseased or damaged.

Male Sterilization
Sterilization in men is less complicated than in women. The procedure, called a **vasectomy**, is frequently done on an outpatient basis, using a local anesthetic (see Figure 7.7b).

In a small percentage of cases, complications occur: formation of a blood clot in the scrotum (which usually disappears without medical treatment), infection, or inflammatory reactions. Because sperm are stored in other areas of the reproductive system besides the ductus deferentia, couples must use alternative methods of birth control for at least one month after the vasectomy. The man must check with his physician (who will do a semen analysis) to determine when unprotected intercourse can take place. The pregnancy rate in women whose partners have had vasectomies, after one year, is 0.15 percent.[7]

Essure   A new, nonsurgical sterilization procedure in which a physician places small microcoils into the uterine tubes in order to block them.

hysterectomy   Removal of the uterus.

vasectomy   Sterilization of the male that involves the cutting and tying off of both ductus deferentia.

intrauterine device (IUD)   A T-shaped device that is implanted in the uterus to prevent pregnancy.

Many men are reluctant to consider sterilization because they fear the operation will affect their sexual performance. However, a vasectomy in no way affects sexual response. Because sperm constitute only a small percentage of the semen, the amount of ejaculate is not changed significantly. The testes continue to produce sperm, but the sperm can no longer enter the ejaculatory duct. After a time, sperm production may diminish. Any sperm that are manufactured disintegrate and are absorbed into the lymphatic system.

Although a vasectomy should be considered permanent, surgical reversal can sometimes restore fertility successfully. Recent improvements in microsurgery techniques have resulted in annual pregnancy rates of 40 to 60 percent for women whose partners have had reversals. The two major factors influencing the success rate of reversal are the doctor's expertise and the time elapsed since the vasectomy.

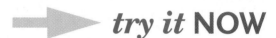 *try it* NOW

Be prepared. Any method of contraception can fail. Take active steps to protect yourself from unplanned pregnancy and STIs at all times. Whether you are on the pill or rely on condoms, always have a backup plan in mind and supplies available in case the condom tears or you forget to take a pill. An extra pack of condoms and spermicidal jelly, foam, or film are good items to have on hand.

Other Methods of Contraception

Intrauterine Devices   Women have been using **intrauterine devices (IUDs)** since 1909, but we still are not certain how they work. Although it was once thought that IUDs act by preventing implantation of a fertilized egg, most experts now believe that they interfere with the sperm's fertilization of the egg.

Two IUDs are currently available. *ParaGard* (copper-T) is a T-shaped plastic device with copper wrapped around the shaft. It does not contain any hormones and can be left in place for ten years before replacement. A newer IUD, *Mirena*, is effective for five years and releases small amounts of the progestin levonorgestrel.

A physician must fit and insert an IUD. The practitioner measures the depth of the uterus with a special instrument and then uses these measurements to place the IUD accurately. One or two strings extend from the IUD into the vagina so the user can check to make sure that her IUD is in place. The device is removed by a practitioner when desired.

Disadvantages of IUDs include discomfort, cost of insertion, and potential complications. The device can cause heavy menstrual flow and severe cramps. Women using IUDs have a higher risk of uterine perforation, ectopic pregnancy, pelvic

TABLE 7.2	Costs of Contraception
Method	**Cost**
Continuous abstinence	None
Outercourse (sex play without vaginal intercourse)	None
Withdrawal	None
Sterilization	
Tubal ligation: permanently blocks female's uterine tubes where sperm join egg	$1,500–$6,000
Vasectomy: permanently blocks male's ductus deferentia that carry sperm	$240–$1,000
Depo-Provera	$20–$40/visits to clinician; $50/injection
IUD (intrauterine device)	$175–$400/exam, insertion, and follow-up visit
Oral contraceptives	$15–$35/monthly pill pack at drugstores, often less at clinics; $35–$125/exam
NuvaRing	$30–$35/ring; $35–$125/exam
Ortho Evra (patch)	$30–$35/monthly supply of patches; $35–$125/exam
Condoms/female condoms and spermicide	50¢ and up/condom—some family planning centers give them away or charge very little; $2.50/female condom; $8–$17/applicator kit of spermicide foam and jelly ($4–$8 refills); similar prices for creams, films, and suppositories
Diaphragm or cervical cap	$15–$75/diaphragm or cap; $50–$125/examination; $4–$8/supplies of spermicide jelly or cream
Fertility awareness methods	$10–$12 for temperature kits; free classes often available in health centers and church

Note: Some family planning clinics charge for services and supplies on a sliding scale according to income.

Source: Reprinted with permission from Planned Parenthood® Federation of America, Inc. © 2006 PPFA. All rights reserved.

inflammatory disease, infertility, and tubal infections. If a pregnancy occurs while the IUD is in place, the chance of miscarriage is 25 to 50 percent; the device should be removed as soon as possible. Doctors often offer therapeutic abortion to women who become pregnant while using an IUD because of the serious risks (including premature delivery, infection, and congenital abnormalities) associated with continuing the pregnancy.

For a comparison of this and other contraceptive option costs, see Table 7.2.

Withdrawal This not very effective method of birth control is most commonly used by people who have not taken the time to consider alternatives. **Withdrawal**, also called coitus interruptus, involves withdrawing the penis from the vagina just prior to ejaculation. Because there can be up to half a million sperm in the drop of fluid at the tip of the penis before ejaculation, this method is unreliable. Timing withdrawal is also difficult, and males concentrating on accurate timing may not be able to relax and enjoy intercourse. In the 2005 American College Health Association-National College Health Assessment, approximately 15 percent of respondents reported that withdrawal was their method of birth control the last time they had sexual intercourse.[8] This statistic is

startlingly high, considering the very high risk of pregnancy or contracting an STI associated with this method of birth control.

Emergency Contraceptive Pills

There are 6.4 million pregnancies every year in the United States. Half of these pregnancies are unintended, and *emergency contraceptive pills (ECPs)* have the potential to reduce this number by at least half. More specifically, researchers estimate that widespread use of ECPs could prevent 1.7 million unintended pregnancies and 800,000 abortions each year in the United States.[9] In a nationwide survey of colleges and universities, 62 percent of all college health centers provide emergency contraception (EC) or prescriptions for EC. On campuses that provide EC, 22 percent are open for at least part of the weekend. Public colleges and

withdrawal A method of contraception that involves withdrawing the penis from the vagina before ejaculation. Also called *coitus interruptus.*

SPOTLIGHT on your health

EMERGENCY CONTRACEPTIVE PILLS: FACTS AND CONTROVERSY

The Centers for Disease Control and Prevention estimate that 86 percent of college students nationwide have had sexual intercourse and that nearly one-third of college women attending four-year institutions have experienced a pregnancy. The 18 to 24-year-old age group has the highest rate of unwanted pregnancies.*

Emergency contraception first became available in 1998; today it is at the center of a hotly contested battle over where it should be available, who should be able to get it, and if it is the same as abortion. Utilization of emergency contraceptive pills (ECPs) can be an effective method of dealing with unwanted pregnancy on college campuses. In fact, the Alan Guttmacher Institute estimates that ECP use prevented 51,000 abortions in 2000 alone. Though no substitute for taking proper precautions before having sex (such as using latex condoms with a spermicide), ECPs' potential for reducing the rate of unintended pregnancy and ultimately abortion is very strong.

However, access to and knowledge of emergency contraception are limited. Emergency contraception is available at only 67 percent of college or university student health centers nationwide. Advocates would like to see this number increase, and the new FDA ruling that makes ECPs available without prescription should improve access substantially. Opponents fear that easy access to emergency contraception will encourage irresponsible sexual activity among young people. Research indicates otherwise: a recent study of women aged 15 to 20 revealed that providing increased access to ECPs does not increase the likelihood of unprotected sex. Nevertheless, the FDA ruling does contain a caveat requiring those under 18 to obtain a prescription. Some opposition also identifies ECP use with abortion, arguing that preventing implantation of an egg into a woman's uterus or fertilization of an egg is equivalent to aborting a growing fetus. Proponents of ECPs do not consider the prevention of implantation or fertilization equivalent to abortion. One thing is clear: the proliferation of emergency

contraceptive pills has opened up a new debate across America about when pregnancy begins.

Emergency contraceptive effectiveness depends on availability. Highest rates of success occur if the pill is taken within 24 to 72 hours after unprotected intercourse. The new FDA ruling that makes Plan B, one brand of ECP, available without prescription to women aged 18 and older should improve success rates.

Source: R. G. Sawyer and E. Thompson, "Knowledge and Attitudes about Emergency Contraception in University Students," *College Student Journal* 4 (December 2003); Alan Guttmacher Institute, "Emergency Contraception Has Tremendous Potential in the Fight to Reduce Unintended Pregnancy," May 2005; L. Miller and R. Sawyer, "Emergency Contraceptive Pills: A 10-Year Follow-Up Survey of Use and Experiences at College Health Centers in the Mid-Atlantic United States," *American Journal of College Health,* (March/April 2006): 249–259. *L. Finer et al., "Disparities in Rates of Unintended Pregnancy in the United States, 1994 and 2001," *Perspectives on Sexual and Reproductive Health* 38, no. 2 (2006).

universities are much more likely to provide EC; only slightly more than half of private college health centers offer EC. A recent study revealed that approximately 11 percent of sexually active college students reported that they or their partner used emergency contraception in the last school year.[10]

Emergency contraception can be used when the chosen method of birth control fails, after a sexual assault, or any time unprotected sexual intercourse occurs. **Emergency contraceptive pills (ECPs)** stop pregnancy in the same way as

Is emergency contraception the same as abortion?

other hormonal contraceptives do: they delay or inhibit ovulation, inhibit fertilization, or block implantation of a fertilized egg, depending on the phase of the woman's menstrual cycle. Although ECPs use the same hormones as birth control pills, not all brands of birth control pills can be used for emergency contraception. When taken within 24 hours EC is up to 95 percent effective; when taken 2 to 5 days later, EC lowers a woman's risk of becoming pregnant by 75 to 88 percent.

Emergency contraceptive pills are now available without a prescription in the United States for women aged 18 and older. For women under 18, a prescription is required. For more on the controversy surrounding ECPs, see the Spotlight on Your Health box.

emergency contraceptive pills (ECPs) Drugs taken within three days after intercourse to prevent fertilization or implantation.

Preven After a woman determines she is not already pregnant, by using the pregnancy test included in the *Preven Emergency Contraception Kit,* the first dose of two light blue emergency pills is taken as soon as possible, within 72 hours after intercourse. The second dose is taken 12 hours later. The most common side effects are nausea, vomiting, menstrual irregularities, breast tenderness, headache, abdominal pain and cramps, and dizziness.

Plan B *Plan B* is more effective than Preven and causes less nausea and vomiting. If taken within 24 hours after intercourse, Plan B may prevent as many as 95 percent of unexpected pregnancies. Overall, Plan B reduces pregnancy risk by about 89 percent, while Preven reduces this risk by about 74 percent. Both are most effective if taken within the first 12 hours.

Emergency Minipills **Emergency minipills** contain progestin only. Like ECPs, minipills can be used up to 72 hours after unprotected intercourse. Emergency minipills are as effective as ECPs, but nausea and vomiting are far less common. Emergency minipills are an excellent alternative for most women who cannot use ECPs that contain estrogen.

Abstinence and "Outercourse"

Strictly defined, abstinence means deliberately avoiding intercourse. This definition would allow one to engage in such forms of sexual intimacy as massage, kissing, and solitary masturbation. However, many people today have broadened the definition of abstinence to include all forms of sexual contact, even those that do not culminate in sexual intercourse.

Couples who go a step further than massage and kissing and engage in activities such as oral–genital sex and mutual masturbation are sometimes said to be engaging in "outercourse." Like abstinence, outercourse can be 100 percent effective for birth control as long as the male does not ejaculate near the vaginal opening. Unlike abstinence, however, outercourse is not 100 percent effective against sexually transmitted infections (STIs). Oral–genital contact can transmit disease, although the practice can be made safer by using a condom on the penis or a dental dam on the vaginal opening.

Fertility Awareness Methods

Methods of fertility control that rely upon the alteration of sexual behavior are called **fertility awareness methods (FAMs)**. These techniques require observing female fertile periods and abstaining from sexual intercourse (penis—vagina contact) during these fertile times.

Two decades ago, the rhythm method was ridiculed because of its low effectiveness rates. However, it was the only method of birth control available to women belonging to religious denominations that forbid the use of oral contraceptives, barrier methods, and sterilization. Our present reproductive knowledge enables women and their partners to use natural methods of birth control with less risk of pregnancy, although these methods remain far less effective than others.

Fertility awareness methods rely upon a knowledge of basic physiology (Figure 7.8, page 212). A released ovum can survive for up to 48 hours after ovulation. Sperm can live for as long as five days in the vagina. Natural methods of birth control teach women to recognize their fertile times. Changes in cervical mucus prior to and during ovulation and a rise in basal body temperature are two frequently used indicators. Another method involves charting a woman's menstrual cycle and ovulation times on a calendar. Women may use any combination of these methods to determine their fertile times more accurately (Figure 7.9, page 213).

Cervical Mucus Method The **cervical mucus method** requires women to examine the consistency and color of their normal vaginal secretions. Prior to ovulation, vaginal mucus becomes gelatinous and stretchy, and normal vaginal secretions may increase. Sexual activity involving penis—vagina contact must be avoided while this mucus is present and for several days afterward.

Body Temperature Method The **body temperature method** relies on the fact that the female's basal body temperature rises between 0.4 and 0.8 degrees after ovulation has occurred. For this method to be effective, the woman must chart her temperature for several months to learn to recognize her body's temperature fluctuations. Abstinence from penis–vagina contact must be observed preceding the temperature rise until several days after the temperature rise was first noted.

---

emergency minipills Contraceptive pills containing only progestin that can be taken up to three days after unprotected intercourse.

fertility awareness methods (FAMs) Several types of birth control that require alteration of sexual behavior rather than chemical or physical intervention in the reproductive process.

cervical mucus method A birth control method that relies upon observation of changes in cervical mucus to determine when the woman is fertile so the couple can abstain from intercourse during those times.

body temperature method A birth control method in which a woman monitors her body temperature for the rise that signals ovulation in order to abstain from intercourse around this time.

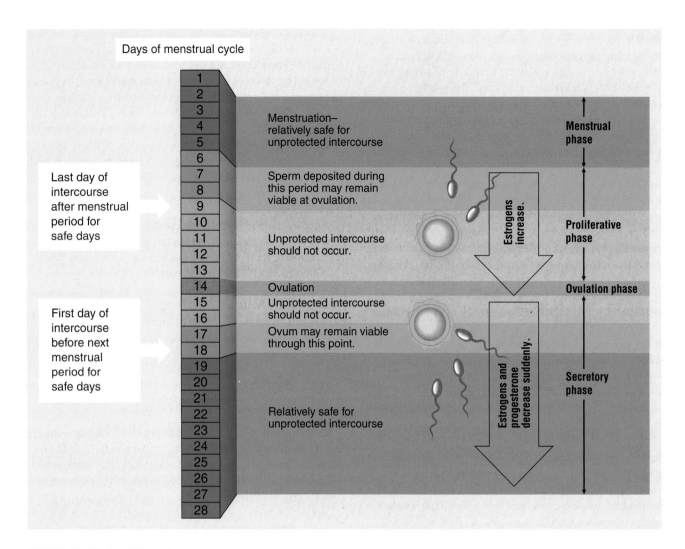

Days of menstrual cycle

1	
2	
3	Menstruation–relatively safe for unprotected intercourse — Menstrual phase
4	
5	
6	
7	Sperm deposited during this period may remain viable at ovulation. — Proliferative phase
8	
9	
10	
11	Unprotected intercourse should not occur. Estrogens increase.
12	
13	
14	Ovulation — Ovulation phase
15	Unprotected intercourse should not occur.
16	
17	Ovum may remain viable through this point. Estrogens and progesterone decrease suddenly. — Secretory phase
18	
19	
20	
21	
22	Relatively safe for unprotected intercourse
23	
24	
25	
26	
27	
28	

Last day of intercourse after menstrual period for safe days →

First day of intercourse before next menstrual period for safe days →

FIGURE 7.8 The Fertility Cycle
Fertility awareness methods (FAMs) can combine the use of a calendar, the cervical mucus method, and body temperature measurements to identify the fertile period. It is important to remember that most women do not have a consistent 28-day cycle.

The Calendar Method   The **calendar method** requires the woman to record the exact number of days in her menstrual cycle. Because few women menstruate with complete regularity, this involves keeping a record of the menstrual cycle for 12 months, during which time some other method of birth control must be used. This method assumes that ovulation occurs during the midpoint of the cycle. The couple must abstain from penis–vagina contact during the fertile time.

Women who wish to use fertility awareness methods of birth control are advised to take classes in their use. Women who are untrained in these techniques run a high risk of unwanted pregnancy.

Abortion

In 1973, the landmark U.S. Supreme Court decision in *Roe v. Wade* stated that the "right to privacy . . . founded on the Fourteenth Amendment's concept of personal liberty . . . is

calendar method   A birth control method in which a woman's menstrual cycle is mapped on a calendar to determine presumed fertile times in order to abstain from penis–vagina contact during those times.

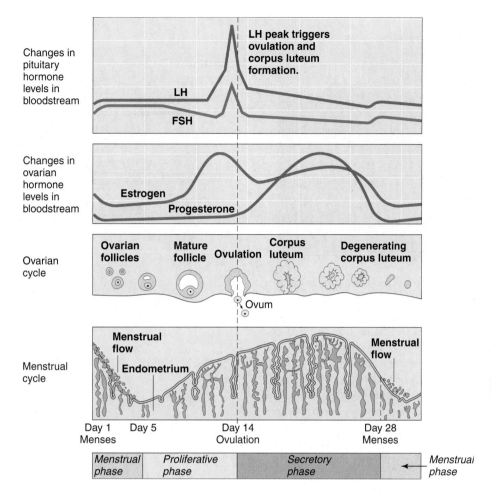

FIGURE 7.9 Changes during the Menstrual Cycle

broad enough to encompass a woman's decision whether or not to terminate her pregnancy."[11] The decision maintained that during the first trimester of pregnancy, a woman and her practitioner have the right to terminate the pregnancy through **abortion** without legal restrictions. It allowed individual states to set conditions for second-trimester abortions. Third-trimester abortions were ruled illegal unless the mother's life or health was in danger.

Prior to the legalization of first- and second-trimester abortions, women wishing to terminate a pregnancy had to travel to a country where the procedure was legal, consult an illegal abortionist, or perform their own abortions. Approximately 480,000 illegal abortions were performed in the United States each year, one-third of them on married women. These procedures sometimes led to death from hemorrhage or infection, or infertility from internal scarring.

Today, nearly half of all pregnancies that occur each year are unplanned, and 50 percent of these pregnancies are terminated by abortion. Although the U.S. abortion rate has declined in recent years, it is still higher than that of many other industrialized nations. Several factors may influence this difference. Many other nations have fewer unwanted pregnancies; early sex education is strongly emphasized, and contraception is easier and cheaper to obtain.[12]

Opponents of abortion believe that the embryo or fetus is a human being with rights that must be protected. The political debate continues as opponents of abortion pressure state and local governments to pass laws prohibiting the use of public funds for abortion and abortion counseling. In recent years, new legislation has given states the right to impose certain restrictions on abortions. Abortions cannot be performed in publicly funded clinics in some states, and other states have laws requiring parental notification before a teenager can obtain an abortion. In 2005 alone, states enacted 98 new sexual and reproductive health laws, over half of which were aimed at restricting abortion access. However, 17 states currently do appropriate public funds for women in poverty who seek an abortion.[13]

On the federal level, the U.S. Congress has banned access to abortion for virtually all women who receive health care through the federal government. This affects Medicaid recipients, women in the military, military dependents stationed overseas, women in federal prison, American Indians, federal

abortion   The medical means of terminating a pregnancy.

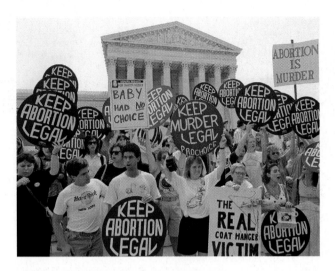

Abortion continues to be a controversial and emotional issue in the United States.

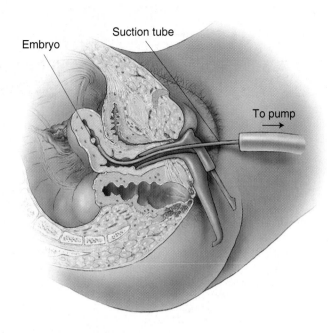

FIGURE 7.10 **Vacuum Aspiration Abortion**

employees, and even Peace Corps volunteers. In early 2006, the Supreme Court agreed to consider the constitutionality of the Federal Abortion Ban. The court struck down an identical law as unconstitutional in 2000, and every court to hear a challenge to this first-ever federal ban on abortion upheld the unconstitutional ruling. The two main reasons are that their broad language could ban abortion as early as the twelfth week in pregnancy, and they lack exceptions to protect women's health.[14] *Roe v. Wade* has not been overturned, but it faces many future challenges.

Although many opponents work through the courts and the political process, attacks on abortion clinics and on doctors who perform abortions are not uncommon. Nearly all clinics have faced some form of threats or acts of violence. Legal protection, such as the Freedom of Access to Clinic Entrance Act (FACE), offers some relief from the harassment and violence directed at abortion clinics. However, because of such acts, the biggest threat to a woman's access to an abortion now is finding a clinic, rather than legal restrictions.

The best birth control methods can fail. Women may be raped. Pregnancies can occur despite every possible precaution. When an unwanted pregnancy does occur, a woman must decide whether to terminate it, carry it to term and keep the baby, or carry it to term and give the baby away. This is a personal decision that each woman must make, based on her personal beliefs, values, and resources, after carefully considering all alternatives. For a discussion on how contraception and abortion are perceived in different countries, see the Health in a Diverse World box.

Methods of Abortion

The choice of abortion procedure is determined by how many weeks the woman has been pregnant. Length of pregnancy is calculated from the first day of her last menstrual period.

Surgical Abortions If performed during the first trimester of pregnancy, abortion presents a relatively low health risk to the mother. The most commonly used method of first-trimester abortion is **vacuum aspiration** (Figure 7.10). The procedure is usually performed under a local anesthetic. The cervix is dilated with instruments or by placing *laminaria,* a sterile seaweed product, in the cervical canal. The laminaria is left in place for a few hours or overnight and slowly dilates the cervix. After it is removed, a long tube is inserted into the uterus through the cervix, and gentle suction removes fetal tissue from the uterine walls.

Pregnancies that progress into the second trimester can be terminated through **dilation and evacuation (D&E)**, a procedure that combines vacuum aspiration with a technique called **dilation and curettage (D&C)**. For this procedure, the cervix is dilated with laminaria for one to two days, and a combination of instruments and vacuum aspiration is used to empty the uterus. Second-trimester abortions may be done under general anesthetic. Both procedures can be performed on an outpatient basis (usually in the physician's office), with

vacuum aspiration   The use of gentle suction to remove fetal tissue from the uterus.

dilation and evacuation (D&E)   An abortion technique that combines vacuum aspiration with dilation and curettage; fetal tissue is both sucked and scraped out of the uterus.

dilation and curettage (D&C)   An abortion technique in which the cervix is dilated and the uterine walls scraped clean.

CONTRACEPTIVE USE HELPS REDUCE THE INCIDENCE OF ABORTION WORLDWIDE

Nearly 80 million pregnancies occur worldwide every year. More than half of these pregnancies end in abortion, often in countries where abortion is illegal and access to contraception is limited. Access to voluntary family planning services, including contraception, is essential in helping to reduce the number of unintended pregnancies and, consequently, the incidence of abortion.

- The primary cause of abortion is unplanned pregnancy. When modern contraceptives are unavailable, women often turn to abortion to end unwanted pregnancy.
- Whether abortion is legal or not has little to do with its overall incidence. In many countries where abortion is illegal or severely restricted (e.g., many Latin American and African countries), abortion rates are higher than in countries where it is legal (e.g., countries in Western Europe).
- Increased use of contraception has been accompanied by significant declines in abortion rates in a number of countries, including Bangladesh, Bulgaria, Chile, Estonia, Hungary, Latvia, Romania, Russia, and Turkey.
- Modern contraceptive use increased in Russia by 74 percent, while abortion rates decreased by 61 percent, between 1988 and 2001.
- Abortion rates declined in the 1990s in tandem with a rise in the use of modern contraception in the republics of Kazakhstan, Uzbekistan, and Kyrgyzstan. In Kazakhstan, contraception prevalence increased by 50 percent in the 1990s and abortion rates decreased by nearly the same amount.

Sources: Adapted from the *Population Action International Fact Sheet,* August 2005; Alan Guttmacher Institute, "Issues in Brief: The Role of Contraception in Reducing Abortion," 2005, available from www.agi-usa.org/pubs/ib19.html; C. Marston and J. Cleland, *The Effects of Contraception on Obstetric Outcomes* (Geneva: World Health Organization, 2004); M. Reynolds, "Abortion Rate Drops to Lowest Level Ever," *The Prague Post,* July 27, 2005, available from www.praguepost.com/P03/2005/Art/0728/news4.php.

---

or without pain medication. Generally, however, the woman is given a mild tranquilizer to help her relax. Both procedures may cause moderate to severe uterine cramping and blood loss.

Two other methods used in second-trimester abortions, though less common than D&E, are prostaglandin or saline **induction abortions**. Prostaglandin hormones or saline solution are injected into the uterus, which kills the fetus and initiates labor contractions. After 24 to 48 hours, the fetus and placenta are expelled from the uterus.

The **hysterotomy**, or surgical removal of the fetus from the uterus, may be used during emergencies, when the mother's life is in danger, or when other types of abortions are deemed too dangerous.

The risks associated with abortion include infection, incomplete abortion (when parts of the placenta remain in the uterus), missed abortion (when the fetus is not actually removed), excessive bleeding, and cervical and uterine trauma. Follow-up and attention to danger signs decrease the chances of long-term problems.

The mortality rate for first-trimester abortions averages one death per every 500,000 procedures at 8 or fewer weeks. The risk of death increases with the length of pregnancy. At 16 to 20 weeks, the mortality rate is 1 per 27,000, and at 21 weeks or more it increases to 1 per 8,000.[15] This higher rate later in the pregnancy is due to the increased risk of uterine perforation, bleeding, infection, and incomplete abortion due to the fact that the uterine wall becomes thinner as the pregnancy progresses.

One surgical method of performing abortion that has been the target of abortion opponents is **intact dilation and extraction (D&X)**, sometimes referred to by the nonmedical term *partial-birth abortion.* This procedure is rarely performed, but is considered when other abortion methods could injure the mother and when there are severe fetal abnormalites. The dilation and extraction procedure is used after 21 weeks of gestation. Two days before the procedure, laminaria is inserted vaginally to dilate the cervix. The water should break on the third day and the woman should return to the clinic. The fetus is rotated to a breech (feet-first) position, and forceps are used

---

induction abortion   A type of abortion in which chemicals are injected into the uterus through the uterine wall; labor begins, and the woman delivers a dead fetus.

hysterotomy   The surgical removal of the fetus from the uterus.

intact dilation and extraction (D&X)   A late-term abortion procedure in which the body of the fetus is extracted up to the head and then the contents of the cranium are aspirated.

to pull the legs, shoulders, and arms through the birth canal. The head is collapsed to allow it to pass through the cervix. Then the fetus is completely removed.

Medical Abortions Unlike surgical abortions, medical abortions are performed without entering the uterus. **Mifepristone**, formerly known as RU-486, is a steroid hormone that induces abortion by blocking the action of progesterone, a hormone produced by the ovaries and placenta that maintains the lining of the uterus. Similar in structure to progesterone, mifepristone binds to cell receptor sites normally occupied by progesterone, causing the uterine lining to break down. As a result, the uterine lining and the embryo are expelled from the uterus, terminating the pregnancy.

Mifepristone's nickname, "the abortion pill," may imply an easy process. However, this treatment actually involves more steps than a surgical abortion, which takes approximately 15 minutes followed by a physical recovery of about one day. A first visit to the clinic involves a physical exam and a dose of three mifepristone tablets, which may cause minor side effects such as nausea, headaches, weakness, and fatigue. The patient returns 2 days later for a dose of prostaglandins (trade name: misoprostol), which cause uterine contractions that expel the fertilized egg. The patient is required to stay under observation at the clinic for 4 hours, and make a follow-up visit 12 days later.[16]

Ninety-six percent of women who take mifepristone and prostaglandins during the first 9 weeks of pregnancy will experience a complete abortion. The side effects of this treatment are similar to those reported during heavy menstruation and include cramping, minor pain, and nausea. Approximately 1 in 1,000 women requires a blood transfusion because of severe bleeding. The procedure does not require hospitalization; women may be treated on an outpatient basis.

Another drug that has been used to induce early-term medical abortions is methotrexate, although it is not approved by the FDA for this purpose. Typically, a woman receives an injection from her clinician and, during an office visit three to seven days later, receives a prostaglandin dose. The pregnancy usually ends within four hours.

Emotional Aspects of Abortion

The emotional aftereffects of abortion have been the subject of much interest. Do women who have had abortions suffer symptoms similar to those of post-traumatic stress disorder? Are they forever haunted by the experience?

Although a variety of feelings, such as regret, guilt, sadness, relief, and happiness, are normal, no evidence has shown that an abortion causes long-term psychological trauma for a woman. In a longitudinal study of over 5,000 women who had had abortions, researchers found that the best predictor of a woman's emotional well-being following an abortion was her emotional well-being prior to the procedure. Even factors such as marital status or affiliation with a religion that is strongly antiabortion were found to have no effect on a woman's later sense of self-esteem and well-being.[17]

A small percentage of women who undergo abortions experience depressive symptoms similar to postpartum blues, but the vast majority express no regrets about their decision and state they would make the choice again if they found themselves in similar circumstances. Certainly the presence of a support network and the assistance of mental health professionals is helpful to any woman who is struggling with the emotional aspects of the abortion decision in her own life.

 what do you THINK?

If you or your partner unexpectedly became pregnant, would you choose to terminate the pregnancy? ■ How might an abortion affect your relationship? ■ What factors would you consider in making your decision? ■ Why do you consider these factors important?

Planning a Pregnancy

The many methods available to control fertility give you choices that did not exist when your parents—and even you—were born. If you are in the process of deciding whether to have children, take the time to evaluate your emotions, finances, and health.

Emotional Health

First and foremost, consider why you want to have a child: To fulfill an inner need to carry on the family? Are there any other reasons? Can you care for this new human being in a loving and nurturing manner? Are you ready to make all the sacrifices necessary to bear and raise a child? If you feel, based on your self-evaluation, that you are ready to be a parent, you can prepare for this change in your life by reading about parenthood, taking classes, talking to parents of children of all ages, and joining a support group. If you choose to adopt, you will find many support groups available to you as well.

mifepristone A steroid hormone that induces abortion by blocking the action of progesterone.

Maternal Health

Before becoming pregnant, a woman should have a thorough medical examination. **Preconception care** should include assessment of potential complications. Medical problems such as diabetes and high blood pressure should be discussed, as should any genetic disorders that run in the family. Additional suggestions for a healthy pregnancy include:

- If you smoke or drink alcohol, stop; reduce or eliminate caffeine intake.
- Avoid X rays and environmental chemicals, such as lawn and garden chemicals.
- Maintain a normal weight; lose weight if necessary.
- Take prenatal vitamins, which are especially important in providing adequate folic acid.

Paternal Health

It is common wisdom that pregnant women should steer clear of toxic chemicals that can cause birth defects. Even women who are trying to conceive are cautioned to avoid toxic environments, eat a nourishing diet, stop smoking and drinking alcohol, and avoid most medications. Now similar precautions are recommended for fathers-to-be. New research suggests that a man's exposure to chemicals influences not only his ability to father a child, but also the future health of his child.

Fathers-to-be have been overlooked in past preconception and prenatal studies for several reasons. Researchers assumed that the genetic damage leading to birth defects and other health problems occurred while a child was in the mother's uterus. After all, they reasoned, that's where embryonic and fetal development take place. Conventional medical wisdom also held that defective-looking sperm (those with misshapen heads, crooked tails, or retarded swimming ability) were incapable of fertilizing an egg. However, scientists have recently discovered that how sperm look has little to do with how they act. Misshapen sperm can penetrate an egg, and they do not necessarily carry defective genetic goods. Moreover, sperm that look healthy and swim well can be the true genetic culprits. DNA fluorescent markers have identified normal-looking, yet genetically flawed, sperm that carry too many or too few chromosomes. Fathers contribute the extra chromosome 21 in about 6 percent of children with Down's syndrome, which causes mental retardation; the extra X chromosome in 50 percent of boys with Klinefelter's syndrome, which causes abnormal sexual development; and the shortened chromosome 15 in about 85 percent of children with Prader-Willi syndrome, a disorder characterized by retardation and obesity.

Although some birth defects are caused by random errors of nature, it now appears that some disorders can be traced to sperm damaged by chemicals. Sperm are naturally vulnerable to toxic assault and genetic damage. Many drugs and ingested chemicals can readily invade the testes from the bloodstream; others ambush sperm after they leave the testes and pass through the epididymides, where they mature and are stored. By one route or another, half of 100 chemicals studied so far (including by-products of cigarette smoke) apparently harm sperm.

Some researchers believe that vitamin C is nature's way of protecting sex cells from damage. Bad diets, exposure to toxic chemicals, cigarette smoking, and not enough foods rich in vitamin C are probably the biggest culprits in sperm damage.[18]

Financial Evaluation

Finances are another important consideration. Are you prepared to go out to dinner with friends less often, forgo a new pair of shoes, or drive an older car? These are important questions to ask yourself when considering the financial aspects of being a parent. Can you afford to give your child the life you would like him or her to enjoy?

First, check your medical insurance: Does it provide pregnancy benefits? If not, you can expect to pay on average $7,000 for a normal delivery, and up $11,450 for a C-section. These costs don't include prenatal medical care, and complications can also impact the average cost substantially. Both partners should investigate their employers' policies concerning parental leave, including length of leave available and conditions for returning to work.

The U.S. Department of Agriculture estimates that it can cost as much as $250,000 for a middle-class married couple to raise a child to the age of 17. (Housing costs and food are the two largest expenditures.)[19] That figure does not include college, which can now run over $40,000 per year with room and board at a private institution. Also consider the cost and availability of quality child care. How much family assistance can you realistically expect with a new baby, and is nonfamily child care available? How much does full-time child care cost? Costs vary by region and type of care. According to statistics gathered in the last U.S. census, families with young children spent 10 percent of their total income on child care in 2002.[20]

Though you may be aware of the federal tax credit available for child care, you may not realize how little assistance it actually provides. For example, a family with an income of over $28,000 can expect to receive a maximum credit of $480 for one child. A second child doubles the credit, but no further assistance is provided for a third child or more children.

preconception care   Medical care received prior to becoming pregnant that helps a woman assess and address potential maternal health.

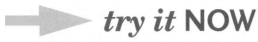

try it NOW

Make a budget! Thinking about starting a family? The financial responsibilities of being a parent go beyond providing basic needs. Make a list of monthly expenses associated with being a parent of a 6-year-old. Consider school supplies and extracurricular activities like piano lessons or Little League. Don't forget basics either, such as food, clothing, and child care. Now look at your monthly income. What types of sacrifices would you have to make to provide the best possible life for a child?

Contingency Planning

A final consideration is how to provide for the child should something happen to you and your partner. If both of you were to die while the child is young, do you have relatives or close friends who would raise the child? If you have more than one child, would they have to be split up or could they be kept together? Though unpleasant to think about, this sort of contingency planning is very important. Children who lose their parents are heartbroken and confused. A prearranged plan of action will smooth their transition into new families.

what do you THINK?

What factors will you consider in deciding whether or when to have children? ■ Is there a certain age at which you feel you will be ready to be a parent? ■ What goals do you hope to achieve before undertaking parenthood? ■ What are your biggest concerns about parenthood?

Pregnancy

Pregnancy is an important event in a woman's life. The actions taken before a pregnancy begins, as well as behaviors during pregnancy, can have a significant effect on the health of both infant and mother.

Prenatal Care

A successful pregnancy depends on the mother taking good care of herself and the fetus. It is essential to have regular medical checkups, beginning as soon as possible (certainly within the first three months). Early detection of fetal abnormalities, identification of high-risk mothers and infants, and a complication-free pregnancy are the major purposes of prenatal care. On the first visit, the practitioner should obtain a complete medical history of the mother and her family and note any hereditary conditions that could put a woman or her fetus at risk.

Regular checkups to measure weight gain and blood pressure and to monitor the size and position of the fetus continue throughout the pregnancy. This early care reduces infant mortality and low birth weight. A study group for the American College of Obstetricians and Gynecologists recommends seven or eight prenatal visits for women who have low-risk pregnancies.

Unfortunately, prenatal care is not available to everyone. Approximately 30 percent of pregnant teenagers and unmarried women do not receive adequate prenatal attention. American Indian and African American women have the lowest rates of prenatal care in the United States.[21] Babies of mothers who received no prenatal care are about ten times more likely to die in the first month of life than babies of mothers who did get prenatal care.

Additional concerns include the mother's physical condition, her level of nutrition, her confidence in her ability to give birth, her use of drugs and medications, and the availability of a skilled practitioner who can oversee the pregnancy and delivery. A woman planning a pregnancy also needs a support system (spouse or partner, family, friends, community groups) willing to provide love and emotional support during and after her pregnancy.

Choosing a Practitioner A woman should carefully choose a practitioner to attend her pregnancy and delivery. If possible, this choice should be made before she becomes pregnant. Recommendations from friends or the family physician are a good starting point.

When choosing a practitioner, parents should ask about credentials, professional qualifications, and experience. Besides this information, a pregnant woman must ask questions specific to her condition. Prospective parents should inquire about the practitioner's experience in handling various complications, commitment to being at the mother's side during delivery, and beliefs and practices concerning the use of anesthesia, fetal monitoring, induced labor, and forceps delivery. What are the practitioner's attitudes toward birth control, abortion, and alternative birthing procedures? The practitioner's approach to nutrition and medication during pregnancy should be similar to the woman's own. Finally, the parents must learn under what circumstances the practitioner would perform a cesarean section.

Two types of physicians can attend pregnancies and deliveries. The *obstetrician-gynecologist (OB-Gyn)* is a medical doctor (MD) who specializes in obstetrics (pregnancy and birth) and gynecology (the care of women's reproductive organs). These practitioners are trained to handle all types of pregnancy- and delivery-related emergencies. A *family practitioner* is a licensed medical doctor who provides comprehensive care for people of all ages. The majority of family practitioners have obstetrical experience but will refer a patient to a specialist if necessary. Unlike the OB-Gyn, the family practitioner can serve as the baby's physician after attending the birth.

Midwives are also experienced practitioners who can attend both pregnancies and deliveries. *Certified nurse-midwives* are registered nurses with specialized training in pregnancy and delivery. Most midwives work in private practice or in conjunction with physicians. Those who work with physicians have access to traditional medical facilities to which they can turn in an emergency. *Lay midwives* may or may not have extensive training in handling an emergency. They may be self-taught or trained through formal certification procedures. Women should carefully evaluate the credentials of a prospective midwife, and be sure access to medical care is available if needed.

Nutrition and Exercise

Pregnant women need additional protein, calories, vitamins, and minerals, so their diets should be carefully monitored by a qualified practitioner. Special attention should be paid to getting enough folic acid (found in dark, leafy greens), iron (dried fruits, meats, legumes, liver, egg yolks), calcium (nonfat or low-fat dairy products, some canned fish), and fluids.

Vitamin supplements can correct some deficiencies, but there is no substitute for a well-balanced diet. Babies born to poorly nourished mothers run high risks of substandard mental and physical development. Folic acid, when consumed before and during early pregnancy, reduces the risk of spina bifida, a common disabling birth condition resulting from failure of the spinal column to close. Manufacturers of breads, pastas, rice, and other grain products are now required to add folic acid to their products to reduce neural tube defects in newborns.

Weight gain during pregnancy helps nourish a growing baby. For a woman of normal weight before pregnancy, the recommended weight gain during pregnancy is 25 to 35 pounds. For obese or overweight women, 15 to 25 pounds is recommended. Underweight women can gain 28 to 40 pounds, and women carrying twins should gain about 35 to 45 pounds. Gaining too much or too little weight can lead to complications. With higher weight gains, women may develop gestational diabetes, hypertension, or increased risk of delivery complications. Gaining too little weight increases the chance of a low–birth weight baby.

Of the total number of pounds gained during pregnancy, about 6 to 8 are the baby. The baby's birth weight is important, because low weight can mean health problems during labor and the baby's first few months. Pregnancy is not the time to think about losing weight—doing so may endanger the fetus.

As in all other stages of life, exercise is an important factor in weight control during pregnancy and overall maternal health. In one study, a balanced 45-minute exercise session three days per week was associated with heavier–birth weight babies, fewer surgical births, and shorter hospital stays after birth. Pregnant women should consult their physicians before starting any exercise program.

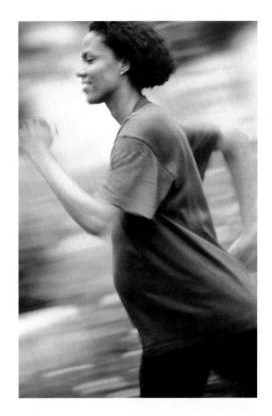

A doctor-approved exercise program during pregnancy can help control weight, make delivery easier, and have a healthy effect on the fetus.

Alcohol and Drugs

A woman should avoid all types of drugs during pregnancy. Even common over-the-counter medications such as aspirin and beverages such as coffee and tea can damage a developing fetus.

During the first three months of pregnancy, the fetus is especially subject to the **teratogenic** (birth defect–causing) effects of some chemical substances. The fetus can also develop an addiction to or tolerance for drugs that the mother takes. Medical professionals are especially concerned about the use of tobacco and alcohol during pregnancy.

Women who are heavy drinkers may have normal first babies but subsequently deliver children having fetal alcohol syndrome. The symptoms of **fetal alcohol syndrome (FAS)**

---

midwives Experienced practitioners who assist with pregnancy and delivery.

teratogenic Causing birth defects; may refer to drugs, environmental chemicals, X rays, or diseases.

fetal alcohol syndrome (FAS) A collection of symptoms, including mental retardation, that can appear in infants of women who drink too much alcohol during pregnancy.

include mental retardation, slowed nerve reflexes, and small head size. The exact amount of alcohol that causes FAS is not known, but researchers doubt that any alcohol is safe. Therefore, they recommend total abstinence from alcohol during pregnancy.

Smoking Tobacco use harms every phase of reproduction. Women who smoke have more difficulty becoming pregnant and have a higher risk of being infertile. Women who smoke during pregnancy have a greater chance of complications, premature births, low–birth weight infants, stillbirth, and infant mortality.[22] Smoking restricts the blood supply to the developing fetus and thus limits oxygen and nutrition delivery and waste removal. It appears to be a significant factor in the development of cleft lip and palate.

Studies are now revealing that secondhand smoke is also detrimental. The exposed fetus is likely to experience low birth weight, increased susceptibility to childhood diseases, and sudden infant death syndrome.[23] Smoking clearly has an influence throughout the pregnancy cycle.

X rays X rays present a clear danger to the fetus. Although most diagnostic tests produce minimal amounts of radiation, even low levels may cause birth defects or other problems, particularly if several low-dose X rays are taken over a short time period. Pregnant women are advised to avoid X rays unless absolutely necessary.

Other Factors A pregnant woman should avoid exposure to toxic chemicals, heavy metals, pesticides, gases, and other hazardous compounds. She should not clean cat-litter boxes because cat feces can contain organisms that cause a disease called **toxoplasmosis**. If a pregnant woman contracts this disease, her baby may be stillborn or suffer mental retardation or other birth defects.

Before becoming pregnant, a woman should be tested to determine if she has had rubella (German measles). If she has not had rubella, she should be immunized for it and wait the recommended length of time before becoming pregnant. A rubella infection can kill the fetus or cause blindness or hearing disorders. Sexually transmitted infections such as genital herpes or HIV are also risk factors. A woman should inform her physician of any infectious condition so proper precautions and treatment can be taken. The physician may want to

---

toxoplasmosis A disease caused by an organism found in cat feces that, when contracted by a pregnant woman, may result in stillbirth or an infant with mental retardation or birth defects.

Down's syndrome A condition characterized by mental retardation and a variety of physical abnormalities.

---

deliver the baby by cesarean section, especially if a woman has active lesions. Contact with an active herpes infection during birth can be fatal to the baby.

what do you THINK?

In looking at your current lifestyle, what behaviors (nutritional choices, fitness, etc.) would you cease or begin in order to promote a healthy pregnancy?
■ What characteristics or skills would you look for in selecting a health care provider during your own or your partner's pregnancy?

A Woman's Reproductive Years

Approximately half of the average American woman's expected life span is spent between menarche (first menses) and menopause (last menses), a period of approximately 40 years. Deciding if and when to have children, as well as how to prevent pregnancy when necessary, is a long-term concern.

Today, a woman over 35 who is pregnant has plenty of company. While births to women in their twenties are declining, the rate of first births to women between the ages of 30 and 39 has doubled in the past decade, and births to women over 39 have increased by more than 50 percent. Many women who wait until their thirties to consider having a child find themselves wondering, "Am I too old to have a baby?" Statistically, the chances of having a baby with birth defects do rise after the age of 35. Researchers believe that there is a decline in both the quality and viability of eggs after this age.

Down's syndrome, a condition characterized by mild to severe mental retardation and a variety of physical abnormalities, is the most common genetic condition. The incidence of Down's syndrome does increase with the mother's age.[24] The incidence for babies born to a mother age 20 is 1 in 10,000 births; it rises to 1 in 400 by age 35, to 1 in 110 by age 40, and to 1 in 35 when she is 45.[25]

Women who delay motherhood until their late thirties also worry about their physical ability to carry and deliver their babies. For these women, a comprehensive exercise program will assist in maintaining good posture and promoting a successful delivery.

Despite these concerns, there are some advantages to having a baby later in life. In fact, many doctors note that older mothers tend to be more conscientious about following medical advice during pregnancy and are more psychologically mature and ready to include an infant in their family than some younger women.

Pregnancy Testing

A woman may suspect she is pregnant before she has any pregnancy tests. A typical sign is a missed menstrual period, yet this is not always an accurate indicator. A woman can

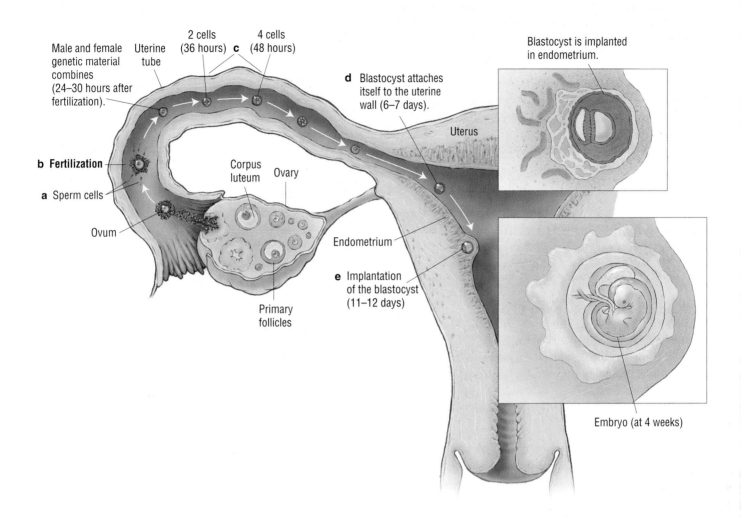

Male and female genetic material combines (24–30 hours after fertilization).

Uterine tube

2 cells (36 hours) **c**

4 cells (48 hours)

d Blastocyst attaches itself to the uterine wall (6–7 days).

Uterus

Blastocyst is implanted in endometrium.

b Fertilization

Corpus luteum

Ovary

a Sperm cells

Ovum

Primary follicles

Endometrium

e Implantation of the blastocyst (11–12 days)

Embryo (at 4 weeks)

FIGURE 7.11 Fertilization

(a) The efforts of hundreds of sperm may allow one sperm to penetrate the ovum's corona radiata, an outer layer of cells, and then the zona pellucida, a thick inner membrane. (b) The sperm nucleus fuses with egg nucleus at fertilization, which produces a zygote. (c) The zygote divides first into two cells, then four cells, and so on. (d) The blastocyst attaches itself to the uterine wall. (e) The blastocyst implants itself in the endometrium.

miss her period for a variety of reasons, including stress, exercise, and emotional upset. A pregnancy test scheduled in a medical office or birth control clinic will confirm the pregnancy. Women who wish to know immediately can purchase home pregnancy test kits, sold over the counter in drugstores. A positive test is based on the secretion of **human chorionic gonadotropin (HCG)**, found in the woman's urine. Home test kits come equipped with a small sample of red blood cells coated with HCG antibodies to which the user adds a small amount of urine (HCG is also detectable in blood). If the concentration of HCG is great enough, it will clump together with the HCG antibodies, indicating that the user is pregnant.

Home pregnancy test kits are about 85 to 95 percent reliable. If done too early in the pregnancy, they may show a false negative. Other causes of false negatives are unclean test tubes, ingestion of certain drugs, and vaginal or urinary

Are home pregnancy testing kits reliable?

tract infections. Accuracy also depends on the quality of the test itself and the user's ability to perform it and interpret the results. Blood tests administered and analyzed by a medical laboratory are more accurate.

The Process of Pregnancy

The process of pregnancy begins the moment a sperm fertilizes an ovum in the uterine tubes (Figure 7.11). From there,

human chorionic gonadotropin (HCG) Hormone detectable in blood or urine samples of a mother within the first few weeks of pregnancy.

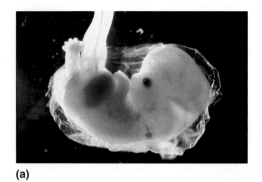

(a)

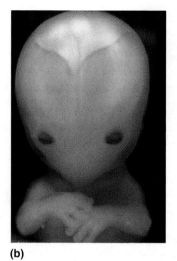

(b)

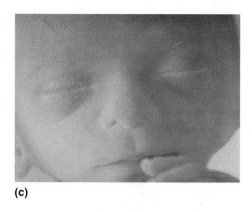

(c)

This series of fetoscopic photographs shows the development of the fetus in the (a) first, (b) second, and (c) third trimesters of pregnancy.

the single cell multiplies, becoming a sphere-shaped cluster of cells as it travels toward the uterus, a journey that may take three to four days. Upon arrival, the embryo burrows into the thick, spongy endometrium and is nourished from this carefully prepared lining.

Early Signs of Pregnancy
The first sign of pregnancy is usually a missed menstrual period (although some women "spot" in early pregnancy, which may be mistaken for a period). Other signs of pregnancy include breast tenderness, emotional upset, extreme fatigue, sleeplessness, and nausea and vomiting (especially in the morning).

Pregnancy typically lasts 40 weeks. The due date is calculated from the expectant mother's last menstrual period. Pregnancy is typically divided into three phases, or **trimesters**, of approximately three months each.

The First Trimester
During the first trimester, few noticeable changes occur in the mother's body. The expectant mother may urinate more frequently and experience morning sickness, swollen breasts, or undue fatigue. These symptoms may not be frequent or severe, so she may not even realize she is pregnant unless she has a pregnancy test.

During the first two months after conception, the **embryo** differentiates and develops its various organ systems, beginning with the nervous and circulatory systems. At the start of the third month, the embryo is called a **fetus**, indicating that all organ systems are in place. For the rest of the pregnancy, growth and refinement occur in each major body system so that it can function independently, yet in coordination with all the others, at birth. The photos above illustrate physical changes during fetal development.

The Second Trimester
At the beginning of the second trimester, physical changes in the mother become more visible. Her breasts swell, and her waistline thickens. During this time, the fetus makes greater demands upon the mother's body. In particular, the **placenta**, the network of blood vessels that carries nutrients and oxygen to the fetus and fetal waste products to the mother, becomes well established.

The Third Trimester
From the end of the sixth month through the ninth is the third trimester. This is the period of greatest fetal growth, when the fetus gains most of its weight. During the third trimester, the fetus must get large amounts of calcium, iron, and nitrogen from the food the mother eats. Approximately 85 percent of the calcium and iron the mother digests goes into the fetal bloodstream.

Although the fetus may live if it is born during the seventh month, it needs the layer of fat it acquires during the eighth month and time for the organs (especially the respiratory and digestive organs) to develop to their full potential. Infants born prematurely usually require intensive medical care.

Emotional Changes
Of course, the process of pregnancy involves much more than the changes in a woman's body. Many important emotional changes occur from the time a woman learns she is pregnant through the **"fourth trimester"** (the first six weeks of an infant's life outside the

trimester A three-month segment of pregnancy; used to describe specific developmental changes that occur in the embryo or fetus.

embryo The fertilized egg from conception until the end of two months' development.

fetus The term for a developing baby from the third month of pregnancy until birth.

placenta The network of blood vessels, connected to the umbilical cord, that carries nutrients to the developing infant and carries wastes away.

fourth trimester The first six weeks of an infant's life outside the uterus.

uterus). Throughout pregnancy women may experience fear of pregnancy complications, anxiety over becoming a parent, and wonder and excitement over the developing baby.

Prenatal Testing and Screening

Throughout pregnancy, women receive routine medical tests as part of prenatal care. Modern technology enables health care providers to detect health defects in a fetus as early as twelve weeks. One common test is *ultrasound,* which uses high-frequency sound waves to create a *sonogram,* or visual image, of the fetus in the uterus. The sonogram is used to determine the size and position of the fetus. Knowing the position of the fetus assists health care providers in performing *amniocentesis* and delivering the infant. Sonograms can also detect birth defects in the central nervous system and digestive system. New three-dimensional ultrasound techniques clarify images and improve doctors' efforts to detect and treat defects prenatally. Ultrasound does not provide any genetic information about the fetus.

The **triple marker screen (TMS)** is a maternal blood test that is used to identify certain birth defects and genetic abnormalities in growing fetuses (e.g., neural tube defects, Down's syndrome). Optimally the test is conducted between the sixteenth and eighteenth weeks of pregnancy. A blood sample is taken and sent to a lab for analysis. The lab analyzes the levels of alpha-fetoprotein (AFP), human chorionic gonadotropin (HCG), and unconjugated estriol (uE_3) in the blood and determines whether they fall in a "normal" range for this stage of the pregnancy, based on age, weight, race, and other factors (such as having diabetes). TMS is a screening test, not a diagnostic test; it can detect susceptibility for a birth defect or genetic abnormality, but is not meant to confirm a diagnosis of any condition. In the case of abnormal TMS results, parents may choose to have further testing such as ultrasound or amniocentesis.

Amniocentesis is a common testing procedure that is strongly recommended for women over 35. This procedure involves inserting a long needle through the mother's abdominal and uterine walls into the **amniotic sac**, the protective pouch surrounding the fetus. The needle draws out 3 to 4 teaspoons of fluid, which is analyzed for genetic information about the baby (Figure 7.12). This test can reveal the presence of 40 genetic abnormalities, including Down's syndrome, Tay-Sachs disease (a fatal disorder of the central nervous system common among Jewish people of Eastern European descent), and sickle cell disease (a debilitating blood disorder found primarily among African Americans). Amniocentesis can also reveal gender, a fact some parents may choose not to know until after birth. Although widely used, amniocentesis is not without risk. The chance of miscarriage as a result of testing is 1 in 200, or less.

A third procedure, *chorionic villus sampling (CVS),* involves snipping tissue from the developing fetal sac. CVS can be used at 10 to 12 weeks of pregnancy, and the test

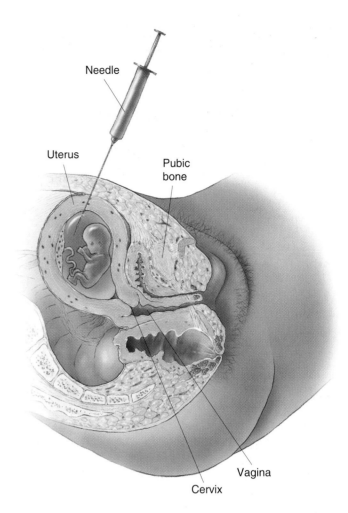

FIGURE 7.12 Amniocentesis

The process of amniocentesis can detect certain congenital problems as well as the sex of the fetus.

results are available in 12 to 48 hours. CVS is an attractive option for couples who are at high risk for having a baby with Down's syndrome or a debilitating hereditary disease.

A fourth procedure, *fetoscopy,* involves making a small incision in the abdominal and uterine walls and inserting an optical viewer into the uterus to view the fetus directly. This device is used with ultrasound to determine fetal age and location of the placenta. This method is still experimental and

---

triple marker screen (TMS)   A maternal blood test that can be used to help identify fetuses with certain birth defects and genetic abnormalities.

amniocentesis   A medical test in which a small amount of fluid is drawn from the amniotic sac to test for Down's syndrome and other genetic diseases.

amniotic sac   The protective pouch surrounding the baby.

HEALTH ETHICS
conflict and controversy

THE SCIENCE OF SEX SELECTION

Parents have wanted the ability to choose the gender of their child since prehistoric times: intense interest in sex selection has been noted in early Chinese, Egyptian, and Greek cultures. Even in today's high-tech times, people try a variety of ways, most based on folklore, to conceive a particular sex. From diet, sexual positioning, and testicle temperature to following the phases of the moon, couples try to defy the odds of nature.

Now science may help couples have the baby they want. Choosing gender may eliminate one of the fundamental mysteries of procreation, but for people who have grown accustomed to seeing three-dimensional ultrasounds of fetuses, learning a baby's sex within weeks of conception, and scheduling convenient delivery dates, it's simply the next logical step.

Currently, an FDA clinical trial of sophisticated sperm-sorting technology is more than half way to completion. FDA approval of the technique would add it to the arse-nal of couples intent on having a baby of a particular sex. The *MicroSort method* is an experimental technique that separates X (female) from Y (male) chromosomes. Sperm are stained with a fluorescent dye that binds to the chromosomes. The sperm are then zapped with a laser that illuminates the dye. X chromosomes are bigger than Y chromosomes and soak up more dye, so they look brighter. Then the dyed sperm pass by an electrode that gives Xs a positive charge and Ys a negative one. Charged plates attract and separate the chromosomes, channeling them into separate receptacles. Separation is not absolutely perfect, but one sample is used to fertilize a woman's eggs, depending upon the requested gender.

Another technique, the *Ericsson method,* has been used for about a decade. In this technique, sperm are poured into a viscous layer of fluid. The heavy head of the sperm makes them swim downward. Sperm carrying the Y (male) chromosome swim faster than those with the X chromosome, reaching the bottom of the tube faster. They can then be extracted and used for insemination. The Ericsson method claims to have a 78 to 85 percent chance of producing a boy, although critics say the odds are not better than 50:50.

Preimplantation genetic diagnosis, a third technique, was originally used to detect genetic diseases. Doctors remove eggs from the woman and fertilize them with sperm in the lab, creating embryos. After three days, technicians extract a cell from each embryo. They can differentiate male and female embryos by examining their chromosomes. After determining the sex of the embryos, doctors implant the desired ones. Though more invasive and costly than other methods, success is virtually guaranteed.

Source: Adapted from K. Springen, "Brave New Babies," *Newsweek,* January 26, 2004, 45–53. © 2004 Newsweek, Inc. All rights reserved. Reprinted by permission.

involves some risk. It causes miscarriage in approximately 5 percent of cases.

If any of these tests reveals a serious birth defect, parents are advised to undergo genetic counseling. In the case of a chromosomal abnormality such as Down's syndrome, the parents are usually offered the option of a therapeutic abortion. Some parents choose this option; others research the disability and decide to go ahead with the birth.

Some prospective parents even undergo procedures aimed at increasing the odds of having a baby of a particular gender; see the Health Ethics: Conflict and Controversy box.

Childbirth

Prospective parents need to make a number of key decisions long before the baby is born. These include where to have the baby, whether to use drugs during labor and delivery, choice of childbirth method, and whether to breast-feed or bottle-feed. Answering these questions in advance will ensure a smoother passage into parenthood.

Choosing Where to Have Your Baby

Today's prospective mothers have many delivery options, ranging from traditional hospital birth to home birth. Parental values are important. Many couples, for instance, feel that the modern medical establishment has dehumanized the birth process; thus they choose to deliver at home or at a *birthing center,* a homelike setting outside a hospital where women can give birth and receive postdelivery care by a team of professional practitioners, including physicians and registered nurses.

However, hospitals have responded to the desire for a more relaxed, less medically oriented birthing process. Many hospitals now offer labor–delivery–postpartum birthing rooms, which allow patients with noncomplicated deliveries to remain in one room during the entire process. In addition, "rooming-in," or keeping the baby in the same room with the mother at all times, is encouraged to facilitate bonding and breast-feeding. Partners are generally encouraged to room-in with the mother and baby as well.

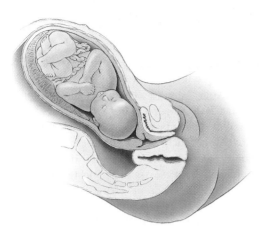

Dilation of the cervix

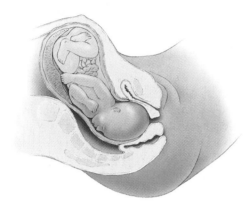

Transition ————————————— **End of Stage I**

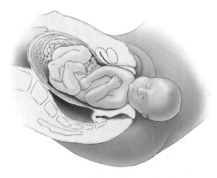

Birth of the baby (Expulsion) ————— **End of Stage II**

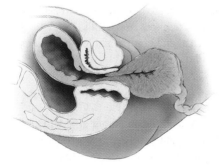

Delivery of the placenta ————— **End of Stage III**

FIGURE 7.13 The Birth Process

Labor and Delivery

The birth process has three stages (Figure 7.13). The exact mechanisms that initiate labor are unknown. During the last few weeks before delivery, the baby normally shifts and turns to a head-down position, and the cervix begins to dilate (widen). The junction of the pubic bones gradually loosens as the third trimester progresses, to permit expansion of the pelvic girdle during birth.

First Stage of Labor In the first stage of labor, the amniotic sac breaks, causing a rush of fluid from the vagina (commonly referred to as "water breaking"). Contractions in the abdomen and lower back also signal the beginning of labor. Early contractions push the baby downward, putting pressure on the cervix and dilating it further. The first stage of labor may last from a couple of hours to more than a day for a first birth but is usually much shorter during subsequent births.

The end of the first stage of labor, called **transition**, is the process during which the cervix becomes fully dilated and the baby's head begins to move into the vagina, or birth canal. Contractions usually come quickly during transition, which generally lasts 30 minutes or less.

Second Stage of Labor The second stage of labor (the *expulsion stage*) follows transition, when the cervix has become fully dilated. Contractions become rhythmic, strong, and more painful as the uterus works to push the baby through the birth canal. The expulsion stage lasts one to four hours and concludes when the infant is finally pushed out of the mother's body. In some cases, the attending practitioner will do an **episiotomy**, a straight incision in the mother's perineum, to prevent the baby's head from tearing vaginal tissues and speed the baby's exit from the vagina. Sometimes women can avoid the need for an episiotomy by exercising and getting good nutrition throughout pregnancy, by trying different birth positions, or by having an attendant massage the perineal tissue. However, the skin's natural elasticity and the baby's size are limiting factors.

After delivery, the attending practitioner cleans the baby's mucus-filled breathing passages, and the baby takes its first breath, generally accompanied by a loud wail. (The traditional slap on the baby's buttocks, often depicted in old movies, is no longer a common practice because of the trauma associated with it.) The umbilical cord is then tied and severed. The stump of cord attached to the baby's navel dries up and drops off within a few days.

transition The process during which the cervix becomes nearly fully dilated and the head of the fetus begins to move into the birth canal.

episiotomy A straight incision in the mother's perineum in the area between the vulva and the anus.

Third Stage of Labor In the meantime, the mother continues into the third stage of labor, during which the placenta, or **afterbirth**, is expelled from the uterus. This stage is usually completed within 30 minutes after delivery.

Most mothers prefer to have their new infants next to them following the birth. Together with their spouse or partner, they feel a need to share this time of bonding with their infant.

Managing Labor: Medical and Nonmedical Approaches

Because painkilling drugs given to the mother during labor can cause sluggish responses in the newborn and other complications, many women choose drug-free labor and delivery—but it is important to keep a flexible attitude about pain relief because each labor is different. Working in partnership with a health care provider to make the best decision for mother and baby is optimal. Use of painkilling medication during a delivery is not a sign of weakness. One person is not a "success" for delivering without medication while another is a "failure" for using medical measures. Remember, pain is to be expected. In fact, many experts say that the pain of labor is the most difficult in the human experience. There is no one right answer for managing that pain.

Birth Alternatives

Expectant parents have several options beyond the traditional hospital setting for the process of their infant's birth and their participation in it. Although several of these methods have decreased in popularity, all continue to be used.

The Lamaze method is the most popular birth alternative in the United States. Prelabor classes teach the mother to control her pain through special breathing patterns, focusing exercises, and relaxation. Lamaze births usually take place in a hospital or birthing center with a physician or midwife in attendance. The partner (or labor coach) assists by giving emotional support, physical comfort (massage and ice chips), and coaching for proper breath control during contractions. Lamaze proponents discourage the use of drugs.

Other methods that prospective parents can research include the Harris method, Childbirth without Fear, the Leboyer method, the Bradley method, and water birth. These vary in their philosophies regarding painkillers, partner participation, and other elements.

afterbirth   The expelled placenta.

postpartum depression   The experience of energy depletion, anxiety, mood swings, and depression that women may feel during the postpartum period.

The Postpartum Period

The postpartum period typically lasts four to six weeks after delivery. During this period many women experience fluctuating emotions. The physical stress of labor, dehydration and blood loss, and other stresses challenge many new mothers' stamina. About 50 to 80 percent of new mothers experience what is called the "baby blues" characterized by periods of sadness, anxiety, headache, sleep disturbances, and irritability. For most women these symptoms disappear. About 10 percent of new mothers experience **postpartum depression**, a more disabling syndrome characterized by mood swings, lack of energy, crying, guilt, and depression. It can happen any time within the first year after childbirth. Mothers who experience postpartum depression should be encouraged to seek professional treatment. Counseling and/or medication are two of the most common types of treatment.[26]

Breast-Feeding

Although the new mother's milk will not begin to flow for two or more days, her breasts secrete a thick yellow substance called *colostrum*. Because this fluid contains vital antibodies to help fight infection, the newborn baby should be allowed to suckle.

The American Academy of Pediatrics strongly recommends that infants should be breast-fed for at least 6 months and ideally for 12 months. Scientific findings indicate there are many advantages to breast-feeding. Breast milk is perfectly suited to a baby's nutritional needs. Breast-fed babies have fewer illnesses and a much lower hospitalization rate because breast milk contains maternal antibodies and immunological cells that stimulate the infant's immune system. When breast-fed babies do get sick, they recover more quickly. They are also less likely to be obese than babies fed on formulas, and they have fewer allergies. They may even be more intelligent: a new study finds that the longer a baby was breast-fed, the higher the IQ in adulthood. Researchers have found that breast milk contains substances that enhance brain development.[27]

This does not mean that breast milk is the only way to nourish a baby. Some women are unable or unwilling to breast-feed. Prepared formulas can provide nourishment that allows a baby to grow and thrive. When deciding whether to breast- or bottle-feed, mothers need to consider their own desires and preferences, too. Both feeding methods can supply the physical and emotional closeness so essential to the parent–child relationship.

Complications

Problems can occur during labor and delivery, even following a successful pregnancy. The mother should discuss these possibilities with her practitioner prior to labor so she understands the medical procedures that may be necessary for her safety and that of her child. Although pregnancy still involves a certain amount of risk, the risk is lower than for many other common activities.

Preeclampsia and Eclampsia

Preeclampsia is a condition that is characterized by high blood pressure, protein in the urine, and edema (fluid retention), which usually causes swelling of the hands and face. This condition complicates approximately 10 percent of pregnancies and is responsible for 18 percent of U.S. maternal deaths each year. Symptoms may include sudden weight gain, headache, nausea or vomiting, changes in vision, racing pulse, mental confusion, and stomach or right shoulder pain. If preeclampsia is not treated, it can cause strokes and seizures, a condition called **eclampsia**. Potential problems can include liver and kidney damage, internal bleeding, stroke, poor fetal growth, and fetal and maternal death.

This condition tends to occur in the late second or third trimesters. The cause is not known; however, the incidence of preeclampsia is higher in first-time mothers, women over 40 or under 18 years of age, women carrying multiple fetuses, and women with a history of chronic hypertension, diabetes or kidney disorder, or previous history of preeclampsia. Family history of preeclampsia is also a risk factor, whether the history is on the male or female side. Treatment for preeclampsia ranges from bed rest and monitoring for those with mild cases to hospitalization and close monitoring for more severe cases, which have the potential to be life-threatening for the woman and her fetus.

Cesarean Section (C-section)

If labor lasts too long or if a baby is presenting wrong (about to exit the uterus any way but head first), a **cesarean section (C-section)** may be necessary. This surgical procedure involves making an incision across the mother's abdomen and through the uterus to remove the baby. A C-section is also performed if labor is extremely difficult, maternal blood pressure falls rapidly, the placenta separates from the uterus too soon, the mother has diabetes, or other problems occur. A C-section can be traumatic for the mother if she is not prepared for it. Risks are the same as for any major abdominal surgery, and recovery from birth takes considerably longer after a C-section.

The rate of delivery by C-section in the United States has increased from 5 percent in the mid-1960s to 29 percent in 2004.[28] Although necessary in certain cases, some physicians and critics, including the Centers for Disease Control and Prevention (CDC), feel that C-sections are performed too frequently in this country.

Miscarriage

One in ten pregnancies does not end in delivery. Loss of the fetus before it is viable is called a **miscarriage** (also referred to as spontaneous abortion). An estimated 70 to 90 percent of women who miscarry eventually become pregnant again.

Reasons for miscarriage vary. In some cases, the fertilized egg has failed to divide correctly. In others, genetic abnormalities, maternal illness, or infections are responsible.

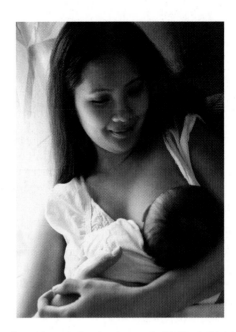

Breast-feeding enhances the development of intimate bonds between mother and child.

Maternal hormonal imbalance may also cause a miscarriage, as may a weak cervix or toxic chemicals in the environment. In most cases, the cause is not known.

Rh Factor

A blood incompatibility between mother and fetus can cause **Rh factor** problems, sometimes resulting in miscarriage. Rh is a blood protein, and problems occur when the mother is Rh-negative and the fetus is Rh-positive. During a first birth, some of the baby's blood passes into the mother's bloodstream. An Rh-negative mother may manufacture antibodies to destroy the Rh-positive blood introduced into her bloodstream at the time of birth. Her first baby will

preeclampsia A complication in pregnancy characterized by high blood pressure, protein in the urine, and edema.

eclampsia Untreated preeclampsia can develop into this potentially fatal complication that involves maternal strokes and seizures.

cesarean section (C-section) A surgical procedure in which a baby is removed through an incision made in the mother's abdominal and uterine walls.

miscarriage Loss of the fetus before it is viable; also called spontaneous abortion.

Rh factor A blood protein related to the production of antibodies. If an Rh-negative mother is pregnant with an Rh-positive fetus, the mother will manufacture antibodies that can kill the fetus, causing miscarriage.

be unaffected, but subsequent babies with positive Rh factor will be at risk for a severe anemia called *hemolytic disease* because the mother's Rh antibodies will attack the fetus's red blood cells.

If prenatal testing reveals Rh incompatibility, intrauterine transfusions can be given or an early delivery by C-section can be done.

Prevention is preferable to treatment. All women with Rh-negative blood should be injected with a medication called RhoGAM within 72 hours of any birth, miscarriage, or abortion. This injection will prevent them from developing the Rh antibodies.

Ectopic Pregnancy
The implantation of a fertilized egg outside the uterus, usually in the fallopian tube or occasionally in the pelvic cavity, is called an **ectopic pregnancy.** Because these structures are not capable of expanding and nourishing a developing fetus, the pregnancy must be terminated surgically, or a miscarriage will occur. Ectopic pregnancy generally is accompanied by pain in the lower abdomen or aching in the shoulders as the blood flows toward the diaphragm. If bleeding is significant, blood pressure drops, and the woman can go into shock. If an ectopic pregnancy goes undiagnosed and untreated, the fallopian tube will rupture, which puts the woman at great risk of hemorrhage, peritonitis (infection in the abdomen), and even death.

Over the past five years, the incidence of ectopic pregnancy has tripled, and no one really understands why. We do know that ectopic pregnancy is a potential side effect of pelvic inflammatory disease (Chapter 17), which has become increasingly common in recent years. The scarring or blockage of the fallopian tubes that is characteristic of this disease prevents the fertilized egg from passing to the uterus.

Stillbirth
One of the most traumatic events a couple can face is a **stillbirth**. A stillborn baby is born dead, often for no apparent reason. The grief experienced following a stillbirth is devastating. Nine months of happy anticipation have been thwarted. Family, friends, and other children may be in a state of shock, needing comfort and not knowing where to turn.

The mother's breasts produce milk, and there is no infant to be fed. A room with a crib and toys is left empty.

The grief can last for years, and partners may blame themselves or each other. In many cases, no amount of reassurance from the attending physician, relatives, or friends can assuage the grief or guilt. Well-intentioned comments such as "Oh, you'll have another baby someday" may bring no comfort.

Some communities have groups called the Compassionate Friends to help parents and other family members through this grieving process. This nonprofit organization is for parents who have lost a child of any age for any reason.

Sudden Infant Death Syndrome
The sudden death of an infant under one year of age, for no apparent reason, is called **sudden infant death syndrome (SIDS)**. Though SIDS is the leading cause of death for children aged one month to one year, affecting about 1 in 1,000 infants in the United States each year, it is not a disease. Rather, it is ruled the cause of death after all other possibilities are ruled out. A SIDS death is sudden and silent; death occurs quickly, often associated with sleep and with no signs of suffering.

Doctors do not know what causes SIDS. However, research done in countries including England, New Zealand, Australia, and Norway has shown that placing children on their backs or sides to sleep cuts the rate of SIDS by as much as half. The American Academy of Pediatrics advises parents to lay infants on their backs and is a sponsor of the Back to Sleep educational campaign urging parents to position babies on their backs. Additional precautions against SIDS include having a firm surface for the infant's bed, not allowing the infant to become too warm, maintaining a smoke-free environment, having regular pediatric visits, breast-feeding, and seeking prenatal care. The use of a pacifier is also recommended, and should be offered to an infant up to 1 year old during daytime naps, and during the night. Research has shown that this practice does reduce the risk of SIDS.[29]

? *what do you* THINK?

What are your thoughts on medical versus natural management of labor and delivery? ■ Do you have strong preferences for how you'd like to manage your own birthing process? If so, what are they? ■ What might be the advantages and disadvantages of breast-feeding?

Infertility

An estimated one in six American couples experiences **infertility**, or difficulties in conceiving. Reasons include the trend toward delaying childbirth (as a woman gets older, she is less likely to conceive), endometriosis, and the rising incidence of pelvic inflammatory disease.

ectopic pregnancy   Implantation of a fertilized egg outside the uterus, usually in a uterine tube; a medical emergency that can end in death from hemorrhage for the mother.

stillbirth   The birth of a dead baby.

sudden infant death syndrome (SIDS)   The sudden death of an infant under one year of age for no apparent reason.

infertility   Difficulties in conceiving.

Causes in Women

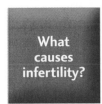

Endometriosis is the leading cause of infertility in women in the United States. With this disorder, parts of the endometrial lining of the uterus implant themselves outside the uterus—in the uterine tubes, lungs, intestines, outer uterine walls or ovarian walls, and/or on the ligaments that support the uterus. The disorder can be treated surgically or with hormonal preparations. Success rates vary.

Another cause of infertility is **pelvic inflammatory disease (PID)**, a serious bacterial infection that scars the fallopian tubes and blocks sperm migration. PID often results from chlamydia or gonorrheal infections that spread to the uterine tubes or ovaries. Symptoms of PID include severe pain, fever, and sometimes vaginal discharge.

The past 30 years have brought a tremendous increase in the annual number of PID cases, from 17,800 to about 1 million per year. One episode of PID causes sterility in 10 to 15 percent of women, and 50 to 75 percent become sterile after three or four infections.[30]

Causes in Men

Among men, the most common fertility problem is **low sperm count**. Although only one viable sperm is needed for fertilization, research has shown that all the other sperm in the ejaculate aid in the fertilization process. There are normally 60 million to 80 million sperm per milliliter of semen. When the count drops below 20 million, fertility declines.

Low sperm count may be attributable to environmental factors such as exposure of the scrotum to intense heat or cold, radiation, or altitude, or even wearing excessively tight underwear or outerwear. However, other factors, such as the mumps virus, can damage the cells that make sperm. Varicose veins above one or both testicles can also render men infertile. Male infertility problems account for around 40 percent of infertility cases.

Treatments

For the couple desperately wishing to conceive, the road to parenthood may be frustrating. Fortunately, medical treatment can identify the cause of infertility in about 90 percent of cases. The chances of becoming pregnant range from 30 to 70 percent, depending on the reason for infertility. The countless tests and the invasion of privacy that characterize some couples' efforts to conceive can put stress on an otherwise strong, healthy relationship. A good physician or fertility team will take the time to ascertain the couple's level of motivation.

Fertility workups can be very expensive, and the costs are not usually covered by insurance companies. Fertility workups for men include a sperm count, a test for sperm motility, and analysis of any disease processes present. Such procedures should be undertaken only by a qualified urologist. Women are thoroughly examined by an obstetrician-gynecologist to determine the composition of cervical mucus and evidence of tubal scarring or endometriosis. Complete fertility workups may take four to five months and can be unsettling. The couple may be instructed to have sex "by the calendar" to increase their chances of conceiving. Sometimes pregnancy can be achieved by collecting the man's sperm from several ejaculations and inseminating the woman at a later time. In some cases, surgery can correct structural problems such as tubal scarring. In others, administering hormones can improve the health of ova and sperm.

Fertility Drugs **Fertility drugs** stimulate ovulation in women who are not ovulating. Ninety percent of women who use these drugs will begin to ovulate, and half will conceive. Fertility drugs can have many side effects, including headaches, irritability, restlessness, depression, fatigue, edema (fluid retention), abnormal uterine bleeding, breast tenderness, vasomotor flushes (hot flashes), and visual difficulties. Women using fertility drugs are also at increased risk of developing multiple ovarian cysts (fluid-filled growths) and liver damage. The drugs sometimes trigger the release of more than one egg. Thus a woman treated with one of these drugs has a one in ten chance of having multiple births. Most such births are twins, but triplets and even quadruplets are not uncommon.

Alternative Insemination Another treatment option is **alternative insemination** of a woman with her partner's sperm. This technique has led to an estimated 250,000 births in the United States, primarily for couples in which the man is infertile. If this procedure fails, the couple may choose insemination by an anonymous donor through a sperm bank. The sperm are medically screened, classified according to the

---

endometriosis A disorder in which uterine lining tissue establishes itself outside the uterus; the leading cause of infertility in the United States.

pelvic inflammatory disease (PID) An infection that scars the uterine tubes and consequently blocks sperm migration, causing infertility.

low sperm count A sperm count below 60 million sperm per milliliter of semen; the leading cause of infertility in men.

fertility drugs Hormones that stimulate ovulation in women who are not ovulating; often responsible for multiple births.

alternative insemination Fertilization accomplished by depositing a partner's or a donor's semen into a woman's vagina via a thin tube; almost always done in a doctor's office.

physical characteristics of the donor (for example, blonde hair, blue eyes), and then frozen for future use. Frozen sperm can survive for up to five years. The woman being inseminated may choose sperm from a man whose physical characteristics resemble those of her partner or match her own personal preferences.

In the last few years, concern has been expressed about the possibility of transmitting the AIDS virus through alternative insemination. As a result, donors are routinely screened for the disease.

In Vitro Fertilization Often referred to as test tube fertilization, **in vitro fertilization** involves collecting a viable ovum from the prospective mother and transferring it to a nutrient medium in a laboratory, where it is fertilized with sperm from the woman's partner or a donor. After a few days, the embryo is transplanted into the mother's uterus, where, it is hoped, it will develop normally. Since 1984, the in vitro process has been responsible for an estimated 60,000 babies.

Gamete Intrafallopian Transfer

In **gamete intrafallopian transfer (GIFT)**, the egg is harvested from the woman's ovary and placed in one of the uterine tubes with the man's sperm. Less expensive and time-consuming than in vitro fertilization, GIFT mimics nature by allowing the egg to be fertilized in the uterine tube and migrate to the uterus according to the normal timetable.

Intracytoplasmic Sperm Injection

In **intracytoplasmic sperm injection (ICSI),** a sperm cell is injected into an egg. First performed successfully in 1992, this procedure required researchers to learn how to manipulate both egg and sperm without damaging them. ICSI can help men with low sperm counts or motility, and even those who cannot ejaculate or have no live sperm in their semen as a result of vasectomy, chemotherapy, or a medical disorder. However, recent studies have found that infants conceived with the use of ICSI or in vitro fertilization have twice the risk of a major birth defect as those conceived naturally.[31]

Nonsurgical Embryo Transfer and Other Techniques In **nonsurgical embryo transfer**, a donor egg is fertilized by the man's sperm and implanted in the woman's uterus. This procedure may also be used to transfer an already fertilized ovum into the uterus of another woman. In **embryo transfer**, an ovum from a donor is artificially inseminated by the man's sperm, allowed to stay in the donor's body for a time, and then transplanted into the woman's body.

Infertile couples have another alternative—**embryo adoption programs**. The adopting couple can experience pregnancy and control prenatal care. The cost is approximately $4,000 for an embryo to be thawed and transferred to an infertile woman's uterus or uterine tubes.

The ethical and moral questions surrounding experimental infertility treatments are staggering. Before moving forward with any of these treatments, individuals need to ask themselves a few important questions. Has infertility been absolutely confirmed? Are reputable infertility counseling services accessible? Have they explored all possible alternatives and considered potential risks? Have all parties examined their attitudes, values, and beliefs about conceiving a child in this manner? Finally, they need to consider what and how they will tell the child about their method of conception.

Surrogate Motherhood

Sixty to seventy percent of infertile couples are able to conceive after treatment. The rest decide to live without children, to adopt, or to attempt surrogate motherhood. In this option, the couple hires a woman to be alternatively inseminated by the male partner. The surrogate then carries the baby to term and surrenders it upon birth to the couple. Surrogate mothers are reportedly paid about $10,000 for their services and are reimbursed for medical expenses. Legal and medical expenses can run as high as $30,000 for the infertile couple.

Couples considering surrogate motherhood are advised to consult a lawyer regarding contracts. Most of these legal documents stipulate that the surrogate mother must undergo amniocentesis and that if the fetus is defective, she must consent to an abortion. In that case, or if the surrogate miscarries, she is reimbursed for her time and expenses. The prospective parents must also agree to take the baby if it is carried to term, even if it is unhealthy or has physical abnormalities.

Adoption

For couples who have decided that biological childbirth is not an option, adoption provides an alternative. Currently, about 50,000 children are available for adoption in the United

---

in vitro fertilization Fertilization of an egg in a nutrient medium and subsequent transfer back to the mother's body.

gamete intrafallopian transfer (GIFT) Procedure in which an egg harvested from the female partner's ovary is placed with the male partner's sperm in her uterine tube, where it is fertilized and then migrates to the uterus for implantation.

intracytoplasmic sperm injection (ICSI) Fertilization accomplished by injecting a sperm cell directly into an egg.

nonsurgical embryo transfer In vitro fertilization of a donor egg by the male partner's (or donor's) sperm and subsequent transfer to the female partner's or another woman's uterus.

embryo transfer Artificial insemination of a donor with the male partner's sperm; after a time, the embryo is transferred from the donor to the female partner's body.

embryo adoption programs A procedure whereby an infertile couple is able to purchase frozen embryos donated by another couple.

States every year. This is far fewer than the number of couples seeking adoptions. By some estimates, only 1 in 30 couples receives the children they want. On average, couples spend two years and $100,000 on the adoption process.

Women who choose adoption come from families who are supportive of the adoption process. If you are pregnant and considering adoption, make sure you think through all the possibilities before you make your decision. Remember: adoption is permanent. People who can help you think through your options include your partner, friends, family, crisis centers, student health services, family planning clinic, family service agency, or adoption agency.

There are two types of adoption: *confidential* and *open.* In confidential adoption the birth parents and the adoptive parents never know each other. Adoptive parents are only given information about the birth parents that they need to take care of the child, such as medical information. In open adoption, birth parents and adoptive parents know something about each other. There are different levels of openness. Both parties must agree to this plan, and it is not available in every state.

Because the number of American children available for adoption is limited, women who consider placing their child for adoption have gained new leverage. Increasingly, couples wishing to adopt have turned to independent adoptions arranged by a lawyer, or they may directly negotiate with the birth mother. Independent adoptions now outnumber those arranged by social service agencies.

Increasingly, couples are choosing to adopt children from other countries. In 2004, U.S. families adopted over 258,000 foreign-born children. The cost of intercountry adoption can range greatly, from approximately $10,000 to more than $30,000, including agency fees, dossier and immigration processing fees, and court costs. However, it may be a good alternative for many couples, especially those who want to adopt an infant.

what do you THINK?

If you found that you or your partner had infertility problems, how much time and money would you be willing to invest in infertility treatments? ▪ Do you think that single women and lesbians should have equal access to alternative methods of insemination? Why or why not? ▪ Do you think single women, single men, gay males, and lesbians should have equal opportunities to adopt? ▪ How do you think society views these types of adoptions?

TAKING charge

Summary

- Latex condoms and the female condom, when used correctly for oral sex or intercourse, provide the most effective protection from sexually transmitted infections. Other contraceptive methods include abstinence, outercourse, oral contraceptives, foams, jellies, suppositories, creams, film, the diaphragm, the cervical cap, Lea's shield, FemCap, skin patches, the vaginal ring, the sponge, intrauterine devices, withdrawal, and Depo-Provera. Whereas all these methods of contraception are reversible, sterilization is considered permanent.
- Abortion is legal in the United States through the second trimester. Abortion methods include vacuum aspiration, dilation and evacuation (D&E), dilation and curettage (D&C), intact dilation and extraction (D&X), hysterotomy, induction abortion, mifepristone, and methotrexate.
- Parenting is a demanding job that requires careful planning. Emotional health, maternal health, paternal health, financial plans, and contingency planning all need to be taken into account.
- Prenatal care includes a complete physical exam within the first trimester and avoidance of all substances that could have teratogenic effects on the fetus, such as alcohol and drugs, smoking, X rays, and harmful chemicals. Full-term pregnancy covers three trimesters.
- Childbirth occurs in three stages. Partners should jointly choose a labor method early in the pregnancy to be better prepared for labor when it occurs. Possible complications of pregnancy and childbirth include preeclampsia and eclampsia, miscarriage, Rh factor problems, ectopic pregnancy, stillbirth, and the need for a cesarean section.
- Infertility in women may be caused by pelvic inflammatory disease (PID) or endometriosis. In men, it may be caused by low sperm count. Treatments may include alternative insemination, in vitro fertilization, gamete intrafallopian transfer (GIFT), intracytoplasmic sperm injection (ICSI), nonsurgical embryo transfer, and embryo transfer. Surrogate motherhood involves hiring a fertile woman to be alternatively inseminated by the male partner. Adoption, including international adoptions, can be a viable option.

Chapter Review

1. Which of the following is *not* a barrier contraceptive?
   a. cervical cap
   b. condom
   c. diaphragm
   d. contraceptive patch

2. Which of the following should *not* be used with any type of latex barrier contraceptive?
   a. oil based lubricant
   b. water based lubricant
   c. vegetable shortening
   d. A and C

3. Which form of birth control offers a 100 percent effective contraceptive rate?
   a. condoms
   b. birth control pill
   c. male sterilization
   d. abstinence

4. What is meant by the *failure rate* of contraceptive use?
   a. the number of times a woman fails to get pregnant when she wanted to
   b. the number of times a woman gets pregnant when she did not want to
   c. the number of pregnancies that occur for women using a particular method of birth control
   d. the reliability of alternative methods of birth control that do not use condoms

5. The birth control patch administers its contraceptive drug through which route into the body?
   a. injection
   b. orally through the mouth
   c. transdermal through the skin
   d. inhalation

6. In an ectopic pregnancy, the fertilized egg grows into the fetus in the woman's
   a. fallopian tube.
   b. uterus.
   c. vagina.
   d. ovaries.

7. In which trimester of a woman's pregnancy is the colostrum milk able to be secreted for the baby's nursing needs?
   a. first trimester
   b. second trimester
   c. third trimester
   d. postpartum

8. Mary uses a method of natural birth control in which she examines the consistency and color of her normal vaginal secretions. What is this method called?
   a. body temperature method
   b. rhythm method
   c. cervical mucus method
   d. calendar method

9. Teratogenic birth defects are mostly likely to occur during which trimester of a woman's pregnancy?
   a. first trimester
   b. second trimester
   c. third trimester
   d. fourth trimester

10. Which of the following is the most common method for preventing unwanted pregnancy in U.S. women?
    a. Norplant
    b. sterilization
    c. calendar method
    d. oral contraceptive pill

Answers to these questions can be found on page A-1.

Questions for Discussion and Reflection

1. List the most effective contraceptive methods. What are their drawbacks? What medical conditions would keep a person from using each one? What are the characteristics of the methods you think would be most effective for you?
2. What are the various methods of abortion? What are the opposing viewpoints concerning abortion? What is *Roe v. Wade,* and what impact has it had on the abortion debate?
3. What are the most important considerations in deciding whether the time is right to become a parent? If you choose to have children, what factors will you consider regarding the number of children to have?

4. Discuss the growth of the fetus through the three trimesters. What medical checkups or tests should be done during each trimester?
5. Discuss the emotional aspects of pregnancy. What types of emotional reactions are common in each trimester and in the postpartum period (the "fourth trimester")?
6. If you and your partner are unable to have children, what alternative methods of conception would you consider? Would you consider adoption?

Accessing Your Health on the Internet

The following websites explore further topics and issues related to personal health. You'll also find links to each organization's website on the Companion Website for *Access to Health, Tenth Edition,* at www.aw-bc.com/donatelle.

1. *The Alan Guttmacher Institute.* This site focuses on sexual and reproductive health research, policy analysis, and public education. www.guttmacher.org
2. *Go Ask Alice.* This website enables you to ask health questions anonymously. It is designed to help visitors make informed decisions about all aspects of their health by providing nonjudgmental, science-based responses to their questions. www.goaskalice.columbia.edu
3. *The American Pregnancy Association.* This national organization offers a wealth of resources to promote reproductive and pregnancy wellness. The website includes

educational materials and information on the latest research. www.Americanpregnancy.org
4. *Dr. Drew.* This site provides answers and advice on sex, relationships, and many other topics of interest to college students. www.DrDrew.com
5. *Planned Parenthood.* This site offers a range of up-to-date information on sexual health issues, such as birth control, the decision of when and whether to have a child, and sexually transmitted infections and safer sex. www.plannedparenthood.org
6. *Sexuality Information and Education Council of the United States.* Information, guidelines, and materials for the advancement of sexuality education are available from this site, which advocates the right of individuals to make responsible sexual choices. www.siecus.org

Further Reading

Boston Women's Health Collective. *Our Bodies, Ourselves: A New Edition for a New Era. New York:* Simon & Schuster, 2005

> Like its earlier editions, this volume contains information about women's health from a decidedly feminist angle. Every aspect of health is covered, including nutrition, emotional health, fitness, relationships, reproduction, contraception, and pregnancy.

Feldt, G. *The War on Choice.* New York: Bantam, 2004.

> A history and analysis of threats to women's reproductive rights. Feldt describes political efforts to outlaw abortion and argues that women should mobilize to support pro-choice causes.

Hatcher, R. A. et al. *Contraceptive Technology.* 18th ed. New York: Ardent Media, 2004.

> Perhaps the best primary reference concerning birth control, for physicians, family planning centers, student health services, and educators. Contributors include staff members from the Centers for Disease Control and Prevention.

Hatcher, R.A. et al. *Safely Sexual.* 2nd ed. New York: Ardent Media, 2005.

> Provides practical recommendations for unplanned pregnancy, as well as the prevention of STIs and HIV.

Kitzinger, S. *The Complete Book of Pregnancy and Childbirth,* 4th ed. New York: Knopf, 2003.

> *The book provides expectant mothers with new insights into having a healthy pregnancy and what happens in today's* birthing rooms. *Offers women and their partners an in-depth look at both the baby's and the mother's physical and emotional development during pregnancy.*

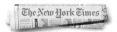

e-themes from *The New York Times*

For up-to-date articles about current health issues, visit www.aw-bc.com/donatelle, select *Access to Health,* Tenth Edition, Chapter 7, and click on "e-themes."

References

1. World Health Organization, "Nonoxynol 9 Ineffective in Preventing HIV Infection," June 8, 2006, www.who.int/mediacentre/notes/release55/en.
2. U.S. Department of Health and Human Services. "FDA Approves Seasonale Oral Contraceptive," FDA Talk Paper TO3–65, September 5, 2003, www.fda.gov.
3. R. A. Hatcher et al., *Contraceptive Technology,* 18th rev. ed. (New York: Ardent Media, 1998), 457.
4. R. A. Hatcher et al., *Contraceptive Technology,* 18th ed. (New York: Ardent Media, 2004); R. Burkman et al., "Safety Concerns and Health Benefits Associated with Oral Contraception," *American Journal of Obstetrics and Gynecology* 190, (4 Suppl. S) (2004): S5–S22.
5. Food and Drug Administration, "FDA Updates Labeling for Ortho Evra Contraceptive Patch," *FDA News,* November 10, 2005, www.fda.gov/bbs/topics/news/2005/NEW01262.html.
6. D. Bensyl et al., "Contraceptive Use—United States and Territories, Behavioral Risk Factor Surveillance System, 2002," *Morbidity and Mortality Weekly Report* 54 (SS6) (November 18, 2005): 1–72.
7. K. N. Anderson, L. E. Anderson, and W. D. Glanze, eds., *Mosby's Medical, Nursing and Allied Health Dictionary* (Philadelphia: W. B. Saunders, 2002); Hatcher, *Contraceptive Technology.*
8. American College Health Association, "American College Health Association-National College Health Assessment Web Summary," updated April 2006, www.acha.org.
9. S. J. Ventura, J. C. Abma, W. D. Mosher, and S. Henshaw, "Estimated Pregnancy Rates for the United States, 1990–2000: An Update," *National Vital Statistic Reports* 52 (2004): 1–2; H. Boonstra, "Emergency Contraception: The Need to Increase Public Awareness," *Guttmacher Rep Public Policy* 5 (2002): 3–6; Planned Parenthood Federation of America, "Emergency Contraception," www.plannedparenthood.org/pp2/portal/files/portalmedicalinfo//ec/fact/fact-emergency-contraception.xml. Accessed June 6, 2006.
10. American College Health Association, Access to Emergency Contraception on College and University Campuses, "American College Health Association-National College Health Assessment (ACHA-NCHA) Spring 2005 Reference Group Data Report," *The Journal of American College Health,* July/August 2006.
11. Boston Women's Health Collective, *Our Bodies, Ourselves: A New Edition for a New Era* (New York: Simon & Schuster, 2005).
12. Ibid.
13. The Alan Guttmacher Institute, "State Policies in Brief: State Funding of Abortion Under Medicaid," June 1, 2006, www.agi-usa.org; The Alan Guttmacher Institute, "Sexual and Reproductive Health Issues in the States: Major Trends in 2005," www.agi-usa.org.
14. NARAL, Pro Choice America, "The Federal Abortion Ban," February 21, 2006, www.prochoiceamerica.org/issues/abortion/abortion-bans/index.html.
15. The Alan Guttmacher Institute, "Facts in Brief: Induced Abortion in the United States," 2005, www.agi-usa.org.
16. Planned Parenthood, "The Difference between Emergency Contraception Pills and Medication Abortion," July 9, 2005, www.plannedparenthood.org.
17. N. F. Russo and A. J. Dabul, "The Relationship of Abortion to Well-Being: Do Race and Religion Make a Difference?" *Professional Psychology: Research and Practice* 28, no. 1 (2000): 23–31.
18. K. Schmidt, "The Dark Legacy of Fatherhood," *U.S. News and World Report* (December 14, 1992): 94–95.
19. Center for Nutrition Policy and Promotion, "Expenditure on Children by Families, 2005 Annual Report," April 2006, www.usda.gov/cnpp/Crc/crc2003.pdf.
20. U.S. Census Bureau, Population Division, Fertility and Family Statistics Branch Survey of Income and Program Participation, "Who's Minding the Kids? Child Care Arrangements: Winter 2002 Household Economic Studies," October 2005.
21. Hatcher et al., *Contraceptive Technology,* 1998; National Center for Health Statistics, "Births: Preliminary Data for 2003" (PHS 2004-1120), *National Vital Statistics Reports* 53, no. 9, 2004.
22. S. Kitzinger, *The Complete Book of Pregnancy and Childbirth,* 4th ed. (New York: Knopf, 2003); U.S. Department of Health and Human Services, "The Health Consequences of Smoking: What It Means to You," in *The 2004 Surgeon General's Report* (Washington, DC: Government Printing Office, 2004).
23. M. Kharrazi et al., "Environmental Tobacco Smoke and Pregnancy Outcome," *Epidemiology* 15, no. 6 (November 2006).
24. National Institute of Child Health and Human Development, "Facts about Down's Syndrome," 2005, www.nichd.nih.gov/publications/downsyndrome.
25. National Down Syndrome Society, 2006, www.ndss.org.

26. National Institute of Mental Health, "Frequently Asked Questions: Depression During and After Pregnancy," April 2005, www .4woman.gov.

27. American Pregnancy Association, "What's in Breast Milk?" June 9, 2006, www.americanpregnancy.org.

28. J. A. Martin et al., *Preliminary Births for 2004: Infant and Maternal Health* (Hyattsville, MD: National Center for Health Statistics, 2006).

29. F. R. Hawk et al., "Do Pacifiers Reduce the Risk of Sudden Infant Death Syndrome? A Meta-Analysis," *Pediatrics,* October 10, 2005.

30. Centers for Disease Control and Prevention, "Pelvic Inflammatory Disease—Fact Sheet," 2006, www.cdc.gov/std/pid.

31. K. Powell, "Fertility Treatments: Seeds of Doubt," *Nature* 422 (2003): 656–658.

Nutrition

EATING FOR OPTIMUM HEALTH

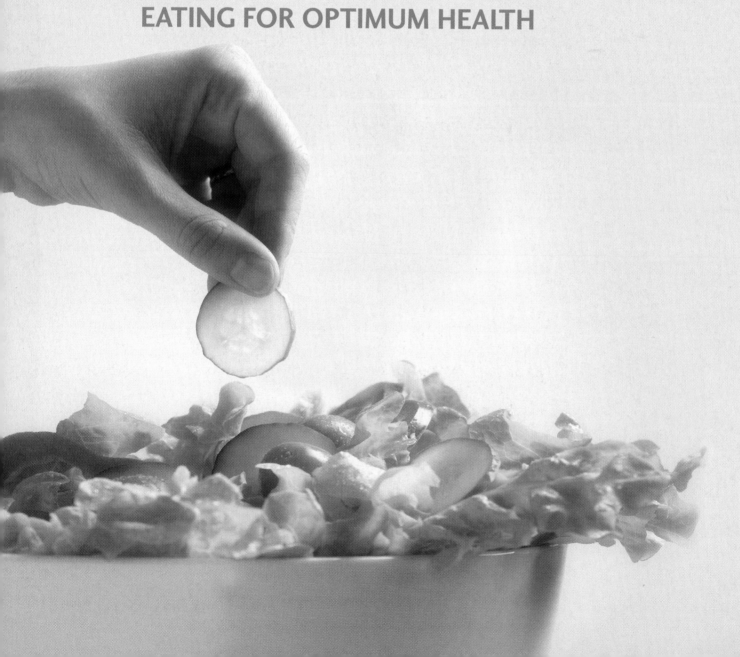

Can I get enough protein in my diet if I'm a **vegetarian**?

Will **energy** bars or drinks improve my athletic performance?

Is there really a way to make a meal from McDonald's **healthy**?

Can I substitute dietary **supplements** for a balanced diet?

How do I know if **organic** food is truly organic?

OBJECTIVES

- Understand the factors that influence dietary choices and the role major essential nutrients play in maintaining our health.
- Discuss how to change old eating habits, improve behaviors, and use the USDA MyPyramid Plan appropriately.
- Discuss the facts related to new trends and research in nutrition, including food supplements, and fads and use this information to make healthy choices.
- Discuss issues that can influence dietary needs, such as pregnancy, illness, and exercise.
- Discuss the unique problems that college students face when trying to eat healthy foods and the actions they can take to eat healthfully.
- Explain food safety concerns facing Americans and people in other regions of the world.

When was the last time you ate something without thinking about how much fat or carbohydrates it had? Did you wonder whether the calories would end up as fat on your hips or stomach, and whether the food was good or bad for you? Knowing what to eat, how much to eat, and how to choose foods that help prevent disease and promote health is not as easy as it was even 50 years ago. Today, we are bombarded with dietary regimens—from low carb to low fat to low glycemic index—that promise quick weight loss, more energy, decreased risk from disease, and other benefits. The trade-off is giving up chocolate, substituting vegetable burgers for hamburgers, tossing high-carb pizza, pasta, and baked potatoes, or adding fiber-rich flax to just about everything we eat. And, if you aren't confused and frustrated enough, you must also be concerned about the safety of the foods you eat. Are they full of preservatives and chemicals, are there pathogens lurking in them, or can you contract deadly diseases from ingesting them?

Clearly, Americans are trying to heed expert advice about how to have a healthy diet. For example, in survey after survey, 60 to 80 percent of food shoppers say they read food labels before selecting products, yet these same surveys reveal frequent misunderstandings and confusion.[1] Nutritionists, fad diet advocates, and media reports of research studies offer an array of claims and warnings (see the New Horizons in Health box on page 240). Although the Food and Drug Administration (FDA) does a remarkable job in helping to protect us, it can't possibly regulate every dietary claim or new food product that comes into the market. That means that the responsibility for making wise dietary decisions is largely yours. The good news is that, according to the American Dietetic Association, more Americans are seeking information on food and nutrition and taking action to improve their habits than ever before.[2] College students especially face nutritional challenges. Finding time to purchase and prepare meals, the cost of many high-nutrient foods, and having a well-equipped kitchen to prepare meals are just three. In addition, some students grew up in homes where their parents did not cook or follow nutrition guidelines, leaving them without the experience needed to prepare healthy meals.

Although numerous studies point to the importance of diet in overall health, many people lack the motivation or knowledge to eat for health. Just how important is sound nutrition? As an example, a hallmark review of over 4,500 research studies concluded that widespread consumption of 5 to 6 servings of fruits and vegetables daily would lower cancer rates by over 20 percent in the global population.[3] Subse-

quent research has emphasized the role of diet and nutrition in cardiovascular disease, diabetes, and a host of other chronic and disabling conditions.[4]

The next three chapters focus on fundamental principles designed to help you eat more healthy foods, avoid the problems that so many people face with their weight, and improve your general fitness. In this chapter, we will discuss basic nutrition science and apply sound principles to lifestyle behaviors. You will also gain an appreciation for why you eat as you do, the role of your family of origin and basic biology in determining your eating patterns and choices, and the resources that can help you change negative patterns while building on the healthy choices you are already making.

Assessing Eating Behaviors: Are You What You Eat?

True **hunger** occurs when there is a lack or shortage of basic foods needed to provide the energy and nutrients that support health.[5] When we are hungry, chemical messages in the brain, especially in the hypothalamus, initiate a physiological response that prompts us to seek food.[6] Although we have all experienced hunger before mealtime, few Americans have experienced the type of hunger that continues for days and threatens survival. Most of us do not eat to sustain physical survival. Instead, we eat because of our **appetite,** a learned desire to eat that may or may not have anything to do with feeling hungry. Time of day, the smell or sight of food, or other triggers often stimulate our appetite, even when we are actually full.

 Many factors influence when we eat, what we eat, and how much we eat. Finding out which triggers influence each of us, and learning to balance eating to maintain body function (eating to live) with eating to satisfy appetite (living to eat), is a constant struggle for many of us. Typical influences that make us head to the kitchen or nearest restaurant include:[7]

- *Cultural and social meanings attached to food.* From our earliest days, we learn to celebrate our family's cultural heritage with special meals or food choices, and this influences our food preferences throughout life. We learn to like the tastes of certain foods, and a yearning for sweet, salty, and high-fat foods can evolve from our earliest days. For your author, spaghetti-and-meatball dinners were a weekly event, and other Italian foods were a form of comfort food that meant family gatherings and sharing. People crave the foods they grew up eating, whether the bratwurst and beer of northern Wisconsin, the Creole and seafood of Louisiana, the hot peppers of Mexican cooking, or the curry spices of Indian dishes.
- *Convenience and availability.* You're driving by and it's right there, or it's the only convenient option.

---

hunger The physiological impulse to seek food, prompted by the lack or shortage of basic foods needed to provide the energy and nutrients that support health.

appetite The desire to eat; normally accompanies hunger but is more psychological than physiological.

- *Habit or values.* Often we select foods because they are familiar.
- *Advertising.* You saw that juicy burger on TV and decide it looks really good. You've got to have it.
- *Economy.* It seems like a good buy for the money, and you can afford it.
- *Emotional comfort.* Eating it makes you feel better—a form of reward and security. We derive pleasure or sensory delight from eating some foods.
- *Weight/body image.* You think a food will help you gain, maintain, or lose weight.
- *Social interaction.* Eating out or having company over for a meal is an enjoyable social event. We also feel pressure to eat what is offered or served.
- *Regional/seasonal trends.* Some foods may be favored in your area by season or overall climate.
- *Nutritional value and health benefits.* You think the food is good or bad for you. A new interest in **functional foods,** foods thought to enhance physiological function and improve health, motivates many people (see Chapter 23).

With all of the factors that influence our dietary choices and the wide array of foods available, the challenge of eating for health increases daily. Fortunately, we have a wealth of solid information that serves as a foundation for our decisions. **Nutrition** is the science that investigates the relationship between physiological function and the essential elements of the foods we eat. With our country's overabundance of food and vast array of choices, media that "prime" us to want the tasty morsels shown in advertisements, and easy access to almost every type of **nutrient** (proteins, carbohydrates, fats, vitamins, minerals, and water), Americans should have few nutritional problems. However, these "diets of affluence" contribute to many major diseases, including obesity-related problems with heart disease (Chapter 15), certain types of cancer (Chapter 16), diabetes (Chapter 18), hypertension (high blood pressure), cirrhosis of the liver, sleep apnea, varicose veins, gout, gallbladder disease, respiratory problems, abdominal hernias, flat feet, complications in pregnancy and surgery, and even higher accident rates, to name but a few.

Eating for Health

Generally, a healthful diet provides the proper combination of energy and nutrients. It is sufficient to keep us functioning well in our daily activities. A healthful diet should be:[8]

- *Adequate.* It provides enough of the energy, nutrients, and fiber to maintain health and essential body functions. Everyone's needs differ: a small woman who has a sedentary lifestyle may only need 1,700 calories of energy to support her body's functions. A professional bicyclist, such as Lance Armstrong, may need several thousand calories of energy to be fit for his competition. (See Table 8.1 for estimates of recommended total calories consumed per day by age and gender.)

TABLE 8.1	Estimated Daily Calorie Needs		
	Calorie Range		
	Sedentary[a]	→	Active[b]
CHILDREN			
2–3 years	1,000	→	1,400
FEMALES			
4–8 years	1,200	→	1,800
9–13	1,600	→	2,200
14–18	1,800	→	2,400
19–30	2,000	→	2,400
31–50	1,800	→	2,200
51+	1,600	→	2,200
MALES			
4–8 years	1,400	→	2,000
9–13	1,800	→	2,600
14–18	2,200	→	3,200
19–30	2,400	→	3,000
31–50	2,200	→	3,000
51+	2,000	→	2,800

[a] A lifestyle that includes only the light physical activity associated with typical day-to-day life.

[b] A lifestyle that includes physical activity equivalent to walking more than 3 miles per day at 3 to 4 miles per hour, in addition to the light physical activity associated with typical day-to-day life.

Source: Center for Nutrition Policy and Promotion, April 2005, www.MyPyramid.gov.

- *Moderate.* It often isn't what you eat that causes you to gain weight—it's the amount you consume. A **calorie** is the unit of measurement used to quantify the amount of energy we obtain from a particular food. Moderate caloric consumption, portion control, and awareness of the total amount of nutrients in the foods you eat are key aspects of dietary health.

(Text continues on page 242)

functional foods   Foods believed to be beneficial and/or to prevent disease.

nutrition   The science that investigates the relationship between physiological function and the essential elements of foods eaten.

nutrients   The constituents of food that sustain humans physiologically: proteins, carbohydrates, fats, vitamins, minerals, and water.

calorie   A unit of measure that indicates the amount of energy obtained from a particular food.

Choose margarine over butter. Choose butter over margarine. Soy products can lower cholesterol. Soy may not control cholesterol and prevent heart disease. Women should take calcium supplements. Calcium supplements might not be that beneficial. Confused by a wide range of conflicting claims? Frustrated by health food discoveries that seem to fizzle as fast as they burst onto the scene? You're not alone. In the last decade, we've been bombarded with a wide variety of conflicting scientific evidence and claims about dietary choices we can make to reduce the risk of certain diseases and promote health.

The good news is that there are positive outcomes in all of this research, and positive health effects can be gained from proper nutrition. The bad news? This plethora of studies produces conflicting reports that leave many of us scratching our heads. There are some promising new results coming out of the latest research. The jury is still out on the absolute validity of these findings, but let's take a closer look at a few.

THE SKINNY ON SOY

Soy, which contains a chemical called isoflavone, has gained considerable attention for its purported role in reducing the risk for various chronic diseases, most notably cardiovascular disease. Not sure if you should add tofu the next time you hit the salad bar? In January 2006, a committee of the American Heart Association completed a meta-analysis of years of studies on the benefits of soy. The following conclusions based on the findings can help you decide if soy is right for you.

WHAT SOY DOESN'T DO

- Soy foods do not lower cholesterol and triglyceride levels as much as previously believed and don't provide much benefit over milk or other protein. In fact, the American Heart Association concludes that soy has no significant effects on HDL cholesterol, triglycerides, lipoprotein a, or blood pressure.
- Soy proteins don't prevent hot flashes and other symptoms in menopausal women.

WHAT SOY MIGHT DO

- Researchers have not reached a conclusion on whether or not soy prevents postmenopausal bone loss in women.
- The efficacy and safety of soy for the prevention of breast, endometrial, and prostate cancer are not established; evidence from clinical trials is "meager and cautionary with regard to possible adverse effects." For this reason, soy supplements are not recommended.

WHAT SOY PROBABLY DOES

- Soy foods are a good alternative to less heart-healthy foods (particularly saturated animal fats). Soy is low in fat overall, and contains an omega-3 fatty acid that has been independently shown to reduce risks for coronary diseases.
- Soy should be beneficial to some degree because of its high polyunsaturated fat, fiber, vitamin, and mineral content.

ARE THE BENEFITS OF FISH, FISHY?

MyPyramid and other health-related statements from the American Heart Association and other professional groups extol the benefits of fish and promote it is an excellent alternative to higher fat meats and protein sources. Fish has been purported to reduce saturated fats and keep cholesterol levels down. In fact, fish is recommended for most people at least 2 times per week in lieu of red meat and other high-fat foods.

ARE THESE CLAIMS TRUE?

For the most part, these claims have been upheld in a variety of studies, particularly those that point to the benefits of the high omega-3s found in many types of fish. However, in 2005 and 2006, several studies cautioned about the risks of eating farm-raised fish because of high levels of cancer-causing PCBs and antibiotics. However, confusion over farmed versus wild fish doesn't stop there. Some studies indicate that levels of PCBs and mercury are high in wild fish as well, due to environmental contamination, and children and women who are pregnant or nursing should consume only small quantities of fish. Should you steer clear of the seafood counter and head for the poultry and meat instead?

According to the Food and Drug Administration (FDA), a variety of fish is part of a healthy diet. Avoid eating swordfish, tuna, or mackerel every day, or eat them once a month and trade off with other fish with lower mercury levels. However, at-risk groups—including pregnant and nursing women and young children—should always avoid swordfish, shark, tilefish, and king mackerel. The FDA's list of safe, low-mercury options includes shrimp, salmon, pollock, farm-raised catfish, and tilapia. Finally, if you are eating any fish, such as fresh tuna or salmon, opt for the smaller sized fish at the market. In general, smaller size means less exposure to ocean contaminants.

BONING UP ON CALCIUM

If you're like millions of Americans who are faithfully consuming calcium to ward off brittle bones, cancer, and cardiovascular disease, new research appears to throw a wrench into years of research supporting its use as a supplement. In a large, randomized, double-blind, placebo-controlled trial of over 32,000 women who received calcium and vitamin D supplements as part of the Women's Health Initiative (WHI) study, the following findings raised eyebrows:

- Women who received the calcium and vitamin D supplements over a 7-year period did not have any significantly lower risk of colorectal cancer than those who received a placebo.
- In the same WHI study, women who received the supplements were assessed to see if their risk of bone fracture was lower than the group that received no calcium or vitamin D supplements. Researchers were very surprised that there was only a slight improvement in hip bone density, but no significant reductions in hip fracture and a significantly increased risk of kidney stones in the group that received the treatment.

What does this mean for consumers? Should you throw out your calcium supplements? Most experts would tell you to continue to obtain calcium in your daily diet, and continue taking supplements. Although this was a large study, it only studied older women and only examined one form of calcium. As with all research, there is a potential for inaccuracy and factors that may skew results. More research is needed before we can change long-established recommendations, but these results pose interesting questions for future researchers.

THE LATEST ON MULTIVITAMIN SUPPLEMENTS

It's likely that most of the 52 percent of American adults who take multivitamins, at an annual cost of over $23 billion, assume that there is solid scientific evidence supporting these supplements' health benefits. However, according to yet another new report issued by a thirteen-member National Institutes of Health panel, "the present evidence is insufficient to recommend either for or against the use of multivitamins and minerals by the American public to prevent chronic diseases." The verdict? There is more to come on this issue. The committee said that much more research must be done to help make sense of the huge amount of seemingly contradictory studies about using supplements individually, or in combination.

WHAT CAN YOU DO TO MAKE SENSE OF CONFLICTING HEALTH INFORMATION?

Most people might not recognize that even the big reports published in highly respected journals are only single blips on a radar screen full of other studies that have proven just the opposite. Here is what you really need to know about reports you hear and read about in the media:

1. Remember that any single study must be viewed with caution. Often, there are other studies that may prove opposite findings, and they are no less reputable.
2. Many of these studies are "meta-analyses." This means they summarize the results of many studies, often without regard to population, study design, age of the population studied, confounders (things that could influence effects), dosage, underlying bias of the population, and many other factors.
3. Information gained from the Women's Health Initiative about diet and exercise is largely based on self-reporting. Many question the validity of some responses.

Others say that because this was such a long study, those who actually followed through and participated over time might have very different health behaviors than the average person. Even randomized, controlled trials have limitations and results should be viewed in light of potential limitations and the results of previous studies.

4. The best studies will conclude that more research must be done. Though this may seem frustrating, and may not give the definitive answers we are looking for, they are the most current and accurate responses that researchers can give.

The most sound advice? Make healthy changes that influence your entire lifestyle. Rather than taking 10 different vitamin supplements each day, eat whole, nutritious foods from each of the MyPyramid categories. Cut down on saturated animal fats, and use some soy and fish as part of a healthy diet.

Sources: F. Sacks et al., "Soy Proteins, Isoflavones, and Cardiovascular Health," *Circulation* 113 (2006):1034–1044; U.S. Food and Drug Administration, "Advisory on Mercury in Fish," March 2004, www.fda.gov; J. Wactawshi-Wende et al., "Calcium Plus Vitamin D Supplementation and the Risk of Colorectal Cancer," *New England Journal of Medicine* 354, no. 7 (2006): 684–696; R. Jackson et al., "Calcium Plus Vitamin D Supplementation and the Risk of Fractures," *New England Journal of Medicine* 354, no. 7 (2006): 669–683; *Tufts University Health and Nutrition Letter* 24, no. 6 (August 2006), 1–2; "NIH State-of-the-Science Conference Draft Statement," www.consensus.nih.gov/2006/MVMDRAFT051706.pdf; D. Mozaffarian, "Low-Fat Diet and Cardiovascular Disease," *Journal of the American Medical Association* 296, (2006): 279–280.

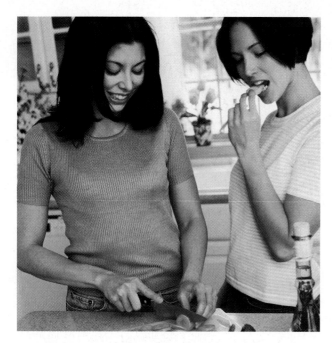

It takes information and planning to make smart menu choices, whether you are eating out, in the dining hall, or at home.

- *Balanced.* Your diet should contain the proper combination of foods from different groups. Following the recommendations for the new MyPyramid Plan, discussed later in the chapter, should help you achieve balance.
- *Varied.* Eat a lot of different foods each day. Variety helps you avoid boredom and can make it easier to keep your diet interesting and in control.

In a 30-year study of changes in consumption, women's overall caloric intake increased by 22 percent and men's by 7 percent.[9] Are we eating more food, or is it what we are eating? Trends indicate that it isn't actual amounts of food, but the amount of calories in the foods we choose to eat (see Figure 8.1). When these trends are combined with our increasingly sedentary lifestyle, it is not surprising that we have seen a dramatic rise in obesity.

Americans typically get approximately 38 percent of their calories from fat, 15 percent from proteins, 22 percent from complex carbohydrates, and 24 percent from simple sugars.[10]

Excess consumption such as this is a factor in our tendency to be overweight. However, it is not so much the quantity of food we eat that is likely to cause weight problems, but the poor nutritional content and lack of physical activity to burn the calories we consume. Nearly one-third of the calories we consume come from junk foods. Sweets and desserts, soft drinks, and alcoholic beverages make up 25 percent of those calories, and another 5 percent come from salty snacks and fruit-flavored drinks. In sharp contrast, healthy foods such as vegetables and fruit make up only 10 percent of our total calories.[11]

How much do *you* know about nutrition and healthy eating? Find out by completing the quiz in the Assess Yourself box on page 244.

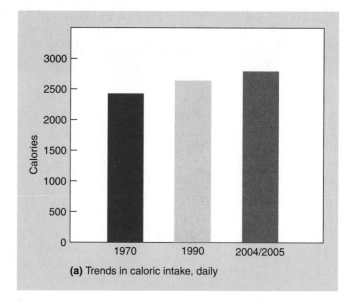

(a) Trends in caloric intake, daily

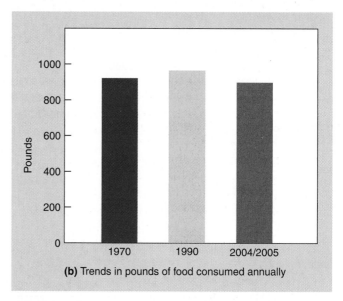

(b) Trends in pounds of food consumed annually

FIGURE 8.1 Trends in Caloric Intake and Food Consumption

Source: U.S. Department of Agriculture, "Food Consumption Patterns: How We've Changed, 1970–2005," December 2005, www.usda.gov/data/foodconsumption.

Obtaining Essential Nutrients

The Digestive Process

Food provides the chemicals we need for energy and body maintenance. Because our bodies cannot synthesize or produce certain essential nutrients, we must obtain them from the foods we eat. Before foods can be utilized properly, the digestive system must break down the larger food particles into smaller, more usable forms. The sequence of functions by which the body breaks down foods and either absorbs or excretes them is known as the **digestive process** (Figure 8.2).

Water: A Crucial Nutrient

If you were to go on a survival trip, which would you take with you—food or water? You may be surprised to learn that you could survive for much longer without food than you could without water. Even in severe conditions, the average person can go for weeks without certain vitamins and minerals before experiencing serious deficiency symptoms. **Dehydration,** however, can cause serious problems within a matter of hours; after a few days without water, death is likely. Too much water can also pose a serious risk to your health. See Chapter 8 for more on water.

Just what functions does water serve in the body? Between 50 and 60 percent of our total body weight is water. The water in our system bathes cells, aids in fluid and electrolyte balance, maintains pH balance, and transports molecules and cells throughout the body. Water is the major component of our blood, which carries oxygen and nutrients to the tissues, removes metabolic wastes, and is responsible for maintaining cells in working order.

Individual needs for water vary drastically according to dietary factors, age, size, environmental temperature and humidity levels, exercise, and the effectiveness of the individual's system. Certain diseases, such as diabetes or cystic fibrosis, cause people to lose fluids at a rate necessitating a higher volume of fluid intake.

Judging by the large number of people sucking at water bottles today, many Americans seem to fear becoming dehydrated. Bottled water has become a multimillion-dollar industry that rivals the soda industry. Is all this water consumption really necessary? See the New Horizons in Health box on page 247 about ongoing research into how much water each of us truly needs.

Is bottled water better for you than tap water? In most instances, when you buy expensive "spring" and bottled water, you are actually purchasing chlorinated city water. Some of the better bottled waters go through a process that removes chemicals. Is it worth the extra cost? Most experts think not. If you are concerned about your current water source, have it tested. Otherwise, spend your slim budget another way.

Proteins

Next to water, **proteins** are the most abundant substances in the human body. Proteins are major components of nearly every cell and have been called the "body builders" because of their role in developing and repairing bone, muscle, skin, and blood cells. Proteins are also the key elements of the antibodies that protect us from disease, of enzymes that control chemical activities in the body, and of hormones that regulate bodily functions. Moreover, proteins aid in the transport of iron, oxygen, and nutrients to all body cells and supply

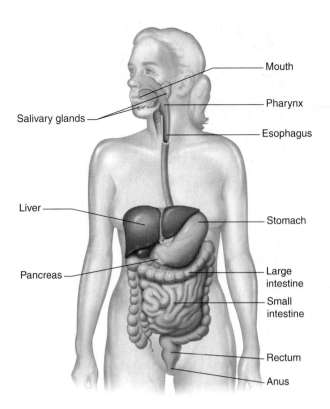

FIGURE 8.2 The Digestive Process
Your mouth prepares for the food by increasing production of saliva, which aids in chewing and swallowing, and contains important enzymes that begin the process of food breakdown. From the mouth, the food passes down the esophagus, a tube that connects the mouth and stomach, and into the stomach. Here, food is mixed by muscular contractions and is broken down with enzymes and stomach acids. Further digestive activity and absorption of nutrients takes place in the small intestine, aided by enzymes from the liver and the pancreas. Next, water and salts are reabsorbed into the system by the large intestine, and then solid waste moves into the rectum and is passed out through the anus. The entire digestive process takes approximately 24 hours.

another source of energy to cells when fats and carbohydrates are not readily available. In short, adequate amounts of protein in the diet are vital to many body functions and ultimately to survival.

(Text continues on page 246)

digestive process The process by which foods are broken down and either absorbed or excreted by the body.

dehydration Abnormal depletion of body fluids; a result of lack of water.

proteins The essential constituents of nearly all body cells; necessary for the development and repair of bone, muscle, skin, and blood; the key elements of antibodies, enzymes, and hormones.

ASSESS yourself

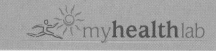

WHAT'S YOUR EQ (EATING QUOTIENT)?

Fill out this assessment online at www.aw-bc.com/myhealthlab or www.aw-bc.com/donatelle.

Keeping up with the latest on what to eat—or not eat—isn't easy. If you think a few facts might have slipped past you, this quiz should help. There's only one correct answer for each question.

	True	False
1. Fresh fruits and vegetables contain more nutrients than canned or frozen varieties.	❏	❏
2. While you are shopping, it makes a difference what area of the store you start in, in terms of keeping your foods safe.	❏	❏
3. Fruit drinks count as a serving from the fruit group in the MyPyramid Plan.	❏	❏
4. Baked potatoes have a higher glycemic index (carbohydrate's ability to raise blood sugar levels quickly) than sweet potatoes or apples.	❏	❏
5. A late dinner is more likely to cause weight gain than eating the same meal earlier in the day.	❏	❏
6. Nuts are okay to eat if you are trying to stick to a low-fat diet.	❏	❏
7. Certain foods, like grapefruit, celery, or cabbage soup, can burn fat and make you lose weight.	❏	❏

8. Which of the following has the most fiber?
   a. chuck roast
   b. dark meat chicken with skin
   c. skinless chicken wing
   d. they are all about the same

9. Which of the following is the strongest predictor of obesity in America today?
   a. region of the country you live in
   b. ethnicity/culture
   c. lack of exercise
   d. low socioeconomic status

10. When you eat a meal, how long does it take for your brain to get the message that you are full?
    a. 10 minutes
    b. 20 minutes
    c. at least an hour
    d. 2 hours or more

11. Which of the following are at the *top* of the list in bacterial levels among domestically grown vegetables?
    a. green onions, cantaloupe, and cilantro
    b. beets, potatoes, and summer squash
    c. celery, leaf lettuce, and parsley
    d. strawberries, apples, and tomatoes

12. Which of the following foods contains the most grams of fiber per serving?
    a. ½ cup of strawberries
    b. ½ cup of kidney beans
    c. 1 cup popcorn
    d. 1 medium banana

13. To insure that you are getting your antioxidants each day, which tip below would be most helpful?
    a. Eat several dark green vegetables and orange, red, and yellow fruits and vegetables.
    b. Eat at least 2 servings of lean red meat per day.
    c. Eat whole-grain foods with at least 2 grams of fiber per serving.
    d. Eat several servings of tuna and salmon per week.

14. Olive oil, one of the heart-healthy monounsaturated fats, is a great source for antioxidants. To reap the most benefits from olive oil, which recommendation should you follow?
    a. Buy it only in amounts that you will use relatively quickly. Nutrients are lost quickly after 12 months sitting on the shelf.
    b. If you buy larger bottles, separate it into smaller bottles and keep the lid on tightly to reduce oxidation from air contact. Refrigerate if possible. Refrigeration causes cloudiness but doesn't affect quality.
    c. Store it in opaque airtight glass bottles or metal tins away from heat and light.
    d. All of the above.

15. Which strategy will help you identify high-fiber breads to maximize your quality carbohydrate intake?
    a. Choose a whole-grain bread that lists a whole grain as the first ingredient.
    b. Try to purchase breads with 1 to 2 grams of fiber per slice.
    c. Look for bread that is dark colored. The darker it is, the greater the chance that it has lots of good quality fiber in its recipe.
    d. All of the above.

Answers

1. *False:* There is usually little difference, depending on how produce is handled and how quickly it reaches your supermarket. Canned and frozen produce is typically picked at its peak and may contain more nutrients than fresh produce that was picked over-ripe or too early, sat in a warehouse, spent days in transit, or sat at improper temperatures for prolonged periods. However, canned or frozen fruits and vegetables may have added salt or sugar, so check labels carefully. Whenever possible, buy produce fresh from local fields or neighboring areas.

2. *True:* As a general rule, milk, meat and other perishables that have been left at room temperature for more than 2 hours have a significant risk of conveying a foodborne illness. Be sure to factor in the time that you spend driving home from the store or running other errands. Start your shopping in the canned and nonrefrigerated sections of the store and save your meat and dairy products and frozen foods until last. Run your other errands before you shop for food, and, if you know it will take time to get home, bring a cooler with ice.

3. *False:* Even if fruit juice is an actual ingredient (often it is not), most fruit drinks are primarily water and high-fructose corn syrup or other sweeteners, colorings, and fruit flavoring. It is always better to eat the whole fruit, as you will get added fiber, more nutrients, and other benefits. Next best are 100 percent fruit juices, preferably with added vitamin C. Lowest on the nutrient quality list are the sweetened, flavored fruit drinks.

4. *True:* Unfortunately we'd probably be better off with a sweet potato or apple instead of substituting baked potatoes for fries if we are trying to keep our blood sugar levels down or control diabetes. For more information, check the glycemic index reference books available at most bookstores or use the handy guide found at www.diabetesnet.com/diabetes_food_diet/glycemic_index.php.

5. *False:* It's not when you eat but what you eat that makes a difference in weight gain. If you ate a 500-calorie salad at 10 PM and it was your only meal, you wouldn't gain weight. However, a 5,000-calorie pizza for breakfast followed by a big lunch and dinner would provide enough total calories to thicken a person's waist.

6. *True:* Although they are high in fat, nuts contain mostly unsaturated (good) fat and are good sources of protein, magnesium, and the antioxidants vitamin E and selenium. Moderation is the key. Be mindful of how many calories you are eating.

7. *False:* No foods can burn fat. Some foods with caffeine may speed up your metabolism for a short time but do not cause weight loss.

8. *D:* There is no fiber in animal foods. Fiber is found only in plants and plant-based foods such as fruits, beans, whole grains, and vegetables.

9. *D:* The greatest single predictor of obesity is low socioeconomic status. Although the other responses play a role, the poor nutritional quality of foods commonly eaten when people are forced to stretch their food budget—high-fat meats, hot dogs, inexpensive white breads and pastries, and other high-calorie, low-fiber foods—often increases the risk of obesity.

10. *B:* It takes about 20 minutes for your brain to get the message that you are full. To make sure you don't gorge yourself, eat slowly, talk with others, put your fork down after taking a bite, or take a drink of water to delay your meal. Let your brain catch up to your fork, and slow it down!

11. *A:* The bad news is that in a recent government study of bacterial levels found in domestic produce, green onions, cantaloupe, and cilantro scored the highest in positive tests for two common bacteria: *Salmonella* or *Shigella*. The good news is that out of nearly 1,100 samples, only 2 to 3 percent were contaminated, but washing your produce is still a must; run a heavy stream of water over the produce while rubbing the outside under the water.

12. *B:* One-half cup of kidney beans provides 4.5 grams of fiber; the medium banana has 2 grams of fiber; strawberries and popcorn each have 1 gram of fiber per serving.

13. *A:* Antioxidants, particularly vitamins C and E, the mineral selenium, and plant pigments known as carotenoids (which include beta-carotene) are found in green leafy vegetables and orange, yellow, and red vegetables and fruit. Eating several servings of these per day helps avoid risks from several health problems.

14. *D:* Olive oil does lose nutrients over time, with one year being the general guesstimate of "use by" time. If the oil smells rancid or if you note mold or other discoloration, discard the bottle.

15. *A:* A true whole-grain bread clearly says so on the label (e.g., "100 percent whole wheat" or "100 percent stone ground whole wheat"). If all the ingredients aren't whole grain, then it's not a true whole-grain bread. The more fiber in each slice the better; look for a minimum of 3 grams. Color is not a good indicator of nutrient value. Dyes and coloring may make even the whitest white bread brown.

(continued)

Scoring

If you answered all of the above correctly, congratulations! You clearly have a good sense of some of the current issues and facts surrounding dietary choices. If you missed one or more questions, read the corresponding section of this chapter to find out more. Don't despair. Nutrition information changes rapidly, and there is a wealth of information available. Check with your instructor for courses you can take to increase your nutritional knowledge. Review the resources that are recommended, and work hard to stay current.

MAKE it happen!

ASSESSMENT: The Assess Yourself activity above gave you the chance to test your knowledge of the health effects of various foods. Now that you have considered these results, you can decide whether you need to do more to keep up on what to eat (and not eat) for long-tern health.

MAKING A CHANGE: In order to change your behavior, you need to develop a plan. Follow these steps below and complete your Behavior Change Contract to take action.

1. Evaluate your behavior and identify patterns and specific things you are doing. What can you change now? What can you change in the near future?

2. Select one pattern of behavior that you want to change.

3. Fill out the Behavior Change Contract found at the front of your book. It should include your long-term goal for change, your short-term goals, the rewards you'll give yourself for reaching these goals, potential obstacles along the way, and strategies for overcoming these obstacles. For each goal, list the small steps and specific actions that you will take.

4. Chart your progress in a journal. At the end of a week, consider how successful you were in following your plan. What helped you be successful? What made change more difficult? What will you do differently next week?

5. Revise your plan as needed: Are the short-term goals attainable? Are the rewards satisfying?

ONE STUDENT'S PLAN: Tara was surprised to see that she had very little idea about what foods to eat and to avoid. She decided to keep track of her normal diet for a week and then to evaluate it in light of some of the guidelines in this chapter. She was surprised to find that she was eating less than 2 servings of vegetables a day, instead of the recommended 3 to 5. Tara looked at her eating patterns and saw several times during the week where she snacked on foods that could be replaced with other, healthier snacks. She decided to carry carrot sticks in her backpack. They stayed fresh all day and made a good snack between classes instead of a candy bar. She also found that her favorite Mexican restaurant offered a vegetarian burrito full of black beans and vegetables; it was even tastier than her usual pork burrito. At the end of the first week, Tara and her friends decided to order pizza. Instead of getting pepperoni or sausage, Tara suggested a pizza with green peppers, spinach, and onions as toppings. Tara did have a setback when she went to a baseball game and ate peanuts and hot dogs all day, but the next day she had a salad for lunch and saw that her vegetable consumption was almost at her goal.

Tara's goal for the next week is to continue to substitute healthy snacks and to look for healthier alternatives when she is eating out. When she is consistently eating the recommended servings of vegetables each week, she will start focusing on other parts of her diet that could use improvement. She is already thinking about how to replace some of the sugary breakfast cereals she eats now with healthier options.

---

amino acids   The building blocks of protein.

essential amino acids   Nine of the basic nitrogen-containing building blocks of protein that must be obtained from foods to ensure health.

complete (high-quality) proteins   Proteins that contain all of the nine essential amino acids.

Whenever you consume proteins, your body breaks them down into smaller molecules known as **amino acids,** which link together like beads in a necklace to form 20 different combinations. Nine of these combinations are termed **essential amino acids,** meaning that the body must obtain them from the diet; the other 11 are produced by the body.

Dietary proteins that supply all of the essential amino acids are called **complete (high-quality) proteins.** Typically,

NEW HORIZONS in health

HOW MUCH WATER DO WE NEED?

How much water do we really need? According to a generation of health experts, we should drink eight 8-ounce glasses per day, not including caffeinated beverages. Not until recently had anyone really questioned what scientific evidence there was for that recommendation. That is when Dr. Heinz Valtin, professor emeritus at Dartmouth Medical School and an expert on how the body maintains fluid balance, began to assess the basis for the 64-ounce/day concept. He determined that the advice probably stems from a muddled interpretation of a 1945 Food and Nutrition Board report that said the body needs about 1 milliliter of water for each calorie consumed—almost 8 cups for a typical 2,000-calorie diet. That advice is probably sound; however, it does not account for the fact that most of this quantity is contained in prepared foods. (Fruits and vegetables are 80 to 95 percent water, meats contain over 50 percent water, and even dry bread and cheese are about 35 percent water.) Dr. Valtin was unable to determine how the report came to be interpreted as recommending eight glasses of pure water per day. Nor did he find any supporting research showing that the average person needs 64 ounces of fluid from any source per day, whether from foods or beverages.

Another key finding of Dr. Valtin's group was that, contrary to popular opinion, caffeinated drinks don't dehydrate the person who consumes them; in fact, coffee, tea, and sodas are actually hydrating for people used to caffeine and, thus, should count toward overall fluid intake.

So, should you continue to pay for all those bottles of water? (See Chapter 21 for information on the environmental effect of the plastic from all those bottles.) If you're drinking water for the health benefits of those eight additional glasses per day, you may be disappointed. For most of us, adding that much water to what we are already getting just means more trips to the bathroom with little harm done—an expensive habit with few rewards. Furthermore, people with certain medical conditions can put undue stress on the bladder and other systems or can excrete more water-soluble vitamins than they would if they had not been drinking so much.

The Food and Nutrition Board has revised its recommendations, and new water-intake guidelines are available on its website at www.iom.edu/board.asp?id=3788. In the meantime, everyone agrees that drinking water is important. The question is whether or not you are already getting close to the right amount with food, juice, milk, soda, coffee, and other fluid sources. Students who aren't eating properly, those who exercise heavily and sweat profusely, and those who aren't getting adequate fluids to compensate for fluid losses may need to pay attention to this. Older people with diminished mental capacity or people on diuretics for heart conditions can also become water depleted and experience serious consequences.

Source: H. Valtin, "Water Consumption Needs: A Look at the Accumulated Evidence," *American Journal of Physiology* 283, no. 5 (2002): 88–94.

---

protein from animal products is complete. When we consume foods that are deficient in some of the essential amino acids, the total amount of protein that can be synthesized from the other amino acids is decreased. For proteins to be complete, they must also be present in digestible form and in amounts proportional to body requirements.

What about plant sources of protein? Proteins from plant sources are often **incomplete proteins** in that they lack one or two of the essential amino acids. Nevertheless, it is relatively easy for the nonmeat eater to combine plant foods effectively and eat complementary sources of plant protein (Figure 8.3 on page 248). An excellent example of this mutual supplementation process is eating peanut butter on whole-grain bread. Although each of these foods lacks certain essential amino acids, eating them together provides high-quality protein.

Plant sources of protein fall into three general categories: legumes (beans, peas, peanuts, and soy products), grains (wheat, corn, rice and oats), and nuts and seeds. Certain vegetables, such as leafy green vegetables and broccoli, also

Can I get enough protein in my diet if I'm a vegetarian?

contribute valuable plant proteins. Mixing two or more foods from each of these categories during the same meal will provide all of the essential amino acids necessary to ensure adequate protein absorption. People who are not interested in obtaining all of their protein from plants can combine incomplete plant proteins with complete low-fat animal proteins such as chicken, fish, turkey, and lean red meat. Low-fat or nonfat cottage cheese, skim milk, egg whites, and nonfat dry milk all provide high-quality proteins and have few calories and little dietary fat. Soy provides an excellent option for many people and is growing in popularity as soy products become more flavorful.

incomplete proteins   Proteins that are lacking in one or more of the essential amino acids.

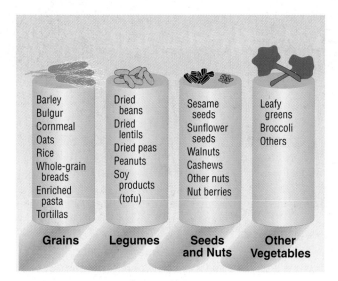

FIGURE 8.3 **Complementary Proteins**

Source: Adapted from J. Thompson and M. Manore, *Nutrition: An Applied Approach* (San Francisco: Benjamin Cummings, 2005).

Group	RDA (g/kg)
Most adults	= 0.8
Nonvegetarian endurance athletes	= 1.2–1.4
Nonvegetarian strength athletes	= 1.6–1.7
Vegetarian endurance athletes	= 1.3–1.5
Vegetarian strength athletes	= 1.7–1.8

40 grams

Calculating Your Protein RDA

1. Determine your body weight.
2. Convert pounds to kilograms (lb ÷ 2.2 lb/kg = kilograms).
3. Multiply by 0.8 g/kg (average adult RDA) to get an RDA in kilograms per day.

Example

1. Weight = 110 lbs
2. 110 ÷ 2.2 lbs/kg = 50 kg
3. 50 kg × 0.8 g/kg average adult = 40 g

Results: a 110-lb person would have an RDA of 40 g of protein.

FIGURE 8.4 **Calculating Your Protein RDA**

Source: Adapted from J. Thompson and M. Manore, *Nutrition: An Applied Approach* (San Francisco: Benjamin Cummings, 2005).

You need to eat enough protein, but make sure you don't overdo it. Eating too much protein, particularly animal protein, can place added stress on the liver and kidneys. Protein-rich foods can also be high-fat foods, contributing to weight gain.

In recent years, several low-calorie diets that practically eliminate carbohydrates and focus on eating large quantities of protein have reemerged in the popular press. Diets that deviate from a balanced nutritional approach are almost certainly flawed. In particular, people who have kidney or liver problems or suffer from fluid imbalances should avoid such diets. For more information, see the following section on carbohydrates and Chapter 9 on weight management.

A person might need to eat extra protein if fighting off a serious infection, recovering from surgery or blood loss, or recovering from burns. In these instances, proteins that are lost to cellular repair must be replaced. There is considerable controversy over whether someone in high-level physical training needs additional protein to build and repair muscle fibers or whether normal daily requirements should suffice.

Although protein deficiency continues to pose a threat to the global population, few Americans suffer from protein deficiencies. In fact, the average American consumes more than 100 grams of protein daily, and about 70 percent of this comes from high-fat animal flesh and dairy products.[12] The recommended protein intake for adults is only 0.8 gram per kilogram of body weight per day. The typical recommendation is that, in a 2,000-calorie diet, 10 to 35 percent of calories should come from protein, for a total average of 50 to 175 grams per day (a 6-ounce steak contains 53 grams of protein—more than the entire daily needs of an average-sized woman!). See Figure 8.4 to determine your daily protein requirement.

Carbohydrates

Although proteins in the body are certainly important, it is **carbohydrates** that supply us with the energy needed to sustain normal daily activity. Carbohydrates can actually be metabolized more quickly and efficiently than proteins and are a quick source of energy for the body, being easily converted to glucose, the fuel for the body's cells. These foods also play an important role in the functioning of internal organs, the nervous system, and the muscles. They are the best fuel for endurance athletics because they provide both an immediate and a timed-release energy source as they are digested easily and then consistently metabolized in the bloodstream.

carbohydrates Basic nutrients that supply the body with glucose, the energy form most commonly used to sustain normal activity.

There are two major types of carbohydrates: **simple sugars,** which are found primarily in fruits, and **complex carbohydrates,** which are found in grains, cereals, dark green leafy vegetables, yellow fruits and vegetables (carrots, yams), *cruciferous* vegetables (such as broccoli, cabbage, and cauliflower), and certain tuberous vegetables, such as potatoes. Most of us do not get enough complex carbohydrates in our daily diets.

A typical American diet contains large amounts of simple sugars. The most common form is *glucose.* Eventually, the human body converts all types of simple sugars to glucose to provide energy to cells; glucose is the only energy form used by the brain. In its natural form, glucose is sweet and is obtained from substances such as corn syrup, honey, molasses, vegetables, and fruits. *Fructose* is another simple sugar found in fruits and berries. Glucose and fructose are **monosaccharides** that contain only one molecule of sugar.

Disaccharides are combinations of two monosaccharides. Perhaps the best-known example is granulated table sugar (known as sucrose), which consists of a molecule of fructose chemically bonded to a molecule of glucose. Lactose, found in milk and milk products, is another form of disaccharide, formed by the combination of glucose and galactose (another simple sugar). Disaccharides must be broken down into simple sugars before they can be used by the body.

Controlling the amount of sugar in your diet can be difficult because it can be hidden in certain foods. Such diverse items as ketchup, Russian dressing, Coffee-mate, and Shake 'n' Bake derive 30 to 65 percent of their calories from sugar. Read food labels carefully and avoid purchasing anything in which the first ingredient is high-fructose corn syrup. Additionally, experts recommend eating whole fruit and avoiding products with corn syrup or fruit juices that are often high in added sugar and low on actual fruit.

Complex carbohydrates, or **polysaccharides,** are formed by long chains of saccharides. Like disaccharides, they must be broken down into simple sugars before the body can utilize them. There are two major forms of complex carbohydrates: *starches* and *fiber,* or **cellulose.**

Starches make up the majority of the complex carbohydrate group. Starches in our diet come from flours, breads, pasta, potatoes, and related foods. They are stored in body muscles and the liver in a polysaccharide form called **glycogen.** When the body requires a sudden burst of energy, it quickly uses up the available store of glucose and then breaks down glycogen into more glucose.

Will energy bars or drinks improve my athletic performance?

Carbohydrates and Athletic Performance Over the past decade, carbohydrates have become the "health food" of many athletes. Some fitness enthusiasts consume concentrated sugary foods, drinks, or sports bars before or during athletic activity, thinking that the sugars will provide extra energy. This may actually be counterproductive.

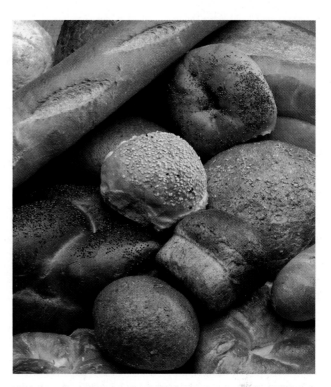

Understanding the role of carbohydrates in your body, and the differences between simple carbohydrates and complex carbohydrates, will help you make wise decisions about your eating patterns.

One possible problem involves the gastrointestinal tract. If your intestines react to activity (like nervousness before competition) by moving material through the small intestine more rapidly than usual, undigested disaccharides and/or unabsorbed monosaccharides will reach the colon, which can result in an inopportune bout of diarrhea.

Consuming large amounts of sugar during exercise can also have a negative effect on hydration. Concentrations exceeding 24 grams of sugar per 8 ounces of fluid can delay stomach emptying and hence absorption of water. Some fruit juices, fruit drinks, and other sugar-sweetened beverages

simple sugars A major type of carbohydrate, which provide short-term energy.

complex carbohydrates A major type of carbohydrate, which provide sustained energy.

monosaccharides Simple sugars that contain only one molecule of sugar.

disaccharides Combinations of two monosaccharides.

polysaccharides Complex carbohydrates formed by the combination of long chains of saccharides.

cellulose Fiber; a major form of complex carbohydrates.

glycogen The polysaccharide form in which glucose is stored in the liver and, to a lesser extent, in muscles.

TABLE 8.2 Artificial Sweeteners

Sweetener	Best Use	Caution
Acesulfame-K (Sunett and Sweet One)	As a tabletop sweetener; also found in thousands of products, such as baked goods and soft drinks	Some people complain of an unpleasant aftertaste.
Aspartame (NutraSweet and Equal)	As a tabletop sweetener; also found in products like gum, cereals, sodas, and a range of other food items	It is not ideal for cooking or baking. Don't use if you have phenylketonuria; the disorder prevents a chemical in aspartame from being metabolized.
Neotame	In foods ranging from frozen desserts to jams and jellies	It is relatively new, so long-term side effects aren't yet known.
Saccharin (Sweet'N Low and Sweet Twin)	As a tabletop sweetener; also found in hard candy, baked goods, soft drinks, and chewing gum	Not ideal for baking.
Sorbitol, mannitol, and maltitol	In sugar-free ice cream, cookies, and other products	These sugar alcohols can cause bloating, gas, and diarrhea when consumed in large amounts.
Stevia	As a tabletop sweetener	It's considered an herbal supplement, so it hasn't been reviewed by the FDA.
Sucralose (sold as Splenda)	As a tabletop sweetener; also found in more than 4,000 food products such as fruit juices and baked goods	Since it's a relative newcomer, long-term side effects are not yet known.
Tagatose	In some 7-Eleven diet Slurpee drinks	It may cause flatulence, bloating, and nausea when consumed in large amounts.

Source: U.S. Food and Drug Administration, "Artificial Sweeteners: No Calories . . . Sweet!" *FDA Consumer Magazine,* July–August 2006, www.fda.gov/fdac.

have more than this amount of sugar. If you use these products, dilute them with ice cubes or water.

Marathon runners and other people who require reserves of energy for demanding tasks often attempt to increase stores of glycogen in the body by *carbohydrate loading.* This process involves modifying the nature of both workouts and diet, usually during the week or so before competition. The athletes train very hard early in the week while eating small amounts of carbohydrates. Right before competition, they dramatically increase their intake of carbohydrates to force the body to store more glycogen, which can then be used during endurance activities (such as the last miles of a marathon).

Is Sugar Addictive?

Although some media reports have suggested that sugar might be addictive, recent research has essentially debunked this myth.[13] Our taste for sweetness is acquired early on in life, based on a preference for sweet or salty foods.

Preference for sweets is also part of our cultural heritage, with indications that we develop a taste for sugar based on learned eating patterns. Culture, genetics, and other factors

appear to be reasons why some of us love sugar far too much. The keys are to monitor sugar intake and eat sweet foods in moderation. Many artificial sweeteners are also available today. See Table 8.2 to see how they compare.

Carbohydrates and Weight Loss The low-carb craze captured the nationwide attention of millions of would-be dieters who started dumping their carbohydrates for programs such as the Atkins Diet, Protein Power, The Zone, South Beach, and other diet plans. As Americans bought into the low-carb diet trend, sales of items such as white bread and pasta took a dive, while an entire low-carb/no-carb industry emerged. Though the interest in extreme carb reduction plans seems to be waning, one positive legacy of these diet plans is that they educated consumers and the food industry on the importance of whole-grain, high-fiber, and low-sugar food choices.

Fiber

Fiber, often referred to as "bulk" or "roughage," is the indigestible portion of plant foods that helps move foods through the digestive system, delays absorption of cholesterol and other nutrients, and softens stools by absorbing water. Fiber also helps to control weight by creating a feeling of fullness without adding extra calories and appears to reduce risk from heart disease.[14] In spite of much advocacy of fiber, the average American consumes between 12 and 17 grams of

fiber The indigestible portion of plant foods that helps move foods through the digestive system and softens stools by absorbing water.

fiber a day, about half the recommended daily amount of 20 to 35 grams.[15]

Insoluble fiber, which is found in bran, whole-grain breads and cereals, and most fruits and vegetables, is associated with gastrointestinal benefits and has also been found to reduce the risk for several forms of cancer. *Soluble fiber* appears to be a factor in lowering blood cholesterol levels and reducing risk for cardiovascular disease. Major sources of soluble fiber in the diet include oat bran, dried beans (such as kidney, garbanzo, pinto, and navy beans), and some fruits and vegetables.

What's the best way to increase your intake of dietary fiber? Eat more complex carbohydrates, such as whole grains, fruits, vegetables, dried peas and beans, nuts, and seeds. As with most nutritional advice, however, too much of a good thing can pose problems. Sudden increases in dietary fiber may cause flatulence (intestinal gas), cramping, or a bloated feeling. Consume plenty of water or other liquids to reduce such side effects.

A few years ago, fiber was thought to be the remedy for just about everything. Much of this hope was probably unrealistic, although research does support many benefits of fiber, such as:[16]

- *Protection against colon and rectal cancer.* One of the leading causes of cancer deaths in the United States, colorectal cancer is much rarer in countries having diets high in fiber and low in animal fat. Several studies have contributed to the theory that fiber-rich diets, particularly those including insoluble fiber, prevent the development of precancerous growths. Whether this is because more fiber helps to move foods through the colon faster (thereby reducing the colon's contact time with cancer-causing substances) or because insoluble fiber reduces bile acids and certain bacterial enzymes that may promote cancer remains in question. Amidst current research, the controversy continues over the mechanics and potential health benefits of fiber alone.

- *Protection against breast cancer.* Research into the effects of fiber on breast cancer risk is inconclusive. However, some studies indicate that wheat bran (rich in insoluble fiber) reduces blood estrogen levels, which may affect the risk for breast cancer. Another theory is that people who eat more fiber have proportionally less fat in their diets and this is what reduces overall risk.

- *Protection against constipation.* Insoluble fiber, consumed with adequate fluids, is the safest, most effective way to prevent or treat constipation. The fiber acts like a sponge, absorbing moisture and producing softer, bulkier stools that are easily passed. Fiber also helps produce gas, which in turn may initiate a bowel movement.

- *Protection against diverticulosis.* About one American in ten over the age of 40 and at least one in three over age 50 suffers from diverticulosis, a condition in which tiny bulges or pouches form on the large intestinal wall. These bulges can become irritated and cause chronic pain if under strain from constipation. Insoluble fiber helps to reduce constipation and discomfort.

- *Protection against heart disease.* Many studies have indicated that soluble fiber (as in oat bran, barley, and fruit pectin) helps reduce blood cholesterol, primarily by lowering LDL ("bad") cholesterol. Whether this reduction is a direct effect or occurs instead through the displacement of fat calories by fiber calories or through intake of other nutrients, such as iron, remains in question.[17]

- *Protection against diabetes.* Some studies suggest that soluble fiber improves control of blood sugar and can reduce the need for insulin or medication in people with diabetes. Exactly why isn't clear, but soluble fiber seems to delay the emptying of the stomach and slow the absorption of glucose by the intestine.

- *Protection against obesity.* Because most high-fiber foods are high in carbohydrates and low in fat, they help control caloric intake. Many take longer to chew, which slows you down at the table, and fiber stays in the digestive tract longer than other nutrients, making you feel full sooner.

Most experts believe that Americans should double their current consumption of dietary fiber—to 20 to 35 grams per day for most people and perhaps to 40 to 50 grams for others. (A large bowl of high-fiber cereal with a banana provides close to 20 grams of fiber.) Tips for increasing your fiber intake include:

- Whenever possible, select whole-grain breads, especially those that are low in fat and sugars. Choose breads with three or more grams of fiber per serving. Read labels—just because bread is brown doesn't mean it is better for you. (See the Skills for Behavior Change box on page 252 for more on whole grains.)

- Eat the fruits and vegetables (with skin) rather than drinking their juices. The fiber in the whole fruit tends to slow blood sugar increases by comparison to juice, and helps us feel full longer.

- Substitute whole-grain pastas, bagels, and pizza crust for the refined, white flour versions.

- Add wheat crumbs, or grains to meat loaf and burgers to increase fiber intake.

- Toast grains to bring out their nutty flavor and make foods more appealing.

- Sprinkle ground flaxseed on cereals, yogurt, and salads, or add to casseroles, burgers, and baked goods. Flaxseeds have a mild flavor and are also high in beneficial omega-3 fatty acids.

Fats

Fats (or *lipids*)—another group of basic nutrients—are perhaps the most misunderstood of the body's required energy

fats Basic nutrients composed of carbon and hydrogen atoms; needed for the proper functioning of cells, insulation of body organs against shock, maintenance of body temperature, and healthy skin and hair.

A CONSUMER GUIDE TO WHOLE-GRAIN GOODNESS

It's hard to beat whole grains. They are packed with vitamins, minerals, and fiber that you just can't find in white bread, processed cereals, or white rice. How can you tell the difference between the various types of bread choices on the supermarket shelves these days? There's multigrain, whole-grain, whole-wheat, sprouted-wheat, cracked-wheat, 12-grain, high-fiber, brown, and now, even white multigrain bread on the shelves.

First, it is important to recognize that a bread's color, texture, and even fiber content may not reflect its whole-grain content. Next, look at the ingredients. Choose the bread with the shortest list of ingredients and be wary of added sugar and sodium. *Whole*-grain kernels (it should actually say whole) should be the first ingredient. These kernels are the unprocessed grain and they pack a nutritional punch of fiber, complex carbohydrates like potassium, vitamin E, the B vitamins (thiamine, riboflavin, niacin, and folate), and minerals (iron, magnesium, and selenium). Be aware that "multigrain" or "7-grain" breads aren't necessarily made from a whole-grain product. Breads that say, "made from whole grain" probably aren't 100 percent whole grain either.

Finally, look at the fiber content (see figure). Your bread of choice should have at least 3 grams of fiber per serving. Now, you can choose bread that truly will fit into your healthful and nutritious meal plan.

Total Carbohydrate 20g

Dietary Fiber 1g

Sugars 4g

INGREGIENTS: **UNBLEACHED ENRICHED WHEAT FLOUR** [FLOUR, MALTED BARLEY FLOUR, REDUCED IRON, NIACIN, THIAMIN MONONITRATE (VITAMIN B1), RIBOFLAVIN (VITAMIN B2), FOLIC ACID], **BUTTERMILK**, HIGH FRUCTOSE CORN SYRUP, SOYBEAN OIL, YEAST, SALT, MONO- AND DIGLYCERIDES, CALCIUM PROPINATE (PRESERVATIVE), **SOY LECITHIN**

(a) Regular white bread label

Total Carbohydrate 18g

Dietary Fiber 5g

Sugars 3g

INGREDIENTS: **WHOLE WHEAT FLOUR**, WATER, SUGAR, INULIN, **SOY FIBER**, WHEAT GLUTEN, YEAST, SOYBEAN OIL, WHEAT BRAN, SALT, MOLASSES, MONO- AND DIGLYCERIDES, CALCIUM PROPIONATE, (PRESERVATIVE), DATEM, CALCIUM CARBONATE, VITAMIN D3, MONOCALCIUM, PHOSPHATE, SOY LECITHIN, **WHEY**, SOY FLOUR*, **NONFAT MILK**
*Trivial amount of soy flour.

(b) 100 percent whole-grain bread label

sources. Fats play a vital role in maintaining healthy skin and hair, insulating body organs against shock, maintaining body temperature, and promoting healthy cell function. Fats make foods taste better and carry the fat-soluble vitamins A, D, E, and K to the cells. They also provide a concentrated form of energy in the absence of sufficient carbohydrates.

So why, if fats perform all these functions, are we constantly urged to cut back on them? Although moderate consumption of fats is essential to health, overconsumption can be dangerous. **Triglycerides,** which make up about 95 percent of total body fat, are the most common form of fat circulating in the blood. When we consume too many calories, the liver converts the excess into triglycerides, which are stored throughout our bodies.

triglycerides The most common form of fat in the body; excess calories consumed are converted into triglycerides and stored as body fat.

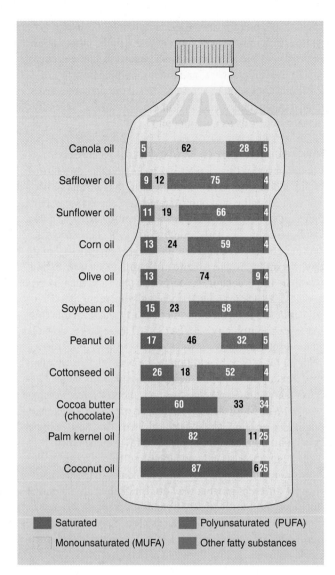

■ Saturated   ■ Polyunsaturated (PUFA)

■ Monounsaturated (MUFA)   ■ Other fatty substances

FIGURE 8.5 Percentages of Saturated, Polyunsaturated, and Monounsaturated Fats in Common Vegetable Oils

The remaining 5 percent of body fat is composed of substances such as **cholesterol,** which can accumulate on the inner walls of arteries, causing a narrowing of the channel through which blood flows. This buildup, called **plaque,** is a major cause of *atherosclerosis* (hardening of the arteries). The ratio of total cholesterol to a group of compounds called **high-density lipoproteins (HDLs)** is important in determining risk for heart disease. Lipoproteins are the transport facilitators for cholesterol in the blood. High-density lipoproteins are capable of transporting more cholesterol than are **low-density lipoproteins (LDLs).** Whereas LDLs transport cholesterol to the body's cells, HDLs apparently transport circulating cholesterol to the liver for metabolism and elimination from the body. People with a high percentage of HDLs therefore appear to be at lower risk for developing cholesterol-clogged arteries. Regular vigorous exercise plays a part in reducing cholesterol by increasing high-density lipoproteins. (See Chapter 15.)

PUFAs and MUFAs: Unsaturated "Good Guys"
Fat cells consist of chains of carbon and hydrogen atoms. Those that are unable to hold any more hydrogen in their chemical structure are labeled **saturated fats.** They generally come from animal sources, such as meats and dairy products, and are solid at room temperature. **Unsaturated fats,** which come from plants and include most vegetable oils, are generally liquid at room temperature and have room for additional hydrogen atoms in their chemical structure. The terms *monounsaturated fat (MUFA)* and *polyunsaturated fat (PUFA)* refer to the relative number of hydrogen atoms that are missing. Peanut and olive oils are high in monounsaturated fats, whereas corn, sunflower, and safflower oils are high in polyunsaturated fats.

There is currently a great deal of controversy about which type of unsaturated fat is most beneficial. Many believe that PUFAs may decrease beneficial HDL levels as well as the harmful LDL. PUFAs come in two forms: omega-3 fatty acids and omega-6 fatty acids. MUFAs, such as olive oil, seem to lower LDL levels and increase HDL levels and thus are currently the "preferred," or least harmful, fats. Nevertheless, one tablespoon of olive oil gives you a hefty 10 grams of MUFAs. For a breakdown of the types of fats in common vegetable oils, see Figure 8.5.

Reducing Total Fat in Your Diet
Want to cut the fat? These guidelines offer a good place to start (for more on low-fat diets, see Chapter 9):

■ *Know what you are putting in your mouth.* Read food labels. No more than 10 percent of your total calories should come from saturated fat, and no more than 30 percent should come from all forms of fat.

■ *Use olive oil for baking and sautéing.* Animal studies have shown that olive oil doesn't raise cholesterol or promote the growth of tumors.

cholesterol A form of fat circulating in the blood that can accumulate on the inner walls of arteries, causing a narrowing of the channel through which blood flows.

plaque Cholesterol buildup on the inner walls of arteries; a major cause of atherosclerosis.

high-density lipoproteins (HDLs) Compounds that facilitate the transport of cholesterol in the blood to the liver for metabolism and elimination from the body.

low-density lipoproteins (LDLs) Compounds that facilitate the transport of cholesterol in the blood to the body's cells.

saturated fats Fats that are unable to hold any more hydrogen in their chemical structure; derived mostly from animal sources; solid at room temperature.

unsaturated fats Fats that do have room for more hydrogen in their chemical structure; derived mostly from plants; liquid at room temperature.

- *Whenever possible, avoid margarine products with trans fatty acids* (see the next section).
- *Choose lean meats, fish, or poultry.* Remove skin. Broil or bake whenever possible. In general, the more well done the meat, the fewer the calories. Drain off fat after cooking.
- *Choose fewer cold cuts, sausages, hot dogs, organ meats, and bacon.* Be careful of products claiming to be "95 percent fat free"—they may still have high levels of fat.
- *Select nonfat dairy products whenever possible.* Part-skim-milk cheeses such as mozzarella, farmer's, lappi, and ricotta are good choices.
- *When cooking, use substitutes for butter, margarine, oils, sour cream, mayonnaise, and salad dressings.* Chicken broth, fresh herbs, wine, vinegar, and low-calorie dressings provide flavor with less fat.
- *Think of your food intake as an average over a day or a couple of days.* If you have a high-fat breakfast or lunch, balance it with a low-fat dinner.

Avoiding *Trans* Fatty Acids

For decades, Americans have shunned saturated fats found in butter, certain cuts of red meat, and a host of other foods. What they didn't know is that foods low in saturated fat, such as margarine, can be just as bad for us. As early as the 1990s, Dutch researchers reported that a form of fat, known as *trans* fats, increased LDL (bad) cholesterol levels while decreasing HDL (good) cholesterol. In a more recent study, researchers concluded that just a 2 percent caloric intake of *trans* fats was associated with an increased risk for CHD of 23 percent and a 47 percent increased chance of sudden cardiac death. Importantly, they estimated that nearly 228,000 coronary and heart disease-related deaths in the United States could be averted each year by reducing Americans' consumption of *trans* fats.[18]

What are **trans fats (*trans* fatty acids)**? *Trans* fats are fatty acids that are produced by adding hydrogen molecules to liquid oil to make the oil into a solid. These "partially hydrogenated" fats (unlike regular fats and oils, they stay solid or semisolid at room temperature) change into irregular shapes at the molecular level, priming them to clog up arteries. *Trans* fats are used in margarines, many commercial baked goods, and restaurant deep-fried foods.

In January 2006, the Food and Drug Administration finally took action and required labeling that tells consumers how much *trans* fat is in that cookie they are putting into their mouths. The evidence against *trans* fats was too overwhelming to ignore any longer. However, keep in mind that the new labels don't require listing *trans* fats for foods containing less than 500 milligrams per serving. If a product claims no *trans* fats, it just contains less than 500 mg.

trans fatty acids (*trans* fats) Fatty acids that are produced when polyunsaturated oils are hydrogenated to make them more solid.

What's the bottom line? Moderation in all fat intake is the best rule of thumb. Whenever possible, opt for other condiments on your bread, such as fresh vegetable spreads, sugar-free jams, fat-free cheese, and other toppings. Be wary of fried foods cooked in restaurants, and avoid prepared cakes, cookies, potato chips, and anything else that lists "partially hydrogenated" oils as an ingredient.

New Fat Advice: Is More Fat Ever Better?

Although most of this chapter has promoted the long-term recommendation to reduce saturated fat, avoid *trans* fatty acids, and eat more monounsaturated fats, some researchers worry that we have gone too far in our antifat frenzy. In fact, according to some experts, our zeal to eat no-fat or low-fat foods may be one of the greatest causes of obesity in America today. According to the American Heart Association, eating fewer than 15 percent of our calories as fat (less than 34 g per day on a 2,000-calorie diet) can actually increase blood triglycerides to levels that promote heart disease, while lowering levels of protective HDLs. See Chapter 15 for new classifications of cholesterol levels.

Not all fat is bad. In addition to the benefits already mentioned, dietary fat supplies the two essential fatty acids (EFAs) that we must receive from our diets, *linoleic acid* and *alpha-linolenic acid*. These two fats are needed to make hormonelike compounds that control immune function, pain perception, and inflammation, to name a few key benefits.[19]

Although linoleic acid and alpha-linolenic acid are both polyunsaturated fats and have similar names, they are actually quite different in what they do. Linoleic acid, a member of the omega-6 family of fats (found in soybeans, peanuts, corn, and sunflower seeds), reduces blood levels of total cholesterol and "bad" cholesterol (LDL) when consumed in reasonable amounts. Alpha-linolenic acid is part of the *omega-3* family of fats and is found in flax, canola oil, sardines, spinach, kale, green leafy vegetables, walnuts, and wheat germ. Alpha-linolenic acid is converted to two other beneficial omega-3 fats in the body, but you get a much bigger dose of those nutrients by eating cold-water fish such as salmon and tuna that have abundant supplies of omega-3. Today, Americans eat 17 times more omega-6 than omega-3 fats, and most experts agree that we need a more balanced approach.[20]

How can you add appropriate amounts of EFAs to your diet?

- Eat fatty fish (bluefish, herring, mackerel, salmon, sardines, or tuna) at least twice weekly.
- Substitute soy and canola oils for corn, safflower, and sunflower oils. Keep using olive oil, too.
- Add healthy doses of green leafy vegetables, walnuts, walnut oil, and ground flaxseed to your diet to increase intake of alpha-linolenic acid.
- Limit processed and convenience foods, because they often contain harmful saturated and *trans* fats.
- Pick the MUFA or PUFA with the least amount of calories and most nutrients.

There is still much research to be done on the benefits versus the risks of consuming large amounts of omega-3s. Stay informed on this issue to be a wise consumer and make wise dietary choices.

Vitamins

Vitamins are potent, essential, organic compounds that promote growth and help maintain life and health. Every minute of every day, vitamins help maintain nerves and skin, produce blood cells, build bones and teeth, heal wounds, and convert food energy to body energy—and they do all of this without adding any calories to your diet.

Age, heat, and other environmental conditions can destroy vitamins in food. Vitamins can be classified as either *fat soluble,* meaning that they are absorbed through the intestinal tract with the help of fats, or *water soluble,* meaning that they are easily dissolved in water. Vitamins A, D, E, and K are fat soluble; B complex vitamins and vitamin C are water soluble. Fat-soluble vitamins tend to be stored in the body, and toxic accumulations in the liver may cause cirrhosis-like symptoms. Water-soluble vitamins are generally excreted and cause few toxicity problems (Table 8.3 on page 256).

Despite media suggestions to the contrary, few Americans will suffer from true vitamin deficiencies if they eat a diet containing all of the food groups at least part of the time. Nevertheless, Americans continue to purchase large quantities of vitamin supplements. For the most part, vitamin supplements are unnecessary and even, in certain instances, harmful. Overusing them can lead to a toxic condition known as **hypervitaminosis.**

Minerals

Minerals are the inorganic, indestructible elements that aid physiological processes within the body. Without minerals, vitamins could not be absorbed. Minerals are readily excreted and are usually not toxic. **Macrominerals** are the minerals that the body needs in fairly large amounts: sodium, calcium, phosphorus, magnesium, potassium, sulfur, and chloride. **Trace minerals** include iron, zinc, manganese, copper, and iodine. Only trace amounts of these minerals are needed, and serious problems may result if excesses or deficiencies occur (see Table 8.4 on page 258).

Although minerals are necessary for body function, there are limits on the amounts we should consume. Americans tend to overuse or underuse certain minerals.

Sodium Sodium is necessary for the regulation of blood and body fluids, transmission of nerve impulses, heart activity, and certain metabolic functions. In general, however, we consume much more than we need. It is estimated that the average adult who does not sweat profusely requires only 250–500 milligrams of sodium (about ¼ teaspoon) per day; yet the average American consumes over 4,000 milligrams of sodium each day. Most professional groups recommend

restricting sodium to 1,200 to 2,300 milligrams per day; less is better.[21]

Why are we consuming all of this excess sodium? A common misconception is that "salt" and "sodium" are the same thing. However, table salt accounts for only 15 percent of sodium intake. In fact, table salt is actually sodium chloride, a mixture that is 40 percent sodium and 60 percent chloride. The majority of sodium in our diet comes from highly processed foods that are infused with sodium to enhance flavor and preservation. Pickles, fast foods, salty snack foods, processed cheeses, many breads and bakery products, and smoked meats and sausages often contain several hundred milligrams of sodium per serving. A sausage and cheese pizza with sauce would put you well on your way to that 4,000 milligram-per-day average!

Many experts believe that there is a link between excessive sodium intake and hypertension (high blood pressure). Although this theory is controversial, researchers recommend that hypertensive Americans cut back on sodium to reduce their risk for cardiovascular disorders.[22] Osteoporosis researchers confirm that high sodium intake may increase calcium loss in urine, increasing your risk for debilitating bone fractures as you age.

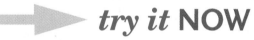

try it NOW

Shake your salt habit! Extra salt can be found in almost everything from cereal to bread to snack foods. Take simple steps today to reduce your overall sodium intake: choose low-sodium or salt-free food products. Order your popcorn without salt. Switch to kosher salt—it has 25 percent less sodium than regular table salt. Instead of adding salt to food you prepare, try using fresh or prepackaged herb blends to season foods. Once you cut your sodium intake, you'll taste the difference the next time you eat a sodium-heavy product.

Calcium The issue of calcium consumption has gained national attention with the rising incidence of osteoporosis

---

vitamins Essential organic compounds that promote growth and reproduction and help maintain life and health.

hypervitaminosis A toxic condition caused by overuse of vitamin supplements.

minerals Inorganic, indestructible elements that aid physiological processes.

macrominerals Minerals that the body needs in fairly large amounts.

trace minerals Minerals that the body needs in only very small amounts.

TABLE 8.3 A Guide to Vitamins

Vitamin	Best Sources	Chief Functions in the Body
WATER-SOLUBLE VITAMINS		
Vitamin B$_1$ (thiamin) 1.5 mg (RDA + RDI)	Meat, pork, liver, fish, poultry, whole-grain and enriched breads, cereals, pasta, nuts, legumes, wheat germ, oats	Helps carbohydrate convert to energy; supports normal appetite and nervous system function
Vitamin B$_2$ (riboflavin) 1.7 mg (RDA + RDI)	Milk, dark green vegetables, yogurt, cottage cheese, liver, meat, whole-grain or enriched breads and cereals	Helps carbohydrates, fat, and protein convert to energy; promotes healthy skin and normal vision
Niacin 20 mg NE (RDA + RDI)	Meat, eggs, poultry, fish, milk, whole-grain and enriched breads and cereals, nuts, legumes, peanuts, nutritional yeast, all protein foods	Helps convert nutrients to energy; promotes health of skin, nerves, and digestive system
Vitamin B$_6$ (pyridoxine) 2.0 mg (RDA + RDI)	Meat, poultry, fish, shellfish, legumes, whole-grain products, green leafy vegetables, bananas	Protein and fat metabolism, formation of antibodies and red blood cells; helps convert tryptophan to niacin
Folate 400 µg (DFE + RDA)	Green leafy vegetables, liver, legumes, seeds	Red blood cell formation; protein metabolism; new cell division; prevents neural tube defects
Vitamin B$_{12}$ (cobalamin) 2.4 mg (RDA)	Meat, fish, poultry, shellfish, milk, cheese, eggs, nutritional yeast	Maintenance of nerve cells; red blood cell formation; synthesis of genetic material
Pantothenic acid 5–7 mg (AI)	Widespread in foods	Coenzyme in energy metabolism
Biotin 30 µg (AI)	Widespread in foods	Coenzyme in energy metabolism; fat synthesis; glycogen formation
Vitamin C (ascorbic acid) (RDI + RDA) 60 mg	Citrus fruits, cabbage-type vegetables, tomatoes, potatoes, dark green vegetables, peppers, lettuce, cantaloupe, strawberries	Heals wounds, maintains bones and teeth, strengthens blood vessels; antioxidant; strengthens resistance to infection; aids iron absorption
FAT-SOLUBLE VITAMINS		
Vitamin A 5,000 IU	Fortified milk and margarine, cream, cheese, butter, eggs, liver, spinach, and other dark leafy greens, broccoli, deep orange fruits and vegetables (carrots, sweet potatoes, peaches)	Vision; growth and repair of body tissues; reproduction; bone and tooth formation; immunity; cancer protection; hormone synthesis
Vitamin D 400–600 IU (RDA + RDI)	Self-synthesis with sunlight, fortified milk, fortified margarine, eggs, liver, fish	Calcium and phosphorus metabolism (bone and tooth formation); aids body's absorption of calcium
Vitamin E 30 IU (RDA + RDI)	Vegetable oils, green leafy vegetables, wheat germ, whole-grain products, butter, liver, egg yolk, milk fat, nuts, seeds	Protects red blood cells; antioxidant; stabilization of cell membranes
Vitamin K 70–140 µg	Liver; green leafy, and cabbage-type vegetables; milk	Bacterial synthesis in digestive tract. Synthesis of blood-clotting proteins and a blood protein that regulates blood calcium

among older adults. Although calcium plays a vital role in building strong bones and teeth, muscle contraction, blood clotting, nerve impulse transmission, regulating heartbeat, and fluid balance within cells, most Americans do not consume the recommended amount of 1,200 milligrams of calcium per day.

Because calcium intake is so important throughout life for maintaining strong bones, it is critical to consume the minimum required amount each day. Over half of our calcium intake usually comes from milk, one of the highest sources. Calcium-fortified orange juice and soy milk provide a good way to get calcium if you do not drink dairy milk. Many green, leafy vegetables are good sources of calcium, but some contain oxalic acid, which makes their calcium harder to absorb. Spinach, chard, and beet greens are not particularly good sources of calcium, whereas broccoli, cauliflower, and many peas and beans offer good supplies (pinto beans and soybeans are among the best). Many nuts, particularly

Deficiency Symptoms	Toxicity Symptoms
Beriberi, edema, heart irregularity, mental confusion, muscle weakness, low morale, impaired growth	Rapid pulse, weakness, headaches, insomnia, irritability
Eye problems, skin disorders around nose and mouth	None reported, but an excess of any of the B vitamins can cause a deficiency of the others
Pellagra: skin rash on parts exposed to sun, loss of appetite, dizziness, weakness, irritability, fatigue, mental confusion, indigestion	Flushing, nausea, headaches, cramps, ulcer irritation, heartburn, abnormal liver function, low blood pressure
Nervous disorders, skin rash, muscle weakness, anemia, convulsions, kidney stones	Depression, fatigue, irritability, headaches, numbness, damage to nerves, difficulty walking
Anemia, heartburn, diarrhea, smooth tongue depression, poor growth	Diarrhea, insomnia, irritability, may mask a vitamin B_{12} deficiency
Anemia, smooth tongue, fatigue, nerve degeneration progressing to paralysis	None reported
Rare; sleep disturbances, nausea, fatigue	Occasional diarrhea
Loss of appetite, nausea, depression, muscle pain, weakness, fatigue, rash	None reported
Scurvy, anemia, depression, frequent infections, bleeding gums, loosened teeth, muscle degeneration, rough skin, bone fragility, poor wound healing	Nausea, abdominal cramps, diarrhea, breakdown of red blood cells in persons with certain genetic disorders; deficiency symptoms may appear at first on withdrawal of high doses
Night blindness, rough skin, susceptibility to infection, impaired bone growth, vision problems	Nosebleeds, abdominal cramps, nausea, diarrhea, weight loss, blurred vision, irritability, bone pain, rashes, cessation of menstruation, growth retardation
Rickets in children; osteomalacia in adults; abnormal growth, joint pain, soft bones	Raised blood calcium, constipation, weight loss, irritability, weakness, nausea, kidney stones, mental and physical retardation
Muscle wasting, weakness, red blood cell breakage, anemia, hemorrhaging, fibrocystic breast disease	Interference with anticlotting medication, general discomfort
Hemorrhaging	Interference with anticlotting medication; may cause jaundice

Note: Values increase among women who are pregnant or lactating.

Source: From J. Thompson and M. Manore, *Nutrition: An Applied Approach* (San Francisco: Benjamin Cummings, 2005). Reprinted by permission of Pearson Education, Inc.

almonds, Brazil nuts, and hazelnuts, and seeds such as sunflower and sesame contain good amounts of calcium. Molasses is fairly high in calcium, and some fruits—citrus, figs, raisins, and dried apricots—have moderate amounts. Bone meal is not a recommended calcium source due to possible contamination.

Do you consume carbonated soft drinks? Be aware that the added phosphoric acid (phosphate) in these drinks can cause you to excrete extra calcium, which may result in calcium being pulled out of your bones. Calcium-phosphorus imbalance may lead to kidney stones and other calcification problems, as well as to increased atherosclerotic plaque.

TABLE 8.4 A Guide to Minerals

Mineral	Significant Sources	Chief Functions in the Body
Calcium AI: 1,000 mg/day (men and women aged 19 to 50); 1,200 mg/day (men and women over 50)	Milk and milk products, small fish (with bones), tofu, greens, legumes	Principal mineral of bones and teeth; involved in muscle contraction and relaxation, nerve function, blood clotting, blood pressure
Phosphorus RDA = 700 mg/day	All animal tissues	Part of every cell; involved in acid-base balance
Magnesium RDA = 400 mg/day (men); 310 mg/day (women)	Nuts, legumes, whole grains, dark green vegetables, seafood, chocolate, cocoa	Involved in bone mineralization, protein synthesis, enzyme action, normal muscular contraction, nerve transmission
Sodium AI: 1.5 g/day	Salt, soy sauce; processed foods; cured, canned, and pickled foods	Helps maintain normal fluid and acid-base balance
Chloride AI: 2.3 g/day	Salt, soy sauce; processed foods	Part of stomach acid, necessary for proper digestion, fluid balance
Potassium AI: 4.7 g/day	All whole foods: meats, milk, fruits, vegetables, grains, legumes	Facilitates many reactions including protein synthesis, fluid balance, nerve transmission, and contraction of muscles
Iodine RDA = 150 µg	Iodized salt, seafood	Part of thyroxine, which regulates metabolism
Iron RDA = 8 mg/day (men; women over 51); 18 mg/day (women aged 19 to 50)	Beef, fish, poultry, shellfish, eggs, legumes, dried fruits	Hemoglobin formation; part of myoglobin; energy use
Zinc RDA = 11 mg/day (men); 8 mg/day (women)	Protein-containing foods: meats, fish, poultry, grains, vegetables	Part of many enzymes; present in insulin; involved in making genetic material and proteins, immunity, vitamin A transport, taste, wound healing, sperm creation, normal fetal development
Fluoride AI: 3 to 4 mg/day	Drinking water (if naturally fluoride-containing or fluoridated), tea, seafood	Formation of bones and teeth; helps make teeth resistant to decay and bones resistant to mineral loss
Selenium RDA = 55 µg	Seafood, meats, grains	Helps protect body compounds from oxidation

We also know that sunlight increases the manufacture of vitamin D in the body and is therefore like having an extra calcium source because vitamin D improves absorption of calcium. Stress, on the other hand, depletes calcium. It is generally best to take calcium throughout the day, consuming it with foods containing protein, vitamin D, and vitamin C for optimum absorption. Experts vary on which type of supplemental calcium is most readily and efficiently absorbed, although aspartate and citrate salts of calcium are often recommended. As with all nutrients, the best way to obtain calcium is to consume it as part of a balanced diet.

anemia Iron-deficiency disease that results from the body's inability to produce hemoglobin.

pica Iron-deficiency disease characterized by a craving for certain foods and substances.

Iron Worldwide, iron deficiency is the most common nutrient deficiency, affecting more than 2 billion people, many of whom are children and women who suffer from *iron-deficiency anemia*. This is nearly 30 percent of the world's population. In the United States, iron-deficiency anemia is less prevalent but is the most common micronutrient deficiency.[23] In addition to suffering from **anemia,** a problem resulting from the body's inability to produce hemoglobin (the bright red, oxygen-carrying component of the blood), people with iron-deficiency anemia may develop a condition known as **pica,** an appetite for ice, clay, paste, and other non-food substances that do not actually contain iron and, in fact, may inhibit iron absorption.

How much iron do we need? Females aged 19 to 50 need about 18 milligrams per day, and males aged 19 to 50 need about 10 milligrams.

When iron deficiency occurs, body cells receive less oxygen, and carbon dioxide wastes are removed less efficiently.

Deficiency Symptoms	Toxicity Symptoms
Stunted growth in children; bone loss (osteoporosis) in adults	Excess calcium is excreted except in hormonal imbalance states
Unknown	Can create relative deficiency of calcium
Weakness, confusion, depressed pancreatic hormone secretion, growth failure, behavioral disturbances, muscle spasms	Pharmacological overuse can cause nausea, cramps, dehydration
Muscle cramps, mental apathy, loss of appetite	Hypertension (in salt-sensitive persons)
Growth failure in children, muscle cramps, mental apathy, loss of appetite	Normally harmless (different from poisonous chlorine gas); disturbed acid-base balance; vomiting
Muscle weakness, paralysis, confusion; can cause death, accompanies dehydration	Causes muscular weakness; triggers vomiting; if given into a vein, can stop the heart
Goiter, cretinism	Very high intakes depress thyroid activity
Anemia: weakness, pallor, headaches, reduced resistance to infection, inability to concentrate	Nausea, vomiting, dizziness, damage to organs, death
Growth failure in children, delayed development of sexual organs, loss of taste, poor wound healing	Fever, nausea, vomiting, diarrhea
Susceptibility to tooth decay and bone loss	Fluorosis (discoloration of teeth)
Impaired immune function, depression, muscle pain	Vomiting, nausea, rash, brittle hair and nails

Note: RDA = Recommended Daily Allowance; AI = Adequate Intakes. Values are for all adults aged 19 and older, except as noted.

Source: From J. Thompson and M. Manore, *Nutrition: An Applied Approach* (San Francisco: Benjamin Cummings, 2005). Reprinted by permission of Pearson Education, Inc.

As a result, the iron-deficient person feels tired and run down. Although iron deficiency in the diet is a common cause of anemia, it can also result from blood loss, cancers, ulcers, and other conditions. Generally, women are more likely to develop iron-deficiency problems because they typically eat less than men and their diets contain less iron. Women having heavy menstrual flow may be at greater risk.

Iron overload (known as **hemochromatosis**), or iron toxicity due to ingesting too many iron-containing supplements, remains the leading cause of accidental poisoning in small children in the United States. Symptoms of toxicity include nausea, vomiting, diarrhea, rapid heartbeat, weak pulse, dizziness, shock, and confusion. Doses as small as five iron tablets containing as little as 200 milligrams of iron have killed dozens of children.

Determining Your Nutritional Needs

Historically, dietary guidelines were developed to reduce the public's risk of diseases from nutrient deficiency. Known as the **Recommended Dietary Allowances (RDAs),** these

hemochromatosis Iron toxicity due to excess consumption.

Recommended Dietary Allowances (RDAs) The average daily intakes of energy and nutrients considered adequate to meet the needs of most healthy people in the United States under usual conditions.

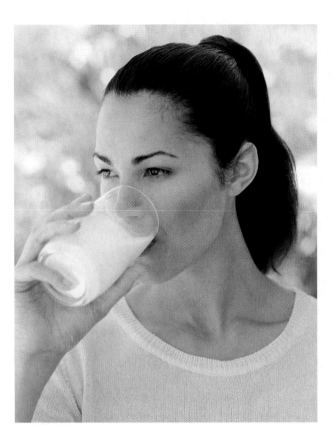

Consuming your RDA of calcium is key to your health not only now, but in the future.

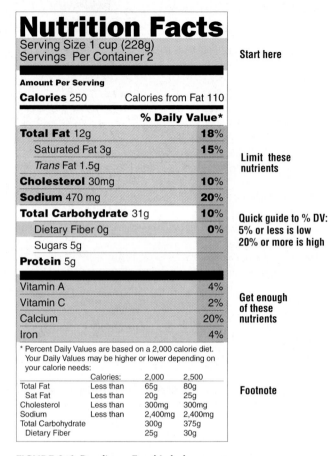

Sample Label for
Macaroni and Cheese

Nutrition Facts

Serving Size 1 cup (228g)
Servings Per Container 2

Start here

Amount Per Serving

Calories 250   Calories from Fat 110

% Daily Value*

Total Fat 12g	**18%**
Saturated Fat 3g	**15%**
Trans Fat 1.5g	
Cholesterol 30mg	**10%**
Sodium 470 mg	**20%**
Total Carbohydrate 31g	**10%**
Dietary Fiber 0g	**0%**
Sugars 5g	
Protein 5g	

Limit these nutrients

Quick guide to % DV:
5% or less is low
20% or more is high

Vitamin A	4%
Vitamin C	2%
Calcium	20%
Iron	4%

Get enough of these nutrients

* Percent Daily Values are based on a 2,000 calorie diet. Your Daily Values may be higher or lower depending on your calorie needs:

	Calories:	2,000	2,500
Total Fat	Less than	65g	80g
Sat Fat	Less than	20g	25g
Cholesterol	Less than	300mg	300mg
Sodium	Less than	2,400mg	2,400mg
Total Carbohydrate		300g	375g
Dietary Fiber		25g	30g

Footnote

FIGURE 8.6 Reading a Food Label

Source: Center for Food Safety and Applied Nutrition, "Questions and Answers about *Trans* Fat Nutrition Labeling," 2004, www.cfsan.fda.gov/~dms/qatrans2.html.

guidelines have provided Americans and Canadians with recommended intake levels necessary to meet the nutritional needs of about 97 percent of healthy individuals. More recently, the U.S. Food and Nutrition Board replaced and expanded upon the RDAs by creating new **Dietary Reference Intakes (DRIs),** a list of 26 nutrients essential to maintaining health. DRIs identify recommended and maximum safe

Dietary Reference Intakes (DRIs)   A set of nutritional values; a new combined listing, including more than 26 essential vitamins and minerals, that applies to healthy people.

U.S. Recommended Daily Allowances (USRDAs)   Dietary guidelines developed by the Food and Drug Administration (FDA) and the U.S. Department of Agriculture.

Adequate Intake (AI)   Best estimates of nutritional needs.

Tolerable Upper Intake Level (UL)   The highest amount of a nutrient that an individual can safely consume every day without risking adverse health effects.

Reference Daily Intakes (RDIs)   Recommended amounts of 19 vitamins and minerals, also known as micronutrients.

Daily Reference Values (DRVs)   Recommended amounts for macronutrients such as total fat, saturated fat, and cholesterol.

intake levels for healthy people, as well as establishing the amount of a nutrient needed to prevent deficiencies or to reduce the risk of chronic disease. DRIs are considered the umbrella guidelines under which the following categories fall:

- **U.S. Recommended Dietary Allowances (USRDAs):** reference standard for intake levels necessary to meet the nutritional needs of 97 to 98 percent of healthy individuals
- **Adequate Intake (AI):** the recommended average daily intake level of a nutrient by healthy people when there is not enough research to determine the full RDA
- **Tolerable Upper Intake Level (UL):** the highest amount of a nutrient an individual can consume daily without the risk of adverse health effects

Reading Labels for Health   In order to help consumers determine the nutritional values of foods, the Food and Drug Administration and the U.S. Department of Agriculture developed the **Reference Daily Intakes (RDIs)** and **Daily Reference Values (DRVs).** RDIs are the recommended

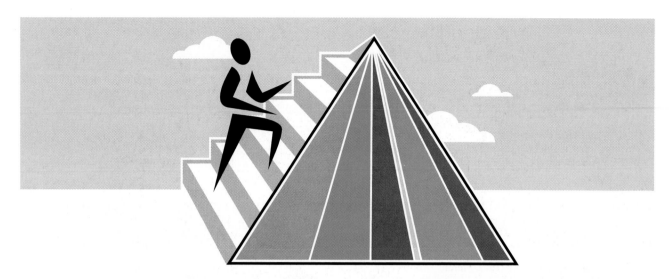

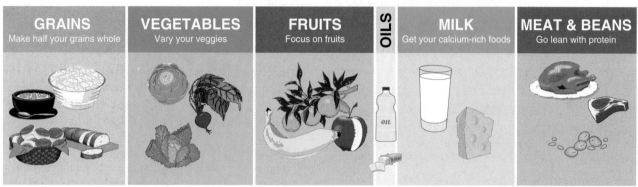

| GRAINS
Make half your grains whole | VEGETABLES
Vary your veggies | FRUITS
Focus on fruits | OILS | MILK
Get your calcium-rich foods | MEAT & BEANS
Go lean with protein |

FIGURE 8.7 The MyPyramid Plan

The USDA MyPyramid Plan takes a new approach to dietary and exercise recommendations. Each colored section of the pyramid represents a food group, with the specific needs of individuals in mind.

Source: U.S. Department of Agriculture, 2005, www.MyPyramid.gov.

amounts of 19 vitamins and minerals, also known as micronutrients, and DRVs are the recommended amounts for macronutrients, such as total fat, saturated fat, cholesterol, total carbohydrates, dietary fiber, sodium, potassium, and protein.

Together, RDIs and DRVs make up the **Daily Values (DVs)** that you will find on food and supplement labels listed as a percentage (% DV); see Figure 8.6 for an example. Other than telling you what percentage of nutrients is found in a serving of food, labels also include information on the serving size, calories and calories from fat per serving, and percentage of *trans* fats in a food.

The New MyPyramid Food Guide

In 2005, the Food Guide Pyramid underwent a significant overhaul in order to better account for the variety of different nutritional needs throughout the U.S. population (Figure 8.7). This new pyramid, called the MyPyramid Plan, replaces the former Food Guide Pyramid promoted since 1993 by the U.S. Department of Agriculture (USDA), and incorporates the *2005 Dietary Guidelines for Americans.*[24] Whereas the former pyramid emphasized variety in daily intake, it did not reflect what we now know about restricting fats, eating more fruits and vegetables, and consuming whole grains. The new pyramid is also significantly improved in that it takes into consideration the various dietary and caloric needs of a variety of individuals (those over 65, children, active adults, etc.) as well as activity levels.

Goals of the MyPyramid Plan

The MyPyramid Plan is meant to encourage consumers to make healthier food choices and to be active every day, and to promote personalized dietary and exercise recommendations

Daily Values (DVs)   The RDIs and DRVs together make up the daily values seen on food and supplement labels.

	1,200	1,400	1,600	1,800	2,000	2,200	2,400	2,600	2,800	3,000
Fruits	1 cup	1.5 cups	1.5 cups	1.5 cups	2 cups	2 cups	2 cups	2 cups	2.5 cups	2.5 cups
Vegetables	1.5 cups	1.5 cups	2 cups	2.5 cups	2.5 cups	3 cups	3 cups	3.5 cups	3.5 cups	4 cups
Grains	4 oz.-eq.	5 oz.-eq.	5 oz.-eq.	6 oz.-eq.	6 oz.-eq.	7 oz.-eq.	8 oz.-eq.	9 oz.-eq.	10 oz.-eq.	10 oz.-eq.
Meat and Beans	3 oz.-eq.	4 oz.-eq.	5 oz.-eq.	5 oz.-eq.	5.5 oz.-eq.	6 oz.-eq.	6.5 oz.-eq.	6.5 oz.-eq.	7 oz.-eq.	7 oz.-eq.
Milk	2 cups	2 cups	3 cups	3 cups	3 cups	3 cups	3 cups	3 cups	3 cup	3 cups
Oils	4 tsp.	4 tsp.	5 tsp.	5 tsp.	6 tsp.	6 tsp.	7 tsp.	8 tsp.	8 tsp.	10 tsp.
Discretionary calorie allowance	171	171	132	195	267	290	362	410	426	512

FIGURE 8.8 Nutritional Needs for Different Groups

Once you've determined your daily calorie requirements (Table 8.1), use this chart to determine how many servings of each food group you need per day to maintain good health.

based upon individual needs.[25] MyPyramid strives to illustrate the following:

- *Personalization* is demonstrated by the MyPyramid website, www.MyPyramid.gov. The website offers personalized recommendation of the kinds and amounts of food to eat each day, tips and ideas for achieving a healthy diet, and interactive assessments based on an individual's gender, age, and activity level.
- *Gradual improvement* encourages individuals to take small steps to improve their diet and lifestyle each day.
- *Physical activity,* represented by the person climbing steps, reminds us about the importance of daily physical activity in maintaining a healthy weight, and improving overall health and disease prevention.
- *Variety* is represented by the six color bands. It is important to eat foods from each group every day in order to receive the proper nutrients for overall health.
- *Moderation* in food intake is represented by the narrowing of each color band from bottom to top. You should select foods with little or no fat or sugar more often to get the most from the foods you eat.
- *Proportionality* is symbolized by the varying width of each color band. A wider band generally suggests you should choose more foods from that group, while a narrow band suggests you limit your intake of foods from the corresponding group.

Using the New MyPyramid Plan

Understanding serving sizes, daily physical activity, and eating a nutritionally balanced diet are key components to using the MyPyramid Plan recommendations successfully. Though these elements are not new to the 2005 pyramid, they have been updated to reflect the latest in nutritional science.

Understanding Serving Sizes How much is one serving? Is it different than a portion? Although these two terms are often used interchangeably, they actually mean very different things, and it is important to understand the difference to be able to use MyPyramid and other nutrition guidelines effectively. A *serving* is the recommended amount you should consume, while a *portion* is the amount you choose to eat at any one time and may be more or less than a serving. Most of us select portions that are much bigger than servings. According to a survey conducted by the American Institute for Cancer Research, respondents were asked to estimate the standard servings defined by the old USDA Food Guide Pyramid for eight different foods. Only 1 percent of those surveyed correctly answered all serving size questions and nearly 65 percent answered five or more of them incorrectly.[26] See the Skills for Behavior Change box on the facing page for tips on recognizing serving sizes.

Unfortunately, we don't always get a clear picture from food producers and advertisers about what a serving really is. Consider a bottle of soda: the food label may list one serving as 8 fluid ounces and 100 calories. However, note the size of the bottle; the bottle may hold 20 ounces and drinking the entire bottle serves up a whopping 250 calories.

Be sure to eat at least the lowest number of servings from the major food groups; you need them for the nutrients they provide. If you eat a large portion, count it as more than one serving. Figure 8.8 lists the suggested daily amount of food from each group for a variety of calorie intake levels. Examples of one serving from each food group in MyPyramid are listed below.

Grains
- 1 slice of bread or ½ English muffin
- ½ cup cooked rice, pasta, or hot cereal
- 1 cup ready-to-eat cereal

SKILLS FOR *behavior change*

GETTING A GRIP ON PORTION DISTORTION

One of the challenges of following a healthy diet is judging how big a portion size should be and how many servings you are really eating each time you put your hand in the potato chip bag or scoop some ice cream into a dish. The American Dietetic Association and other experts have developed some tips for getting a grip.

SERVING SIZES

- A deck of playing cards = 1 serving (3 ounces) of meat, poultry, or fish

- Half a baseball (not a softball!) = 1 serving (½ cup) of fruit, vegetables, pasta, or rice
- Pair of dice = 1 serving (1 ounce) of cheese
- A tennis ball = 1-cup serving of fresh greens

MANAGING YOUR PORTIONS

- Before eating, visualize the serving sizes recommended above. Putting one of these servings onto a smaller plate may help it look bigger.
- Don't eat out of a bag or a carton. There can be a lot hidden in there, and it's very difficult to compare it to a serving size. Try to purchase snack items that come in a single-serving size package (check the label!).
- Use measuring cups or a small scale at home until you can accurately assess the size of a serving.
- Buffets and restaurant meals served "family style" make it difficult to gauge servings. Try to avoid these situations unless you can really pay attention to how much food ends up on your plate.

Fruits
- 1 small apple or 1 large banana
- 1 cup of raw, cooked, or canned fruit
- 1 cup of fruit juice
- ½ cup dried fruit

Vegetables
- 1 cup raw greens or 2 cups cooked greens
- 1 cup beans, peas, or carrots (raw or cooked)
- 1 medium baked potato

Meat and Beans
- 1 ounce lean meat, poultry, or fish
- 1 tablespoon peanut butter
- ¼ cup tofu or cooked beans
- 1 egg

Milk
- 1 cup milk or yogurt
- 1½ ounces natural cheese or ⅓ cup shredded cheese
- 2 ounces processed cheese

Oil
- 1 tablespoon margarine or mayonnaise equals 2½ teaspoons of oil
- ½ avocado equals 3 teaspoons of oil
- 2 tablespoons Italian dressing equals 2 teaspoons oil

Discretionary Calories Every day you must consume a certain number of nutrient-rich foods in order to maintain health. *Discretionary calories* are those obtained from foods that do not provide a significant amount of nutritional value. Most of us have a very small discretionary calorie allowance at the end of the day. For example, suppose you are on a 2,000-calorie diet, and you've eaten wisely all day, choosing whole-grain, low-fat, and low-sugar food items, and your calorie balance for the day is at 1,800. This means you can spend the remaining 200 calories on what might be considered luxury indulgences. This might include a soda, a small serving of ice cream, or a higher fat cheese or meat than you would normally consume.

Physical Activity Strive to be physically active for at least 30 minutes daily, preferably with moderate to vigorous activity levels on most days. Physical activity does not mean you have to go to the gym, jog three miles a day, or hire a personal trainer. Any activity that gets your heart pumping such as gardening, playing basketball, heavy yard work, and dancing the night away are all examples of ways to get moving. For more on physical fitness, see Chapter 10.

Eating "Nutrient-Dense" Foods Although eating the proper number of servings from MyPyramid is important, it is also important to recognize that there are large

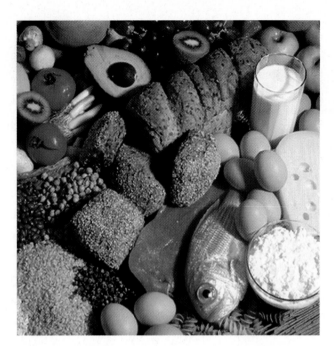

Eating a variety of foods is a key goal of the MyPyramid Plan.

caloric, fat, and energy differences between foods within a given food group. For example, fish and hot dogs provide vastly different fat and energy levels per ounce, with fish providing better energy and calorie value per serving. Nutrient density is even more important for someone who is ill and unable to keep food down. It is important to eat foods that have a high nutritional value for their calorie content. Avoid empty calories, or high-calorie foods that have little nutritional value.

Making the Pyramid Work For You

Creating a dietary plan that meets all of the recommendations discussed in this chapter can be overwhelming. First, think about the simple changes you can make to your diet today. What foods do you eat plenty of now? What can you get more of? You can also visit the MyPyramid website (www.MyPyramid.gov) and use the MyPyramid Tracker. This tool allows you to enter in the foods you eat and your

vegetarian A term with a variety of meanings: vegans avoid all foods of animal origin; lacto-vegetarians avoid flesh foods but eat dairy products; ovo-vegetarians avoid flesh foods but eat eggs; lacto-ovo-vegetarians avoid flesh foods but eat both dairy products and eggs; pesco-vegetarians avoid meat but eat fish, dairy products, and eggs; semivegetarians eat chicken, fish, dairy products, and eggs.

physical activity level to give you a personalized idea of how balanced your diet is.

Vegetarianism: Eating for Health

For ethical, economic, personal, health, cultural, or religious reasons, some people choose specialized diets. Today, between 5 and 15 percent of all Americans identify themselves as vegetarians. Normally, vegetarianism provides a superb alternative to our high-fat, high-calorie, meat-based cuisine, but without proper information and food choices, vegetarians can also develop serious dietary problems.

The term **vegetarian** means different things to different people. Strict vegetarians, or *vegans,* avoid all foods of animal origin, including dairy products and eggs. Vegans must be careful to obtain all of the necessary nutrients. Far more common are *lacto-vegetarians,* who eat dairy products but avoid flesh foods. Their diet can be low in fat and cholesterol but only if they consume skim milk and other low-fat or non-fat products. *Ovo-vegetarians* add eggs to their diet, while *lacto-ovo-vegetarians* eat both dairy products and eggs. *Pesco-vegetarians* eat fish, dairy products, and eggs, while *semivegetarians* eat chicken, fish, dairy products, and eggs. Some people in the semivegetarian category prefer to call themselves "non–red meat eaters."

Generally, people who follow a balanced vegetarian diet weigh less and have better cholesterol levels, fewer problems with irregular bowel movements (constipation and diarrhea), and a lower risk of heart disease than do nonvegetarians. The benefits of vegetarianism also include a reduced risk of some cancers, particularly colon, and a lower risk of kidney disease.[27]

Although in the past vegetarians often suffered from vitamin deficiencies, the vegetarian of the new millennium is usually extremely adept at combining the right types of foods to ensure proper nutrient intake. People who eat dairy products and small amounts of chicken or fish are seldom nutrient deficient; in fact, while vegans typically get 50 to 60 grams of protein per day, lacto-ovo-vegetarians normally consume between 70 and 90 grams per day, well beyond the RDA. Vegan diets may be deficient in vitamins B_2 (riboflavin), B_{12}, and D. Riboflavin is found mainly in meat, eggs, and dairy products; but broccoli, asparagus, almonds, and fortified cereals are also good sources. Vitamins B_{12} and D are found only in dairy products and fortified products such as soy milk. Vegans are also at risk for deficiencies of calcium, iron, zinc, and other minerals but can obtain these nutrients from supplements. Strict vegans have to pay much more attention to what they eat than the average person does; but, by eating complementary combinations of plant products, they can receive adequate amounts of essential amino acids. Examples of complementary combinations are corn and beans, and peanut

Eating Pattern	DASH[a]	TLC[b]	Serving Sizes
Grains[c]	6 to 8 servings per day	7 servings[d] per day	1 slice bread; 1 oz dry cereal;[e] $\frac{1}{2}$ cup cooked rice, pasta, or cereal
Vegetables	4 to 5 servings per day	5 servings[d] per day	1 cup raw leafy vegetable, $\frac{1}{2}$ cup cut up raw or cooked vegetable, $\frac{1}{2}$ cup vegetable juice
Fruits	4 to 5 servings per day	4 servings[d] per day	1 medium fruit; $\frac{1}{4}$ cup dried fruit; $\frac{1}{2}$ cup fresh, frozen, or canned fruit; $\frac{1}{2}$ cup fruit juice
Fat-free or low-fat milk and milk products	2 to 3 servings per day	2 to 3 servings per day	1 cup milk, 1 cup yogurt, $1\frac{1}{2}$ oz cheese
Lean[f] meats, poultry, and fish	<6 oz per day	≤5 oz per day	
Nuts, seeds, and legumes	4 to 5 servings per week	Counted in vegetable servings	$\frac{1}{3}$ cup ($1\frac{1}{2}$ oz), 2 Tbsp peanut butter, 2 Tbsp or $\frac{1}{2}$ oz seeds, $\frac{1}{2}$ cup dry beans or peas
Fats and oils	2 to 3 servings[g] per day	Amount depends on daily calorie level	1 tsp soft margarine, 1 Tbsp mayonnaise, 2 Tbsp salad dressing, 1 tsp vegetable oil
Sweets and added sugars	5 or fewer servings per week	No recommendation	1 Tbsp sugar, 1 Tbsp jelly or jam, $\frac{1}{2}$ cup sorbet and ices, 1 cup lemonade

[a] Dietary Approaches to Stop Hypertension. For more information, please visit www.nhlbi.nih.gov/health/public/heart/hbp/dash.

[b] Therapeutic Lifestyle Changes. For more information, please visit www.nhlbi.nih.gov/cgi-bin/chd/step2intro.cgi.

TLC includes two therapeutic diet options: plant stanol/sterol (add 2 g per day) and soluble fiber (add 5 to 10 g per day).

[c] Whole-grain foods are recommended for most grain servings to meet fiber recommendations.

[d] This number can be less or more depending on other food choices to meet 2,000 calories.

[e] Equals $\frac{1}{2}$ to $1\frac{1}{4}$ cups, depending on cereal type. Check the product's Nutrition Facts label.

[f] Lean cuts include sirloin tip, round steak, and rump roast; extra lean hamburger; and cold cuts made with lean meat or soy protein. Lean cuts of pork are center-cut ham, loin chops, and pork tenderloin.

[g] Fat content changes serving counts for fats and oils: For example, 1 Tbsp of regular salad dressing equals 1 serving; 1 Tbsp of low-fat dressing equals $\frac{1}{2}$ serving; 1 Tbsp of fat-free dressing equals 0 servings.

butter and whole-grain bread. Eating a full variety of grains, legumes, fruits, vegetables, and seeds each day will keep even the strictest vegetarian in excellent health. Pregnant women, the elderly, the sick, and children who are vegans need to take special care to ensure that their diets are adequate. People who take part in heavy aerobic exercise programs (over three hours per week) may need to increase their protein consumption. In all cases, seek advice from a health care professional if you have questions.

Adapting MyPyramid for Vegetarians

As mentioned above, vegetarian diets can easily meet all of the recommendations for nutrient needs. By focusing on non-meat sources of protein, iron, calcium, zinc, and vitamin B_{12}, and paying attention to personalized serving size and physical activity guidelines, vegetarians can be just as healthy as omnivores.

 what do you THINK?

Why are so many people today becoming vegetarians? ■ How easy is it to be a vegetarian on your campus? ■ What concerns about vegetarianism would you be likely to have, if any?

Can Food Have Medicinal Value?

The old adage "you are what you eat" is indeed a motto to live by. Beneficial foods are termed *functional foods* based on the ancient belief that eating the right foods may not only prevent disease, but also actually cure it. This perspective is gaining credibility within the scientific community. The American Heart Association recommends dietary changes to reduce cholesterol and control diabetes (see Table 8.5). This is just the beginning of the functional food trend.

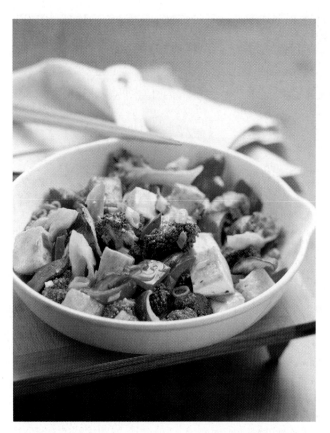

Meals like this tofu and vegetable stir-fry provide the vegetarian with essential vitamins and protein. Adding a whole grain, such as brown rice, would further enhance this meal by making use of complementary plant proteins.

Antioxidants and Your Health

Many people today believe that **antioxidants** are wonder nutrients that will prevent just about anything. Whereas these substances do appear to protect people from the ravages of oxidative stress and resultant tissue damage at the cellular level, you may want to take a step back and consider all of the evidence. First, it is important to understand what *oxidative stress* really is. This damage occurs in a complex process in which *free radicals* (molecules with unpaired electrons that are produced in excess when the body is overly stressed through exposure to toxic substances or events) either damage or kill healthy cells, cell proteins, or genetic material in the cells. Antioxidants produce enzymes that destroy excess free radicals by scavenging free radicals, slowing their formation, and/or actually repairing oxidative stress damage.

antioxidants Substances believed to protect active people from oxidative stress and resultant tissue damage at the cellular level.

carotenoids Fat-soluble compounds with antioxidant properties.

Thus, the theory goes that if you consume lots of antioxidants, you will nullify or greatly reduce the negative effects of oxidative stress. Among the more commonly cited nutrients touted as providing a protective effect are vitamin C, vitamin E, beta-carotene and other carotenoids, and the mineral selenium.

How valid is the theory? To date, many claims about the benefits of antioxidants in reducing the risk of heart disease, improving vision, and slowing the aging process have not been fully investigated, and conclusive statements about their true benefits aren't available. Studies do indicate that when people's diets include foods rich in vitamin C, they seem to develop fewer cancers, but other studies detect no effect from dietary vitamin C.[28]

Possibilities of vitamin E are even more controversial. It has long been theorized that because many cancers result from DNA damage, and vitamin E appears to protect against DNA damage, it would also reduce cancer risk. Surprisingly, the great majority of studies demonstrate no effect.[29] The American Heart Association cautions people to get their antioxidants from a balanced diet, rather than from supplements in pill form.

Some minerals, including selenium, copper, zinc, iron, and magnesium, also have shown promising results in trials where they are linked to a variety of health benefits. But as with vitamins, much of this research continues to be controversial.

Carotenoids are part of the red, orange, and yellow pigments found in fruits and vegetables. They are fat soluble, transported in the blood by lipoproteins, and stored in the fatty tissues of the body. Beta-carotene, the most researched carotenoid, is a precursor of vitamin A. This means that vitamin A can be produced in the body from beta-carotene; like vitamin A, beta-carotene has antioxidant properties.[30]

Although there are over 600 carotenoids in nature, two that receive the most attention are *lycopene* (found in tomatoes, papaya, pink grapefruit, and guava) and *lutein* (found in green, leafy vegetables such as spinach, broccoli, kale, and brussels sprouts). Both are believed to be more beneficial than beta-carotene in preventing disease.

The National Cancer Institute and the American Cancer Society have endorsed lycopene as a possible factor in reducing the risk of cancer. An influential study assessing the effects of tomato-based foods reported that men who ate 10 or more servings of lycopene-rich foods per week had a 45 percent reduced risk of prostate cancer.[31] Subsequent research has questioned the benefits of lycopene and some professional groups are modifying their endorsements of tomato-based products.

Lutein is most often touted as a means of protecting the eyes, particularly from age-related macular degeneration (ARMD), a leading cause of blindness for people aged 65 and over. Researchers speculate that oxidative damage may contribute to ARMD, and thus, antioxidants may be a means of prevention.[32] Researchers at the National Eye Institute found that those with the highest blood levels of lutein and other antioxidants found in foods were 70 percent less likely to develop ARMD than those with the lowest levels. Researchers in the Nurses Health Study found that eating spinach more than five days a week lowered risk by 47 percent and also lowered risk of cataracts.[33]

"Antioxidants should always be taken as part of a well-balanced mixture, either as a diet or as a supplement, and not singly," says Dr. John R. Smythies, a researcher at the University of California–San Diego and author of *Every Person's Guide to Antioxidants*.[34] Smythies, like other experts, advocates balance in intake and advises that adults take 500 milligrams of vitamin C and 400 to 800 IUs of vitamin E daily, plus 10 milligrams of beta-carotene. Researchers agree that intake should vary based on physical activity levels and overall health. According to Dr. Balz Frei at the Linus Pauling Institute, the "200 rule" might be the best option. This recommendation calls for fruits and vegetables in the diet and a supplement of 200 milligrams of vitamin C, 200 IUs of vitamin E, and 200 micrograms of selenium, along with 400 micrograms of folate and 3 milligrams of vitamin B_6 daily.[35] Until research conclusively proves the benefit or harm, a moderate intake as part of a vegetable- and fruit-abundant diet is desirable.

Probiotics are currently receiving much attention as natural healers. Probiotics are live microorganisms found in, or added to, fermented foods, which optimize the bacterial environment in our intestines. Commonly, they are found in fermented milk products such as yogurt, and you will see them labeled as *Lactobacillus* or *Bifidobacterium* in a product's list of ingredients. Although thousands of studies of various supplements and functional foods have been done, no single supplement has been proven effective in a compelling way.[36] Probiotics do not typically pose harm to healthy humans. However, it is possible that someone with a compromised immune system could have complications over time.

Folate

In 1998, the FDA began requiring *folate* fortification of all bread, cereal, rice, and pasta sold in the United States. This practice, which boosts folate intake by an average of about 100 µg daily, is expected to decrease the number of infants born with spina bifida and other neural tube defects.

Folate is a form of vitamin B that is believed to protect against cardiovascular disease and decrease blood levels of *homocysteine,* an amino acid that has been linked to vascular diseases.[37] Homocysteine results from the breakdown of methionine, an amino acid found in meat and other protein-laden foods. Two B vitamins—folate and B_6—are believed to control homocysteine levels.[38] When intake of folate and B_6 is low, homocysteine levels rise in the blood. Recent studies indicate that when the level of homocysteine rises, arterial walls and blood platelets become sticky, which encourages clotting. (*Note:* Homocysteine levels tend to rise with age, smoking, and menopause.) When clots develop in areas already narrowed by atherosclerosis, a heart attack or stroke can result.

Although the amount of folate needed to protect the heart has not been determined, many people have jumped on the

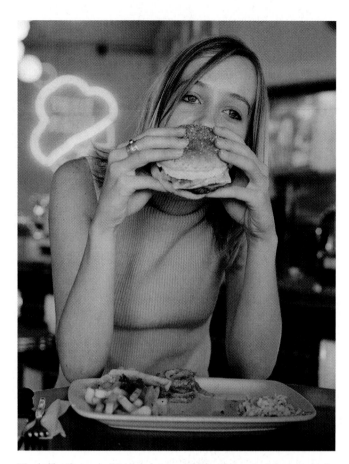

Meals like the one pictured above might be convenient, but are high in fat and calories. It is possible to make healthier choices when you are short on time and money.

folate bandwagon, taking daily folate supplements of up to 800 µg. Recently, a new *dietary folate equivalent (DFE)* was established to distinguish folate in food from its synthetic counterpart, *folic acid*. As a food additive or a supplement, folic acid is absorbed about twice as efficiently as folate. The DFE for folate in women aged 19 or over is approximately 400 µg, with higher levels for pregnant or lactating women. (See Table 8.3 for daily recommended amounts of other B vitamins.) Potential dangers of taking too much folate include masking of B_{12} (cobalamin) deficiencies and resulting problems ranging from nerve damage, immunodeficiency problems, anemia, fatigue, and headache to constipation, diarrhea, weight loss, gastrointestinal disturbances, and a host of neurological symptoms.[39]

probiotics   Live microorganisms found in or added to fermented foods; they optimize the bacterial environment in our intestines.

folate   A type of vitamin B that is believed to decrease levels of homocysteine, an amino acid that has been linked to vascular diseases.

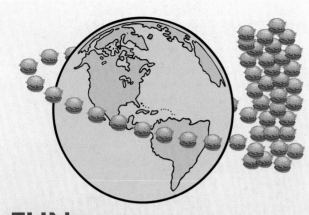

FUNfact

U.S. college students consume an estimated 2 billion hamburgers each year. That's enough burgers to circle the earth nearly 5 times.

FIGURE 8.9 How Many Hamburgers Do U.S. College Students Eat Each Year?

Source: Based on an estimated 14 million college students in the United States, consuming an average of 3 hamburgers per week. *Cornell Hotel and Restaurant Administration Quarterly,* June 2000.

Gender and Nutrition

Men and women differ in body size, body composition, and overall metabolic rates. Not surprisingly, they have differing needs for most nutrients throughout the life cycle and face unique difficulties in keeping on track with their dietary goals. We have already discussed some of these differences. However, there are some factors that need further consideration. Have you ever wondered why men can eat more than women without gaining weight? Although there are many possible reasons, one factor is that women have a lower ratio of lean body mass to adipose (fatty) tissue at all ages and stages of life. Also, after sexual maturation, the rate of metabolism is higher in men, meaning that they will burn more calories doing the same activities.

Different Cycles, Different Needs

In addition to these differences, women have many more "milestone" times in life when their nutritional needs vary significantly from requirements at other times. From menarche to menopause, women undergo cyclical physiological changes that can exert dramatic effects on metabolism and nutritional needs. For example, during pregnancy and lactation, women's nutritional requirements increase substantially. Those who are unable to follow the strict dietary recommen-

dations of their doctors may find themselves gaining much weight during pregnancy and retaining it afterward. During the menstrual cycle, many women report significant food cravings. Later in life, with the advent of menopause, nutritional needs again change rather dramatically. With depletion of the hormone estrogen, the body's need for calcium to ward off bone deterioration becomes pronounced. Women must pay closer attention to exercising and getting enough calcium through diet or dietary supplements, or they run the risk of osteoporosis (see Chapter 19).

Changing the "Meat-and-Potatoes" American

Since our earliest agrarian years, many Americans, especially men, have relied on a "meat-and-potatoes" diet. What's wrong with all those hamburgers and french fries? Heart disease, stroke, and cancer are probably the greatest threats. Add increased risk for colon and prostate cancers, and the rationale for dietary change becomes even more compelling.

Consider the following points:

- Heavy red meat eaters are more than twice as likely to get prostate cancer and nearly five times more likely to develop colon cancer.
- For every three servings of fruits or vegetables they consume per day, men can expect a 22 percent lower risk of stroke.
- Diets high in fruit and vegetables may lower the risk of lung cancer in smokers from 20 times the risk of nonsmokers to "only" 10 times the risk. They may also protect against oral, throat, pancreatic, and bladder cancers, all of which are more common among smokers.
- The fastest rising malignancy in the United States is cancer of the lower esophagus, particularly among white men. Though obesity seems to be a factor, fruits and vegetables are the protectors. (The average American male eats fewer than three servings per day, although five to nine servings are recommended. Women average three to seven servings per day.)

Does something in meat make it inherently bad? The fat content of meat and fried potatoes and the potential carcinogenic substances produced through cooking have been implicated. Probably something more basic is also involved. By eating so much protein, a person fills up sooner and never gets around to the fruits and vegetables. Thus, the potential protective value of consuming these foods is lost. Use the information in the Skills for Behavior Change box on page 270 to incorporate more salads into your diet.

Improved Eating for the College Student

College students often face a challenge when trying to eat healthy foods. Some students live in dorms and do not have their own cooking or refrigeration facilities. Others live in crowded apartments where everyone forages in the refrigerator for everyone else's food. Still others eat at university food services where food choices may be limited. And nearly all of them have financial and time constraints that make buying, preparing, and eating healthy food a difficult task. What's a student to do?

When Time Is Short: Eating on the Run

Is there really a way to make a meal from McDonald's healthy?

Many college students may find it hard to fit a well-balanced meal into the day, but eating breakfast and lunch are important in order to keep energy levels up and get the most out of your classes. If your campus is like many others, you've probably noticed a distinct move toward fast-food restaurants in your student unions, in order to meet students' needs for a fast bite of food at a reasonable price between classes.

Eating a complete breakfast that includes complex carbohydrates and protein, and bringing a small healthy snack such as carrots, an apple, or even a small sandwich on whole-grain bread to class are all ways to ensure you fit meals into your day. Bringing food with you to munch on throughout the day is also a lot easier on your wallet (see Figure 8.9). If you must eat fast food, follow the tips below.

- Ask for nutritional analyses of items. Most fast-food chains now have them.
- Order salads, and be careful how much dressing you add. Many people think they are being health-smart by eating salad, only to load it with calorie- and fat-laden dressing. Try the vinegar and oil or low-fat alternative dressings or get your dressing on the side. Stay away from eggs and other high-fat add-ons such as bacon bits.
- If you must have fries, check to see what type of oil is used to cook them. Avoid lard-based or other saturated fat products. Oven-baked fries are usually best.
- Avoid giant sizes and refrain from ordering extra sauce, butter, bacon, and other such items high in additional calories and fat.
- Order one single hamburger, and ask the server to hold the cheese.

For more tips on eating healthfully at a restaurant, see the Spotlight on Your Health box on page 272.

When Funds Are Short

Maintaining a nutritious diet within the confines of student life can be challenging. However, if you take the time to plan healthy meals, you will find that you are eating better, enjoying it more, and actually saving money. Follow these steps to ensure a healthy

TABLE 8.6	Eating Well in the Dining Hall

- Choose lean meats, grilled chicken, fish, or vegetable dishes. Avoid fried chicken, fatty cuts of red meat, or meat dishes smothered in creamy or oily sauce.
- Hit the salad bar and load up on leafy greens, beans, tuna, or tofu. Choose items such as avocado or nuts for a little "good" fat, and go easy on the dressing.
- Get creative: Choose items such as a baked potato with salsa, or add a grilled chicken breast to your salad. Toast some bread, and top it with veggies, hummus, or grilled chicken or tuna.
- When choosing foods from a made-to-order food station, ask the preparer to hold the butter or oil, mayonnaise, sour cream, or a cheese- or cream-based sauce. Do ask for extra servings of veggies and lean meat or white-meat chicken.
- Avoid going back for seconds and consuming large portions. Many colleges limit the number of visits you make each day to the dining hall, but don't view this as a reason to overeat.
- If there is something you'd like, but you don't see it in your dining hall, or you are vegetarian and feel like your food choices are limited, speak to your food services manager and provide suggestions.
- Pass on high-calorie, low-nutrient foods such as sugary cereals, soft-serve ice cream, waffles, and other sweet treats. Choose fruit or low-fat yogurt to satisfy your sweet tooth.

but affordable diet, and see Table 8.6 for ideas on how to eat healthily in the dining hall.

- Buy fruits and vegetables in season whenever possible for their lower cost, higher nutrient quality, and greater variety. As soon as you get home, wash them, cut them up, and put them in small bags. You are more likely to eat them if they are quickly available.
- Use coupons and specials to get price reductions.
- Shop at discount warehouse food chains; capitalize on volume discounts and no-frills products.
- Plan ahead to get the most for your dollar and avoid extra trips to the store; extra trips usually mean extra purchases. Make a list and stick to it.
- Purchase meats and other products in volume, freezing portions for future needs. Or purchase small amounts of meat and combine it with beans and plant proteins for lower cost, calories, and fat.
- Cook large meals, and freeze small portions for later.
- Drain off extra fat after cooking. Save juices and broths to use in soups and other dishes.
- If you find that you have no money for food, talk to staff at your county or city health department. They may know of ways for you to get assistance.

ADDING MORE SALADS TO YOUR DIET

Salads and healthful salad toppings add variety to your diet and balance out the average American's meat-and-potatoes diet. Use this information to choose healthful salad greens and toppings.

NUTRITIONAL COMPARISON OF SALAD GREEN SERVINGS

Salad Green (1 cup)	Calories	Vitamin A (IU)	Vitamin C (mg)	Potassium (mg)	Calcium (mg)
Arugula (rocket, roquette)	5	480	3	74	32
Butterhead lettuce (Boston, Bibb)	7	534	4	141	18
Cabbage, red	19	28	40	144	36
Endive	8	1,025	3	157	26
Iceberg lettuce	7	182	2	87	10
Leaf lettuce	10	1,064	10	148	38
Romaine lettuce	8	1,456	13	162	20
Spinach	7	2,015	8	167	30*

NUTRITIONAL COMPARISON OF HEALTHFUL SALAD TOPPINGS

Topping	Serving Size	Calories	Bonus Nutrients
Artichoke hearts, in olive oil	1 heart	40	Fiber, folate, potassium, calcium
Avocado, California	¼ of whole fruit	77	Monounsaturated fats, vitamin E, folate, fiber
Beets	½ cup boiled	37	Folate, potassium
Broccoli	½ cup raw	12	Vitamins A and C, calcium, potassium, fiber

 try it NOW

Eating for health and convenience. Eating while you are short on time shouldn't mean you have to compromise on nutrition. Make it a habit to purchase items like small bags of carrots and salad-in-a-bag. If you have to eat at McDonald's, order a happy meal or get a grilled chicken sandwich and toss half the bun. Try choosing one day of the week to prepare a quick, big, healthy meal with your roommates. Make enough for leftovers and you'll be eating well for lunch the next day too!

dietary supplements   Vitamins and minerals taken by mouth that are intended to supplement existing diets.

Supplements: New Research on the Daily Dose

In 2002, sales of dietary supplements increased to nearly $20 billion, with projections for rapid increases over the next decade.[40] **Dietary supplements** are usually vitamins and minerals taken by mouth and are intended to supplement existing diets. Ingredients range from vitamins and minerals to enzymes and organ tissues. They can come in tablet, capsule, liquid, or other forms. An important thing to remember about all dietary supplements is that they are regulated differently than other food and drug products. Currently, there are no formal guidelines for their sale and safety, and supplement

Topping	Serving Size	Calories	Bonus Nutrients
Carrots	½ cup raw	31	Vitamin A, beta-carotene, fiber
Cauliflower	½ cup raw	13	Vitamin C
Celery	½ cup raw	6	Vitamin C, potassium
Chicken breast	3 ounces white meat	173	Protein, niacin, vitamin B_6
Chickpeas (garbanzo beans)	½ cup boiled or canned	135	Protein, folate, calcium, potassium, zinc, fiber
Egg, hard boiled	1 whole	78	Vitamins A, E, B_{12}, and D, riboflavin, folate, selenium, zinc. Limit to one egg.
Mushrooms	½ cup	9	Riboflavin, niacin, potassium, selenium
Olives	5 small	20	Monounsaturated fats
Peppers, red, yellow, orange	½ cup raw	14	Vitamins A and C, beta-carotene, fiber
Sunflower seeds	1 ounce	160	Vitamins E, B_6, niacin, folate, copper, magnesium, zinc, fiber, linoleic acid
Tofu, processed with calcium sulfate	½ cup	94	Protein, calcium, iron, manganese
Tomatoes	½ tomato	13	Vitamins A, C, potassium, lycopene
Tuna, canned, in water	3 ounces	99	Protein, niacin, omega-3 fatty acids

Note: IU = international units, mg = milligrams

*Much not available to body for use.

Source: From A. Platzman, "Salads: Going Beyond the Green to Boost Nutrition," and "Nutrition Comparison of Healthful Salad Toppings." Reprinted with permission from *Environmental Nutrition* (August 2002), 52 Riverside Drive, Suite 15A, New York, NY 10024. For subscription information: (800) 829-5384, www.environmentalnutrition.com.

manufacturers are responsible for self-monitoring their activities. The United States Food and Drug administration is developing guidelines for their sale. Nevertheless, consumers are using them for a wide variety of health-promoting reasons, from improving performance and energy to preventing colds and flu.

For years, health experts touted the benefits of eating a balanced diet over popping a vitamin or mineral supplement. So eyebrows were raised when an article in the esteemed *Journal of the American Medical Association (JAMA)* recommended that "a vitamin/mineral supplement a day just might be important in keeping the doctor away, particularly for some groups of people."[41] The article indicated that elderly people, vegans, alcohol-dependent individuals, and patients with malabsorption problems may be at particular risk for deficiency of several vitamins. Although it acknowledged that there may be a risk if you overdose on fat-soluble vitamins, it noted that preliminary research has linked inadequate amounts of nutrients such as vitamins B_6, B_{12}, D, and E to chronic diseases, including coronary heart disease, cancer, and osteoporosis. As a result of this study, JAMA advised that all adults should take a basic multivitamin. Yet, the scientific debate doesn't stop there.

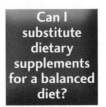
Can I substitute dietary supplements for a balanced diet?

If you are in doubt about which supplements might be best for you, make sure you eat from the major food groups. If you are facing extreme stressors on the body from physical endurance events, illness, or other nutrient-depleting events, supplements might be beneficial, and in general, a multivitamin added to a balanced diet is likely to do more good than harm. In all cases, beware of megadoses and overdosing on ultravitamin supplements.

WHAT'S GOOD ON THE MENU?

Although some restaurants offer hints for health-conscious diners, you're on your own most of the time. To help you order wisely, here are lighter options and high-fat pitfalls. "Best" choices contain fewer than 30 grams of fat, a generous meal's worth for an active, medium-sized woman. "Worst" choices have up to 100 grams of fat.

FAST FOOD

Best	Grilled chicken sandwich
	Roast beef sandwich
	Single hamburger
	Salad with light vinaigrette
Worst	Bacon burger
	Double cheeseburger
	French fries
	Onion rings
Tips	Order sandwiches without mayo or "special sauce." Avoid deep-fried items like fish fillets, chicken nuggets, and french fries.

ITALIAN

Best	Pasta with red or white clam sauce
	Spaghetti with marinara or tomato-and-meat sauce
Worst	Eggplant parmigiana
	Fettuccine Alfredo
	Fried calamari
	Lasagna
Tips	Stick with plain bread instead of garlic bread made with butter or oil. Ask for the waiter's help in avoiding cream- or egg-based sauces. Try vegetarian pizza, and don't ask for extra cheese.

MEXICAN

Best	Bean burrito (no cheese)
	Chicken fajitas
Worst	Beef chimichanga
	Chile relleno
	Quesadilla
	Refried beans
Tips	Choose soft tortillas (not fried) with fresh salsa, not guacamole. Special-order grilled shrimp, fish, or chicken. Ask for beans made without lard or fat and for cheeses and sour cream provided on the side or left out altogether.

CHINESE

Best	Hot-and-sour soup
	Stir-fried vegetables
	Shrimp with garlic sauce
	Szechuan shrimp
	Wonton soup
Worst	Crispy chicken
	Kung pao chicken
	Moo shu pork
	Sweet-and-sour pork
Tips	Share a stir-fry; help yourself to steamed rice. Ask for vegetables steamed or stir-fried with less oil. Order moo shu vegetables instead of pork. Avoid fried rice,

Food Safety: A Growing Concern

As we become increasingly worried that the food we put in our mouths may be contaminated with bacteria, insects, worms, or other substances, the food industry has come under fire. To convince us that their products are safe, some manufacturers have come up with "new and improved" ways of protecting our foods. How well do they work?

Foodborne Illnesses

Are you concerned that the chicken you are buying doesn't look pleasingly pink, or that your "fresh" fish smells a little *too* fishy or has a grayish tinge? Are you sure that your apple juice is free of animal waste? You may have good reason to be worried. In increasing numbers, Americans are becoming sick from what they eat, and many of these illnesses are life-threatening. Scientists estimate, based on several studies conducted over the past ten years, that foodborne pathogens sicken over 76 million people and cause some 400,000 hospitalizations and 5,000 deaths in the United States annually.[42] Because most of us don't go to the doctor every time we feel ill, we may not make a connection between what we eat and later symptoms.

Signs of foodborne illnesses vary tremendously and usually include one or several symptoms: diarrhea, nausea, cramping, and vomiting. Depending on the amount and virulence of the pathogen, symptoms may appear as early as 30 minutes after eating contaminated food or as long as several days or weeks later. Most of the time, symptoms occur five to eight hours after eating and last only a day or two. For certain populations, however, such as the very young, the elderly, or people with severe illnesses such as cancer, diabetes, kidney disease, or AIDS, foodborne diseases can be fatal.

breaded dishes, egg rolls and spring rolls, and items loaded with nuts. Avoid high-sodium sauces.

JAPANESE

Best   Steamed rice and vegetables

Tofu as a substitute for meat

Broiled or steamed chicken and fish

Worst   Fried rice dishes

Miso (very high in sodium)

Tempura

Tips   Avoid soy sauces. Use caution in eating sashimi and sushi (raw fish) dishes to avoid possible bacteria or parasites.

THAI

Best   Clear broth soups

Stir-fried chicken and vegetables

Grilled meats

Worst   Coconut milk

Peanut sauces

Deep-fried dishes

Tips   Avoid coconut-based curries. Ask for steamed, not fried, rice.

BREAKFAST

Best   Hot or cold cereal with 2% milk

Pancakes or French toast with syrup

Scrambled eggs with hash browns and plain toast

Worst   Belgian waffle with sausage

Sausage and eggs with biscuits and gravy

Ham-and-cheese omelette with hash browns and toast

Tips   Ask for whole-grain cereal or shredded wheat with 1% milk or whole-wheat toast without butter or margarine. Order omelettes without cheese, fried eggs without bacon or sausage.

SANDWICHES

Best   Ham and Swiss cheese

Roast beef

Turkey

Worst   Tuna salad

Reuben

Submarine

Tips   Ask for mustard; hold the mayo and cheese. See if turkey-ham is available.

SEAFOOD

Best   Broiled bass, halibut, or snapper

Grilled scallops

Steamed crab or lobster

Worst   Fried seafood platter

Blackened catfish

Tips   Order fish broiled, baked, grilled, or steamed—not pan-fried or sauteed. Ask for lemon instead of tartar sauce. Avoid creamy and buttery sauces.

Sources: American Dietetic Association, 2002, www.eatright.org.

Several factors may be contributing to the increase in foodborne illnesses. The movement away from a traditional meat-and-potato American diet to "heart-healthy" eating—increasing consumption of fruits, vegetables, and grains—has spurred demand for fresh foods that are not in season most of the year. This means that we must import fresh fruits and vegetables, thus putting ourselves at risk for ingesting exotic pathogens or even pesticides that have been banned in the United States for safety reasons. Depending on the season, up to 70 percent of the fruits and vegetables consumed in the United States come from Mexico alone. The upshot is that a visit to developing countries isn't necessary to be stricken with foodborne "traveler's diarrhea," because the produce does the traveling. Although we are told when we travel to developing countries, "boil it, peel it, or don't eat it," we bring these foods into our kitchens and eat them, often without even washing them. Food can become contaminated by being watered with contaminated water, fertilized with "organic" fertilizers (animal manure), hand picked by people who have not washed their hands properly after using the toilet, or by not being subjected to the same rigorous pesticide regulations as American-raised produce. To give you an idea of the implications, studies have shown that *Escherichia coli* (*E. coli*, a lethal bacterial pathogen) can survive in cow manure for up to 70 days and can multiply in foods grown with manure unless heat or additives such as salt or preservatives are used to kill the microbes.[43] There are no regulations that prohibit farmers from using animal manure to fertilize crops. Turkey manure, pig manure, and other agribusiness by-products are often sprayed on fields that ultimately grow foods for consumers. *E. coli* O157:H7 actually increases in summer months in cows awaiting slaughter in crowded, overheated pens. This increases the chances of meat coming to market already contaminated.[44] Key factors associated with the increasing spread of foodborne diseases include the following:[45]

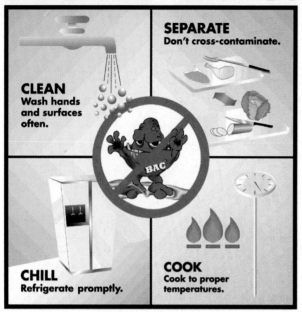

FIGHT BAC!

CLEAN Wash hands and surfaces often.

SEPARATE Don't cross-contaminate.

CHILL Refrigerate promptly.

COOK Cook to proper temperatures.

Keep Food Safe From Bacteria™

FIGURE 8.10 The USDA's Fight BAC!
This logo reminds consumers how to prevent foodborne illness.

- *Globalization of the food supply.* Because food is distributed worldwide, the possibility of exposure to pathogens native to remote regions of the world is greater. For example, a large outbreak of *Shigella* occurred in Norway, Sweden, and the United Kingdom from lettuce that originated in southern Europe.
- *Climate change and global warming.* These may increase the incidence of infectious diseases and certain types of toxins. Extreme weather may cause flooding, which contaminates food supplies.
- *Inadvertent introduction of pathogens into new geographic regions.* Cholera may have been introduced into waters off the coast of the southern United States when a cargo ship discharged contaminated ballast as it came into harbor. Other pathogens may enter into aquatic life in a similar manner.
- *Exposure to unfamiliar foodborne hazards.* Travelers, refugees, and immigrants who move through foreign countries are exposed to foodborne hazards and bring them home.
- *Changes in microbial populations.* Changing microbial populations can lead to the evolution of new pathogens. As a result, old pathogens develop new virulence factors or become resistant to antibiotics, making diseases more difficult to treat.
- *Increased susceptibility of varying populations.* People are becoming more vulnerable to disease. The numbers of highly susceptible persons are expanding worldwide because of aging populations, HIV infection, and other

underlying medical conditions, such as malnutrition and the compromised health status that results from the use of immunosuppressive drugs. In developing countries, poor hygiene and inadequate sanitation facilities and food preparation areas also increase risk.

- *Insufficient education about food safety.* Increased urbanization, industrialization, and travel, combined with more people eating out, raise the risk of unsafe food handling and illness.

Know what the typical foodborne hazards are, how you can contract them, and what you can do to prevent infection. Table 8.7 lists common foodborne illnesses and their symptoms.

Responsible Use: Avoiding Risks in the Home

Part of the responsibility for preventing foodborne illness lies with consumers (see Figure 8.10 for the USDA's food safety recommendations). Over 30 percent of all such illnesses result from unsafe handling of food at home.

- When shopping, pick up packaged and canned foods first, and save frozen foods and perishables such as dairy, meat, poultry, and fish till last. Place these foods in separate plastic bags so drippings don't run onto other foods in your cart and contaminate them. When you get home, store foods in separate areas so that meat drippings don't contaminate fresh vegetables, fruits, and water or ice.
- Check for cleanliness at the salad bar, and meat and fish counters. For instance, cooked shrimp lying on the same small bed of ice as raw fish can easily be contaminated.
- When shopping for fish, buy from markets that get their supplies from state-approved or organic sources; stay clear of vendors who sell shellfish from roadside stands or the back of trucks. If you're planning to harvest your own shellfish, check the safety of the water in the area.
- Most cuts of meat, fish, and poultry should be kept in the refrigerator no more than one or two days. They shouldn't be in the grocery store meat counter beyond their dated shelf life, either. Check the shelf life of all products before buying. If expiration dates are close, freeze or eat the product immediately.
- Avoid preparing food if you are ill. Wear latex gloves if you have cuts or burns on your hands. Keep your hands away from your nose, mouth, and eyes. Thoroughly wash your hands after bathroom trips.
- Eat leftovers within three days. Store leftovers in small containers to ensure they cool faster, and heat up easily all the way through. This will prevent bacterial growth.
- Keep hot foods hot and cold foods cold.
- Use a thermometer to ensure that meats are completely cooked. Beef and lamb steaks and roasts should be cooked to at least 145°F; ground meat, pork chops, ribs, and egg dishes to 160°F; ground poultry and hot dogs to 165°F; chicken and turkey breasts to 170°F; and chicken and turkey legs, thighs, and whole birds to 180°F.

TABLE 8.7 Recognizing the Common Foodborne Illnesses

Illness	Symptoms/Related Problems
Campylobacteriosis	Diarrhea (can be severe), abdominal pain, fever. Incubation period is 2–5 days, and illness usually lasts 2–10 days. Can be fatal in the very young, the very old, or the immunocompromised.
Clostridium perfringens	Typically occurs 6–24 hours after ingestion of food. Mild gastrointestinal distress lasting a day. Deaths are uncommon.
Escherichia coli O157:H7	Mild gastrointestinal illness that occurs 3–5 days after eating contaminated foods. If there is sudden onset of severe abdominal cramps, little or no fever, and diarrhea that may become grossly bloody, contact doctor or go to the emergency room.
Listeria monocytogenes	Characterized by sudden onset of fever, severe headache, vomiting, and other flulike symptoms. Listeriosis may appear mild in healthy adults and more severe in fetuses, older adults, those with kidney disease, or the immunocompromised.
Salmonella	Usually occurs 6–72 hours after eating contaminated foods and lasts for a day or two. Nausea, diarrhea, stomach pain and vomiting are hallmark symptoms.
Staphylococcus aureus	Usually occurs within 1–6 hours following consumption of toxins; may occur within 30 minutes. Severe nausea and vomiting, cramps, and diarrhea are common. Illness lasts longer than 1–2 days typically.
Toxoplasmosis	Mild flulike symptoms or no symptoms. Undercooked meat or cat feces often the cause. Can cause stillbirths and birth defects.

Source: Centers for Disease Control and Prevention, "Foodborne Illnesses," 2003, www.cdc.gov/health/foodill.htm.

- Fish is done when the thickest part becomes opaque and the fish flakes easily when poked with a fork. If you have any concerns, skip seafood such as sushi and raw oysters.
- Never leave cooked food standing on the stove or table for more than two hours. Disease-causing bacteria grow in temperatures between 40°F and 140°F. Cooked foods that have been left standing in this temperature range for more than two hours should be thrown away.
- Never bring your grilled meat into the house on the same plate you took it out on when it was uncooked. Raw meat juices are hotbeds for deadly bacteria.
- Never thaw frozen foods at room temperature. Put them in the refrigerator for a day to thaw or thaw in cold water, changing the water every 30 minutes.
- Wash your hands with soap and water between courses when preparing food, particularly after handling meat, fish, or poultry. Use warm (not hot) water and soap. Don't use antibacterial soap, which only contributes to antibacterial resistance. To wash, rub hands vigorously together for 15 to 20 seconds. Wash the countertop and all utensils before using them for other foods.

Food Irradiation: How Safe Is It?

Each year, thousands of people get sick from largely preventable diseases such as those caused by *E. coli* and other bacteria such as *Salmonella* and *Listeria* (Chapter 17). In response to these concerns, the USDA approved large-scale irradiation of beef, lamb, poultry, pork, and other raw animal foods. It has also approved irradiation of wheat, potatoes, flour, spices, fruits, and vegetables for the purpose of eliminating insects and inhibiting spoilage.

Food irradiation is a process that involves treating foods with invisible waves of energy that damage microorganisms. These energy waves are actually low doses of radiation, or ionizing energy, which breaks chemical bonds in the DNA of harmful bacteria, destroying the pathogens and keeping them from replicating. The rays essentially pass through the food without leaving any radioactive residue.[46]

The minimal costs of irradiation should result in lower overall costs to consumers, in addition to reducing the need for toxic chemicals now used to preserve foods and prevent foodborne illnesses from external pathogens. Some environmentalists and consumer groups have raised concerns; however, food irradiation is now common in over 40 countries. Foods that have been irradiated are marked with the "radura" logo.

Food Additives

Additives (such as nitrates added to cured meats) generally reduce the risk of foodborne illness, prevent spoilage, and enhance the way foods look and taste. Additives can also enhance nutrient value, especially to benefit the general public. Good examples include the fortification of milk with vitamin

food irradiation Treating foods with gamma radiation from radioactive cobalt, cesium, or some other source of X rays to kill microorganisms.

D and of grain products with folate. Although the FDA regulates additives according to effectiveness, safety, and ability to detect them in foods, questions have been raised about additives put into foods intentionally and those that get in unintentionally before or after processing. Whenever such products are added, consumers should take the time to determine what the substances are and if there are alternatives. As a general rule of thumb, the fewer chemicals, colorants, and preservatives, the better. Also, it should be noted that certain foods and additives can interact with medications. To be a smart consumer, be aware of these potential dietary interactions. Examples of common additives include:

- *Antimicrobial agents.* Substances such as salt, sugar, nitrates, and others tend to make foods less hospitable for microbes.
- *Antioxidants.* Substances that preserve color and flavor by reducing loss due to exposure to oxygen. Vitamins C and E are among the antioxidants believed to reduce the risk of cancer and cardiovascular disease. BHA and BHT are additives that also are antioxidant in action.
- *Artificial colors.*
- *Nutrient additives.*
- *Flavor enhancers such as MSG (monosodium glutamate)*
- *Sulfites.* Used to preserve vegetable color; some people have severe allergic reactions.
- *Dioxins.* Found in coffee filters, milk containers, and frozen foods.
- *Methylene chloride.* Found in decaffeinated coffee.
- *Hormones.* Bovine growth hormone (BGH) is found in some animal meat.

Food Allergy or Food Intolerance?

At some point in time, nearly everyone will experience a *food allergy* or *food intolerance*. You eat something, develop gas or have an unpleasant visit to the bathroom, and then assume that it is a food allergy. One out of every three people today either say they have a food allergy or avoid something in their diet because they think they are allergic; in fact, only 2 percent of adults and 5 percent of all children experience genuine allergic reactions to what they eat.[47] Surprised? Most people are when they hear this.

food allergy Overreaction by the body to normally harmless proteins, which are perceived as allergens. In response, the body produces antibodies, triggering allergic symptoms.

food intolerance Adverse effects resulting when people who lack the digestive chemicals needed to break down certain substances eat those substances.

organic Foods that are grown without use of pesticides, chemicals, or hormones.

A **food allergy,** or hypersensitivity, is an abnormal response to a food that is triggered by the immune system. Reactions range from minor rashes to severe swelling in the mouth, tongue, and throat, to violent vomiting and diarrhea and occasionally death.

In 2004, Congress passed the Food Allergies Labeling and Consumer Protection Act (FALCPA), which requires food manufacturers to clearly label foods containing ingredients that are common allergens, or foods that could have been contaminated by a major allergen. The most common allergens are milk, eggs, fish and shellfish, nuts, wheat, and soybeans.[48]

In contrast to allergies, in cases of **food intolerance** you may have symptoms of gastric upset, but they are not the result of an immune system response. Probably the best example of a food intolerance is *lactose intolerance,* a problem that affects about 1 in every 10 adults. Lactase is an enzyme in the lining of the gut that degrades lactose, which is in dairy products. If you don't have enough lactase, lactose cannot be digested and remains in the gut to be used by bacteria. Gas is formed, and you experience bloating, abdominal pain, and sometimes diarrhea. Food intolerance also occurs in response to some food additives, such as the flavor enhancer MSG, certain dyes, sulfites, gluten, and other substances. In some cases the food intolerance may have psychological triggers.

If you suspect that you have an actual allergic reaction to food, see an allergist to be tested to determine the source of the problem. Because there are several diseases that share symptoms with food allergies (ulcers and cancers of the gastrointestinal tract can cause vomiting, bloating, diarrhea, nausea, and pain), you should have persistent symptoms checked out as soon as possible. If particular foods seem to bother you consistently, look for alternatives or modify your diet. In true allergic instances, you may not be able to consume even the smallest amount safely. For example, people have had severe allergic reactions to peanuts from ingesting as little as a crumb or an airborne particle.

Is Organic for You?

Due to mounting concerns about food safety, many people refuse to buy processed foods and mass-produced agricultural products. Instead, they purchase foods that are **organic**—foods and beverages developed, grown, or raised without the use of synthetic pesticides, chemicals, or hormones. Less than a decade ago, buying organic foods meant going to a specialty store and paying premium prices for produce that was wilted, wormy, and smaller than its nonorganic alternative. People who bought these foods did so out of a desire to eat "healthier" produce and avoid the chemicals that they were increasingly being told caused cancer, immune system problems, and a host of other ailments.

Enter the organics of the twenty-first century—larger, more attractive, and fresher looking but still carrying a hefty price tag. The market for organics has been increasing by over 20 percent per year—five times faster than food sales in general. Nearly 40 percent of U.S. consumers now reach occasionally for something labeled organic, with sales topping $14 billion in 2005; by 2010, organic food sales are expected to rise to $23.8 billion.[49]

Is buying organic really better for you? Perhaps if we could put a group of people in a pristine environment and ensure that they never ate, drank, or were exposed to chemicals, we could test this hypothesis; however, it is difficult, if not impossible, to assess the overall impact of organic versus nonorganic food in terms of health outcomes. Organic farming is better for the environment, though.

How do I know if organic food is truly organic?

As of 2002, any food sold as organic has to meet criteria set by the U.S. Department of Agriculture under the National Organic Rule and can carry a new USDA seal verifying that it is "certified organic." Under this rule, something that is certified may carry one of the following terms: 100 Percent Organic (100 percent compliance with organic criteria), Organic (must contain at least 95 percent organic materials), Made with Organic Ingredients (must contain at least 70 percent organic ingredients), or Some Organic Ingredients (contains less than 70 percent organic ingredients—usually listed individually). In order to be certified and use any of the above terms, the foods must be produced without hormones, antibiotics, herbicides, insecticides, chemical fertilizers, genetic modification, or germ-killing radiation. However, reliable monitoring systems to ensure credibility are still under development.

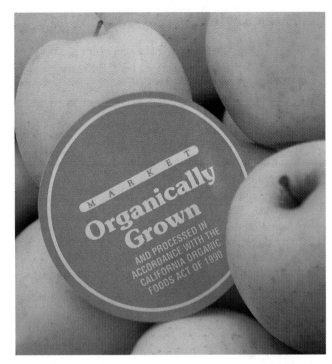

When buying organic foods at the grocery store, look for signs indicating that the foods you choose are in fact organic.

TAKING charge

Summary

- Recognizing that we eat for more reasons than just survival is the first step toward changing our dietary habits.
- The major nutrients that are essential for life and health include water, proteins, carbohydrates, fiber, fats, vitamins, and minerals. MyPyramid provides guidelines for healthy eating.
- Vegetarianism can provide a healthy alternative for those wishing to cut fat from their diets or reduce animal consumption. The vegetarian pyramid provides dietary guidelines to help vegetarians obtain needed nutrients.
- Men and women have differing needs for most nutrients throughout the life cycle because of different body size and composition.

- Experts are interested in the role of food as medicine and in the benefits of "functional foods." These foods may play an important role in improving certain conditions, such as hypertension.
- College students face unique challenges in eating healthfully. Learning to make better choices at fast-food restaurants, eat healthfully when funds are short, and eat nutritionally in the dorm are all possible when you use the knowledge in this chapter.
- Foodborne illnesses, food irradiation, food allergies, organic foods, and other food safety and health concerns are becoming increasingly important to healthwise consumers. Recognizing potential risks and taking steps to prevent problems are part of a sound nutritional plan.

Chapter Review

1. Which type of carbohydrates are found in grains, cereals, and potatoes?
   a. simple sugars
   b. complex carbs
   c. disaccharides
   d. cellulose

2. Which of the following foods would be considered a healthy, *nutrient-dense* food?
   a. nonfat milk
   b. cheddar cheese
   c. soft drink
   d. potato chips

3. Which of the following foods is not an example of a saturated fat?
   a. red meat
   b. dairy products
   c. egg yolks
   d. canola oil

4. What is a function of the nutrient water?
   a. It lubricates the joints of the body.
   b. It helps with the digestive process.
   c. It maintains body temperature.
   d. All of the above.

5. Which of the following nutrients are required for the repair and growth of body tissue?
   a. carbohydrates
   b. proteins
   c. vitamins
   d. fats

6. Foods containing *trans* fats are known as
   a. unsaturated fats.
   b. saturated fats.
   c. a liquid form of fat oils.
   d. polyunsaturated fats.

7. Which of the following is *not* a true statement of the new *Dietary Guidelines*?
   a. Consume a variety of foods within and among the basic food groups.
   b. Be physically active every day to stay in shape.
   c. Drink as many alcoholic beverages as you wish since alcohol is not part the nutritional guidelines.
   d. Choose fats wisely, and don't eat a lot of saturated fats.

8. Typically, when away from home and living on their own, college students change their diet by
   a. eating poorly.
   b. not eating enough servings of fruits and vegetables each day.
   c. not calculating their portion sizes accurately.
   d. All of the above are true.

9. A vegetarian person who consumes only dairy, eggs, and vegetables is known as a
   a. lacto-ovo-pesco vegetarian.
   b. lacto-vegetarian.
   c. vegan.
   d. laco-ovo vegetarian.

10. The healthier fat to include in the diet is
    a. *trans* fat.
    b. saturated fat.
    c. unsaturated fat.
    d. hydrogenated fat.

Answers to these questions can be found on page A-1.

Questions for Discussion and Reflection

1. Which factors influence the dietary patterns and behaviors of the typical college student? What factors have been the greatest influences on your eating behaviors? Why is it important to recognize influences on your diet as you think about changing eating behaviors?

2. What are the six major food groups in MyPyramid? From which groups do you eat too few servings? What can you do to increase or decrease your intake of selected food groups? How can you remember the six groups?

3. What are the major types of nutrients that you need to obtain from the foods you eat? What happens if you fail to get enough of some of them? Are there significant differences between the sexes in particular areas of nutrition?

4. Distinguish between the different types of vegetarianism. Which types are most likely to lead to nutrient deficiencies? What can be done to ensure that even the strictest vegetarian receives enough of the major nutrients?

5. What are functional foods? What are the major functional foods discussed in this chapter? What are their reported benefits, if any?

6. What are the major problems that many college students face when trying to eat the right foods? List five actions that you and your classmates could take immediately to improve your eating.

7. What are the potential benefits and risks of food irradiation? Why is it being used? What are the major risks for foodborne illnesses, and what can you do to protect yourself? How do food illnesses differ from food allergies?

Accessing Your Health on the Internet

The following websites explore further topics and issues related to personal health. You'll also find links to each organization's website on the Companion Website for *Access to Health*, Tenth Edition, at www.aw-bc.com/donatelle.

1. *American Dietetic Association (ADA).* Provides information on a full range of dietary topics, including sports nutrition, healthful cooking, and nutritional eating; also links to scientific publications and information on scholarships and public meetings. www.eatright.org

2. *American Heart Association (AHA).* Includes information about a heart-healthy eating plan and an easy-to-follow guide to healthy eating. www.americanheart.org

3. *Food and Nutrition Information Center.* Offers a wide variety of information related to food and nutrition. http://fnic.nal.usda.gov

4. *National Institutes of Health: Office of Dietary Supplements.* Site of the International Bibliographic Database of Information on Dietary Supplements (IBDIDS), updated quarterly. http://dietary-supplements.info.nih.gov

5. *U.S. Department of Agriculture (USDA).* Offers a full discussion of the USDA's *Dietary Guidelines for Americans.* www.usda.gov

6. *U.S. Food and Drug Administration (FDA).* Provides information for consumers and professionals in the areas of food safety, supplements, and medical devices and links to other sources of nutrition and food information. www.fda.gov

7. *National Center for Complementary and Alternative Medicine.* Includes information on new research results for supplements and functional foods. http://nccam.nih.gov

Further Reading

Center for Science in the Public Interest. *Nutrition Action Healthletter.* Washington, DC.

This newsletter, published ten times a year, contains up-to-date information on diet and nutritional claims and current research issues. The newsletter can be obtained by writing to the Center for Science in the Public Interest, 1501 16th St. NW, Washington, DC 20036.

Kaufman, F. *Diabesity: The Obesity Epidemic That Threatens America and What We Must Do to Stop It.* New York: Bantam Books, 2005.

Written by a past president of the American Diabetic Association who has a family history of diabetes, this book outlines a plan for changing lifestyle and slowing the course of diabetes in America.

Nutrition Today. Baltimore, MD: Williams & Wilkins.

An excellent magazine for the interested nonspecialist. Covers controversial issues and provides a forum for conflicting opinions. Six issues per year. Order from Williams & Wilkins, 351 West Camden Street, Baltimore, MD 21201-2436.

Schlosser, E. *Chew on This.* Boston: Houghton Mifflin, 2006.

Overview of fast foods and their effect on health and well-being in America, with a special focus on children.

Thompson, J. and M. Manore, *Nutrition: An Applied Approach.* San Francisco: Benjamin Cummings, 2005.

An introductory college health text that provides an outstanding overview of nutritional information in a highly accessible, easy-to-read format.

Tufts University Health and Nutrition Letter. Medford, MA: Tufts University.

An excellent source for quick "fixes" on current nutritional topics. Reputable sources and information. E-mail: tufts@tiac.net. Phone: (800) 274-7581. The Tufts Nutrition Navigator website (http://navigator.tufts.edu) rates nutrition-related websites for information and accuracy.

U.S. Department of Agriculture.

For information on the proper handling of meat and poultry and other information, call the USDA's Meat and Poultry Hotline at the toll-free number (800) 535-4555 between 10:00 AM and 4:00 PM on weekdays. Write to the Meat and Poultry Hotline, USDA-FSIS, Room 1165-S, Washington, DC, 20250 for a new booklet, A Quick Consumer's Guide to Safe Food Handling.

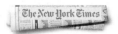

e-themes from *The New York Times*

For up-to-date articles about current health issues, visit
www.aw-bc.com/donatelle, select *Access to Health,* Tenth
Edition, Chapter 8, and click on "e-themes."

References

1. Centers for Disease Control and Prevention, "Behavioral Risk Factor Surveillance System," 2004, www.cdc.gov/brfss.
2. Ibid.
3. American Institute of Cancer Research, *Food, Nutrition and the Prevention of Cancer: A Global Perspective* (Washington, DC: American Institute of Cancer Research, 1997).
4. K. Flegal et al., "Excess Death Associated with Underweight, Overweight, and Obesity," *Journal of the American Medical Association* 293 (2005): 1861–1867.
5. J. Thompson, M. Manore, and L. Vaughn, *The Science of Nutrition* (San Francisco: Benjamin Cummings, 2008).
6. Ibid.
7. Ibid.
8. Ibid.
9. U.S. Department of Agriculture, "Food Consumption Patterns: How We've Changed, 1970–2005," December 2005, www.usda.gov/data/foodconsumption.
10. Thompson et al., *The Science of Nutrition.*
11. G. Block, "Foods Contributing to Energy Intake in the U.S.: Data from NHANES III and NHANES 1999–2000," *Journal of Food Composition and Analysis* 17, nos. 3–4 (2004): 439–447.
12. FAO Global and Regional Food Trends and Consumption Patterns, 2003, www.fao.org/documents/show_cdr.asp?url_file=/DOCREP/005/AC911E/ac911e05.htm12.
13. "Is Sugar Really Addictive?" *Tufts University Health and Nutrition Letter: Special Report* 20, no. 8 (2002): 1–4.
14. M. Pereira et al., "Dietary Fiber and Risk of Coronary Heart Disease: A Pooled Analysis of Cohort Studies," *Archives of Internal Medicine* 164, no. 4 (2004): 370–376.
15. Ibid.
16. Ibid.
17. Ibid.
18. D. Mozaffarian et al., "Trans Fatty Acids and Cardiovascular Disease," *The New England Journal of Medicine* 354 (2006): 1601–1613.
19. B. McKevith, "Review: Nutritional Aspects of Oilseeds," *Nutrition Bulletin* 30, no. 1 (2005): 13–14.
20. "MUFAs and PUFAs," *Food and Fitness Advisor* 9, September 2002, www.foodandfitnessadvisor.com.
21. Institute of Medicine, "Dietary Reference Intake for Water, Potassium, Sodium, Chloride, and Sulfate," March 4, 2004, www.nap.edu.
22. "American Heart Association Position Statement," 2005, www.americanheart.org.
23. World Health Organization, "Miconutrient Deficiencies," 2006, www.who.int/nutrition/topics/ida/en/index.html.
24. U.S. Department of Health and Human Services and U.S. Department of Agriculture, *Dietary Guidelines for Americans, 2005* (Washington, DC: Government Printing Office, 2005).
25. U.S. Department of Agriculture, "Johanns Reveals USDA's Steps to a Healthier You," Press Release, April 19, 2005.
26. B. Black, "Healthgate: Just How Much Food Is on That Plate? Understanding Portion Control," 2004, http://community.healthgate.com/getcontent.asp?siteid=contentupdate&docid.
27. J. Thompson and M. Manore, *Nutrition: An Applied Approach* (San Francisco: Benjamin Cummings, 2005).
28. Ibid.
29. C. M. Hasler et al., "Position Statement of the American Dietetic Association: Functional Foods," *Journal of the American Dietetic Association* 104, no. 5 (2004): 814–818.
30. M. Manore and J. Thompson, *Sport Nutrition for Health and Performance* (Champaign, IL: Human Kinetics Publishing, 2000), 283.
31. J. Chan and E. Giovannucci, "Vegetables, Fruits, Associated Micronutrients and Risk of Prostate Cancer," *Epidemiology Review* 23, no. 1 (2001): 82–86.
32. C. Golub "Kale, Collards and Spinach Beat Carrots for Protecting Aging Eyes," *Environmental Nutrition* 24, no. 4 (2001).
33. Ibid.
34. J. Smythies, *Every Person's Guide to Antioxidants* (Newark, NJ: Rutgers University Press, 1998).
35. B. Frie, Linus Pauling Institute Seminar Series (Portland, OR, 2000).
36. Ibid.
37. A. Chait et al., "Increased Dietary Micronutrients Decrease Serum Homocysteine Concentrations in Patients at High Risk of Cardiovascular Disease," *American Journal of Clinical Nutrition* 70, no. 5: 881–887.
38. R. Malinow, "Homocysteine, Folic Acid and CVD," Linus Pauling Institute International Conference on Diet and Optimum Health (Portland, OR, May 2001).
39. Thompson et al., *The Science of Nutrition.*
40. National Institutes of Health, "Biologically Based Practices: An Overview," *NCCAM Backgrounder,* 2004, http://nccam.nih.gov/health/backgrounds/biobasedprac.htm.
41. K. M. Fairfield and R. H. Fletcher, "Vitamins for Chronic Disease Prevention in Adults: Scientific Review," *Journal of the American Medical Association* 287, no. 23 (2001): 3116–3126.
42. Center for Infectious Diseases, "Food-Borne Illnesses," 2006, www.cdc.gov.
43. National Center for Infectious Diseases, "*E. Coli,*" 2006, www.cdc.gov/ncid/facts.htm
44. Ibid.

45. National Center for Infectious Diseases, "*E. Coli,*" 2006; G. Hall et al., "Food-Borne Disease in the New Millennium," *The Medical Journal of Australia* 177, no. 11 (2002): 614–618; M. Glavin, "A Single Microbial Sea: Food Safety as a Global Concern," *SAIS Review* 23, no. 1 (2003): 203–220.

46. Iowa State University, "Food Irradiation: What Is It?" *Iowa State University Extension Newsletter,* 2004, www.extension.iastate.edu/foodsafety/irradiation.

47. U.S. Food and Drug Administration, "Center for Food Safety and Applied Nutrition, Information for Consumers: Food Allergy Labeling," 2006, www.cfsan.fda.gov/.

48. Ibid.

49. Economic Research Service, "Food Consumption," 2006, www.ers.usda.gov/briefing/consumption.

9

Managing Your Weight

FINDING A HEALTHY BALANCE

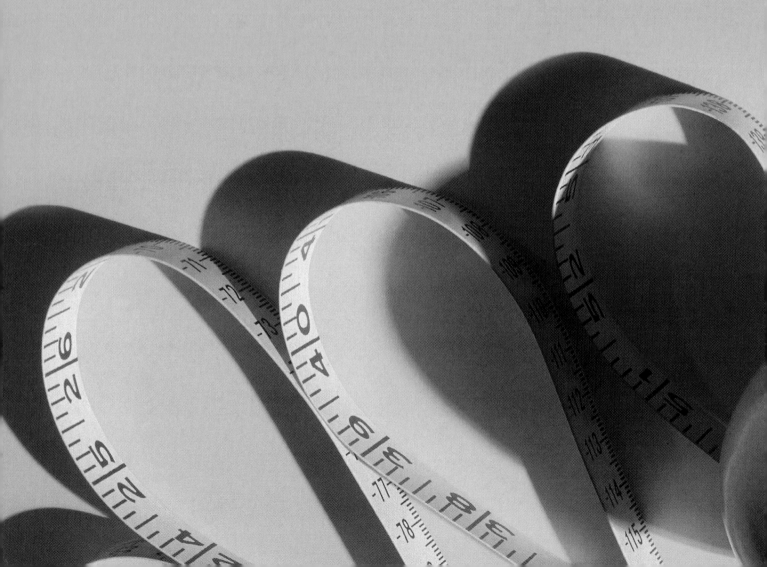

How can I determine my **ideal** body weight?

I **exercise** and eat right, but I can't seem to lose any more weight. Why?

What's the best way to lose weight or **maintain** my current weight?

Do **men** ever have eating disorders?

How can I control my weight without resorting to **fad** diets?

OBJECTIVES

- Define obesity, describe the current epidemic of obesity in the United States, and understand risk factors associated with obesity.
- Explain why so many people are obsessed with thinness and how to determine the right weight for you.
- Discuss reliable options for determining body fat content.
- Describe factors that place people at risk for problems with obesity. Distinguish between factors that can and cannot be controlled.
- Discuss the roles of exercise, dieting, nutrition, lifestyle modification, fad diets, and other strategies of weight control, and which methods are most effective.
- Describe major eating disorders, explain the health risks related to these conditions, and indicate the factors that make people susceptible to these disorders.

Over the past 20 years, the United States has become known as one of the fattest nations on earth. From young children who find it difficult to walk even short distances because of severe obesity to seniors who can't perform daily activities such as cleaning their homes because of crippling weight-related joint problems or obesity-related diseases, virtually no segment of the populace is immune to the epidemic of overweight and obesity (Figure 9.1). Soaring rates of obesity-related diseases such as hypertension and diabetes have caused health professionals to sound the alarm about potentially devastating individual and societal health care burdens that will result from our **obesogenic** society. Just how serious is the problem?

According to a national survey of health behaviors and nutrition, the National Heath and Nutrition Examination Survey (NHANES), 66 percent of American adults are considered overweight and an additional 32 percent are obese.[1] The trend does not seem to be reversing: obesity rates have continued to rise dramatically in nearly every state. In a recent report, Mississippi ranked as the heaviest state and Colorado ranked as the least heavy state. The heaviest states tended to be in the southeastern United States. Experts predict that, at the current pace, 50 percent of Americans will be obese by the year 2025.[2]

What does all of this excess weight really mean to the health of our population? Recent studies indicate that obesity is one of the top underlying preventable causes of death in the United States. Like tobacco, obesity and inactivity increase the risks from three of our leading killers: heart disease, cancer, and cerebrovascular ailments, including strokes.[3] Other associated health risks (see Table 9.1) include diabetes, gallstones, sleep apnea, osteoarthritis, and several cancers. For example, some experts predict that the numbers of Americans diagnosed with diabetes, a major obesity-associated problem, will increase by a whopping 165 percent, from 15 million in 2005 to 30 million in 2030; since 1990 there has been a 49 percent increase in the number of Americans who have diabetes.[4]

Short- and long-term health consequences of obesity are not our only concern: the estimated annual cost of obesity in the United States exceeds $152 billion in medical expenses and lost productivity.[5] As much of the population ages, these costs will increase proportionally. Of course, it is impossible to place a dollar value on a life lost prematurely due to diabetes, stroke, or heart attack or assess the cost of social isolation and discrimination against overweight individuals. Of growing importance is the recognition that obese individuals suffer significant disability during their lives, in terms of both mobility and activities of daily living.[6]

obesogenic The presence of several factors that make people more prone to obesity.

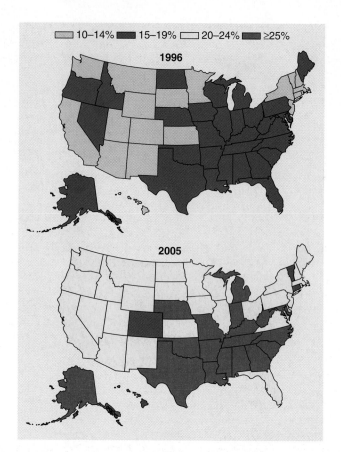

FIGURE 9.1 Obesity Trends Among U.S. Adults, 1996 and 2005

Source: Centers for Disease Control and Prevention, "U.S. Obesity Trends: 1985–2005, Obesity Trend Maps," www.cdc.gov/nccdphp/dnpa/obesity.

This chapter will help you understand why we have such a weight problem in America today and provide simple strategies to help you manage your weight. (See the Assess Yourself box on page 288 to obtain a better understanding of your own dietary habits.) It will also help you understand what *underweight, normal weight, overweight,* and *obesity* really mean, and why managing your weight is essential to overall health and well-being.

Determining the Right Weight for You

How can I determine my ideal body weight?

What weight is best for you? Each person's optimal weight depends on a wide range of variables, including body structure, height, weight distribution, and the ratio of fat to lean tissue. In fact, your weight can be a deceptive indicator.

Many extremely muscular athletes would be considered overweight based on traditional height–weight charts, while many young women think that they are the right weight based on charts, only to be shocked to discover that 35 to 40 percent of their weight is body fat!

TABLE 9.1	Selected Health Consequences of Overweight and Obesity

PREMATURE DEATH

- Obese individuals have a 50–100% increased risk of death from all causes compared with people of normal weight. Among 25- to 35-year-olds, severe obesity increases the risk of death by a factor of 12.
- At least 300,000 deaths per year may be attributable to obesity.
- The risk of death rises with increasing weight.
- Even moderate excess weight (10–20 pounds for a person of average height) increases risk of death.

CARDIOVASCULAR DISEASE

- High blood pressure is twice as common in obese adults as it is for those who are at healthy weights.
- Incidence of all forms of heart disease is increased among overweight and obese people.
- Obesity is associated with elevated triglycerides and decreased HDLs ("good" cholesterol).

DIABETES

- A weight gain of 11–18 pounds increases a person's risk of developing type 2 diabetes to twice that of individuals who have not gained weight.
- More than 80% of people with diabetes are overweight or obese.

CANCER

- Overweight and obesity are associated with increased risk of endometrial, colon, gallbladder, prostate, kidney, uterine, and postmenopausal breast cancer.
- Women gaining more than 20 pounds between age 18 and midlife double their risk of postmenopausal breast cancer compared with women whose weight remains stable.

ADDITIONAL HEALTH CONSEQUENCES

- Sleep apnea and asthma are both associated with obesity.
- For every 2-pound increase in weight, the risk of developing arthritis increases by 9–13%.
- Obesity-related complications during pregnancy include increased risk of fetal and maternal death, labor and delivery complications, and increased risk of birth defects.
- Increased risk of osteoarthritis, especially in weight-bearing joints like knees and hips.

Sources: Mayo Clinic, "Obesity Consequences," 2006, www.mayoclinic.com; National Institutes of Health, "Summary of Obesity," 2005; S. J. Olshansky et al., "A Potential Decline in Life Expectancy in the U.S. in the 21st Century," *New England Journal of Medicine* 352 (2005): 1103–1110.

In general, weights at the lower end of the range on traditional charts are recommended for individuals with a low ratio of muscle and bone to fat; those at the upper end are advised for people with more muscular builds. However, since actual body composition is hard to determine, most charts today simply give a general range for men and women.

Overweight or Obese?

Most of us cringe at the thought of being labeled with one of the "O" words. What is the distinction between the two? **Overweight** refers to increased body weight in relation to height, when compared to a standard such as the height–weight charts in Table 9.2 on page 286. The excess weight may come from muscle, bone, fat, and/or water. Historically, health experts have defined overweight as being 1 to 19 percent above one's ideal weight and obese as over 19 percent.

Another measurement of overweight and obesity is a mathematical formula known as **body mass index (BMI)**, which represents weight levels associated with the lowest overall risk to health (see the next section to calculate your BMI). Desirable BMI levels may vary with age.[7] You would be classified as being overweight if you have a BMI of 25.0 to 29.9. About 34 percent of all Americans fit this category.

It is important to remember that BMI is a good—but not perfect—indicator of your percentage of body fat. According to the standards, a person could be classified as overweight

even if the weight gain is due to an increase in lean muscle mass. For example, as just described, an athlete may be very lean and muscular, with very little body fat, yet she may weigh a lot more than others of the same height who have little muscle tissue. For those who have lost muscle mass, such as older adults, people with anorexia, or those who are seriously disabled or bedridden, BMI estimates must be carefully considered for accuracy, taking body composition into account. Conversely, a person may proudly proclaim that he weighs the same amount that he did in high school but carry a much greater proportion of body fat, particularly in the hips, buttocks, or thighs, than he did at a younger age. Therefore, BMI is a useful guideline, but by itself is not diagnostic of a person's overall fitness and health status.[8]

Obesity is defined as an excessively high amount of body fat (adipose tissue) in relation to lean body mass or a BMI of 30 or more. Over 31 percent of all Americans are obese. It is

overweight Increased body weight in relation to height.

body mass index (BMI) A technique of weight assessment based on the relationship of weight to height.

obesity A weight disorder generally defined as an accumulation of fat beyond that considered normal for a person based on age, sex, and body type.

TABLE 9.2	Healthy Weight Ranges*
Height without Shoes	**Weight† without Clothes**
4'10"	91–119
4'11"	94–124
5'0"	97–128
5'1"	101–132
5'2"	104–137
5'3"	107–141
5'4"	111–146
5'5"	114–150
5'6"	118–155
5'7"	121–160
5'8"	125–164
5'9"	129–169
5'10"	132–174
5'11"	136–179
6'0"	140–184
6'1"	144–189
6'2"	148–195
6'3"	152–200
6'4"	156–205
6'5"	160–211
6'6"	164–216

*Each data entry applies to both men and women.

†In pounds

Source: Center for Nutrition Policy and Promotion, "Dietary Guidelines for Americans, 2005," 2005, www.usda.gov/cnpp/Pubs.

important to consider both the distribution of fat throughout the body and the size of the adipose tissue deposits. Body fat distribution can be estimated by skinfold measures, waist-to-hip circumference ratios, or techniques such as ultrasound, computed tomography, magnetic resonance imaging, or others. Using traditional standards, people 20 to 40 percent above their ideal weight are labeled as *mildly obese* (90 percent of the obese fall into this category). Those 41 to 99 percent above their ideal weight are described as *moderately obese* (about 7 to 8 percent of the obese fit into this category), and 2 to 3 percent are in the *severely, morbidly,* or *grossly obese* category, meaning that they are 100 percent or more above their ideal weight. In the last decade, more and more people have attained moderate and severe levels of obesity, meaning increased risks at all ages and stages of their lives.[9]

The difficulty with defining obesity lies in determining what is normal. To date, there are no universally accepted standards for the most desirable or ideal body weight or *body composition* (the ratio of lean body mass to fat body mass). Although sources vary slightly, men's bodies should contain

between 11 and 15 percent total body fat, and women should be within the range of 18 to 22 percent body fat. At various ages and stages of life, these ranges also vary, but generally, when men exceed 20 percent body fat and women exceed 30 percent body fat, they have slipped into obesity.

Why the difference between men and women? Much of it may be attributed to the normal structure of the female body and to sex hormones. Lean body mass consists of the structural and functional elements in cells, body water, muscle, bones, and other body organs such as the heart, liver, and kidneys. Body fat is composed of two types: essential fat and storage fat. Essential fat is necessary for normal physiological functioning, such as nerve conduction. Essential fat makes up approximately 3 to 7 percent of total body weight in men and approximately 15 percent of total body weight in women. Storage fat, the part that many of us try to shed, makes up the remainder of our fat reserves. It accounts for only a small percentage of total body weight for very lean people and between 5 and 25 percent of the body weight of most American adults. Female bodybuilders, who are among the leanest of female athletes, may have body fat percentages ranging from 8 to 13 percent, nearly all of which is essential fat.

Too Little Fat?

A certain amount of body fat is necessary for insulating the body, cushioning parts of the body and vital organs, and maintaining body functions. In men, this lower limit is approximately 3 to 4 percent. Women should generally not go below 8 percent. Excessively low body fat in females may lead to amenorrhea, disruption of the normal menstrual cycle. The critical level of body fat necessary to maintain normal menstrual flow is believed to be between 8 and 13 percent, but there are many additional factors that affect the menstrual cycle. Under extreme circumstances, such as extreme diets and certain diseases, the body utilizes all available fat reserves and begins to break down muscle tissue as a last-ditch effort to obtain nourishment.

The fact is that too much fat and too little fat are both potentially harmful. The key is to find a healthy level at which you are comfortable with your appearance and your ability to be as active as possible. Many options are available for determining your body fat and weight.

Assessing Fat Levels

Today, most authorities believe that getting on the scale to determine your weight and then looking at where you fall on some arbitrary chart may not be helpful. A number of other measures exist for calculating body fat content, and some provide a very precise reading or calculation of body fat. They include body mass index, waist circumference, waist-to-hip ratio, and various measures of body fat.

		Healthy Weight						Overweight					Obese					
	BMI	19	20	21	22	23	24	25	26	27	28	29	30	31	32	33	34	35
		Weight in Pounds																
	4'10"	91	96	100	105	110	115	119	124	129	134	138	143	148	153	158	162	167
	4'11"	94	99	104	109	114	119	124	128	133	138	143	148	153	158	163	168	173
	5'	97	102	107	112	118	123	128	133	138	143	148	153	158	163	158	174	179
	5'1"	100	106	111	116	122	127	132	137	143	148	153	158	164	169	174	180	185
	5'2"	104	109	115	120	126	131	136	142	147	153	158	164	169	175	180	186	191
	5'3"	107	113	118	124	130	135	141	146	152	158	163	169	175	180	186	191	197
	5'4"	110	116	122	128	134	140	145	151	157	163	169	174	180	186	192	197	204
Height	5'5"	114	120	126	132	138	144	150	156	162	168	174	180	186	192	198	204	210
	5'6"	118	124	130	136	142	148	155	161	167	173	179	186	192	198	204	210	216
	5'7"	121	127	134	140	146	153	159	166	172	178	185	191	198	204	211	217	223
	5'8"	125	131	138	144	151	158	164	171	177	184	190	197	203	210	216	223	230
	5'9"	128	135	142	149	155	162	169	176	182	189	196	203	209	216	223	230	236
	5'10"	132	139	146	153	160	167	174	181	188	195	202	209	216	222	229	236	243
	5'11"	136	143	150	157	165	172	179	186	193	200	208	215	222	229	236	243	250
	6'	140	147	154	162	169	177	184	191	199	206	213	221	228	235	242	250	258
	6'1"	144	151	159	166	174	182	189	197	204	212	219	227	235	242	250	257	265
	6'2"	148	155	163	171	179	186	194	202	210	218	225	233	241	249	256	264	272
	6'3"	152	160	168	176	184	192	200	208	216	224	232	240	248	256	264	272	279

- BMI of 18.5 or lower is underweight
- BMI of 25 defines the upper boundary of healthy weight
- BMI of higher than 25 to 30 defines overweight
- BMI of higher than 30 defines obesity

FIGURE 9.2 Body Mass Index: Are You at a Healthy Weight?

Find your height along the left side of the chart, and follow that row until you get to the weight closest to your own. Follow that line straight up to the top for your BMI.

Source: National Heart, Lung, and Blood Institute, "Evidence Report of Clinical Guidelines on the Identification, Evaluation, and Treatment of Overweight and Obesity in Adults, 1998."

Body Mass Index

A useful index of the relationship between height and weight, BMI is a standard measurement used by obesity researchers and health professionals. It is not gender specific, and although it does not directly measure percentage of body fat, it does provide a more accurate measure of overweight and obesity than weight alone.[10]

We find BMI by dividing a person's weight in kilograms by height in meters squared. The mathematical formula is:

$$\text{BMI} = \text{weight (kg)/height squared (m}^2\text{)}$$

To determine BMI using pounds and inches, see Figure 9.2. The BMI calculator also is available at the National Heart, Lung, and Blood Institute website at http://nhlbisupport.com/bmi/bmicalc.htm.

Healthy weights are defined as those associated with BMIs of 19 to 25, the range of lowest statistical health risk.[11] The desirable range for females falls between 21 and 23; for males, between 22 and 24.[12] A BMI greater than 25 indicates overweight and potentially significant health risks. A body mass index of 30 or more is considered obese.[13] Many experts believe that this number is too high, particularly for younger adults.

Calculating BMI is simple, quick, and inexpensive—but it does have limitations. One problem with using BMI as a measurement is that very muscular people may fall into the overweight category when they are actually healthy and fit. As well, certain population groups, such as Asians, tend to have higher-than-healthy body fat at normal BMI levels, while Polynesians have somewhat lower body fat than other populations at the same BMI.[14] Another problem is that, as previously described, people who have lost muscle mass such as older adults may be in the healthy weight category according to BMI, but actually have reduced nutritional reserves.

These standards may seem almost impossible for people who consistently exceed the target weights and who have difficulty keeping off any lost weight. Constant failure may lead them to stop trying. The secret lies in establishing a healthful weight at a young age and maintaining it—a task easier said than done. The *U.S. Dietary Guidelines for Americans* encourage a weight gain of no more than ten pounds after reaching adult height and endorse small weight losses of one-half to one pound per week, if needed, as well as smaller weight losses of 5 to 10 percent to make a difference toward health.[15]

(Text continues on page 292)

ASSESS yourself

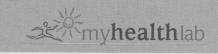

READINESS FOR WEIGHT LOSS

Fill out this assessment online at
www.aw-bc.com/myhealthlab or
www.aw-bc.com/donatelle.

How well do your attitudes equip you for a weight-loss program? For each question, circle the answer that best describes your attitude. As you complete each section, tally your score and analyze it according to the scoring guide.

I. GOALS, ATTITUDES, AND READINESS

1. Compared to previous attempts, how motivated are you to lose weight this time?

1	2	3	4	5
Not at all motivated	Slightly motivated	Somewhat motivated	Quite motivated	Extremely motivated

2. How certain are you that you will stay committed to a weight-loss program for the time it will take to reach your goal?

1	2	3	4	5
Not at all certain	Slightly certain	Somewhat certain	Quite certain	Extremely certain

3. Considering all outside factors at this time in your life—stress at work, family obligations, and so on—to what extent can you tolerate the effort required to stick to a diet?

1	2	3	4	5
Cannot tolerate	Can tolerate somewhat	Uncertain	Can tolerate well	Can tolerate easily

4. Think honestly about how much weight you hope to lose and how quickly you hope to lose it. Figuring a weight loss of one to two pounds per week, how realistic is your expectation?

1	2	3	4	5
Very unrealistic	Somewhat unrealistic	Moderately unrealistic	Somewhat realistic	Very realistic

5. While dieting, do you fantasize about eating a lot of your favorite foods?

1	2	3	4	5
Always	Frequently	Occasionally	Rarely	Never

6. While dieting, do you feel deprived, angry, and/or upset?

1	2	3	4	5
Always	Frequently	Occasionally	Rarely	Never

Analyzing This Section

6 to 16: This may not be a good time for you to start a diet. Inadequate motivation and commitment and unrealistic goals could block your progress. Think about what contributes to your unreadiness, and consider changing these factors before undertaking a diet.

17 to 23: You may be close to being ready to begin a program but should think about ways to boost your readiness.

24 to 30: The path is clear: you can decide how to lose weight in a safe, effective way.

II. HUNGER AND EATING CUES

7. When food comes up in conversation or in something you read, do you want to eat, even if you are not hungry?

1	2	3	4	5
Never	Rarely	Occasionally	Frequently	Always

8. How often do you eat for a reason other than physical hunger?

1	2	3	4	5
Never	Rarely	Occasionally	Frequently	Always

9. Do you have trouble controlling your eating when your favorite foods are around the house?

1	2	3	4	5
Never	Rarely	Occasionally	Frequently	Always

Analyzing This Section

3 to 6: You might occasionally eat more than you should, but it does not appear to be due to high responsiveness to environmental cues. Controlling the attitudes that make you eat may be especially helpful.

7 to 9: You may have a moderate tendency to eat just because food is available. Losing weight may be easier for you if you try to resist external cues and eat only when you are physically hungry.

10 to 15: Some or much of your eating may be in response to thinking about food or exposing yourself to temptations to eat. Think of ways to minimize your exposure to temptations so you eat only in response to physical hunger.

III. CONTROLLING OVEREATING

If the following situations occurred while you were on a diet, would you be likely to eat more or less immediately afterward and for the rest of the day?

10. Although you planned to skip lunch, a friend talks you into going out for a midday meal.

1	2	3	4	5
Would eat much less	Would eat somewhat less	Would make no difference	Would eat somewhat more	Would eat much more

11. You "break" your plan by eating a fattening, "forbidden" food.

1	2	3	4	5
Would eat much less	Would eat somewhat less	Would make no difference	Would eat somewhat more	Would eat much more

12. You have been following your diet faithfully and decide to test yourself by eating something you consider a treat.

1	2	3	4	5
Would eat much less	Would eat somewhat less	Would make no difference	Would eat somewhat more	Would eat much more

Analyzing This Section

3 to 7: You recover rapidly from mistakes. However, if you frequently alternate between eating that is out of control and dieting very strictly, you may have a serious eating problem and should get professional help.

8 to 11: You do not seem to let unplanned eating disrupt your program. This is a flexible, balanced approach.

12 to 15: You may be prone to overeat after an event breaks your control or throws you off track. Your reaction to these problem-causing events can be improved.

(continued)

IV. BINGE EATING AND PURGING

13. Aside from holiday feasts, have you ever eaten a large amount of food rapidly and felt afterward that this eating incident was excessive and out of control?

2	0
Yes	No

14. If you answered yes to question 13, how often have you engaged in this behavior during the past year?

1	2	3	4	5	6
Less than once a month	About once a month	A few times a month	About once a week	About 3 times a week	Daily

15. Have you purged (used laxatives or diuretics, or induced vomiting) to control your weight?

5	0
Yes	No

16. If you answered yes to question 15, how often have you engaged in this behavior during the past year?

1	2	3	4	5	6
Less than once a month	About once a month	A few times a month	About once a week	About 3 times a week	Daily

Analyzing This Section

0: It appears that binge eating and purging are not problems for you.

2 to 11: Pay attention to these eating patterns. Should they arise more frequently, get professional help.

12 to 19: You show signs of having a potentially serious eating problem. See a counselor experienced in evaluating eating disorders right away.

V. EMOTIONAL EATING

17. Do you eat more than you would like to when you have negative feelings such as anxiety, depression, anger, or loneliness?

1	2	3	4	5
Never	Rarely	Occasionally	Frequently	Always

18. Do you have trouble controlling your eating when you have positive feelings—do you celebrate feeling good by eating?

1	2	3	4	5
Never	Rarely	Occasionally	Frequently	Always

19. When you have unpleasant interactions with others in your life or after a difficult day at work, do you eat more than you'd like?

1	2	3	4	5
Never	Rarely	Occasionally	Frequently	Always

Analyzing This Section

3 to 8: You do not appear to let your emotions affect your eating.

9 to 11: You sometimes eat in response to emotional highs and lows. Monitor this behavior to learn when and why it occurs, and be prepared to find alternate activities.

12 to 15: Emotional ups and downs can stimulate your eating. Try to deal with the feelings that trigger the eating and find other ways to express them.

VI. EXERCISE PATTERNS AND ATTITUDES

20. How often do you exercise?

1	2	3	4	5
Never	Rarely	Occasionally	Somewhat frequently	Frequently

21. How confident are you that you can exercise regularly?

1	2	3	4	5
Not at all confident	Slightly confident	Somewhat confident	Highly confident	Completely confident

22. When you think about exercise, do you develop a positive or negative picture in your mind?

1	2	3	4	5
Completely negative	Somewhat negative	Neutral	Somewhat positive	Completely positive

23. How certain are you that you can work regular exercise into your daily schedule?

1	2	3	4	5
Not at all certain	Slightly certain	Somewhat certain	Quite certain	Extremely certain

Analyzing This Section

4 to 10: You're probably not exercising as regularly as you should. Determine whether attitude about exercise or your lifestyle is blocking your way, then change what you must and put on those walking shoes!

11 to 16: You need to feel more positive about exercise so you can do it more often. Think of ways to be more active that are fun and fit your lifestyle.

17 to 20: It looks as if the path is clear for you to be active. Now think of ways to get motivated. After scoring yourself in each section of this questionnaire, you should be able to better judge your dieting strengths and weaknesses. Remember that the first step in changing eating behavior is to understand the conditions that influence your eating habits.

Source: K. D. Brownell, "When and How to Diet," *Psychology Today,* June 1989, 41–46. Reprinted with permission from *Psychology Today Magazine*. Copyright © 1989, Sussex Publishers, Inc.

MAKE it happen!

ASSESSMENT: The Assess Yourself activity identifies six areas of importance in determining your readiness for weight loss. If you should lose weight to improve your health, understanding your attitudes about food and exercise will help you succeed in your plan.

MAKING A CHANGE: In order to change your behavior, you need to develop a plan. Follow these steps below and complete your Behavior Change Contract to take action.

1. Evaluate your behavior, and identify patterns and specific things you are doing. What can you change now? What can you change in the near future?

2. Select one pattern of behavior that you want to change.

3. Fill out the Behavior Change Contract found at the front of your book. It should include your long-term goal for change, your short-term goals, the rewards you'll give yourself for reaching these goals, potential obstacles along the way, and strategies for overcoming these obstacles. For each goal, list the small steps and specific actions that you will take.

4. Chart your progress in a journal. At the end of a week, consider how successful you were in following your plan. What helped you be successful? What made change more difficult? What will you do differently next week?

5. Revise your plan as needed. Are the short-term goals attainable? Are the rewards satisfying?

ONE STUDENT'S PLAN: Shannon had gained the "freshman 15" and wanted to put together a weight management plan. She assessed her readiness for weight loss and saw that her scores in certain areas highlighted where improvement was needed for success. Shannon saw that she was not always

(continued)

aware of the eating cues and emotions that caused her to overeat (sections II, III, and V). Although she hadn't realized it, she tended to do most of her snacking while she was studying at night. No matter what else she had eaten during the day, she would end up eating candy and chips from the vending machines. Especially when she was anxious about an upcoming test or bored by her reading, she would eat even though she was already full. Shannon also noted her strengths: She had never binged and purged (section IV), she had strong motivation (section I), and she already had an enjoyable, regular exercise program (section VI).

Shannon made a plan that would help her manage her weight by controlling snacking. She set up a series of small steps to help her become aware of what she was eating and how it was contributing to her weight gain. First, she went through her cupboards and got rid of any unhealthy snacks. Then she bought some study snacks that were healthier

choices than chips and candy, such as grapes and low-fat granola. She then drew up a daily exercise plan, and created a schedule that included mealtimes and snack times. Shannon planned to note if she was eating out of hunger or mindlessly on this schedule. If she was snacking because she was bored or anxious, she would try to restrict her snack to a predetermined amount or to wait until she really was hungry. Shannon tried this plan for two weeks. At the end of two weeks she saw that she had lost 4 pounds. She decided she wanted to address another of her eating habits, which was ordering pizza with her roommates when they watched their favorite TV shows during the week. Even after she had eaten a full dinner, Shannon found herself eating two or three pieces of pizza in front of the TV. Shannon suggested to her roommates that, if they already had eaten dinner, they pop some popcorn to eat instead of the pizza. Not only was this healthier, but it cost less than having a pizza delivered.

Circumference and Ratio Measurements

Waist circumference measurement is a useful tool for assessing abdominal fat. Research indicates that a waistline greater than 40 inches (102 cm) in men and 35 inches (88 cm) in women may indicate greater health risk. If a person has a short stature (under 5 feet tall) or has a BMI of 35 or above, waist circumference standards used for the general population might not apply.[16] Measure waist circumference by wrapping a tape measure comfortably around the smallest area below the rib cage and above the belly button.

The **waist-to-hip ratio** measures regional fat distribution. A waist-to-hip ratio greater than 1.0 in men and 0.8 in women indicates increased health risks.[17] Therefore, knowing where your fat is carried may be more important than knowing your total fat

content. Men and postmenopausal women tend to store fat in the upper regions of their body, particularly in the abdominal area. Premenopausal women usually store their fat in lower regions of their bodies, particularly the hips, buttocks, and thighs.

Measures of Body Fat

There are numerous ways of assessing whether your body fat levels are too high besides BMI calculations. One low-tech way is simply to look in the mirror or consider how your clothes fit compared with how they fit the last season you wore them. Of course, we've all seen people who appear to have a disconnect between how they look and the size of clothing they are wearing or their body image. More accurate ways of determining body fat are available for those who really are interested in having a precise measurement. Before undergoing any procedure, make sure you understand the expense, potential for accuracy, risks, and training of the tester.

Hydrostatic Weighing Techniques From a clinical perspective, **hydrostatic weighing techniques** offer the most accurate method of measuring body fat. This method measures the amount of water a person displaces when completely submerged. Because fat tissue is less dense than muscle or bone tissue, a relatively accurate indication of actual body fat can be computed by comparing underwater and out-of-water weights.

Skinfold Caliper Technique One of the most common methods of assessing body fat is the **skinfold caliper technique**. In this method a handheld caliper is used to measure the skinfold thickness at several points on the body (usually between 3 and 7 spots). The technician grasps the skin

waist circumference measurement Assessment of healthy weight by measurement of the circumference of the waist.

waist-to-hip ratio Ratio that indicates increased risks due to unhealthy fat distribution.

hydrostatic weighing techniques Method of determining body fat by measuring the amount of water displaced when a person is completely submerged.

skinfold caliper technique A method of determining body fat whereby folds of skin and fat at various points on the body are grasped between thumb and forefinger and measured with calipers.

and underlying tissue, shakes it slightly to make sure that muscle is not part of the grab, and pinches the remaining skin and fat in the grips of the caliper, which provides a measure. Measurements are added, and a percentage is calculated. Although it is a good rough indicator of fatness, the skill of the technician is key. In general, the more overweight or obese a person is, the more difficult it is to get accurate measures.

Dual Energy X-Ray Absorptiometry
One of the newer technologies available for assessing body fat, **dual energy X-ray absorptiometry (DEXA)** is also among the most accurate and precise. DEXA is based on a three-compartment model that divides the body into total body mineral, fat-free soft (lean) mass, and fat tissue mass. Essentially, DEXA is a whole-body scanning technique that has two low-dose X rays that read bone and soft tissue mass at the same time. DEXA scans are also used for assessing osteoporosis risk. It takes about 20 minutes to perform as the scanner slowly passes over your body while you lie on a table. DEXA is more precise than other methods and is relatively easy for anyone to have done. The downside is that it isn't as accurate for extremely obese individuals and it is expensive because of the high cost of the machines. Many universities have DEXA machines in their exercise physiology or biomechanics labs. If you have one on your campus, you may be able to participate in a research study and obtain free testing for your willingness to participate.

Near-Infrared Interactance
Another newer technique is **near-infrared interactance (NIR)**, in which a fiber-optic probe is connected to a digital analyzer that indirectly measures tissue composition (both fat and water). Usually, the biceps are used to assess fatness; once measures are taken, an equation that includes your height, weight, frame size, and level of activity is used to calculate body fat. Often you will see this technique used outside of the laboratory. It is relatively inexpensive and fast, but it is not nearly as accurate as the other methods described above. Very fat and very lean, muscular people are likely to have inaccurate measures. Numerous studies have indicated that more research must be done to determine if this technique is accurate and if it is better than caliper methods and other simple strategies.

Magnetic Resonance Imaging
This is a technique that has been around for a long time, but its cost typically prohibits its use for simple body fat calculations. **Magnetic resonance imaging (MRI)** uses magnetic fields to accurately assess how much fat a person has and where it is deposited. If you were having a full-body MRI for diagnosis of other illnesses, it is possible that you could ask the technician to determine your body fat.

Total Body Electrical Conductivity
Much like an MRI, **total body electrical conductivity (TOBEC)** requires a person to lie in a cylinder that generates a very weak electromagnetic field. It is based on the assumption that lean tissue is a better conductor of electricity than fat; and, as it takes a series of readings, it provides data on fat versus lean

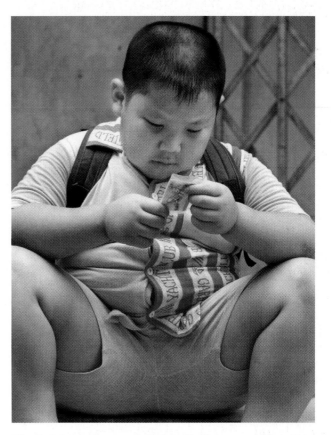

Obesity is increasing especially dramatically among children. Being overweight or obese from an early age can have devastating physical and emotional consequences.

tissue in your body. Like MRI, it is very expensive and not practical for many people.

Computed Tomography
This method provides a cross-sectional scan of the body, using radiation as in a typical X ray. **Computed tomography (CT)** is good for assessing intraabdominal fat as compared to fat under the skin and in other body areas. CTs are costly, and the added risk of radiation exposure makes it less than desirable.

dual energy X-ray absorptiometry (DEXA)   Technique using low-dose X rays that read bone and soft tissue mass at the same time.

near-infrared interactance (NIR)   Fiber-optic measurement of tissue composition.

magnetic resonance imaging (MRI)   Diagnostic technique using magnetic fields, which can be used to measure body fat.

total body electrical conductivity (TOBEC)   Technique using an electromagnetic force field to assess relative body fat.

computed tomography (CT)   Use of X ray for a cross-section of the body, which can reveal intraabdominal fat.

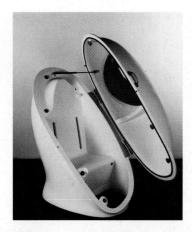

The Bod Pod is a new fat assessment machine with a chamber in which a person sits, and the air displaced by the body is measured to determine body fat.

The Bod Pod (Adults) and Pea Pod (Children)
The **Bod Pod** and **Pea Pod** are relative newcomers on the body fat assessment scene. This egg-shaped chamber requires the person to sit inside, then it is closed with a tight seal so that the machine can measure the amount of air your body displaces. Bod Pods use this air displacement measure, along with your body weight, to assess your overall body fat.

Bioelectrical Impedance Analysis
This is the only method based on measuring electrical signals as they pass through fat, lean mass, and water in the body, rather than estimating fat from other measures. Essentially, **bioelectrical impedance analysis (BIA)** measures how lean you are, rather than how fat you are, yet the net results are just as informative. BIA reliability is related to the sophistication of the machine doing the testing and the knowledge of the technician. Be wary of mail-order BIA equipment or very inexpensive offers.

Risk Factors for Obesity

In spite of massive efforts to keep Americans fit and in good health, obesity is the most common nutritional disorder in the United States, with rates that have increased dramatically among children and adults in recent decades.[18] The prevalence of obesity and overweight (defined as a BMI of 25 or higher) is generally higher among minorities, especially minority women.[19] These rates are especially noteworthy when

Bod Pod/Pea Pod   A method of body fat assessment that measures the air your body displaces in a sealed chamber.

bioelectrical impedance analysis (BIA)   A technique of body fat assessment in which electrical currents are passed through fat and lean tissue.

compared with obesity trends in the rest of the world (see the Health in a Diverse World box).

In a major report on strategies to combat overweight and obesity, the Surgeon General stated it quite plainly: "Overweight and obesity result from an energy imbalance. This means eating too many calories and not getting enough exercise."[20] However, many have criticized such a simplistic view. If it were that simple, many Americans would merely reevaluate their diets, reduce the amount they eat, and exercise more. Unfortunately, it's not that easy.

What are some of these factors that influence our collective trends toward overweight and obesity? We know that body weight is a result of genes, metabolism, behavior, environment, culture, and socioeconomic status. Of these, behavior and environment are the easiest to change.

Key Environmental Factors

With the advent of all our twenty-first century conveniences, environmental factors play a large role in weight maintenance. Automobiles, remote controls, office jobs where we sit all day, and spending time on the Internet all cause us to move less, and this lack of physical activity causes a decrease in energy expenditure.[21] Time our grandparents spent going for a walk after dinner is now spent watching our favorite television shows. Not only has our culture urged us to move less, but also to eat more. A long list of environmental factors that encourages us to increase our consumption includes the following.

- Bombardment with advertising designed to increase energy intake—ads for high-calorie foods at a low price, marketing super-sized portions. Prepackaged meals, fast food, and soft drinks are all increasingly widespread. High-calorie drinks such as coffee lattes and energy drinks add to daily caloric intake.[22]
- Changes in the number of working women, leading to greater use of restaurant meals, fast foods, and convenience foods. Women now consume, on average, nearly 350 calories per day more than they did in the 1970s.[23]
- Bottle-feeding of infants, which may increase energy intake relative to breast-feeding.[24]
- Misleading food labels that confuse consumers about portion and serving sizes.

 what do you THINK?

In addition to those listed, can you think of other environmental factors that contribute to obesity? ▪ What actions could you take to reduce your risk for each of these factors?

Heredity and Genetic Factors

Are some people born to be fat? Several factors appear to influence why one person becomes obese and another remains thin; genes seem to interact with many of these factors. In

GLOBESITY: AN EPIDEMIC OF GROWING PROPORTIONS

It's not just Americans today who are bigger and less fit than at any time in history. A similar trend is emerging around the world in both developed and developing regions. According to estimates from the World Health Organization (WHO), over 75 percent of women over the age of 30 in countries such as Barbados, Egypt, Mexico, South Africa, and Turkey (not to mention the United States) are overweight. This epidemic is not specific to women; globally, there are over 1 billion overweight adults, and at least 300 million of them are obese. In Pacific Island nations, the epidemic is even more pronounced, with 9 out of 10 adults overweight.

Although there is growing concern about the epidemic in adults, even more disturbing is the enormous jump in obesity rates among children. Rates of childhood obesity have increased 66 percent in the United States in past decades—and a whopping 240 percent during the same period in Brazil. Worldwide, the WHO estimates that 22 million children under the age of 5 are overweight.

Among the consequences is the parallel rise in type 2 diabetes in the global population; it is now nearly five times more prevalent than it was 18 years ago. The dual impact of diabetes and obesity is sure to demand increasing attention to the global health consequences and disease burden.

Dietary excesses and sedentary lifestyles are key contributors to the increase in obesity. However, according to Donna Eberwine, editor of the Pan American Health Organization's *Perspectives in Health*, "The growing body of public health literature on the 'globesity' epidemic places the bulk of the blame not on individuals, but on globalization and development, with poverty as an exacerbating factor." As entire cultures move away from traditional diets, with raw fruits and vegetables and fewer fats, to diets heavy in highly processed, high-fat, and high-calorie fast food and packaged products, the same thing that happened to Americans during the move from the farms to cities is occurring. The world population has become super-sized along with the products we consume.

Another factor is the increasingly sprawling infrastructure in which people travel only by car, and walking or bicycling is difficult. Lack of health education about the risks of obesity also contributes to its increase.

The challenge is daunting, and there is no simple solution. Nations must work together in the decades ahead to educate their populations, promote nutritious diets, and encourage physical activity.

Sources: International Diabetes Federation, "World Health Organization Issues Warning on World Heart Day," 2005, www.globalnews.idf .org/2005/09/who_issues_warning.html; World Health Organization, "Obesity and Overweight, 2006," www.who.int/dietphysicalactivity/ publications/facts/obesity/en/print.html.

---

fact, over 250 gene markers have shown positive association to obesity in over 400 separate studies.[25]

Body Type and Genes In some animal species, the shape and size of the individual's body are largely determined by its parents' shape and size. Many scientists have explored the role of heredity in determining human body shape. You need only look at your parents and then glance in the mirror to see where you got your own body type. Children whose parents are obese also tend to be overweight. In fact, a family history of obesity has long been thought to increase one's chances of becoming obese. Researchers have found that adopted individuals tend to be similar in weight to their biological parents, and that identical twins are twice as likely to weigh the same as are fraternal twins, even if they are raised separately.[26] Genes play a significant role in how the body balances calories and energy. Also, by influencing the amount of body fat and fat distribution, genes can make a person more susceptible to gaining weight.[27]

Although the exact mechanism remains unknown, it is believed that genes set metabolic rates, influencing how the body handles calories. Other genes, such as the *CD36* gene, may influence our cravings for fatty foods.[28] However, there is still much research to be done on the role of specific genes and obesity.

Specific Obesity Genes? In the past decade, more and more research has pointed to the existence of a "fat gene." Rather than inheriting a particular body type that predisposes us to overweight, it may be that our genes predispose us toward certain satiety and feeding behaviors. This "I need to eat" gene may account for up to one-third of our risk for obesity.[29] The most promising candidate is the *GAD2* gene. For some individuals, a variation in this gene increases the production of a chemical that boosts appetite and signals us to eat. Researchers hope that discovery of this gene and others may one day help those predisposed to obesity take steps to prevent becoming obese.[30]

Another gene getting a lot of attention is an *Ob* gene (for obesity), which is believed to disrupt the body's "I've had enough to eat" signaling system and may prompt individuals to keep eating past the point of being comfortably full. Research on Pima Indians, who have an estimated 75 percent obesity rate (nine out of ten are overweight), points to an *Ob*

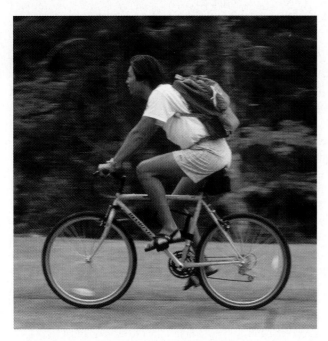

Modern conveniences support a sedentary lifestyle. Small changes to your daily activities, like biking to class, can help to increase your activity level and impact your health positively.

gene that is a "thrifty gene." It is theorized that because their ancestors struggled through centuries of famine, their basal metabolic rates slowed, allowing them to store precious fat for survival. Survivors may have passed these genes on to their children, which would explain the lower metabolic rates found in Pimas today and their tendency toward obesity.[31]

Endocrine Influence: The Hungry Hormones

Some researchers are focusing on the hormone *leptin,* which scientists believe signals the brain when you are full and need to stop eating.[32] When levels of leptin in the blood rise, appetite levels drop. Although obese people have adequate amounts of leptin and leptin receptors, they do not seem to work properly. It was believed that if leptin levels in the blood could be enhanced, people would find it easier to control their hunger urges. However, in a huge leptin study sponsored by a pharmaceutical company, few participants lost weight. In fact, the inability of leptin to trigger weight loss was so pronounced in this study that the trial ended early.

hunger An inborn physiological response to nutritional needs.

appetite A learned response that is tied to an emotional or psychological craving for food and is often unrelated to nutritional need.

satiety The feeling of fullness or satisfaction at the end of a meal.

However, researchers still believe leptin does play a role in hunger and satiety, and studies continue.[33]

Another hormone researchers suspect may play a role in our ability to keep weight off is *ghrelin,* which is produced in the stomach. Researchers at the University of Washington studied a small group of obese people who had lost weight over a six-month period.[34] They noted that ghrelin levels rose before every meal and fell drastically shortly afterward, suggesting that the hormone plays a role in appetite stimulation. Though ghrelin doesn't seem to be a cause of obesity, researchers believe that it may make it more difficult to lose weight once you gain it due to its influence on appetite and eating cues. Subsequent studies will test the impact of ghrelin-blocking drugs in controlling appetite as a form of intervention.

Other scientists have isolated a hormone called *GLP-1,* which is known to slow down the passage of food through the intestines to allow the absorption of nutrients. Research suggests that the GLP-1 hormone may be a key factor in stimulating insulin production and may eventually be a key factor in diabetes and obesity prevention and control.[35]

It is speculated that leptin and GLP-1 might play complementary roles in weight control. Leptin and its receptors may regulate body weight over the long term, calling upon fast-acting appetite suppressants like GLP-1 when necessary.

Over the years, many people have attributed obesity to problems with their thyroid gland. They believed that an underactive thyroid impeded their ability to burn calories. However, most authorities agree that less than 2 percent of the obese population have a thyroid problem and can instead trace their weight problems to another metabolic issue or to a hormone imbalance.[36]

Hunger, Appetite, and Satiety

Scientists distinguish between **hunger,** an inborn physiological response to nutritional needs, and **appetite,** a learned response to food that is tied to an emotional or psychological craving and is often unrelated to nutritional need. Obese people may be more likely than those at a healthy weight to satisfy their appetite and eat for reasons other than nutrition.

In some instances, the problem with overconsumption may be more related to **satiety** than to appetite or hunger. People generally feel satiated, or full, when they have satisfied their nutritional needs and their stomach signals "no more." For undetermined reasons, obese people may not feel full until much later than thin people. The leptin and GLP-1 studies seem to support this theory.

Theories abound concerning the mechanisms that regulate hunger, appetite, and satiety. The hypothalamus (the part of the brain that regulates appetite) closely monitors levels of certain nutrients in the blood. When these levels fall, the brain signals us to eat. According to one theory, in the obese person the monitoring system does not work properly and the cues to eat are more frequent and intense than they are in people of normal weight.

Another theory is that thin people send more effective messages to the hypothalamus. This concept, known as

adaptive thermogenesis, states that thin people can consume large amounts of food without gaining weight because the appetite center of their brains speeds up metabolic activity to compensate for the increased consumption.

Developmental Factors

Some obese people may have excessive numbers of fat cells. This type of obesity, **hyperplasia**, usually appears in early childhood and perhaps, due to the mother's dietary habits, even prior to birth. The most critical periods for the development of hyperplasia seem to be the last two to three months of fetal development, the first year of life, and between the ages of 9 and 13. Parents who allow their children to eat without restrictions and become overweight may be setting them up for a lifelong excess of fat cells. Central to this theory is the belief that the number of fat cells in a person's body does not increase appreciably during adulthood. However, the ability of each of these cells to swell (**hypertrophy**) and shrink does carry over into adulthood. Weight gain may be tied to both the number of fat cells in the body and the capacity of individual cells to enlarge.

An average-weight adult has approximately 25 billion to 35 billion fat cells, a moderately obese adult 60 billion to 100 billion, and an extremely obese adult as many as 200 billion.[37] People who add large numbers of fat cells to their bodies in childhood may be able to lose weight by decreasing the size of each cell in adulthood, but the total number of cells will remain the same. With the next calorie binge, the cells swell and sabotage weight-loss efforts (Figure 9.3). Additional research is needed to test these theories.

Setpoint Theory

I exercise and eat right, but I can't seem to lose any more weight. Why?

Nutritional researchers William Bennett and Joel Gurin developed the original **setpoint theory**, which stated that a person's body has a setpoint of weight at which it is programmed to be comfortable. If your setpoint is around 160 pounds, you will gain and lose weight fairly easily within a given range of that point. For example, if you gain 5 to 10 pounds on vacation, it will be fairly easy to lose that weight and remain around the 160-pound mark. Through adaptive thermogenesis, the body actually tries to maintain this weight. Some people equate this point with the **plateau** that dieters sometimes reach after losing a certain amount of weight. The setpoint theory proposes that after losing a predetermined amount of weight, the body will actually sabotage additional weight loss by slowing down metabolism. In extreme cases, the metabolic rate will decrease to a point at which the body will maintain its weight on as little as 1,000 calories per day.

Although it is recognized that a plateau does exist when one tries to lose weight, current research on genes, hormones, and other theories have superceded the setpoint theory. However, some researchers still believe that there is some type of setpoint mechanism at work.

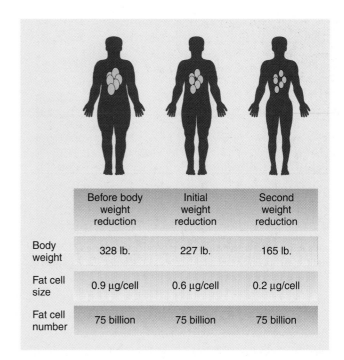

	Before body weight reduction	Initial weight reduction	Second weight reduction
Body weight	328 lb.	227 lb.	165 lb.
Fat cell size	0.9 µg/cell	0.6 µg/cell	0.2 µg/cell
Fat cell number	75 billion	75 billion	75 billion

FIGURE 9.3 One Person at Various Stages of Weight Loss
Note that, according to the hyperplasia theory, the number of fat cells remains constant but their size decreases when weight is lost.

Psychosocial Factors

The relationship of weight problems to deeply rooted emotional insecurities, needs, and wants remains uncertain. Food is often used as a reward for good behavior in childhood. As adults face unemployment, broken relationships, financial uncertainty, fears about health, and other problems, the bright spot in the day is often "what's on the table for dinner" or "we're going to that restaurant tonight." Again, the research underlying theories linking obesity with psychosocial factors is controversial. What is certain is that eating tends to be a focal point of people's lives, and the comfort foods of childhood may provide a salve for painful social pressures. Eating is essentially a social ritual associated with companionship, celebration, and enjoyment. For many people, the social emphasis on the eating experience is a major

adaptive thermogenesis Theoretical mechanism by which the brain regulates metabolic activity according to caloric intake.

hyperplasia A condition characterized by an excessive number of fat cells.

hypertrophy The ability of cells to swell.

setpoint theory A theory of obesity causation that suggests that fat storage is determined by a thermostatic mechanism in the body that acts to maintain a specific amount of body weight.

plateau That point in a weight-loss program at which the dieter finds it difficult to lose more weight.

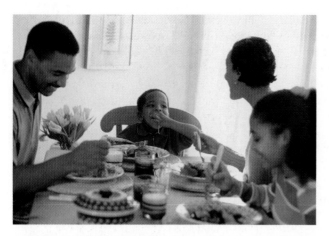

Many factors help determine body type, including heredity and genetic makeup, environmental factors, and learned eating patterns, which are often connected to family habits.

obstacle to successful dieting. Although some restaurants offer menu items designed to aid dieters, many people have difficulty choosing responsibly when confronted with an entire menu of delicious, fattening foods.

Some theorists contend that obese people ignore internal cues of hunger and are more likely to use the clock as a guide for "time to eat" than real hunger cues. Other studies refute this hypothesis.

Early Sabotage: Obesity in Youth

Another major factor is the pressure placed on us by the food industry's sophisticated marketing campaigns. There may be salad bars at the local fast-food joints, but customers have to run the gauntlet of starchy, beefy delights and high-fat fries to find them. The food and restaurant industries spend billions each year on ads to entice hungry people to forgo fresh fruit and sliced vegetables for Ring Dings and Happy Meals (see the Health Ethics box on page 300). Children are among the most vulnerable to these ads.

Children's impulses to eat junk food haven't changed much in recent decades. However, as noted earlier, they are eating larger portions. Social forces mentioned earlier, including the decline of home cooking, increased production of calorie- and fat-laden fast foods, and video technology that encourages kids to surf the Internet rather than ride their bicycles, have converged to increase the number of overweight young Americans. As a direct consequence, over 17 percent of American children and adolescents are now overweight or obese enough to endanger their health. Millions of others are on the threshold, and the problem is growing more extreme daily. Obese children suffer both physically and emotionally

basal metabolic rate (BMR) The energy expenditure of the body under resting conditions at normal room temperature.

throughout childhood, and those who stay heavy in adolescence tend to stay fat as adults.[38]

Dietary Myths and Misperceptions

An early and revealing study compared the self-reported and actual caloric intakes and amounts of exercise among a group of overweight adults. The researchers carefully followed obese people who had been unsuccessful on as many as 20 diets but claimed that they consumed fewer than 1,200 calories per day. They blamed their failure to lose weight on metabolism. It turned out that their metabolism levels were normal, but they were actually eating nearly twice as much as they thought they were and exercising only three-quarters as much as they reported.[39] This misperception of dietary intakes and exercise behaviors is pervasive today, with widespread underestimating of actual calorie consumption common.

Other studies have shown that obese individuals do not eat much more than their normal-weight counterparts. However, it should be noted that they do exercise less. The majority of overweight individuals are less active than nonobese people. Of course, it could be argued that their obesity leads to their sedentary lifestyle. Much more research is necessary before scientists have a clear profile of both the obese and the nonobese.

Metabolic Rates and Weight

Even at rest, the body consumes a certain amount of energy. The amount of energy your body uses at complete rest is your **basal metabolic rate (BMR)**. About 60 to 70 percent of all the calories you consume on a given day go to support your basal metabolism: heartbeat, breathing, maintaining body temperature, and so on. So if you consume 2,000 calories per day, between 1,200 and 1,400 of those calories are burned without your doing any significant physical activity. However, unless you exert yourself enough to burn the remaining 600 to 800 calories, you will gain weight.

Your BMR can fluctuate considerably, with several factors influencing whether it slows down or speeds up. In general, the younger you are, the higher your BMR, partly because in young people cells undergo rapid subdivision, which consumes a good deal of energy. BMR is highest during infancy, puberty, and pregnancy, when bodily changes are most rapid.

BMR is also influenced by body composition. Muscle tissue is highly active—even at rest—compared with fat tissue. In essence, the more lean tissue you have, the greater your BMR, and the more fat tissue you have, the lower your BMR. Men have a higher BMR than women do, at least partly because of their greater proportion of lean tissue. (This is another reason why developing muscular strength and endurance is so important to weight-loss and obesity-reduction plans.)[40]

Age is another factor. After age 30, BMR slows down by about 1 to 2 percent a year. Therefore, people over 30 commonly find that they must work harder to burn off an extra helping of ice cream than they did when in their teens. "Middle-aged spread," a reference to the tendency to put on weight later in life, is partly related to this change. A slower BMR, coupled with less activity, shifting priorities (family and career become more important than fitness), and loss in muscle mass, puts the weight of many middle-aged people in jeopardy.

In addition, the body has a number of self-protective mechanisms that signal BMR to speed up or slow down. For example, when you have a fever, the energy needs of your cells increase, which generates heat and speeds up your BMR. In starvation situations, the body protects itself by slowing down BMR to conserve precious energy. Thus, when people repeatedly resort to extreme diets, it is believed that their bodies reset their BMRs at lower rates. **Yo-yo diets**, in which people repeatedly gain weight and then starve themselves to lose it, are doomed to failure. When dieters resume eating after their weight loss, their BMR is set lower, making it almost certain that they will regain the pounds they just lost. After repeated cycles of dieting and regaining weight, these people find it increasingly hard to lose weight and increasingly easy to regain it, so they become heavier and heavier.

New research also supports the theory that by increasing your muscle mass, you will increase your metabolism and burn more calories each time you exercise (Chapter 10).

Lifestyle

Of all the factors affecting obesity, perhaps the most critical is the relationship between activity level and calorie intake. Obesity rates are rising. But how can this be happening? Aren't more people exercising than ever before?

Though the many advertisements for sports equipment and the popularity of athletes may give the impression that Americans love a good workout, the facts are not so positive. Data from the National Health Interview Survey show that four in ten adults in the United States never engage in any exercise, sports, or physically active hobbies in their leisure time.[41] Women (43.2 percent) were somewhat more likely than men (36.5 percent) to be sedentary, a finding that was consistent across all age groups. Among both men and women, black and Hispanic adults were more sedentary than white adults.[42] Leisure-time physical activity was also strongly associated with level of education. About 72 percent of adults who never attended high school were sedentary, declining steadily to 45 percent among high school graduates and about 24 percent among adults with graduate-level college degrees.[43]

Do you know people who seemingly can eat whatever they want without gaining weight? With few exceptions, if you were to follow them around for a typical day and monitor the level and intensity of their activity, you would discover the reason. Even if their schedule does not include jogging or intense exercise, it probably includes a high level of activity. Walking up a flight of stairs rather than taking the elevator, speeding up the pace while mowing the lawn, getting up to change the TV channel rather than using the remote, and doing housework all burn extra calories.

Actually, it may even go beyond that. In studies of calorie burning by individuals placed in a controlled respiratory chamber environment where calories consumed, motion, and overall activity were measured, it was found that some people are better fat burners than others. It is possible that low fat burners may not produce as many of the enzymes needed to convert fat to energy. Or they may not have as many blood vessels supplying fatty tissue, making it tougher for them to deliver fat-burning oxygen. Or perhaps in subtle ways, high fat burners burn more calories through extra motions. Clearly, any form of activity that burns additional calories helps maintain weight.

Smoking Women who smoke tend to weigh six to ten pounds less than nonsmokers. After quitting, weight generally increases to the level found among nonsmokers. Weight gain after smoking cessation may be partly due to nicotine's ability to raise metabolic rate. When smokers stop, they burn fewer calories. Another reason former smokers often gain weight is that they generally eat more after they quit in order to satisfy free-floating cravings.[44]

what do you THINK?

Why do you think men and women differ so much in their physical activity patterns? ■ Why are certain minority groups less likely to exercise than other groups? ■ What might be done in terms of policies, programs, and services to change these statistics?

Gender and Obesity

Throughout our lives, issues of appearance and attractiveness are constantly in the foreground. Only recently have researchers begun to understand just how significant, especially for women, the quest for beauty and the perfect body really is.

Researchers have determined that being severely overweight in adolescence may influence one's social and economic future—particularly for females. Researchers found that obese women complete about half a year less schooling, are 20 percent less likely to get married, and earn thousands of dollars less on average per year than their slimmer counterparts. Obese women also have rates of household poverty 10 percent higher than those of women who are not overweight. In contrast, the study found that overweight men are 11 percent less likely to be married than thinner men but suffer few adverse economic consequences.[45]

It may be that women suffer such negative consequences because the social stigma of being overweight is more severe for women than for men. Women are also disadvantaged

yo-yo diets   Cycles in which people repeatedly gain weight, and then starve themselves to lose weight. This lowers their BMR, which makes regaining weight even more likely.

HEALTH ETHICS
conflict and controversy

ARE SUPER-SIZED MEALS SUPER-SIZING AMERICANS?

Today, super-sized meals are the norm at many restaurants. Biscuits and gravy, huge steaks, and plate-filling meals are popular fare. Consider the 25-ounce prime rib dinner served at a local steak chain. At nearly 3,000 calories and 150 grams of fat for the meat alone, this meal both slams shut arteries and adds on pounds. Add a baked potato with sour cream and/or butter, a salad loaded with creamy salad dressing, and fresh bread with real butter, and the meal may surpass the 5,000-calorie mark and ring in at close to 300 grams of fat. In other words, it exceeds what most adults should eat in two days!

And this is just the beginning. Soft drinks, once commonly served in 12-ounce portions, now come in "big gulps" and 1-liter bottles. Cinnamon buns at local chains now come in giant, butter-laden, 700-calorie portions. What is the result? Super-sized portions consumed by super-sized Americans. A quick glance at the fattening of Americans provides growing evidence of a significant health problem. According to Donna Skoda, a dietitian and chair of the Ohio State University Extension Service, "People are eating a ton of extra

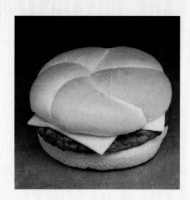

20 YEARS AGO

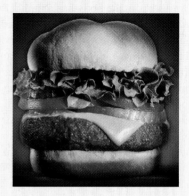

TODAY

calories. For the first time in history, more people are overweight in America than are underweight. Ironically, although the U.S. fat intake has dropped in the past 20 years from an average of 40 to 33 percent of calories, the daily calorie intake has risen from 1,852 calories per day to over 2,000 per day. In theory, this translates into a weight gain of 15 pounds a year." Skoda and others say that the main reason that Americans are gaining weight is that people no longer know what a normal serving size is. In a recent U.S. Department of Agriculture survey, only 1 percent of the respondents could correctly identify the serving sizes recommended in the Food

Guide Pyramid, the visual dietary aid developed by the USDA.

The National Heart, Lung, and Blood Institute, part of the National Institutes of Health, has developed a "Portion Distortion" quiz that shows how today's portions compare with those of 20 years ago. Test yourself online at http://hin.nhlbi.nih.gov/portion to see if you can recognize the differences between today's super-sized meals and those once considered normal. Just one example is the difference between an average cheeseburger 20 years ago (left photo) and the typical cheeseburger of today (right photo).

---

biologically when it comes to losing weight. Compared to men, they have a lower ratio of lean body mass to fatty mass, in part due to differences in bone size and mass, muscle size, and other variables. Because men have more muscle, and muscle uses more energy than fat, they burn 10 to 20 percent more calories than women do during rest.[46] (See Chapter 10 for an overview of the role that increased muscle mass has on weight reduction.) After sexual maturity, men have higher metabolic rates, making it easier for them to burn off excess calories. Women also face greater potential for weight fluctuation due to hormonal changes, pregnancy, and other conditions that increase the likelihood of weight gain. Also,

as a group, men are more socialized into physical activity from birth. Strenuous work and play are encouraged for men, whereas women's roles have typically been more sedentary and required a lower level of caloric expenditure.

Not only are women more vulnerable to weight gain, but also pressures to maintain and/or lose weight make them more likely to take dramatic measures to lose weight. For example, eating disorders are more prevalent among women, and more women than men take diet pills.

However, males experience these pressures too, and are becoming more preoccupied with their own physical form (see Chapter 10). Thus, eating disorders, exercise addictions, and other maladaptive responses are on the increase among men as well.

Of increasing interest is an emerging problem seen in both young men and women, known as **social physique anxiety (SPA)**, in which the desire to "look good" has a destructive and sometimes disabling effect on one's ability to function

social physique anxiety (SPA) A desire to look good that has a destructive effect on a person's ability to function effectively socially.

How can you reduce your own risk of super-sizing? Follow these strategies:

- Avoid super-sizing anything. Order the smallest size available when dining out. Focus on taste, not quantity. Get used to eating less and enjoying what you are eating.
- Chew your food, and avoid the urge to wash it down with high-calorie drinks. Take time, and let your fullness indicator have a chance to kick in while there is still time to quit.
- Serve food on a small or medium plate. Put those big platter-size dinner plates on the top shelf of your cupboard, and leave them there.
- Always order dressings, gravies, and sauces on the side. Sprinkle these added calories on carefully, rather than washing your foods down with them. Remember that a tablespoon of gravy could mean an hour on the treadmill to burn off its 200+ calories!
- If you order a large muffin or bagel, share it with a friend, or eat only half and wrap up the rest. Carry a small zip-lock bag, and use it to take home part of those big portions for another day.

- Avoid appetizers in restaurants. They are expensive, in terms of money, calories, and fat content.
- Share your dinner with a friend, and order a side salad for each of you. Alternatively, eat only half of your dinner and save the rest for another day.
- Measure portions. Before ordering, ask for the size of servings, and always order a size smaller than you really want. When the server tells you it is a "rich dish" or "a lot of food," avoid it.
- Avoid buffets and all-you-can-eat establishments. Most of us can eat two to three times what we need—or more.

Who's to blame for this portion distortion? Are we as consumers succumbing to slick advertising that entices us to eat even when we are full? Or are we truly an overindulgent and sedentary culture, to which food manufacturers are merely responding?

According to Carrie Wiatt, a Los Angeles dietitian and author of the recently released book *Portion Savvy,* a telling marker of the big-food trend is that restaurant plates have grown from an average of 9 inches to 13 inches in the past decade.

Studies show that people eat 40 to 50 percent more than they normally would now that large portions are available.

In fact, alarming statistics such as these are part of the growing controversy over who is liable for our overfat and sedentary populace. Lawsuits have been brought against companies like McDonald's, only to be thrown out by judges, and experts are examining our behaviors and weighing in on who is to blame for our overindulgence. However, any kind of real change is unlikely in the near future. For now, it is up to us to take personal action.

Are restaurants to blame for luring us in with gigantic, more-bang-for-your-buck portions? Should the government regulate fast-food companies to reign in high-calorie meals and advertisements that target children? Should candy- and soda-vending machines be outlawed in school cafeterias and dormitories nationwide?

Sources: E. J. Fried, "The Potential for Policy Initiatives to Address the Obesity Epidemic in the United States," in D. Crawford and R. W. Jeffrey, eds., *Obesity Prevention and Public Health* (New York: Oxford University Press, 2005); K. D. Brownell et al., "Does a Toxic Environment Make Obesity Inevitable?" *Obesity Management* (2005): 52–55.

---

effectively in relationships and interactions with others. People suffering from SPA may spend a disproportionate amount of time fixating on their bodies, working out, and performing tasks that are ego-centered and self-directed, rather than focusing on interpersonal relationships and general tasks.[47] Incessant worry about their bodies and their appearance permeates their lives. Overweight and obesity are clear risks for these people, and experts speculate that this anxiety may contribute to eating-disordered behaviors.

Individuality

Although researchers have learned a great deal in recent years about the factors that predispose people to gain or lose weight, controversy remains. Perhaps the most overlooked element is the individual. Just as no two people are exactly alike physiologically, we are not psychologically identical.

Each person is a unique result of genetic background, environment, lifestyle, and emotional responses to a lifetime of experiences.

It is highly possible that the causes of obesity are as varied as the people who are obese. If this is so, there can be no universal cure for weight problems. Instead, we must look for a mechanism of prevention or intervention for each individual that is based upon appropriate cultural, social, environmental, and other factors.

 what do you THINK?

Can you think of other reasons why men and women may differ in how much weight they gain and how easily they are able to lose it? ■ What historical patterns may have contributed to this?

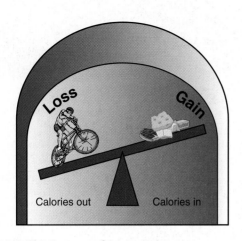

FIGURE 9.4 The Concept of Energy Balance
How many calories do you need each day? If you consume more calories than you burn, you will gain weight. If you burn more than you consume, you will lose weight, and if both are equal, your weight will not change, according to this concept.

Managing Your Weight

What's the best way to lose weight or maintain my current weight?

At some point in our lives, almost all of us will decide to go on a diet, and many will meet with mixed success. The problem is probably related to the fact that we think in terms of dieting rather than adjusting lifestyle and eating behaviors. It has been well documented that hypocaloric (low-calorie) diets produce only temporary losses and may actually lead to disordered binge eating or related problems. Repeated bouts of restrictive dieting may be physiologically harmful, and the sense of failure that we get each time we try and fail can exact far-reaching psychological costs. Drugs and intensive counseling can contribute to positive weight loss, but even then, many people regain weight after treatment.

Keeping Weight Control in Perspective

Although experts say that losing weight simply requires burning more calories than are consumed, putting this principle into practice is far from simple (Figure 9.4). Sure, calories in minus calories out equals weight, but people of the same age, sex, height, and weight can have differences of as much as 1,000 calories a day in resting metabolic rate—this may explain why one person's gluttony is another's starvation, even if it results in the same readout on the scale. And while peo-

ple of normal weight average 25 billion to 35 billion fat cells, obese people can inherit a billowing 135 billion. Other factors such as depression, stress, culture, and available foods can also play a role.

Weight loss is more difficult for some people and may require supportive friends, relatives, and community resources, plus extraordinary efforts to prime the body for burning extra calories. Being overweight does not mean people are weak-willed or lazy. As scientists unlock the many secrets of genetic messengers that influence body weight and learn more about the role of certain foods in the weight-loss equation, dieting may not be the same villain in the future that it is today.

To reach and maintain the weight at which you will be healthy and feel best, you need to develop a program of exercise and healthy eating behaviors that will work for you now and in the long term. See the Skills for Behavior Change box on page 304 for strategies to make your weight management program succeed. To become a wise food consumer, you also need to become familiar with important concepts in weight control.

Understanding Calories

A **calorie** is a unit of measure that indicates the amount of energy we obtain from a particular food. One pound of body fat contains approximately 3,500 calories. So each time you consume 3,500 calories more than your body needs to maintain weight, you gain a pound. Conversely, each time your body expends an extra 3,500 calories, you lose a pound. So if you drink an extra can of soft drink (140 calories) every single day and make no other changes in diet or activity, you would gain one pound in 25 days (3,500 calories ÷ 140 calories/day = 25 days). Conversely, if you walk for 30 minutes each day at a pace of 15 minutes per mile (172 calories burned), you would lose one pound in 20 days (3,500 calories ÷ 172 calories/day = 20.3 days). Remember, too, that the number of calories you burn is also related to your weight. The heavier you are, the more energy (calories) it takes to move.

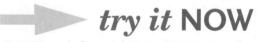

The two ways to lose weight, then, are to lower caloric intake (through better eating habits) and to increase exercise (thereby expending more calories). Don't forget, it took time to gain weight; it will take time to lose it.

➡ ***try it* NOW**

Set SMART goals for weight loss. Give your goals a reality check: Are they **S**pecific, **M**easurable, **A**chievable, **R**elevant, and **T**ime specific? For example, rather than aiming to lose 15 pounds this month (which probably wouldn't be healthy or achievable) set a comfortable goal to lose 5 pounds in a month. Realistic goals will encourage weight-loss success by boosting your confidence in your ability to make lifelong healthy changes.

calorie A unit of measurement indicating the energy obtained from a particular food.

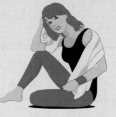

What Triggers Your "Eat" Response?

- Time of day
- Mood
- Boredom

- Nervousness/anxiety/stress
- Hormonal fluctuations
- Peer/family pressure
- Inattentiveness
- Habit
- Hunger/appetite
- Low self-esteem
- Environment/social setting
- Sight and smell of favorite foods

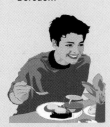

What Stops Your "Eat" Response?

- Acting responsibly in assessing foods
- Practicing stress management
- Breaking the habit
- Remaining active
- Analyzing emotional problems
- Making a conscious effort
- Recognizing true hunger
- Avoiding environment that causes "eat" response

- Selecting alternatives
- Recognizing triggers
- Planning

FIGURE 9.5 The "Eat" Response
Learn to understand what triggers and stops your "eat" response by keeping a daily log.

Adding Exercise

Approximately 90 percent of the daily caloric expenditures of most people occurs as a result of the **resting metabolic rate (RMR)**. Slightly higher than the BMR, the RMR includes the BMR plus any additional energy expended through daily sedentary activities such as food digestion, sitting, studying, or standing. The **exercise metabolic rate (EMR)** accounts for the remaining 10 percent of all daily caloric expenditures; it refers to the energy expenditure that occurs during physical exercise. For most of us, these calories come from light daily activities, such as walking, climbing stairs, and mowing the lawn. If we increase the level of physical activity to moderate or heavy, however, our EMR may be 10 to 20 times greater than typical resting metabolic rates and can contribute substantially to weight loss.

Increasing BMR, RMR, or EMR levels will help burn calories. Any increase in the intensity, frequency, and duration of daily exercise levels can have a significant impact on total calorie expenditure.

Physical activity makes a greater contribution to BMR when it involves large muscle groups. The energy spent on physical activity is the energy used to move the body's muscles—the muscles of the arms, back, abdomen, legs, and so on—and the extra energy used to speed up heartbeat and respiration rate. The number of calories spent depends on three factors:

1. The amount of muscle mass moved
2. The amount of weight moved
3. The amount of time the activity takes

An activity involving both the arms and legs burns more calories than one involving only the legs; an activity performed by a heavy person burns more calories than one performed by a lighter individual; and an activity performed for 40 minutes requires twice as much energy than one performed for only 20 minutes. Thus, obese persons walking for one mile burn more calories than slim people walking the same distance. It may also take overweight people longer to walk the mile, which means that they are burning energy for a longer time and therefore expending more overall calories than the thin walkers.

Improving Your Eating Habits

At any given time, many Americans are trying to lose weight. Given the hundreds of different diets and endless expert advice available, why do we find it so difficult?

Determining What Triggers an Eating Behavior Before you can change a behavior, you must first determine what causes it.

Many people have found it helpful to keep a chart of their eating patterns: when they feel like eating, where they are when they decide to eat, the amount of time they spend eating, other activities they engage in during the meal (watching television or reading), whether they eat alone or with others, what and how much they consume, and how they felt before they took their first bite. If you keep a detailed daily log of the triggers listed in Figure 9.5 for at least a week, you will discover useful clues about what in your environment or your emotional makeup causes you to want food. Typically, these dietary triggers center on problems in everyday living rather than on real hunger pangs. Many people find that they eat compulsively when stressed or when they have problems in their

resting metabolic rate (RMR)   The energy expenditure of the body under BMR conditions plus other daily sedentary activities.

exercise metabolic rate (EMR)   The energy expenditure that occurs during exercise.

TIPS FOR SENSIBLE AND SAFE WEIGHT MANAGEMENT

TIPS FOR SENSIBLE WEIGHT MANAGEMENT

How can I control my weight without resorting to fad diets?

Rather than thinking about the best diet, the key to successful weight management is finding a sustainable way to control food that will work for you. Combine the following strategies with a Behavior Change Contract to develop a weight management plan that is right for you. Remember, you are not going on a diet that you will quit someday. You are making lifelong changes that will result in weight loss.

BEFORE YOU BEGIN YOUR PLAN

- *Talk with your health care provider.* Tell your health care provider that you would like to lose weight. Be sure to discuss any medical condition you have or medicines you take. Ask questions, and be sure you understand everything your doctor is saying.
- *Ask yourself some key questions.* Why do you want to make this change? Is your weight affecting your health and quality of life? What are your weight-loss goals? Are you ready to change your eating habits and incorporate physical activity into your lifestyle?
- *Assess where you are.* Monitor your eating habits for 2 or 3 days, taking careful note of the good things you are doing and the things that need improvement.

MAKING A PLAN

- *Think of it as a way of life.* This is a way of improving your body and your health rather than a punishment or a diet.
- *Set realistic goals.* No matter what you do, you may not have a perfect body. Establish short-term goals on the way to the final goal. Make changes that you can stick with and that are comfortable for you (parking farther from a destination and walking, eating cereal and juice for breakfast, walking 3 days per week, and so on). Set a schedule for exercise and try to stick to it, with an alternative time each day in case your plans change. Always have a fallback option for your scheduled exercise.
- *Establish a plan.* What are three dietary changes you can make today? What exercise will you do tomorrow, the next day, and sustain for one week? Once you do one week, plot a course for two weeks. Jot down how you feel after each week's activity.
- *Look for balance in what you do.* Remember that it's more about balance than about giving things up. If you must have that piece of chocolate cake, enjoy it, but then be responsible for doing the extra exercise it takes to burn off the calories or for limiting caloric intake the next day. Remember that it's calories taken in and burned over time that makes the difference.
- *Stay positive.* Focus on the positive steps you are taking and the healthy things you do each week rather than the less healthy things.
- *Be patient and persistent.* You didn't develop a weight problem overnight. Don't expect instant results. Assess other gains that you make each week:

relationships. For other people, the same circumstances diminish their appetite, causing them to lose weight.

Changing Your Triggers Once you recognize the factors that cause you to eat, removing the triggers or substituting other activities for them will help you develop more sensible eating patterns. Here are some examples of substitute behaviors:

- When eating dinner, turn off all distractions, including phones, computers, the television, and radio.
- Replace snack breaks or coffee breaks with exercise breaks.
- Instead of gulping your food, chew each bite slowly and savor it.
- Vary mealtimes. Instead of eating by the clock, do not eat until you are truly hungry. Allow yourself only a designated amount of time for eating—but do not rush. Try to become more aware of true feelings of hunger.

- If you find that you generally eat all that you can cram on a plate, use smaller plates. Put your dinner plates away, and use the salad plates instead.
- Stop buying high-calorie foods that tempt you to snack, or store them in an inconvenient place. (Having to run upstairs for the potato chips will force you to think twice before munching them.)

These are just suggestions. After recording your daily intake for one week, you will be able to devise a list of substitutes that are geared toward your particular eating behaviors. Table 9.3 on page 306 lists some ideas for sensible snacking.

what do you THINK?

If you wanted to lose weight, what strategies would you most likely choose? ■ Which strategies offer the lowest health risk and the greatest chance for success? ■ What factors might serve to support or sabotage your weight-loss efforts?

gains in energy level, the fit of your clothes, and how you feel in your body.

- *Reward success.* Set short-term goals and reward yourself when you've reached them—new shoes, a new CD, whatever it takes to keep you motivated.

CHANGING YOUR DIET

- *Be adventurous.* Diversify your usual meals and snacks with a wide variety of different options. Focus on the quality of the food rather than the amount you get. Avoid buffets that allow you to replenish your plate several times.
- *Do not constantly deprive yourself of favorite foods or set unrealistic guidelines.* If you slip and eat something you know you shouldn't, just be more careful the next day. Balance over a week's time is important. Allow slips and reward successes.
- *Be sensible with your knife and fork.* Enjoy all foods, just don't overdo. When you eat out, eat slowly, cut food into smaller pieces, and think about taking some home for tomorrow's lunch or

dinner. Share entrées with a friend and order salads with dressings on the side.

- *Eat on a regular schedule.* Do not skip meals or let yourself get too hungry.
- *Eat breakfast.* This will prevent you from being too hungry and overeating at lunch.
- *Plan ahead and be prepared for when you might get hungry.* Always have good food available when and where you get hungry.

CHANGING YOUR LEVEL OF ACTIVITY

- *Be active and slowly increase activity.* If you stick to something, it will gradually take less and less effort to walk that mile, for example. Gradually increase your speed and/or distance (see Chapter 10). Move more, sit less. Remember, every step counts. Purchasing an inexpensive pedometer and recording your daily steps is an excellent way to monitor and improve your level of activity.
- *Be creative with your physical activity.* Find activities that you really love and stick to them. If you hate to walk in the

rain but love to shop, walk in a covered mall and then shop! Try things you haven't tried before. Today, options such as yoga, Pilates, dancing, swimming, skiing, and gardening are available.

- *Pick an activity that is inexpensive and does not require fancy equipment.* This means you will maintain your fitness program even when you are traveling away from home.
- *Find an exercise partner to help you stay motivated.* Don't pick your fittest friend. Find someone who is patient, understanding, and supportive. Choose people who need help and commit to helping them. It will also help you get through the difficult days until exercise is part of your lifestyle.

Sources: Adapted in part from M. Manore and J. Thompson, "Table 15.3: Techniques to Help an Active Individual Identify and Maintain a Healthy Body Weight Throughout the Life Cycle," in *Sport Nutrition for Health and Performance* (Champaign, IL: Human Kinetics Publishing, 2000), 417; Weight Control Information Network, "Choosing a Safe and Successful Weight-Loss Program," NIH Publication No. 03-3700, February 2006.

Selecting a Nutritional Plan

Seek assistance from reputable sources in selecting a dietary plan that is nutritious and easy to follow, such as the MyPyramid Plan discussed in Chapter 8. Registered dietitians, some physicians (not all doctors have a strong background in nutrition), health educators and exercise physiologists with nutritional training, and other health professionals can provide reliable information. Beware of people who call themselves nutritionists. There is no such official designation, which leaves the door open for just about anyone to call himself or herself a nutritional expert. Avoid weight-loss programs that promise quick, "miracle" results. See the Spotlight on Your Health box on page 308 for a summary of popular weight-loss plaus.

For any weight-loss program, ask about the credentials of the adviser; assess the nutrient value of the prescribed diet; verify that dietary guidelines are consistent with reliable nutrition research; and analyze the suitability of the diet to your tastes, budget, and lifestyle. Any diet that requires radical be-

havior changes is doomed to failure. The most successful plans allow you to make food choices and do not ask you to sacrifice everything you enjoy.

Reward yourself when you lose pounds. If you binge and go off your nutrition plan, get right back on it the next day. Remember that you did not gain 40 pounds in eight weeks, so it is unrealistic to punish your body by trying to lose that amount of weight in that short a time.

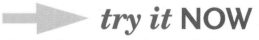 *try it* NOW

Healthy substitutions at mealtime are the key to weight maintenance success! The next time you make dinner, take a look at the proportions on your plate. Veggies and whole grains should take up the most space; if not, substitute 1 cup of the meat, pasta, or cheese on your plate with 1 cup of legumes, salad greens, or a favorite vegetable. You'll reduce the number of calories in your meal while eating the same amount of food!

TABLE 9.3 Tips for Sensible Snacking

According to the American Heart Association and other professional groups focused on nutrition, these healthy snacks can help curb your hunger pangs, keep your blood glucose from spiking, and will stay with you for longer periods of time.

- **Keep healthy munchies around.** Buy whole-wheat breads and if you need something to spice that up, buy low-fat or soy cheese, low-fat cream cheese, or other healthy favorites and use them.
- **Keep crunchies on hand.** Apples, pears, green pepper sticks, popcorn, carrots, and celery all are good choices. Wash them and cut them up to carry with you or eat when you feel a snack attack coming on.
- **Quench your thirst with hot drinks.** Hot tea, heated milk, decaffeinated coffee, hot chocolate made with nonfat milk or water, or soup broths will help keep you satisfied.
- **Choose natural beverages.** Drink plain water, natural 100% juice drinks, tomato juice, or other low-sugar choices to satisfy your thirst.
- **Eat nuts instead of candy.** If you have to have a piece of chocolate, keep that piece small, preferably DARK chocolate.
- **Avoid high-calorie energy bars** unless you are really exercising hard and don't have an opportunity to eat normal food. If you buy energy bars, look for a good mixture of fiber, protein, low-fat, and low-calorie options.

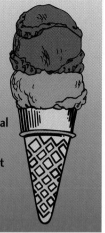

FUNfact

Want to avoid the "freshman 15"? Skip dessert. There are 130 calories in a typical half-cup serving of ice cream. You could gain 14 pounds if you indulge in this treat every day for a year.

FIGURE 9.6 Are You on Your Way to the Freshman 15?

Determining a Reasonable Rate for Weight Loss

Once you have discovered what factors tend to sabotage your weight-loss efforts, you will be well on your way to healthy weight control. To succeed, however, you must plan for success. By setting goals that are unrealistic, you will doom yourself to failure. Do not try to lose 40 pounds in two months. Try, instead, to lose a healthy 1 to 2 pounds during the first week, and stay with this slow and easy regimen. Supplements and other fads that promise anything faster may be appealing, but not only are the goals unrealistic, so is the expectation that you will maintain that weight loss. However, making permanent changes to your lifestyle by adding exercise and cutting back on calories for a total deficit of 500 calories per day will put you on the path to a weight-loss rate of 1 pound per week, and diet success.

Considering Drastic Weight-Loss Measures

When nothing seems to work, people often become willing to take significant risks in order to lose weight. Dramatic weight loss may be recommended in high-risk cases of hypertension, cardiac strain, imperiled lung capacity, gastrointestinal difficulties, crippling strain on bones and joints, surgical risk, and other problems. Even in such situations, drastic dietary, pharmacological, or surgical measures should be considered carefully and discussed with several knowledgeable health professionals and with full awareness of potential adverse effects.

Fad Diets Fasting, starvation diets, and other forms of **very low-calorie diets (VLCDs)** have been shown to cause significant health risks. Typically, depriving the body of food for prolonged periods forces it to make adjustments to prevent the shutdown of organs. The body depletes its energy reserves to obtain necessary fuels. One of the first reserves the body turns to in order to maintain its supply of glucose is lean, protein tissue. As this is consumed, weight is lost rapidly because protein contains only half as many calories per pound as fat. At the same time, significant water stores are lost. Over time, the body begins to run out of liver tissue, heart muscle, and so on, as these readily available substances are burned to supply energy. Only after depleting the readily available proteins from these sources does the body begin to burn fat reserves. In this process, known as **ketosis**, the body adapts to prolonged fasting or carbohydrate deprivation by converting body fat to ketones, which can be used as fuel for some brain cells. Within about ten days after the typical adult begins a complete fast, the body will have used many of its energy stores, and death may occur.

In VLCDs, powdered formulas are usually given to patients under medical supervision. These formulas have daily values of 400 to 700 calories plus vitamin and mineral supplements. Although

---

very low-calorie diets (VLCDs) Diets with a daily caloric value of 400 to 700 calories.

ketosis A condition in which the body adapts to prolonged fasting or carbohydrate deprivation by converting body fat to ketones, which can be used as fuel for some brain activity.

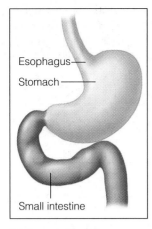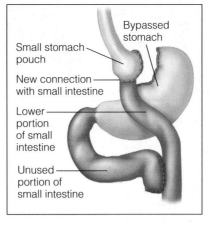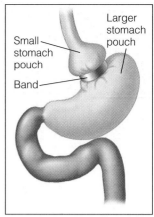

(a) Normal stomach   (b) Gastric bypass   (c) Gastric banding

FIGURE 9.7 Weight-Loss Surgery Alters the Normal Anatomy of Your Stomach

these diets may be beneficial for people who have failed at all conventional weight-loss methods and who face severe health risks due to obesity, they should never be undertaken without strict medical supervision. Problems associated with fasting, VLCDs, and other forms of severe caloric deprivation include blood sugar imbalance, cold intolerance, constipation, decreased BMR, dehydration, diarrhea, emotional problems, fatigue, headaches, heart irregularity, ketosis, kidney infections and failure, loss of lean body tissue, weakness, and eventual weight gain due to the yo-yo effect and other variables.

Also consider the nutritional quality of packaged "low-fat" foods commonly used as part of a low-calorie diet. Many of these foods have a high sugar and sodium content to make the food taste better. They might be low fat, but generally, they are full of empty calories from sugar, and lots of salt. For more on low-fat diets, see the New Horizons in Health box on page 311.

Drug Treatment When used as part of a long-term, comprehensive weight-loss program, drugs can help those who are severely obese lose up to 10 percent of their weight and maintain this. The challenge is to develop an effective drug that can be used over time without adverse effects or abuse, and no such drug currently exists.

A classic example of supposedly safe drugs that later were found to have dangerous side effects are Pondimin and Redux, known as *fen-phen* (from their chemical names fenfluramine and phentermine), two of the most widely prescribed diet drugs in U.S. history.[48] When they were found to damage heart valves and contribute to pulmonary hypertension, a massive recall and lawsuit occurred.

Other diet drugs that you should view with caution include:

■ *Sibutramine (Meridia)*. Suppresses appetite by inhibiting the uptake of serotonin. It works best with a reduced-calorie diet and exercise, but side effects are not to be taken lightly. They include dry mouth, headache, constipation, insomnia, and high blood pressure. Newer research does show a positive effect on blood glucose control.[49]

■ *Orlistat (Xenical)*. Works by inhibiting the action of lipase, an enzyme that helps digest fats. About 30 percent of fats consumed pass through the system undigested, leading to reduced overall caloric intake. Known side effects include oily spotting; gas with watery fecal discharge; fecal urgency; oily stools; frequent, often unexpected, bowel movements; and possible deficiencies of fat-soluble vitamins.

■ *Herbal Weight-Loss Aids*. In attempts to fight the battle of the bulge, many people turn to potentially unsafe herbal remedies (see Chapter 23). Products containing *Ephedra* can cause rapid heart rate, tremors, seizures, insomnia, headaches, and raised blood pressure, all without significant effects on long-term weight control. *St. John's Wort (SJW)* and other alternative medicines reported to enhance serotonin and suppress appetite, as well as reduce the side effects of depression, have not been shown to be effective in weight loss, either.

Surgery When all else fails, particularly for those who are severely overweight and have weight-related diseases such as diabetes or hypertension, a person may be a candidate for one of the various forms of weight-loss surgery. Generally, these surgeries fall into one of two major categories: *restrictive surgeries,* such as *gastric banding,* or *malabsorption surgeries,* such as *gastric bypass* (Figure 9.7). In gastric banding and other restrictive surgeries, the surgeon uses an inflatable band to partition off part of the stomach. The band is wrapped around that part of the stomach and is pulled tight, like a belt, leaving only a small opening between the two parts of the stomach. The upper part of the stomach is smaller, so one feels full more quickly, and food digestion slows so that you also feel full longer. Although the bands are designed to stay in place, they can be removed surgically. Weight loss is slower than with gastric bypass surgery, but risks are fewer, particularly since it is a less invasive surgical procedure. In contrast, gastric bypass is designed to drastically restrict the

(Text continues on page 310)

ANALYZING POPULAR DIETS

Eighty-three percent of college-aged women report dieting, regardless of their current weight. Dieting behaviors include skipping meals, eating less, using artificial sweeteners, and smoking to suppress appetite.* College students, like all Americans, are in an ongoing quest to lose weight. However, not only do many college-aged women choose unhealthy options like skipping breakfast or smoking cigarettes to control hunger, but they must also negotiate a myriad of seemingly reputable diets. Are any of these diet plans really the miracles they often claim to be? Don't count on it. Some are quite good, but others produce no long-term effects and may even be dangerous.

Virtually anyone can write a book making diet claims. Arguments or claims may be based on unproven science or faulty scientific reasoning. Although health claims should only be published after solid research has proven the results repeatedly with different populations, this happens all too infrequently.

Below we summarize some of the most popular diets and the consensus opinions of the U.S. Department of Agriculture, the American Heart Association, the Center for Science in the Public Interest, and several other professional groups and individuals regarding the effectiveness and safety of these diets.

Book/Program and Author	Premise of the Diet	How It Claims to Work	Experts' Opinions	Comments
The Atkins Diet, Robert Atkins, MD	Says overweight people eat too many carbohydrates. High-protein diet allows you to eat all the protein you want (meat, eggs, cheese, and more) and restricts refined sugar, milk, white rice, and white flour	Restrict carbohydrates and body goes into ketosis. In ketosis, body gets energy from ketones, little carbon fragments that are the fuel created by breakdown of fat stores. You feel less hungry.	Highly controversial. Low intake of fruits and vegetables a problem. High intake of animal fats unhealthy.	Possible side effects: nausea, fatigue, low blood pressure, elevated uric acid/kidney problems, bad breath, constipation, fetal harm if pregnant
Dean Ornish Diet, Dean Ornish, MD	Diet and exercise are important. Watch what you eat; there are foods you should eat all of the time, some of the time, and none of the time. Less than 10% of your calories should come from fat. Eat lots of little meals.	Metabolism is a result of our ancestors. We need to change old metabolic patterns. Meditation is a part of this: when your soul is fed, you have less need to overeat.	Mostly positive for highly restrictive diet and healthy lifestyle regimen. Documented studies show heart blockage reversal. Drawbacks are that it is tough to stick to this diet and new eating patterns must be learned. Only the most committed will stick to this rigid diet.	May be tough for all but strict vegans to adhere to this plan. Eating smaller, more frequent meals may be difficult. Otherwise a good model.
Eating Well for Optimum Health, Andrew Weil, MD	Eat less, exercise more. Take a more Eastern than Western approach. Avoid quick fixes and set realistic goal of 1–2 pounds of weight loss per week. Balance the amount and type of food. Describes meats as "flesh foods." Minimize dairy and take a Mediterranean dietary approach.	Keeps it simple. Criticizes high-protein diets because of rise in cholesterol and calcium depletion. Moderation is key.	A more holistic approach to dieting than most. Considers exercise and stress as factors.	May not be sustainable for those who are used to diets high in dairy or meat. Nutrition experts support this common-sense approach. Vegetarian emphasis substantiated as healthy by numerous studies.

Book/Program and Author	Premise of the Diet	How It Claims to Work	Experts' Opinion	Comments
The Pritikin Principle, Robert Pritikin	Concern not for calories, but for density of calories. Eat more foods that are not calorie dense, such as apples and oatmeal.	Fill up on foods that have fewer calories. Large volume of fiber and water will keep you full. Emphasis on vegetables, fruits, beans, unprocessed grains; exercise strongly recommended.	Weight loss will occur, but so will frequent feelings of hunger. Weight will usually creep back. Low in fat so healthy in general, except when taken to extreme or for certain groups of people.	Strict limitations of animal products a plus. Incorporates exercise and stress management. Not an easy plan to stick to.
The South Beach Diet, Arthur Agatston, MD	Similar to other low-carb diets, but with more emphasis on glycemic index.	Carbohydrates lead to overeating and cravings. Advocates combining small amounts of undesirable carbs with vegetables and proteins.	As with other low-carb diets, research is still being conducted into effectiveness of this style of dieting.	Does not include recommendations to incorporate exercise into program, a key to any weight loss. Less restrictive on portion sizes than other diets.
Eat Right 4 Your Type Peter D'Adamo, MD	Claims that people will be healthier overall, and have better weight management success, if they tailor their diet according to blood type.	The main blood types, A, B, AB, and O, are predisposed to certain medical conditions, including weight loss/gain. You should eat foods that will prevent these conditions.	No reliable clinical research has been carried out to date on this type of diet.	Difficult to eat a meal with others, if all have different blood types. Eliminates certain food groups, and can cause nutrient deficiency. Does not account for changing nutritional needs throughout life. Will lose weight due to restricting food intake.
Weight Watchers	Eat from food groups, tally points to monitor intake. Based on weight and dietary goals. Eat what you want, but use discretion in amount.	Based on calories in, calories out. Includes exercise and social support.	Life focus rather than diet focus. Has support of most national organizations. One of the most highly recommended diets.	Works well for many people, particularly those for whom social support is important.
The Zone, Barry Sears, PhD	Offers a wellness philosophy to develop a metabolic state in which the body works efficiently. Recommends eating different calories than you do now and a small amount of protein. Identifies favorable vs. unfavorable carbohydrates.	Claims that his percentages of fat, protein, and carbohydrates are the best ratios for health.	Superiority of given ratios is unsubstantiated by research. Mixed reviews from experts: easy to follow, but don't count on results. Some recommendations (eating high-fat ice cream) are questionable.	Not a lot of do's and don'ts. Dieters may find it easy to follow.

Sources: U.S. Department of Agriculture, "The Great Nutrition Debate," 2000, www.usda.gov/cnpp/publications.html; *B. M. Malinauskas et al., "Dieting Practices, Weight Perceptions, and Body Composition: A Comparison of Normal Weight, Overweight, and Obese College Females," *Nutrition Journal* 5, no. 11 (2006).

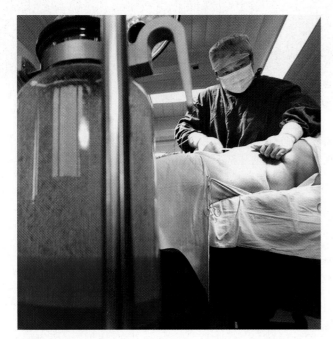

Liposuction is a surgical procedure that removes fat cells from specific areas of the body. It is not a good solution for long-term weight loss.

TABLE 9.4	Putting on the Pounds: Tips for Gaining Weight

- Eat at regularly scheduled times, whether hungry or not.
- Eat more frequently, spend more time eating, eat the high-calorie foods first if you fill up fast, and always start with the main course. Take time to shop, to cook, to eat slowly. Put extra spreads such as peanut butter, cream cheese, or cheese on your foods. Make your sandwiches with extra-thick slices of bread, and add more filling. Take seconds whenever possible, and eat high-calorie snacks during the day.
- Supplement your diet. Add high-calorie drinks that have a healthy balance of nutrients.
- Try to eat with people you are comfortable with. Avoid people who you feel are analyzing what you eat or make you feel like you should eat less.
- If you are sedentary, be aware that exercise can increase appetite. If you are exercising, or exercising to extremes, moderate your activities until you've gained some weight.
- Avoid diuretics, laxatives, and other medications that cause you to lose body fluids and nutrients.
- Relax. Many people who are underweight operate at high gear most of the time. Slow down, get more rest, and control stress.

amount of food you can eat and absorb. It is done with general anesthesia, hospitalization is required, and it is irreversible. Results are fast and dramatic, but there are many risks, including death, blood clots in the legs, a leak in a staple line in the stomach, pneumonia, or infection. Because the stomach pouch that remains after surgery is so small (about the size of a lime), you can only drink a few tablespoons of liquid, and consume only a very small amount of food at a time. For this reason, possible side effects include nausea and vomiting (if you eat or drink too much), or vitamin and mineral deficiencies and dehydration (if you cannot eat or drink enough).

Keep in mind that it is always best to lose weight through a healthy diet and regular physical activity. Ironically, even after going through surgery, people must learn to eat healthy foods and exercise or they can continue to gain weight, even returning to their original weight. There are no quick fixes for weight-control problems.

Liposuction is another surgical procedure for spot reducing, but there are risks and it may not be a permanent solution. Although this technique has garnered much attention, it, too, is not without risk: infections, severe scarring, and even death have resulted. In many cases, people who have liposuction regain fat in those areas or require multiple surgeries to repair lumpy, irregular surfaces from which the fat was removed.

Trying to Gain Weight

For some, trying to gain weight is a challenge for a variety of metabolic, hereditary, psychological, and other reasons. If you are one of these individuals, the first priority is to determine why you cannot gain weight. For example, among older adults, senses of taste and smell may decline, which makes food taste differently and be less pleasurable. Visual problems and other disabilities may make food more difficult to prepare, and dental problems may make eating certain foods more difficult. People who engage in extreme sports that require extreme nutritional supplementation may be at risk for nutritional deficiencies, which can lead to immune system problems and organ dysfunction, weakness that leads to falls and fractures, slower recovery from diseases, and a host of other problems. Table 9.4 details some weight-gaining strategies.

Thinking Thin: Body Image and Eating Disorders

Today, waiflike celebrities such as Kate Moss and Nicole Richie dominate fashion and the media. These images set the standard for what we find attractive, and people will go to impossible extremes to be the perfect size 0, or have the biggest biceps. Most of us think of this obsession with weight control as a recent phenomenon. However, an obsession with being thin has long been part of our culture. During the Victorian era, women wore corsets to achieve unrealistically tiny waists. By the 1920s, it was common knowledge that obesity was linked to poor health. In the 1960s supermodel Twiggy emerged on the scene.

NEW HORIZONS in health

DECIPHERING NEW RESEARCH ON "GOOD FATS" AND "BAD FATS"

In February 2005 results from a massive study that is part of the Women's Health Initiative (WHI) were released and you couldn't miss the headlines: "Low-Fat Diet Does Not Cut Health Risks" and "Eating Lean Doesn't Cut Risk." Newspapers nationwide trumpeted what seemed to be a contradiction of long-standing wisdom and medical advice, proclaiming that the study determined that fat wasn't so bad for us after all. However, looking a bit closer at the actual results of the study should stop you on your way to McDonald's for a celebratory Big Mac and fries. This study was not meant to evaluate the effectiveness of low-fat diets on overall health for the entire population, but rather, it focused on women between ages 50 and 79 and whether or not a low-fat diet could reduce the risk of breast cancer.

This study and its treatment by the news media may leave us wondering what to believe. Are low-fat diets really necessary? Or should we eat what we want?

Actually, there are good fats and bad fats, but that was not the focus of the WHI study, so headlines touting the fact that fat isn't so bad for you weren't entirely wrong, but there is more to it. Here's a look at some of the current findings on "good fats."

Nuts. At the height of the low-fat diet craze, in the 1980s and 1990s, nuts were shunned by the health conscious everywhere. However, current research has found that nuts actually contain good fat—unsaturated fat. They are also high in fiber and protein. Nuts can make an excellent snack a few times a week—just beware of their high calorie content.

Eggs. Eggs are high in cholesterol: however, research shows that eggs in moderation are not a major contributor to high cholesterol and heart disease. One egg a day can be part of a healthy meal or snack.

Olive Oil. There is some evidence suggesting that 2 tablespoons of olive oil daily may reduce risk for heart disease, if it is

consumed in place of foods high in saturated fat, while at the same time not increasing the total number of calories consumed daily. Use olive oil in salad dressing, and when cooking, instead of vegetable oil.

Avocados. Like olive oil, avocados are high in monounsaturated fats and omega-3 fatty acids, and can be a healthy substitute for saturated fats. Studies show that this type of fat can help reduce levels of bad LDL cholesterol. Avocados are also high in antioxidants. Use avocados like a condiment, instead of mayonnaise on sandwiches, as a dip, or in salads.

Sources: B. Kantrowitz and C. Kalb, "Food News Blues," *Newsweek,* March 13, 2006; FDA News "FDA Allows Qualified Health Claim to Decrease Risk of Coronary Heart Disease," November 1, 2004, www.fda.gov/bbs/topics/news/2004/NEW01129.html; N. Unlu et al., "Carotenoid Absorption from Salad and Salsa by Humans Is Enhanced by the Addition of Avocado or Avocado Oil," *Journal of Nutrition* 135 (2005): 431–436.

Today more than ever before, underweight models and celebrities exemplify desirability and success, delivering the subtle message that thin is best. Some of these distorted views of self-image arise from misinterpreting height–weight charts, making some people strive for the lower readings stipulated for a light-boned person when determining their own normal weight. Increasing numbers of adolescents, teens, and adults are so preoccupied with trying to be "model thin" that they make themselves ill. Being overweight has become socially unacceptable in many circles and obese people are increasingly stigmatized in our society.[50]

Americans are looking for fast answers: Should we count calories or carbohydrates? Is dietary fat your biggest enemy? Is Pritikin, Atkins, Weight Watchers, or something else your best weight-control strategy? Sadly, many people end up answering these questions with disordered eating patterns such as anorexia, bulimia, and binge eating.

Eating Disorders

For an increasing number of people, particularly young women, an obsessive relationship with food develops into

anorexia nervosa, a persistent, chronic eating disorder characterized by deliberate food restriction and severe, life-threatening weight loss. **Bulimia nervosa,** another eating disorder, involves frequent bouts of binge eating followed by purging (self-induced vomiting), laxative abuse, or excessive exercise. **Binge eating disorder (BED)** also involves episodes of binge eating, but unlike bulimics, binge eaters do not purge after a binge episode.

anorexia nervosa Eating disorder characterized by excessive preoccupation with food, self-starvation, and/or extreme exercising to achieve weight loss.

bulimia nervosa Eating disorder characterized by binge eating followed by inappropriate measures to prevent weight gain.

binge eating disorder (BED) Eating disorder characterized by recurrent binge eating, without excessive measures to prevent weight gain.

• I am not concerned about what others think regarding what and how much I eat. • I feel no guilt or shame no matter how much I eat or what I eat. • Food is an important part of my life but only occupies a small part of my time. • I trust my body to tell me what and how much to eat.	• I pay attention to what I eat in order to maintain a healthy body. • I may weigh more than what I like, but I enjoy eating and balance my pleasure in eating with my concern for a healthy body. • I am moderate and flexible in goals for eating well. • I try to follow the *Dietary Guidelines* for healthy eating.	• I think about food a lot. • I feel I don't eat well most of the time. • It's hard for me to enjoy eating with others. • I feel ashamed when I eat more than others or more than what I feel I should be eating. • I am afraid of getting fat. • I wish I could change how much I want to eat and what I am hungry for.	• I have tried diet pills, laxatives, vomiting, or extra time exercising in order to lose or maintain my weight. • I have fasted or avoided eating for long periods of time in order to lose or maintain my weight. • I feel strong when I can restrict how much I eat. • Eating more than I wanted to makes me feel out of control.	• I regularly stuff myself and then exercise, vomit, use diet pills or laxatives to get rid of the food or calories. • My friends/family tell me I am too thin. • I am terrified of eating fat. • When I let myself eat, I have a hard time controlling the amount of food I eat. • I am afraid to eat in front of others.
FOOD IS NOT AN ISSUE	CONCERNED WELL	FOOD PREOCCUPIED/OBSESSED	DISRUPTIVE EATING PATTERNS	EATING DISORDERED
BODY OWNERSHIP	BODY ACCEPTANCE	BODY PREOCCUPIED/OBSESSED	DISTORTED BODY IMAGE	BODY HATE/DISASSOCIATION
• Body image is not an issue for me. • My body is beautiful to me. • My feelings about my body are not influenced by society's concept of an ideal body shape. • I know that the significant others in my life will always find me attractive. • I trust my body to find the weight it needs to be so I can move and feel confident of my physical body.	• I base my body image equally on social norms and my own self-concept. • I pay attention to my body because it is important to me, but it only occupies a small part of my day. • I nourish my body so it has the strength and energy to achieve my physical goals. • I am able to assert myself and maintain a healthy body without losing my self-esteem.	• I spend a significant time viewing my body in the mirror. • I spend a significant time comparing my body to others. • I have days when I feel fat. • I am preoccupied with my body. • I accept society's ideal body shape and size as the best body shape and size. • I'd be more attractive if I was thinner, more muscular, etc...	• I spend a significant amount of time exercising and dieting to change my body. • My body shape and size keeps me from dating or finding someone who will treat me the way I want to be treated. • I have considered changing or have changed my body shape and size through surgical means so I can accept myself. • I wish I could change the way I look in the mirror.	• I often feel separated and distant from my body—as if it belongs to someone else. • I hate my body and I often isolate myself from others. • I don't see anything positive or even neutral about my body shape and size. • I don't believe others when they tell me I look OK. • I hate the way I look in the mirror.

FIGURE 9.8 The Eating Issues and Body Image Continuum

Individuals whose responses to these questions fall to the far left side of the continuum have normal eating patterns, and are not at risk for an eating disorder. Individuals whose answers fall to the far right of this continuum likely suffer from an eating disorder. Where do you fall?

Source: C. Shlaalak, *Preventive Medicine and Public Health.* Copyright © 1997. Arizona Board of Regents. Used with permission.

In the United States more than 10 million women meet the established criteria for one of these disorders, and their numbers appear to be increasing.[51] In addition, it is estimated that 10 percent of all female college students suffer from an eating disorder.[52] Some suffer from lesser forms of these conditions—not enough for a true diagnosis, but dangerously close to the precipice that will ultimately lead to life-threatening results. Physical complications associated with eating disorders include osteoporosis, heart attack, seizures, anemia, electrolyte imbalances, and tooth erosion. The severity of these conditions varies with the degree and duration of the eating disorder.[53]

Anorexia Nervosa

Anorexia involves self-starvation motivated by an intense fear of gaining weight along with an extremely distorted body image. Nearly 1 percent of girls in late adolescence meet the full criteria for anorexia; many others suffer from significant symptoms.

Initially, most people with anorexia lose weight by reducing total food intake, particularly of high-calorie foods, eventually leading to restricted intake of almost all foods. What they do eat, they often purge through vomiting or using laxatives. Although they lose weight, people with anorexia never seem to feel "thin enough" and constantly identify body parts that are "too fat." Anorexia has the highest death rate (20 percent) of any psychological illness.

Bulimia Nervosa

People with bulimia often binge and then take inappropriate measures, such as secret vomiting (purging), to lose the calories they have just acquired. Up to 3 percent of adolescents and young female adults are bulimic, with male rates being

TABLE 9.5	Does Someone Close to You Have an Eating Disorder?

Although every situation is different, there are several things that you can do if you suspect someone is struggling with an eating disorder.

- Learn as much as you can about eating disorders ahead of time.
- Check out resources on your campus and in your local community. Talk to professionals about what approaches and treatments have been most successful. Have a list of referrals ready to give to the person. Be armed with information.
- Set up a time to meet and share your concerns openly, honestly, and in a caring and supportive way. Be a good listener, and don't give advice unless asked.
- Provide examples of why you think there might be a disordered eating problem. Talk about health, relationships, and changes in behaviors.
- Avoid conflicts or a battle of the wills with this person. If he or she denies that there is a problem or minimizes it, repeat your concerns in a nonjudgmental way. You want the person to feel comfortable talking to you—not to drive him or her away.

- Never nag, plead, beg, bribe, threaten, or manipulate. Be straightforward, acknowledge it will be hard but that you know he or she can work through this.
- Don't get involved in endless conversations about diet, fatness, or exercise.
- Don't talk about how thin they are or focus on weight, diets, or exercise. Remember that the person wants to hear he or she is thin, and if you say it's good he or she is gaining weight, he or she will try to lose it.
- If the person is nervous about seeing a counselor, offer to go along as a support.
- Avoid placing shame, guilt, or accusations. Use "I" words (such as, "I am worried that you won't be able to do such and such if you don't eat,") rather than, "you need to eat or you are going to make yourself really sick."
- Stay calm and realize your own limitations. Be patient and supportive and be there in an emergency if the person asks for your help.

Sources: Adapted from "Anorexia Nervosa and Related Eating Disorders. When You Want to Help Someone You Care About," October 2003; National Eating Disorders Association, "Communication: What Should I Say?" 2002, www.nationaleatingdisorders.org/p.asp?WebPage-ID=322 &Profile-ID=41174.

about 10 percent of the female rate. People with bulimia are also obsessed with their bodies, weight gain, and how they appear to others. Unlike those with anorexia, people with bulimia are often "hidden" from the public eye because their weight may vary only slightly or fall within a normal range. Also, treatment appears to be more effective for bulimia than for anorexia.

One of the more common symptoms of bulimia is tooth erosion, a result of the excessive vomiting associated with this disorder. Chronic regurgitation causes hydrochloric acid (stomach acid) to break down the enamel of the teeth.[54]

Binge Eating Disorder

Individuals with binge eating disorder binge like their bulimic counterparts, but do not take excessive measures to lose the weight that they gain. Often they are clinically obese, and they tend to binge much more often than the typical obese person. Binge eating episodes are often characterized by eating rapidly, eating large amounts of food, even if one does not feel hungry, and feeling guilty or depressed after overeating.[55]

Who's at Risk?

Do men ever have eating disorders?

There's no simple explanation for why intelligent, often highly accomplished people spiral downward into the destructive behaviors associated with eating disorders. Obsessive-compulsive disorder, depression, and anxiety can all play a role, as can a desperate need to win social

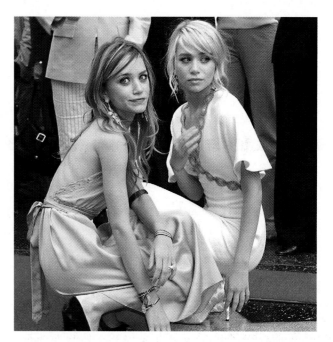

Pressures from society, especially on women, can have a detrimental effect on body image. Mary-Kate Olsen is one Hollywood actress struggling with an eating disorder.

approval or gain control of their lives through food. Figure 9.8 details the characteristics of those at risk for an eating disorder.

Women aren't the only ones at risk: eating disorders are on the rise among young men. About 15 percent of people affected are males.[56] Certain athletic competitions appear to put males at much greater risk. Jockeys, bodybuilders, wrestlers, dancers, swimmers, rowers, gymnasts, and runners are at highest risk. At the other end of the continuum are men and women who are so obsessed with bulking up and obtaining "six-pack abs" that they are willing to do just about anything to get "the look."[57]

Some studies have shown possible associations between identical twins, and others point to the large numbers of eating-disordered persons who have a parent or sibling with the disease. Many people with disordered eating patterns also suffer from other problems: many are clinically depressed, suffer from obsessive-compulsive disorder, and have other health problems. One recent study of college-aged women who purge regularly indicated that this group is also at high risk for alcohol abuse and other negative consequences from alcohol.[58]

Treatment for Eating Disorders

Because eating disorders result from many factors, spanning many years of development, there are no quick or simple solutions. Table 9.5 on the previous page details what you can do to help a friend or family member who has an eating disorder.

Treatment often focuses first on reducing the threat to life; once the patient is stabilized, long-term therapy involves family, friends, and other significant people in the individual's life. Therapy focuses on the psychological, social, environmental, and physiological factors that have led to the problem. Finding a therapist who really understands the multidimensional aspects of the problem is a must. Therapy allows the patient to focus on building new eating behaviors, recognizing threats, building self-confidence, and finding other ways to deal with life's problems. Support groups often help the family and the individual gain understanding and emotional support and learn self-development techniques designed to foster positive reactions and actions. Treatment of underlying depression may also be a focus.

what do you THINK?

Which groups or individuals on your campus appear to be at greatest risk for eating disorders? ■ What social factors might encourage this? ■ Why do you think society tends to overlook eating disorders in males? ■ What programs or services on your campus are available for someone with an eating disorder?

TAKING charge

Summary

- Overweight, obesity, and weight-related problems are on the rise in the United States. Obesity is now defined in terms of fat content rather than in terms of weight alone.
- There are many different methods of assessing body fat. Body mass index (BMI) is one of the most commonly accepted measures of weight based on height. Body fat percentages more accurately indicate how fat or lean a person is.
- Many factors contribute to one's risk for obesity, including genetics, developmental factors, setpoint, endocrine influences, psychosocial factors, eating cues, lack of awareness, metabolic changes, lifestyle, and gender. Women often have considerably more difficulty losing weight.

- Exercise, dieting, diet pills, surgery, and other strategies are used to maintain or lose weight. However, sensible eating behavior and adequate exercise offer the best options.
- Eating disorders consist of severe disturbances in eating behaviors, unhealthy efforts to control body weight, and abnormal attitudes about body and shape. Anorexia nervosa, bulimia nervosa, and binge eating disorder are the three main eating disorders. Though prevalent among white women of upper- and middle-class families, eating disorders affect women of all backgrounds and increasing numbers of men.

Chapter Review

1. The Body Mass Index (BMI) is an index of the relationship between
   a. fat tissue and muscle tissue.
   b. age and weight.
   c. height and weight.
   d. gender and weight.

2. Which of the following reasons has contributed to the rise in obesity in the United States?
   a. People are consuming more calories per day.
   b. Larger portions of food are being consumed.
   c. People are living a more sedentary lifestyle.
   d. All of the above.

3. At what body mass index (BMI) is a person considered to be overweight?
   a. 18–24
   b. 25–29
   c. 30–39
   d. greater than 40

4. The main difference between compulsive binge eating and bulimia is that
   a. both conditions use vomiting as a way of purging the body of excess calories.
   b. bulimia usually resorts to vomiting or laxatives to rid the body of excess calories whereas with binge eating, there is no purging.
   c. both conditions can lead to anorexia.
   d. None of the above.

5. Which of the following is not a characteristic of women suffering from anorexia?
   a. increased sensitivity to cold
   b. absence of menstruation
   c. gaining more weight
   d. abnormal sense of taste

6. What percentage of American children today are considered to be overweight or obese?
   a. 5–10 percent
   b. 17–20 percent
   c. 40–50 percent
   d. 60–70 percent

7. Which of the following is *not* a reason for the increase in overweight people today?
   a. More technology has made people have less of a need for physical activity.
   b. Many people are "supersizing" meals at fast food restaurants.
   c. People who live in poverty tend to be overweight or obese.
   d. Portions of food are much smaller than they were two decades ago.

8. To effectively lose weight, one should
   a. employ either a dieting or exercise program, but not both at the same time.
   b. increase exercise without decreasing food intake.
   c. employ a combination of both dietary change and moderate to high-level intensity exercise.
   d. eat less but don't exercise.

9. The diet plan that appears to be the safest and feasible for losing the maximum amount of weight and maintaining the weight loss long-term is
   a. a low carbohydrate diet.
   b. a low-fat diet.
   c. a low calorie diet.
   c. None of these are long term ways to maintain or lose weight.

10. In designing a safe and healthy weight-loss plan, one should
    a. avoid *trans* and saturated fats.
    b. eat fewer simple carbohydrates such as white bread.
    c. consume more low-fat dairy products.
    d. All of the above.

Answers to these questions can be found on page A-1.

Questions for Discussion and Reflection

1. Discuss the pressures, if any, you feel to improve your personal body image. Do these pressures come from media, family, friends, and other external sources, or from concern for your personal health?

2. What type of measurement would you choose in order to assess your fat levels? Why?

3. List the risk factors for obesity. Evaluate which seem to be most important in determining whether you will be obese in middle age.

4. Create a plan to help someone lose the "freshman 15" over the summer vacation. Assume that the person is male, 180 pounds, and has 15 weeks to lose the excess weight.

5. Differentiate among the three eating disorders. Then give reasons why females might be more prone to anorexia and bulimia than males are.

Accessing Your Health on the Internet

The following websites explore further topics and issues related to personal health. You'll also find links to each organization's website on the Companion Website for *Access to Health,* Tenth Edition, at www.aw-bc.com/donatelle.

1. *American Dietetic Association.* Recommended dietary guidelines and other current information about weight control. www.eatright.org
2. *Duke University Diet and Fitness Center.* Information about one of the best programs in the country focused on helping people live healthier, fuller lives through weight control and lifestyle change. www.cfl.duke.edu/ (qtn2mx45ckgvcw2spmzsrb45)/dfc/home
3. *Helping to End Eating Disorders (HEED).* The website of an organization dedicated to fighting eating disorders and helping individuals through the ordeal. Includes a chat room for people to exchange thoughts and share support. www.helpingendeatingdisorders.org
4. *Weight Control Information Network.* Excellent resource for diet and weight-control information. Offers practical strategies and current information on research. http://win.niddk.nih.gov/index.htm
5. *Yale Center for Eating and Weight Disorders.* Operated by the Yale University psychology department, this center offers services to those who experience problems with weight and food. A good source of information on eating disorders. www.yale.edu/ycewd/index.html
6. *The Rudd Center for Foods Policy and Obesity.* Website for the research center at Yale University. Provides excellent information on the latest in obesity research, public policy, and ways to put a stop to the obesity epidemic at the community level. www.yaleruddcenter.org

Further Reading

Brownell, K. and K. Horgen, *Food Fight: The Inside Story of the Food Industry, America's Obesity Crisis—and What We Can Do About It.* New York: McGraw-Hill, 2004.

> *Director of the Yale Center for Eating and Weight Disorders, Brownell critiques the way that food is marketed and sold to children, placing much of the blame for childhood obesity on advertising and unhealthy foods being offered in schools.*

K. D. Brownell et al., (eds.) *Weight Bias: Nature, Consequences and Remedies.* (New York: Guilford Press, 2005).

> *Expert review of issues surrounding weight stigma, bias, and discrimination, as well as possible solutions to these problems.*

Piscatella, J. *The Fat-Gram Guide to Restaurant Food,* 3rd ed. New York: Workman Press, 2000.

> *Useful guide to fast foods and restaurant fat content.*

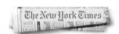

e-themes from *The New York Times*

For up-to-date articles about current health issues, visit www.aw-bc.com/donatelle, select *Access to Health,* Tenth Edition, Chapter 9, and click on "e-themes."

References

1. National Center for Health Statistics, *National Health and Nutrition Examination Survey (NHANES) 2003–2004* (Hyattsville, MD: U.S. Department of Health and Human Services, 2005); C. L. Ogden et al., "Prevalence of Overweight and Obesity in the U.S., 1999–2004," *Journal of the American Medical Association* 295, no. 13 (April 2006): 1549–1555.
2. Specific information about how your state ranks is available at www.healthyamericans.org; Department of Health and Children, *Obesity—The Policy Challenges: The Report of the National Task-force on Obesity* (Dublin, Ireland: Department of Health and Children, 2005), www.dohc.ie/publications.
3. K. Flegal et al., "Excess Deaths Associated with Underweight, Overweight and Obesity," *Journal of the American Medical Association* 293 (2005): 1861–1867.
4. S. Wild et al., "Global Prevalence of Diabetes," *Diabetes Care* 27 (2004): 1047–1053.
5. E. Finkelstein et al., "Economic Causes and Consequences of Obesity," *Annual Reviews of Public Health* 26 (2005): 239–257.
6. A. Peeters et al., "Adult Obesity and the Burden of Disability Throughout Life," *Obesity Research* 12 (2004): 1145–1151.
7. U.S. Department of Health and Human Services and U.S. Department of Agriculture, *Dietary Guidelines for Americans 2005,* 2005, www.healthierus.gov/dietaryguidelines.
8. Weight-Control Information Network, "Statistics Related to Overweight and Obesity," 2006, www.niddk.nih.gov/health/nutrit/pubs/statobes.htm.
9. Ibid.
10. Ibid.

11. American Obesity Association (AOA), "AOA Fact Sheets: What Is Obesity?" May 2005, www.obesity.org.

12. National Center for Health Statistics, *Prevalence of Overweight and Obesity Among Adults: United States, 1999–2002, 2004* (Hyattsville, MD: NCHS).

13. American Obesity Association, "What Is Obesity?"

14. D. Eberwine, "Globesity: The Crisis of Growing Proportions," *Perspectives in Health* 7, no. 3 (2003): 9.

15. U.S. Department of Health and Human Services, *Dietary Guidelines for Americans 2005.*

16. Eberwine, "Globesity: The Crisis of Growing Proportions."

17. Rush University, "Waist to Hip Ratio Calculator," 2005, www.rush.edu/itools/hip/hipcalc.html.

18. S. Kautiainen et al., "Use of Information and Communication Technology and Prevalence of Overweight and Obesity Among Adolescents," *International Journal of Obesity* 29 (2005): 925–933.

19. Ibid.

20. U.S. Department of Health and Human Services, *Surgeon General's Call to Action to Prevent and Decrease Overweight and Obesity* (Washington, DC: USOHHS, 2005).

21. American Obesity Association, "Obesity: A Global Epidemic," May 2005, www.obesity.org.

22. A. Drewnowski and N. Darmon, "Food Choices and Diet Costs: An Economic Analysis," *Journal of Nutrition* 135 (2005): 900–990; L. Young and M. Nestle, "Expanding Portion Sizes in the U.S. Marketplace: Implications for Nutrition Counseling," *Journal of the American Dietetic Association* 103 (2003): 231–234.

23. J. D. Wright et al., "Trends in Intake of Energy and Macronutrients—United States, 1971–2000," *Morbidity and Mortality Weekly Report* 53, no. 4 (February 6, 2004): 80

24. T. Harder et al., "Duration of Breast-Feeding and Risk of Overweight," *American Journal of Epidemiology* 162, no. 5 (2005): 397–403.

25. T. Rankinen et al., "The Human Obesity Gene Map: 2005 Update," *Obesity* 14 (2006): 529–644.

26. D. Cummings and M. Schwartz, "Genetics and Pathophysiology of Human Obesity," *Annual Review of Medicine* 54 (2003): 453–471.

27. C. Bell et al., "The Genetics of Obesity," *Nature Reviews Genetics* 6 (2005): 221–234.

28. N. Abumad, "*CD36* May Determine Our Desire for Dietary Fats," *Journal of Clinical Nutrition* 115 (2005): 2965–2967.

29. Rankinen et al., "The Human Obesity Gene Map."

30. Ibid.

31. R. J. Loos and C. Bouchard, "Obesity—Is It a Genetic Disorder?" *Journal of Internal Medicine* 254 (2003): 401–425.

32. S. G. Bouret et al., "Trophic Action of Leptin on Hypothalamic Neurons That Regulate Feeding," *Science* 304 (April 2, 2004): 110–115.

33. Howard Hughes Medical Institute, "Leptin's Legacy," *Howard Hughes Medical Institue Bulletin* 16, no. 1 (2003): 24–27.

34. D. E. Cummings et al., "Plasma Ghrelin Levels After Diet-Induced Weight Loss or Gastric Bypass Surgery," *New England Journal of Medicine* 346, no. 21 (2002): 1623–1630.

35. M. Bodman and J. Flier, "The Gut and Energy Balance: Visceral Allies in the Obesity Wars," *Science* 307 (2005): 1909–1914.

36. Mayo Clinic, "Special Report: Weight Control," 2005, www.mayo clinic.com.

37. L. K. Mahan and S. Escott-Stump, *Krause's Food, Nutrition, and Diet Therapy* (New York: W.B. Saunders Company, 2000).

38. Ogden et al., "Prevalence of Overweight and Obesity."

39. S. Lichman et al., "Discrepancy between Self-Reported and Actual Caloric Intake and Exercise in Obese Subjects," *New England Journal of Medicine* 327 (1992): 1894–1897.

40. Centers for Disease Control and Prevention, "Growing Stronger: Strength Training for Older Adults: Why Strength Training?" April 2005, www.cdc.gov/nccdphpdnpa/physical/growing_stronger/why.htm.

41. National Center for Health Statistics, "Prevalence of Sedentary Leisure Time Behavior Among Adults in the United States," February 2005, www.cdc.gov/nchs.

42. Ibid.

43. Ibid.

44. National Institute of Diabetes and Digestive and Kidney Diseases, "You Can Control Your Weight as You Quit Smoking," 2005, www.pueblo.gsa.gov.

45. I. Rashad and M. Grossman, "Economics of Obesity," *The Public Interest* 156 (2004), www.thepublicinterest.com/previous/article3.html.

46. Mayo Clinic, "Special Report: Weight Control."

47. G. Flett and P. Hewitt, "The Perils of Perfectionism in Sports and Exercise," *Current Directions in Psychological Science* 14, no. 1 (2005): 14–22; P. Crocker et al., "Examining Current Ideal Discrepancy Scores and Exercise Motivations as Predictors of Social Physique Anxiety in Exercising Females," *Journal of Sport Behavior* 28 (2005): 63–72.

48. "Fen-Phen Legal Resources," 2002, www.fen-phen-legal-resources.com.

49. R. Vettor et al., "Effect of Sibutramine on Weight Management and Metabolic Control in Type 2 Diabetes: A Meta-Analysis," *Diabetes Care* 28 (2005): 942–949.

50. R. M. Puhl, "Coping with Weight Stigma," in *Weight Bias: Nature, Consequences and Remedies*, K. D. Brownell et al., eds. (New York: Guilford Press, 2005).

51. National Eating Disorder Association, "Statistics: Eating Disorders and Their Precursors," 2002, www.nationaleatingdisorders.org.

52. M. Spearing, *Eating Disorders: Facts About Eating Disorders and the Search for Solutions* (Bethesda, MD: National Institute of Mental Health, NIH Publication No. 01-4901, 2001).

53. The Renfrew Center Foundation for Eating Disorders, "Eating Disorders 101 Guide: A Summary of Issues, Statistics, and Resources," October 2003, www.renfrew.org.

54. M. P. Faine, "Recognition and Management of Eating Disorders in the Dental Office," *The Dental Clinics of North America* 42, no. 9: 395–410.

55. J. Manwaring et al., "Risk Factors and Patterns of Onset in Binge Eating Disorder," *International Journal of Eating Disorders* 39, no. 2 (2005): 101–107.

56. Ibid.

57. J. Mond et al., "An Update on the Definition of Excessive Exercise," *Eating Disorders Research* 39, no. 2 (2005): 147–153.

58. T. Adams and T. Araas, "Purging and Alcohol-Related Effects in College Women," *International Journal of Eating Disorders* 39, no. 3 (2006): 240–244.

10

Personal Fitness

IMPROVING HEALTH THROUGH EXERCISE

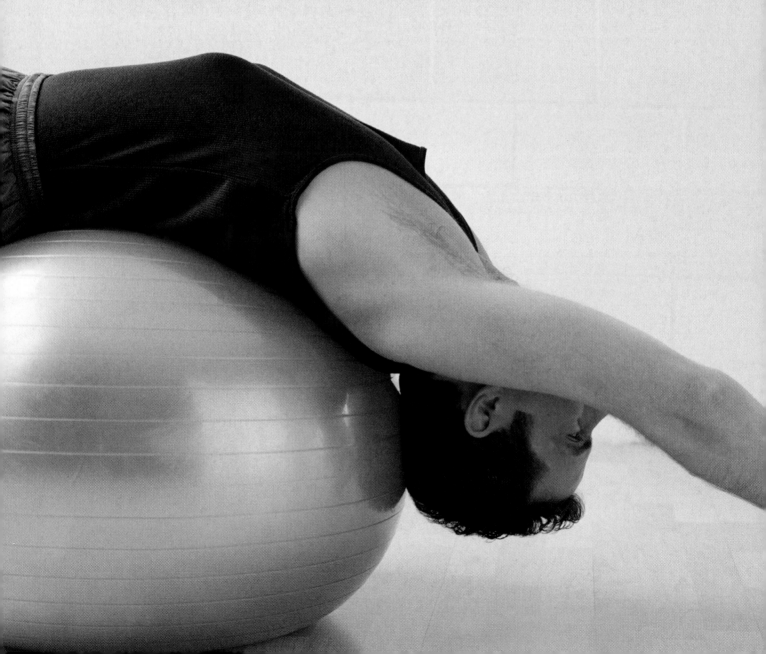

Can I lose **weight** through exercise alone?

What types of exercises can I do to **improve** my muscular strength?

Which factors should I think about as I develop a **fitness** plan?

How do I choose a good **running** shoe?

What can I do to charge up my **exercise** routine and prevent boredom?

OBJECTIVES

- Distinguish between physical activity for health, for fitness, and for performance.
- Describe the benefits of regular physical activity, including improvements in physical health, mental health, stress management, and life span.
- Explain the components of an aerobic exercise program and a stretching and strength training program.
- Summarize ways to prevent and treat common fitness injuries.
- Discuss the factors that contribute to obsessive exercise patterns, and suggest strategies for preventing them.
- Summarize the key components of a personal fitness program, and design a program that works for you.

A century ago in the United States, simple survival required performing heavy physical labor on a daily basis. A trip to the store meant hitching up the horses or walking, without the benefit of special walking shoes. Today, taking a walk is something we do for recreation rather than necessity. Motorized vehicles provide our transportation, and even bicycles are designed to minimize rider effort.

Today most people in our country lead sedentary lifestyles and perform little physical labor or exercise. About 24 percent of U.S. adults aged 18 and over do no physical activity at all. College-aged students fare no better. A 2005 survey indicated that 31 percent of college women and 22 percent of college men participate in no moderate or vigorous physical activities.[1] The growing percentage of Americans who live sedentary lives has been linked to dramatic increases in the incidence of obesity, diabetes, and other chronic diseases.[2] More than 108 million Americans are overweight or obese, 65 million have high blood pressure, 7.2 million suffer a heart attack in any given year, 21 million have diabetes, and approximately 41 million have "prediabetes."[3]

Do these statistics look grim? There is something we can do to improve them. Decades of research show that physical activity has tremendous health-promoting and disease-preventing benefits.[4] Now is an excellent time to develop exercise habits that will improve the quality and duration of your own life.

Physical Activity for Health, Fitness, and Performance

Generally speaking, **physical activity** is defined as any bodily movement that is produced by the contraction of skeletal muscles and that substantially increases energy expenditure.[5] Walking, swimming, heavy lifting, and housework are all examples of physical activity. Physical activities also may vary by intensity. For example, walking to class may require little

physical activity Any bodily movement that is produced by the contraction of skeletal muscles and that substantially increases energy expenditure.

exercise Planned, structured, and repetitive bodily movement done to improve or maintain one or more components of physical fitness.

physical fitness The ability to perform moderate to vigorous levels of physical activity on a regular basis without excessive fatigue.

TABLE 10.1	Components of Physical Fitness
Cardiorespiratory fitness	Ability to sustain moderate-intensity whole-body activity for extended time periods
Flexibility	Range of motion at a joint or series of joints
Muscular strength and endurance	Maximum force applied with single muscle contraction; ability to perform repeated high-intensity muscle contractions
Body composition	A composite of total body mass, fat mass, fat-free mass, and fat distribution

Source: American College of Sports Medicine, "ACSM Position Stand on the Recommended Quantity and Quality of Exercise for Developing and Maintaining Cardiorespiratory and Muscular Fitness and Flexibility in Adults," *Medicine and Science in Sports and Exercise* 30 (1998): 975–991. http://lww.com.

effort but walking to class up a hill while carrying a heavy backpack makes the activity more intense. There are three general categories of physical activity defined by the purpose for which they are done.

Physical Activity for Health

Research shows that just about everyone can improve general health by increasing overall physical activity, even if it doesn't involve going to the gym. Just adding more physical movement to your day can benefit your health. A physically active lifestyle might include choices such as parking further away from your destination, taking walking breaks while studying, or choosing to take the stairs instead of the elevator. In addition to these incidental ways to increase activity, there are lots of ways you can enjoy being physically active in recreation. Going dancing, playing frisbee, or walking your dog are all good examples of recreational physical activity. The good thing about lifestyle physical activity is that you don't necessarily have to sustain your activity for an extended period of time to get a health benefit. Research shows that accumulating activity throughout the day can contribute to overall health and well-being.

Physical Activity for Fitness

The term **exercise** is a bit more specific than physical activity. Whereas all exercise is physical activity, all physical activity may not be exercise. For example, walking from your car to class is physical activity, but going for a brisk 30-minute walk would be considered exercise. Exercise is defined as planned, structured, and repetitive bodily movement done to improve or maintain one or more components of physical fitness, such as endurance, flexibility, and strength.[6] **Physical fitness** is the ability to perform moderate to vigorous levels of physical activity on a regular basis without excessive fatigue. Table 10.1 identifies the major health-related components of physical fitness.

If you want to become physically fit, you'll need to do more than make physically active lifestyle choices. You'll need to increase the frequency, intensity, and duration of your exercise. Both the Centers for Disease Control and Prevention (CDC) and the American College of Sports Medicine (ACSM) recommend that adults engage in moderate-intensity physical activities for at least 30 minutes on most days of the week.[7] This amount of physical activity will not prepare you for running a marathon, but it can improve your overall health and can result in some cardiovascular improvements. The ACSM and CDC recommend that if you want to improve your cardiorespiratory fitness even more, you need to perform vigorous physical activities (for example, jogging or running, walking hills, circuit weight training, singles tennis) at least three days per week for at least 20 minutes at a time; if losing weight is your goal, you must add moderate to vigorous exercise for 60 to 90 minutes to your daily routine. See the Spotlight on Your Health box on page 322 for more on physical activity guidelines.

Some people have physical limitations that make achieving these recommendations difficult, but they can still be physically active and reap the benefits of a regular exercise program. For example, a woman with arthritis in the knee and hip joints might not be able to jog without extreme pain, but she can engage in water exercise in a swimming pool. The water will help relieve much of the stress on her joints and she can improve her range of motion. Similarly, a man who uses a wheelchair may be unable to walk or run, but he can stay physically fit by playing wheelchair basketball.

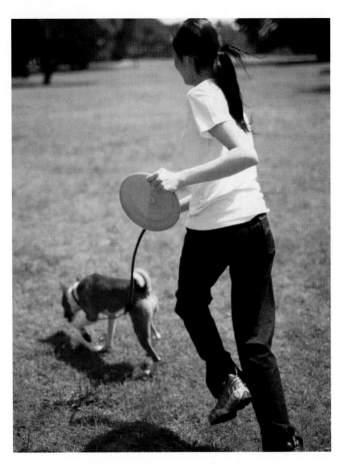

Exercise does not have to be in the form of going to the gym; activities such as playing with your dog do count toward your daily physical activity.

Physical Activity for Performance

People who want to take their fitness level one step further can add exercise to improve performance. Specific programs can be designed to increase speed, strength, or overall performance. One example of a common activity used in performance training programs is plyometrics. *Plyometrics* are exercises that contract muscles in a certain order to increase power. An example of a plyometric activity would be a push-up with a clap in between each push-up. It can help improve body control and the speed at which you physically change directions. Additionally, recreational exercisers and athletes alike utilize interval training to improve speed and cardiovascular fitness (see the New Horizons in Health box on page 324).

Performance training is meant for those who already have a high level of physical fitness, and are training to enhance some aspect of their ability. Those who engage in this level of activity will achieve a high level of fitness, but are also more prone to risk of injury and overtraining.

Benefits of Regular Physical Activity

Regular physical activity has been shown to improve more than 50 different physiological, metabolic, and psychological aspects of human life. There is no better time than now to develop an exercise plan that will enable you to reap these benefits.[8]

Improved Cardiorespiratory Fitness

Cardiorespiratory fitness refers to the ability of the circulatory and respiratory systems to supply oxygen to the body during sustained physical activity.[9] Regular exercise makes

(Text continues on page 324)

cardiorespiratory fitness   The ability of the heart, lungs, and blood vessels to supply oxygen to skeletal muscles during sustained physical activity.

HOW MUCH IS ENOUGH? A CLOSER LOOK AT EXERCISE GUIDELINES

In 2005, the USDA released not only the new *Dietary Guidelines for Americans,* but also recommendations for physical activity. These guidelines, which recommend 60 minutes of exercise each day to maintain current weight or as much as 90 minutes to sustain significant weight loss, conflict with older exercise guidelines that recommend at least 30 minutes of sustained physical activity daily to ward off chronic disease and cancer. These conflicting recommendations can be confusing for most. How can you navigate the myriad of recommendations on physical activity? The best way to clear the confusion is to look at the intended outcome of each guideline. For example, are you trying to maintain your recent weight loss but hate to work up a sweat? You might try the recommendation for a longer duration of moderate exercise. Or do you want to improve overall health and prevent heart disease and diabetes? Then 30 minutes of moderate activity might be suitable. Finally, realize that all guidelines are just that. Think of them as a general goal, rather than strict rules you must follow. The bottom line is that no matter which recommendation you choose, you will improve your health with exercise.

The chart below summarizes older and more recent guidelines for exercise, and can help you determine which prescription will help you meet your goals.

Agency and Year	Guideline	Facts to Consider	Who Should Follow This Recommendation?
National Institutes of Health, 1995	Children and adults should accumulate at least 30 minutes of moderate-intensity physical activity on most, and preferably all, days of the week.	• OK to accumulate your 30 minutes of activity over the day, rather than complete it all at once • Probably not enough for weight loss or improvement in physical fitness for some people	Anyone who wants to increase their lifestyle physical activity for overall improvement in health and well-being. This is a good step toward a more ambitious exercise program.
Centers for Disease Control and Prevention/American College of Sports Medicine, 1996	Adults should engage in moderate-intensity activity for at least 30 minutes, 5 or more days of the week OR vigorous activity for at least 20 minutes, 3 or more days per week.	• Manageable time frame • Activity can be completed all at once (at moderate level) or in increments (vigorous level) • May help control weight and develop lean muscle • More sedentary people should start at the lower end of the recommendation	Anyone who wants to increase their lifestyle physical activity for overall improvement in health, cardiovascular health, and well-being. Individuals can build on this recommendation to reach a desired goal.
U.S. Department of Agriculture, 2005	In addition to activities of daily living (ADLs), engage in at least 30 minutes of moderate-intensity physical activity most days of the week. Can increase duration and intensity for greater health benefits.	• Looks at overall energy balance with diet and exercise • Manageable time frame • Probably not enough for weight loss	Anyone who wants to reduce the risk of chronic disease in adulthood. Provides a good start for someone who is inactive.

Agency and Year	Guideline	Facts to Consider	Who Should Follow This Recommendation?
U.S. Department of Agriculture, 2005	Engage in approximately 60 to 90 minutes of moderate- to vigorous-intensity activity on most days of the week while not exceeding caloric intake requirements.	■ Based on nutrition science ■ Time commitment may be difficult for many people ■ Less fit individuals should build up to this exercise program ■ Results require a combination of exercise and appropriate food intake	Anyone who is trying to lose weight, maintain weight loss, or prevent weight gain. Will also improve overall cardiorespiratory endurance.
Food and Agriculture Organization of the United Nations/World Health Organization, 2003	One hour per day of moderate-intensity activity, such as walking, on most days of the week, is needed to maintain a healthy body weight.	■ Based on review of evidence on diet, nutrition, and their effects on chronic diseases ■ Time commitment may be a challenge	Anyone who wants to maintain a healthy body weight by controlling energy balance. Suitable for those starting a weight management program, or trying to maintain weight loss.
Institute of Medicine/International Association for the Study of Obesity, 2005	Children and adults should engage in a minimum of 60 minutes per day of moderately intense exercise.	■ Nutrition report based on evidence in energy balance ■ Time commitment may be difficult for many ■ Less fit individuals should build up to this exercise program	Anyone who wants to lose weight or keep it off. Also a suitable program for overall improvement of health.

Sources: National Institutes of Health, "Physical Activity and Cardiovascular Health: Consensus Statement," 1995, http://consensus.nih.gov/1995/1995activitycardiovascularhealth101html.htm; R. Pate et al., "Physical Activity and Public Health: A Recommendation from the Centers for Disease Control and Prevention and the American College of Sports Medicine," *Journal of the American Medical Association* 273(5): 402–7, 1995; Food and Nutrition Board, Institutes of Medicine, *Dietary Reference Intakes for Energy Carbohydrates, Fiber, Fat, Protein, and Amino Acids* (Washington DC: National Academy Press, 2002); Food and Agriculture Organization and World Health Organization, "Diet, Nutrition, and the Prevention of Chronic Diseases," (Geneva, Switzerland: World Health Organization, 2003); U.S. Department of Agriculture, *Dietary Guidelines for Americans 2005,* www.health.gov/dietaryguidelines/dga2005/recommendations.htm.

INTERVAL TRAINING BOOSTS MOTIVATION AND PERFORMANCE

Want to give your workout and your motivation a boost? Try adding interval training to your regime. Interval training involves alternating short bursts of intense activity with what is called "active recovery," which

What can I do to charge up my exercise routine and prevent boredom?

is typically a less intense form of the original activity. For example, jogging the "straights" on a track and walking the "curves" would be an example of interval training. Spinning classes also utilize this form of training.

Researchers in Sweden are credited for discovering this type of training. They call it *Fartlek* training, which means "speed play." Although this type of training has been used by athletes for many years, it is becoming more popular among those who exercise to achieve general fitness or

weight management goals. This type of training can not only increase your performance and endurance, but also helps you avoid injuries that can result from continuous heavy activity. Intervals can also break up the boredom of working out. Smaller increments of work seem to make time pass more quickly. Also, you burn more calories with higher intensity work.

In its most basic form, interval training might involve walking for two minutes, then jogging for two minutes, and alternating these for the duration of the workout. By doing this, the overall intensity of your workout will be greater than if you just sustained a brisk walk for the whole time. Four variables to keep in mind when planning your interval training program include:

- Intensity of your work interval
- Duration (distance or time) of your work interval
- Duration of rest or recovery interval
- Number of repetitions of each interval

As you get more fit or would like to spice up your interval training sequence, you can mix it up a bit. Try doing harder work intervals for shorter time periods, or giving yourself less recovery time in between hard intervals. If you are on a treadmill, increase the incline for your work interval. Instead of walking or jogging, try jumping rope for the work interval. The possibilities for variety are endless.

If you want to make sure you are doing the best interval workout for your fitness goals, consult an athletic trainer, coach, or personal trainer.

Sources: E. Quinn, "About Interval Training," 2006, www.sportsmedicine.about.com; American Council on Exercise, "ACE Fit Facts, Interval Training," 2006, www.acefitness.org; G. Mirkin, "Interval Training Is the Key to Speed in Competition," *The Washington Times,* August 2004.

---

these systems more efficient by enlarging the heart muscle, enabling more blood to be pumped with each stroke, and increasing the number of *capillaries* (small blood vessels that allow gas exchange between blood and surrounding tissues) in trained skeletal muscles, which supply more blood to working muscles. Exercise also improves the respiratory system by increasing the amount of oxygen that is inhaled and distributed to body tissues.[10]

Reduced Risk of Heart Disease
Your heart is a muscular organ made up of highly specialized tissue. Because muscles become stronger and more efficient with use, regular exercise strengthens the heart, enabling it to pump more blood with each beat. This increased efficiency means that the heart requires fewer beats per minute to circulate blood throughout the body. A stronger, more efficient heart is better able to meet the ordinary demands of life.

Prevention of Hypertension
Blood pressure refers to the force exerted by blood against blood vessel walls, generated by the pumping action of the heart. *Hypertension,* the medical term for abnormally high blood pressure, is a significant risk factor for cardiovascular disease and stroke. Hypertension is particularly prevalent in adult African Americans.[11] People with consistently elevated blood

pressure are two to four times more susceptible to heart disease than people with normal blood pressure.[12] Studies report that moderate exercise can reduce both diastolic and systolic blood pressure by 7 mmHg.[13] (See Chapter 15 for blood pressure guidelines.)

Improved Blood Lipid and Lipoprotein Profile
Lipids are fats that circulate in the bloodstream and are stored in various places in the body. Regular exercise is known to increase the number of high-density lipoproteins (HDLs, or "good" cholesterol) in the blood.[14] Higher HDL levels are associated with lower risk for arterial disease because they remove some of the "bad" cholesterol from arterial walls and hence reduce clogging. The bottom line: regular exercise lowers the risk of cardiovascular disease. (For more on cholesterol and blood pressure, see Chapter 15.)

Reduced Cancer Risk

Regular physical activity appears to lower the risk for some types of cancer. There is strong evidence that physical activity reduces the risk of breast and colon cancer. Research on exercise and breast cancer risk has found that the earlier in life a woman starts to exercise, the greater the reduction in breast cancer risk.[15] One theory on how exercise reduces colon cancer risk has to do with intestinal transit time. Experts say that because physical activity makes food move more quickly through your digestive system, there is less time for the body to absorb potential carcinogens and for potential carcinogens to be in contact with the digestive tract. Physical activity also decreases the levels of prostaglandins, substances found in cells of the large intestine that are implicated in cancer.[16]

Improved Bone Mass

A common affliction among older adults is **osteoporosis**, a disease characterized by low bone mass and deterioration of bone tissue, which increase fracture risk. Bone, like other human tissues, responds to the demands placed upon it. Women (and men) have much to gain by remaining physically active as they age—bone mass levels are significantly higher among active than among sedentary women.[17] New research indicates that by "surprising" bone (by jumping and other sudden activities), young children may improve their bone density.[18] Regular weight-bearing exercise, when combined with a balanced diet containing adequate calcium, helps keep bones healthy.[19] (See Chapter 19 for more on osteoporosis.)

Improved Weight Control

Can I lose weight through exercise alone?

Many people start exercising because they want to lose weight. Level of physical activity has a direct effect upon metabolic rate and can raise it for several hours following a vigorous workout. An effective method for losing weight combines regular endurance-type exercises with a moderate decrease in food intake. In addition to helping you lose weight, increased physical activity also improves your chances of keeping the weight off once you have lost it.[20]

The ACSM recommends 30 minutes of moderate physical activity daily with an intake between 1,500 and 2,000 calories per day.[21] Cutting daily caloric intake beyond this range ("severe dieting") actually decreases metabolic rate by up to 20 percent and makes weight loss more difficult. Though exercise and dietary changes work best for weight loss, research shows that exercise alone can be used for obesity reduction. For example, in a study of obese men, those who exercised at a moderate intensity for 60 minutes 5 times a week with no dietary changes significantly decreased their body fat and increased muscle mass.[22] However, remember that if you want to lose weight only through physical activity, you will have to spend more time exercising than if you reduce your calories at the same time.

Improved Health and Life Span

Prevention of Diabetes

Noninsulin-dependent diabetes (type 2 diabetes) is a complex disorder that affects millions of Americans, many of whom have no idea that they

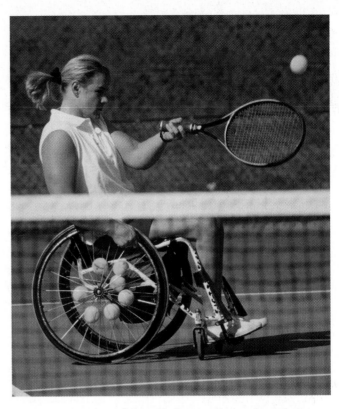

Everyone can attain cardiovascular fitness and muscular endurance.

have the disease (see Chapter 18). Risk factors for diabetes include obesity, high blood pressure, and high cholesterol, as well as a family history of the disease.[23] Physicians suggest exercise combined with weight loss and a healthy diet to help prevent diabetes. In a recent study, individuals who increased their moderate to vigorous physical activity the most were nearly 65 percent less likely to develop diabetes than those who did not increase their physical activity.[24] Exercise also helps manage the disease. It is reported that walking for 30 to 60 minutes a day lowers a diabetic's risk of dying from cardiovascular disease by 40 to 50 percent.[25]

Longer Life Span

Several large studies that followed groups of people over time found that those who exercised or were more fit lived longer.[26] In a study of over 5,000 middle-aged and older Americans, researchers found that those who had moderate to high levels of activity lived 1.3 to 3.7 years longer than those who got little exercise. Study subjects who exercised at a more intense level outlived sedentary subjects by 3.5 to 3.7 years.[27]

Improved Immunity to Disease

Regular, consistent exercise promotes a healthy immune system. Research shows that moderate exercise gives the immune system a

osteoporosis A disease characterized by low bone mass and deterioration of bone tissue, which increase risk of fracture.

WHEN EXERCISE BECOMES AN OBSESSION

In a quest to be thin, muscular, and achieve the ideal body, many men and women, particularly those who are physically active, are at risk for a group of often-unrecognized disorders. In women, these disorders frequently are a combination of conditions: disordered eating, amenorrhea (lack of menstrual periods), and osteoporosis. For men, obsessive exercise disorders are often characterized by bingeing and purging, excessive exercise, steroid abuse, and overuse of nutritional and dietary supplements in an effort to obtain perfect but unrealistic physiques.

THE FEMALE ATHLETE TRIAD

Women who are athletes in a competitive sport often strive for perfection. In an effort to be the best, they often do more damage than good. Women who have what is often termed "anorexia athletica" exhibit disordered eating behaviors (anorexia, bulimia, or other forms of bingeing, purging, or restricted eating) combined with excessive exercise. Why is this dangerous? A regular pattern of disordered eating and too much exercise can alter normal body functions. If the disordered eating is prolonged or without effective intervention, serious calcium depletion, changes in body hormones, and other negative effects may weaken bones and cause other problems. Severe cases can lead to disability or even death.

Not all athletes are equally prone to this syndrome; this problem is particularly prevalent in women who participate in highly competitive sports that value self-discipline and perfection. Gymnasts, ice skaters, cross-country runners, swimmers, and ballet dancers are at the highest risk for the female athlete triad.

Physical Warning Signs

- Fatigue
- Anemia
- Tendency toward stress fractures and injury

- Cold intolerance
- Sore throat
- Eroded dental enamel from frequent vomiting
- Abdominal pain and bloating
- Constipation
- Dry skin
- Lightheadedness/fainting
- Chest pain
- Irregular or absent menstrual periods
- Lanugo (fine, downy hair covering the body)
- Changes in endurance, strength, or speed

Behavioral Warning Signs

- Use of weight-loss products and/or laxatives
- Depression
- Decreased ability to concentrate
- Excessive and compulsive exercise
- Preoccupation with food and weight
- Trips to bathroom during or after eating
- Increasing self-criticism and hostility to self

Playing sports and being active is part of a healthy lifestyle. However, groups such as the American College of Sports Medicine (ACSM) are noticing a growing incidence of the female athlete triad in physically active girls and women who don't compete athletically. Young girls and women who exercise and watch what they eat to remain fit or lose a few pounds might take it too far.

EXERCISE OBSESSION AND MEN

It's not just women who suffer from the physiological and psychological problems of exercise obsession. Millions of boys and men are experiencing an obsession about their looks, too. Whereas women often strive to be thin, men want to be muscular and gain weight. Male television and movie heroes, video game characters, and even GI Joe dolls sport buff bodies and bulging biceps. Men trying to achieve an unrealistic level of fitness can experience muscle dys-

morphia, or "bigarexia," a damaging body perspective that perpetuates their obsession. Researchers refer to this disorder as the "Adonis Complex." Men with muscle dysmorphia have a distorted perception of their muscularity, and may go to extreme measures to build muscle.

Warning Signs

- Distortion of body image
- Exercise interferes with other areas of life
- Adherence to a rigid exercise routine

Men suffering from the Adonis Complex are also prone to use steroids and other muscle-building supplements in order to achieve the perfect physique they seek. The abuse of steroids can introduce a range of health issues, often complicating the physical harm already caused by an obsessive exercise pattern.

TREATING OBESSIVE EXERCISE DISORDERS

If you wonder whether a friend or family member may be experiencing the symptoms of the female athlete triad or muscle dysmorphia, ask her or him about their behavior. If symptoms are present, a multidisciplinary approach involving parents, coaches, friends, physicians, dietitians, and mental health professionals is warranted. Some counselors specialize in working with athletes who have a distorted body image. You can also consult a trusted health care provider, as a source for referrals to other health professionals. If you, or someone you know, has an obsession with exercise that interferes with overall health and enjoyment of life, seek help.

Sources: K. Birch, 2005, "Female Athlete Triad," *British Medical Journal* 330: 244–246; Center for Young Women's Health, The Female Triad, Children's Hospital Boston, 2006, www.youngwomenshealth.org/triad.html; H. G. Pope et al, 2002, *The Adonis Complex. How to Identify, Treat, and Prevent Body Obsession in Men and Boys* (New York: Free Press, 2002).

temporary boost in the production of cells that attack bacteria.[28] But whereas moderate amounts of exercise can be beneficial, extreme exercise may actually be detrimental. For example, athletes engaging in marathon-type events or very intense physical training have an increased risk of colds and flu.[29]

Just how exercise alters immunity is not well understood. We do know that brisk exercise temporarily increases the number of white blood cells (WBCs), the blood cells responsible for fighting infection.[30] The largest changes in immunity are seen in people who are sedentary and begin a moderately energetic program. These individuals gain a large number of WBCs due to their low fitness level when embarking on an exercise program. Interestingly, those who participate in regular, long-term heavy exercise, such as marathon runners, experience a decrease in their immune function. If you are feeling worn down, this could be your body trying to tell you to take a break and prevent overtraining. In general, however, the more vigorous the exercise, the more gains in WBCs.[31]

Improved Mental Health and Stress Management

People who engage in regular physical activity also notice psychological benefits. Exercise can "burn off" the chemical by-products of the stress response and increase endorphins, giving your mood a natural boost. Improvements in physical appearance that come with exercise can also improve mental state: a fitter, stronger, leaner body can boost self-esteem. Also, mastering new skills and developing increased abilities in favorite recreational activities can improve self-esteem. At the same time, as people come to appreciate the improved strength, conditioning, and flexibility that accompany fitness, they often become less obsessed with physical appearance.[32] For some, however, the quest for fitness can lead to obsessive exercise patterns (see the Women's Health/Men's Health box).

? *what do you* THINK?

Among the many benefits to be derived from physical activity, which two are most important to you? Why? ■ After exercising regularly for several weeks, what benefits do you notice?

Improving Cardiorespiratory Fitness

"Aerobics," a term coined by Dr. Kenneth Cooper, was first used in the 1970s to describe the type of exercise that improves cardiovascular endurance. The term **aerobic** means "with oxygen" and describes any type of exercise, typically performed at moderate levels of intensity for extended periods of time, that increases your heart rate. A person said to be in good shape has

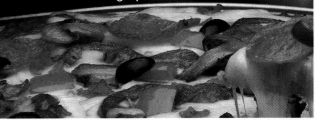

FUNfact
One-quarter of all college students do not participate in any vigorous or moderate-intensity exercise. Jogging for just 30 minutes 3 times a week can help you burn approximately 580 calories, enough to burn off about 3 slices of that late-night pizza break.

FIGURE 10.1 How Much Exercise Do You Get?

Source: American College Health Association-National College Health Assessment, *Reference Group Report, Spring 2005.*

an above-average **aerobic capacity**—a term used to describe the functional status of the cardiorespiratory system (heart, lungs, blood vessels). Aerobic capacity (commonly written as VO_{2max}) is defined as the maximum volume of oxygen consumed by the muscles during exercise. Vigorous endurance activities enhance VO_{2max}. Distance runners and cross-country skiers have the highest VO_{2max} of all athletes.

To measure your maximal aerobic capacity, an exercise physiologist or physician will typically perform a **graded exercise test**. A graded exercise test, sometimes called a stress test, is a diagnostic exam used to evaluate your level of fitness, heart rate, and blood pressure response to activity and the adequacy of blood supply to your heart. The test is performed on a treadmill or a stationary bicycle. Participants start out slowly and gradually increase the speed, resistance, or elevation. The end result is an accurate assessment of the body's capability to do physical work. Generally, the higher your cardiorespiratory endurance level, the more oxygen you can transport to exercising muscles and the longer you can exercise without becoming exhausted. In other words, the higher the VO_{2max} value, the higher your level of aerobic fitness.

You can test your own aerobic capacity by using either the 1.5-mile run or the 12-minute run endurance test described in the Assess Yourself box on page 328. However, do not take

(Text continues on page 330)

aerobic exercise   Any type of exercise that increases heart rate.

aerobic capacity   The current functional status of a person's cardiovascular system; measured as VO_{2max}.

graded exercise test   A test of aerobic capacity administered by a physician, exercise physiologist, or other trained person; two common forms are the treadmill running test and the stationary bike test.

ASSESS yourself

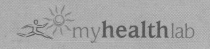

EVALUATING YOUR CARDIORESPIRATORY ENDURANCE

Fill out this assessment online at www.aw-bc.com/myhealthlab or www.aw-bc.com/donatelle.

After you have exercised regularly for several months, you might want to assess your cardiorespiratory endurance level. Find a local track, typically one quarter mile per lap, to perform your test. You may either run or walk for 1.5 miles and measure how long it takes to reach that distance or run or walk for 12 minutes and determine the distance you covered in that time. Use the chart below to estimate your cardiorespiratory fitness level based upon your age and sex. Note that women have lower standards for each fitness category because they have higher levels of essential fat than men do.

Age	1.5-Mile Run/Walk (min:sec)		12-Minute Run/Walk (miles)	
	Women (min:sec)	Men (min:sec)	Women (miles)	Men (miles)
GOOD				
18–29	<13:24	<11:27	>1.3	>1.5
30–39	<14:03	<12:06	>1.2	>1.4
40–49	<14:29	<12:32	>1:1	>1.4
50+	<15:21	<13:50	>1.0	>1.2
ADEQUATE FOR MOST ACTIVITIES				
18–29	13:25–14:55	11:28–12:58	1.1–1.3	1.3–1.5
30–39	14:04–15:21	12:07–13:37	1.1–1.2	1.3–1.45
40–49	14:30–15:47	12:33–14:03	0.99–1.11	1.25–1.4
50+	15:22–16:39	13:25–15:21	0.87–1.0	1.0–1.3
BORDERLINE				
18–29	14:56–15:22	12:59–13:25	0.96–1.2	1.2–1.4
30–39	15.22–15:48	13:38–14:04	0.95–1.05	1.2–1.3
40–49	15:48–16:14	14:04–14:30	0.9–1.0	1.14–1.24
50+	16:40–17:06	15:22–15:48	0.78–0.93	0.87–1.16
NEED EXTRA WORK ON CARDIOVASCULAR FITNESS				
18–29	>15:22	>13:25	<1.0	<1.3
30–39	>15:48	>14:04	<0.94	<1.18
40–49	>16:14	>14:30	<0.88	<1.14
50+	>17:06	>15:48	<0.84	<1.0

If you are now at the good level, congratulations! Your emphasis should be on maintaining this level for the rest of your life. If you are currently at lower levels, set realistic goals for improvement.

Source: Reprinted by permission from E. T. Howley and B. D. Franks, *Health Fitness Instructor's Handbook,* 3rd ed. (Champaign, IL: Human Kinetics Publishers, 1997), 85.

MAKE it happen!

ASSESSMENT: Complete the Assess Yourself activity to determine your current cardiorespiratory endurance level. Your results may indicate that you should take steps to improve this component of your physical fitness.

MAKING A CHANGE: In order to change your behavior, you need to develop a plan. Follow the steps below and complete your Behavior Change Contract to take action.

1. Evaluate your behavior and identify patterns and specific things you are doing. What can you change now? What can you change in the near future?

2. Select one pattern of behavior that you want to change.

3. Fill out the Behavior Change Contract found at the front of your book. It should include your long-term goal for change, your short-term goals, the rewards you'll give yourself for reaching these goals, potential obstacles along the way, and strategies for overcoming these obstacles. For each goal, list the small steps and specific actions that you will take.

4. Chart your progress in a journal. At the end of a week, consider how successful you were in following your plan. What helped you be successful? What made change more difficult? What will you do differently next week?

5. Revise your plan as needed: Are the short-term goals attainable? Are the rewards satisfying?

ONE STUDENT'S PLAN: Chris decided to measure how long it took him to run 1.5 miles around the school track to determine his level of cardiorespiratory endurance. It took him 13.0 minutes, which, as a 20-year-old, put him into the "borderline" category. Chris had played sports in high school and considered himself in good physical shape. However, he realized he had stopped exercising regularly in his freshman year when he didn't make the baseball team.

Chris decided to start by incorporating more activity into his daily routine. He tended to drive even to places that he could walk or bicycle to as easily. His friends had invited him to join in the pick-up basketball games they played on Saturday afternoons, but he had turned them down in order to play Playstation with his roommate. Chris filled out a Behavior Change Contract with a goal of riding his bicycle the three miles to and from campus three times a week and to play basketball every Saturday. If he did this consistently every week, he would reward himself with a new CD. After a month of this increased activity, Chris was already feeling more fit and was ready to add another aerobic activity. With winter weather coming, he thought he should add an indoor activity and started swimming laps at the school pool. He found swimming boring, so when he realized he was making excuses not to go, Chris switched to using a stair-climbing machine, which he could do while reading *Sports Illustrated* or watching ESPN. He was able to stick to doing this three times a week and made a commitment to go a fourth time whenever he missed his Saturday basketball game.

6	No exertion at all
7	Extremely light (7.5)
8	
9	Very light
10	
11	Light
12	
13	Somewhat hard
14	
15	Hard (heavy)
16	
17	Very hard
18	
19	Extremely hard
20	Maximal exertion

FIGURE 10.2 Rating of Perceived Exertion (RPE) Scale

Source: G. Borg, *Borg's Perceived Exertion and Pain Scales* (Champaign, IL: Human Kinetics, 1998), 47. Used with permission of Borg Products USA, Inc. www.acc.org/clinical/guidelines/exercise/tablea1.htm

these endurance-run tests if you are just starting to exercise. Progress slowly through a walking/jogging program at low intensities before measuring your aerobic capacity with one of these tests. If you're new to exercise or have any medical conditions such as asthma, diabetes, heart disease, or obesity, consult your physician before beginning any exercise program.

Aerobic Fitness Programs

The most beneficial aerobic exercises are total body activities involving all the large muscle groups of your body; for example, swimming, cross-country skiing, and rowing. If you have been sedentary for quite a while, simply initiating a physical activity program may be the hardest task you'll face. Don't be put off by the next-day soreness you are likely to feel. The key is to begin at a very low intensity, progress slowly, and stay with it!

There are three main components of an aerobic exercise program: frequency, intensity, and duration. The characteristics of these components vary by individual exercise goal and beginning fitness level. You can remember them with the acronym FIT (frequency, intensity, and time/duration).

target heart rate Calculated as a percentage of maximum heart rate (220 minus age); heart rate (pulse) is taken during aerobic exercise to check if exercise intensity is at the desired level (e.g., 60 percent of maximum heart rate).

Determining Exercise Frequency To best improve your cardiovascular endurance, you will need to vigorously exercise at least three times a week. If you are a newcomer to exercise, you can still make improvements by doing less intense exercise but doing it more days a week, following the Centers for Disease Control and Prevention and the American College of Sports Medicine recommendations for moderate physical activity five days a week (see the Spotlight on your Health box earlier in this chapter).

Determining Exercise Intensity There are several ways of measuring exercise intensity. One of the main ways is using your **target heart rate**. To calculate target heart rate, start by subtracting your age from 220 to find your maximum heart rate. Your target heart rate is a desired percentage of this maximum heart rate, often 60 percent. Thus, if you are a 20-year-old, your 60 percent target heart rate would be $(220 - 20) \times 0.60$, or 120 beats per minute (bpm).

For moderate-intensity physical activity, you should work out at 50 to 70 percent of your maximum heart rate. For more vigorous activities (such as running), you should work within 70 to 85 percent of your maximum heart rate. People in poor physical condition should set a target heart rate between 40 and 50 percent of maximum. As your condition improves, you can gradually increase your target heart rate. Increases should be made in small increments of 5 percent, from 40 to 45 percent, then from 45 to 50 percent.

Once you know your target heart rate, you can take your pulse to determine how close you are to this value during your workout. As you exercise, lightly place your index and middle fingers (don't use your thumb) on your radial artery (inside your wrist, on the thumb side). Using a watch or clock, take your pulse for six seconds and multiply this number by 10 (just add a zero to your count) to get the number of beats per minute. Your pulse should be within a range of 5 bpm above or below your target heart rate. If necessary, adjust the pace or intensity of your workout to achieve your target heart rate.

Another way of determining intensity is to use the Borg rating of perceived exertion (RPE) scale, as shown in Figure 10.2. Perceived exertion is how hard you feel you are working, based on your heart rate, increased breathing rate, sweating, and muscle fatigue. This scale uses a rating from 6 (no exertion at all) to 20 (maximal exertion). This method corresponds to heart rate for most people. Experts agree that RPE ratings of 3 to 4 correspond to moderate-intensity activity and 5 to 7 for vigorous activity.

The easiest but least scientific method of measuring exercise intensity is the "talk test." If you are exercising moderately, you should be able to carry on a conversation comfortably. If you are too out of breath to carry on a conversation, you are exercising vigorously.

Determining Exercise Duration Duration refers to the number of minutes of activity performed during any one session. It is recommended that vigorous activities be performed for at least 20 minutes at a time, and moderate activities for at least 30 minutes at a time.

The lower the intensity of your activity, the longer duration you'll need to get the same caloric expenditure. The number of calories burned increases for a person who weighs more and is less for those who weigh less.[33] Aim to expend 300 to 500 calories per exercise session, with an eventual weekly goal of 1,500 to 2,000 calories. As you progress, add to your exercise load by increasing duration or intensity, but not both at the same time. From week to week, don't increase duration or intensity by more than 10 percent.

Many of the health benefits associated with cardiorespiratory fitness (such as lower blood pressure) may take several months to achieve; don't expect improvements overnight.[34] However, any physical activity of low to moderate intensity will benefit your overall health almost from the start (Figure 10.3).

Are you having trouble getting started? See the Skills for Behavior Change box on page 332 for strategies.

Improving Muscular Strength and Endurance

To get a sense of what resistance training is about, do a resistance exercise. Start by holding your right arm straight down by your side, then turn your hand palm up and bring it up toward your shoulder. That's a resistance exercise: using a muscle, your biceps, to move a resistance, in this case just the weight of your hand—not very much resistance. Resistance training usually involves more weight or tension than this. You don't get to look like Arnold Schwarzenegger doing these exercises empty handed. Free weights, such as dumbbells and barbells, and all sorts of tension-producing machines are usually part of resistance training. It's not just bodybuilding that uses this type of exercise, either. Fitness programs and many sports employ resistance training to improve strength and endurance. Also, resistance exercises are an integral part of rehabilitation programs to help patients recover from muscle and joint injury. Many college students are incorporating strengthening exercises into their physical fitness program. In a 2005 survey, 45 percent of college-aged men and 27 percent of women reported doing exercises to strengthen or tone muscles at least 3 times a week.[35]

Strength and Endurance

In the field of resistance training, **muscular strength** refers to the amount of force a muscle or group of muscles is capable of exerting. The most common way to assess strength in a resistance exercise program is to measure the **one repetition maximum (1 RM)**, which is the maximum amount of weight a person can move one time (and no more) in a particular exercise. For example, 1 RM for the simple exercise done at the beginning of this section is the maximum weight you lift to your shoulder one time. In order to calculate your maximum,

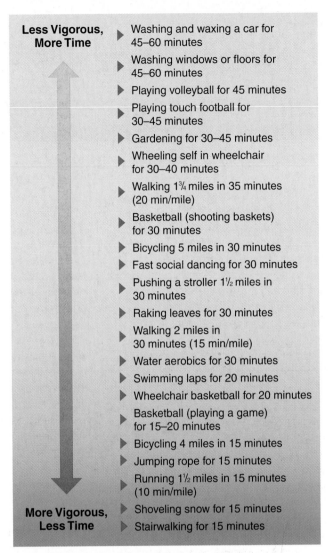

Less Vigorous, More Time
- Washing and waxing a car for 45–60 minutes
- Washing windows or floors for 45–60 minutes
- Playing volleyball for 45 minutes
- Playing touch football for 30–45 minutes
- Gardening for 30–45 minutes
- Wheeling self in wheelchair for 30–40 minutes
- Walking 1¾ miles in 35 minutes (20 min/mile)
- Basketball (shooting baskets) for 30 minutes
- Bicycling 5 miles in 30 minutes
- Fast social dancing for 30 minutes
- Pushing a stroller 1½ miles in 30 minutes
- Raking leaves for 30 minutes
- Walking 2 miles in 30 minutes (15 min/mile)
- Water aerobics for 30 minutes
- Swimming laps for 20 minutes
- Wheelchair basketball for 20 minutes
- Basketball (playing a game) for 15–20 minutes
- Bicycling 4 miles in 15 minutes
- Jumping rope for 15 minutes
- Running 1½ miles in 15 minutes (10 min/mile)
- Shoveling snow for 15 minutes
- Stairwalking for 15 minutes

More Vigorous, Less Time

FIGURE 10.3 Levels of Physical Activity

A moderate amount of physical activity is roughly equivalent to physical activity that uses approximately 150 calories of energy per day, or 1,000 calories per week. Some activities can be performed at various intensities; the suggested durations correspond to expected intensity of effort.

Source: U.S. Department of Health and Human Services, *Physical Activity and Health: A Report of the Surgeon General* (Atlanta: Centers for Disease Control, National Center for Chronic Disease Prevention and Health Promotion, 1996).

begin with a weight that you can lift easily. Rest for 2 to 3 minutes between lifts, then add 5 to 10 lbs of weight until you can no longer complete a successful lift. This muscle strength assessment is a good way to help create an effective weight-training program and monitor progress.

muscular strength The amount of force that a muscle is capable of exerting.

one repetition maximum (1 RM) The amount of weight or resistance that can be lifted or moved once, but not twice; a common measure of strength.

SKILLS FOR behavior change

ESTABLISHING AND MAINTAINING A SUCCESSFUL EXERCISE PROGRAM

STARTING AN EXERCISE ROUTINE

The most successful exercise program is one that is realistic and appropriate for your skill level and needs. Be realistic about the amount of time you will need to get into good physical condition. Perhaps the most significant factor early on in an exercise program is personal comfort. Experiment and find an activity that you truly enjoy. Be open to exploring new activities and new exercise equipment.

- *Start slow.* For the sedentary, first-time exerciser, any type and amount of physical activity will be a step in the right direction. If you are extremely overweight or out of condition, you might be able to walk for only five minutes at a time. Don't be discouraged; you're on your way!
- *Make only one life change at a time.* Success with one major behavioral change will encourage you to make other positive changes.
- *Set reasonable expectations for yourself and your fitness program.* Many

people become exercise dropouts because their expectations were too high to begin with. Allow sufficient time to reach your fitness goals.

- *Choose a specific time to exercise and stick with it.* Learning to establish priorities and keeping to a schedule are vital steps toward improved fitness. Experiment by exercising at different times of the day to learn what schedule works best for you.
- *Make exercise a positive habit.* Usually, if you are able to practice a desired activity for three weeks, you will be able to incorporate it into your lifestyle.
- *Keep a record of your progress.* Include various facts about your physical activities (duration, intensity) and chronicle your emotions and personal achievements as you progress.
- *Take lapses in stride.* Physical deconditioning—a decline in fitness level—occurs at about the same rate as physical conditioning. Renew your commitment to fitness, and restart your exercise program.

OVERCOMING COMMON OBSTACLES TO EXERCISE

There are many reasons why people do not exercise. These reasons range from personal ("I don't have time") to environmental ("I don't have a safe place to exercise"). You may be reluctant to start exercising if you are overweight or out of shape. Overcoming these barriers is an important part of starting and maintaining a regular exercise program.

In order to evaluate your obstacles to physical activity, you have to ask yourself what keeps you from being more active. Is it time? Do you lack a support group of family and friends to encourage your new plan? Is the gym or fitness center inconvenient or do you lack money for a membership or equipment? Perhaps you're even ready to begin, but just can't get over that final hurdle of just getting started. Once you've evaluated why you don't move more, look at the chart below to determine how you can overcome your hurdle.

Obstacles to Physical Activity	Possible Solutions
Lack of Time	- Take a good look at your schedule. Can you find three 30-minute time slots in your week? - Multitask. Read while riding an exercise bike or listen to lecture tapes while walking. - Exercise during your lunch breaks or between classes. - Select activities that require minimal time, such as brisk walking or jogging.
Social Influence	- Invite family and friends to exercise with you. - Join a class to meet new people who share your exercise interests. - Explain the importance of exercise to people who may not support your efforts.
Lack of Motivation/Willpower/Energy	- Write your planned workout time in your schedule book. - Enlist the help of an exercise partner to make you accountable for working out. - Give yourself an incentive. - Schedule your workouts when you feel most energetic. - Remind yourself that exercise can give you more energy.
Lack of Resources	- Select an activity that requires minimal equipment, such as walking, jogging, jumping rope, or calisthenics. - Identify inexpensive resources on campus or in the community.

Source: National Center for Chronic Disease Prevention and Health Promotion, "How Can I Overcome Barriers to Physical Activity?" 2003, www.cdc.gov/nccdphp/dnpa/physical/life/overcome.htm.

Muscular endurance is the ability of muscle to exert force repeatedly without fatiguing. If you can perform the exercise described earlier holding a five-pound weight in your hand and lifting 10 times, you will have greater endurance than someone who attempts that same exercise but is only able to lift the weight seven times. There are two categories of muscle endurance. The first is static endurance, or a force that is held as long as possible. An example of static abdominal endurance would be a measure of how long you can hold a double leg lift. The second is dynamic, or maximum repetitions completed at a determined rate. Timed sit-up or push-up tests are an example of dynamic muscle endurance.

Principles of Resistance

An effective **resistance exercise program** involves three key principles: tension, overload, and specificity of training.[36]

The Tension Principle
The key to developing strength is to create tension within a muscle or group of muscles. Tension is created by resistance provided by weights such as barbells or dumbbells, specially designed machines, or the weight of the body.

The Overload Principle
The overload principle is the most important of the three key principles. Overload doesn't mean forcing a muscle or group of muscles to do too much, which could result in injuries. Rather, overload in resistance training requires muscles to do more than they are used to. Everyone begins a resistance training program with an initial level of strength. To become stronger, you must regularly create a degree of tension in your muscles that is greater than you are accustomed to. This overload will cause your muscles to adapt to a new level. As your muscles respond to a regular program of overloading by getting larger, they become stronger.

Remember that resistance training exercises cause microscopic damage (tears) to muscle fibers, and the rebuilding process that increases the size and capacity of the muscle takes about 24 to 48 hours. Thus, resistance training exercise programs should include at least one day of rest and recovery between workouts before overloading the same muscles again.

The Specificity-of-Training Principle
According to the specificity principle, the effects of resistance exercise training are specific to the muscles being exercised. Only the muscle or muscle group that you exercise responds to the demands placed upon it. For example, if you regularly do curls, the muscles involved—your biceps—will become larger and stronger, but the other muscles in your body won't change. It is important to note that only exercising certain muscle groups may put opposing muscle groups at increased risk for injury. For example, overworking your quadriceps muscles, but neglecting your hamstrings, can put you at risk for a hamstring muscle pull or strain.

Gender Differences in Weight Training

The results of resistance training in men and women are quite different. Women don't normally develop muscle to the same extent that men do. The main reason for this difference is that men and women have different levels of the hormone testosterone in their blood. Before puberty, testosterone levels are similar for both boys and girls. During adolescence, testosterone levels in boys increase dramatically, about tenfold, while testosterone levels in girls remain unchanged. Muscles will become larger (**hypertrophy**) as a result of resistance training exercise, but typically this change is less dramatic in women. To enhance muscle bulk, some bodybuilders (both men and women) take synthetic hormones (anabolic steroids) that mimic the effects of testosterone. However, using anabolic steroids is a dangerous and illegal practice. (See Chapter 14.)

Types of Muscle Activity

In the past, the term "contraction" was used to define the tension a muscle produces as it shortens. Because tension develops as muscles lengthen, the term "muscle action" is a better descriptor. Your skeletal muscles act in three different ways: isometric, concentric, and eccentric.[37] In **isometric muscle action** (Figure 10.4a on page 334), force is produced through tension and muscle contraction, not movement. A **concentric muscle action** (Figure 10.4b) causes joint movement and a production of force while the muscle shortens. The empty-hand curl we did at the beginning of this section is a concentric exercise, with joint movement occurring at the elbow. In general, concentric muscle actions produce movement in opposition to the downward pull of gravity.

Eccentric muscle action describes the ability of a muscle to produce force while lengthening. Typically, eccentric muscle actions occur when movement is in the same direction as the pull of gravity (see Figure 10.4c). Once you've brought a weight up during a curl, an eccentric muscle action would be to lower your hand and the weight back to their original position.

---

muscular endurance A muscle's ability to exert force repeatedly without fatiguing.

resistance exercise program A regular program of exercises designed to improve muscular strength and endurance in the major muscle groups.

hypertrophy Increased size (girth) of a muscle.

isometric muscle action Force produced without any resulting joint movement.

concentric muscle action Force produced while the muscle is shortening.

eccentric muscle action Force produced while the muscle is lengthening.

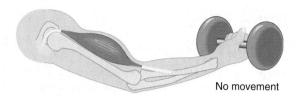

No movement

(a) Isometric muscle action
Muscle contracts
but does not shorten

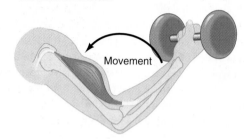

Movement

(b) Concentric muscle action

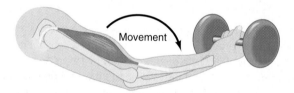

Movement

(c) Eccentric muscle action

FIGURE 10.4 Isometric, Concentric, and Eccentric Muscle Actions

Source: S. Powers and E. Howley, *Exercise Physiology: Theory and Application to Fitness and Performance.* Copyright © 1998 Lippincott, Williams & Wilkins. Used with permission.

Methods of Providing Resistance

What types of exercises can I do to improve my muscular strength?

There are four commonly used resistance exercise methods: body weight resistance and fixed, variable, and accommodating resistance devices.

Body Weight Resistance (Calisthenics)

Strength and endurance training doesn't have to rely on equipment. You can use your own body weight to develop skeletal muscle fitness. Calisthenics (such as push-ups and chin-ups) use part or all of your body weight to offer resistance during exercise. Though less effective than other resistance methods in developing large muscle mass and strength, calisthenics are quite adequate for improving general muscular fitness and are generally sufficient to improve muscle tone and maintain a level of muscular strength.

Fixed Resistance

Fixed-resistance exercises provide a constant amount of resistance throughout the full range of movement. Free weights, such as barbells and dumbbells, and some machines provide fixed resistance because their weight, or the amount of resistance, does not change during an exercise. Fixed-resistance equipment has the potential to strengthen all the major muscle groups in the body. Fixed-resistance exercise machines are commonly available at college recreation/fitness facilities, health clubs, and many resorts and hotels.

There are several advantages of using free weights. First, free weights require more balance and coordination. Also, free weights tend to recruit more muscle groups for action and promote more activity of the joint and stabilizer muscles. From a financial perspective, free weights are relatively inexpensive and can provide a great muscle workout.

Variable Resistance

Variable-resistance equipment alters the resistance encountered by a muscle during a movement, so that the effort by the muscle is more consistent throughout the full range of motion. Variable-resistance equipment provides a more controlled motion and specifically isolates certain muscle groups and is often used for rehabilitation of muscle injuries. Although some of these machines are expensive and too big to move easily, others are affordable and more portable. Many forms of variable-resistance devices are sold for home use.

Accommodating-Resistance Devices

These machines, sometimes called isokinetic machines, adjust the resistance according to the amount of force generated by the person using the equipment. The exerciser performs at a maximal level of effort, while the device controls the speed of the exercise. The machine is set to a particular speed, and muscles being exercised must move at a rate faster than or equal to that speed in order to encounter resistance.[38]

Core Strength Training

The body's core muscles are the foundation for movement. These muscles are deep back and abdominal muscles that attach to the spine and pelvis. The contraction of these muscles provides the basis of support for movements of the upper and lower body and powerful movements of the extremities. A weak core increases your chances for poor posture, lower back pain, and muscle injuries. A strong core gives you a more stable center of gravity and a more stable platform for movements, thus reducing the chance of injury.

Core strength can be developed by simple calisthenics, using fitness equipment such as a fitness ball, or taking an exercise class like yoga or Pilates. Holding yourself in a plank or "up" push-up position and doing abdominal curl-ups are two examples of calisthenic exercises to increase core strength. Exercising with a fitness ball requires using core muscles for support.

Experts recommend doing core-strengthening activities at least three times per week.[39] It's a good idea to get started with the help of a professional (e.g., a personal trainer or physical therapist) because body alignment and positioning are crucial.

Benefits of Strength Training

Does strength training offer any benefits beyond simply getting stronger? Indeed, regular strength training can reduce the occurrence of lower back pain and joint and muscle injuries. It can also postpone loss of muscle tissue due to aging and a sedentary lifestyle and help prevent osteoporosis. People of all ages, including children and older adults, can benefit from strength training.

Strength training enhances muscle definition and tone and improves personal appearance. This, in turn, enhances self-esteem. Strength training even has a hidden benefit: muscle tissue burns calories faster than most other tissues, even when it is resting. So, increasing your muscle mass can help boost your metabolism and maintain a healthy weight.

 what do you THINK?

What types of resistance equipment can you currently access? ▪ Based on what you've read, what actions can you take to increase your muscular strength? ▪ Muscular endurance? ▪ How would you measure your improvement?

Improving Flexibility

Stretching Exercises and Well-Being

Who would guess that improved flexibility can give you a sense of well-being, help you deal with stress better, and stop your joints from hurting as much as they used to? Stretching exercises are the main way to improve **flexibility**, a measure of the range of motion, or the amount of movement possible, at a particular joint. Improving the range of motion enhances efficiency, extent of movement, and posture. Today, stretching exercises are extremely popular, both because they are effective and because people can begin them at virtually any age and enjoy them for a lifetime. Flexibility exercises have been shown to be effective in reducing the incidence and severity of lower back problems and muscle or tendon injuries that can occur during sports and everyday physical activities.[40] Improved flexibility also means less tension and pressure on joints, resulting in less joint pain and joint deterioration.[41]

Flexibility is enhanced by the controlled stretching of muscles and muscle attachments that act on a particular joint. Each muscle involved in a stretching exercise is attached to our skeleton by tendons. The goal of stretching is to decrease the resistance of a muscle and its tendons to tension, that is, to reduce resistance to being stretched. Stretching exercises gradually result in greater flexibility. They involve stretching a muscle or group of muscles to a point of slight discomfort and holding that position for up to 30 seconds or more. For many people a regular program of stretching exercises enhances psychological as well as physical well-being.

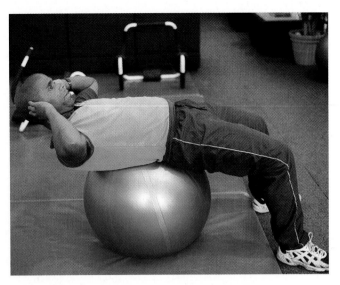

Equipment such as an exercise ball is excellent for increasing core body strength.

Types of Stretching Exercises

Static stretching techniques involve the slow, gradual stretching of muscles and their tendons, then holding them at a point. During this holding period—the stretch—participants may feel mild discomfort and a warm sensation in the stretched muscles. Static stretching exercises involve specialized tension receptors in our muscles. When done properly, such stretching slightly lessens the sensitivity of tension receptors, which allows the muscle to relax and be stretched to greater length.[42] The stretch is followed by a slow return to the starting position. Correct body positioning is critical for safe and effective static stretching. See Figure 10.5 on page 336 for some tips on how to minimize the risk of injury.

Dynamic stretching is a technique that has recently been deemed an effective way of preparing muscles for intense aerobic activity such as running, soccer, or dance.[43] Dynamic stretching involves moving parts of your body and gradually increasing reach, speed of movement, or both. This is not the old "ballistic" type of stretching that was popular decades ago that promoted bouncy, jerky movements to stretch. Dynamic stretching consists of controlled leg and arm swings that take you (gently!) to the limits of your range of motion. An example of dynamic stretching would be slow, controlled leg swings, arm swings, or torso twists.[44]

flexibility The measure of the range of motion, or the amount of movement possible, at a particular joint.

static stretching Techniques that gradually lengthen a muscle to an elongated position (to the point of discomfort) and hold that position for 10 to 30 seconds.

dynamic stretching Moving parts of your body in a gradual and controlled manner, taking you to the limits of your range of motion.

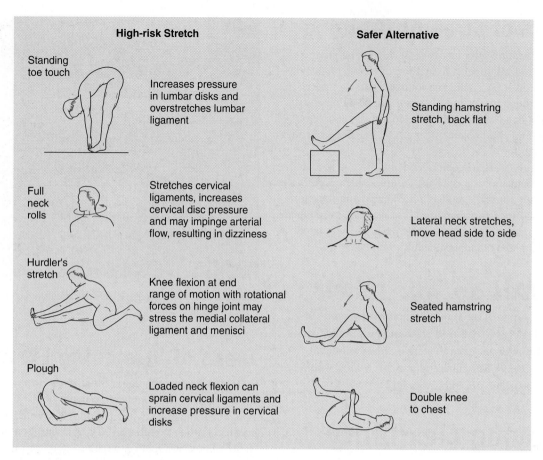

High-risk Stretch		Safer Alternative	

Standing toe touch — Increases pressure in lumbar disks and overstretches lumbar ligament

Standing hamstring stretch, back flat

Full neck rolls — Stretches cervical ligaments, increases cervical disc pressure and may impinge arterial flow, resulting in dizziness

Lateral neck stretches, move head side to side

Hurdler's stretch — Knee flexion at end range of motion with rotational forces on hinge joint may stress the medial collateral ligament and menisci

Seated hamstring stretch

Plough — Loaded neck flexion can sprain cervical ligaments and increase pressure in cervical disks

Double knee to chest

FIGURE 10.5 Common High-Risk Stretches and Recommended Alternatives

Source: American College of Sports Medicine, *Resource Manual for Guidelines for Exercise Testing and Prescription,* 3rd ed. Copyright © 1998 Lippincott Williams and Wilkins. Used by permission.

Yoga, Tai Chi, and Pilates

Three major styles of exercise that include static stretching have become widely practiced in the United States and other Western countries: yoga, tai chi, and Pilates. All three emphasize a joining of mind and body as a result of intense concentration on breathing and body position. As mentioned in the strength training section elsewhere in this chapter, these styles of exercise are also an excellent way to improve core body strength.

Yoga One of the most popular fitness and static stretching activities, **yoga** originated in India about 5,000 years ago. Yoga blends the mental and physical aspects of exercise, a union of mind and body that participants find relaxing and

satisfying. Done regularly, its combination of mental focus and physical effort improves flexibility, vitality, posture, agility, and coordination.

The practice of yoga focuses attention on controlled breathing as well as purely physical exercise. In addition to its mental dimensions, yoga incorporates a complex array of static stretching exercises expressed as postures (*asanas*). Over 200 postures exist, but only about 50 are commonly practiced. During a session, participants move to different asanas and hold them for 30 seconds or more. Yoga not only enhances flexibility, it has the great advantage of being flexible itself. Asanas and combinations of asanas can be changed and adjusted for young and old and to accommodate people with physical limitations or disabilities. Asanas can also be combined to provide even conditioned athletes with challenging sessions.

A typical yoga session will move the spine and joints through their full range of motion. Yoga postures lengthen, strengthen, and balance musculature, leading to increased flexibility, stamina, and strength—and many people report a psychological sense of general well-being, too. Table 10.2 details the three most popular styles of yoga.

yoga A variety of Indian traditions geared toward self-discipline and the realization of unity; includes forms of exercise widely practiced in the West today that promote balance, coordination, flexibility, and meditation.

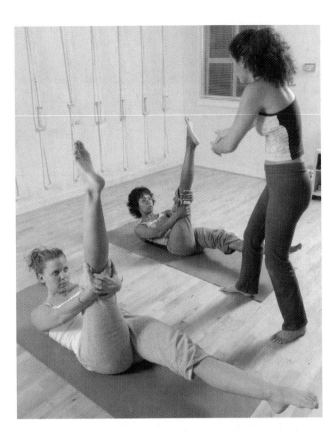
Pilates and other styles of exercise that strengthen core body muscles also enhance flexibility and lower stress levels.

Tai chi
Tai chi is an ancient Chinese form of exercise that, like yoga, combines stretching, balance, coordination, and meditation. It is designed to increase range of motion and flexibility while reducing muscular tension. Based on Chi Kung, a Taoist philosophy dedicated to spiritual growth and good health, tai chi was developed about 1000 AD by monks to defend themselves against bandits and warlords. It involves a series of positions called *forms* that are performed continuously. Both yoga and tai chi are excellent for improving flexibility and muscular coordination.

Pilates
Compared with yoga and tai chi, **Pilates** is the new kid on the exercise block. It was developed by Joseph Pilates, who came from Germany to New York City in 1926. Shortly after his arrival, he introduced his exercise methodology, which emphasizes flexibility, coordination, strength, and tone. Pilates combines stretching with movement against resistance, which is aided by devices such as tension springs or heavy rubber bands.

Pilates differs from yoga and tai chi because it includes a component designed specifically to increase strength. The method consists of a sequence of carefully performed movements. Some are carried out on specially designed equipment, while others are performed on mats. Each exercise stretches and strengthens the muscles involved and has a specific breathing pattern associated with it. A Pilates class focuses on strengthening specific muscle groups, using equipment that provides resistance.

TABLE 10.2 Popular Yoga Styles

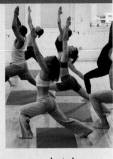

- Iyengar yoga focuses on precision and alignment in the poses. Standing poses are basic to this style, and are often held longer than in other styles.
- Ashtanga yoga in its pure form is based on a specific flow of poses with an emphasis on strength and agility that creates internal heat. *Power yoga,* a style growing in popularity, is a derivative of ashtanga yoga.
- Bikram yoga, or hot yoga, is similar to power yoga but does not incorporate a specific flow of poses. Literally the hottest yoga going, it is performed in temperatures of 100°F, or even a bit higher. Proponents say that the heat increases the body's ability to move and stretch without injury.

try it NOW

Stretching and improved flexibility are important both in the gym and in the classroom and library. Sitting hunched over a pile of books for an extended period of time can be a pain in the neck! Be sure to stretch every 20 minutes or so by doing shoulder rolls, shrugs, and neck stretches to help work out the kinks. These mini stretch breaks will ease your muscles and your mind.

Body Composition

Body composition is the fourth and final component of a comprehensive fitness program. Body composition describes the relative proportions of lean tissue (muscle, bone, water, organs) and fat tissue in the body. Body composition parameters that can be influenced by regular physical activity include total body mass, fat mass, fat-free mass, and regional fat distribution. Aerobic activities that improve cardiovascular endurance also help improve body composition because they expend calories and contribute to weight loss and help with weight-loss maintenance.

There are many ways to assess body composition. These range from simple (e.g., height–weight charts) to complex (e.g., underwater weighing). See the Assessing Fat Levels section in Chapter 9.

---

tai chi An ancient Chinese form of exercise widely practiced in the West today that promotes balance, coordination, stretching, and meditation.

Pilates Exercise programs that combine stretching with movement against resistance, aided by devices such as tension springs and heavy rubber bands.

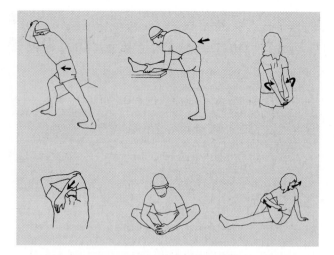

FIGURE 10.6 Stretching Exercises to Improve Flexibility

These diagrams show how simple stretching can be. Use these stretches as part of your warm-up and cool-down. Hold each one for 10 to 30 seconds, and repeat four times on each side. After only a few weeks of regular stretching, you'll begin to have more flexibility.

Source: Excerpted from *Stretching, 20th Anniversary Revised Edition.* © 2000 Shelter Publications, Box 279, Bolinas, CA 94924. Reprinted by permission.

TABLE 10.3	Resistance Training Program Guidelines

- Resistance training should be an integral part of an adult fitness program and be of sufficient intensity to enhance strength and muscular endurance and to maintain fat-free mass.
- Resistance training should be progressive in nature, individualized, and provide a stimulus (overload) to all major muscle groups in the body.
- The exercise sequence should include large before small muscle group exercises, multiple-joint exercises before single-joint exercises, and higher intensity before lower intensity exercises.
- Performing a minimum of 8 to 10 exercises that train the major muscle groups two to three days per week is recommended.
- The amount of weight used and number of repetitions vary by individual's target goal, physical capacity, and training status.

Source: W. J. Kraemer et al, "American College of Sports Medicine Position Stand on Progression Models in Resistance Training for Healthy Adults," *Medicine and Science in Sports and Exercise* 34, no. 2 (2002): 364–380. Reprinted by Permission of Lippincott Williams & Wilkins.

Creating Your Own Fitness Program

Identify Your Fitness Goals

The first step in creating your own fitness program is to identify your fitness goals. Do you want to improve your quality of life? Lose weight? Train for an upcoming 5K race? Think about a timeline for your goals. Do you want to be able to jog 3 miles before spring break? Hike across campus next semester, with a heavy backpack, and not be out of breath? Once you develop a specific goal, you can create a plan to help you achieve that goal.

When you become committed to regular physical activity and exercise, you will observe gradual improvements in your functional abilities and note progress toward your goals. Perhaps your most vital goal will be to become committed to fitness for the long haul—to establish a realistic schedule of diverse exercise activities that you can maintain and enjoy throughout your life.

Designing Your Program

Which factors should I think about as I develop a fitness plan?

Now that you know the fundamentals of fitness, you can design your own personalized fitness program. There are several factors to consider that will boost your chances of successfully achieving your goals. First, choose an activity that is appropriate for you. For example, don't plan on swimming if the pool is difficult to access. Also, choose activities that you like to do. If you hate to run, don't choose running as your exercise. Be creative in your activity choice; try something new! There are many different classes (e.g., Salsa Aerobics, Boot Camp Classes) that can keep you motivated and if you don't like one activity, you can always try another.

Your plan should include very specific ways to incorporate physical activity into your lifestyle. When will you exercise? For how long? It is best to write out these goals and put them in your daily planner as you would any other scheduled activity. Lack of time is the number-one reason given for not exercising. By looking at your weekly schedule, you can identify segments of time that work for you.

Reevaluate your fitness goal and action plan after 30 days. This time period should allow you to know whether the program is working for you. Make changes if necessary, and then make a plan to reevaluate after another 30-day period.

Fitness Program Components

The amount and type of exercise required to yield beneficial results vary with the age and physical condition of the exerciser. Men over age 40 and women over age 50 should consult their physicians before beginning any fitness program.

Good fitness programs are designed to improve or maintain cardiorespiratory fitness, flexibility, muscular strength and endurance, and body composition. A comprehensive program could include a warm-up period of easy walking, followed by stretching activities to improve flexibility, then selected strength development exercises, followed by an aerobic activity for 20 minutes or more, and concluding with a cool-down period of gentle flexibility exercises.

TABLE 10.4 Picking Your Workout Machine

Machine	Advantages	Best Use
Elliptical machine	This machine is designed for nonimpact cardiovascular exercise. Some machines are equipped with handles for arm action that improve the overall workout.	For machines without arm action, pump arms at your sides as you would if you were running. If the machine has arm handles, use resistance by pushing and pulling along with the handles.
Stair climber	This machine is a great low-impact lower body workout and most can be adjusted from very easy to very difficult.	Since the degree of workout depends on working against your body weight, stay upright and don't lean on the console. Try not to touch the handrails other than for balance. Keep your steps shallow (no deeper than 6 inches).
Stationary bike	This machine provides an excellent lower body workout. It is generally easy to use and most come with varied resistance programs. Recumbent bikes offer less strain on the back and knees.	Adjust the seat so your leg is almost fully extended when the pedal is at its lowest. Don't grip the handles too tightly or lean on the handlebars.
Treadmill	This machine offers a great lower body workout and improves cardiovascular fitness. It is relatively easy to use and burns more calories than bikes or a stair climber.	Most come with an emergency shut-off clip. Be sure to use this for safety. Start gradually and progress to either faster pace or increased incline. Arms should naturally swing at your sides.

Source: Adapted from S. Eyler, StarTrac Fitness, "Comparison of Workout Machines, 2006."

Warming Up and Stretching Warming up prepares your body for physical activity and provides a transition from rest to exercise. A 5-minute warm-up may start with a 5-minute brisk walk to ease your cardiovascular system into more vigorous activity and to increase blood flow to the exercising muscles. This 5-minute warm-up can increase the temperature and elasticity of muscles and connective tissue, making stretching more effective. Add 5 to 10 minutes of stretching after your warm-up to your fitness routine and you'll be ready to go! Figure 10.6 shows a selection of exercises that will stretch the major muscle groups of your body and can be used as a warm-up for other physical activities and exercise programs.

Resistance Training When beginning a resistance exercise program, always consider your age, fitness level, and personal goals. Strength training exercises are done in a set, or a single series of multiple repetitions using the same resistance. For both men and women under the age of 50, the ACSM recommends working major muscle groups with at least one set of eight to ten different exercises two to three days per week.[45] Weight loads should be at a level to allow up to 8 to 12 repetitions. Beginners should use lighter weights and complete 10 to 15 repetitions. Table 10.3 presents essential information for a program to build muscular strength and endurance. Remember, experts suggest allowing at least one day of rest and recovery between workouts.

Cardiorespiratory Training The greatest proportion of exercise time should be spent developing cardiovascular fitness. Choose an aerobic activity you think you will like. Many people find cross training—alternate-day participation in two or more aerobic activities (such as jogging and swimming)—less monotonous and more enjoyable than long-term participation in only one activity. Cross training is also beneficial because it strengthens a variety of muscles, thus helping you avoid overuse injuries to muscles and joints. Jogging, walking, cycling, rowing, step aerobics, and cross-country skiing are all excellent activities for developing cardiovascular fitness. Most colleges have recreation centers where students can use stair-climbing machines, stationary bicycles, treadmills, rowing machines, and ski-simulators.

Table 10.4 describes these and other popular workout tools and provides tips for their use.

Cooling Down and Stretching Just as you ease into a workout with a warm-up, you should slowly transition from activity to rest. At least 5 minutes of your workout should be devoted to a gradual slowdown, decreasing the intensity of your activity. For example, if you jog, walk briskly, then slowly, before stretching. This allows your breathing and heart rate to return to normal. Be sure to stretch the major muscle groups to help reduce the amount of soreness from exercise.

Choosing the Right Exercise Equipment

If you have a treadmill that you use as a clothes hanger or belong to a gym you haven't visited in months, you are not alone. Many people buy great equipment and don't get motivated to get moving, but others buy services and equipment

TABLE 10.5	Evaluating Fitness Products

Fitness products are a multimillion-dollar industry, but some may make fantastic claims that sound too good to be true. To get the most out of your investment, choose wisely and consider the following:

- Ignore claims that an exercise machine or device can provide lasting, "no sweat" results in a short time.
- Disbelieve claims that a product can burn fat off a particular part of the body.
- Read the fine print. Advertised results may be based on more than just using a machine; they may also be based on caloric restriction.
- Be skeptical of testimonials and before and after pictures from "satisfied" customers.
- Get details on warranties, guarantees, and return policies.
- Check out the company's customer support and service sections. Call the number to see how helpful the person on the other end really is.

There are other things to consider before investing in any fitness equipment, even products with proven benefits. Here are some more consumer tips:

- **Ask around.** Get tips from friends or store personnel.
- **Try before you buy.** You may be able to try out items at a gym or borrow one from someone before you invest in it.
- **Do your research.** Check out consumer reports or online resources for the best product ratings and reviews.

Source: Federal Trade Commision, www.ftc.gov/bcp/conline/pubs/alerts/musclealrt.htm, 2003.

that don't have a ghost's chance of being useful. Evaluate advertising claims for fitness products carefully. (See Table 10.5.)

Popular and Practical Exercise Equipment

There are many useful exercise products that can be used to take your exercise program to the next level. Here, we'll look at some of the most popular—and effective—equipment.

Heart Rate Monitors
Fitness enthusiasts use heart rate monitors to become aware of their heart rate and training intensity and push performance higher. These monitors usually have a strap with a sensor for placing around the chest and a watchlike readout on the wrist. Monitors cost between $50 and $200 and can provide instant feedback about the intensity of your workouts. If you want a more technical way to measure heart rate than the fingers-to-the-wrist method, a heart rate monitor is for you.

Pedometers
Pedometers offer features such as monitoring your calories, counting number of steps, and keeping track of distance and speed. They are usually small, easy to use, and can help you figure out how far you've gone on your daily walk/run or measure how many steps you take on an average day. They can be an excellent motivator. Before you buy a pedometer, make sure it's simple to use and has an easy-to-read display. The unit should be accurate in its count when you wear it correctly—you may have to experiment with where to wear it. Distance accuracy depends on setting your stride length correctly. Some pedometers even come with a computer program to upload your step and distance records. Prices range from $20 to $100.

Exercise (Fitness) Balls
Stabilizing yourself on a ball strengthens core muscles. If you sit on the ball and do arm or shoulder exercises, you work your abdominals as well as your arms and shoulders. High-quality balls are made of burst-resistant vinyl and are independently tested to withstand as much as 600 pounds while still retaining their shape and usefulness.

Choose a ball that is suited to both your weight and height. To determine if the ball is right for you, sit on it. Your feet should be flat on the floor, your weight distributed evenly, and your knees should be at a 90-degree or slightly greater angle. Be sure to inflate it to the right height and use it properly—for safety reasons and to ensure maximum workout results. Read the package carefully to be certain that if the ball is punctured, it will not drop you to the ground (high-quality balls are designed to deflate slowly if punctured, to minimize the risk of injury). Prices range from $25 to $50.

Balance Boards
By doing strengthening moves on the balance board, your core muscles contract, thus it works your abs as well as other muscle groups. Athletes who regularly train with balance boards improve agility and reaction skills and ankle strength. This greatly decreases the risk of ankle injury during play, while improving coordination and overall athletic ability. For less-athletic types, working out on the balance board can reduce your chances of tripping and falling in everyday life. The cost is $40 to $80.

Resistance Bands
These bands are usually rubber or elastic material with handles that can be used to work the muscles without weights. The bands can provide various ways to improve muscular endurance and strength, flexibility, and range of motion. They are lightweight, portable, and can add variety to gym workouts. They are also compact and easy to pack when traveling. You can buy bands in varying degrees of resistance, depending on your fitness level or exercise goal, for $5 to $15.

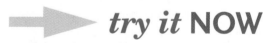 *try it* NOW

Boost daily exercise today with small changes. For example, when you have a choice between elevator and stairs, choose the stairs. Walking up a few flights of stairs a day can be beneficial to your health, especially when you add the weight of a backpack or books. Walking stairs can help strengthen your legs, gets your heart pumping, and contributes to your daily activity level.

Fitness Injuries

Overtraining is the most frequent cause of injuries associated with fitness activities, affecting up to 20 percent of all athletes. Enthusiastic but out-of-shape beginners can injure themselves by doing too much too soon. Experienced athletes can develop overtraining syndrome by engaging in systematic and progressive increases in training without getting enough rest and recovery time. Eventually, performance declines and training sessions become increasingly difficult. Adequate rest, good nutrition, and rehydration are important to sustain or improve fitness levels.

Pay attention to your body's warning signs. To avoid injuring a particular muscle group or body part, vary your fitness activities throughout the week to give muscles and joints a rest. Set appropriate short-term and long-term training goals. Establishing realistic but challenging fitness goals can help you stay motivated without overdoing it. Overtraining injuries occur most often in repetitive activities like skiing, running, bicycling, and step aerobics. However, use common sense and you're likely to remain injury-free.

Causes of Fitness-Related Injuries

There are two basic types of injuries stemming from fitness-related activities: overuse and traumatic injuries. **Overuse injuries** occur because of cumulative, day-after-day stresses placed on tendons, bones, and ligaments during exercise. These injuries occur most often in repetitive activities like swimming, running, bicycling, and step aerobics. The forces that occur normally during physical activity are not enough to cause a ligament sprain or muscle strain, but when these forces are applied daily for weeks or months, they can result in an injury. Common sites of overuse injuries are the leg, knee, shoulder, and elbow joints.

Traumatic injuries occur suddenly and violently, typically by accident. Typical traumatic injuries are broken bones, torn ligaments and muscles, contusions, and lacerations. Some traumatic injuries occur quickly and are difficult to avoid—for example, spraining your ankle by landing on another person's foot after jumping up for a rebound in basketball. If your traumatic injury causes a noticeable loss of function and immediate pain or pain that does not go away after 30 minutes, consult a physician.

Preventing Injuries

How do I choose a good running shoe?

Appropriate Footwear Shoes are made to protect the foot from sport-specific movements. Proper footwear can decrease the likelihood of foot, knee, or back injuries.

When you purchase running shoes, look for several key components (see Figure 10.7). Biomechanics research has revealed that run-

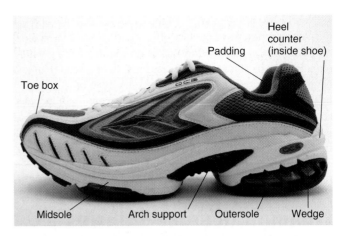

FIGURE 10.7 Anatomy of a Running Shoe
The midsole of your shoe is one of the most important factors in comfort. To evaluate the flexibility of the midsole, hold the shoe lengthwise between the index fingers of your right and left hand. When you push on both ends of the shoe, it should bend easily at the midsole. If the force exerted by your index fingers cannot bend the shoe, its midsole is probably too rigid and will be painful.

ning is a collision sport—with each stride, the runner's foot collides with the ground with a force three to five times the runner's body weight.[46] The force not absorbed by the running shoe is transmitted upward into the foot, leg, thigh, and back. Our bodies are able to absorb forces such as these but may be injured by the cumulative effect of repetitive impacts (such as running 40 miles per week). Therefore, the ability of running shoes to absorb shock is critical. Proper fit is also important.

Basketball, tennis, and other sport enthusiasts can also buy shoes specific to their sport. A cross-training shoe can be used for several different fitness activities by the novice or recreational athlete.

Appropriate Protective Equipment Some activities require special protective equipment to reduce chances of injury. Eye injuries can occur in virtually all fitness-related activities, although some sports are more risky than others. As many as 90 percent of the eye injuries resulting from racquetball and squash could be prevented by wearing appropriate eye protection—for example, goggles with polycarbonate lenses.[47]

overuse injuries Injuries that result from the cumulative effects of day-after-day stresses placed on tendons, muscles, and joints.

traumatic injuries Injuries that are accidental in nature, which occur suddenly and violently (including fractured bones, ruptured tendons, and sprained ligaments).

Nearly 100 million people in the United States ride bikes for pleasure, fitness, or competition. Wearing a helmet while bicycle riding is an important safety precaution. Riding without a helmet significantly increases the risk of a head injury. Nonhelmeted riders are 14 times more likely to be involved in a fatal crash than helmeted riders; 85 percent of all bicycle accident fatalities are due to head or brain injury, many of which could have been prevented by helmet usage.[48] Look for helmets that meet the standards established by the American National Standards Institute and the Snell Memorial Foundation.

Common Overuse Injuries

Three of the most common overuse injuries are plantar fasciitis, shin splints, and runner's knee.

Plantar Fasciitis
Plantar fasciitis is an inflammation of the plantar fascia, a broad band of tissue (fascia) that protects the nerves, blood vessels, and muscles of the foot from injury. Repetitive weight-bearing fitness activities such as walking and running can inflame the plantar fascia. Common symptoms are pain and tenderness under the ball of the foot, at the heel, or at both locations.[49]

This injury can often be prevented by regularly stretching the plantar fascia prior to exercise and by wearing athletic shoes with good arch support and shock absorbency. Stretch the plantar fascia by slowly pulling all five toes upward toward your head, holding for 10 to 15 seconds. Repeat this three to five times on each foot prior to exercise.

Shin Splints
A general term for any pain that occurs below the knee and above the ankle is *shin splints*. This broad description includes more than 20 different medical conditions. Pain can be due to muscles, bones, or attachments from muscle to bone. Typically, there is pain and swelling along the middle third of the posteromedial tibia in the soft tissues, not the bone.

Sedentary people who start a new weight-bearing exercise program are at the greatest risk for shin splints, though even well-conditioned athletes who rapidly increase their distance or pace may also develop them.[50] Running is the most frequent cause of shin splints, but those who do a great deal of walking (such as mail carriers and restaurant workers) may also develop this injury.

To help prevent shin splints, wear athletic shoes with good arch support and shock absorbency. Also, gradually increase training intensity and vary your routine. If the pain continues,

see your physician. You may be advised to substitute a non-weight-bearing activity such as swimming during your recovery period.

Runner's Knee
Runner's knee describes a series of problems involving the muscles, tendons, and ligaments around the knee. The main symptom of this kind of runner's knee is the pain experienced when downward pressure is applied to the kneecap after the knee is straightened fully. Symptoms include pain, swelling, redness, and tenderness around the kneecap.[51] If you have these symptoms, your physician will probably recommend that you stop running for a few weeks and reduce activities that compress the kneecap (for example, exercise on a stair-climbing machine or doing squats with heavy resistance) until you no longer feel any pain.

Treatment

First-aid treatment for virtually all personal fitness injuries involves **RICE: r**est, **i**ce, **c**ompression, and **e**levation. *Rest,* the first component of this treatment, is required to avoid further irritation of the injured body part. *Ice* is applied to relieve pain and constrict the blood vessels to stop any internal or external bleeding. Never apply ice cubes, reusable gel ice packs, chemical cold packs, or other forms of cold directly to your skin. Instead, place a layer of wet toweling or elastic bandage between the ice and your skin. Ice should be applied to a new injury for approximately 20 minutes every hour for the first 24 to 72 hours. *Compression* of the injured body part can be accomplished with a 4- or 6-inch-wide elastic bandage; this applies indirect pressure to damaged blood vessels to help stop bleeding. Be careful, though, that the compression wrap does not interfere with normal blood flow. A throbbing, painful hand or foot indicates that the compression wrap should be loosened. *Elevation* of an injured extremity above the level of your heart also helps to control internal or external bleeding by making the blood flow uphill to reach the injured area.

Exercising in the Heat

Heat stress, which includes several potentially fatal illnesses resulting from excessive body core temperature, is a concern when exercising in warm, humid weather. In these conditions, your body's rate of heat production can exceed its ability to cool itself.

You can help prevent heat stress by following certain precautions. First, proper acclimatization to hot and/or humid climates is essential. The process of heat acclimatization, which increases your body's cooling efficiency, requires about 10 to 14 days of gradually increased activity in the hot environment. Second, avoid dehydration by replacing the fluids you lose during and after exercise. Third, wear clothing appropriate for your activity and the environment. And finally, use common sense—for example, on an 85°F,

---

RICE Acronym for the standard first-aid treatment for virtually all traumatic and overuse injuries: rest, ice, compression, and elevation.

80 percent humidity day, postpone your usual lunchtime run until the cool of evening.

The three different heat stress illnesses—heat cramps, heat exhaustion, and heatstroke—are progressive in severity. **Heat cramps** (heat-related muscle cramps), the least serious problem, can usually be prevented by warm-ups, adequate fluid replacement, and a diet that includes the electrolytes lost during sweating (sodium and potassium). **Heat exhaustion** is caused by excessive water loss resulting from prolonged exercise or work. Symptoms of heat exhaustion include nausea, headache, fatigue, dizziness and faintness, and, paradoxically, "goosebumps" and chills. If you are suffering from heat exhaustion, your skin will be cool and moist. Heat exhaustion occurs when the body's cooling system falters and circulation slows. **Heatstroke**, often called sunstroke, is a life-threatening emergency with a 20 to 70 percent death rate.[52] Heatstroke occurs during vigorous exercise when the body's heat production significantly exceeds its cooling capacities. Body core temperature can rise from normal (98.6°F) to 105°F to 110°F within minutes after the body's cooling mechanism shuts down. With no cooling taking place, a rapidly increasing core temperature can cause brain damage, permanent disability, and death. Common signs of heatstroke are dry, hot, and usually red skin; very high body temperature; and rapid heart rate.

If you experience any of the symptoms mentioned here, stop exercising immediately. Move to the shade or a cool spot to rest and drink large amounts of cool fluids. Be aware that heat stress can strike in situations in which the danger is not obvious. Serious or fatal heatstroke may result from prolonged sauna, hot tub, or steam bath exposure, or performing activity in lots of heavy clothing and equipment, such as a football uniform.[53]

How much fluid do you need to stay well hydrated and avoid heat stress? The ACSM, along with the National Athletic Trainers Association, recommend consuming 14 to 22 ounces of fluid two hours prior to exercise. Drinking fluids during exercise is also important. For intense exercise, you should drink about 6 to 12 ounces per 15 to 20 minutes. On a daily basis, drink enough fluid so you have to urinate every two to four hours. Your urine should be pale, and there should be lots of it.[54] What are the best fluids to drink? For exercise sessions lasting less than one hour, plain water is sufficient for rehydration. If your exercise session exceeds one hour, consider a sport drink. Athletes such as marathon runners use sport drinks to maintain their electrolyte balance.[55] For athletes in endurance events lasting over 4 hours, the overconsumption of plain water can dilute the sodium concentration in the blood with fatal results, an effect called **hyponatremia**.

Exercising in the Cold

When you exercise in cool weather, especially in windy conditions, your body's rate of heat loss is frequently greater than its rate of heat production. These conditions may lead to **hypothermia**—a potentially fatal condition resulting from abnormally low body core temperature, which occurs when

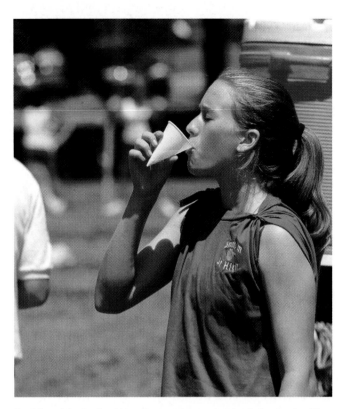

Avoiding dehydration is important when exercising in hot and cold weather, whether to avoid heat exhaustion, heatstroke, or hypothermia.

body heat is lost faster than it is produced. Temperatures need not be frigid for hypothermia to occur; it can also result from prolonged, vigorous exercise (as in snowboarding or rugby) in 40°F to 50°F temperatures, particularly if there is rain, snow, or a strong wind.

In mild cases of hypothermia, as body core temperature drops from the normal 98.6°F to about 93.2°F, you will begin to shiver. Shivering—the involuntary contraction of nearly every muscle in the body—increases body temperature by using the heat given off by muscle activity. During this first

heat cramps Muscle cramps that occur during or following exercise in warm or hot weather.

heat exhaustion A heat stress illness caused by significant dehydration resulting from exercise in warm or hot conditions; frequent precursor to heatstroke.

heat stroke A deadly heat stress illness resulting from dehydration and overexertion in warm or hot conditions; can cause body core temperature to rise from normal to 105°F to 110°F in just a few minutes.

hyponatremia The overconsumption of plain water, which leads to a dilution of sodium concentration in the blood and can have fatal results.

hypothermia Potentially fatal condition caused by abnormally low body core temperature.

stage of hypothermia, you may also experience cold hands and feet, poor judgment, apathy, and amnesia. Shivering ceases in most hypothermia victims as body core temperatures drop to between 87°F and 90°F, a sign that the body has lost its ability to generate heat. Death usually occurs at body core temperatures between 75°F and 80°F.[56]

To prevent hypothermia, follow these commonsense guidelines:

- Analyze weather conditions and your risk of hypothermia before you undertake an outdoor physical activity. Remember that wind and humidity are as significant as temperature.
- Use the "buddy system"—have a friend join you for cold weather outdoor activities.
- Wear layers of appropriate clothing to prevent excessive heat loss (polypropylene or woolen undergarments, a windproof outer garment, and wool hat and gloves). Keep your head, hands, and feet warm.
- Finally, don't allow yourself to become dehydrated. Drink plenty of fluids. Thirst is suppressed in cold environments.[57]

Preventing Cramps

Although most of us have experienced the quick, intense pain of muscle cramps, they are poorly understood. A cramp is an involuntary and forcibly contracted muscle that does not relax. Cramps in legs, feet, arms, abdomen, and along the rib cage are common. A cramp can last a few seconds to 15 minutes or longer. There are several theories about cramping. According to the overexertion theory, when a muscle gets tired, the numerous muscle fibers that comprise it fail to contract in a synchronized rhythm, probably due to overstimulation from the nerves that trigger the muscles to contract.[58] Other theories relate cramping to dehydration. Dehydration may occur simply if someone doesn't consume sufficient liquids to compensate for loss in urine and sweat.

Even if dehydration is not the only cause, it is clearly a problem for those who exercise and perspire heavily. Drinking enough fluids before, during, and after such activity is important.

If you get cramps, what should you do? Generally massage, stretching, putting pressure on the muscle that is cramping, and deep breathing are useful remedies.

TAKING charge

Summary

- The physiological benefits of regular physical activity include (1) reduced risk of heart attack, some cancers, hypertension, and diabetes and (2) improved blood profile, skeletal mass, weight control, immunity to disease, mental health and stress management, and physical fitness. Regular physical activity can also increase life span.
- For general health benefits, it is recommended that every adult participate in moderate-intensity activities for 30 minutes at least 5 days a week. For improvements in cardiorespiratory fitness, you should work out aerobically for at least 20 minutes, a minimum of 3 days per week. The longer the exercise period, the more calories burned and the bigger the improvement in cardiovascular fitness.
- The key principles for developing muscular strength and endurance are the tension principle, the overload principle, and the specificity-of-training principle. The different types of muscle actions include isometric, concentric, and eccentric. Resistance training programs include body weight resistance (calisthenics), fixed resistance, variable resistance, and use of accommodating-resistance devices.
- Flexibility exercises should involve static stretching exercises performed in sets of four or more repetitions held for 15 to 30 seconds, at least two to three days a week. Dynamic stretching is another form of effective stretching. Popular forms of stretching exercise include yoga, tai chi, and Pilates.
- Planning a fitness program involves setting goals and designing a program to achieve these goals. A comprehensive program would include a warm-up period, stretching activities, strength development exercises, an aerobic activity, and a cool-down period.
- Fitness injuries are generally caused by overuse or trauma; the most common are plantar fasciitis, shin splints, and runner's knee. Proper footwear and equipment can help prevent injuries. Exercise in the heat or cold requires special precautions.

Chapter Review

1. What is physical fitness?
   a. The ability to respond to routine physical demands.
   b. Having enough reserves after working out to cope with a sudden challenge.
   c. It is both aerobic and muscular strength.
   d. All of the above.

2. An example of aerobic exercise is
   a. brisk walking.
   b. bench pressing weights.
   c. stretching exercises.
   d. yoga breathing.

3. Flexibility is the range of motion around
   a. specific bones.
   b. specific joints.
   c. the hips and pelvis.
   d. the muscles.

4. The number one obstacle college students cite for not staying physically fit is
   a. lack of money to pay for physical fitness programs.
   b. lack of motivation to work out.
   c. lack of time.
   d. inability to find a workout partner.

5. Which of the following describes a benefit of exercise?
   a. It improves one's mood and reduces stress.
   b. It improves digestion and fat metabolism.
   c. It strengthens bones and increases flexibility.
   d. All of the above.

6. An example of an anaerobic physical activity is
   a. weight lifting.
   b. Pilates step dancing.
   c. bowling.
   d. both A and C.

7. The best example of an *isometric* muscle exercise is
   a. pushing against an immovable object such as a wall.
   b. weight lifting and holding it in place above your head.
   c. forcing your leg muscles to push on the pedals of a stationary bicycle faster.
   d. None of the above.

8. Abby is a cross-country runner and is therefore able to sustain moderate-intensity, whole-body activity for extended periods of time. This ability relates to what component of physical fitness?
   a. flexibility
   b. body composition
   c. cardiorespiratory fitness
   d. muscular strength and endurance

9. In resistance training, the most important key principle for improved muscular endurance is
   a. tension.
   b. overload.
   c. specificity of training.
   d. core strength.

10. Which of the following *best* defines the major difference between muscular strength and muscular endurance?
    a. Muscular strength refers to the amount of force a muscle is capable of exerting.
    b. Muscular endurance is how long one can hold a heavy weight without collapsing.
    c. Muscular endurance is only of a static nature.
    d. None of the above.

Answers to these questions can be found on page A-1.

Questions for Discussion and Reflection

1. How do you define physical fitness? What are the key components of a physical fitness program? What might you need to consider when beginning a fitness program?
2. How would you determine the proper intensity and duration of an exercise program? How often should exercise sessions be scheduled?
3. Why is stretching vital to improving physical flexibility?
4. Identify at least four physiological and psychological benefits of physical fitness. How would you promote these benefits to nonexercisers?
5. Describe the different types of resistance employed in an exercise program. What are the benefits of each type of resistance?
6. Your roommate has decided to start running first thing in the morning in an effort to lose weight, tone muscles, and improve cardiorespiratory fitness. What advice would you give to make sure your roommate gets off to a good start and doesn't get injured?
7. What key components would you include in a fitness program for yourself?

Accessing Your Health on the Internet

The following websites explore further topics and issues related to personal health. You'll also find links to each organization's website on the Companion Website for *Access to Health*, Tenth Edition, at www.aw-bc.com/donatelle.

1. *ACSM Online.* A link with the American College of Sports Medicine and all its resources. www.acsm.org
2. *American Council on Exercise.* Information on exercise and disease prevention. www.acefitness.org
3. *Just Move.* The American Heart Association's fitness website has the latest information on heart disease and exercise, plus a guide to local, regional, and national fitness events. www.justmove.org
4. *Centers for Disease Control and Prevention, National Center for Chronic Disease Prevention and Health Promotion, Division of Nutrition and Physical Activity.* A resource for current information on exercise and health. www.cdc.gov/nccdphp/dnpa
5. *National Strength and Conditioning Association.* A resource for personal trainers and others interested in conditioning and fitness. www.nsca-lift.org
6. *Presidents Council on Physical Fitness and Sports.* Provides information on fitness programs. www.fitness.gov

Further Reading

Fahey, T. D. *Super Fitness for Sports, Conditioning, and Health.* Boston: Allyn & Bacon, 2000.

> *A brief guide to developing fitness that emphasizes training techniques for improving sports performance.*

Powers, S. K., S. L. Dodd, and V. J. Noland. *Total Fitness and Wellness,* 4th ed. San Francisco: Benjamin Cummings, 2006.

> *A complete guide to improving all areas of fitness, including being a smart health consumer, interviews with fitness specialists, and the links between nutrition and fitness.*

Schlosberg, S. *The Ultimate Workout Log: An Exercise Diary and Fitness Guide.* Boston: Houghton Mifflin, 1999.

> *A six-month log that also provides fitness definitions, training tips, and motivational quotes.*

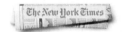

e-themes from *The New York Times*

For up-to-date articles about current health issues, visit www.aw-bc.com/donatelle, select *Access to Health,* Tenth Edition, Chapter 10, and click on "e-themes."

References

1. American College Health Association (ACHA), *American College Health Association-National College Health Assessment Reference Group Data Report, 2005* (Baltimore: ACHA, 2006).
2. Ibid.; National Center for Chronic Disease Prevention and Health Promotion, *Physical Activity for Everyone: The Importance of Physical Activity* (Atlanta: Centers for Disease Control and Prevention, 2006), www.cdc.gov/nccdphp/dnpa/physical/importance/index.htm.
3. American Heart Association, "Cardiovascular Disease Rates, 2006," www.americanheart.org/presenter.jhtml?identifier=4478; Centers for Disease Control and Prevention, "Fact Sheet: Number of Americans with Diabetes Continues to Rise," 2006, www.cdc.gov/od/oc/media/pressrel/fs051026.htm.
4. National Center for Chronic Disease Prevention and Health Promotion, *Physical Activity for Everyone.*
5. U.S. Department of Health and Human Services, *Physical Activity and Health: A Report of the Surgeon General* (Atlanta: Centers for Disease Control, National Center for Chronic Disease Prevention and Health Promotion, 1996.
6. Ibid.
7. National Center for Chronic Disease Prevention and Health Promotion, "Nutrition and Physical Activity Recommendations," 2004, www.cdc.gov/nccdphp/dnpa/physical/recommendations/index.htm.
8. Ibid.
9. C. B. Corbin et al., *Concepts of Physical Fitness,* 13th ed. (Boston: McGraw-Hill, 2006).
10. A. Colin et al., "Cardiorespiratory Fitness, Physical Activity, and Arterial Stiffness: The Northern Ireland Young Hearts Project," *Hypertension* 44 (2004): 721–726.
11. American Heart Association, "The Number of Adults in the U.S. with High Blood Pressure Rose in the Last Decade," 2004, www.americanheart.org/presenter.jhtml?identifier=3024254.
12. W. Wang et al., "A Longitudinal Study of Hypertension Risk Factors and Their Relation to Cardiovascular Disease," *Hypertension* 47 (2006): 403.
13. American College of Sports Medicine, *ACSM's Certification Review,* 2nd ed. (Lippincott Williams & Wilkins, 2006).
14. American Stroke Association, "American Heart Association: Cholesterol," 2006, www.strokeassociation.org.

15. G. A. Colditz et al., "Physical Activity and Risk of Breast Cancer in Premenopausal Women," *British Journal of Cancer* 89, no. 5 (2003): 847–851; A. K. Samad et al., "A Meta-Analysis of the Association of Physical Activity with Risk of Colorectal Cancer," *Colorectal Disease* 7, no. 3 (2005): 204–213; L. Bernstein et al., "Lifetime Recreational Exercise Activity and Breast Cancer Risk Among Black and White Women," *Journal of the National Cancer Institute* 77, no. 22 (2005): 1671–1679.

16. T. J. Key et al., "Diet, Nutrition, and the Prevention of Cancer," *Public Health Nutrition,* no. 1A (February 7, 2004): 187–200.

17. K. J. Stewart et al., "Exercise Effects on Bone Mineral Density Relationships to Changes in Fitness and Fatness," *American Journal of Preventive Medicine* 28, no. 5 (2005): 453–460.

18. Ibid.

19. W. McArdle, F. Katch, and V. Katch, *Exercise Physiology,* 6th ed. (Philadelphia: Lippincott Williams and Wilkins, 2006), 60–65.

20. University of Colorodo Health Sciences Center, "National Weight Control Registry," www.uchsc.edu/nutrition/WyattJortberg/nwcr.html.

21. American College of Sports Medicine, "Exercise Recommendations," *Guidelines for Physical Activity,* www.acsm.org/pdf/Guidelines.pdf.

22. S. Lee et al., "Exercise Without Weight Loss Is an Effective Strategy for Obesity Reduction in Obese Individuals With or Without Type 2 Diabetes," *Journal of Applied Physiology* 99, no. 3 (2005): 1220–1225.

23. American Diabetes Association, "Diabetes Risk Test," 2004, www.diabetes.org/risk-test.jsp.

24. D. E. Laaksonen et al., "Physical Activity in the Prevention of Type 2 Diabetes: The Finnish Diabetes Prevention Study," *Diabetes* 54, no. 1 (2005): 158–165.

25. J. Shaw, "The Deadliest Sin," *Harvard Magazine,* March/April 2004.

26. National Center for Chronic Disease Prevention and Health Promotion, "Physical Activity and Health."

27. O. H. Franco et al., "Effects of Physical Activity on Life Expectancy with Cardiovascular Disease," *Archives of Internal Medicine,* 165, no. 20 (2005): 2355–2360.

28. E. Quinn, "Exercise and Immunity," *Sports Medicine,* 2004, http://sportsmedicine.about.com/cs/exercisephysiology/a/aa100303a.htm.

29. E. Tiollier et al., "Intense Training: Mucosal Immunity and Incidence of Respiratory Infections," *European Journal of Applied Physiology* 93, no. 4: 421–428, 2006.

30. B. F. Burke, "Exercise and Immunity," *MedLine Plus,* National Institutes of Health, April 19, 2004, www.nlm.nih.gov/medlineplus/ency/article/007165.htm.

31. Ibid.

32. L. M. Hays, T. M. Damush, and D. O. Clark, "Relationships Between Exercise Self-Definitions and Exercise Participation among Urban Women in Primary Care," *Journal of Cardiovascular Nursing* 20, no. 1 (2005): 9–17.

33. Centers for Disease Control and Prevention, "Calories Per Hour," 2006, www.cdc.gov/nccdphp/dnpa/spotlights/calories_per_hour_table.htm.

34. J. Gavin, *Life Fitness Coaching* (Champaign, IL: Human Kinetics, 2005).

35. American College Health Association (ACHA), *American College Health Association-National College Health Assessment Reference Group Data Report.*

36. J. Orvis, "Weight Training Workouts That Work," Volume II (Farmington, MN: Ideal Publishing, 2004).

37. S. J. Fleck and W. I. Kraemer, *Designing Resistance Training Programs,* 3rd ed. (Champaign, IL: Human Kinetics, 2004).

38. American Council on Exercise, *Personal Trainer Manual: Resource for Fitness Professionals,* 3rd ed. (Indianapolis: American College of Sports Medicine, 2003).

39. Mayo Clinic, "Core Exercises: Beyond Your Average Abs Routine," October 6, 2005, www.mayoclinic.com/health/core-exercises/SM00071.

40. P. A. Adler and B. L. Roberts, "The Use of Tai Chi to Improve Health in Older Adults," *Orthopedic Nursing* 25, no. 2 (2006): 122–126.

41. Arthritis Foundation, "Exercise and Arthritis," 2004, www.arthritis.org/conditions/exercise.

42. J. W. Smith, "Flexibility Basics: Physiology, Research, and Current Guidelines" *ACSM Certified News* 14, no. 3 (2004): 7–9.

43. T. Little, "Effects of Differential Stretching Protocols During Warm-Ups on High-Speed Motor Capacities of Professional Soccer Players," *Journal of Strength and Conditioning Research* 20, no. 1 (2006): 203–207.

44. International Fitness Association, "Types of Stretching," 2004, www.ifafitness.com/stretch/stretch4.htm#SEC2.

45. American College of Sports Medicine, *ACSM Certification Review, 2006* (Philadelphia: Lippincott Williams and Wilkins, 2005).

46. U. G. Kersting and G. P. Bruggemann, "Midsole Material-Related Force Control During Heel-Toe Running," *Research in Sports Medicine* 14, no. 1 (2006): 1–17.

47. American Academy of Ophthalmology, "Play Sports Safely—Use Eye Protection," 2003, www.medem.com/search/article-detailb.cfm?article-id=222egmlpkc850bcat=32

48. Bicycle Helmet Safety Institute, "A Compendium of Statistics," 2004, www.bhsi.org/stats.htm.

49. D. Ritchie, "Plantar Fasciitis: Treatment Pearls," American Academy of Podiatric Sports Medicine, www.aapsm.org/plantar_fasciitis.html.

50. J. Cluett, "About Shin Splints," 2006, www.orthopedics.about.com/cs/sportsmedicine/a/shinsplint-2.htm.

51. American Academy of Orthopaedic Surgeons, "Runner's Knee," 2003, http://orthoinfo.aaos.org/fact/thr_report.cfm?Thread_ID=417&topcategory=Knee.

52. N. M. Lugo-Amador, T. Rothenhaus, and P. Mover, "Heat-Related Illness," *Emergency Medical Clinics of North America* 22, no. 2 (2004): 315–327.

53. International Fitness Association, *Aerobics and Fitness Institute Certification Coursebook* (Orlando, FL: International Fitness Association, 2004), http://ifafitness.com/book1.

54. Dieticians in Sports and Exercise Nutrition, "Fluid and Hydration in Sport," 2004, www.disen.org/nutrition/pages-to-edit/fluids.htm.

55. S. M. Shirreffs et al., "Fluid and Electrolyte Needs for Preparation and Recovery from Training and Competition," *Journal of Sports Science* 22, no. 1 (2004): 57–63.

56. R. Curtis, *Outdoor Action Guide to Hypothermia and Cold Weather Injuries* (Atlanta: Centers for Disease Control and Prevention, 2006).

57. American Council on Exercise, *Exercising in the Cold, 2006* (Indianapolis: American Council on Exercise, 2006).

58. N. Clark, "Muscle Cramps: Do They Cramp Your Style?" *Newsletter of the American College of Sports Medicine,* no. 7 (Summer 2001).

11

Addictions and Addictive Behavior

THREATS TO WELLNESS

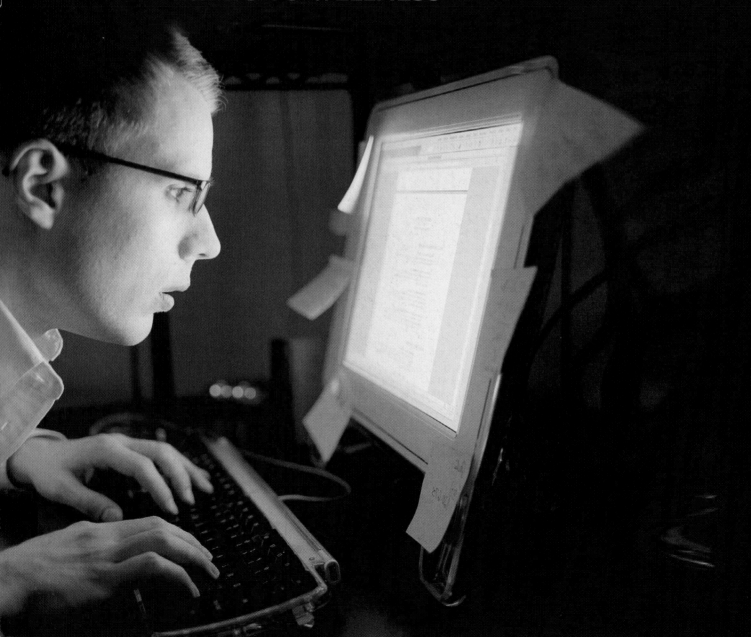

What makes **addiction** different from a habit?

How can I recognize **addiction** in a loved one or even myself?

Do some people have more **addictive** personalities than others?

Is my roommate's **obsessive** video-game playing an addiction?

How can I **approach** someone who needs help and treatment?

OBJECTIVES

- Define addiction.
- Distinguish addictions from habits, and identify the signs of addiction.
- Discuss the addictive process, the physiology of addiction, and the biopsychosocial model of addiction.
- Describe types of addictions, including gambling, work, exercise, sexual, and Internet addictions, as well as codependence.
- Evaluate treatment and recovery options for addicts, including individual therapy, group therapy, family therapy, and 12-step programs.

It isn't difficult these days to find high-profile cases of compulsive and destructive behavior. Stories of celebrities and politicians struggling with addictions to alcohol, drugs, and sex are splashed in the headlines and profiled on television news programs. But millions of "everyday" people throughout the world are staging their own battles with addiction as well. Addictions can be perplexing, because many potentially addictive activities may actually enhance the lives of those who engage in them moderately. In addition to alcohol and drugs, the most commonly recognized objects of addiction include food, sex, relationships, spending money, work, exercise, gambling, and using the Internet.

Defining Addiction

Addiction is continued involvement with a substance or activity despite ongoing negative consequences. Addictive behaviors initially provide a sense of pleasure or stability that is beyond the addict's power to achieve in other ways. Eventually, the addicted person needs to be involved in the behavior in order to feel normal.

In this chapter, *addiction* is used interchangeably with *physiological addiction.* However, **physiological dependence**, the adaptive state that occurs with regular addictive behavior and results in withdrawal syndrome, is only one indicator of addiction. Psychological dynamics play an important role, which explains why behaviors not related to the use of chemicals—gambling, for example—may also be addictive. A person who possesses a strong desire to continue engaging in a particular activity is said to have developed a psychological dependence. In fact, psychological and physiological dependence are so intertwined that it is not really possible to separate the two. For every psychological state, there is a corresponding physiological state. In other words, everything you feel is tied to a chemical process occurring in your body.[1] Thus, addictions once thought to be entirely psychological in nature are now understood to have physiological components.

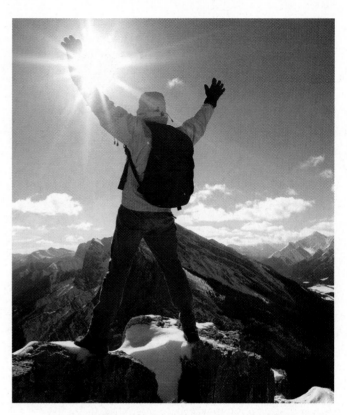

The euphoric feeling we have after successfully completing an achievement or experiencing joy is mimicked by addictive substances and the chemical reactions they trigger in our brain.

To be addictive, a behavior must have the potential to produce a positive mood change. Chemicals are responsible for the most profound addictions, not only because they produce dramatic mood changes, but also because they cause cellular changes to which the body adapts so well that it eventually requires the chemical in order to function normally. Yet other behaviors, such as gambling, spending money, working, and sex, also create changes at the cellular level along with positive mood changes. Although the mechanism is not well understood, all forms of addiction probably reflect dysfunction of certain biochemical systems in the brain.[2]

Traditionally, diagnosis of an addiction was limited to drug addiction and was based on four criteria, as defined by the American Psychological Association:

1. Use for the purpose of relieving **withdrawal** symptoms—a series of temporary physical and psychological symptoms that occurs when the addicted person abruptly stops using the drug.

2. Continued use of the substance despite knowledge of the harm it causes yourself and others (deterioration in work performance, relationships, and social interaction).

3. Unsuccessful efforts to cut down or cease using the drug, including **relapse,** the tendency to return to the addictive behavior after a period of abstinence.

addiction Continued involvement with a substance or activity despite ongoing negative consequences.

physiological dependence The adaptive state that occurs with regular addictive behavior and results in withdrawal syndrome.

withdrawal A series of temporary physical and biopsychosocial symptoms that occur when the addict abruptly abstains from an addictive chemical or behavior.

relapse The tendency to return to the addictive behavior after a period of abstinence.

4. **Tolerance,** or an acquired reaction to a drug in which continued intake of the same dose has diminished effects. In response to tolerance, drug users must increase the dose in order to achieve the desired effect.

Until recently, health professionals were unwilling to diagnose an addiction until medical symptoms appeared in the patient. Now we know that although withdrawal, pathological behavior, relapse, and medical symptoms are valid indicators of addiction (we'll examine these more closely later in the chapter), they do not characterize all addictive behavior.

Habit versus Addiction

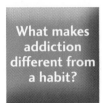
What makes addiction different from a habit?

How do we distinguish between a harmless habit and an addiction? The stereotypical image of the addict is of someone desperately seeking a fix 24 hours a day. People have the notion that if you aren't doing the behavior every day, you're not addicted. The reality is somewhere between these two extremes.

Addiction certainly involves elements of **habit,** a repeated behavior in which the repetition may be unconscious. A habit can be annoying, but it can be broken without too much discomfort by simply becoming aware of its presence and choosing not to do it. Addiction also involves repetition of a behavior, but the repetition occurs by **compulsion,** and considerable discomfort is experienced if the behavior is not performed. An addiction is a habit that has gotten out of control and has negative health effects.

To understand addiction, we need to look beyond the amount and frequency of the behavior, for what happens when a person is involved in the behavior is far more meaningful. For example, someone who drinks only rarely, and then in moderation, may experience personality changes, blackouts (drug-induced amnesia), and other negative consequences (for example, failing a test, missing an important appointment, getting into a fight) that would never have occurred had the person not taken a few drinks. On the other hand, someone who has a few martinis every evening may never do anything out of character while under the influence of alcohol but may become irritable, manipulative, and aggressive without those regular drinks. For both of these people, alcohol appears to perform a function (mood control) that people should be able to perform without the aid of chemicals, which is a possible sign of addiction. Habits are behaviors that occur through choice and typically do not cause negative health consequences. In contrast, no one decides to become addicted, even though people make choices that contribute to the development of an addiction.

Signs of Addiction

If you asked ten people to define addiction, you would quite possibly get ten different responses. Studies show that all animals share the same basic pleasure and reward circuits in the brain that turn on when they come into contact with addictive substances or engage in something pleasurable, such as eating or orgasm. We all engage in potentially addictive behaviors to some extent because some are essential to our survival and are highly reinforcing, such as eating, drinking, and sex. At some point along the continuum, however, some individuals are not able to engage in these or other behaviors moderately and become addicted.

How can I recognize addiction in a loved one or even myself?

Although different opinions exist as to the cause of addiction, most experts agree on some universal signs of it. All addictions are characterized by four common symptoms: (1) compulsion, which is characterized by **obsession**, or excessive preoccupation with the behavior and an overwhelming need to perform it; (2) **loss of control,** or the inability to predict reliably whether any isolated occurrence of the behavior will be healthy or damaging; (3) **negative consequences**, such as physical damage, legal trouble, financial problems, academic failure, and family dissolution, which do not occur with healthy involvement in any behavior; and (4) **denial**, or the inability to perceive that the behavior is self-destructive.

These four components are present in all addictions, whether chemical or behavioral.

what do you THINK?

Have you ever seen signs of addiction in a friend or family member? ■ What types of negative consequences have you witnessed? ■ Can you think of any habits you have that could potentially become addictive?

---

tolerance   Phenomenon in which progressively larger doses of a drug or more intense involvement in a behavior are needed to produce the desired effects.

habit   A repeated behavior in which the repetition may be unconscious.

compulsion   Obsessive preoccupation with a behavior and an overwhelming need to perform it.

obsession   Excessive preoccupation with an addictive object or behavior.

loss of control   Inability to predict reliably whether a particular instance of involvement with the addictive object or behavior will be healthy or damaging.

negative consequences   Physical damage, legal trouble, financial problems, academic failure, family dissolution, and other severe problems associated with addiction.

denial   Inability to perceive or accurately interpret the effects of the addictive behavior.

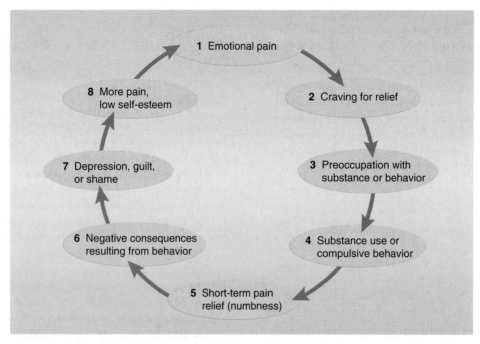

FIGURE 11.1 Cycle of Psychological Addiction

Source: From R. Goldberg, *Drugs Across the Spectrum,* 5th ed. Copyright 2006. Reprinted with permission of Brooks/Cole, a division of Thomson Learning: www.thomsonrights.com. Fax 800-730-2215.

The Addictive Process

Addiction is a process that evolves over time. It begins when a person repeatedly seeks the illusion of relief to avoid unpleasant feelings or situations. This pattern is known as **nurturing through avoidance** and is a maladaptive way of taking care of emotional needs. As a person becomes increasingly dependent on the addictive behavior, there is a corresponding deterioration in relationships with family, friends, and coworkers; in performance at work or school; and in personal life. Eventually, addicts do not find the addictive behavior pleasurable but consider it preferable to the unhappy realities they are seeking to escape. Figure 11.1 illustrates the cycle of psychological addiction.

The Physiology of Addiction

Virtually all intellectual, emotional, and behavioral functions occur as a result of biochemical interactions between nerve cells in the body. Biochemical messengers, called **neurotransmitters,** exert their influence at specific receptor sites on nerve cells. Drug use and chronic stress can alter these receptor sites and cause the production and breakdown of neurotransmitters.

Mood-altering chemicals, for example, fill up the receptor sites for the body's natural "feel-good" neurotransmitters (endorphins) so that nerve cells are fooled into believing they have enough neurotransmitters and shut down production of these substances temporarily. When the drug use stops, those receptor sites empty, resulting in uncomfortable feelings that remain until the body resumes normal neurotransmitter production or the person consumes more of the drug. Some people's bodies naturally produce insufficient quantities of these neurotransmitters, so they are predisposed to seek out chemicals such as alcohol as substitutes or pursue behaviors such as exercise that increase natural production. Thus, some may be "wired" to seek out substances or experiences that increase pleasure or reduce discomfort.

Mood-altering substances and experiences produce *tolerance,* defined earlier as a phenomenon in which progressively larger doses of a drug or more intense involvement in an experience are needed to obtain the desired effects. All of us develop some degree of tolerance to any mood-altering experience. But because addicts tend to seek intense mood-altering experiences, they eventually increase the amount and intensity to the point of causing negative side effects.

Withdrawal is another phenomenon associated with mood-altering experiences. The drug or activity replaces or causes

nurturing through avoidance Repeatedly seeking the illusion of relief to avoid unpleasant feelings or situations, a maladaptive way of taking care of emotional needs.

neurotransmitters Biochemical messengers that exert influence at specific receptor sites on nerve cells.

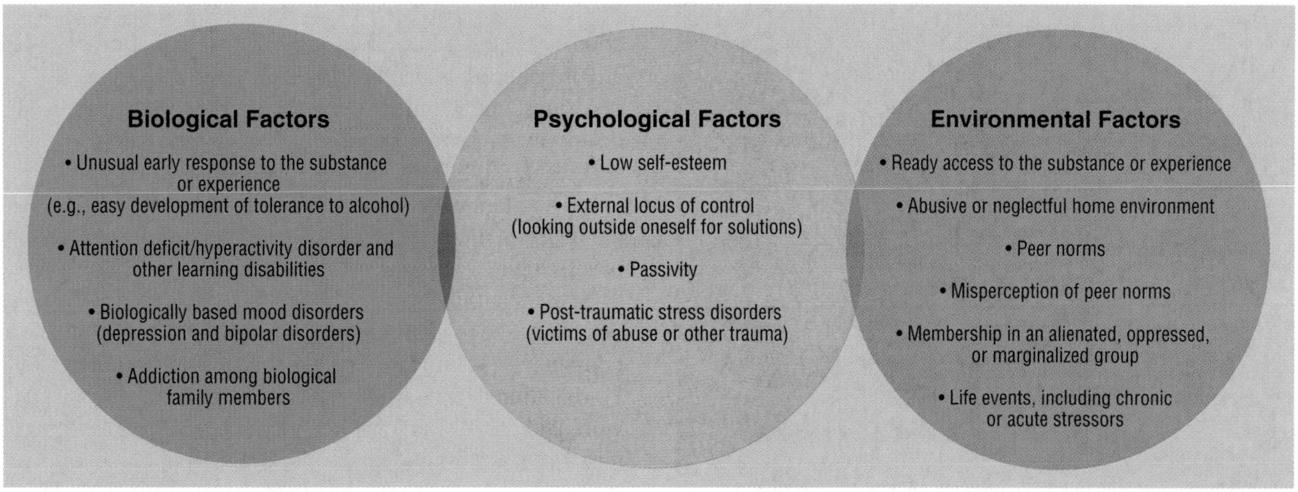

FIGURE 11.2 Risk Factors for Addiction

an effect that the body should normally provide on its own. If the experience is repeated often enough, the body adjusts: it starts to require the drug or experience to obtain the effect. Stopping the behavior will cause a withdrawal syndrome because the body cannot naturally create the same effect as the drug.

Withdrawal symptoms of chemical dependencies are generally the opposite of the effects of the drug being withdrawn. For example, a cocaine addict experiences a characteristic "crash" (depression and lethargy), while a barbiturate addict experiences trembling, irritability, and convulsions upon withdrawal. Withdrawal symptoms for addictive behaviors are usually less dramatic. They usually involve psychological discomfort such as anxiety, depression, irritability, guilt, anger, and frustration, with an underlying preoccupation with or craving for another exposure to the behavior.

Withdrawal syndromes range from mild to severe. The most severe form of withdrawal syndrome is delirium tremens (DTs), which occurs in approximately 5 percent of dependent individuals withdrawing from alcohol.

Psychological Factors

Do some people have more addictive personalities than others?

A person's individual psychological makeup also factors into the potential for addiction. People with low self-esteem, a tendency toward risk-taking behavior, or poor coping skills are more likely to develop addictive patterns of behavior. Individuals who consistently look outside themselves (who have an external locus of control) for solutions and explanations for life events are more likely to experience addiction.

The complexity of addiction and consistent evidence of multiple contributing factors lead us to conclude that addiction is not the result of a single influence, but rather of a variety of influences working together. Biological, psychological,

and environmental factors all contribute to its development. Although one factor may play a larger role than another in a specific individual, a single factor is rarely sufficient to explain an addiction. Figure 11.2 lists risk factors for addiction.

A Model of Addiction

Biological or disease models of addiction have been proposed since ancient times. However, it has become clear through time that psychological and environmental factors may also be involved in the development of addiction. The most effective treatment today is being provided by those who rely on the **biopsychosocial model of addiction**, which proposes that addiction is caused by a variety of factors operating together, thereby lending credibility to all the other theories. The biopsychosocial model is not a compromise solution to a theoretical controversy. Rather, it represents a reasonable comprehension of all that we have learned about addiction.

Biological or Disease Influences Addiction for many is thought to be based in the brain, involving memory, motivation, and emotional state. The processes involved in these aspects of brain function have thus become logical targets for gene research into assessing the underlying risk for addiction, in particular addiction to alcohol and other substances. Studies show that people addicted to mood-altering substances metabolize these substances differently than nonaddicted people. Research does suggest that genes affecting the activity of the neurotransmitters serotonin and

biopsychosocial model of addiction Theory of the relationship between an addict's biological (genetic) nature and psychological and environmental influences.

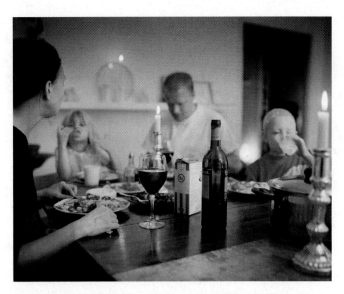

One predisposing factor for developing an addiction might be environmental influences such as how we are raised. For example, in other cultures, alcohol is treated as a normal part of life, and is not abused as it is by young people in the United States.

GABA (gamma-aminobutyric acid) are likely candidates for involvement in the risk for alcoholism.[3] For example, a study found that college students with a particular variant of the serotonin transporter gene consumed more alcohol per occasion, drank expressly to become inebriated more often, and engaged more frequently in heavy drinking than students with another variant of the gene. The relationships between neurotransmitters and alcoholism are complex, however; not all studies have shown a connection between alcoholism risk and these genes.[4]

Studies also support a genetic influence on addiction. It has been known for centuries that alcoholism runs in families. Studies in recent years have confirmed that identical twins, who share the same genes, are about twice as likely as fraternal twins, who share an average of 50 percent of their genes, to resemble each other in terms of the presence of alcoholism. Studies also show that 50 to 60 percent of the risk for alcoholism is genetically determined for both men and women.[5]

Environmental Influences
Cultural expectations and mores help determine whether people engage in certain behaviors. For example, although many native Italians use alcohol abundantly, there is a low incidence of alcoholism

in this culture. Low rates of alcoholism typically exist in countries such as Italy and France, where children are gradually introduced to alcohol in diluted amounts, on special occasions, and within a strong family group. There is deep disapproval of intoxication, which is not viewed as socially acceptable, stylish, or funny.[6] Such cultural traditions and values are less widespread in the United States, where the incidence of alcohol addiction and alcohol-related problems is very high.

Societal attitudes and messages also influence addictive behavior. The media's emphasis on appearance and the ideal body plays a significant role in exercise addiction. Societal glorification of money and material achievement can lead to work addiction, which is often admired. Societal changes, in turn, influence individual norms. People living in cities characterized by rapid social change or social disorganization often feel less connected to social, religious, and civic institutions. The resulting disenfranchisement leads to increased destructive behaviors, including addiction.[7]

Social learning theory proposes that people learn behaviors by watching role models—parents, caregivers, and significant others. The effects of modeling, imitation, and identification with behavior from early childhood on are well documented. Modeling is especially influential when it involves behavior that is mood altering. Many studies show that modeling by parents and by idolized celebrities exerts a profound influence on young people.[8]

On an individual level, major stressful life events, such as marriage, divorce, change in work status, and death of a loved one, may trigger addictive behaviors. The death of a spouse is the most common trigger event for excessive drinking among the elderly. Traumatic events in general often instigate addictive behaviors, as traumatized people seek to medicate their pain—pain they may not even be aware of because they've repressed it. One thing that makes addictive behaviors so powerfully attractive is that they reliably alleviate personal pain, at least for a short time. However, this relief of pain through addictive behaviors is only temporary; addictive behaviors actually cause more pain than they relieve. Family members whose needs for love, security, and affirmation are not consistently met; who are refused permission to express their feelings, desires, or needs; and who frequently submerge their personalities to "keep the peace" are prone to addiction. Children whose parents are not consistently available to them (physically or emotionally); who are subjected to sexual abuse, physical abuse, neglect, or abandonment; or who receive inconsistent or disparaging messages about their self-worth may experience psychosocial or physical illness and addiction in adulthood.

social learning theory Theory that people learn behaviors by watching role models—parents, caregivers, and significant others.

 what do you THINK?

Which factors discussed in this section do you think play the biggest role in addiction? ■ Do you think some addictions have a biological basis? Why?

Types of Addiction

It is difficult to document the incidence of addictions of any kind because involvement with a chemical or a behavior does not, by itself, indicate addiction. Nevertheless, many studies on morbidity and mortality associated with a substance or behavior provide reasonable estimates.

Clearly, tobacco, alcohol, and other drugs are addictive, and addictions to these drugs create multiple problems for addicted individuals as well as their families and society. Later chapters in this book will discuss specific substance-related addictions. In this chapter we examine the fundamental concepts and process of addiction, as well as its associated problems. We will also look at what are commonly called **process addictions**—behaviors known to be addictive because they are mood altering. Examples include compulsive shopping, gambling, work, exercise, Internet use, and sexual addictions.

Compulsive or Pathological Gambling

Gambling is a form of recreation and entertainment for millions of Americans. Most people who gamble do so casually and moderately to experience the excitement of anticipating a win.

However, over 3 million Americans are **compulsive, or pathological, gamblers** (addicted to gambling), and 15 million more are considered at risk for developing a gambling addiction.[9] The American Psychiatric Association (APA) recognizes pathological gambling as a mental disorder and lists ten characteristic behaviors including preoccupation with gambling, unsuccessful efforts to cut back or quit, using gambling to escape problems, and lying to family members to conceal the extent of involvement with gambling.

Gamblers and drug addicts describe many similar cravings and highs. A recent study supports what many experts believe to be true: that compulsive gambling is like drug addiction. Compulsive gamblers in this study were found to have decreased blood flow to a key section of the brain's reward system. Much like those who abuse drugs, it is thought that compulsive gamblers compensate for this deficiency in their brain's reward system by overdoing it and getting hooked.[10] Most compulsive gamblers state that they seek excitement even more than money. They place progressively larger bets to obtain the desired level of excitement. See the gambling portion of the Assess Yourself box on page 356 to evaluate your gambling behavior.

Who is at risk for getting hooked on the rush of gambling? Men are more likely to have gambling problems than women are. Gambling prevalence is also higher among lower-income individuals, those who are divorced, African Americans, older adults, and individuals residing within 50 miles of a casino. Residents in southern states, where opportunities to gamble have increased significantly over the past 20 years, also have higher gambling rates.[11]

College student gambling appears to be on the rise on college campuses across the nation. In a telephone poll conducted by University of Pennsylvania's Annenburg Public Policy Center, it was reported that in 2005, 15.5 percent of college students reported gambling once a week, up from 8.3 percent in 2002, an 87 percent increase. Males were dominant in the gambling scene; 26 percent reported gambling each week, while 5.5 percent of females reported gambling weekly.[12]

What accounts for this trend? College students have easier access to gambling opportunities than ever before with the advent of online gambling, a growing number of casinos, scratch tickets, lotteries, and sports-betting networks. In particular, the largest boost has been from the increasing popularity of poker. Access to poker on the Internet and poker tournaments that are frequently televised have brought a resurgence of the game, with many young people spending an unhealthy amount of time and money participating in online poker tournaments.

Other characteristics associated with gambling among college students include spending more time watching TV, using computers for nonacademic purposes, less time studying, lower grades, participation in intercollegiate athletics, and more likelihood of engaging in heavy, episodic drinking and use of illicit drugs in the past year.[13] See the Spotlight on Your Health box on page 360 for more on college students and gambling.

Whereas casual gamblers can stop anytime they wish and are capable of seeing the necessity to do so, compulsive gamblers are unable to control the urge to gamble even in the face of devastating consequences: high debt, legal problems, and the loss of everything meaningful, including homes, families, jobs, health, and even their lives. Gambling can have a detrimental effect on health: cardiovascular problems affect 38 percent of compulsive gamblers, and their suicide rate is 20 times higher than that of the general population.

Compulsive Shopping and Borrowing

Although compulsive spending has been a pervasive problem in the United States for some time, a more insidious form of the addiction lurks in the new "plastic generation." Credit

(Text continues on page 360)

> **process addictions** Behaviors such as money addiction, work addiction, exercise addiction, and sex addiction that are known to be addictive because they are mood altering.
>
> **compulsive (pathological) gambler** A person addicted to gambling.

ASSESS yourself

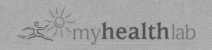

ARE YOU ADDICTED?

Fill out this assessment online at www.aw-bc.com/myhealthlab or www.aw-bc.com/donatelle.

We may not always recognize addictive behaviors in ourselves or even our closest friends. This simple exercise will help you in two ways: (1) if you already know or strongly believe you are addicted to one of the behaviors below, this guide will assist you in identifying the areas in your life most impacted by your compulsive behavior and (2) if you're not sure whether you are addicted, this will help you determine the answer and assess the damage. When answering, consider only the time you spend participating in the behavior at the expense of academic, work, and social responsibilities.

INTERNET ADDICTION

Internet addiction is not simply a matter of time spent online. Some people indicate they are addicted with only 20 hours in a given period of time such as per week of Internet use, while others who spend much more time online insist it is not a problem for them. It's more important to measure how your Internet use affects your life. Have any conflicts emerged in family, relationships, work, or school?

Circle the answer that most closely describes your behavior.

	Rarely	Occasionally	Frequently	Often	Always
1. How often do you find that you stay online longer than you intended?	1	2	3	4	5
2. How often do you neglect household chores to spend more time online?	1	2	3	4	5
3. How often do you prefer the excitement of the Internet to intimacy with your partner?	1	2	3	4	5
4. How often do you form new relationships with fellow online users?	1	2	3	4	5
5. How often do others in your life complain to you about the amount of time you spend online?	1	2	3	4	5
6. How often do your grades or school work suffer because of the amount of time you spend online?	1	2	3	4	5
7. How often do you check your e-mail before something else that you need to do?	1	2	3	4	5
8. How often does your job performance or productivity suffer because of the Internet?	1	2	3	4	5
9. How often do you become defensive or secretive when anyone else asks you what you do online?	1	2	3	4	5
10. How often do you block out disturbing thoughts about your life with soothing thoughts about the Internet?	1	2	3	4	5
11. How often do you find yourself anticipating when you will go online again?	1	2	3	4	5
12. How often do you fear that life without the Internet would be boring, empty, and joyless?	1	2	3	4	5
13. How often do you snap, yell, or act annoyed if someone bothers you while you are online?	1	2	3	4	5
14. How often do you lose sleep to late-night log-ons?	1	2	3	4	5
15. How often do you feel preoccupied with the Internet when offline or fantasize about being online?	1	2	3	4	5
16. How often do you find yourself saying "just a few more minutes" when online?	1	2	3	4	5

	Rarely	Occasionally	Frequently	Often	Always
17. How often do you try to cut down the amount of time you spend online and fail?	1	2	3	4	5
18. How often do you try to hide how long you've been online?	1	2	3	4	5
19. How often do you choose to spend more time online over going out with others?	1	2	3	4	5
20. How often do you feel depressed, moody, or nervous when you are offline? Do these feelings go away once you are back online?	1	2	3	4	5

Interpreting Your Scores for This Section

After you have answered all the questions, add the numbers you selected for each response to obtain a final score. The higher your score, the greater your level of addiction and the problems your Internet usage causes.

20–49 points: You are an average Internet user. You may surf the Web a bit too long at times, but you have control over your usage.

50–79 points: You are experiencing occasional or frequent problems because of the Internet. You should consider the Internet's full impact on your life.

80–100 points: Your Internet usage is causing significant problems in your life. You should evaluate the impact of the Internet on your life and address the problems directly caused by your Internet usage.

COMPULSIVE GAMBLING

Answer Yes or No to the following questions:

	Yes	No
1. Do you ever lose time at school or work due to gambling?	❏	❏
2. Did you ever gamble to get money with which to pay debts or otherwise solve financial difficulties?	❏	❏
3. After losing did you feel you must return to gambling as soon as possible to win back your losses?	❏	❏
4. Do you often gamble until your last dollar is gone?	❏	❏
5. Do you ever borrow to finance your gambling?	❏	❏
6. Have you ever sold anything to finance your gambling?	❏	❏
7. Did you ever gamble longer than you had planned?	❏	❏
8. Have you ever gambled to escape worry or trouble?	❏	❏
9. Has gambling ever made your life unhappy?	❏	❏
10. Has gambling ever made you careless of the welfare of yourself or your family?	❏	❏
11. Has gambling ever affected your reputation?	❏	❏
12. Do arguments, disappointments, or frustrations give you the urge to gamble?	❏	❏
13. Have you ever felt remorse after gambling?	❏	❏
14. After a win did you have a strong urge to return and win more?	❏	❏
15. Did gambling ever cause you to have difficulty sleeping?	❏	❏

(continued)

ASSESS yourself

	Yes	No
16. Did you ever have an urge to celebrate any good fortune by going gambling?	❑	❑
17. Have you ever committed, or considered committing, an illegal act to finance gambling?	❑	❑
18. Have you ever felt self-destructive or suicidal as a result of gambling losses?	❑	❑
19. Has gambling ever caused a decrease in your ambition or efficiency?	❑	❑
20. Have you ever been reluctant to use "gambling money" for normal expenditures?	❑	❑

Interpreting Your Scores for This Section

If you answered Yes to any of these questions, we would encourage you to consider your potential for problem gambling.

3–7: If you answered Yes to three of these questions, you are involved in problem gambling.

8 or more: If you answered Yes to seven or more, you may be a compulsive gambler.

COMPULSIVE SHOPPING

Answer True or False to each of the following questions:

	True	False
1. I often return items—at least one out of every four purchases.	❑	❑
2. I've lied to my spouse, friends, or colleagues about the cost of things.	❑	❑
3. I've had guilt, insomnia, fatigue, or a sense of hopelessness about my spending.	❑	❑
4. I can correlate my overspending with overeating.	❑	❑
5. My closet has over four unworn items with the tags still hanging from them.	❑	❑
6. I'm having trouble making ends meet.	❑	❑
7. I screen my calls so I don't have to talk to creditors.	❑	❑
8. Shopping is my antidote to feeling bored, lonely, angry, or frustrated.	❑	❑
9. When I shop, I can't return home empty-handed.	❑	❑
10. I've made false statements to creditors to get new lines of credit.	❑	❑
11. My shopping habits have interfered with my work.	❑	❑
12. My spending has caused problems in my marriage or my primary relationship.	❑	❑
13. I feel uneasy if I've not shopped in a week.	❑	❑
14. I spend over 30 percent of my income on nonmortgage debt.	❑	❑
15. I have considered illegal or questionable means to raise money to support my shopping habits.	❑	❑
16. I've had issues with eating disorders or sexual, drug, or alcohol addictions.	❑	❑
17. I repeatedly resolve not to spend, only to relapse and bingeshop.	❑	❑
18. I have to drive or wear status initials (BMW, DKNY, LV).	❑	❑

Interpreting Your Scores for This Section

Total your True responses and find your corresponding score below.

1–3: You have an indicator or two that trouble could be brewing around the corner, but you know your issues and are in a strong position to keep a check on things. Keep your good habits going!

4–6: Congratulations for admitting you're imperfect! However, you're within shouting distance of the slippery slope. Make note of any marked changes in your shopping habits. Cognizance of your behavior is your most effective tool for keeping your spending in check.

7–12: Uh-oh! You're teetering on the edge of that slippery slope and could tip over with the next sale. Take a good look at the motivations driving your behavior. Know what money will buy for you, and get clear about what it won't. Don't rule out seeking advice from a credit counselor or a therapist.

13–18: Red alert! Okay, well, there's some serious slippage, but now is not the time to berate yourself. Chin up. Deep breath. Got to kick in some action because your previous attempts at control aren't working! Don't lose hope—thousands have been here before you and recovered from their shopping scourges. Check out www.debtorsanonymous.org. Relief is only a meeting away.

Source: Reprinted by permission of Dr. K. S. Young, director of the Center for Online and Internet Addiction, 2004, www.netaddiction .com; Gamblers Anonymous, "Twenty Questions," 2006, www .gamblersanonymous.org; S. Durling, "Am I a Compulsive Shopper?" www.womenswallstreet.com, March 1, 2006.

MAKE it happen!

ASSESSMENT: The Assess Yourself activity above gave you a chance to evaluate signs of Internet, gambling, and spending addictions. Depending on your results, you may need to take steps toward changing certain behaviors that may be detrimental to your health.

MAKING A CHANGE: In order to change your behavior, you need to develop a plan. Follow the steps below and complete your Behavior Change Contract to take action.

1. Evaluate your behavior and identify patterns and specific things you are doing. What can you change now? What can you change in the near future?

2. Select one pattern of behavior that you want to change.

3. Fill out the Behavior Change Contract found at the front of your book. It should include your long-term goal for change, your short-term goals, the rewards you'll give yourself for reaching these goals, potential obstacles along the way, and strategies for overcoming these obstacles. For each goal, list the small steps and specific actions that you will take.

4. Chart your progress in a journal. At the end of a week, consider how successful you were in following your plan. What helped you be successful? What made change more difficult? What will you do differently next week?

5. Revise your plan as needed: Are the short-term goals attainable? Are the rewards satisfying?

ONE STUDENT'S PLAN: Taylor is a freshman living on campus. He came to school from out of state and has not really developed a close group of friends or even met many of the students living in his dorm. He does not have a roommate, which he likes because it allows him to do whatever he wishes when he wishes. However, Taylor was surprised to score 90 points on the Internet addiction self-assessment. He had been spending many hours online and in chat rooms but had never realized how much of his days and nights it was consuming. Taylor also admitted that rather than study or socialize with other students, he preferred being online. His grades and social life had deteriorated from his high school days, however, and he decided one cure was to spend less time on the Internet.

Taylor decided to develop a plan to cut back on his Internet use and to give himself some rewards for staying offline. He also decided to anticipate and write down some times that might make it difficult to stay off the Internet (when he was feeling lonely, for example) and some strategies for those situations (meeting other students in the hall or going to a location away from his computer to study). Taylor also decided to keep a log of the time he was on the computer and set a daily time limit. He would also record when he went over the time limit and consider how to avoid the situation the next time. Over time, Taylor spent much less time online and developed friendships with other students living in his dorm.

GAMBLING AND COLLEGE STUDENTS

Although many people gamble occasionally without it ever becoming a problem, many otherwise "model" students can find themselves caught up in the rush of making big bets and winning even bigger money. Consider the story of John,* a Lehigh University sophomore, who is the son of a Baptist minister, a fraternity member, a cellist in the university orchestra, and the sophomore class president—the epitome of a responsible student active in the community and serving as a role model to the student body. When John was arrested for allegedly robbing the Wachovia Bank branch in Allentown, Pennsylvania, making off with $2,781, many wondered why such a good kid would be driven to such an act. According to the Associated Press, his lawyer stated that his client had run up about $5,000 in debt playing online poker. In a desperate move to feed his compulsive gambling addiction, John turned to bank robbery.

Compulsive gambling on college campuses has become a big concern for college administrators as gambling grows ever more popular among students. The National Collegiate Athletic Association (NCAA) estimates that each year during March Madness (the men's college basketball tournament) there are over 1.2 million active gambling pools, with over 2.5 billion dollars gambled. More and more of these dollars come from the pockets of college students. There is growing evidence, in fact, that betting on college campuses is interfering with students' financial and academic futures. In a recent survey, approximately 26 percent of students reported gambling in the past week. Consider the following:

- Almost 53 percent of college students have participated in most forms of gambling, including casino gambling, lottery tickets, racing, and sports betting in the past month.
- At least 78 percent of youths have placed a bet by the age of 18.
- It is estimated that roughly 18 percent of men and 4 percent of women on college campuses could be classified as problem gamblers.
- The three most common reasons college students give for gambling are risk, excitement, and the chance to make money.

Although most college students who gamble are able to do so without developing a problem, warning signs of problem gambling include:

- Frequent talk about gambling
- Spending more time or money on gambling than can be afforded
- Borrowing money to gamble

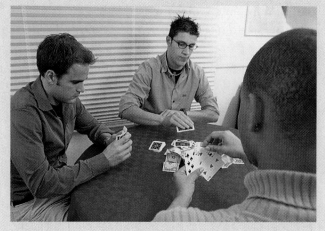

- Encouraging or challenging others to gamble
- Selling sports-betting cards or organizing sports pools
- Possession of gambling paraphernalia such as lottery tickets or poker items
- Missing or being late for school, work, or family activities due to gambling
- Feeling sad, anxious, fearful, or angry about gambling losses

*Not his real name

Sources: W. DeJong et al., "Gambling: The New Addiction Crisis in Higher Education," *Prevention Profile* (March 2006): 11–13; The Annenburg Public Policy Center, "Card-Playing Trend in Young People Continues," www.annenberg publicpolicycenter.org, Press Release, September 28, 2005; Massachusetts Council on Compulsive Gambling, "Students Know the Limits," www.masscompulsivegambling.org.

card companies entice you with fantasies of having it all, right now—whether or not you can afford it.

The credit card companies seem to be succeeding. There are 400 million MasterCards and Visas out there. Add to that cable shopping stations, catalog shopping, and shopping over the Internet, and the opportunity to overspend is greater than ever before. The resulting debt from all this spending is phenomenal. Bankruptcies, formerly a last resort, have become almost run of the mill—approximately 2 million were recorded for 2005. On average, compulsive spenders are $23,000 in debt, usually in the form of credit card debt or mortgages against their homes.[14]

Although most people can manage debt with careful planning, some spend money to meet emotional needs they can't fulfill elsewhere. Anxiety, self-doubt, and anger all lead to spending as a way of coping with daily stressors. College students may be particularly vulnerable to spending problems because advertisers and credit card companies heavily target them.

Compulsive gambling and shopping can frequently lead to compulsive borrowing to help support the addiction. Irresponsible investments and purchases lead to debts that the addict tries to repay by borrowing more. Compulsive debtors borrow money repeatedly from family, friends, or institutions in spite of the problems this causes. Although most people incur overwhelming debt through a combination of hardship and ignorance about financial management, compulsive debtors incur debt primarily as a result of buying or gambling behaviors in which they have engaged to relieve painful feelings.

Work Addiction

In order to understand work addiction, we need to understand the concept of healthy work. Healthy work provides a sense of identity, helps develop our strengths, and is a means of satisfaction, accomplishment, and mastery of problems. Healthy workers may work passionately for long hours. Although they have occasional projects that keep them away from family, friends, and personal interests for short periods of time, they generally maintain balance in their lives and full control of their schedules. Healthy work does not "consume" the worker.

Conversely, **work addiction** is the compulsive use of work and the work persona to fulfill needs of intimacy, power, and success. It is characterized by obsession, perfectionism, rigidity, fear, anxiety, feelings of inadequacy, low self-esteem, and alienation. Work addiction is more than being unable to relax when not doing something considered "productive." It is the pursuit of the "work persona"—the image that work addicts wish to project onto others. Work addiction is found among all age, racial, and socioeconomic groups, but it typically develops in people in their forties and fifties. Male work addicts outnumber female work addicts, but women are catching up fast as they gain more equality in the workforce.

Although work addicts tend to be admired in our society, the effects on individuals and those around them are far reaching. Work addiction is a major source of marital discord and family breakup. In fact, most work addicts come from homes that were alcoholic, rigid, violent, or otherwise dysfunctional.

Whether or not they lose their families, work addicts do compromise their emotional and physical health. They may become emotionally crippled, losing the communication and human interaction skills critical to living and working with other people. They are often riddled with guilt and chronic fear—of failure, boredom, laziness, persecution, or being found out. Because they are unable to relax and play, they commonly suffer from chronic fatigue. The excessive pumping of adrenaline that is part of the addiction causes fatigue, hypertension and other cardiovascular diseases, nervousness, trembling, and increased sweating. Work addicts commonly suffer from disorders of the gastrointestinal tract, and they often report a feeling of pressure in the chest, constricted

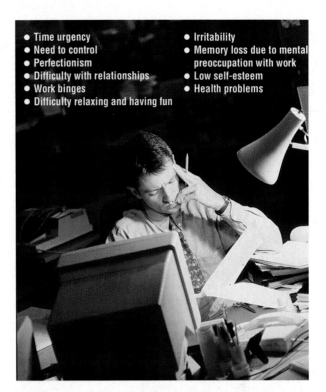

- Time urgency
- Need to control
- Perfectionism
- Difficulty with relationships
- Work binges
- Difficulty relaxing and having fun
- Irritability
- Memory loss due to mental preoccupation with work
- Low self-esteem
- Health problems

FIGURE 11.3 Signs of Work Addiction

breathing, dizziness, and lightheadedness. Figure 11.3 identifies other typical signs of work addiction.

Exercise Addiction

It may seem odd that a personal health text that advocates exercise would also identify it as a potential addiction. Yet, as a powerful mood enhancer, exercise can be addictive. Statistics on the incidence of this addiction are not available, but one indication of its prevalence is that a large portion of America's 2 million people with anorexia and/or bulimia use exercise to purge instead of or in addition to self-induced vomiting.

Addictive exercisers abuse exercise in the same way that alcoholics abuse alcohol or addictive spenders abuse money. They use it compulsively to try to meet needs—for nurturance, intimacy, self-esteem, and self-competency—that cannot truly be met by an object or activity. As a result, addictive exercise results in negative consequences similar to those found in other addictions: alienation of family and friends, injuries from overdoing it, and a craving for more.

work addiction The compulsive use of work and the work persona to fulfill needs for intimacy, power, and success.

addictive exercisers People who exercise compulsively to try to meet needs of nurturance, intimacy, self-esteem, and self-competency.

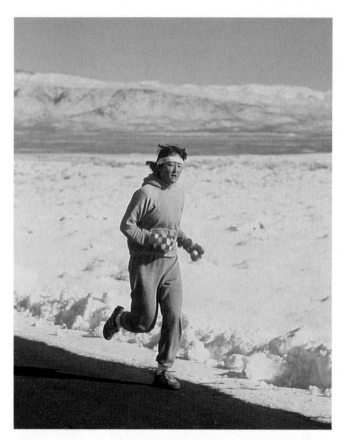
Obsession with a substance or behavior, even a generally positive activity such as exercise, can eventually develop into an addiction.

Traditionally, women have been perceived as more at risk for exercise addiction. However, evidence is growing that more men are developing unhealthy exercise patterns. Media images promoting "six-pack abs" and lean, muscular male bodies have influenced society's view of the masculine ideal. However, that body type is as unrealistic for most men as the stick-thin fashion model figure is for most women. Meanwhile, more men are abusing steroids and overexercising to attain the desired frame. **Muscle dysmorphia**, sometimes referred to as "bigarexia," is a pathological preoccupation with being larger and more muscular.[15] Sufferers view themselves as small and weak even though they may be quite the opposite.[16] Consequences of muscle dysmorphia include excessive weight lifting and exercising as well as steroid or supplement abuse (for more on problems associated with too much exercise, see Chapter 10).

muscle dysmorphia Sometimes referred to as "bigarexia," a pathological preoccupation with being larger and more muscular, which can lead to exercise addiction.

Internet addiction Compulsive use of computer activities such as fantasy games, online shopping, and chat rooms.

sexual addiction Compulsive involvement in sexual activity.

Internet Addiction

Have you ever opened up your Web browser to quickly check something out, and an hour later you were still online? Our access to the Internet continues to expand; we can now get online via our cell phones, PDAs, and Blackberries. With this practically unlimited access to the Internet, recent research has found that surfing the World Wide Web can be addictive. It is estimated that 5 to 10 percent of Internet users will likely experience Internet addiction.[17] **Internet addiction** is a blanket term that encompasses five problematic issues: cybersex addiction, cyber relationship addiction, Net compulsions, information overload, and addiction to interactive computer games.[18]

Men and women experience Internet addiction differently. Men are interested in information seeking, games, and cybersex (see Chapter 5). Women, on the other hand, use the Internet more for support and friendship, and romance.

> **Is my roommate's obsessive video-game playing an addiction?**

Internet addicts have multiple signs and symptoms, such as general disregard for one's health, sleep deprivation, neglecting family and friends, lack of physical activity, euphoria when online, lower grades in school, and poor job performance. Approximately 15 percent of college students reported that Internet use and computer games interfered with their academic performance.[19] Internet addicts may feel moody or uncomfortable when they are not online. As with other addictive behaviors, online addicts may be using their behavior to compensate for feelings of loneliness, marital or work problems, a poor social life, or financial problems. See the Assess Yourself box to analyze your own Internet use.

Sexual Addiction

Everyone needs love and intimacy, but the sexual practices of people addicted to sex involve neither. In **sexual addiction**, people confuse the intensity of physical arousal with intimacy.[20] They do not feel nurtured by the person with whom they have sex but by the activity itself. Likewise, they are incapable of nurturing another because sex, not the person, is the object of their affection. In fact, people with sexual addictions do not necessarily seek partners to obtain sexual arousal; they may be satisfied by masturbation, whether alone or during phone sex or while reading or watching erotica. They may participate in a wide range of sexual activities, including affairs, sex with strangers, prostitution, voyeurism, exhibitionism, cross-dressing, rape, incest, and pedophilia.

People addicted to sex frequently experience crushing episodes of depression and anxiety, fueled by the fear of discovery. Suicide is high among people who have problems with sexual control. The toll that sexual addiction exacts is most clearly seen in loss of intimacy with loved ones, which frequently leads to family disintegration.

No group of people is more or less likely than another to become involved in sexual addictions. They affect men and women of all ages, including married and single people, and people of any sexual preference. Most people with sexual addictions share a similar background: a dysfunctional childhood family, often characterized by chemical dependency or other addictions. Many were physically and emotionally abused. People addicted to sex tend to have a history of sexual abuse.

what do you THINK?

We have used a broad definition of the concept of addiction in this text. Do you think any behavior can be addictive? ■ Can one be a chocolate addict or a study addict? ■ What potential dangers lie in using the term addiction too loosely?

Multiple Addictions

Treatment centers for addiction often find that addicts depend on more than one chemical and/or behavior. Though addicts tend to have a drug or behavior of choice—one that they prefer because it is more effective at meeting their needs—as many as 60 percent of people in treatment have problems with more than one addiction. The figure may be as high as 75 percent for people addicted to chemicals. For example, alcohol addiction and eating disorders are commonly paired in women. Chemically dependent women and men frequently resort to compulsive eating to keep themselves abstinent from drugs. Though multiple addictions certainly complicate recovery, they do not make it impossible. As with single addictions, recovery begins with the recognition that there is a problem.

How Addiction Affects Family and Friends

The family and friends of an addicted person also suffer many negative consequences. Often they struggle with **codependence**, a self-defeating relationship pattern in which a person is "addicted to the addict." It is the primary outcome of dysfunctional relationships or families.

Codependence is not accurately defined by isolated incidents, but rather by a pattern of behavior. Codependents find it hard to set healthy boundaries and often live in the chaotic, crisis-oriented mode that naturally occurs around addicts. They assume responsibility for meeting others' needs to the point that they subordinate or even cease being aware of their own needs. They may be unable to perceive their needs because they have repeatedly been taught that their needs are inappropriate or less important than someone else's. Their

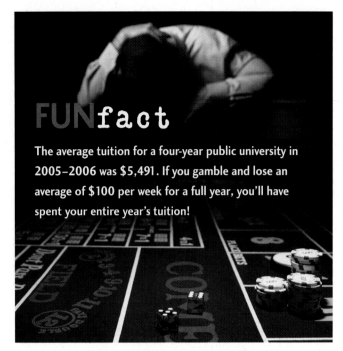

FUNfact

The average tuition for a four-year public university in 2005–2006 was $5,491. If you gamble and lose an average of $100 per week for a full year, you'll have spent your entire year's tuition!

FIGURE 11.4 Understanding the Cost of Addiction
Source: Annual Survey of Colleges, 2006. The College Board, New York, NY.

behavior goes far beyond performing kind services for another person. Codependents feel less than human if they fail to respond to the needs of someone else, even when their help was not requested. Although the term codependent is used less frequently today, treatment professionals still recognize the importance of helping addicts recognize how their behavior affects those around them and of working with family and friends to establish healthier relationships and boundaries.

Family and friends can play an important role in getting an addict to seek treatment. They are most helpful when they refuse to be enablers. **Enablers** are people who knowingly or unknowingly protect addicts from the natural consequences of their behavior. If they don't have to deal with the consequences, addicts cannot see the self-destructive nature of their behavior and will therefore continue it. Codependents are the primary enablers of their addicted loved ones, although anyone who has contact with an addict can be an enabler and thus contribute (perhaps powerfully) to continuation of the

codependence A self-defeating relationship pattern in which a person is "addicted to the addict."

enablers People who knowingly or unknowingly protect addicts from the natural consequences of their behavior.

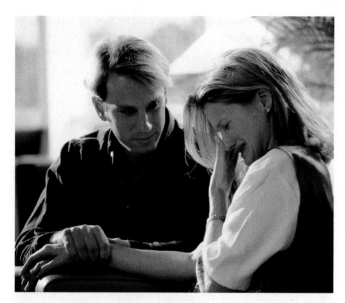

The process of acknowledging and overcoming an addiction is a long and difficult journey for everyone involved.

addictive behavior. Enablers are generally unaware that their behavior has this effect. In fact, enabling is rarely conscious and certainly not intentional.

 what do you THINK?

Why do we tend to protect others from the natural consequences of their destructive behaviors? ■ Have you ever confronted someone you were concerned about? If so, was the confrontation successful? ■ What tips would you give someone who wants to confront a loved one about an addiction?

Treatment for and Recovery from Addiction

A key step in the recovery process is to recognize the addiction. This can be difficult because of the power of denial. Denial—the inability to see the truth—is the hallmark of addiction. It can be so powerful that intervention is sometimes necessary to break down the addict's defenses against recognizing the problem.

intervention   A planned process of confronting an addict; carried out by significant others.

Intervention

How can I approach someone who needs help and treatment?

Intervention is a planned process of confrontation by people who are important to the addict, including spouse, parents, children, boss, and friends. Its purpose is to break down the denial compassionately so that the addict can see the destructive nature of the addiction. It is not enough to get the person to admit that he or she is addicted. The addict must come to perceive that the addiction is destructive and requires treatment.

Individual confrontation is difficult and often futile. However, an addict's defenses generally crumble when significant others collectively share their observations and concerns about the addict's behavior. It is critical that those involved in the intervention clarify how they plan to end their enabling. For example, a wife may state that she will no longer cover bounced checks or make excuses for her compulsive gambling husband's antisocial behavior. She may even close their joint bank account and open a personal account so she will not be legally responsible for his irresponsible acts. All parties involved in the intervention must choose consequences they are ready to actually stick to in the event that the addict refuses treatment. Significant others must also be ready to give support if the addict is willing to begin a recovery program.

Components of effective intervention include the following:

- Emphasizing care and concern for the addicted person
- Describing the behavior that is the cause for concern
- Expressing how the behavior affects the addict, each person taking part in the intervention, and others
- Outlining specifically what you would like to see happen

Intervention is a serious step toward helping someone who probably does not want help. It should therefore be well planned and rehearsed. Most addiction treatment centers have specialists on staff who can help plan an intervention. In addition, books on the subject are available for families and friends who are concerned about someone who may be addicted. Once the problem has been recognized, recovery can begin.

 try it NOW

Addiction can be an obstacle to goals. On a piece of paper, identify one long-term goal you would like to achieve, such as going on to law school after college, and becoming a lawyer. Be sure your goal is specific. Next, write down three steps you need to take to reach the goal (e.g., an internship with the District Attorney, passing the Bar exam). Finally, think about an addictive behavior you may be prone too, its consequences, and how these factors will make your goal difficult to achieve or prevent you from reaching it at all.

Treatment

Treatment and recovery for any addiction generally begin with **abstinence**—refraining from the addictive behavior. Whereas literal abstinence is possible for people addicted to chemicals, it obviously is not for people addicted to behaviors like work and sex. For these addicts, abstinence means restoring balance to their lives through noncompulsive engagement in the behaviors, such as avoiding certain activities.

Detoxification refers to the early abstinence period during which an addict adjusts physically and cognitively to being free from the influence of the addiction. It occurs in virtually every recovering addict; and, whereas it is uncomfortable for all addicts, it can be dangerous for some. This is primarily true for those addicted to chemicals, especially alcohol, heroin, and painkillers such as OxyContin. For these people, early abstinence may involve profound withdrawal symptoms that require medical supervision. Therefore, most inpatient treatment programs provide a pretreatment component of supervised detoxification to achieve abstinence safely before treatment begins.

Abstinence alone does little to change the psychological, biological, and environmental dynamics that underlie the addictive behavior. Without recovery, an addict is apt to relapse time and again or simply to change addictions. Recovery involves learning new ways of looking at oneself, others, and the world. It may require exploring a traumatic past so that psychological wounds can be healed. It also involves learning interdependence with significant others and new ways of taking care of oneself, physically and emotionally—and it involves developing communication skills and new ways of having fun.

Recovery programs are the fuel that gives addicts the energy to resist relapsing. For a large number of addicts, recovery begins with a period of formal treatment. A good treatment program includes the following characteristics:

- Professional staff familiar with the specific addictive disorder for which help is being sought
- A flexible schedule of both inpatient and outpatient services
- Access to medical personnel who can assess the addict's health and treat all medical concerns as needed
- Medical supervision of addicts who are at high risk for a complicated detoxification
- Involvement of family members in the treatment process
- A team approach to treating addictive disorders (for example, medical personnel, counselors, psychotherapists, social workers, clergy, educators, dietitians, and fitness counselors)
- Both group and individual therapy options
- Peer-led support groups that encourage the addict to continue involvement after treatment ends
- Structured aftercare and relapse-prevention programs
- Accreditation by the Joint Commission on Accreditation of Healthcare Organizations (JCAHO) and a license from the state in which it operates

Most programs apply a combination of family, individual, and group counseling, supplemented with attendance at a 12-step support group. Individuals may also wish to explore alternatives to 12-step groups. Organizations such as Rational Recovery and the Secular Organization for Sobriety provide support without the spiritual emphasis of 12-step groups such as Alcoholics Anonymous.

Choosing a Treatment The National Institute on Alcohol Abuse and Alcoholism (NIAAA) completed Project MATCH (Matching Alcoholism Treatment to Client Heterogeneity), a large-scale study designed to determine if certain types of patients respond better to particular treatments.

The investigators studied three strategies: cognitive-behavior therapy, motivational psychology, and a facilitated 12-step program with sessions run by a therapist. Results showed that patients did equally well in each of the treatment approaches. This outcome was somewhat surprising, given that it has been common practice for treatment professionals to match patients to certain approaches. Researchers concluded that the focus, therefore, should simply be on selecting a competently run treatment program. Large-scale studies on other addictions have yet to occur.[21]

The Women's Health/Men's Health box on page 366 describes factors that are important to address when treating female addicts.

Relapse

Relapse is an isolated occurrence of or full return to addictive behavior. It is one of the defining characteristics of addiction. A person who does not relapse or have powerful urges to do so was probably not addicted in the first place. Relapse is proof that a person is addicted and has abandoned the practice of an ongoing recovery program. Addicts are set up to relapse long before they actually do so because of their tendency to meet change and other forms of stress in their lives with the same kind of denial they once used to justify their addictive behavior (for example, thinking "I don't have a problem, I can handle this"). This sets off a series of events involving immediate or gradual abandonment of structured recovery plans. For example, the addict may quit attending support group meetings and slip into situations that previously triggered the addictive behavior.

Because treatment programs recognize this strong tendency to relapse, they routinely teach clients and significant others concepts of relapse prevention. Relapse prevention teaches people to recognize the signs of imminent relapse and to develop a plan for responding to these signs.

> **abstinence** Refraining from an addictive behavior.
>
> **detoxification** The early abstinence period during which an addict adjusts physically and cognitively to being free from the influences of the addiction.

ADDICTION TREATMENT FOR WOMEN: STILL CONFRONTING BARRIERS

The addiction treatment industry has been based on a male model and has only recently begun to address the unique needs of women. Studies support the need for greater prevention efforts targeted specifically at women at risk and gender-specific treatment for drug and alcohol dependence. Unfortunately, significant barriers remain for women seeking addiction treatment.

Although women entering treatment generally have fewer addiction-related legal problems (arrests for public intoxication or drug dealing, for example) than men do, they face more psychological issues and family, financial, and medical problems. Studies consistently indicate that the two primary barriers women face in successfully completing treatment are child care and transportation. One study found that women who were able to bring their children to inpatient treatment were more likely to remain healthy at six months after treatment. Additional barriers for women

seeking addiction treatment include the following factors.

INDIVIDUAL

- Lack of insurance or inadequate coverage
- Fear of losing child custody
- Low self-esteem
- Low feelings of self-efficacy

FAMILY

- Too many responsibilities
- Lack of family support for treatment
- Abuse in the family environment

COMMUNITY

- Lack of support from employer
- Lack of gender-sensitive treatment options

A "women-friendly" treatment center should offer the following:

- Educational programs on self-worth, assertiveness, family issues, parenting, and anger management

- Women-only groups, especially for addressing issues of rape, incest, and abuse
- Networking with and support from other women in recovery
- Housing and day care

Clearly, many women have different treatment needs than men do. Finding a program that addresses these needs improves the likelihood of long-term success and recovery.

Sources: W. Weschberg, S. Craddock, and R. Hubbard, "How Are Women Who Enter Substance Abuse Treatment Different Than Men? A Gender Comparison from the Drug Abuse Treatment Outcome Study," in *Women and Substance Abuse: Gender Transparency,* eds. S. Stevens and H. Wexler (New York: Haworth, 1998); C. A. Hernandez-Avila, B. J. Rounsaville, and H. R. Kranzler, "Opioid-, Cannabis-, and Alcohol-Dependent Women Show More Rapid Progression to Substance-Abuse Treatment," *Journal of Drug and Alcohol Dependence* 74, no. 3 (2004): 265–272.

Without such a plan, recovering addicts are likely to relapse more frequently, more completely, and perhaps permanently.

Relapse should not be interpreted as failure to change or lack of desire to stay well. The appropriate response to relapse is to remind addicts that they are addicted and to redirect them to the recovery strategies that have previously worked for them.

In addition to teaching skills, relapse prevention may involve aftercare planning such as connecting the recovering person with support groups, career counselors, or community services.

what do you THINK?

Why do you think people with addictions resist seeking treatment, even when they may admit they have a problem? ▪ What factors need to be considered in helping addicted individuals prevent relapse?

TAKING charge

Summary

- Addiction is the continued involvement with a substance or activity despite ongoing negative consequences.
- Habits are repeated behaviors, whereas addiction is behavior resulting from compulsion; without the behavior, the addict experiences withdrawal. All addictions share four common symptoms: compulsion, loss of control, negative consequences, and denial.
- Addiction is a process, evolving over time through a pattern known as nurturing through avoidance. Mood-altering substances and experiences produce biochemical reactions that make the body feel good; when absent, the person feels a withdrawal effect. The biopsychosocial model of addiction takes into account biological (genetic) factors as well as psychological and environmental influences in understanding the addiction process.
- Addictions include compulsive gambling, spending, and borrowing, work addiction, exercise addiction, sexual addiction, Internet addiction, and codependence. Codependents are "addicted to the addict." These behaviors are all addictive because they are mood altering.
- Treatment begins with abstinence from the addictive behavior or substance, usually instituted through intervention by significant others. Treatment programs may include individual, group, or family therapy, as well as 12-step programs.

Chapter Review

1. What is the most common characteristic of an addictive personality?
   a. denial
   b. tolerance
   c. codependency
   d. enabling

2. Jason is addicted to the Internet. He is so preoccupied with talking in chat rooms that he skips classes. What symptom of addiction does his preoccupation characterize?
   a. denial
   b. obsession and compulsion
   c. loss of control
   d. negative consequences

3. Which of the following is an example of *tolerance*?
   a. The human body's rejection to a drug or chemical.
   b. The need to consume more of a drug to achieve the same high as was previously able to be achieved with a lesser amount.
   c. The need to consume a lesser amount of the chemical or drug.
   d. A person's ability to handle a larger amount of drugs in their body.

4. Chemical dependency *relapse* refers to
   a. a person who is experiencing a blackout memory loss.
   b. a gap in one's drinking or drugging patterns.
   c. a full return to addictive behavior.
   d. the failure to change one's behavior.

5. People who excessively exercise or work out compulsively to meet needs of nurturance, intimacy, and self-esteem have a(n)
   a. money addiction.
   b. work addiction.
   c. shopping addiction.
   d. exercise addiction.

6. When a person repeatedly seeks the illusion of relief to avoid unpleasant feelings, this pattern is known as
   a. neurotransmitter-deficiency.
   b. nurturing through avoidance.
   c. a bad habit.
   d. compulsive behavior.

7. The current theory of addiction relies on the biopsychosocial model of addiction. This model proposes that most addictive conditions were influenced by
   a. biological or disease influences.
   b. genetic influences.
   c. environmental influences.
   d. All of the above.

8. Chris was obsessed with his weight-lifting program and constantly checking to see if his "6-pack abs" and lean muscles were nicely sculpted. He suffers from
   a. anorexia.
   b. muscle dysmorphia.
   c. exercise addiction.
   d. tolerance.

9. An example of a *process addiction* is
   a. alcohol addiction.
   b. marijuana addiction.
   c. sexual addiction.
   d. adrenaline addiction.

10. An individual who knowingly tries to protect an addict from natural consequences of his or her destructive behaviors is
    a. enabling.
    b. coddling.
    c. practicing intervention.
    d. controlling.

Answers to these questions can be found on page A-1.

Questions for Discussion and Reflection

1. What factors distinguish a habit from an addiction? Is it possible for you to tell whether someone else is really addicted?
2. Explain why the biopsychosocial model of addiction is a more effective model for treatment than a single-factor model.
3. Explain the potential genetic, environmental, and psychological risk factors for addiction.

4. Discuss how addiction affects family and friends. What role do family and friends play in helping the addict get help and maintain recovery?
5. What are some key components of an effective treatment program? Do the components vary for men and women? Why or why not?

Accessing Your Health on the Internet

The following websites explore further topics and issues related to personal health. You'll also find links to each organization's website on the Companion Website for *Access to Health,* Tenth Edition, at www.aw-bc.com/donatelle.

1. *Addiction Support.Net.* A comprehensive drug and alcohol addiction site with information on recognizing addiction, confronting a loved one, referral for rehabilitation programs, and information on postrehabilitation support. www.addictionsupport.net
2. *Center for Online and Internet Addiction.* Information and assistance for those dealing with Internet addiction. www.netaddiction.com

3. *National Council on Problem Gambling.* Provides information and help for people with gambling problems and their families, including a searchable directory for counselors. www.ncpgambling.org
4. *Web of Addictions.* This site is dedicated to providing accurate information about alcohol and other drug addictions. www.well.com/user/woa
5. *Society for the Advancement of Sexual Health.* Provides information, resources, and a self-quiz relating to sexual addiction. www.ncsac.org

Further Reading

Elster, J. (ed.). *Addiction: Entries and Exits*. New York: Russell Sage Foundation, 2000.

> Addresses current addiction controversies from an international perspective, with authors from the United States and Norway. Topics include whether addicts have a choice in their behavior and current addiction theories.

Hurley, J. (ed.). *Addiction: Opposing Viewpoints*. San Diego: Greenhaven Press, 2000.

> Part of the Opposing Viewpoints series; addresses addiction theories, treatment approaches, and risk factors, among other topics.

Nakken, C. *The Addictive Personality*. Center City, MN: Hazelden, 1996.

> A very down-to-earth overview of addiction, including non-substance addictions.

Frey, J. *A Million Little Pieces*. New York: Random House/Doubleday, 2003.

> A controversial book exploring the consciousness of an addict.

Shaw, B. *Addiction and Recovery for Dummies*. Hoboken: Wiley Publishing Co., 2005.

> This compassionate guide helps you identify the problem and work toward a healthy, realistic approach to recovery, explaining the latest clinical and self-help treatments for both adults and teens.

Peele, S. *Seven Tools to Beat Addiction*. New York: Three Rivers Press, 2004.

> A hands-on, practical guide to overcoming addiction of any kind.

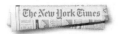

e-themes from *The New York Times*

For up-to-date articles about current health issues, visit
www.aw-bc.com/donatelle, select *Access to Health,* Tenth
Edition, Chapter 11, and click on "e-themes."

References

1. H. F. Doweiko, *Concepts of Chemical Dependency,* 6th ed. (Belmont, CA: Wadsworth, 2005), 11.
2. R. Goldberg, *Drugs Across the Spectrum* (Pacific Grove, CA: Brooks/Cole, 2002), 17.
3. National Institute on Alcohol Abuse and Alcoholism, "Alcohol Alert 60: The Genetics of Alcoholism," July 2003, www.niaaa.nih.
4. A. I. Herman et al., "Serotonin Transporter Promoter Polymorphism and Differences in Alcohol Consumption Behavior in a College Student Population," *Alcohol and Alcoholism* 38 (2003): 446–449.
5. National Institute on Alcohol Abuse and Alcoholism, "Alcohol Alert."
6. J. Kinney, *Loosening the Grip* (Boston: McGraw-Hill, 2005), 106.
7. G. Hansen and P. Venturelli, *Drugs and Society,* 7th ed. (Sudbury, MA: Jones and Bartlett, 2002), 49.
8. Ibid., 4.
9. National Council on Problem Gambling, "Fact Sheets," September 1, 2004, www.ncpgambling.org.
10. *Science,* 307, no. 5708 (2005).
11. J. W. Welte et al., "Gambling Participation and Pathology in the United States,"*Addictive Behaviors* 29, no. 5 (2004): 983–989.
12. The Annenburg Public Policy Center, "Card-Playing Trend in Young People Continues," www.annenbergpublicpolicycenter.org, Press Release, September 28, 2005.
13. W. DeJong et al., "Gambling: The New Addiction Crisis in Higher Education," *Prevention Profile* (March 2006): 11–13.
14. American Bankruptcy Institute, "Quarterly Non-Business Filings by Year, 2005," www.abiworld.org; Women's Wall Street, "Conquer the Compulsive Shopping Blues," June 19, 2004.
15. J. Leone et al., "Recognition and Treatment of Muscle Dysmorphia and Related Body Image Disorders," *Journal of Athletic Training* 40, no. 4 (2005): 352–359.
16. M. Maine, *Body Wars: Making Peace with Women's Bodies* (Carlsbad, CA: Gurze, 2000), 282.
17. D. M. Wieland, "Computer Addiction: Implications for Nursing Psychotherapy Practice," *Perspectives in Psychiatric Care* 41, no. 4 (2005): 153–161.
18. Ibid.
19. American College Health Association, "American College Health Association-National College Health Assessment Spring 2005 Reference Group Data Report," *The Journal of American College Health,* July/August 2006.
20. C. Nakken, *The Addictive Personality* (Center City, MN: Hazelden, 1996).
21. S. Maisto, P. Clifford, and J. S. Tonigan, "Initial and Long-Term Alcohol Treatment Success: A 10-Year Study of the Project MATCH Albuquerque Sample," *Alcoholism: Clinical and Experimental Research* 26, no. 5 (supplement), 2003.

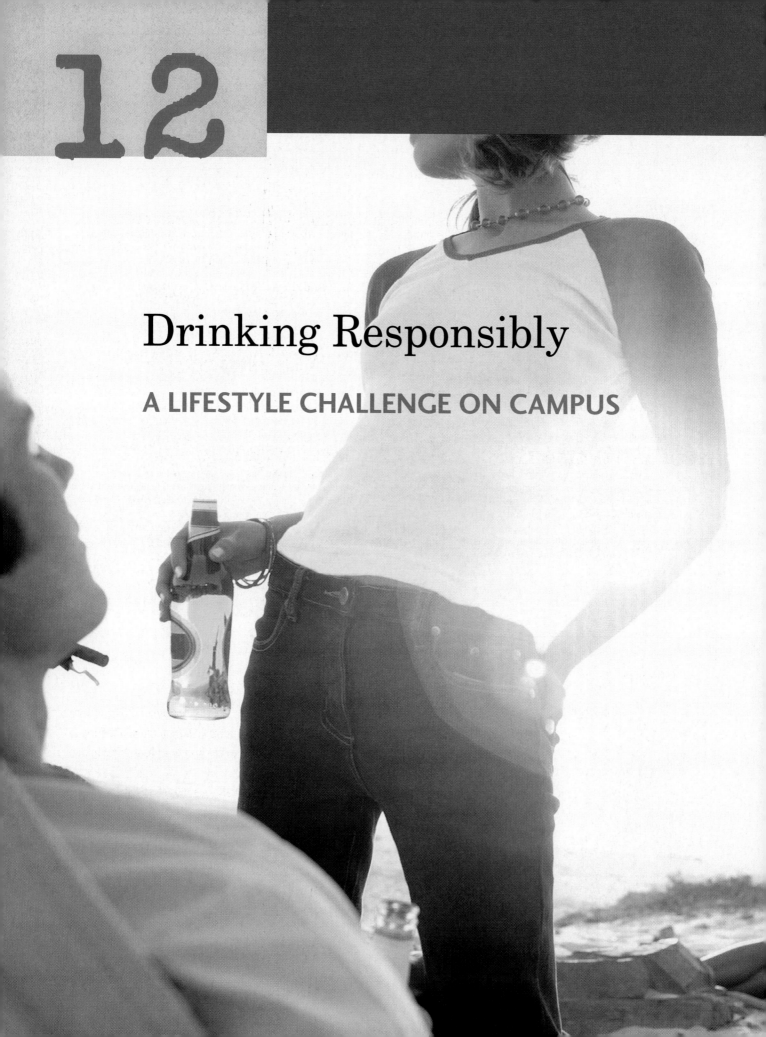

12

Drinking Responsibly

A LIFESTYLE CHALLENGE ON CAMPUS

Aren't the majority of college students **heavy** drinkers?

Is the **alcohol** in beer the same as in vodka?

Is there any cure for a **hangover**?

What's the legal limit for **drinking** and driving?

How can I approach a friend with a drinking **problem**?

OBJECTIVES

- Discuss the alcohol use patterns of college students and overall trends in consumption.
- Explain the physiological and behavioral effects of alcohol, including blood alcohol concentration, absorption, metabolism, and the immediate and long-term effects of alcohol consumption.
- Learn practical strategies for drinking responsibly and coping effectively with campus pressures to drink.
- Explain the symptoms and causes of alcoholism, its cost to society, and its effects on the family.
- Explain the treatment of alcoholism, including the family's role, varied treatment methods, and whether or not alcoholics can be cured.

The consumption of alcoholic beverages is interwoven with many traditions. Moderate use of alcohol can enhance celebrations or special times. Research shows that very low levels of drinking may actually lower some health risks. We may also consume alcohol to help ease the pain caused by rejection or loss. We are certainly not unique in this regard; people all over the world and throughout history have used alcohol for everything from social gatherings to religious ceremonies.

However, always remember that alcohol is a chemical substance that affects your physical and mental behavior. The fact is, alcohol is a drug, and if it is not used responsibly, it can become dangerous. In this chapter we will discuss the composition of alcohol and its effects on the body. We will also look at the hallmarks of responsible consumption, signs of alcohol dependency, and the health risks of irresponsible use.

Alcohol: An Overview

An estimated 65 percent of Americans consume alcoholic beverages regularly, though consumption patterns are unevenly distributed throughout the drinking population. Ten percent are heavy drinkers, and they account for half of all the alcohol consumed. The remaining 90 percent of the drinking population is composed of infrequent, light, or moderate drinkers.

Alcohol and College Students

Alcohol is the most widely used and abused recreational drug in our society. It is also the most popular drug on college campuses, where approximately 90 percent of students have consumed alcoholic beverages in the past 30 days.[1] About one-third of all college students are classified as heavy episodic drinkers or binge drinkers. **Heavy episodic ("binge") drinking** is typically defined as five or more drinks in a row for men, and four or more in a row for women. Therefore a student classifies as a heavy episodic drinker by drinking four drinks (female) or five drinks (male) during that occasion. Another trend that is occurring on college campuses is a rise in women's alcohol consumption; today, it is close to or equaling men's consumption of alcohol. (See the Spotlight on Your Health box for more on alcohol and college students.)

College is a critical time to become aware of and responsible for drinking. There is little doubt that drinking is a part of campus culture and tradition. Many students are away from home, often for the first time, and are excited by their

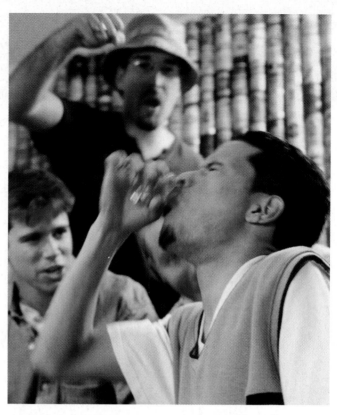

Deciding when to drink, and how much, is no small matter. Irresponsible consumption of alcohol can easily result in disaster.

newfound independence. For some students, this independence and the rite of passage into the college culture are symbolized by the use of alcohol. It provides the answer to one of the most commonly heard statements on any college campus: "There is nothing to do." Additionally, many students say they drink to have fun. Having fun, which often means drinking simply to get drunk, may really be a way of coping with stress, boredom, anxiety, or pressures created by academic and social demands.

Aren't the majority of college students heavy drinkers?

Statistics about college students' drinking may not always reflect actual consumption. Many colleges and universities are trying a social norms approach, sending a consistent message to students about the actual norms of drinking behaviors on campus. There is growing research that college students' drinking behavior is strongly influenced by the incorrect perception of peer drinking norms. Many students misperceive that their peers drink more than they actually drink. This misperception is true not only for students' drinking, but actual consequences students experience as a result of their drinking. For example, at a large midwestern university, 42 percent of students reported not having a hangover in the past six months. Yet the same group of surveyed students perceived that only 3 percent of their peers had not had a hangover in the past month.

---

heavy episodic (binge) drinking Drinking for the express purpose of becoming intoxicated; five drinks or more on a single occasion for men and four drinks or more for women.

THE FACTS ABOUT COLLEGE STUDENTS AND DRINKING

College administrators estimate that alcohol is involved with 29 percent of dropouts, 38 percent of academic failures, and 64 percent of violent behaviors.* Perhaps you've heard conflicting reports in the media about the prevalence and effects of drinking on campus. What are the facts? The statistic above is just one of many that detail the risks, and the complete scope, of the problem. Consider the following facts about students and alcohol consumption:

- Alcohol kills more people below age 21 than cocaine, marijuana, and heroin combined.
- Half a million students between ages 15 and 24 are unintentionally injured each year while intoxicated.
- Eight percent of students reported alcohol use as one of their top ten impediments to academic performance in the previous year.
- Nearly 40 percent of students reported consuming 5 or more drinks in one sitting at least once during the previous two weeks. Over 10 percent did this 3 to 5 times during the previous two weeks.

- Students reported drinking on average 4.5 drinks over a three-hour period the last time they partied or socialized.
- Of today's first-year college students, 159,000 will drop out of school next year for alcohol or other drug-related reasons.
- Over the past decade, there has been a threefold increase in the number of college women who report having been drunk on ten or more occasions in the previous month.
- Areas of a college campus offering cheap beer prices have more crime, including trouble between students and police or other campus authorities, arguments, physical fighting, property damage, false fire alarms, and sexual misconduct.
- Alcohol is involved in more than two-thirds of suicides among college students, 90 percent of campus rapes and sexual assaults, and 95 percent of violent crime on campus.
- Seventy-five percent of male students and 55 percent of female students involved in acquaintance rape had been drinking or using drugs at the time.
- Each year, more than 100,000 students between the ages of 18 and 24 report

having been too intoxicated to know if they consented to having sex.
- College students under the age of 21 are more prone to binge drinking and pay less for their alcohol than their older classmates do. Though underage students drink less often, they consume more per occasion than students age 21 and older who are allowed to drink legally.

Source: Data were compiled from the numerous studies cited throughout this chapter and from M. Mohler-Kuo, et al., "College Rapes Linked to Binge-Drinking Rates," *Journal of Studies on Alcohol* 65, no. 1 (2004); H. Wechsler, "Watering Down the Drinks: The Moderating Effect of College Demographics on Alcohol Use in High-Risk Groups," *American Journal of Public Health* 93, no. 11 (2003): 1929–1933; T. F. Nelson et al., "Alcohol and Collegiate Sports Fans," *Addictive Behaviors* 28, no. 1 (2003): 1–11; R. W. Hingson et al., "Magnitude of Alcohol-Related Mortality and Morbidity among U.S. College Students Ages 18–24," *Journal of Studies on Alcohol* 63, no. 2 (2002): 136–144; American College Health Association, "American College Health Association-National College Health Assessment Spring 2005 Reference Group Data Report," *Journal of American College Health,* July/August 2006; *Facts on Tap, "The College Experience: Alcohol and Student Life," 2006, www.factsontap.org.

Today, many campuses are working to change misperceptions of normal drinking behavior. There has been significant reduction of heavy episodic alcohol consumption—"binge drinking"—at various campuses across the country (see Table 12.1 on page 374).

"Binge" Drinking and College Students

There are, however, some students who do indulge in binge drinking. The stakes of binge drinking are high because of the increased risk for alcohol-related injuries and death. According to a 2005 study, 1,700 college students die each year due to alcohol-related unintentional injuries, including car

accidents. Binge drinking is the number-one cause of preventable death among undergraduate college students in the United States today.[2]

A study by the Harvard School of Public Health found that 44.4 percent of students were binge drinkers, and, of those, 22.8 percent were frequent bingers (people who binge drink three times or more in a two-week period).[3] (See Table 12.2 on page 375) Compared with nonbingers, frequent binge drinkers are 16 times more likely to miss class, 8 times more likely to get behind in their schoolwork, and more apt to get into trouble with campus or local police.[4] Unfortunately, recent studies confirm what students have been experiencing for a long time—binge drinkers cause problems not only for themselves, but also for those around them.

TABLE 12.1   Reported Change in Alcohol Use as a Result of Social Norms Campaigns

The statistics below represent a small number of institutions using social norms campaigns to reduce alcohol consumption among college students, and their reported results.

University or College with a Social Norms Campaign	Reduction in Heavy Episodic Alcohol Consumption Due to Social Norms Campaign
Northern Illinois University (NIU)	44% over 10 years
Hobart & William Smith Colleges (HWS)	40% over 5 years
Rowan University (Rowan)	23% over 5 semesters
University of Missouri-Columbia (MU)	21% over 2 years
University of North Carolina (UNC)	30% over 5 years
University of Arizona (UA)	29% over 3 years
Western Washington University (WWU)	20% over 3 years
Florida State University (FSU)	22% over 3 years
Michigan State University (MSU)	26% over 3 years

Source: National Social Norms Resource Center, July 17, 2006, www.socialnorms.org.

Although everyone is at some risk for alcohol-related problems, college students seem to be particularly vulnerable, for the following reasons:

- Alcohol exacerbates their already high risk for suicide, automobile crashes, and falls.
- Many college and university customs, norms, traditions, and mores encourage certain dangerous practices and patterns of alcohol use.
- University campuses are heavily targeted by advertising and promotions from the alcoholic beverage industry.
- It is more common for college students than their noncollegiate peers to drink recklessly and to engage in drinking games and other dangerous drinking practices.
- College students are particularly vulnerable to peer influence and have a strong need to be accepted by their peers.
- There is institutional denial by college administrators that alcohol problems exist on their campuses.

Binge drinking is especially dangerous because it often involves drinking a lot of alcohol in a very short period of time. This type of consumption can quickly lead to extreme intoxication, including unconsciousness, alcohol poisoning, and even death. Often, drinking competitions or games, and hazing rituals encourage this type of drinking. To see if your alcohol consumption is a problem, complete the Assess Yourself box on page 376.

There is also significant evidence that campus rape is linked to binge drinking. Women from colleges with medium to high binge drinking rates are 1.5 times more at risk of being raped than those from schools with a low binge drinking rate. Seventy-two percent of campus rapes occur when the victim is so intoxicated that she is unable to consent or refuse.[5] For more on rape, see Chapter 4.

Binge drinking also affects those who do not participate in binge drinking behavior. A recent study indicates that each year over 696,000 students between the ages of 18 and 24 are assaulted by another student who has been drinking.[6] Other students report sleep and study disruptions, experiencing sexual abuse and other unwanted sexual advances, and vandalism of personal property.

To curb binge drinking and alcohol abuse, many schools are instituting strong policies against drinking. University presidents have formed a leadership group to help curb the problem of alcohol abuse. Many fraternities have elected to have dry houses. At the same time, schools are making more help available to students with drinking problems. Today, both individual and group counseling are offered on most campuses, and more attention is being directed toward the prevention of alcohol abuse. Student organizations such as BACCHUS (Boost Alcohol Consciousness Concerning the Health of University Students) promote responsible drinking and party hosting. See the Health Ethics box on page 378 to learn about another aspect of colleges' response to alcohol.

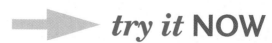 *try it* **NOW**

Cutting back on or abstaining from alcohol will improve your life and health. Here are some harm reduction strategies you can practice when you drink: Determine in advance not to exceed a set number of drinks and keep track of how many you've had; choose not to drink alcohol, but if you feel you must have a drink in your hand, choose soda with a lemon or lime; use a designated driver and never ride with a driver who has been drinking; eat before or during drinking; avoid drinking games.

| TABLE 12.2 | The Frequency and Effects of Binge Drinking among College Students | | | | | | |

College Students' Patterns of Alcohol Use, 2001				Alcohol-Related Problems			
Category	Total (%)	Men (%)	Women (%)	Problem Reported	Nonbinge Drinkers (%)	Frequent Binge Drinkers (%)	
Abstainer (past year)	19.3	20.1	18.7	Did something regrettable	18	62	
Nonbinge drinker	36.3	31.3	40.4	Missed a class	9	63	
Occasional binge drinker	21.6	23.4	20.0	Forgot where they were or what they did	10	54	
Frequent binge drinker	22.8	25.2	20.9	Got behind in schoolwork	10	46	
				Argued with friends	10	43	
				Got hurt or injured	4	27	
				Damaged property	2	23	
				Engaged in unplanned sexual activities	8	42	
				Drove after drinking	19	57	

Sources: H. Wechsler et al., "Trends in College Binge Drinking During a Period of Increased Prevention Efforts: Findings from Four Harvard School of Public Health College Study Surveys: 1993–2001," *Journal of American College Health* 50, no. 5 (2002): 207; H. Wechsler et al., "College Binge Drinking in the 1990s: A Continuing Problem," *Journal of American College Health* 48 (2002): 207. Reprinted with permission of Helen Dwight Reid Educational Foundation. Published by Heldref Publications, 1319 18th St. NW, Washington, DC 20036. Copyright 2002.

Trends in Consumption

In general, alcohol consumption levels among Americans have declined steadily since the late 1970s. In 2003, the estimated per capita consumption was the equivalent of 2.2 gallons of pure alcohol per person.[7] This represents a substantial decline from 2.64 gallons in 1977. (This measure indicates the amount of alcohol that a person would obtain by drinking approximately 50 gallons of beer, 20 gallons of wine, or more than 4 gallons of distilled spirits.)

This downward trend has been tied to a growing attention to weight, personal health, and physical activity. The alcohol industry has responded by introducing beers and wines with fewer calories and carbohydrates and with reduced alcohol content.

what do you THINK?

Why do some college students drink excessive amounts of alcohol? ■ Are there particular traditions or norms related to when and why students drink on your campus? ■ Have you ever had your sleep or studies interrupted or have you had to babysit a friend because he or she had been drinking? ■ Did you say anything about it to your friend? ■ How did the person respond?

Physiological and Behavioral Effects of Alcohol

The Chemical Makeup of Alcohol

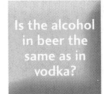

Is the alcohol in beer the same as in vodka?

The intoxicating substance found in beer, wine, liquor, and liqueurs is **ethyl alcohol, or ethanol.** It is produced during a process called **fermentation,** whereby yeast organisms break down plant sugars, yielding ethanol and carbon dioxide.

(Text continues on page 378)

ethyl alcohol (ethanol) An addictive drug produced by fermentation and found in many beverages.

fermentation The process whereby yeast organisms break down plant sugars to yield ethanol.

ASSESS yourself

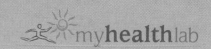

ALCOHOL ABUSE: EVALUATING YOUR RISK

Fill out this assessment online at
www.aw-bc.com/MyHealthLab or
www.aw-bc.com/donatelle.

For each question choose the answer that is correct for you.

1. How often do you have a drink containing alcohol?

   | Never | Monthly or less | Two to four times a month | Two to three times a week | Four or more times a week |

2. How many drinks containing alcohol do you have on a typical day when you are drinking?

   | 1 or 2 | 3 or 4 | 5 or 6 | 7 to 9 | 10 or more |

3. How often do you have six drinks or more on one occasion?

   | Never | Less than monthly | Monthly | Weekly | Daily or almost daily |

4. How often during the last year have you found that you were not able to stop drinking once you had started?

   | Never | Less than monthly | Monthly | Weekly | Daily or almost daily |

5. How often during the last year have you failed to do what was normally expected from you because of drinking?

   | Never | Less than monthly | Monthly | Weekly | Daily or almost daily |

6. How often during the last year have you needed a first drink in the morning to get yourself going after a heavy drinking session?

   | Never | Less than monthly | Monthly | Weekly | Daily or almost daily |

7. How often during the last year have you had a feeling of guilt or remorse after drinking?

   | Never | Less than monthly | Monthly | Weekly | Daily or almost daily |

8. How often during the last year have you been unable to remember what happened the night before because you had been drinking?

   | Never | Less than monthly | Monthly | Weekly | Daily or almost daily |

9. Have you or someone else been injured as a result of your drinking?

   | No | Yes, but not in the last year | Yes, during the last year |

10. Has a relative or friend or a doctor or other health worker been concerned about your drinking or suggested you cut down?

   | No | Yes, but not in the last year | Yes, during the last year |

Analyzing Your Answers

Each question has a unique scoring system. Assign yourself the correct number of points as indicated below, based on your answers above.

Question 1: 0 = never; 1 = monthly or less; 2 = 2–4 times/month; 3 = 2–3 times/week; 4 = four or more times/week

Question 2: 0 = 1–2 drinks; 1 = 3–4 drinks; 2 = 5–6 drinks; 3 = 7–9 drinks; 4 = 10 or more drinks

Questions 3–8: 0 = never; 1 = less than monthly; 2 = monthly; 3 = weekly; 4 = daily or almost daily

Questions 9 and 10: 0 = no; 1 = yes, but not in the last year; 2 = yes, during the last year

Scores below 6: Congratulations! You are in control of your drinking behaviors and do a good job of consuming alcohol responsibly and in moderation.

Scores between 6 and 8: Your alcohol consumption is possibly risky. Try to take steps to change your drinking behavior. It might be hard when you are surrounded by friends who participate in the same risky actions, but try to make some positive changes for your health and safety.

Scores above 8: Your drinking patterns are putting you at high risk for illness, unsafe sexual situations, or alcohol-related injuries, and may even affect your academic performance. Look back at how you answered each question, and identify some changes you can make to reduce your risk.

Source: K. Bush et al., "The AUDIT Alcohol Consumption Questions (Audit-C)," *Archives of Internal Medicine* 158, no. 16 (1998): 1789–1795, 1998; World Health Organization, Division of Mental Health and Prevention of Substance Abuse, "Alcohol Use Disorders Identification Test (AUDIT)," 2006, www.who.net.

MAKE it happen!

ASSESSMENT: The Assess Yourself activity above gave you the chance to evaluate your alcohol consumption and determine if it is harmful to you and those around you. If you were surprised by some of your answers, or couldn't be sure how to answer some of the questions, you may want to take steps to change your behavior.

MAKING A CHANGE: In order to change your behavior, you need to develop a plan. Follow the steps below and complete your Behavior Change Contract to take action.

1. Evaluate your behavior and identify patterns and specific things you are doing. What can you change now? What can you change in the near future?

2. Select one pattern of behavior that you want to change.

3. Fill out the Behavior Change Contract found at the front of your book. It should include your long-term goal for change, your short-term goals, the rewards you'll give yourself for reaching these goals, potential obstacles along the way, and strategies for overcoming these obstacles. For each goal, list the small steps and specific actions that you will take.

4. Chart your progress in a journal. At the end of a week, consider how successful you were in following your plan. What helped you be successful? What made change more difficult? What will you do differently next week?

5. Revise your plan as needed: Are the short-term goals attainable? Are the rewards satisfying?

ONE STUDENT'S PLAN: After completing the Assess Yourself box, Mark was surprised to discover that he drank much more often than he thought. In particular, he was surprised to realize that he was a heavy episodic drinker. During his three years in college, Mark had grown used to consuming five or more drinks once a week, and he had never seen this as a problem before he completed this questionnaire. He decided to address his concerns about his alcohol use in several steps.

First, Mark kept a log of his alcohol consumption over two weeks. He saw that he was drinking almost every night of the week, and drinking very heavily at least once a week. Mark decided that he wanted to reduce his drinking and set two goals: taking a break from drinking altogether for three weeks, and after that, drinking only 3 drinks on Friday and Saturday nights for the rest of the semester. Mark explained to his friends that he was taking a break and invited them to go with him on hikes, to the movies, and to other alcohol-free environments. After successfully taking this break, Mark decided to set some goals and limits for himself on the alcohol he would consume in the future. He went to a fraternity party on a Friday night and drank two beers, his predetermined limit. He was happy to realize when he woke up the next morning that he felt refreshed, not hung over. When he went out for dinner with his friends Saturday night, they wanted to go barhopping afterward. He volunteered to be the designated driver, and the bar gave him free sodas for the night. The next weekend, Mark found he had extra money that he hadn't spent on beer during the week and bought himself a new DVD.

SHOULD COLLEGES CALL PARENTS WITHOUT STUDENT CONSENT?

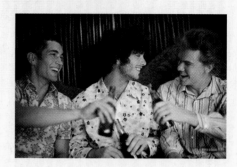

Students' right to privacy versus parents' right to know is at the heart of a debate over a federal law that allows school administrators to disclose a student's academic or probationary record to parents without the student's consent. Legally, universities have the option of telling a student's parents about underage drinking and illicit drug violations. Some college officials are taking a wait-and-see approach, whereas others are embracing the law, saying it gives them a chance to respond to early warning signs to curb alcohol and drug abuse on campus.

What is your campus's policy on parental notification? What are some of the issues surrounding this amendment? Do you think this is a good idea? Explain your answer.

Fermentation continues until the solution of plant sugars (called mash) reaches a concentration of 14 percent alcohol. At this point, the alcohol kills the yeast and halts the chemical reactions that produce it.

For beers and ales, which are fermented from malt barley, manufacturers then add other ingredients that dilute the alcohol content of the beverage. Other alcoholic beverages are produced through further processing called **distillation,** during which alcohol vapors are released from the mash at high temperatures. The vapors are then condensed and mixed with water to make the final product.

The **proof** of an alcoholic drink is a measure of the percentage of alcohol in the beverage. "Proof" comes from "gunpowder proof," a reference to the gunpowder test, whereby potential buyers would test the distiller's product by pouring it on gunpowder and attempting to light it. If the alcohol content was at least 50 percent, the gunpowder would burn; otherwise the water in the product would put out the flame. Thus, alcohol percentage is 50 percent of the given proof. For example, 80 proof whiskey or scotch is 40 percent alcohol by volume, and 100 proof vodka is 50 percent alcohol by volume. The proof of a beverage indicates its strength. Lower-proof drinks will produce fewer alcoholic effects than the same amount of higher-proof drinks.

Most wines are between 12 and 15 percent alcohol, and ales are between 6 and 8 percent. The alcoholic content of beers is between 2 and 6 percent, varying according to state laws and type of beer (Figure 12.2).

Absorption and Metabolism

Unlike the molecules found in most other ingestible foods and drugs, alcohol molecules are sufficiently small and fat soluble to be absorbed throughout the entire gastrointestinal system. A negligible amount of alcohol is absorbed through the lining of the mouth. Approximately 20 percent of ingested alcohol diffuses through the stomach lining into the bloodstream, and nearly 80 percent passes through the linings of the upper third of the small intestine. Absorption into the bloodstream is rapid and complete.

Several factors influence how quickly your body will absorb alcohol: the alcohol concentration in your drink, the amount of alcohol you consume, the amount of food in your stomach, pylorospasm (spasm of the pyloric valve in the digestive system), your metabolism, weight, and body mass index, and your mood. The higher the concentration of alcohol in your drink, the more rapidly it will be absorbed in your

distillation The process whereby mash is subjected to high temperatures to release alcohol vapors, which are then condensed and mixed with water to make the final product.

proof A measure of the percentage of alcohol in a beverage.

FUNfact

Every year, undergraduate students in America consume 4 billion cans of beer, or the equivalent of 48 billion gallons. That's enough beer to fill the Pacific Ocean 748 times.

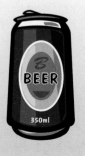

FIGURE 12.1 How Much Beer Do College Students Consume Each Year?

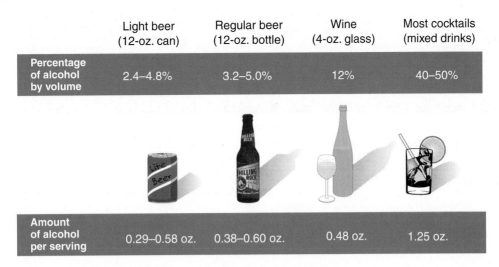

	Light beer (12-oz. can)	Regular beer (12-oz. bottle)	Wine (4-oz. glass)	Most cocktails (mixed drinks)
Percentage of alcohol by volume	2.4–4.8%	3.2–5.0%	12%	40–50%
Amount of alcohol per serving	0.29–0.58 oz.	0.38–0.60 oz.	0.48 oz.	1.25 oz.

FIGURE 12.2 Alcoholic Beverages and Their Alcohol Equivalencies

digestive tract. As a rule, wine and beer are absorbed more slowly than distilled beverages. Carbonated alcoholic beverages—such as champagne and carbonated wines—are absorbed more rapidly than those containing no sparkling additives, or fizz. Carbonated beverages and drinks served with mixers cause the pyloric valve—the opening from the stomach into the small intestine—to relax, thereby emptying the contents of the stomach more rapidly into the small intestine. Because the small intestine is the site of the greatest absorption of alcohol, carbonated beverages increase the rate of absorption. On the other hand, if your stomach is full, absorption slows because the surface area exposed to alcohol is smaller. A full stomach also retards the emptying of alcoholic beverages into the small intestine.

In addition, the more alcohol you consume, the longer absorption takes. Alcohol can irritate the digestive system, causing a spasm in the pyloric valve (pylorospasm). When the pyloric valve is closed, nothing can move from the stomach to the upper third of the small intestine, which slows absorption. If the irritation continues, it can cause vomiting.

Mood is another factor, because emotions affect how long it takes for the contents of the stomach to empty into the intestine. Powerful moods, such as stress and tension, are likely to cause the stomach to dump its contents into the small intestine. That is why alcohol is absorbed much more rapidly when people are tense than when they are relaxed.

Alcohol is metabolized in the liver, where it is converted by the enzyme *alcohol dehydrogenase* to *acetaldehyde*. It is then rapidly oxidized to *acetate,* converted to carbon dioxide and water, and eventually excreted from the body. Acetaldehyde is a toxic chemical that can cause immediate symptoms such as nausea and vomiting, as well as long-term effects such as liver damage. A very small portion of alcohol is excreted unchanged by the kidneys, lungs, and skin.

Like food, alcohol contains calories. Proteins and carbohydrates (starches and sugars) each contain 4 kilocalories (kcal) per gram. Fat contains 9 kcal per gram. Alcohol, although similar in structure to carbohydrates, contains 7 kcal per gram. The body uses the calories in alcohol in the same manner as it uses calories from carbohydrates: for immediate energy or for storage as fat if not immediately needed.

When compared to the variable breakdown rates of foods and other beverages, the breakdown of alcohol occurs at a fairly constant rate of 0.5 ounce per hour. This amount of alcohol is equivalent to 12 ounces of 5 percent beer, 8 ounces of malt liquor, 4 ounces of 12 percent wine, or 1.5 ounces of 40 percent (80 proof) liquor.

Blood Alcohol Concentration

Blood alcohol concentration (BAC) is the ratio of alcohol to total blood volume. It is the primary method of measuring the amount of alcohol one has consumed and to gauge the physiological and behavioral effects of alcohol. At low concentrations, alcohol tends to make people feel relaxed and more outgoing; at higher blood alcohol levels, people may feel angry, irritable, or sleepy. Despite individual differences, alcohol produces some general behavioral effects depending on BAC (Table 12.3 on page 380). At a BAC of 0.02 percent, a person feels slightly relaxed and in a good mood. At 0.05 percent, relaxation increases, there is some motor impairment, and a willingness to talk becomes apparent. At 0.08 percent, the person feels euphoric, and there is further motor impairment. At 0.10 percent, the depressant effects of alcohol become apparent, drowsiness sets in, and motor skills are further impaired, followed by a loss of judgment. Thus, a driver may not be able to estimate distance or speed, and some

blood alcohol concentration (BAC) The ratio of alcohol to total blood volume; the factor used to measure the physiological and behavioral effects of alcohol.

Number of Drinks†	Blood Alcohol Concentration (%)	Psychological and Physical Effects
2	0.05–0.06	Feeling of relaxation, warmth; slight decrease in reaction time and in fine-muscle coordination
3	0.08–0.09	Balance, speech, vision, and hearing slightly impaired; feelings of euphoria, increased confidence; loss of motor coordination
3–4	0.08	Legal intoxication in most states
4	0.11–0.12	Coordination and balance becoming difficult; distinct impairment of mental faculties, judgment
5	0.14–0.15	Major impairment of mental and physical control; slurred speech, blurred vision, lack of motor skills
7	0.20	Loss of motor control—must have assistance in moving about; mental confusion
>10	>0.30	Severe intoxication; minimal conscious control of mind and body
14	0.40	Unconsciousness, coma, death

*For each hour elapsed since the last drink, subtract 0.015 percent blood alcohol concentration, or approximately one drink.

† One drink = one beer (4% alcohol, 12 ounces), one highball (1.25 ounces whiskey), or one glass table wine (5 ounces).

Source: Modified from data given in Ohio State Police Driver Information Seminars and the National Clearinghouse for Alcohol and Alcoholism Information, Rockville, MD.

drinkers lose their ability to make value-related decisions and may do things they would not do when sober. As BAC increases, the drinker suffers increased physiological and psychological effects. All these changes are negative. Alcohol ingestion does not enhance any physical skills or mental functions.

A drinker's BAC depends on weight and body fat, the water content in body tissues, the concentration of alcohol in the beverage consumed, the rate of consumption, and the volume of alcohol consumed. Heavier people have larger body surfaces through which to diffuse alcohol; therefore, they have lower concentrations of alcohol in their blood than do thin people after drinking the same amount. Because alcohol does not diffuse as rapidly into body fat as into water, the BAC is higher in a person with more body fat. Because a woman is likely to have more body fat and less water in her body tissues than a man of the same weight, she will be more intoxicated than a man after drinking the same amount of alcohol.

Both breath analysis (Breathalyzer tests) and urinalysis are used to determine whether an individual is legally intoxicated, but blood tests are more accurate measures of BAC. An increasing number of states are requiring blood tests for people suspected of driving under the influence of alcohol. In some states, refusal to take the breath or urine test results in immediate revocation of the person's driver's license. A driver whose level of BAC exceeds the state's legal limit is considered legally intoxicated.

 People can acquire physical and psychological tolerance of the effects of alcohol through regular use. The nervous system adapts over time, so greater amounts of alcohol are required to produce the same physiological and psychological effects. Some people can learn to modify their behavior so that they appear to be sober even when their BAC is quite high. This ability is called **learned behavioral tolerance.**

Physiological and Behavioral Effects

Alcohol and Injuries
The use of alcohol plays a significant role in the types of injuries people experience. Thirteen percent of emergency room visits by undergraduates are related to alcohol, and of this total, 34 percent were the result of acute intoxication. A recent study found that injured patients treated in emergency rooms with a BAC of over 0.08 percent were 3.2 times more likely to have a violent injury than an unintentional injury.[8] Men 21 years or older are the most common emergency room admittees, mostly as the result of accidents or fights, where alcohol was involved.[9]

Alcohol Poisoning
Alcohol poisoning occurs much more frequently than people realize, and all too often it can be fatal. Drinking large amounts of alcohol in a short period of time can cause the blood alcohol level to reach the lethal range quickly. Alcohol, used either alone or in combination

learned behavioral tolerance The ability of heavy drinkers to modify behavior so that they appear to be sober even when they have high BAC levels.

Number of drinks consumed in:

Body weight (pounds)	1 hour					2 hours					3 hours					4 hours				
	1	2	3	4	5	1	2	3	4	5	1	2	3	4	5	1	2	3	4	5
100																				
120																				
140																				
160																				
180																				
200																				

■ (0.00%) Not impaired   ■ (0.05–0.07%) Usually impaired

■ (0.01–0.04%) Sometimes impaired   ■ (0.08% and up) Always impaired

FIGURE 12.3 Approximate Blood Alcohol Concentration Based on Body Weight and Number of Drinks
This represents the BAC of an average individual, considering weight and number of drinks consumed. Remember that there are many variables that can affect BAC, so is just a rough estimate of what your BAC would be.

with other drugs, is responsible for more toxic overdose deaths than any other substance. An all-too-common scenario on college campuses occurs when inexperienced drinkers play drinking games or try to see who can drink the most. A college student might try to consume 21 drinks for his or her twenty-first birthday; in real life, college students have died as a result of such challenges.

Death from alcohol poisoning can be caused by either central nervous system (CNS) and respiratory depression or the inhalation of vomit or fluid into the lungs. The amount of alcohol it takes for a person to become unconscious is dangerously close to the lethal dose. Signs of alcohol poisoning include inability to be roused; a weak, rapid pulse; an unusual, slow, or irregular breathing pattern; mental confusion; vomiting; seizures; and cool (possibly damp), pale, or bluish skin.

What should you do if you suspect someone has alcohol poisoning? Make sure you know the warning signals, and don't wait for all of the symptoms to be present before calling for help. If you are with someone who has been drinking heavily and who exhibits symptoms, or if you are unsure about the person's condition, call 911 for emergency help right away. Don't wait for the individual to become unconscious; by then, the risk of death increases tenfold.

Alcohol and Sexual Decision Making
Alcohol has a clear influence on one's abilities to make good decisions about sex, because it lowers your inhibitions, and you may do things you might not do when sober. Seventy percent of college students admit to having engaged in sexual activity primarily as a result of being under the influence of alcohol. Students who are intoxicated are less likely to use safer sex practices, and are more likely to engage in other high-risk sexual activity. The risk of acquiring an STI or an unplanned

pregnancy also increases among those who drink more heavily, compared with those who drink moderately or not at all.

Women and Alcohol
Body fat is not the only contributor to the differences in alcohol's effects on men and women. Compared with men, women appear to have half as much *alcohol dehydrogenase,* the enzyme that breaks down alcohol in the stomach before it has a chance to get to the bloodstream and the brain. Therefore, if a man and a woman drink the same amount of alcohol, the woman's BAC will be approximately 30 percent higher than the man's, leaving her more vulnerable to slurred speech, dangerous driving, and other drinking-related impairments.

Hormonal differences can also affect a woman's BAC. Certain times in the menstrual cycle and oral contraceptives are likely to contribute to longer periods of intoxication. This prolonged peak appears to be related to estrogen levels.

Women who consume alcohol need to pay close attention to how much they consume. It is possible that a woman matching her male friend drink for drink could become twice as intoxicated. For example, if a 180-pound college-aged man and a 120-pound college-aged woman each have three drinks, the BAC for the male would be 0.06 percent and for the female 0.11 percent, almost double that of her male friend. Figure 12.3 compares blood alcohol levels by weight and consumption. Although this table can provide an estimate of probable BAC levels, many additional factors may cause considerable variation in these rates.

what do you THINK?
Have you noticed that some types of alcoholic beverages affect people more quickly than others? ■ What factors affect BAC levels? ■ Are these factors different for men and women? If so, how?

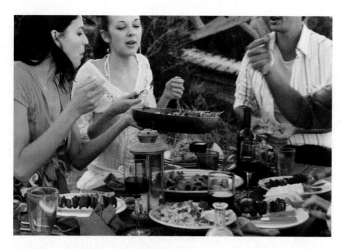

Many factors influence how rapidly your body absorbs alcohol. For example, eating while drinking is a safe habit to practice, as it slows down the absorption of alcohol into your bloodstream.

Immediate Effects of Alcohol

The most dramatic effects produced by ethanol occur within the central nervous system (CNS). Alcohol depresses CNS functions, with resulting decreases in respiratory rate, pulse rate, and blood pressure. As CNS depression deepens, vital functions become noticeably depressed. In extreme cases, coma and death can result.

Alcohol is a diuretic, causing increased urinary output. Although this effect might be expected to lead to automatic **dehydration** (loss of water from body tissues), the body actually retains water, most of it in the muscles or in cerebral tissues. This is because water is usually pulled out of the **cerebrospinal fluid** (fluid within the brain and spinal cord), leading to what is known as mitochondrial dehydration at the cellular level within the nervous system. Mitochondria are miniature organs within cells that are responsible for specific functions, and they rely heavily upon fluid balance. When mitochondrial dehydration occurs from drinking, the mitochondria cannot carry out their normal functions, resulting in symptoms that include the "morning-after" headaches suffered by some drinkers.

Alcohol irritates the gastrointestinal system and may cause indigestion and heartburn if taken on an empty stomach. In addition, people who engage in brief drinking sprees during which they consume unusually high amounts of alcohol put

---

dehydration Loss of fluids from body tissues.

cerebrospinal fluid Fluid within and surrounding the brain and spinal cord tissues.

hangover The physiological reaction to excessive drinking, including symptoms such as headache, upset stomach, anxiety, depression, diarrhea, and thirst.

congeners Forms of alcohol that are metabolized more slowly than ethanol and produce toxic by-products.

---

themselves at risk for irregular heartbeat or even total loss of heart rhythm, which can disrupt blood flow and damage the heart muscle.

Is there any cure for a hangover?

Hangover A **hangover** is often experienced the morning after a drinking spree. The symptoms of a hangover are familiar to most people who drink: headache, muscle aches, upset stomach, anxiety, depression, diarrhea, and thirst. Congeners are thought to play a role in the development of a hangover. **Congeners** are forms of alcohol that are metabolized more slowly than ethanol and are more toxic. The body metabolizes the congeners after the ethanol is gone from the system, and their toxic by-products may contribute to the hangover. Alcohol also upsets water balance in the body, resulting in excess urination and thirst the next day. Increased production of hydrochloric acid can irritate the stomach lining and cause nausea. It usually takes 12 hours to recover from a hangover. Bed rest, solid food, and aspirin may help relieve its discomforts, but the only cure for a hangover is abstaining from excessive alcohol use.

Drug Interactions When you use any drug (and alcohol is a drug), you need to be aware of its possible interactions with other drugs, whether prescription or over the counter. If you are taking any medication, ask your doctor or pharmacist if alcohol consumption is safe while taking the medication. Avoid using alcohol when taking antihistamines, antibiotics, analgesics, antidepressants, and antianxiety medications due to the potential for hazardous interactions. Note that alcohol may cause a negative interaction even with aspirin.

Long-Term Effects

Alcohol is distributed throughout most of the body and may affect many different organs and tissues. Problems associated with long-term, habitual abuse of alcohol include diseases of the cardiovascular system, nervous system, and liver, and some cancers.

Effects on the Nervous System The nervous system is especially sensitive to alcohol. Even people who drink moderately experience shrinkage in brain size and weight and a loss of some degree of intellectual ability.

New research suggests that developing brains in adolescents are much more prone to brain damage than was previously thought. Alcohol appears to damage the frontal areas of the adolescent brain, which are crucial for controlling impulses and thinking through consequences of intended actions.[10] In addition, researchers suggest that people who begin drinking at an early age face enormous risks of becoming alcoholics: 47 percent of those who begin drinking alcohol before age 14 become alcohol dependent at some time in their lives, compared with 9 percent of those who wait until at least age 21.[11]

Cardiovascular Effects Alcohol affects the cardiovascular system in a number of ways. Numerous studies have associated light-to-moderate alcohol consumption (no more than two drinks a day) with a reduced risk of coronary artery disease. Several mechanisms have been proposed to explain how this might happen. The strongest evidence favors an increase in high-density lipoprotein (HDL) cholesterol, which is known as the "good" cholesterol. Studies have shown that drinkers have higher levels of HDL. Another factor that might help is an *antithrombotic effect.* Alcohol consumption is associated with a decrease in clotting factors that contribute to the development of atherosclerosis.

However, this does not mean that alcohol consumption is recommended as a preventive measure against heart disease—it causes many more cardiovascular health hazards than benefits. Alcohol contributes to high blood pressure and slightly increased heart rate and cardiac output. Those who report drinking three to five drinks a day, regardless of race or sex, have higher blood pressure than those who drink less.

Liver Disease One of the most common diseases related to alcohol abuse is **cirrhosis** of the liver. It is among the top ten causes of death in the United States. One result of heavy drinking is that the liver begins to store fat—a condition known as fatty liver. If there is insufficient time between drinking episodes, this fat cannot be transported to storage sites, and the fat-filled liver cells stop functioning. Continued drinking can cause a further stage of liver deterioration called fibrosis, in which the damaged area of the liver develops fibrous scar tissue. Cell function can be partially restored at this stage with proper nutrition and abstinence from alcohol. If the person continues to drink, however, cirrhosis results. At this point, the liver cells die and the damage becomes permanent.

Alcoholic hepatitis is a serious condition resulting from prolonged use of alcohol. A chronic inflammation of the liver develops, which may be fatal in itself or progress to cirrhosis.

Cancer The repeated irritation caused by long-term use of alcohol has been linked to cancers of the esophagus, stomach, mouth, tongue, pancreas, and liver. There is substantial evidence that breast cancer risk is elevated for women consuming high levels of alcohol (more than three drinks per day) compared with abstainers.[12] It is unclear how alcohol exerts its carcinogenic effects. In a recent study, a team of scientists from the National Institute of Alcohol Abuse and Alcoholism discovered a possible link between acetaldehyde and DNA damage. Scientists suspect that the results of this study could help to explain the connection between drinking and certain types of cancer.[13]

Other Effects Alcohol abuse is a major cause of chronic inflammation of the pancreas, the organ that produces digestive enzymes and insulin. Drinking alcohol can also block the absorption of calcium, a nutrient that strengthens bones. This should be of particular concern to women, for as women age their risk for osteoporosis increases.

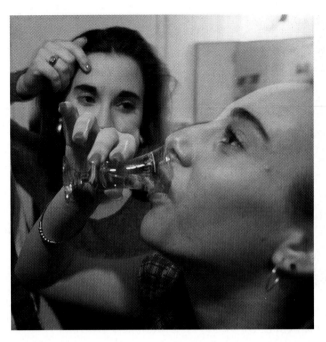

Increasing numbers of women on college campuses are trying to keep up with their male peers when binge drinking. The results can be dangerous; a woman's BAC will be higher than a man's after the same number of drinks.

Evidence also suggests that alcohol impairs the body's ability to recognize and fight foreign bodies such as bacteria and viruses. The relationship between alcohol and AIDS is unclear, especially as some of the populations at risk for AIDS are also at risk for alcohol abuse. But any stressor like alcohol, with a known effect on the immune system, would probably contribute to the development of the disease.

Alcohol and Pregnancy

Recall from Chapter 7 that *teratogenic* substances cause birth defects. Of the 30 known teratogens in the environment, alcohol is one of the most dangerous and common. Alcohol can harm fetal development. More than 10 percent of all children have been exposed to high levels of alcohol in utero. All will suffer varying degrees of effects, ranging from mild learning disabilities to major physical, mental, and intellectual impairment. A disorder called **fetal alcohol syndrome (FAS)**

cirrhosis The last stage of liver disease associated with chronic heavy use of alcohol during which liver cells die and damage becomes permanent.

alcoholic hepatitis A condition resulting from prolonged use of alcohol in which the liver is inflamed; it can result in death.

fetal alcohol syndrome (FAS) A disorder that may affect the fetus when the mother consumes alcohol during pregnancy. Among its effects are mental retardation, small head, tremors, and abnormalities of the face, limbs, heart, and brain.

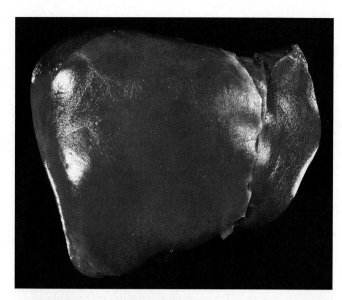

(a) A normal liver.

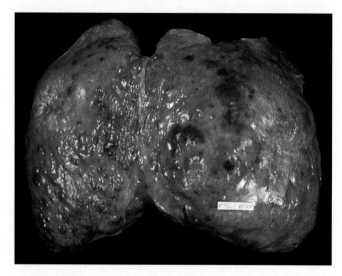

(b) A liver with cirrhosis.

is associated with alcohol consumption during pregnancy. Alcohol consumed during the first trimester poses the greatest threat to organ development; exposure during the last trimester, when the brain is developing rapidly, is most likely to affect CNS development. FAS is the third most common birth defect and the second leading cause of mental retardation in the United States. The incidence of FAS is estimated to be 1 to 2 of every 1,000 live births. It is the most common preventable cause of mental impairment in the Western world.

fetal alcohol effects (FAE) A syndrome describing children with a history of prenatal alcohol exposure but without all the physical or behavioral symptoms of FAS. Among its symptoms are low birth weight, irritability, and possible permanent mental impairment.

If a woman ingests alcohol while pregnant, it will pass through the placenta and enter the growing fetus's bloodstream. It is recommended that women do not consume any alcohol during pregnancy. Among the symptoms of FAS are mental retardation, small head, tremors, and abnormalities of the face, limbs, heart, and brain. Children with FAS may experience problems such as:[14]

■ Difficulty in structuring work time
■ Poor social judgment and memory, and impaired learning
■ Reduced attention span, impulsive behaviors, and fearlessness
■ Differences in sensory awareness (hyposensitive or hypersensitive)
■ Poor problem-solving strategies

Some children may have fewer than the full physical or behavioral symptoms of FAS and can be categorized as having **fetal alcohol effects (FAE).** FAE is estimated to occur three to four times more often than FAS, although it is much less recognized. The signs of FAE in newborns are low birth weight and irritability, and there may be permanent mental impairment. Infants whose mothers habitually consumed more than three ounces of alcohol (approximately six drinks) in a short time period when pregnant are at high risk for FAS. Risk levels for babies whose mothers consume smaller amounts are uncertain.

 what do you THINK?

Why do we hear so little about FAS in this country when it is the third most common birth defect and second leading cause of mental retardation? ■ Is this a reflection of our society's denial of alcohol as a dangerous drug?

Drinking and Driving

Traffic accidents are the leading cause of death for all age groups from 5 to 45 years old (including college students). Approximately 39 percent of all traffic fatalities in 2004 were alcohol related.[15] Unfortunately, college students are overrepresented in alcohol-related crashes. In the hallmark College Alcohol Study, findings indicated that 20 percent of non-bingers, 43 percent of occasional bingers, and 59 percent of frequent bingers reported driving while intoxicated.[16] Furthermore, it estimated that three out of every ten Americans will be involved in an alcohol-related accident at some time in their lives.[17]

What's the legal limit for drinking and driving?

In 2004, there were 16,694 alcohol-related traffic fatalities (ARTFs), a 5 percent reduction from 1982.[18] Over the past 20 years, intoxication rates (BAC of 0.10 percent or greater) decreased for drivers of all age groups involved in fatal crashes (Figure 12.4). This number represents an average of one alcohol-related fatality approximately every 30 minutes.[19] Several factors probably contributed to

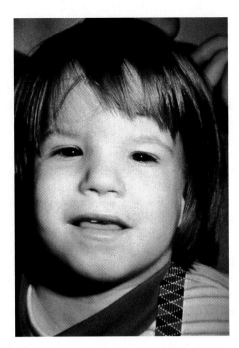

The effects of fetal alcohol syndrome on a child are irreversible.

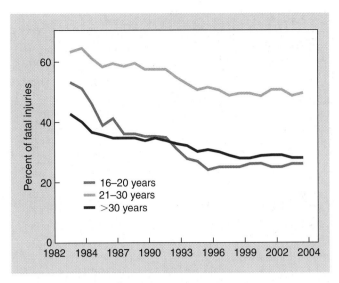

FIGURE 12.4 Percentage of Fatally Injured Passenger Vehicle Drivers with BACs ≥ 0.08 Percent, by Driver Age
The highest intoxication rates in fatal crashes were recorded for drivers 21 to 30 years old.

Source: Insurance Institute for Highway Safety, "Fatality Facts: Alcohol 2002," 2003, www.iihs.org.

these reductions in ARTFs: laws that raised the drinking age to 21; stricter law enforcement; increased emphasis on zero tolerance (laws prohibiting those under 21 from driving with any detectable BAC); and educational programs designed to discourage drinking and driving. In 2005, the legal limit for BAC in all states was 0.08 percent. Furthermore, many states have zero-tolerance laws, and the penalty usually is a suspended driver's license.[20]

Laboratory and test track research shows that the vast majority of drivers, even experienced drinkers, are impaired even at 0.08 percent with regard to critical driving tasks. Braking, steering, lane changing, judgment, and attention, among other measures, are all affected significantly at 0.08 percent BAC. National groups such as MADD (Mothers Against Drunk Driving) and SADD (Students Against Destructive Decisions) try to educate their peers about the dangers of drinking and driving.

Despite all these measures, the risk of being involved in an alcohol-related automobile crash remains substantial. Researchers have shown a direct relationship between the amount of alcohol in a driver's bloodstream and the likelihood of a crash. A driver with a BAC level of 0.10 percent is approximately ten times more likely to be involved in a car accident than a driver who has not been drinking. At a BAC of 0.15 percent on weekend nights, the likelihood of dying in a single-vehicle crash is more than 380 times higher than for nondrinkers. Only 27 percent of fatally injured drivers involved in nighttime single-vehicle crashes had no alcohol in their blood.[21]

Not only does the time of day increase risk of being involved in an alcohol-related crash, but it also makes a difference whether it is a weekday or weekend. In 2002, 25 percent of all fatal crashes during the week were alcohol related, compared with 44 percent on weekends.[22]

 what do you THINK?

What do you think the legal BAC for drivers should be? ■ What should the penalty be for people arrested for driving under the influence of alcohol (DUI) for the first offense? The second offense? The third offense?

Alcohol Abuse and Alcoholism

Alcohol use becomes **alcohol abuse** when it interferes with work, school, or social and family relationships or when it entails any violation of the law, including driving under the influence (DUI). **Alcoholism,** or **alcohol dependency,** results when personal and health problems related to alcohol use are severe and stopping alcohol use results in withdrawal symptoms; some 6 million Americans can be described as alcoholics.

alcohol abuse Use of alcohol that interferes with work, school, or personal relationships or that entails violations of the law.

alcoholism (alcohol dependency) A condition in which personal and health problems related to alcohol use are severe and stopping alcohol use results in withdrawal symptoms.

Identifying a Problem Drinker

As in other drug addictions, tolerance, psychological dependence, and withdrawal symptoms must be present to qualify a drinker as an addict (Chapter 11). Irresponsible and problem drinkers, such as people who get into fights or embarrass themselves or others when they drink, are not necessarily alcoholics. Ninety-five percent of alcoholics live in some type of extended family unit. Alcoholics can be found at all socioeconomic levels and in all professions, ethnic groups, geographical locations, religions, and races.

Studies suggest that the lifetime risk of alcoholism in the United States is about 10 percent for men and 3 percent for women. Moreover, almost 25 percent of the American population (50 million people) is affected by the alcoholism of a friend or family member.[23]

Recognizing and admitting the existence of an alcohol problem is often extremely difficult. Alcoholics themselves deny their problem, often making statements such as, "I can stop any time I want to. I just don't want to right now." Their families also tend to deny the problem, saying things like, "He really has been under a lot of stress lately. Besides, he only drinks beer." The fear of being labeled a "problem drinker" often prevents people from seeking help.

Alcoholics tend to have a number of symptoms in common. People who recognize one or more of these behaviors in themselves may wish to seek professional help to determine whether alcohol has become a controlling factor in their lives. The Skills for Behavior Change box on the facing page gives tips for cutting down on drinking.

Women are the fastest growing population of alcohol abusers. They tend to become alcoholic at a later age and after fewer years of heavy drinking than do male alcoholics. Women at highest risk for alcohol-related problems are those who are unmarried but living with a partner, are in their twenties or early thirties, or have a husband or partner who drinks heavily.

College Students and Problem Drinking

A recent study shows that 6 percent of college students meet the criteria for a diagnosis of alcohol dependence (also referred to as alcoholism) and 31 percent meet the criteria for alcohol abuse. Students who attend colleges with heavy drinking environments are more likely to be diagnosed with abuse or dependence. Despite the prevalence of alcohol disorders on campus, very few students seek treatment.[24]

The Causes of Alcohol Abuse and Alcoholism

We know that alcoholism is a disease with biological and social/environmental components, but we do not know what role each component plays in the disease.

Biological and Family Factors Research into the hereditary and environmental causes of alcohol abuse and alcoholism have found higher rates of alcoholism among children of alcoholics than in the general population. In fact, alcoholism is four to five times more common among children of alcoholics than in the general population. These children may be strongly influenced by the behavior they see in their parents.[25]

Scientists continue to work toward understanding the role of genes responsible for putting people at increased risk for alcoholism. Despite these efforts, no specific gene has been identified. However, studies have shown evidence of heredity's role. Studies of identical twins (twins who share the same genes) and fraternal twins (share about half of their genes, like other siblings) suggest that heredity accounts for two-thirds of the risk for becoming alcoholic in both men and women.[26]

Social and Cultural Factors Social and cultural factors may trigger the affliction for many people who are not genetically predisposed to alcoholism. Some people begin drinking as a way to dull the pain of an acute loss or an emotional or social problem. For example, college students may drink to escape the stress of college life, disappointment over unfulfilled expectations, or loss of the security of home, loved ones, and close friends. Unfortunately, the emotional discomfort that causes many people to turn to alcohol also ultimately causes them to become even more uncomfortable as the depressant effect of the drug begins to take its toll. Thus, the person who is already depressed may become even more depressed, antagonizing friends and other social supports until they turn away. Eventually, the drinker becomes physically dependent on the drug.

Family attitudes toward alcohol also seem to influence whether or not a person will develop a drinking problem. It has been clearly demonstrated that people who are raised in cultures in which drinking is a part of religious or ceremonial activities or in which alcohol is a traditional part of the family meal are less prone to alcohol dependency. In contrast, in societies in which alcohol purchase is carefully controlled and drinking is regarded as a rite of passage to adulthood, the tendency for abuse appears to be greater.

Apparently, then, some combination of heredity and environment plays a decisive role in the development of alcoholism. Certain ethnic and racial groups also have special alcohol abuse problems.

Effects of Alcoholism on the Family

Only recently have we recognized that it is not only the alcoholic, but the alcoholic's entire family that suffers. Although most research focuses on family effects during the late stages of alcoholism, the family unit actually begins to react early on as the person starts to show symptoms of the disease.

SKILLS FOR behavior change

HOW TO CUT DOWN ON YOUR DRINKING

If you are drinking too much, you can improve your life and health by cutting down. How do you know if you drink too much? Read these questions and answer yes or no.

- Do you drink alone when you feel angry or sad?
- Does your drinking ever make you late for class?
- Does your drinking worry your family?
- Do you ever forget what you did while you were drinking?
- Do you get headaches or have a hangover after you have been drinking?

If you answered "yes" to any of these questions, you may drink too much and this could be a problem. Talk with a counselor or a clinician at your student health center to be sure. Either one of these professionals will be able to tell you whether you should cut down or abstain. If you have a severe drinking problem, alcoholism in your family, or other medical problems, you should not just cut down on your drinking—you should stop drinking completely. Your counselor or clinician will advise you about what is right for you.

If you need to cut down on your drinking, these steps can help you:

1. *Write your reasons for cutting down or stopping.* There are many reasons why you may want to cut down or stop drinking. You may want to improve your health, sleep better, or get along better with your family or friends. Make a list of the reasons you want to drink less.
2. *Set a drinking goal.* Choose a limit for how much you will drink. You may

choose to cut down or to not drink at all. If you aren't sure what goal is right for you, talk with your counselor. He or she can help you determine a safe level of alcohol consumption. Once you determine your goal, write it down on a piece of paper. Put it where you can see it, such as on your refrigerator or bathroom mirror.

3. *Keep a "diary" of your drinking.* To help you reach your goal, keep a "diary" of your drinking. For example, write down every time you have a drink for 1 week. Try to keep your diary for 3 or 4 weeks. This will show you how much you drink and when. You may be surprised. How different is your goal from the amount you drink now?

These tips can help you moderate your drinking and achieve your goal:

1. *Watch it at home.* Keep a small amount or no alcohol at home. Don't keep temptations around.
2. *Drink slowly.* When you drink, sip your drink slowly. Take a break of 1 hour between drinks. Drink soda, water, or juice after a drink with alcohol. Do not drink on an empty stomach! Eat food when you are drinking.
3. *Take a break from alcohol.* Pick a day or two each week when you will not drink at all. Then, try to stop drinking for 1 week. Think about how you feel physically and emotionally on these days. When you succeed and feel better, you may find it easier to cut down for good.
4. *Learn how to say NO.* You do not have to drink when other people drink, or

take a drink when offered one. Practice ways to say no politely. For example, you can tell people you feel better when you drink less. Stay away from people who give you a hard time about not drinking.

5. *Stay active.* Use the time and money once spent on drinking to do something fun with your family or friends. Go out to eat, see a movie, or play sports or a game.
6. *Get support.* Cutting down on your drinking may be difficult at times. Ask your family and friends for support to help you reach your goal. Talk to your counselor if you are having trouble cutting down. Get the help you need to reach your goal.
7. *Watch out for temptations.* Watch out for people, places, or times that make you drink, even if you do not want to. Plan ahead of time what you will do to avoid drinking when you are tempted. Do not drink when you are angry or upset or have a bad day. These are habits you need to break if you want to drink less.
8. *Remember, do not give up!* Most people do not cut down or give up drinking all at once. Just like a diet, it is not easy to change. That is okay. If you do not reach your goal the first time, try again. Remember, get support from people who care about you and want to help.

Source: National Institute on Alcohol Abuse and Alcoholism, "How to Cut Down on Your Drinking," 2005, www.collegedrinkingprevention .gov/OtherAlcoholInformation/cutDownOn Drinking.aspx.

An estimated 77 million Americans (about 43 percent of the U.S. adult population) have been exposed to alcoholism in the family.[27] Twenty-two million members of alcoholic families are age 18 or older, and many have carried childhood emotional scars into adulthood. Approximately one in four children under age 18 lives in an atmosphere of anxiety, tension, confusion, and denial.[28]

In dysfunctional families, children learn certain "rules" from a very early age: don't talk, don't trust, and don't feel. These unspoken rules allow the family to avoid dealing with real problems and real issues, and help keep the alcoholic drinking. Children in such dysfunctional families generally assume at least one role listed on the next page.

- *Family hero.* Tries to divert attention from the problem by being too good to be true.
- *Scapegoat.* Draws attention away from the family's primary problem through delinquency or misbehavior.
- *Lost child.* Becomes passive and quietly withdraws from upsetting situations.
- *Mascot.* Disrupts tense situations by providing comic relief.

For children in alcoholic homes, life is a struggle. They have to deal with constant stress, anxiety, and embarrassment. It is not uncommon for these children to be victims of violence, abuse, neglect, or incest. As we have seen, when such children grow up, they are much more prone to alcoholic behaviors themselves than are children from nonalcoholic families.

In the past decade, we have come to recognize the unique problems of adult children of alcoholics whose difficulties in life stem from a lack of parental nurturing during childhood. Fortunately, not all individuals who have grown up in alcoholic families are doomed to have lifelong problems. As many of these people mature, they develop resiliency in response to their families' problems.

 what do you THINK?

How was alcohol used in your family when you were growing up? ■ Was alcohol used only on special occasions or not at all? ■ How much do you think your family's attitudes and behaviors toward alcohol have shaped your behavior?

Costs to Society

It is estimated that alcohol-related costs to society are well over $184.6 billion when health insurance, criminal justice costs, treatment costs, and lost productivity are factored in. Reportedly, alcoholism is directly or indirectly responsible for over 25 percent of the nation's medical expenses and lost earnings.[29]

The Cost of Underage Drinking A recent study detailed the societal costs of underage "teen" drinking. These costs take into consideration crashes, violence, property crime, suicide, burns, drowning, fetal alcohol syndrome, high-risk sex, poisoning, psychosis, and dependency treatment. It is estimated that underage drinking costs society $61.9 billion annually. The largest costs were related to violence ($34.7 billion) and drunken driving accidents ($13.5 billion). The next highest estimated costs were high-risk sex (nearly $5 billion), property crime ($3 billion), and addiction treatment programs (nearly $2 billion). When you divide the cost of underage drinking by the estimated number of underage drinkers, the study estimated that every underage drinker costs society an average of $4,680 a year.[30]

Women and Alcoholism

Studies indicate that there are now almost as many female as male alcoholics. Women get addicted faster with less alcohol use and then suffer the consequences more profoundly. Women alcoholics have death rates 50 to 100 percent higher than male alcoholics, including deaths from suicide, alcohol-related accidents, heart disease and stroke, and cirrhosis.[31]

Risk factors for drinking problems among *all women* include:

- A family history of drinking problems
- Pressure to drink from a peer or spouse
- Depression
- Stress

Drinking patterns among different age groups also differ in these ways:

- Younger women drink more overall, and experience more alcohol-related problems, such as drinking and driving, assaults, suicide attempts, and difficulties at work.
- Middle-aged women are more likely to develop drinking problems in response to a traumatic or life-changing event, such as divorce, surgery, or death of a significant other.
- Older women are more likely than older men to have developed drinking problems within the past ten years.[32]

It is estimated that only 14 percent of women who need treatment get it. In one study, women cited potential loss of income, not wanting others to know they may have a problem, inability to pay for treatment, and fear that treatment would not be confidential as reasons for not seeking treatment.[33]

Alcohol and Ethnic or Racial Differences

Different ethnic and racial minority groups have their own patterns of alcohol consumption and abuse. Among American Indian populations, alcohol is the most widely used drug; the rate of alcoholism in this population is 2 to 3 times higher than the national average, and the death rate from alcohol-related causes is 8 times higher than the national average. Possible factors for the alcoholism problem in the American Indian population are poor economic conditions and the cultural belief that alcoholism is a spiritual problem, not a physical disease.

African American and Latino populations also exhibit distinct patterns of abuse. As a group, African Americans drink less than the average white American; however, those who do drink tend to be heavy drinkers. Among Latinos, males have a higher than average rate of alcohol abuse and alcohol-related health problems. Cirrhosis and drunk driving are the most common causes of alcohol-related death or injury for Latino men. Latino women often abstain. Many researchers agree that a major factor for alcohol problems in this ethnic group is the key role that drinking plays in Latino culture.

Asian Americans have a very low rate of alcoholism. Social and cultural influences, such as strong kinship ties, are thought to discourage heavy drinking in Asian groups. Asians also have a genetic predisposition that might influence their low risk for alcohol abuse: for many, a defect in the gene that manufactures aldehyde dehydrogenase, a key enzyme in alcohol metabolism, makes drinking a less pleasurable experience due to unpleasant side effects.[34]

Despite growing recognition of our national alcohol problem, few receive any care. Factors contributing to this include an inability or unwillingness to admit to an alcohol problem; the social stigma attached to alcoholism; breakdowns in referral and delivery systems (failure of physicians or psychotherapists to follow up on referrals, client failure to follow through with recommended treatments, or failure of rehabilitation facilities to give quality care); and failure of the professional medical establishment to recognize and diagnose alcoholic symptoms among patients.

 what do you THINK?

Why do you think women appear to be drinking more heavily today than they did in the past? ■ Does society look at men's and women's drinking habits in the same way? ■ Can you think of ways to increase support for women in their recovery process?

Recovery

Most alcoholics and problem drinkers who seek help have experienced a turning point: flunking out of school, getting arrested for drunk driving, or having a spouse walk out or a boss issue an ultimatum to dry out or ship out. The alcoholic ready for treatment has, in most cases, reached a low point. Devoid of hope, physically depleted, and spiritually despairing, the person has finally recognized that alcohol controls his or her life. The first step on the road to recovery is to regain that control and assume responsibility for personal actions.

The Family's Role

Members of an alcoholic's family sometimes take action before the alcoholic does. They may go to an organization or a treatment facility to seek help for themselves and their relative.

As we saw in Chapter 11, *intervention*—a planned confrontation with the alcoholic that involves friends, family members, and professional counselors—is an effective method of helping an alcoholic to recognize the problem. Intervention is the turning point for a growing number of alcoholics. If you feel that you need to talk to a friend or family member about that person's drinking, see the Skills for Behavior Change box pn page 391 for some guidelines for this challenging task.

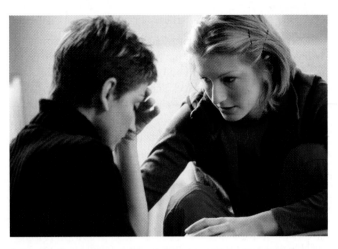

Often, family members or friends have to confront the alcohol-dependent person to help him or her take the first steps toward recovery.

Treatment Programs

The alcoholic who is ready for help has several avenues of treatment: psychologists and psychiatrists specializing in the treatment of alcoholism, private treatment centers, hospitals specifically designed to treat alcoholics, community mental health facilities, and support groups such as Alcoholics Anonymous.

Private Treatment Facilities
Private treatment facilities have made concerted efforts to attract patients through radio and television advertising. Upon admission to the treatment facility, the patient receives a complete physical exam to determine whether underlying medical problems will interfere with treatment.

Alcoholics who decide to quit drinking will experience *detoxification,* the process by which addicts end their dependence on a drug, and withdrawal symptoms such as hyperexcitability, confusion and agitation, sleep disorders, convulsions, tremors of the hands, depression, headache, and seizures. For a small percentage of people, alcohol withdrawal results in a severe syndrome known as **delirium tremens (DTs).** Delirium tremens is characterized by confusion, delusions, agitated behavior, and hallucinations.

Shortly after detoxification, alcoholics begin their treatment for psychological addiction. Most treatment facilities keep their patients from three to six weeks. Treatment at private treatment centers costs several thousand dollars, but some insurance programs or employers will assume most of this expense.

delirium tremens (DTs) A state of confusion brought on by withdrawal from alcohol. Symptoms include hallucinations, anxiety, and trembling.

Family Therapy, Individual Therapy, and Group Therapy

In family therapy, the person and family members gradually examine the psychological reasons underlying the addiction. In individual and group therapy with fellow addicts, alcoholics learn positive coping skills for situations that have regularly caused them to turn to alcohol.

On some college campuses, the problems associated with alcohol abuse are so great that student health centers are opening their own treatment programs. The University of Texas offers a new support service called "Complete Recovery 101," and at other schools, students in recovery live together in special housing. Because it can be difficult to recover from an alcohol abuse problem in college, support programs such as these hope to provide the support and comfortable environment recovering students need.

Other Types of Treatment

Two other treatments are drug therapy and group support. Disulfiram (trade name: Antabuse) is the drug of choice for treating alcoholics. If alcohol is consumed, the drug causes unpleasant effects such as headache, nausea, vomiting, drowsiness, and hangover. These symptoms discourage the alcoholic from drinking.

Alcoholics Anonymous (AA) is a private, nonprofit, self-help organization founded in 1935. The organization, which relies upon group support to help people stop drinking, currently has branches all over the world and more than 1 million members. At meetings, last names are never used, and no one is forced to speak. Members are taught to believe that their alcoholism is a lifetime problem and that they may never use alcohol again. They share their struggles with each other and talk about the devastating effects alcoholism has had on their personal and professional lives. All members are asked to place their faith and control of the habit into the hands of a "higher power." The road to recovery is taken one step at a time. AA offers specialized meetings for Spanish speakers, gays, atheists, people with HIV, and a variety of other people with alcohol problems.

Alcoholics Anonymous also has auxiliary groups to help spouses or partners, friends, and children of alcoholics. *Al-Anon* is the group dedicated to helping adult relatives and friends of alcoholics understand the disease and how they can contribute to the recovery process. Spouses and other adult loved ones often play an unwitting role in perpetuating the alcoholic's problems. For example, they may call the alcoholic's boss and lie about why the alcoholic missed work. At

---

alcoholics anonymous (AA) An organization whose goal is to help alcoholics stop drinking; includes auxiliary branches such as Al-Anon and Alateen.

Al-Anon, these people examine their roles in their loved one's drinking and explore alternative behaviors.

Alateen, another AA-related organization, helps adolescents live with alcoholic parents. They are taught that they are not at fault for their parents' problems. They develop their self-esteem to overcome their guilt and function better socially.

The support gained from talking with others who have similar problems is one of the greatest benefits derived from self-help groups. Many members learn to exert greater control over their own lives and rid themselves of the guilt they feel about their participation in their loved one's alcoholism.

Other self-help groups include Women for Sobriety and Secular Organizations for Sobriety (SOS). Women for Sobriety addresses the differing needs of female alcoholics, who often have more severe problems than males. Unlike AA meetings, where attendance can be quite large, each group has no more than 10 members. Secular Organizations for Sobriety was founded to help people who are uncomfortable with AA's spiritual emphasis.

Relapse

Success in recovery varies with the individual. Roughly 60 percent of alcoholics relapse (resume drinking) within the first three months of treatment. Why is the relapse rate so high? Treating an addiction requires more than getting the addict to stop using a substance; it also requires getting the person to break a pattern of behavior that has dominated his or her life. Many alcoholics refer to themselves as "recovering" throughout their lifetime; they never use the word *cured.*

People who are seeking to regain a healthy lifestyle must not only confront their addiction, but also guard against the tendency to relapse. Drinkers with compulsive personalities need to learn to understand themselves and take control. To succeed, a recovery program must offer the alcoholic ways to increase self-esteem and resume personal growth.

Can Recovering Alcoholics Take a Drink?

Research conducted over a period of 5 to 10 years has shown that fewer than 1 percent of recovering alcoholics are able to resume drinking on a limited basis. To prevent the return to the bottle, abstinence is the safest and sanest path.

A comprehensive approach that includes drug therapy, group support, family therapy, and personal counseling designed to improve living and coping skills is usually the most effective course of treatment. The alcoholics most likely to recover completely are those who developed their dependencies after the age of 20, those with intact and supportive family units, and those who have reached a high level of personal disgust coupled with strong motivation to recover.

SKILLS FOR behavior change

TALKING TO A FRIEND ABOUT ALCOHOL USE

It's difficult to know when to say something when you're worried about a friend's alcohol use. Ask yourself...

HOW DOES IT AFFECT YOU?

How can I approach a friend with a drinking problem?

- Have you lost time from classes, studying, or a job in order to help your friend cope with problems caused by her drinking?
- Is your friend's drinking making you unhappy in any aspect of your life?
- Is your friend's behavior affecting your reputation in a way you don't like?
- Have you ever felt embarrassed or hurt by something he said or did while intoxicated?
- Have you ever had to take care of your friend because of his alcohol use?

HOW DOES IT AFFECT YOUR FRIEND?

- Does your friend "slam" drinks or drink to get drunk?
- Is your friend doing dangerous things because of alcohol?
- Has your friend ever wanted to cut down on drinking?
- Does your friend ever have to drink to steady his nerves or get rid of a hangover?
- Has your friend ever been in trouble because of drinking?
- Does your friend find it necessary to drink or get high to enjoy a party?
- Is alcohol affecting your friend's academic performance?
- Does your friend drink to escape from or cope with problems or stress? Does she use drugs or alcohol to avoid painful feelings?
- Has your friend even been unable to remember things she said or did while drinking (blacked out)?

- Is your friend annoyed when people criticize his drinking?
- Has your friend ever received medical care for something related to drinking?
- Have you noticed a decline in his personal health or appearance?

The more questions you answer yes to, and the more frequently each factor is true, the more likely it is that your friend has a problem. A caring conversation will help your friend learn how his behavior affects others and can help him get the help he needs. Some people just need the wake-up call of your honest opinion; others can benefit from professional help to make changes or maintain abstinence.

BEFORE YOU TALK TO YOUR FRIEND

- Learn about alcohol abuse.
- Prepare a list of specific problems that have occurred because of your friend's drinking or drug use. Keep these items as concrete as possible. "You're so antisocial when you drink" will not mean as much as, "When you were drunk, you made fun of me and were mean to me. You hurt me." Bring the list with you and keep the conversation focused.
- Choose a private location where you can talk without embarrassment or interruption.

HOW TO TALK TO YOUR FRIEND

- Talk to your friend when she is sober. The sooner you can arrange this after a bad episode, the better.
- Restrict your comments to what you feel and what you have experienced of your friend's behavior. Express statements that cannot be disputed. Remarks like, "Everyone's disgusted with you," or, "Lily thinks you have a real problem," will probably lead to arguments about Lily's problems or who "everyone" is. Avoid such generalizations.

- Convey your concern with specific statements: "I want to talk to you because I am worried about you," or "Our friendship means a lot to me. I don't like to see what's been happening."
- It is important to openly discuss the negative consequences of your friend's drinking or drug use. Use concrete examples from your list. "At the party I was left standing there while you threw up. The next day you were too hung over to write your paper. It makes me sad that these things are happening in your life."
- Emphasize the difference between sober behavior that you like and drinking behavior that you dislike. "You have the most wonderful sense of humor, but when you drink it turns into cruel sarcasm, and you're not funny any more. You're mean."
- Be sure to distinguish between the person and the behavior. "I think you're a great person, but the more alcohol you drink, the less you seem to care about anything."
- Encourage your friend to consult a professional about his or her alcohol problem. You can offer to help find resources or go with your friend to an appointment.
- Talk to people you trust (other friends or relatives) about your concerns. Their involvement may help.

WHAT NOT TO DO

- Don't accuse or argue.
- Don't lecture or moralize. Remain factual, listen, and be nonjudgmental.
- Don't give up. If your friend seems resistant, you can bring it up later or make it clear that you're available if he or she ever wants to talk.

Source: Brown University Health Education, "Talking to a Friend about Drinking or Drug Use," 2005, www.brown.edu/Student_Services/Health_Services/Health_Education/atod/help afriend.htm.

TAKING charge

Summary

- Alcohol is a central nervous system depressant used by 70 percent of all Americans and 90 percent of all college students; over one-third of all college students are binge drinkers. Although consumption trends are slowly creeping downward, college students are under extreme pressure to consume alcohol.
- Alcohol's effect on the body is measured by the blood alcohol concentration (BAC), the ratio of alcohol to total blood volume. The higher the BAC, the greater the impaired judgment and coordination and drowsiness.
- Negative consequences associated with alcohol use by college students are lower grade point averages, academic problems, dropping out of school, unplanned sex, hangovers, alcohol poisoning, and injury. Long-term effects of alcohol overuse include damage to the nervous system, cardiovascular damage, liver disease, and increased risk for cancer. Drinking during pregnancy can cause fetal alcohol effects (FAE) or fetal alcohol syndrome (FAS). Alcohol is also a causative factor in many traffic accidents.

- Drinking large amounts of alcohol in a short amount of time can cause a rapid rise in BAC, resulting in a coma or even death.
- Alcohol use becomes alcoholism when it interferes with school, work, or social and family relationships or entails violations of the law. Causes of alcoholism include biological, family, social, and cultural factors. Alcoholism has far-reaching effects on families, especially on children. Children of alcoholics have problematic childhoods and may take those problems into adulthood.
- Recovery is problematic for alcoholics. Most alcoholics do not admit to a problem until reaching a major life crisis or having their families intervene. Treatment options include detoxification at private medical facilities, therapy (family, individual, or group), and self-help programs such as Alcoholics Anonymous. Most alcoholics relapse (60 percent within three months) because alcoholism is a behavioral addiction as well as a chemical addiction.

Chapter Review

1. What does the term *proof* represent with alcohol?
   a. It is an expression of alcohol content.
   b. It is a number that represents twice the percentage of alcohol by volume.
   c. It is used to determine the strength of alcohol.
   d. All of the above.

2. Which of the following is a *true* statement regarding how one can metabolize alcohol faster to lower one's blood alcohol level?
   a. Drink black coffee.
   b. Take a cold shower.
   c. Engage in vigorous exercise.
   d. Only time can metabolize and rid the body of high alcohol content.

3. What does BAC measure?
   a. The percentage of alcohol in the blood.
   b. It is used to determine if someone is legally intoxicated to be driving a vehicle.
   c. It is based on body weight and number of drinks consumed and is different for men and women.
   d. All of the above.

4. What are some "self-protective" strategies you could take to avoid drinking too much?
   a. Alternate alcoholic beverages with nonalcoholic drinks.
   b. Eat before and during drinking.
   c. Pace your drinks to one or fewer per hour.
   d. All of the above.

5. Which of the following statements is *not* true?
   a. College students drink less often than older students but drink more heavily.
   b. More underage students report drinking just to get drunk.
   c. Binge-drinking students usually continue to binge drink after graduating from college.
   d. Students living in fraternity or sorority houses are more likely to binge drink.

6. Which of the following is *not* a typical defect of a child born with fetal alcohol syndrome?
   a. a small head
   b. normal growth and height for age
   c. delayed speech
   d. abnormal facial features

7. Which ethnic group has a genetic physiological reaction to alcohol that causes facial flushing, rapid heart rate, and low blood pressure that makes them less likely to drink alcohol?
   a. Jewish
   b. Asian
   c. Native American
   d. African American

8. When Amanda goes out with her friends on the weekends, she usually has four to five beers in a row. This type of high-risk drinking is called
   a. tolerance.
   b. alcoholic addiction.
   c. alcohol over-consumption.
   d. binge drinking.

9. Drinking large amounts of alcohol in a short period of time that leads to passing out is known as
   a. learned behavioral tolerance.
   b. alcoholic unconsciousness.
   c. acute alcohol poisoning.
   d. acute metabolism syndrome.

10. Jake was raised in an alcoholic family. To adapt to his father's alcoholic behavior, he played the obedient and good son to his parents. What role did Jake assume?
    a. family hero
    b. mascot
    c. scapegoat
    d. lost child

Answers to these questions can be found on page A-1.

Questions for Discussion and Reflection

1. When it comes to drinking alcohol, how much is too much? How can you avoid drinking amounts that will affect your judgment? When you see a friend having "too many" drinks at a party, what actions do you normally take? What actions could you take?
2. What are some of the most common negative consequences college students experience as a result of drinking? What are secondhand effects of binge drinking? Why do students tolerate the negative behaviors of students who have been drinking?
3. Determine what your BAC would be if you drank four beers in two hours (assume they are spaced at equal intervals). What physiological effects will you feel after each drink? Would a person of similar weight show greater effects after having four gin and tonics instead of beer? Why or why not? At what point in your life should you start worrying about the long-term effects of alcohol abuse?
4. Describe the difference between a problem drinker and an alcoholic. What factors can cause someone to slide from responsibly consuming alcohol to becoming an alcoholic? What effect does alcoholism have on an alcoholic's family?
5. Does anyone ever recover from alcoholism? Why or why not? Do you think society's views on drinking have changed over the years? Explain your answer.

Accessing Your Health on the Internet

The following websites explore further topics and issues related to personal health. You'll also find links to each organization's website on the Companion Website for *Access to Health,* Tenth Edition, at www.aw-bc.com/donatelle.

1. *College Drinking: Changing the Culture.* This online resource center is based on a series of reports published by the Task Force of the National Advisory Council on Alcohol Abuse and Alcoholism. It targets students and the alcohol-dependent drinker. www.collegedrinking prevention.gov
2. *Had Enough.* This entertaining website is designed for college students who have suffered the secondhand effects (babysitting a roommate who has been drinking, having sleep interrupted, etc.) of other students' drinking. It offers suggestions for taking action and being proactive about policy issues on your campus. http://gbgm-umc.org/mission_programs/cim/hadenough/home/index.html
3. *Higher Education Center for Alcohol and Other Drug Prevention.* This website is funded through the U.S. Department of Education and provides information relevant to colleges and universities. A specific site exists for students who are seeking information regarding alcohol. www.higheredcenter.org
4. *Alcoholics Anonymous (AA).* This website provides general information about AA and the 12-step program. www.alcoholics-anonymous.org

Further Reading

Jersild, D. *Happy Hours: Alcohol in a Woman's Life.* New York: HarperCollins, 2001.

This book, a combination of cutting-edge research and personal stories of women who have struggled with alcohol problems, examines the role that alcohol plays in women's lives.

Kuhn, C., S. Swartzwelder, W. Wilson, J. Foster, and L. Wilson. *Buzzed: The Straight Facts About the Most Used and Abused Drugs from Alcohol to Ecstasy.* New York: W. W. Norton & Company, 2003.

A series of publications containing the results of a number of studies conducted by research scientists under the auspices of NIAAA through 2002. These monographs address issues such as alcohol use among older adults, occupational alcoholism, social drinking, and the relationship between heredity and alcoholism.

Sperber, M. *Beer and Circus: How Big-Time College Sports Is Crippling Undergraduate Education.* New York: Henry Holt, 2000.

Sperber's book is an indictment of the attraction of undergraduates to schools based on the school's sports success and party reputations. He links student drinking behaviors to sports programs and argues that such an atmosphere shortchanges undergraduates' education.

Wechsler, H. and B. Wuethrich. *Dying to Drink: Confronting Binge Drinking on College Campuses.* Emmaus, PA: Rodale, 2002.

A report of the widespread alcohol culture that exists on many campuses.

Zailckas, K. *Smashed: A Story of a Drunken Girlhood.* New York: Viking, 2005.

A 24-year-old woman writes about her own experiences of drinking through high school and college.

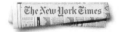

e-themes from *The New York Times*

For up-to-date articles about current health issues, visit www.aw-bc.com/donatelle, select *Access to Health,* Tenth Edition, Chapter 12, and click on "e-themes."

References

1. American College Health Association, "American College Health Association-National College Health Assessment (ACHA-NCHA) Spring 2005 Reference Group Data Report," *Journal of American College Health,* July/August 2006.
2. R. Hingson et al., "Magnitude of Alcohol-Related Mortality and Morbidity among U.S. College Students Ages 18–24: Changes from 1998 to 2001," *Annual Review of Public Health* 26 (2005): 259–279.
3. H. Wechsler et al., "Trends in College Binge Drinking During a Period of Increased Prevention Efforts: Findings from Four Harvard School of Public Health College Study Surveys: 1993–2001," *Journal of American College Health* 50, no. 5 (2002): 207.
4. H. Wechsler et al., "College Binge Drinking in the 1990s: A Continuing Problem," *Journal of American College Health* 48, no. 10 (2000): 199–210.
5. M. Mohler-Kuo et al., "Correlates of Rape While Intoxicated in a National Sample of College Women," *Journal of Studies on Alcohol* 65, no. 1 (2004): 37.
6. Hingson et al., "Magnitude of Alcohol-Related Mortality and Morbidity."
7. N. E. Lakins et al., "Apparent Trends in per Capita Alcohol Consumption: National, State, and Regional Trends, 1977–2003," *Surveillance Report,* no. 73 (2005), www.niaaa.nih.gov/publications/surveillance73/CONS03.htm.
8. S. MacDonald, "The Criteria for Causation of Alcohol in Violent Injuries in Six Countries," *Addictive Behaviors* 30, no. 1 (2005): 103–113.
9. J. Turner et al., "Serious Health Consequences Associated with Alcohol Use among College Students: Demographic and Clinical Characteristics of Patients Seen in the Emergency Department," *Journal of Studies on Alcohol* 65, no. 2 (2004): 179.
10. K. Butler, "The Grim Neurology of Teenage Drinking," *The New York Times,* July 4, 2006, www.nytimes.com/2006/7/04/04/health.
11. R. W. Hingson et al., "Age at Drinking Onset and Alcohol Dependence," *Archives of Pediatric and Adolescent Medicine* 160 (2006): 739–746.
12. National Institutes of Health, "Alcohol: A Women's Health Issue," 2003, www.niaaa.nih.gov/publications/brochurewomen/women.htm.
13. J. Theruvathu et al., "Polyamines Stimulate the Formation of Mutagenic 1, N2-Propanodeoxyguanosine Adducts from Acetaldehyde," *Nucleic Acids Research* 33, no. 11 (2005): 3513–3520.
14. National Organization on Fetal Alcohol Syndrome, 2005, www.nofas.org.
15. National Highway Traffic Safety Administration, "Traffic Safety Facts, 2004: A Compilation of Motor Vehicle Crash Data from the Fatal Analysis Reporting System and General Estimates System," 2005, www.nrd.nhtsa.dot.gov.

16. H. Wechsler et al., "Changes in Binge Drinking and Related Problems Among American College Students between 1993 and 1997," *Journal of American College Health* 47, no. 2 (1998): 57–68.

17. National Highway Traffic Safety Administration, *Traffic Safety Facts, 1996—Alcohol* (Washington, DC: National Center for Statistics and Analysis, 1997.)

18. National Highway Traffic Safety Administration, "Crash Stats: Alcohol-Related Fatalities by State, 2004," www.nhtsa.dot.gov.

19. Ibid.

20. Ibid.

21. Insurance Institute for Highway Safety, "Fatality Facts: Alcohol 2004," 2005, www.iihs.org.

22. Ibid.

23. Substance Abuse and Mental Health Services Administration, "Results from the 2003 National Survey on Drug Use and Health: National Findings" (Office of Applied Studies, NHSDA Series H-24, DHHS Publication No. SMA 04–3963), (U.S. Department of Health and Human Services, Rockville, MD: 2004).

24. J. Knight et al., "Alcohol Abuse and Dependence."

25. C. Wilson and J. Knight, "When Parents Have a Drinking Problem," *Contemporary Pediatrics* 18, no. 1 (January 2001): 67.

26. Ibid.

27. Ibid.

28. B. F. Grant, "Estimates of U.S. Children Exposed to Alcohol Abuse and Dependence in the Family," *American Journal of Public Health* 90, no. 1 (2000).

29. National Institute on Alcohol Abuse and Alcoholism, *Alcohol Alert,* no. 51, January 2001.

30. T. R. Miller et al., "Societal Costs of Underage Drinking," *Journal of Studies on Alcohol* 67, no. 4 (2006): 519–528.

31. National Institute on Alcohol Abuse and Alcoholism, "Alcohol: A Women's Health Issue," NIH Pub. N. 04-4956.

32. F. Blow et al., "Use and Misuse of Alcohol among Older Women," *Alcohol Research and Health* 26, no. 4 (2002): 308.

33. National Institute on Drug Abuse, "Info Facts: Treatment Methods for Women," August 30, 2004, www.nida.nih.gov/Infofax/treatwomen.html.

34. T. Wall and C. Ehlers, "Genetic Influences Affecting Alcohol Use among Asians," *Alcohol Health and Research World* 19, no. 3: 184–189.

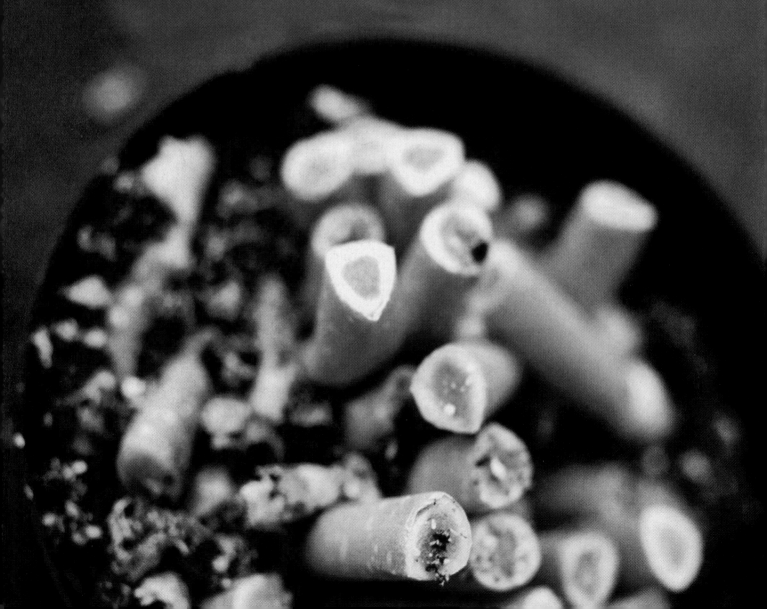

13

Tobacco and Caffeine

DAILY PLEASURES, DAILY CHALLENGES

Are **cigars** as bad for you as cigarettes?

Is chewing tobacco **addictive**?

Is secondhand smoke a **risk** to my health?

Will **quitting** smoking reverse the damage I've already done?

Is **caffeine** really addictive?

OBJECTIVES

- Discuss the social and political issues involved in tobacco use.
- Explain how the chemicals in tobacco products affect a tobacco user's body.
- Review how smoking and the use of smokeless tobacco affect one's risk for cancer, cardiovascular disease, and respiratory diseases and how it adversely affects a fetus's health.
- Evaluate the risks to nonsmokers associated with environmental tobacco smoke.
- Describe strategies people adopt to quit using tobacco products, including strategies aimed at breaking the nicotine addiction, as well as habit.
- Compare the benefits and risks associated with caffeine, and summarize the health consequences of long-term caffeine use.

obacco use is the single most preventable cause of death in the United States.[1] While tobacco companies continue to publish full-page advertisements refuting the dangers of smoking, nearly 438,000 Americans die each year of tobacco-related diseases (Figure 13.1).[2] This is 50 times as many as will die from all illegal drugs combined. In addition, 10 million people will suffer from disorders caused by tobacco. To date, tobacco is known to cause about 25 diseases, and one in every five deaths in the United States is smoking related. About half of all regular smokers die of smoking-related diseases. Therefore, any contention by the tobacco industry that tobacco use is not dangerous is irresponsible and ignores the scientific evidence.

Our Smoking Society

In 1991, the Youth Risk Behavior Surveillance (YRBS), which includes only middle and high school students, indicated that 27.5 percent of teenagers smoked; by 2005, 23 percent were current smokers. Though this recent survey indicates a downward trend in numbers of adolescent smokers (Figure 13.2), this does not mean teens are not becoming smokers altogether. Every day, 6,000 teens under the age of 18 smoke their first cigarette and more than 3,000 become daily smokers.[3] Cigarette use among teens is attributed in part to the ready availability of tobacco products through vending machines and the aggressive drive by tobacco companies to entice young people to smoke.

Cigarette smoking results in untold loss of human potential, with thousands of Americans dying prematurely each year. As you can see in Table 13.1 on page 400, the rate of smoking between groups is very similar. Factors contributing to this include heavy advertising that targets the 18- to 24-year-old age group, and, among the older age groups, habits developed 20 years ago or more, when the practice of smoking was more common and the public was not educated about the health risks associated with tobacco use.

Tobacco and Social Issues

The production and distribution of tobacco products in the United States and abroad involve many political and economic issues. Tobacco-growing states derive substantial income from tobacco production, and federal, state, and local governments benefit enormously from cigarette taxes.

More recently, nationwide health awareness has led to a decrease in the use of tobacco products among U.S. adults. To compensate for revenue losses, many major tobacco companies have merged with or purchased other corporations that market food and beverage products and have aggressively expanded their marketing worldwide.

Advertising According to estimates, the tobacco industry spends $18 million per day on advertising and promo-

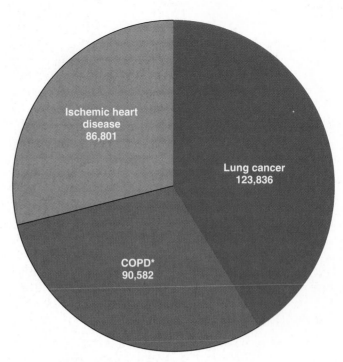

FIGURE 13.1 Annual Deaths Attributable to Smoking in the United States

*Chronic obstructive pulmonary disease

Source: Centers for Disease Control and Prevention, "Annual Smoking-Attributable Mortality, Years of Potential Life Lost, and Productivity Losses," *Morbidity and Mortality Weekly Report* 54, no. 25 (2005): 625–628.

tional materials. With the number of smokers declining by about 1 million each year, the industry must actively recruit new smokers. Campaigns are directed at all age, social, and ethnic groups, but because children and teenagers constitute 90 percent of all new smokers, much of the advertising has been directed toward them. Evidence of product recognition among underage smokers is clear: 86 percent of underage smokers prefer one of the three most heavily advertised brands—Marlboro, Newport, or Camel. One of the most blatant campaigns aimed at young adults was the popular Joe Camel ad campaign. After R. J. Reynolds introduced the cartoon figure, Camel's market share among underage smokers jumped from 3 to 13.3 percent in three years.

Advertisements in women's magazines imply that smoking is the key to financial success, independence, and social acceptance. Many brands also have thin spokeswomen pushing "slim" and "light" cigarettes to cash in on women's fear of gaining weight. These ads have apparently been working. From the mid-1970s through the early 2000s, cigarette sales to women increased dramatically. Not coincidentally, by 1987 cigarette-induced lung cancer had surpassed breast cancer as the leading cancer killer among women.

Women are not the only targets of gender-based cigarette advertisements. Males are depicted in locker rooms, charging over rugged terrain in off-road vehicles, or riding stallions into the sunset in blatant appeals to a need to feel and appear masculine. Minorities also are often targeted.

Apparently, 18- to 24-year-olds have become the new target for tobacco advertisers. The tobacco industry has set up

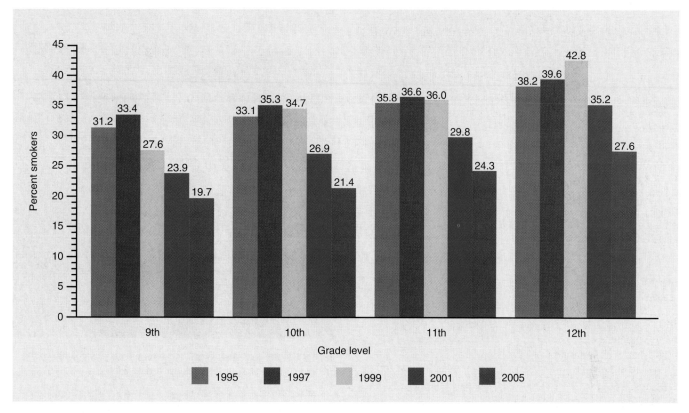

FIGURE 13.2 Cigarette Smoking by Grade Level

Source: Centers for Disease Control and Prevention, "Youth Risk Behavior Surveillance, 2005," *Morbidity and Mortality Weekly Report* 55, supplement, 2006.

aggressive marketing promotions at bars, music festivals, and the like, specifically targeted to this age group. Additionally, modeling and peer influence have an impact on smoking initiation. This potential impact is heightened by the fact that, although over half of campuses are considered smoke-free, they do permit smoking in residence hall rooms, student centers, and cafeterias, and many sell tobacco products in campus stores and student lounges. See the Health Ethics box on page 401 for more on the tobacco industry.

Financial Costs to Society The use of tobacco products is costly to all of us in terms of lost productivity and lost lives. Estimates show that tobacco use caused over $167 billion in annual health-related economic losses from 1997 to 2001. The economic burden of tobacco use totaled more than $75.5 billion in medical expenditures (these costs include hospital, physician, and nursing home expenditures; prescription drugs; and home health care expenditures) and $92 billion in indirect costs (absenteeism, added cost of fire insurance, training costs to replace employees who die prematurely, disability payments, and so on). The economic costs of smoking are estimated to be about $3,391 per smoker per year.[4]

College Students and Smoking

College students are especially vulnerable when they are placed in a new, often stressful social and academic environ-

ment. For many, the college years are their initial taste of freedom from parental supervision. College students are also subject to heavy tobacco marketing and advertising campaigns directed at them (see the Spotlight on Your Health box on page 402). Smoking may begin earlier, but most university students are a part of the significant age group in which people start smoking and become hooked.

Cigarette smoking among U.S. college students has decreased slightly in recent years. About 22 percent of college students report smoking cigarettes in the past 30 days. This is down from about 30 percent in 1999. College men and women have nearly identical rates of cigarette smoking, but men use more cigars and smokeless tobacco.[5]

Social Smoking Many smokers identify themselves as "social smokers." A recent study defined *social smoking* as smoking when you are with people, rather than alone. Fifty-one percent of past-30-day smokers were identified as social smokers. What else differentiates a social smoker from a smoker? Social smokers smoke less often, and less intensely, and are less dependent on nicotine. Social smokers do not view themselves as being addicted to cigarettes, and are less likely to quit the habit or have any intention to quit.[6]

However, even occasional smoking is not without risks. Social smoking in college can lead to a complete dependence on nicotine, and thus, all of the same health risks as smoking regularly. So why do college students become smokers? A survey identified four factors that contribute to smoking in

TABLE 13.1	Percentage of Population That Smokes (age 18 and older) among Select Groups in the United States

	Percentage
United States overall	20.4
RACE	
American Indian/Alaska Native	33.4
Asian/Pacific Islander	11.3
Black	20.2
Hispanic	15.0
White	22.2
AGE	
18–24	23.6
25–44	23.8
45–64	22.4
65+	8.8
SEX	
Male	23.4
Female	18.5
EDUCATION	
Undergraduate	11.7
Some college	22.2
High school	24.0
9–11 years	34.0
INCOME LEVEL	
Below poverty level	29.1
At or above poverty level	20.6

Source: Centers for Disease Control, "Cigarette Smoking Among Adults—United States 2002," *Morbidity and Mortality Weekly Report 53*, no. 20 (2004): 427–431.

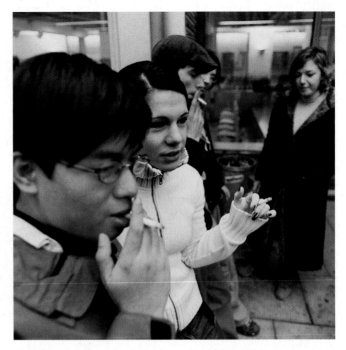

Despite all we know about the long-term effects of smoking, young people continue to put their health at risk. Why?

college: a tendency toward risk-taking, depression, social norms that tolerate or encourage smoking, and a lack of self-efficacy to resist peer pressure.[7]

Unlike social smokers, students who smoke regularly and are nicotine dependent do want to stop smoking. One study reported that 70 percent of cigarette smokers had tried to quit smoking. Unfortunately, three out of four were still smokers.[8] It is important that colleges and universities engage in anti-smoking efforts, strictly control tobacco advertising, provide

nicotine   The primary stimulant chemical in tobacco products.

smoke-free residence halls, and offer greater access to smoking cessation programs. See the Assess Yourself box on page 406 to determine whether you are dependent on tobacco.

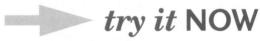 *try it* NOW

Why do you smoke? Visit www.utoronto.ca/health/ healthtips/smkrprfl/smkrprfl.htm and take the quiz to get a handle on why you light up. Determining the type of smoker you are is the first step in breaking the habit.

Tobacco and Its Effects

The chemical stimulant **nicotine** is the major psychoactive substance in all tobacco products. In its natural form, nicotine is a colorless liquid that turns brown upon oxidation (removal of electrons, often by exposure to oxygen). When tobacco leaves are burned in a cigarette, pipe, or cigar, nicotine is released and inhaled into the lungs. Sucking or chewing a quid (a pinch of snuff typically tucked between the gum and lower lip) of tobacco releases nicotine into the saliva, and the nicotine is then absorbed through the mucous membranes in the mouth.

Smoking is the most common form of tobacco use. Smoking delivers a strong dose of nicotine to the user, along with an additional 4,700 chemical substances (Table 13.2 on page 403). Among these chemicals are various gases and vapors that carry particulate matter in concentrations that are 500,000 times greater than those of the most air-polluted cities in the world.[9]

Philip Morris is the world's largest producer and marketer of consumer packaged goods and the largest food company in the nation. It is also the world's largest and most profitable tobacco corporation. To many Americans, Philip Morris, which owns Kraft Foods, is firmly linked to the more than 400,000 people in the United States and 3.4 million worldwide who die each year from smoking-related illnesses. This company has also led the way, in the United States and internationally, in spreading the tobacco epidemic, in particular to girls and women in regions where they traditionally have not smoked. In addition, Philip Morris and other tobacco companies have been convicted of lying, deliberately deceiving the public regarding the safety of tobacco, and creating and marketing a chemical addiction for profit.

However, a visit to the Philip Morris headquarters in New York paints a different picture. The company aggressively promotes its charitable work, in particular its youth smoking-prevention program. It houses the Whitney Museum exhibit of an Indian artist and sponsors the Thurgood Marshall Scholars. Furthermore, Philip Morris employees are involved in efforts to fight hunger and combat domestic violence. The company donates $60 million a year to charity and spends another $100 million in advertising to inform the public about its good deeds. The advertising campaign is a concerted strategy to improve Philip Morris's corporate image and build credibility. In addition to the advertising campaign, the company has established a speakers' bureau where top company executives go on the road to address PTA meetings and other groups about the company's charitable work.

What is a tobacco company's ethical obligation to society? Should it be any different from the ethical obligations of companies in other industries? Do you think Philip Morris is attempting to do the right thing, or are these initiatives a public relations effort? Consider that smokers choose to start smoking. Is it fair to blame Philip Morris if they develop tobacco-related health problems?

Particulate matter condenses in the lungs to form a thick, brownish sludge called **tar.** Tar contains various carcinogenic (cancer-causing) agents such as benzo[*a*]pyrene and chemical irritants such as phenol. Phenol has the potential to combine with other chemicals to contribute to the development of lung cancer.

In healthy lungs, millions of tiny hairlike tissues called cilia sweep foreign matter back toward the throat, to be expelled from the lungs by coughing. Nicotine impairs the cleansing function of the cilia by paralyzing them for up to one hour following the smoking of a single cigarette. This allows tars and other solids in tobacco smoke to accumulate and irritate sensitive lung tissue.

Tar and nicotine are not the only harmful chemicals in cigarettes. In fact, tar accounts for only 8 percent of tobacco smoke. The remaining 92 percent consists of various gases, the most dangerous of which is **carbon monoxide.** In tobacco smoke, the concentration of carbon monoxide is 800 times higher than the level considered safe by the U.S. Environmental Protection Agency (EPA). In the human body, carbon monoxide reduces the oxygen-carrying capacity of the red blood cells by binding with the receptor sites for oxygen. Carbon monoxide binds better than oxygen and is more difficult to remove, so carbon monoxide in the blood causes oxygen deprivation in many body tissues.

The heat from tobacco smoke, which can reach 1,616°F, is also harmful. Inhaling hot gases exposes sensitive mucous membranes to irritating chemicals that weaken the tissues and contribute to cancers of the mouth, larynx, and throat.

Tobacco Products

Tobacco comes in several forms. Cigarettes, cigars, pipes, and bidis are used for burning and inhaling tobacco. Smokeless tobacco is inhaled or placed in the mouth.

Cigarettes
Filtered cigarettes designed to reduce levels of gases such as hydrogen cyanide and hydrocarbons may actually deliver more hazardous carbon monoxide to the user than do nonfiltered brands. Some smokers use low-tar and low-nicotine products as an excuse to smoke more cigarettes. This practice is self-defeating because these users wind up exposing themselves to more harmful substances than they would with regular-strength cigarettes. People smoking low-tar cigarettes also tend to inhale more often and more deeply than people smoking regular cigarettes.

Clove cigarettes contain about 40 percent ground cloves (a spice) and about 60 percent tobacco. Many users mistakenly believe that these products are made entirely of ground cloves and that smoking them eliminates the risks associated with

---

tar A thick, brownish substance condensed from particulate matter in smoked tobacco.

carbon monoxide A gas found in cigarette smoke that binds at oxygen receptor sites in the blood.

TOBACCO, COLLEGE STUDENTS, AND PROMOTIONAL ADVERTISING

According to a recent Harvard University survey, tobacco companies often give away cigarettes at college bars and campus social events. Undergraduates who take advantage of the giveaways are three times more likely to start smoking. The survey found that free cigarettes were handed out on 109 of 119 campuses.*

Surprised by the above statistic? Though the research doesn't definitively link the promotions to smoking, it suggests that tobacco companies are clearly targeting college students, said study co-author Henry Wechsler, director of the College Alcohol Studies Program at the Harvard School of Public Health. "These are very important years, " says Wechsler. "They're also the earliest years that the tobacco industry can legally try to get new customers."

Of the students surveyed, 8.5 percent said they had attended a bar or social event during the previous six months where free cigarettes were given out. Most of those students said they ran into the giveaways off campus. But 3.2 percent said the promotions took place on campus at bars (many colleges have pubs designed for faculty, staff, and students of drinking age) or social events. The events reinforce brand visibility, allow the industry to reach specific target groups, and generate names for future marketing efforts. Promotions at social events have the potential to increase tobacco use by encouraging nonsmokers to try cigarettes, by encouraging experimental smokers to develop regular use, and by discouraging current smokers from quitting.

The researchers found that the students exposed to the giveaways were three times more likely to start smoking or use smokeless tobacco by age 19. But Wechsler said the study's design made it impossible to confirm that there's a "cause-and-effect" relationship. However, he added, "From my perspective, people wouldn't be giving all this stuff away if they didn't think it had some effect."

The tobacco industry is very interested in convincing college-aged people to smoke, according to Stanton A. Glantz, director of the Center for Tobacco Control Research at the University of California, San Francisco. "Historically, if you go far enough back to the '30s, '40s, '50s and even '60s, a lot of smoking initiation occurred in that age group, " Glantz says. "In World War I and World War II, a lot of people started smoking when they were in the Army."

Tobacco companies turned to even younger potential smokers in the 1970s and 1980s, Glantz says, but they remained interested in college-aged people because many develop permanent smoking habits during that stage of their lives. About one-third of people who experiment with cigarettes as young adults go on to become smokers.

What should be done? One solution noted by Wechsler is for colleges to not permit this kind of marketing on their property. Glantz agrees and states, "It's totally irresponsible of colleges to do it because they're basically complicit with the tobacco industry. They're allowing these tobacco companies to prey on their students." Wechsler added that "we should redouble our efforts at having smoke-free establishments that will be much less likely to have these kinds of events."

Dana Bolden, a spokesman for Philip Morris, the largest tobacco company in the world, said not all tobacco companies distribute free cigarettes. Philip Morris, he added, doesn't engage in giveaways and wants the federal government to ban the practice by other companies. Bolden added that his company, which makes Marlboro, Virginia Slims, and other brands, does hold invitation-only music events for customers who sign up to receive information about its products. As for the charge that tobacco companies are trying to entice college students to smoke, Bolden said his company only markets to adults 21 and older, even though it could legally pursue potential customers as young as 18.

Sources: R. Dotinga, "Tobacco Promotions Woo College Crowd," *Lifespan Health News,* December 28, 2004; *N. Rigotti et al., "U.S. College Students' Exposure to Tobacco Promotions: Prevalence and Association with Tobacco Use," *American Journal of Public Health* 94, no. 12 (2004): 1–7.

---

tobacco. In fact, clove cigarettes contain higher levels of tar, nicotine, and carbon monoxide than do regular cigarettes. In addition, the numbing effect of eugenol, the active ingredient in cloves, allows smokers to inhale the smoke more deeply.

Cigars Those big stogies that we see celebrities and government figures puffing on these days are nothing more than tobacco fillers wrapped in more tobacco. Since 1991, cigar sales in the United States have increased dramatically. The fad, especially popular among young men and women, is fueled in part by the willingness of celebrities to be photographed puffing on a cigar. Among some women, cigar smoking symbolizes an impulse to be slightly outrageous and liberated.

Many people believe that cigars are safer than cigarettes, when in fact nothing could be further from the truth.[10] Cigar smoke contains 23 poisons and 43 carcinogens. Smoking as little as one cigar per day can double the risk of several cancers, including cancer of the oral cavity (lip, tongue, mouth, and throat), esophagus, larynx,

Are cigars as bad for you as cigarettes?

TABLE 13.2 What's in Cigarette Smoke?

Cigarette smoke contains more than 4,000 chemicals, including these:

Cancer-Causing Agents	Metals	Other Chemicals	
Benzo[a]pyrene	Aluminum	Acetic acid (vinegar)	Hydrogen cyanide (gas chamber poison)
beta-Naphthylamine	Copper	Acetone (nail polish remover)	Methane (swamp gas)
Cadmium	Gold	Ammonia (floor/toilet cleaner)	Methanol (rocket fuel)
Crysenes	Lead	Arsenic (poison)	Naphthalene (mothballs)
Diberiz acidine	Magnesium	Butane (cigarette lighter fluid)	Nicotine (insecticide/addictive drug)
Nickel	Mercury	Cadmium (rechargeable batteries)	Nitrobenzene (gasoline additive)
Nitrosamines	Silicon	Carbon monoxide (car exhaust fumes)	Nitrous oxide phenols (disinfectant)
N-nitrosonornicotine	Silver	DDT/dieldrin (insecticides)	Stearic acid (candle wax)
PAHs (polycydic aromatic hydrocarbon)	Titanium	Ethanol (alcohol)	Toluene (industrial solvent)
Polonium 210	Zinc	Formaldehyde (preserver of body tissue and fabric)	Vinyl chloride (makes PVC)
Toluidine		Hexamine (barbecue lighter)	

and lungs. The risks increase with the number of cigars smoked per day. Daily cigar smoking, especially for people who inhale the smoke, also increases the risk of heart disease (cigar smokers double their risk of heart attack and stroke) and a type of lung disease known as chronic obstructive pulmonary disease (COPD (Chapter 18).

A common question is whether cigars are addictive. Most cigars contain as much nicotine as several cigarettes, and nicotine is highly addictive. When cigar smokers inhale the smoke, nicotine is absorbed as rapidly as it is with cigarettes. For those who don't inhale, nicotine is still absorbed through the mucous membranes in the mouth.

Bidis Bidis are small hand-rolled, flavored cigarettes, generally made in India or Southeast Asia. They come in a variety of flavors, such as vanilla, chocolate, and cherry, and cost $2 to $4 for a pack of 20. Bidis resemble a marijuana joint or a clove cigarette and have become increasingly popular with college students, who view them as safer, cheaper, and easier to obtain than cigarettes. However, they are far more toxic than cigarettes. A study by the Massachusetts Department of Health found that bidis produced three times more carbon monoxide and nicotine and five times more tar than cigarettes. The tendu leaf wrappers are nonporous, meaning that smokers have to pull harder to inhale and inhale more often to keep the bidi lit. During testing, it took an average of 28 puffs to smoke a bidi, compared to 9 puffs for a regular cigarette. This results in much more exposure to the higher amounts of tar, nicotine, and carbon monoxide, and bidis lack any sort of filter to lessen the levels. Research clearly indicates that bidi smokers are at the same, if not higher, risk for coronary heart disease and cancer due to smoking.[11]

Smokeless Tobacco Approximately 5 million U.S. adults use smokeless tobacco. Most of them are teenage (20 percent of male high school students) and young adult

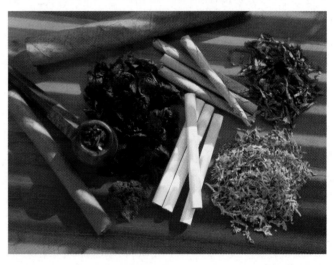

Tobacco is available in a variety of forms, from smokeless tobacco to bidis, but they are all harmful.

males, who are often emulating a professional sports figure or family member. There are two types of smokeless tobacco—chewing tobacco and snuff.

Chewing tobacco is placed between the gums and teeth for sucking or chewing. It comes in three forms: loose leaf, plug, or twist. Chewing tobacco contains tobacco leaves treated with molasses and other flavorings. The user places a "quid" of tobacco in the mouth between the teeth and gums

bidis Hand-rolled flavored cigarettes.

chewing tobacco A stringy type of tobacco that is placed in the mouth and then sucked or chewed.

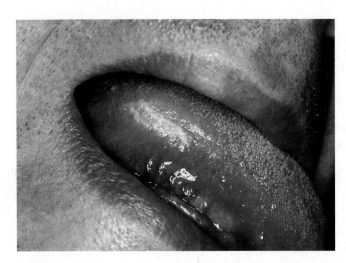

Leukoplakia can appear in the mouth or on the tongue, as shown here.

and then sucks or chews the quid to release the nicotine. Once the quid becomes ineffective, the user spits it out and inserts another. **Dipping** is another method of using chewing tobacco. The dipper takes a small amount of tobacco and places it between the lower lip and teeth to stimulate the flow of saliva and release the nicotine. Dipping releases nicotine rapidly into the bloodstream.

Snuff is a finely ground form of tobacco that can be inhaled, chewed, or placed against the gums. It comes in dry or moist powdered form or sachets (tea bag–like pouches). Usually snuff is placed inside the cheek.

Is chewing tobacco addictive?

Smokeless tobacco is just as addictive as cigarettes because of its nicotine content. There is nicotine in all tobacco products, but smokeless tobacco contains even more than cigarettes. Holding an average-sized dip or chew in the mouth for 30 minutes delivers as much nicotine as smoking four cigarettes. A two-can-a-week snuff dipper gets as much nicotine as a ten-pack-a-week smoker. Smokeless tobacco contains 10 times the amount of cancer-producing substances found in cigarettes and 100 times more than the U.S. Food and Drug Administration allows in foods and other substances used by the public.

A major risk of chewing tobacco is **leukoplakia,** a condition characterized by leathery white patches inside the mouth that are produced by contact with irritants in tobacco juice. Three to 17 percent of diagnosed leukoplakia cases develop into oral cancer.

It is estimated that 75 percent of the 30,990 oral cancer cases in 2006 resulted from either smokeless tobacco or cigarettes.[12] Users of smokeless tobacco are 50 times more likely to develop oral cancers than are nonusers. Warning signs include lumps in the jaw or neck; color changes or lumps inside the lips; white, smooth, or scaly patches in the mouth or on the neck, lips, or tongue; a red spot or sore on the lips or gums or inside the mouth that does not heal in two weeks; repeated bleeding in the mouth; and difficulty or abnormality in speaking or swallowing.

The lag time between first use and contracting cancer is shorter for smokeless tobacco users than for smokers because absorption through the gums is the most efficient route of nicotine administration. A growing body of evidence suggests that long-term use of smokeless tobacco also increases the risk of cancer of the larynx, esophagus, nasal cavity, pancreas, kidney, and bladder. Moreover, many smokeless tobacco users eventually "graduate" to cigarettes and further increase their risk for developing additional problems.

The stimulant effects of nicotine may create the same circulatory and respiratory problems for chewers as for smokers. Chronic smokeless tobacco use also delays wound healing and promotes peptic ulcers.

Like smoked tobacco, smokeless tobacco impairs the senses of taste and smell, causing the user to add salt and sugar to food, which may contribute to high blood pressure and obesity. Some smokeless tobacco products contain high levels of sodium (salt), which also promotes high blood pressure. Dental problems are common among users of smokeless tobacco. Contact with tobacco juice causes receding gums, tooth decay, bad breath, and discolored teeth. Damage to both the teeth and jawbone can contribute to early loss of teeth. Users of any tobacco products may not be able to absorb the vitamins and other nutrients in food effectively.

what do you THINK?

Should smokeless tobacco be banned in all venues that also ban smoking? ■ What is attractive about the use of smokeless tobacco? ■ Why do you think that it is popular with many athletes and males?

Physiological Effects of Nicotine

Nicotine is a powerful central nervous system stimulant that produces a variety of physiological effects. In the cerebral cortex, its stimulant action produces an aroused, alert mental state. Nicotine also stimulates the adrenal glands, increasing the production of adrenaline. The physical effects of nicotine stimulation include increased heart and respiratory rate,

---

dipping   Placing a small amount of chewing tobacco between the lower lip and front teeth for rapid nicotine absorption.

snuff   A powdered form of tobacco that is sniffed and absorbed through the mucous membranes in the nose or placed inside the cheek and sucked.

leukoplakia   A condition characterized by leathery white patches inside the mouth; produced by contact with irritants in tobacco juice.

constricted blood vessels, and subsequent increased blood pressure because the heart must work harder to pump blood through the narrowed vessels.

Nicotine decreases blood sugar levels and the stomach contractions that signal hunger. These factors, along with decreased sensation in the taste buds, reduce appetite. For this reason, many smokers eat less than nonsmokers do and weigh, on average, seven pounds less than nonsmokers.

Beginning smokers usually feel the effects of nicotine with their first puff. These symptoms, called **nicotine poisoning,** include dizziness, lightheadedness, rapid and erratic pulse, clammy skin, nausea, vomiting, and diarrhea. The effects of nicotine poisoning cease as soon as tolerance to the chemical develops. Medical research indicates that tolerance develops almost immediately in new users, perhaps after the second or third cigarette. In contrast, tolerance to most other drugs, such as alcohol, develops over a period of months or years. Regular smokers often do not experience the effects of smoking in the same way as beginning smokers do. They continue to smoke simply because stopping is too difficult.

Tobacco Addiction

Smoking is a complicated behavior. Somewhere between 60 and 80 percent of people have tried or taken at least a puff on a cigarette. Why is it that some walk away from cigarettes while most get hooked? For one thing, smoking is a very efficient drug delivery system. It gets the drug to the brain in just a few seconds, much faster than it would travel if injected. A pack-a-day smoker experiences 300 "hits," or pairings, a day, or 109,500 pairings per year. In pairing, an environmental cue triggers a craving for nicotine.[13] Simple **pairings,** such as drinking a cup of coffee, sitting in a car, finishing a meal, or sipping a beer, induce nicotine craving. Even college students who only smoke occasionally can find it hard to quit because of these paired associations. The brain gets used to these pairings and cries out in displeasure when the association is missing. It is easy to see how stopping even occasional use can be very difficult.

Why does this association occur? One explanation might lie in a person's genes. Two different twin studies found genetic factors to be more influential than environmental factors in smoking initiation and nicotine dependence. Two specific genes may influence smoking behavior by affecting the action of the brain chemical dopamine.[14] Understanding the influence of genetics on nicotine addiction will be crucial to developing more effective treatments for smoking cessation.

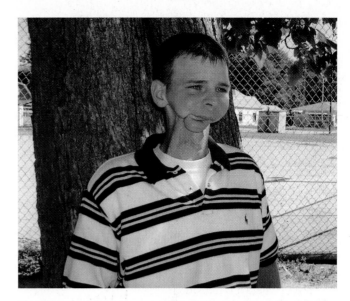

This 25-year-old cancer survivor has undergone almost 30 disfiguring surgeries. One operation removed half his neck muscles, lymph nodes, and tongue. He first tried smokeless tobacco at age 13; by age 17, he was diagnosed with squamous cell carcinoma. He now educates others about the dangers of smokeless tobacco.

Health Hazards of Smoking

Cigarette smoking adversely affects the health of every person who smokes, as well as the health of everyone nearby. Each day cigarettes contribute to over 1,000 deaths from cancer, cardiovascular disease, and respiratory disorders.

Cancer

The American Cancer Society estimates that tobacco smoking causes 85 to 90 percent of all cases of lung cancer; fewer than 10 percent of cases occur among nonsmokers.[15] Lung cancer is the leading cause of cancer deaths in the United States. There were an estimated 174,470 *new* cases of lung cancer in the United States in 2006 alone, and an estimated 162,460 Americans died from the disease in 2006.[16] Figure 13.3 on page 408 illustrates how tobacco smoke damages the lungs.

Lung cancer can take 10 to 30 years to develop, and the outlook for its victims is poor. Most lung cancer is not diagnosed until it is fairly widespread in the body; at that

what do you THINK?

Because nicotine is highly addictive, should it be regulated as a controlled substance? ■ How could tobacco be regulated effectively? ■ Should more resources be used for research into nicotine addiction? Why or why not?

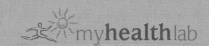
No one who starts smoking intends to become hooked. Imagine making a conscious decision to reduce your oxygen intake and deposit gooey tar on your lungs. It wouldn't be a very wise decision, would it? Smoking usually begins inno- cently enough, as an experiment or a dare or perhaps an attempt to fit in. Could you give it up right now without any problem? Or do you have a dependency? Take the following test to see.

	0 Points	1 Point	2 Points	3 Points
1. How soon after you wake up do you smoke your first cigarette?	After 60 minutes	31–60 minutes	6–30 minutes	Within 5 minutes
2. Do you find it difficult to refrain from smoking in places where it is forbidden?	No	Yes	—	—
3. Which cigarette would you hate most to give up?	The first one in the morning	Any other	—	—
4. How many cigarettes a day do you smoke?	10 or less	11–20	21–30	31 or more
5. Do you smoke more frequently during the first hours after awakening than during the rest of the day?	No	Yes	—	—
6. Do you smoke if you are so ill that you are in bed most of the day?	No	Yes	—	—

Interpreting Your Score

If you scored over 7 points, your level of nicotine dependence is high. You and your doctor should consider various medications to help you stop smoking.

If you scored under 4 points, you probably will be able to succeed in stopping smoking without medication.

Source: T. F. Heatherton, L. T. Kozlowski, R. C. Frecker, and K. O. Fagerstrom, "The Fagerstrom Test for Nicotine Dependence: A Revision of the Fagerstrom Tolerance Questionnaire," *British Journal of Addictions* 86 (1991): 1119–1127. Reprinted by permission of Dr. Karl Fagerstrom.

point, the five-year survival rate is only 13 percent. When a malignancy is diagnosed and recognized while still localized, the five-year survival rate rises to 47 percent.

If you are a smoker, your risk of developing lung cancer depends on several factors. First, the number of cigarettes you smoke per day is important. Someone who smokes two packs a day is 15 to 25 times more likely to develop lung cancer than a nonsmoker. If you started smoking in your teens, you have a greater chance of developing lung cancer than people who started later. If you inhale deeply when you smoke, you also increase your chances. Occupational or domestic exposure to other irritants, such as asbestos and radon, will also increase your likelihood of developing lung cancer.

Tobacco is linked to other cancers as well. The rate of pancreatic cancer is more than twice as high for smokers as non-smokers. Typically, people diagnosed with pancreatic cancer live about 3 months after their diagnosis. Smokers can reduce those odds by 30 percent if they quit for 11 years or more.[17] Cancers of the lip, tongue, salivary glands, and esophagus are five times more likely to occur among smokers than among nonsmokers. Smokers are also more likely to develop kidney, bladder, and larynx cancers.

Cardiovascular Disease

One-third of all tobacco-related deaths occur as a result of some form of heart disease.[18] Smokers have a 70 percent higher death rate from heart disease than nonsmokers do, and heavy smokers have a 200 percent higher death rate than moderate smokers. In fact, smoking cigarettes poses as great a risk for developing heart disease as high blood pressure and high cholesterol levels do.

Smoking contributes to heart disease by adding the equivalent of ten years of aging to the arteries.[19] One explanation

MAKE it happen!

ASSESSMENT: Complete the Assess Yourself Activity to determine if you are nicotine dependent, and the steps you need to take to kick the habit.

MAKING A CHANGE: In order to change your behavior, you need to develop a plan. Follow the steps below and complete your Behavior Change Contract to take action.

1. Evaluate your behavior and identify patterns and specific things you are doing. What can you change now? What can you change in the near future?

2. Select one pattern of behavior that you want to change.

3. Fill out the Behavior Change Contract found at the front of your book. It should include your long-term goal for change, your short-term goals, the rewards you'll give yourself for reaching these goals, potential obstacles along the way, and strategies for overcoming these obstacles. For each goal, list the small steps and specific actions that you will take.

4. Chart your progress in a journal. At the end of a week, consider how successful you were in following your plan. What helped you be successful? What made change more difficult? What will you do differently next week?

5. Revise your plan as needed: Are the short-term goals attainable? Are the rewards satisfying?

ONE STUDENT'S PLAN: After completing the Assess Yourself activity, Jana was surprised to find that her score for nicotine dependence was 10 points. She had convinced herself over the past few semesters that her cravings for cigarettes really were not harmful, but her score made her stop and think. Reflecting back over the last couple of years, she realized her smoking had progressed from occasional cigarettes with friends when they went out to having one or two while studying, to now pretty much smoking throughout the day. Knowing the health risks associated with smoking and the hassle of hiding her habit from family and friends, Jana decided it was time to quit.

First, Jana kept a daily journal for two weeks to record when and where she smoked and who she was with at the time. She wrote down how she felt and how important the cigarette was to her at the time on a scale of one to five. Then she decided to set some goals. The first goal was the date she would begin tapering off her cigarettes, and the second goal was a quit date. She outlined potential obstacles for achieving each goal and ways she could overcome the obstacles. For example, during the tapering phase, Jana decided she would buy only packs of cigarettes, instead of a carton. To assist her after her quit date, she decided she would tell her friends she was quitting and needed their support. She included all of this in her Behavior Change Contract.

Jana kept up her journal throughout her quitting process. She kept track of difficult moments and ways that were helpful to her in overcoming those moments. Also built into her contract were weekly rewards for her success. Jana would go out for dinner with friends or purchase new clothes with the money she was saving by not buying cigarettes.

---

is that smoking encourages atherosclerosis, the buildup of fatty deposits in the heart and major blood vessels. For unknown reasons, smoking decreases blood levels of HDLs (high-density lipoproteins), the "good" cholesterol that helps protect against heart attacks. Smoking also contributes to **platelet adhesiveness,** the sticking together of red blood cells that is associated with blood clots. The oxygen deprivation associated with smoking decreases the oxygen supplied to the heart and can weaken tissues. Smoking also contributes to irregular heart rhythms, which can trigger a heart attack. Both carbon monoxide and nicotine in cigarette smoke can precipitate angina attacks (pain spasms in the chest when the heart muscle does not get the blood supply it needs).

The number of years a person has smoked does not seem to bear much relation to cardiovascular risk. If a person quits smoking, the risk of dying from a heart attack is reduced by half after only one year without smoking and declines steadily thereafter. After about 15 years without smoking, the ex-smoker's risk of cardiovascular disease is similar to that of people who have never smoked.[20]

Stroke Smokers are twice as likely to suffer strokes as nonsmokers are.[21] A stroke occurs when a small blood vessel in the brain bursts or is blocked by a blood clot, denying oxygen and nourishment to vital portions of the brain. Depending on the area of the brain supplied by the vessel, stroke can result in paralysis, loss of mental function, or death. Smoking contributes to strokes by raising blood pressure, thereby increasing the stress on vessel walls. Platelet adhesiveness

platelet adhesiveness Stickiness of red blood cells associated with blood clots.

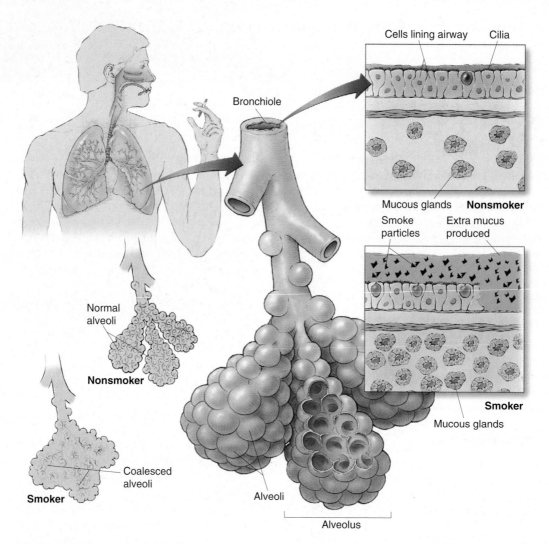

FIGURE 13.3 How Cigarette Smoking Damages the Lungs
Smoke particles irritate the lung pathways, which causes mucus production. They also indirectly destroy the walls of the lungs' alveoli, which coalesce. Both factors reduce lung efficiency. In addition, tar in tobacco smoke has a direct cancer-causing action.

contributes to clotting. However, 5 to 15 years after they stop smoking, the risk of stroke for ex-smokers is the same as that for people who have never smoked.[22]

Respiratory Disorders

Smoking quickly impairs the respiratory system. Smokers can feel its impact in a relatively short period of time—they are more prone to breathlessness, chronic cough, and excess phlegm than nonsmokers their age. Smokers tend to miss work one-third more often than nonsmokers do, primarily because of respiratory diseases, and they are up to 18 times more likely to die of lung disease.[23]

emphysema   A chronic lung disease in which the tiny air sacs in the lungs are destroyed, making breathing difficult.

Chronic bronchitis is the presence of a productive cough that persists or recurs frequently. It may develop in smokers because their inflamed lungs produce more mucus and constantly try to rid themselves of this mucus and foreign particles. This results in "smoker's hack," the persistent cough most smokers experience. Smokers are more prone than nonsmokers to respiratory ailments such as influenza, pneumonia, and colds.

Emphysema is a chronic disease in which the alveoli (the tiny air sacs in the lungs) are destroyed, impairing the lungs' ability to obtain oxygen and remove carbon dioxide. As a result, breathing becomes difficult. Whereas healthy people expend only about 5 percent of their energy in breathing, people with advanced emphysema expend nearly 80 percent of their energy. A simple movement such as rising from a seated position becomes painful and difficult for the emphysema patient. Because the heart has to work harder to do even the simplest tasks, it may become enlarged, and the person may die from heart damage. There is no known cure for emphysema.

Approximately 80 percent of all cases are related to cigarette smoking.

Sexual Dysfunction

Despite attempts by tobacco advertisers to make smoking appear sexy, research shows just the opposite: it can cause impotence in men. A number of recent studies have found that male smokers are about two times more likely than nonsmokers to suffer from some form of impotence. Toxins in cigarette smoke damage blood vessels, reducing blood flow to the penis and leading to an inadequate erection. It is thought that impotence could indicate oncoming cardiovascular disease.

Other Health Effects of Smoking

Gum disease is 3 times more common among smokers than among nonsmokers, and smokers lose significantly more teeth.[24] Nicotine and the other ingredients in cigarettes also interfere with the metabolism of drugs: nicotine speeds up the process by which the body uses and eliminates drugs, so that medications become less effective. There are also health effects of special concern to women (see the Women's Health/Men's Health box on page 410).

 what do you THINK?

Most people are very aware of the long-term hazards associated with tobacco use, yet despite prevention efforts, people continue to smoke. Why do you think this is so? ■ What strategies might be effective to reduce the number of people who begin smoking?

Environmental Tobacco Smoke

Although fewer than 30 percent of Americans are smokers, air pollution from smoking in public places continues to be a problem. **Environmental tobacco smoke (ETS)** is divided into two categories: mainstream and sidestream smoke (commonly called secondhand smoke). **Mainstream smoke** refers to smoke drawn through tobacco while inhaling; **secondhand smoke** (sidestream smoke) refers to smoke from the burning end of a cigarette or smoke exhaled by a smoker. People who breathe smoke from someone else's smoking product are said to be *involuntary,* or *passive* smokers. Nearly nine out of ten nonsmoking Americans are exposed to environmental tobacco smoke. In fact, measurable levels of nicotine were found in the blood of 88 percent of all nontobacco users.

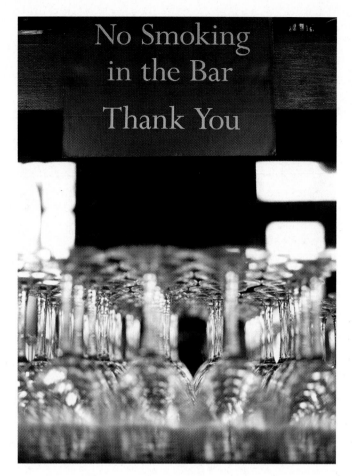

In recent years state lawmakers have taken action to protect nonsmokers from ETS. In many states, smoking is not permitted in public establishments.

Risks from Environmental Tobacco Smoke

Although involuntary smokers breathe less tobacco than active smokers do, they still face risks from exposure to tobacco smoke. Secondhand smoke actually contains more carcinogenic substances than the smoke that a smoker inhales. According to the American Lung Association, secondhand smoke has about 2 times more tar and nicotine, 5 times more carbon monoxide, and 50 times more

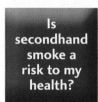

Is secondhand smoke a risk to my health?

environmental tobacco smoke (ETS) Smoke from tobacco products, including secondhand and mainstream smoke.

mainstream smoke Smoke that is drawn through tobacco while inhaling.

secondhand smoke (sidestream smoke) The cigarette, pipe, or cigar smoke breathed by nonsmokers.

WOMEN AND SMOKING

Cigarette smoking was rare among women in the early twentieth century and became prevalent among women long after it did among men. In 2004 in the United States, 21.5 million (18.5 percent of) women smoked. Women have been extensively targeted in tobacco marketing dominated by themes of an association between social desirability, independence, weight control, and smoking messages conveyed through advertisements featuring slim, attractive, and athletic models. Today, men's and women's smoking rates are nearly equal, and accordingly women have a much larger burden of smoking-related diseases than they have in the past.

- One of every five women in America is a smoker. Twenty-three percent of all adult Americans and 21 percent of American women are currently smokers.
- Smoking among women differs by race and ethnicity. Twenty-two percent of white American women smoke, as do 21 percent of African American women, 13 percent of Hispanic women, and 8 percent of Asian American women. A whopping forty-three percent of American Indian/Alaska Native women are smokers.
- Smoking is associated with education. Among U.S. women who earned a GED, 44 percent are smokers. Among college graduates, 12 percent are smokers, while only 8 percent of those who completed graduate work smoke. Women with a high school education

are twice as likely to smoke as women with an undergraduate degree.
- Smoking is associated with poverty. Twenty-nine percent of women who are below the poverty line smoke.

Despite recent declines in smoking, the prevalence of tobacco-related disease continues to increase, especially among women.

- Every year, tobacco-related disease kills over 178,000 women, making it the largest preventable cause of death among women in the United States.
- Smoking has been responsible for the premature deaths of approximately 3 million women since 1985.
- Women who die of a smoking-related disease lose, on average, 14.5 years of potential life. Men who die of a smoking-related disease lose 13 years of life, on average.
- Women who begin smoking at an early age (within 5 years of their first period) are at higher risk of developing breast cancer.
- Evidence suggests that breast cancer is more likely to spread to the lungs in women who smoke than in women with breast cancer who do not smoke.
- Recent CDC data indicate that smoking-related cancer deaths are decreasing among men, while for women they are increasing.
- Some studies suggest that smoking cigarettes dramatically increases the risk of heart disease among younger

women who are also taking birth control pills.
- Women who smoke have an increased risk for ischemic stroke and subarachnoid hemorrhage. Constant exposure to others' tobacco smoke (secondhand smoke) at work or at home also increases the risk, even for nonsmokers.
- Coronary heart disease and lung cancer caused by exposure to a spouse's secondhand smoke is a cause of death among women who do not smoke.
- Women who smoke increase their risk for infertility, ectopic pregnancy, spontaneous abortion, and stillbirth.
- Smoking during pregnancy accounts for 20 to 30 percent of low–birth weight babies, up to 14 percent of preterm deliveries, and about 10 percent of all infant deaths.
- Postmenopausal women who smoke have lower bone density than women who never smoked. Cigarette smoking also causes skin to age prematurely.

Sources: American Lung Association, "Women and Smoking Fact Sheet", March 2006. www.lungusa.org.; American Cancer Society, "Women and Smoking: A Silent Epidemic," February 13, 2006, www.cancer.org; American Legacy Foundation, "Tobacco and Your Health," 2006, www.americanlegacy.org/facts/index.cfm?id=2; American Heart Association, "Women, Heart Disease, and Stroke," 2006, www.americanheart.org; Office on Smoking and Health, "Cigarette Smoking Among Adults—United States, 2004," *Tobacco Information and Prevention Source (TIPS)* 54, no. 44 (2005).

ammonia than mainstream smoke. Every year, ETS is estimated to be responsible for approximately 3,000 lung cancer deaths, 46,000 coronary and heart disease deaths, and 430 deaths in newborns from sudden infant death syndrome.[25]

The Environmental Protection Agency (EPA) has designated secondhand smoke as a known carcinogen (group A carcinogen). The Surgeon General's Report, *The Health*

Consequences of Involuntary Exposure to Tobacco Smoke, finds that there are more than 50 cancer-causing agents found in secondhand smoke.[26] The most likely cause of lung cancer from secondhand smoke is continuous exposure to the carcinogens over time. There is also strong evidence that secondhand smoke interferes with normal functioning of the heart, blood, and vascular systems, significantly increasing the risk for heart disease and having immediate effects on the cardiovascular system.[27] A study found that nonsmokers exposed to secondhand smoke were 25 percent more likely to have coronary heart disease compared with nonsmokers not exposed to smoke.[28]

Children and ETS Exposure to ETS among children increases their risk of infections of the lower respiratory tract. An estimated 300,000 children are at greater risk of pneumonia and bronchitis as a result.[29] Children exposed to secondhand smoke have a greater chance of developing other respiratory problems such as coughing, wheezing, asthma, and chest colds, along with a decrease in lung function. The greatest effects of secondhand smoke are seen in children under the age of five. Children exposed to secondhand smoke daily in the home miss 33 percent more school days and have 10 percent more colds and acute respiratory infections than those not exposed.

Secondhand smoke impacts not only children's physical health, but also their cognitive abilities and academic success. A recent study discovered that children exposed to high levels of secondhand smoke had lower standardized test scores in reading, math, and problem solving.[30] Additionally, children exposed to secondhand smoke are twice as likely to become smokers during adolescence than children who are not exposed to secondhand smoke.[31]

Despite these facts, children continue to be exposed to secondhand smoke in their homes. It is estimated that 23 percent of children under the age of 18 are exposed to cigarette smoke in the home.[32]

ETS and Additional Health Problems

Cigarette, cigar, and pipe smoke in enclosed areas presents other hazards. Ten to 15 percent of nonsmokers are extremely sensitive (hypersensitive) to cigarette smoke. These people experience itchy eyes, difficulty in breathing, painful headaches, nausea, and dizziness in response to minute amounts of smoke. The level of carbon monoxide in cigarette smoke contained in enclosed places is 4,000 times higher than that allowed in the clean air standard recommended by the EPA.

Action to Reduce ETS Efforts to reduce the hazards associated with secondhand smoke have gained momentum in recent years. Groups such as GASP (Group Against Smokers' Pollution) and ASH (Action on Smoking and Health) have been working since the early 1970s to reduce smoking in public places. In response to their efforts, some 44 states have enacted laws restricting smoking in public places such as restaurants, theaters, and airports. Of those 44 states, 14 have laws that make private workplaces smoke free. The Surgeon General has concluded that smoke-free workplace policies are the only effective way to eliminate secondhand smoke exposure in the workplace. Separating smokers from nonsmokers, cleaning the air, and ventilating buildings is not enough to eliminate exposure.[33] Table 13.3 details measures

TABLE 13.3	Protecting Yourself and Others from Secondhand Smoke

Opening a window, sitting in a separate area, or using ventilation, air conditioning, or a fan cannot eliminate secondhand smoke exposure.

You can protect yourself and others by:

- Making your home and car smoke free.
- Asking people not to smoke around you and your children.
- Making sure that your children's day care center or school is smoke free.
- Choosing smoke-free restaurants and other businesses. Thanking businesses for being smoke free. Letting owners of businesses that are not smoke free know that secondhand smoke is harmful to your health and the health of others.
- Teaching children to stay away from secondhand smoke.
- Avoiding secondhand smoke exposure if you or your children have respiratory conditions, you have heart disease, or you are pregnant.
- Talking to your doctor or health care provider more about the dangers of secondhand smoke.

If you are a smoker, the single best way to protect your family from secondhand smoke is to quit smoking. In the meantime, you can protect your family by making your home and vehicles smoke free and only smoking outside. A smoke-free home rule can also help you quit smoking.

Source: Office on Smoking and Health, *The Health Consequences of Involuntary Exposure to Tobacco Smoke: A Report of the Surgeon General— Executive Summary.* (Washington DC: U.S. Department of Health and Human Services, 2006.)

you can take to protect yourself and others from secondhand smoke.

The hospitality industry has also taken steps to protect the health of nonsmokers. Hotels and motels now set aside rooms for nonsmokers, and many hotels are now becoming 100 percent smoke free. Car rental agencies designate certain vehicles for nonsmokers. Smoking is banned on all U.S. airlines and many other countries ban smoking on their airlines as well.

 what do you THINK?

What rights, if any, should smokers have with regard to smoking in public places? ■ Does your campus allow smoking in residence halls? ■ Does your community have nonsmoking restaurants, or only nonsmoking sections in restaurants? ■ Do you think your community would support nonsmoking restaurants and bars? Why or why not?

Tobacco and Politics

It has been 40 years since the government began warning that tobacco use was hazardous to the health of the nation. Despite the fact that there is much education on the health hazards of tobacco use, public health spending associated with smoking is over $75.5 billion a year for health care costs.[34] So, more than four decades after the Surgeon General began to warn the public of the dangers of smoking, tobacco still remains a hot topic. A survey recently found that a majority of U.S. adults support tobacco control strategies, including creation of smoke-free work environments, an increase in tobacco excise taxes, more funds to help prevent people from smoking and to help people stop smoking, and restriction of youth access to tobacco.[35]

After many years of contentious negotiation between the tobacco industry and the U.S. Attorney General, 46 states sued to recover health care costs related to treating smokers. In 1998, the tobacco industry reached a Master's Settlement Agreement with 40 states. Key provisions included the following:

- The tobacco payments will total approximately $206 billion, to be paid over 25 years nationwide.
- The industry will pay $1.5 billion over ten years to support antismoking measures, including education and advertising. An additional $250 million will fund research to determine the most effective ways to stop kids from smoking.
- The industry is barred from billboard advertising, including advertisements on transit systems. In-store ads are still permitted but will be limited in size.
- All outdoor advertising is banned, including billboards, signs, and placards larger than a poster, in arenas, stadiums, shopping malls, and video arcades.
- The agreement bans youth access to free samples, proof-of-purchase gifts, and sale and distribution of "branded" merchandise, such as T-shirts, hats, and other items bearing tobacco brand names or logos.
- There is a ban on the use of cartoon characters in advertising. (Such advertising is considered particularly appealing to young children.)
- Tobacco company sponsorship of concerts, athletic events, or any event in which a significant portion of the audience is young people is forbidden.
- The industry agreed not to market cigarettes to children and not to misrepresent the health effects of cigarettes.

However, funds from the settlement that were supposed to add a strong kick to antismoking initiatives have had trouble doing so. The majority of the funding has not been spent on anything related to smoking; facing budget woes, many states have drastically cut spending on antismoking programs. In the few states that have spent the settlement money on smoking cessation programs, there has been some reported success in decreasing cigarette use.[36]

Quitting

Quitting smoking isn't easy. Smokers must break the physical addiction to nicotine—and they must break the habit of lighting up at certain times of the day.

From what we know about successful quitters, quitting is often a lengthy process involving several unsuccessful attempts before success is finally achieved. Even successful quitters suffer occasional slips, emphasizing the fact that stopping smoking is a dynamic process that occurs over time (Figure 13.4).

Approximately 70 percent of adult smokers in the United States want to quit smoking and up to 40 percent make a serious attempt to quit each year. However, fewer than 5 percent succeed.[37]

The person who wishes to quit smoking has several options. Most people who are successful at quitting quit "cold turkey"—that is, they decide simply not to smoke again. Others resort to short-term programs, such as those offered by the American Cancer Society, which are based on behavior modification and a system of self-rewards. Still others turn to treatment centers that are part of large franchises, a local medical clinic's community outreach plan, or a telephone quit line. Finally, some people work privately with their physicians to reach their goal.

Prospective quitters must decide which method or combination of methods will work best for them. Programs that combine several approaches have shown the most promise. Financial considerations, personality characteristics, and level of addiction are all factors to consider.

Breaking the Nicotine Addiction

Nicotine addiction may be one of the toughest addictions to overcome. Many must try several times to quit before they finally succeed for good.[38] Smokers' attempts to quit lead to withdrawal symptoms. Symptoms of **nicotine withdrawal** include irritability, restlessness, nausea, headaches, and intense cravings for tobacco.

Nicotine Replacement Products
Nontobacco products that replace depleted levels of nicotine in the bloodstream have helped some people stop using tobacco (see Table 13.4 on page 414). The two most common are nicotine chewing gum and the nicotine patch, both of which are available over the counter. The FDA has also approved a nicotine nasal spray and a nicotine inhaler.

Some patients use Nicorette, a prescription chewing gum containing nicotine, to reduce nicotine consumption over

---

nicotine withdrawal Symptoms, including nausea, headaches, irritability, and intense tobacco cravings, suffered by addicted smokers who cease using tobacco.

time. Under the guidance of a physician, the user chews 12 to 24 pieces of gum per day for up to six months. Nicorette delivers about as much nicotine as a cigarette does but is absorbed through the mucous membrane of the mouth. Users experience no withdrawal symptoms and fewer cravings for nicotine as the dosage is reduced until they are completely weaned.

Some controversy surrounds the use of nicotine replacement gum. Opponents believe that it substitutes one addiction for another. Successful users counter that it is a valid way to help break a deadly habit without suffering the unpleasant cravings that often lead to relapse.

The nicotine patch, first marketed in 1991, is generally used in conjunction with a comprehensive smoking-behavior cessation program. A small, thin, 24-hour patch placed on the smoker's upper body delivers a continuous flow of nicotine through the skin, helping to relieve cravings. The patch is worn for 8 to 12 weeks under the guidance of a clinician. During this time, the dose of nicotine is gradually reduced until the smoker is fully weaned from the drug. Occasional side effects include mild skin irritation, insomnia, dry mouth, and nervousness. The patch costs less than a pack of cigarettes—about four dollars—and some insurance plans will pay for it.

The nasal spray, which also requires a prescription, is much more powerful and delivers nicotine to the bloodstream faster than gum or the patch. Patients are warned to be careful not to overdose; as little as 40 milligrams of nicotine taken at once could be lethal. The spray is somewhat unpleasant to use. The FDA has advised that it should be used for no more than three months and never for more than six months so that smokers don't find themselves as dependent on nicotine in spray form as they were on cigarettes. The FDA also advises that no one who experiences nasal or sinus problems, allergies, or asthma should use it.

The nicotine inhaler, also available by prescription, consists of a mouthpiece and cartridge. By puffing on the mouthpiece, the smoker inhales air saturated with nicotine, which is absorbed through the lining of the mouth, not the lungs. This nicotine enters the body much more slowly than the nicotine in cigarettes does. Using the inhaler mimics the hand-to-mouth actions used in smoking and causes the back of the throat to feel as it would when inhaling tobacco smoke. Each cartridge lasts for 80 long puffs, and each cartridge is designed for 20 minutes of use.

Approved in 1997 by the FDA, Zyban, the smoking cessation pill, offers hope to many who thought they could never quit. Zyban is thought to work on dopamine and norepinephrine receptors in the brain to decrease craving and withdrawal symptoms. Because of the way this prescription medication works, it is important to start the pills one to two weeks before the targeted quit date; it requires planning ahead.

A radical new way to help smokers quit is NicVAX, an antismoking vaccine due out on the market very soon. The vaccination prevents nicotine from reaching the brain, making smoking less pleasurable and therefore easier to give up. A small amount that may get to the brain eases the discomfort

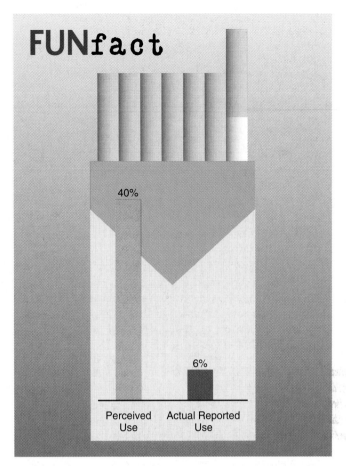

FIGURE 13.4 How Much Do Your Peers Smoke Daily?
This data looks at the actual percentage of students who smoke cigarettes daily, versus how many students are perceived to smoke daily by other students. Surprised?

Source: American College Health Association, *National College Health Assessment: Reference Group Executive Summary, Fall 2005* (Baltimore, MD: American College Health Association, 2006)

of withdrawal. The vaccine differs from conventional cessation treatments by attacking the dependence in the brain, instead of just replacing the nicotine. One of the advantages of the vaccine over other forms of cessation methods is that it will reduce relapses by making the cigarette much less enjoyable when the quitter tries a cigarette again.[39]

How effective are these therapies? The evidence is strong that consistent pharmacological treatments can help a smoker quit, with estimated abstinence after use ranging from 17 to 30 percent.[40]

Breaking the Habit

For some smokers, the road to quitting includes antismoking therapy. Two common techniques are operant conditioning and self-control therapy. Pairing the act of smoking with an external stimulus is a typical example of an operant strategy. For example, one technique requires smokers to carry a timer that sounds a buzzer at different intervals. When the buzzer sounds, the patient is required to smoke a cigarette. Once the

Therapy	Duration	
BUPROPRION (ZYBAN) A nonnicotine-based antidepressant, helps reduce nicotine withdrawal symptoms and urge to smoke. Common side effects are dry mouth, difficulty sleeping, dizziness, and skin rash. Contraindicated if smoker has a history of seizures. *Availability:* Prescription only with a doctor consultation	7–12 weeks; maintenance up to 6 months; start 1–2 weeks before the quit date	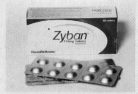
NICOTINE GUM A chewing gum that releases nicotine into the bloodstream through the lining of mouth; might not be appropriate for people with temporomandibular joint disease or those with dentures or other dental work. Up to 2 mg dose if less than 25 cigarettes/day; 4 mg dose if ≧ 25 cigarettes/day *Availability:* Over the counter (OTC)	Up to 12 weeks	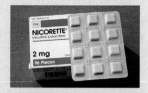
NICOTINE INHALER This device delivers a vaporized form of nicotine to mouth through a mouthpiece attached to a plastic cartridge. Nicotine travels to the mouth and throat, and is absorbed through the mucous membranes. Common side effects include throat and mouth irritation and coughing. Anyone with bronchial problems should use caution. *Availability:* Prescription only with a doctor consultation	Up to 6 months	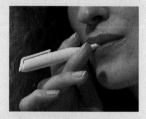
NICOTINE NASAL SPRAY Comes in a pump bottle containing nicotine that tobacco users can inhale when they have urge to smoke. Not recommended for people with nasal or sinus conditions, allergies, or asthma, or for young tobacco users. *Availability:* Prescription only with a doctor consultation	3–6 months	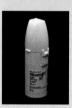
NICOTINE PATCH Patch supplies a steady amount of nicotine to the body through the skin. Is sold in varying strengths as an 8-week smoking cessation treatment. Doses can be regularly lowered as treatment progresses or given as a steady dose during treatment. May not be a good choice for people with skin problems or allergies to adhesive tape. *Availability:* Either OTC or by prescription with a doctor consultation	4 weeks; then 2 weeks; then 2 weeks (8 weeks total)	

Notes: This table contains brief descriptions and was adapted from published medical articles.

Source: American Cancer Society, in "Recommended Therapies for Smoking Cessation," *Cancer Facts & Figures, 2004.* For complete data, see American Cancer Society website www.cancer.org. Used by permission of the American Cancer Society.

smoker is conditioned to associate the buzzer with smoking, the buzzer is eliminated, and, one hopes, so is the smoking. Self-control strategies view smoking as a learned habit associated with specific situations. Therapy is aimed at identifying these situations and teaching smokers the skills necessary to resist smoking.

The Skills for Behavior Change box on page 416 presents one of the American Cancer Society's approaches.

Benefits of Quitting

Will quitting smoking reverse the damage I've already done?

According to the American Cancer Society, many tissues damaged by smoking can repair themselves. As soon as smokers stop, the body begins the repair process (Figure 13.5). Within eight hours, carbon monoxide and oxygen levels return to normal, and "smoker's breath"

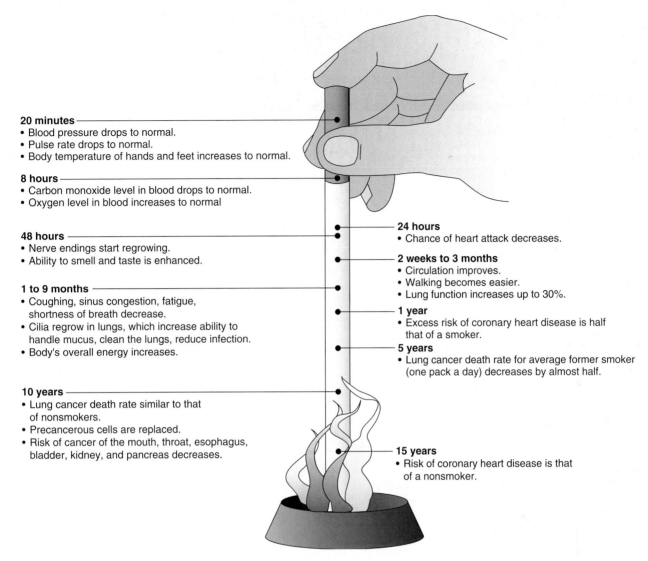

20 minutes
- Blood pressure drops to normal.
- Pulse rate drops to normal.
- Body temperature of hands and feet increases to normal.

8 hours
- Carbon monoxide level in blood drops to normal.
- Oxygen level in blood increases to normal

48 hours
- Nerve endings start regrowing.
- Ability to smell and taste is enhanced.

1 to 9 months
- Coughing, sinus congestion, fatigue, shortness of breath decrease.
- Cilia regrow in lungs, which increase ability to handle mucus, clean the lungs, reduce infection.
- Body's overall energy increases.

10 years
- Lung cancer death rate similar to that of nonsmokers.
- Precancerous cells are replaced.
- Risk of cancer of the mouth, throat, esophagus, bladder, kidney, and pancreas decreases.

24 hours
- Chance of heart attack decreases.

2 weeks to 3 months
- Circulation improves.
- Walking becomes easier.
- Lung function increases up to 30%.

1 year
- Excess risk of coronary heart disease is half that of a smoker.

5 years
- Lung cancer death rate for average former smoker (one pack a day) decreases by almost half.

15 years
- Risk of coronary heart disease is that of a nonsmoker.

FIGURE 13.5 When Smokers Quit

Within 20 minutes of smoking that last cigarette, the body begins a series of changes that continues for years. However, by smoking just one cigarette a day, the smoker loses all of these benefits, according to the American Cancer Society.

Source: G. Hanson and P. Venturelli, *Drugs and Society,* 9th ed. (Sudbury, MA: Jones and Bartlett, 2006). © Jones and Bartlett, www.jbpub.com. Reprinted with permission.

disappears. Often, within a month of quitting, the mucus that clogs airways is broken up and eliminated. Circulation and the senses of taste and smell improve within weeks. Many ex-smokers say they have more energy, sleep better, and feel more alert. By the end of one year, the risk for lung cancer and stroke decreases. In addition, ex-smokers reduce considerably their risk of developing cancers of the mouth, throat, esophagus, larynx, pancreas, bladder, and cervix. They also cut their risk of peripheral arterial disease, chronic obstructive lung disease, coronary heart disease, and ulcers. Women are less likely to bear babies with low birth weight. Within two years, the risk for heart attack drops to near normal. At the end of ten smoke-free years, the ex-smoker can expect to live out his or her normal life span.

 what do you THINK?

Do you know people who have tried to quit smoking? ■ What was this experience like for them? ■ Were they successful? ■ If not, what factors contributed to relapse?

Caffeine

What is the most popular and widely consumed drug in the United States? Caffeine. Almost half of all Americans drink coffee every day, and many others use caffeine in some other form, mainly for its well-known "wake-up" effect. Drinking

SKILLS FOR *behavior change*

DEVELOPING A PLAN TO KICK THE TOBACCO HABIT

There is no magic cure that can help you stop. Take the first step by answering this question: Why do I want to stop smoking?

Write your reasons in the space below. Once you have prepared your list, carry a copy of it with you. Memorize it. Every time you are tempted to smoke, go over your reasons for stopping.

MY REASONS FOR STOPPING

1. _____
2. _____
3. _____
4. _____
5. _____

DEVELOP A PLAN; CHANGE SOME HABITS

Over time, smoking becomes a strong habit. Daily events such as finishing a meal, talking on the phone, drinking coffee, and chatting with friends trigger the urge to smoke. Breaking the link between the trigger and the smoking will help you stop. Think about the times and places you usually smoke. What could you do instead of smoking at those times?

THINGS TO DO INSTEAD OF SMOKING

1. _____
2. _____
3. _____

THE BOTTOM LINE: COMMIT YOURSELF

There comes a time when you have to say good-bye to your cigarettes.

- Pick a day to stop smoking.
- Fill out the Behavior Change Contract.
- Have a family member or friend sign the contract.

Then

- Throw away all your cigarettes, lighters, and ashtrays at home and at work. You will not need them again.
- Be prepared to feel the urge to smoke. The urge will pass whether or not you smoke. Use the four Ds to fight the urge:
  Delay
  Deep breathing
  Drink water
  Do something else

- Keep "mouth toys" handy: lifesavers, gum, straws, and carrot sticks can help.
- If you've had trouble stopping before, ask your doctor about nicotine chewing gum, patches, nasal sprays, inhalers, or pills.
- Tell your family and friends that you've stopped smoking.
- Put "no smoking" signs in your car, work area, and house.
- Give yourself a treat for stopping. Go to a movie, go out to dinner, or buy yourself a gift.

FOCUS ON THE POSITIVES

Now that you have stopped smoking, your mind and your body will begin to feel better. Think of the good things that have happened since you stopped. Can you breathe more easily? Do you have more energy? Do you feel good about what you've done?

Make a list of the good things about not smoking. Carry a copy with you, and look at it when you have the urge to smoke.

---

coffee is legal, even socially encouraged. Many people believe caffeine is not a drug and not really addictive. Coffee, soft drinks, and other caffeine-containing products seem harmless; with no cream or sugar added, many are calorie free and therefore a good way to fill up if you are dieting. If you share these attitudes, you should think again, because research in the past decade has linked caffeine to certain health problems.

Caffeine is a drug derived from the chemical family called **xanthines.** Two related chemicals, *theophylline* and *theobromine,* are found in tea and chocolate, respectively. The xanthines are mild central nervous system stimulants that enhance mental alertness and reduce feelings of fatigue. Other stimulant effects include increased heart muscle contractions, oxygen consumption, metabolism, and urinary output. These effects are felt within 15 to 45 minutes of ingesting a product that contains caffeine.

Side effects of the xanthines include wakefulness, insomnia, irregular heartbeat, dizziness, nausea, indigestion, and sometimes mild delirium. Some people also experience heartburn. As with some other drugs, the user's psychological outlook and expectations will influence the effects.

Different products contain different concentrations of caffeine. A five-ounce cup of coffee contains anywhere from 65 to 115 milligrams of caffeine. Caffeine concentrations vary with the brand of the beverage and the strength of the brew. Small chocolate bars contain up to 15 milligrams of caffeine and theobromine. Table 13.5 compares various caffeine-containing products.

caffeine A stimulant found in coffee, tea, chocolate, and some soft drinks.

xanthines The chemical family of stimulants to which caffeine belongs.

Caffeine Addiction

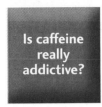

Is caffeine really addictive?

As the effects of caffeine wear off, users may feel let down—mentally or physically depressed, exhausted, and weak. To counteract this, they commonly choose to drink another cup of coffee. Habitually engaging in this practice leads to tolerance and psychological dependency. Until the mid-1970s, caffeine was not medically recognized as addictive. Chronic caffeine use and its attendant behaviors were dismissed as "coffee nerves." This syndrome is now recognized as *caffeine intoxication,* or **caffeinism.**

Symptoms of caffeinism include chronic insomnia, jitters, irritability, nervousness, anxiety, and involuntary muscle twitches. Withdrawing the caffeine may compound the effects and produce severe headaches. (Some physicians ask their patients to take a simple test for caffeine addiction: don't consume anything containing caffeine, and if you get a severe headache within four hours, you are addicted.) Because caffeine meets the requirements for addiction—tolerance, psychological dependency, and withdrawal symptoms—it can be classified as addictive.

Although you would have to drink 67 to 100 cups of coffee in a day to produce a fatal overdose of caffeine, you may experience sensory disturbances after consuming only ten cups of coffee within a 24-hour period. These symptoms include tinnitus (ringing in the ears), spots before the eyes, numbness in arms and legs, poor circulation, and visual hallucinations. Because ten cups of coffee is not an extraordinary amount to drink in one day, caffeine use clearly poses health threats.

The Health Consequences of Long-Term Caffeine Use

Long-term caffeine use has been suspected of being linked to a number of serious health problems, ranging from heart disease and cancer to mental dysfunction and birth defects. However, no strong evidence exists to suggest that moderate caffeine use (less than 300 milligrams daily, approximately three cups of coffee) produces harmful effects in healthy, nonpregnant people.

It appears that caffeine does not cause long-term high blood pressure, and it has not been linked to strokes. Nor is there any evidence of a relationship between coffee and heart disease.[41] However, people who suffer from irregular heartbeat are cautioned against using caffeine because the resultant increase in heart rate might be life-threatening. Both decaffeinated and caffeinated coffee products contain ingredients that can irritate the stomach lining and be harmful to people with stomach ulcers.

For years, caffeine consumption was linked with fibrocystic breast disease, a condition characterized by painful, noncancerous lumps in the breast. Although these conclusions have been challenged, many clinicians advise patients

TABLE 13.5	Caffeine Content of Various Products	
Product	**Caffeine Content (Average mg per Serving)**
Coffee (5-oz. cup)	
Regular brewed	65–115
Decaffeinated brewed	3
Decaffeinated instant	2
Tea (6-oz. cup)	
Hot steeped	36
Iced	31
Bottled (12 oz.)	15
Soft Drinks (12-oz. servings)	
Jolt Cola	100
Dr. Pepper	61
Mountain Dew	54
Coca-Cola	46
Pepsi Cola	36–38
Chocolate	
1 oz. baking chocolate	25
1 oz. chocolate candy bar	15
1/2 cup chocolate pudding	4–12
Over-the-Counter Drugs	
No-Doz (2 tablets)	200
Excedrin (2 tablets)	130
Midol (2 tablets)	65
Anacin (2 tablets)	64

Source: Department of Health and Welfare, October 2001.

with mammillary cysts to avoid caffeine. In addition, some reports indicate that very high doses of caffeine given to pregnant laboratory animals can cause stillbirths or offspring with low birth weights or limb deformations. Studies have found that moderate consumption of caffeine (less than 300 milligrams per day) did not significantly affect human fetal development.[42] However, women are usually advised to avoid or at least reduce caffeine use during pregnancy.

 what do you THINK?

How much caffeine do you consume? ■ What is your pattern of caffeine consumption for the day? ■ Why do you consume it? ■ Have you ever experienced any ill effects after going without caffeine for a period of time?

caffeinism Caffeine intoxication brought on by excessive use; symptoms include chronic insomnia, irritability, anxiety, muscle twitches, and headaches.

TAKING charge

Summary

- The use of tobacco involves many social issues, including advertising targeted at youth and women, the fastest growing populations of smokers. Health care and lost productivity resulting from smoking cost the nation as much as $167 billion per year.
- Tobacco is available in smoking and smokeless forms, both containing addictive nicotine (a psychoactive substance). Smoking also delivers 4,000 other chemicals to the lungs of smokers.
- The health hazards of smoking include markedly higher rates of cancer, heart and circulatory disorders, respiratory diseases, and gum diseases. Smoking while pregnant presents risks for the fetus, including miscarriage and low birth weight.
- Smokeless tobacco contains more nicotine than do cigarettes and dramatically increases risks for oral cancer and other oral problems.

- Environmental tobacco smoke (secondhand smoke) puts nonsmokers at risk for elevated rates of cancer and heart disease.
- For almost 40 years the government has been warning consumers of the dangers associated with tobacco use. In a landmark legal settlement, the tobacco industry agreed to reimburse states for health care costs related to smoking and to finance various antismoking initiatives.
- Quitting is complicated by the dual nature of smoking: smokers must kick a chemical addiction as well as a habit. Nicotine replacement products or Zyban can help wean smokers off nicotine. The new smoking vaccine makes tobacco less pleasurable. Therapy methods can also help smokers break the habit.
- Caffeine is a widely used central nervous system stimulant. No long-term ill-health effects have been proven, although chronic users who try to quit may experience withdrawal.

Chapter Review

1. What are bidis?
   a. a type of clove cigarette
   b. an Indian-made sweet, flavored cigarette
   c. a type of cigar made in India
   d. tobacco rolled with marijuana

2. What is secondhand or sidestream smoke?
   a. The smoke that is inhaled by the smoker.
   b. The smoke emitting from a burning cigarette in an ashtray.
   c. The smoke from a lower tar cigarette.
   d. None of the above.

3. What does carbon monoxide do to smokers?
   a. It makes it difficult for a smoker to breathe.
   b. It causes dizzy spells and light headedness.
   c. It interferes with the ability of hemoglobin in the blood to adequately carry oxygen.
   d. It impairs cleansing function of the lung's cilia hairs.

4. What age group is most targeted by tobacco advertisers?
   a. 14–17 year old teenagers
   b. 18–24 year old college students
   c. 25–30 year old young adults
   d. 31–35 year old married men

5. The major psychoactive ingredient in tobacco products is
   a. carbon monoxide.
   b. tar.
   c. formaldehyde.
   d. nicotine.

6. What does nicotine do to the cilia hairs found in the lungs?
   a. It instantly destroys the cilia hairs.
   b. It thickens the cilia hairs so they can't function properly.
   c. It impairs the cleaning function of the cilia by paralyzing them.
   d. It accumulates nicotine on the cilia hairs.

7. Which type of tobacco product contains the ingredient eugenol that allows smokers to inhale the smoke more deeply?
   a. bidis
   b. cigars
   c. snuff
   d. clove cigarettes

8. Chewing tobacco is generally placed between the gums and teeth for chewing, whereas snuff is
   a. also placed between the gums and teeth for sucking.
   b. usually placed inside the cheek.
   c. placed between the lower lip and teeth.
   d. None of the above.

9. A major health risk of chewing tobacco is
   a. lung cancer.
   b. leukoplakia.
   c. heart disease.
   d. emphysema.

10. Whenever Jake has a cup of coffee, he also craves a cigarette. This is called
    a. joining.
    b. pairing.
    c. tolerance.
    d. replacement.

Answers to these questions can be found on page A-1.

Questions for Discussion and Reflection

1. New research suggests that genetic factors might be more influential than environmental factors in smoking initiation and nicotine dependence. How might this information change current prevention efforts? How would you design smoking prevention strategies targeted at adolescents?
2. Discuss the varied ways in which tobacco is used. Is any method less addictive or hazardous to health than another?
3. Discuss short-term and long-term health hazards associated with smoking. How will increased tobacco use among adolescents and college students impact the medical system in the future? Who should be responsible for the medical expenses of smokers? Insurance companies? Smokers themselves?
4. Do you believe that the tobacco companies could develop a "safe" cigarette? What would it take for you to consider a cigarette "safe"? Consider the claims for safety previously made by tobacco companies as you give your answer.
5. Discuss the various risks of smokeless tobacco use.
6. Restrictions on smoking are increasing in our society. Do you think these restrictions are fair? Do they infringe on people's rights? Are the restrictions too strict or not strict enough?
7. Describe the pros and cons of each method of quitting smoking. Which would be most effective for you? Explain why.
8. Discuss problems related to the ingestion of caffeine. How much caffeine do you consume? Why?

Accessing Your Health on the Internet

The following websites explore further topics and issues related to personal health. You'll also find links to each organization's website on the Companion Website for *Access to Health,* Tenth Edition, at www.aw-bc.com/donatelle.

1. *American Lung Association.* This site offers a wealth of information regarding smoking trends, environmental smoke, and advice on smoking cessation. www.lungusa.org
2. *ASH (Action on Smoking and Health).* The nation's oldest and largest antismoking organization, ASH regularly takes hard-hitting legal actions and does other work to fight smoking and protect the rights of nonsmokers. ASH provides nonsmokers with legal forms and valuable information about protecting their rights and about the problems and costs of smoking to nonsmokers. ASH's actions have helped prohibit cigarette commercials; ban smoking on planes, buses, and in many public places; and lower insurance premiums for nonsmokers. www.ash.org
3. *TIPS (Tobacco Information and Prevention Source).* This website provides access to a variety of information regarding tobacco use in the United States, with specific information for and about young people. www.cdc.gov/tobacco

Further Reading

Gately, I. *Tobacco: A Cultural History of How an Exotic Plant Seduced Civilization.* New York: Grove Press, 2003.

Tobacco has a sweeping history as the world's prevalent addiction. The book begins with pre-Columbian America and continues through the tobacco litigation of the 1990s.

Gilman, R. L., ed. *Smoke: A Global History of Smoking.* London: Reaktion Books, 2004.

An informative book that reviews human preoccupation with smoking over the past six centuries, and explores issues relating to art, culture, and gender.

Glantz, S. A. and E. D. Balbach. *The Tobacco War: Inside the California Battles.* Berkeley: University of California Press, 2000.

> Charts the dramatic and complex history of tobacco politics in California over the past quarter century. Shows how the accomplishments of tobacco-control advocates have changed how people view the tobacco industry and its behavior.

Kluger, R. *Ashes to Ashes: America's Hundred-Year Cigarette War, the Public Health, and the Unabashed Triumph of Philip Morris.* New York: Vintage Books, 1997.

> A definitive history of America's controversial tobacco industry, focusing on Philip Morris. Traces the development of the cigarette, revelations of its toxicity, and the impact of political and corporate shenanigans on the battle over smoking.

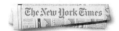

e-themes from *The New York Times*

For up-to-date articles about current health issues, visit www.aw-bc.com/donatelle, select *Access to Health,* Tenth Edition, Chapter 13, and click on "e-themes."

References

1. Centers for Disease Control and Prevention, "Tobacco Information and Prevention Source: Fast Facts," March 2006, www.cdc.gov.
2. Ibid.
3. Office on Smoking and Health, *The Health Consequences of Smoking: What It Means to You* (Washington, DC: U.S. Department of Health and Human Services, 2004).
4. Centers for Disease Control and Prevention, "Annual Smoking-Attributable Mortality, Years of Potential Life Lost, and Productivity Losses—United States, 1997–2001," *Morbidity and Mortality Weekly Report* 54, no. 25 (2005): 625–628.
5. American College Health Association, "National College Health Assessment: Spring 2005 Reference Group Data," *Journal of American College Health* 55, no. 1 (2006): 5–16.
6. S. Moran et al., "Social Smoking Among U.S. College Students," *Pediatrics* 114 (2004): 1028–1034.
7. M. E. Kear, "Psychosocial Determinants of Cigarette Smoking Among College Students," *Journal of Community Health Nursing* 19, no. 4 (2002): 245.
8. S. A. Everett et al., "Smoking Initiation and Smoking Patterns Among U.S. College Students," *Journal of American College Health* 48 (1999): 55.
9. American Cancer Society, "The Facts About Secondhand Smoke," 2004, www.cancer.org.
10. American Cancer Society, "Cigar Smoking," August 2006, www.cancer.org.
11. S. Hansen, "Bidis," University of Iowa's Student Health Service/Health Iowa, 2006, www.uiowa.edu/~shs.
12. American Cancer Society, *Cancer Facts & Figures, 2006* (Atlanta: American Cancer Society, 2006).
13. National Institute on Drug Abuse Research Report Series, "Nicotine Addiction" (USDHHS Publication No. 01-4342) (Bethesda, MD, National Institute on Drug Abuse, 2001).
14. W. Hall, "Will Nicotine Genetics and a Nicotine Vaccine Prevent Cigarette Smoking and Smoking-Related Diseases?" *PLoS Med* 2, No. 9 (2005).
15. American Cancer Society, *Cancer Facts & Figures, 2006.*
16. Ibid.
17. Ibid.
18. American Heart Association, "Heart Disease and Stroke Statistics, 2006 Update," 2006, www.americanheart.org.
19. Ibid.
20. American Lung Association, "Quit Smoking: Benefits," 2005, www.lungusa.org.
21. American Heart Association, "Risk Factors for a Stroke," 2005, www.americanheart.org.
22. Office on Smoking and Health, *The Health Consequences of Smoking.*
23. American Cancer Society, *Cancer Facts & Figures, 2006.*
24. American Academy of Periodontology, "Tobacco Use and Periodontal Disease," 2004, www.perio.org.
25. Office on Smoking and Health, *The Health Consequences of Involuntary Exposure to Tobacco Smoke: A Report of the Surgeon General—Executive Summary* (Washington, DC: U.S. Department of Health and Human Services, 2006).
26. American Lung Association, "U.S. Surgeon General Releases Report on Health Consequences of Secondhand Smoke," 2006, www.lungusa.org.
27. National Center for Chronic Disease Prevention and Health Promotion, *"The Health Consequences of Involuntary Exposure to Tobacco Smoke: A Report of the Surgeon General—Executive Summary"* (Washington, D.C.: U.S. Department of Health and Human Services 2006.)
28. American Lung Association, "LungUSA," 2006, www.lungusa.org.
29. Office on Smoking and Health, *The Health Consequences of Involuntary Exposure to Tobacco Smoke.*
30. K. Yolton et al., "Exposure to Environmental Tobacco Smoke and Cognitive Abilities among U.S. Children and Adolescents," *Environmental Health Perspectives* 113, no. 1 (2005): 9–103.
31. M. R. Becklake et al., "Childhood Predictors of Smoking in Adolescence: A Follow-Up Study of Montreal School Children," *Canadian Medical Association Journal* 173, no. 4 (2005): 377–379.
32. Office on Smoking and Health, *The Health Consequences of Involuntary Exposure to Tobacco Smoke.*
33. Ibid.
34. Centers for Disease Control and Prevention, "Annual Smoking-Attributable Mortality."
35. American Lung Association Action Network, "Public Supports Tobacco Control Strategies Outlined by the American Lung Association," February 2, 2003, www.lungaction.org.
36. M. Fogarty, "Public Health and Smoking Cessation," *The Scientist* 17, no. 6 (2003): 23; Tobacco Control Research Center, Tobacco Litigation Documents, "Multistate Settlement with Tobacco Industry,"

2004, www.library.ucsf.edu/tobacco/litigation; L. Robbins, "Balancing Smokers, Nonsmokers, and Health Concerns: Delaware and California Have Banned All Public Smoking," *State Legislatures* 29, no. 1 (2003): 27.

37. U.S. Department of Health and Human Services, "Effective Strategies for Tobacco Cessation Underused," *National Institutes of Health News,* June 2006.

38. E. Brender, "Smoking Cessation," *The Journal of the American Medical Association* 296, no. 1 (2006): 130.

39. M. Marchione, "Doctors Test Stop-Smoking Vaccine," *Corvallis Gazette Times,* Friday, July 28, 2006.

40. American Cancer Society, *Cancer Facts & Figures, 2006.*

41. Your Nutrition and Food Safety Resource, "Questions and Answers about Caffeine and Health," January 2003, http://ific.org.

42. Ibid.

14

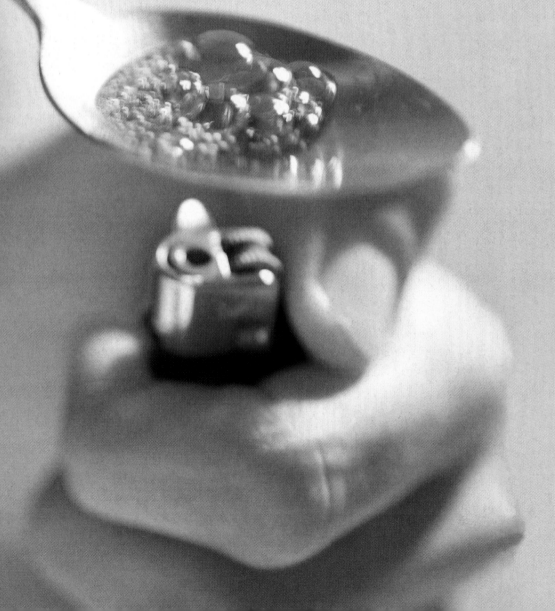

Illicit Drugs

USE, MISUSE, AND ABUSE

How do **drugs** work in the body to make us feel high?

How are drugs **classified?**

Are there any **negative** long-term effects from marijuana use?

Is it **legal** for employers to require employees to take a drug test?

Why is **prescription drug** abuse growing in popularity?

OBJECTIVES

- Discuss the six categories of drugs and their routes of administration.
- Discuss patterns of illicit drug use, including who uses illicit drugs and why.
- Discuss the use and abuse of controlled substances, including cocaine, amphetamines, marijuana, opiates, hallucinogens, designer drugs, inhalants, and steroids.
- Profile illegal drug use in the United States, including frequency, financial impact, arrests for drug offenses, and impact on college campuses and the workplace.

rug misuse and abuse are problems of staggering proportions in our society. Each year drug and alcohol abuse contributes to the deaths of over 120,000 Americans. They cost taxpayers more than $294 billion in preventable health care costs, extra law enforcement, auto crashes, crime, and lost productivity.[1] It's impossible to put a dollar amount on the pain, suffering, and dysfunction that drugs cause in our everyday lives. Although overall use of drugs in the United States has fallen by 50 percent in the last 20 years, the past 10 years have shown an increase in the use of certain drugs by adolescents.[2]

It is important to understand how these drugs work and why people use them. Human beings appear to have a need to alter their consciousness, or mental state. We like to feel good, to escape, and feel different. Consciousness can be altered in many ways: children spinning until they become dizzy and adults enjoying the rush of thrilling high-intensity activities are examples. To change our awareness, many of us listen to music, skydive, ski, read, daydream, meditate, pray, or have sexual relations. Others turn to drugs to alter consciousness.

Drug Dynamics

How do drugs work in the body to make us feel high?

Drugs work because they physically resemble the chemicals produced naturally within the body (Figure 14.1). For example, many painkillers resemble the endorphins (meaning "morphine within") that are manufactured in the body. Most bodily processes result from chemical reactions or from changes in electrical charge. Because drugs possess an electrical charge and a chemical structure similar to those of chemicals that occur naturally in the body, they can affect physical functions in many different ways.

A current explanation of drug actions is the *receptor site theory,* which suggests that drugs bind to specific **receptor sites** in the body. These sites are specialized cells to which, because of their size, shape, electrical charge, and chemical properties, drugs can attach themselves. Most drugs bind to multiple receptor sites located throughout the body in places such as the heart and blood system and the lungs, liver, kidneys, brain, and gonads (testicles or ovaries).

Types of Drugs

Scientists divide drugs into six categories: prescription, over-the-counter (OTC), recreational, herbal, illicit, and commercial drugs. These classifications are based primarily on drug action, although some are based on the source of the chemical in question. Each category includes some drugs that stimulate the body, some that depress body functions, and others that produce hallucinations, images (auditory or visual) that are perceived but are not real. Each category also includes **psychoactive drugs,** which have the potential to alter a person's mood or behavior.

- **Prescription drugs** can be obtained only with the written prescription of a licensed physician. Over 10,000 types of prescription drugs are sold in the United States, at an annual cost of over $200 billion to consumers.[3]
- **Over-the-counter (OTC) drugs** can be purchased without a prescription. Each year, Americans spend more than $20 billion on OTC products, and the market is increasing at the rate of 20 percent annually. More than 300,000 OTC products are available through stores, pharmacies, and the Internet. An estimated three out of four people routinely self-medicate with them.
- **Recreational drugs** belong to a somewhat vague category whose boundaries depend upon how you define recreation. Generally, these substances contain chemicals used to help people relax or socialize. Most of them are legally sanctioned even though they are psychoactive. Alcohol, tobacco, coffee, tea, and chocolate products are usually included in this category.
- **Herbal preparations** form another vague category. Included among these approximately 750 substances are herbal teas and other products of botanical origin that are believed to have medicinal properties. (See Chapter 23 for more on herbal preparations.)
- **Illicit (illegal) drugs** are the most notorious type of drug. Although laws governing their use, possession, cultivation, manufacture, and sale differ from state to state, illicit drugs are generally recognized as harmful. All of them are psychoactive.
- **Commercial preparations** are the most universally used yet least commonly recognized chemical substances. More

receptor sites Specialized cells to which drugs can attach themselves.

psychoactive drugs Drugs that have the potential to alter mood or behavior.

prescription drugs Medications that can be obtained only with the written prescription of a licensed physician.

over-the-counter (OTC) drugs Medications that can be purchased without a physician's prescription.

recreational drugs Drugs that contain chemicals that help people relax or socialize; most, but not all, drugs in this category are legal.

herbal preparations Substances of plant origin that are believed to have medicinal properties.

illicit (illegal) drugs Drugs whose use, possession, cultivation, manufacture, and/or sale are against the law because they are generally recognized as harmful.

commercial preparations Commonly used chemical substances including cosmetics, household cleaning products, and industrial by-products.

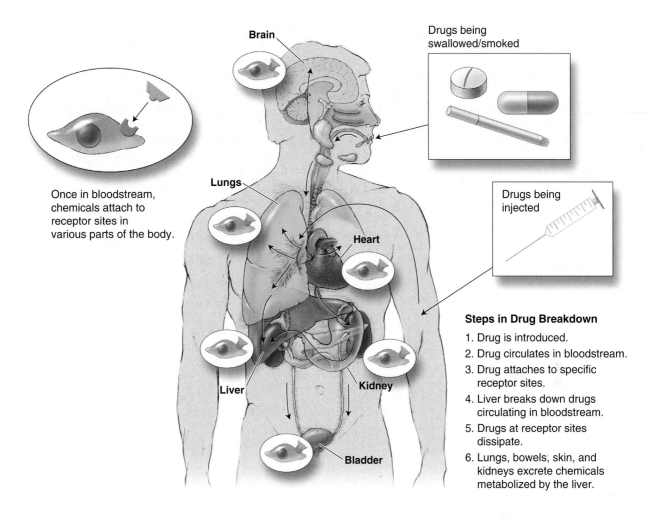

Brain

Drugs being swallowed/smoked

Once in bloodstream, chemicals attach to receptor sites in various parts of the body.

Lungs

Drugs being injected

Heart

Steps in Drug Breakdown

1. Drug is introduced.
2. Drug circulates in bloodstream.
3. Drug attaches to specific receptor sites.
4. Liver breaks down drugs circulating in bloodstream.
5. Drugs at receptor sites dissipate.
6. Lungs, bowels, skin, and kidneys excrete chemicals metabolized by the liver.

Liver

Kidney

Bladder

FIGURE 14.1 How the Body Metabolizes Drugs

than 1,000 of these substances exist, including seemingly benign items such as perfumes, cosmetics, household cleansers, paints, glues, inks, dyes, gardening chemicals, pesticides, and industrial by-products.

Routes of Administration of Drugs

Route of administration refers to the way in which a given drug is taken into the body. The most common methods include by mouth (**oral ingestion**); **inhalation,** which is the administration of drugs through the nostrils via sniffing or smoking; or **injection** into the muscles, bloodstream, or just under the skin. **Intravenous injection,** which involves the insertion of a hypodermic syringe directly into a vein, is the most common method of injection for drug misusers, due to the rapidity with which a drug's effect is felt. It is also the most dangerous method of administration due to the risk of contracting HIV and damage to blood vessels. Drugs can also be absorbed through the skin (**inunction**)—the nicotine patch is a common example of a drug that is administered in this

manner—or through the vagina or anus (**suppositories**). Suppositories are typically mixed with a waxy medium that melts at body temperature so the drug can be released into the bloodstream. However the drug enters the system, most drugs remain active in the body for several hours.

route of administration   The manner in which a drug is taken into the body.

oral ingestion   Intake of drugs through the mouth.

inhalation   The introduction of drugs through the nostrils.

injection   The introduction of drugs into the body via a hypodermic needle.

intravenous injection   The introduction of drugs directly into a vein.

inunction   The introduction of drugs through the skin.

suppositories   Mixtures of drugs and a waxy medium designed to melt at body temperature that are inserted into the anus or vagina.

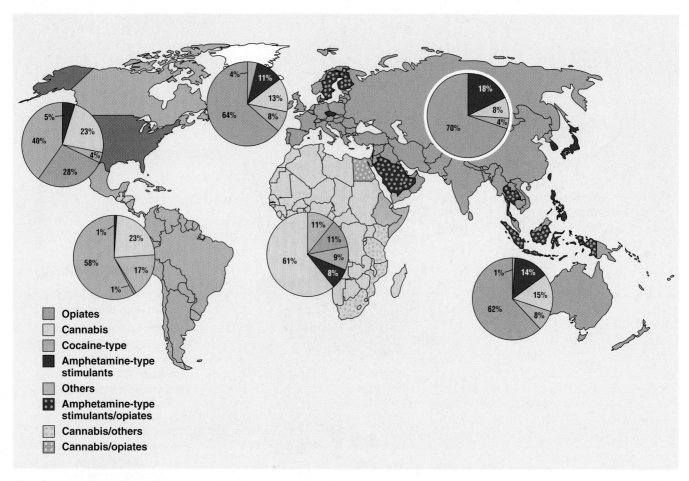

FIGURE 14.2 Global Use of Illicit Drugs, 2003

The main problem drugs in the world, as reflected in demand for treatment, remain the opiates, followed by cocaine. Reports of demand are based on an average from most, but not all, countries in a region over a period of years.

Source: United Nations Office on Drugs and Crime, "Executive Summary: Global Illicit Drug Trends: 2003," 2004, www.unodc.org/unodc/en/global_illicit _drug_trends.html.

Using, Misusing, and Abusing Drugs

Although drug abuse is usually referred to in connection with illicit psychoactive drugs, many people abuse and misuse prescription and OTC medications. **Drug misuse** involves the use of a drug for a purpose for which it was not intended. For example, taking a friend's high-powered prescription painkiller for your headache is a misuse of that drug. This is not too far removed from **drug abuse,** or the excessive use of any drug.

> **drug misuse** Use of a drug for a purpose for which it was not intended.
>
> **drug abuse** Excessive use of a drug.
>
> **illicit drugs** Drugs that are illegal to possess, produce, or sell.

The misuse and abuse of any drug may lead to addiction, the habitual reliance on a substance or behavior to produce a desired mood. Both risks and benefits are involved in the use of any type of chemical substance. Intelligent decision making requires a clear-headed evaluation of these risks and benefits. If, after considering all the facts, you feel that the benefits outweigh the potential problems associated with a particular drug, you may decide to use it—but sometimes unforeseeable reactions or problems arise even after the most careful deliberation.

Illicit Drugs

Some people become addicted to prescription drugs and painkillers; others use **illicit drugs**—those drugs that are illegal to possess, produce, or sell. The problem of illicit drug use touches us all. We may use illicit substances ourselves, watch someone we love struggle with drug abuse, or become the victim of a drug-related crime. At the very least, we are forced to pay increasing taxes for law enforcement and drug rehabilitation. When our coworkers use drugs, the effectiveness of our own work is diminished. If the car we drive was assembled by drug-using workers at the plant, we are in danger. A drug-using bus driver, train engineer, medical professional, or pilot jeopardizes our safety.

The good news is that the use of illicit drugs has declined significantly in recent years in most segments of society. Use of most drugs increased from the early 1970s to the late 1970s, peaked between 1979 and 1986, and declined until 1992, from which point it has not changed. In 2003, an estimated 19.2 million Americans were illicit drug users, about three-quarters the 1979 peak level of 25 million users. Among youth, however, illicit drug use, notably of marijuana, has been rising in recent years.[4]

Who Uses Illicit Drugs?

Many of us have stereotypes in our minds of who uses illicit drugs, but it is difficult to generalize. Illicit drug users span all age groups, ethnicities, occupations, and socioeconomic groups. What can be said is that illicit drug use has a devastating effect on users and their families in the United States and in many other countries (Figure 14.2).

After more than a decade of declining use on American college campuses, illicit drugs have reappeared. In 2004, the number of college students nationwide who had tried any drug stood at almost 52 percent; over a third had smoked pot in the past year, and 20 percent had done so in the past month. Daily use of marijuana was at its highest point since 1989.[5] Cocaine use is down sharply, but LSD use has more than doubled. These figures vary from school to school.

Patterns of drug use vary only slightly by age. For example, a nationwide study of college campuses reported that approximately 33.3 percent of students had tried marijuana during the previous year (Table 14.1), and that number is nearly the same when considering all Americans under the age of 45 who used marijuana during that time, at 33.7 percent. Approximately 6.6 percent of college students surveyed reported using cocaine in the past year, whereas 8.5 percent of all Americans under age 45 said they had used cocaine during the previous year.[6]

Most antidrug programs have not been effective because they have focused on only one aspect of drug abuse, rather than examining all factors that contribute to the problem. The pressures to take drugs are often tremendous, and the reasons for using them are complex. People who develop drug problems generally begin with the belief that they can control their drug use. Initially, they often view taking drugs as a fun and manageable pastime. Peer influence is a strong motivator, especially among adolescents, who greatly fear not being accepted as part of the group. Other people use drugs to cope with feelings of worthlessness and despair or to battle depression and anxiety. But most illegal drugs produce physical and psychological dependency, so it is unrealistic to think that a person can use them regularly without becoming addicted. Consider whether you are controlled by drugs or a drug user by answering the questions in the Assess Yourself box.

TABLE 14.1	Annual Prevalence of Use for Various Types of Drugs, 2004: Full-Time College Students vs. Respondents 1–4 Years beyond High School

	Full-Time College (%)	Others (%)
Any illicit drug	36.2	38.8
Any illicit drug other than marijuana	18.6	23.7
Marijuana	33.3	33.7
Inhalants	2.7	2.4
Hallucinogens	5.9	7.3
LSD	1.2	1.7
Cocaine	6.6	8.5
Crack	1.3	2.3
MDMA (Ecstasy)	2.2	4.7
Heroin	0.4	0.5
Other narcotics	8.2	12.3
OxyContin	2.5	4.3
Vicodin	7.4	12.9
Amphetamines, adjusted	7.0	8.5
Ritalin	4.7	1.6
Methamphetamine	2.9	5.1
Ice	1.1	3.3
Sedatives (barbiturates)	4.2	6.7
Tranquilizers	6.7	9.9
Rohypnol	0.3	0
GHB	0.7	0.2
Ketamine	1.5	0.5
Alcohol	81.2	80.1
Cigarettes	36.7	47.6
Approximate weighted N =	*1,400*	*900*

Source: L. D. Johnson et al., *Monitoring the Future National Survey Results on Drug Use, 1975–2004: Volume II, College Students and Adults* (Bethesda, MD: National Institute on Drug Abuse, 2006).

what do you THINK?

What factors do you believe influence trends of illicit drug use in the United States? ▪ What is the attitude toward drug use on your college campus? ▪ Are some drugs considered more acceptable than others? ▪ Is drug use considered more acceptable at certain times or occasions? Explain your answer.

(Text continues on page 430)

ASSESS yourself

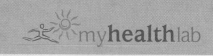

RECOGNIZING A DRUG PROBLEM

Fill out this assessment online at
www.aw-bc.com/myhealthlab or
www.aw-bc.com/donatelle.

ARE YOU CONTROLLED BY DRUGS?

How do you know whether you are chemically dependent? A dependent person can't stop using drugs. This abuse hurts the user and everyone around him or her. Take the following assessment. The more "yes" checks you make, the more likely you have a problem.

	Yes	No
1. Do you use drugs to handle stress or escape from life's problems?	❑	❑
2. Have you unsuccessfully tried to cut down on or quit using your drug?	❑	❑
3. Have you ever been in trouble with the law or been arrested because of your drug use?	❑	❑
4. Do you think a party or social gathering isn't fun unless drugs are available?	❑	❑
5. Do you avoid people or places that do not support your usage?	❑	❑
6. Do you neglect your responsibilities because you'd rather use your drug?	❑	❑
7. Have your friends, family, or employer expressed concern about your drug use?	❑	❑
8. Do you do things under the influence of drugs that you would not normally do?	❑	❑
9. Have you seriously thought that you might have a chemical dependency problem?	❑	❑

ARE YOU CONTROLLED BY A DRUG USER?

Is your life controlled by a chemical abuser? Your love and care (codependence) may actually be enabling the person to continue the abuse, hurting you and others. Try this assessment; the more "yes" checks you make, the more likely there's a problem.

	Yes	No
1. Do you often have to lie or cover up for the chemical abuser?	❑	❑
2. Do you spend time counseling the person about the problem?	❑	❑
3. Have you taken on additional financial or family responsibilities?	❑	❑
4. Do you feel that you have to control the chemical abuser's behavior?	❑	❑
5. At the office, have you done work or attended meetings for the abuser?	❑	❑
6. Do you often put your own needs and desires after the user's?	❑	❑
7. Do you spend time each day worrying about your situation?	❑	❑
8. Do you analyze your behavior to find clues to how it might affect the chemical abuser?	❑	❑
9. Do you feel powerless and at your wit's end about the abuser's problem?	❑	❑

Source: Reprinted by permission of Krames Communications, 1100 Grundy Lane, San Bruno, CA 94066–3030. www.krames.com.

MAKE it happen!

ASSESSMENT: The Assess Yourself activity describes signs of being controlled by drugs or by a drug user. Depending on your results, you may need to change certain behaviors that may be detrimental to your health.

MAKING A CHANGE: In order to change your behavior, you need to develop a plan. Follow the steps below and complete your Behavior Change Contract to take action.

1. Evaluate your behavior and identify patterns and specific things you are doing. What can you change now? What can you change in the near future?

2. Select one pattern of behavior that you want to change.

3. Fill out the Behavior Change Contract found at the front of your book. It should include your long-term goal for change, your short-term goals, the rewards you'll give yourself for reaching these goals, potential obstacles along the way, and strategies for overcoming these obstacles. For each goal, list the small steps and specific actions that you will take.

4. Chart your progress in a journal. At the end of a week, consider how successful you were in following your plan. What helped you be successful? What made change more difficult? What will you do differently next week?

5. Revise your plan as needed: Are the short-term goals attainable? Are the rewards satisfying?

ONE STUDENT'S PLAN: Tranh was surprised to find he had several yes answers to the self-assessment section about being controlled by a drug user. He realized that his girlfriend Kim's drug use was hurting their relationship and negatively affecting his well-being. Kim smoked marijuana almost every day and took club drugs at least twice a month. Tranh often had to lie to Kim's employer if she was too incapacitated to go to work. Recently, she had been in a car accident after smoking pot for several hours, which damaged Tranh's car and increased his insurance rate. And he worried whenever she went out for an evening that she was taking Ecstasy and would find herself in a compromising situation.

These worries, financial consequences, and pressure to lie all made Tranh resolve to take steps to make a change in his responses to Kim's behavior. His first step was to plan what he wanted to say to Kim about her drug use and how it affected both of them. He also started investigating drug counseling resources at school and in the community, both for Kim and for himself to help him cope with the issues raised by Kim's drug use. Finally, he began talking to Kim's friends who, it turned out, also were concerned about her behavior. They worked together to develop strategies to help Kim and provide alternatives to her drug use; Tranh also felt less alone and more supported as soon as he started reaching out to his peers.

TABLE 14.2　How Drugs Are Scheduled

Schedule	Characteristics	Examples	
Schedule I	High potential for abuse and addiction; no accepted medical use	Heroin LSD Marijuana	
Schedule II	High potential for abuse and addiction; restricted medical use	Cocaine Amphetamine (DMA, STP) Methadone OxyContin Ritalin	
Schedule III	Some potential for abuse and addiction; currently accepted medical use	Anabolic steroids Nalorphine Vicodin	
Schedule IV	Low potential for abuse and addiction; currently accepted medical use	Xanax Minor tranquilizers	
Schedule V	Lowest potential for abuse; accepted medical use	Robitussin AC OTC preparations	

Source: National Institute on Drug Abuse, "Commonly Abused Drugs," 2006, www.drugabuse.gov/DrugPages/DrugsofAbuse.html.

Controlled Substances

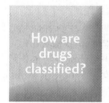

How are drugs classified?

To counteract the increased use of illegal drugs and the overuse of certain prescription drugs, Congress passed the Controlled Substances Act of 1970. This law created categories for both prescription and illegal substances that the federal government felt required strict regulation. The Drug Enforcement Administration (DEA) was founded within the Department of Justice to administer the law.

The law classified drugs into five schedules, or categories, based on their potential for abuse, their medical uses, and accepted standards of safe use (Table 14.2). Schedule I drugs, those with the highest potential for abuse, are considered to have no valid medical uses. Although Schedule II, III, IV, and V drugs have known and accepted medical applications, many of them present serious threats to health when abused or misused. Penalties for illegal use are tied to the drugs' schedule level. Despite the 1970 law, however, manufacturing of and trafficking in illegal drugs in the United States have not diminished.

Hundreds of illegal drugs exist. For general purposes, they can be divided into seven categories: *stimulants,* such as cocaine; marijuana and its derivatives; *depressants,* such as the opiates; *hallucinogens/psychedelics; designer drugs; inhalants;* and *steroids.*

cocaine A powerful stimulant drug made from the leaves of the South American coca shrub.

Stimulants

Cocaine

A white crystalline powder derived from the leaves of the South American coca shrub (not related to cocoa plants), **cocaine** ("coke") has been described as one of the most powerful naturally occurring stimulants.

Methods of Cocaine Use Cocaine can be taken in several ways. The powdered form of the drug is "snorted" through the nose. When cocaine is snorted, it can damage mucous membranes in the nose and cause sinusitis. It can destroy the user's sense of smell, and occasionally it even eats a hole through the septum.

Smoking (known as freebasing) and intravenous injections are even more dangerous means of taking cocaine. Freebasing has become more popular than injecting in recent years because people fear contracting diseases such as AIDS and hepatitis by sharing contaminated needles. But freebasing involves other dangers. Because the volatile mixes it requires are very explosive, some people have been killed or seriously burned. Smoking cocaine can also cause lung and liver damage.

Many cocaine users still occasionally "shoot up," which introduces large amounts into the body rapidly. Within seconds, a sense of euphoria sets in. This intense high lasts for 15 to 20 minutes, and then the user heads into a "crash." To prevent the unpleasant effects of the crash, users must shoot up frequently, which can severely damage veins. Injecting users place themselves at risk not only for AIDS and hepatitis, but also for skin infections, inflamed arteries, and infection of the lining of the heart.

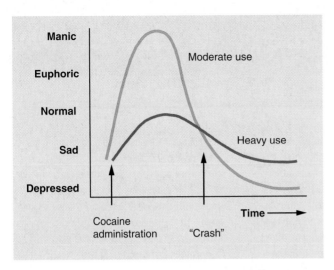

FIGURE 14.3 Ups and Downs of a Typical Dose of Cocaine

Source: C. Levinthal, *Drugs, Behavior, and Modern Society,* 4th ed. (Boston: Allyn & Bacon, 2005). © Pearson Education. Reprinted by permission of the publisher.

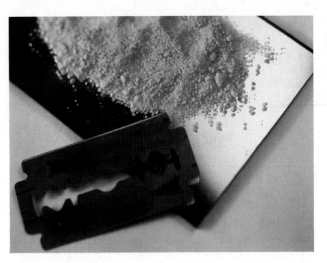

Although cocaine abuse has declined from its peak in the 1980s, it continues to be a commonly abused illicit drug.

Physical Effects of Cocaine The effects of cocaine are felt rapidly. Snorted cocaine enters the bloodstream through the lungs in less than one minute and reaches the brain in less than three minutes. When cocaine binds at its receptor sites in the central nervous system, it produces intense pleasure. The euphoria quickly abates, however, and the desire to regain the pleasurable feelings makes the user want more cocaine (Figure 14.3).

Cocaine is both an anesthetic and a central nervous system stimulant. In tiny doses, it can slow heart rate. In larger doses, the physical effects are dramatic: increased heart rate and blood pressure, loss of appetite that can lead to dramatic weight loss, convulsions, muscle twitching, irregular heartbeat, and even eventual death due to overdose. Other effects of cocaine include temporary relief of depression, decreased fatigue, talkativeness, increased alertness, and heightened self-confidence. However, as the dose increases, users become irritable and apprehensive, and their behavior may turn paranoid or violent.

Types of Cocaine Freebase is a form of cocaine that is more powerful and costly than powder or crack. Street cocaine (cocaine hydrochloride) is converted to pure base by using ether to remove the hydrochloride salt and many of the "cutting agents" used to dilute the drug. (The use of ether, which is flammable, adds to the danger.) The end product, freebase, is smoked through a water pipe.

Because freebase cocaine reaches the brain within seconds, it is more dangerous than snorted cocaine. It produces a quick, intense high that disappears quickly, leaving an intense craving for more. Freebasers typically increase the amount and frequency of the dose. They often become severely addicted and experience serious health problems.

Side effects of freebasing cocaine include weight loss, increased heart rate and blood pressure, depression, paranoia, and hallucinations. Freebase is an extremely dangerous drug

and is responsible for a large number of cocaine-related hospital emergency room visits and deaths.

The street name **crack** is given to freebase cocaine processed from cocaine hydrochloride by using ammonia or sodium bicarbonate (baking soda), water, and heat to remove the hydrochloride. The mixture (90 percent pure cocaine) is then dried. The soapy-looking substance that results can be broken into "rocks" and smoked. These rocks are approximately five times as strong as cocaine. Crack gets its name from the popping noises it makes when burned. In 2004, 2 percent of college students reported using crack during their lives.[7]

Crack is also sometimes called "rock," which is not the same as rock cocaine. Rock cocaine is a cocaine hydrochloride substance that is primarily sold in California. White in color, it is about the shape of a pencil eraser and is typically snorted.

Because crack is such a pure drug, it takes much less time to achieve the desired high. One puff of a pebble-size rock produces an intense high that lasts for approximately 20 minutes. The user can usually get three or four hits off a rock before it is used up. Crack is typically sold in small vials, folding papers, or heavy tinfoil containing two or three rocks, and costing between $10 and $20.

A crack user can become addicted quickly. Addiction is accelerated by the speed at which crack is absorbed through the lungs (it hits the brain within seconds) and by the intensity of the high. It is not uncommon for crack addicts to spend over $1,000 a day on the habit.

Cocaine-Affected Babies Because cocaine rapidly crosses the placenta (as virtually all drugs do), the fetus is vulnerable when a pregnant woman uses cocaine. It is

freebase The most powerful distillate of cocaine.

crack A distillate of powdered cocaine that comes in small, hard "chips" or "rocks"; not the same as rock cocaine.

WOMEN AND DRUG ABUSE

According to the 2004 National Survey on Drug Use and Health, approximately 51 million women report using an illicit drug at some point in their lives, representing 41.1 percent of all females aged 12 and older. Approximately 12.2 percent of females aged 12 and older reported past-year use of an illicit drug and 6.1 percent reported past-month use of an illicit drug.

Many women who use drugs have had troubled lives. Studies show that at least 70 percent of them have been sexually abused by the age of 16. Most of them had at least one parent who abused alcohol or drugs. Furthermore, they often have little self-esteem or self-confidence. They frequently feel lonely, powerless, and isolated from support networks.

Unfortunately, many female drug users are unable to seek help. Some may be unable to find or afford child care during treatment, while others worry that the courts will take away their children once the drug problem is known. Others may fear violence from their husbands, boyfriends, or partners.

Research has shown that female drug abusers have a better chance of recovery when treatment takes care of their basic needs. Some women need the basic services of food, shelter, and clothing. Others also need transportation, child care, and training in parenting. The most successful treatments also teach reading, basic education, and the skills needed to find a job. As a woman's self-esteem increases, so do her chances of remaining drug free.

Source: Office of National Drug Control Policy, *Drug Facts: Women and Drugs,* 2006, www.whitehousedrugpolicy.gov/drugfact/women/index.html.

---

estimated that 2.4 to 3.5 percent of pregnant women between the ages of 12 and 34 abuse cocaine. It is difficult to gauge how many newborns have been exposed to cocaine because pregnant users are reluctant to discuss their drug habit with health care providers for fear of prosecution. The most threatening problem during pregnancy is the increased risk of a miscarriage. (See the Women's Health/Men's Health box.)

Fetuses exposed to cocaine in the womb are more likely to suffer a small head, premature delivery, reduced birth weight, increased irritability, and subtle learning and cognitive deficits. Research suggests that a significant number of these children develop problems with learning and language skills that require remedial attention.[8] It is critical to identify these children early so they can receive immediate intervention. For both financial and humane reasons, prenatal care and education programs for mothers at risk should be considered a priority for state and local government.[9]

Cocaine Addiction and Society Cocaine addicts often suffer both physiological damage and serious disruption in lifestyle, including loss of employment and self-esteem. It is estimated that the annual cost of cocaine addiction in the United States exceeds $3.8 billion. However, there is no way to measure the cost in wasted lives. In 2004, 34.2 million Americans aged 12 and over reported lifetime use of cocaine, and 7.8 million reported using crack. About 5.6 million reported annual use of cocaine, and 1.3 million reported using crack. An estimated 2 million Americans reported current use of cocaine, 467,000 of whom reported using crack. There were an estimated 1 million new users of cocaine in 2004 (approximately 2,700 per day), and most were aged 18 or older although the average age of first use was 20.0 years.[10]

Cocaine has been called unpredictable by drug experts, deadly by coroners, dangerous by former users, and disastrous by the media. Yet, to date there has not been a successful weapon to combat its use in the United States. Apparently, the risks do not override users' desire to experience its effects.

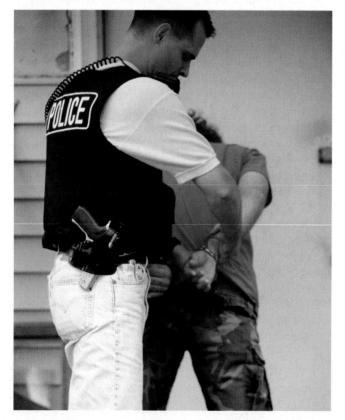

A high percentage of violent and nonviolent crime is linked to drug abuse, affecting not only the abuser, but entire communities.

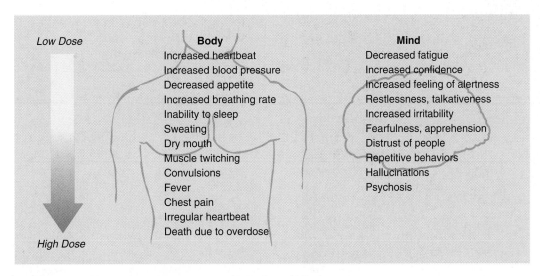

FIGURE 14.4 **Effects of Amphetamines on the Body and Mind**

Because cocaine is illegal, a complex underground network has developed to manufacture and sell the drug. Buyers may not always get the product they think they are purchasing. Cocaine marketed for snorting may be only 60 percent pure. Usually, it is mixed, or "cut," with other white powdery substances such as mannitol or sugar, though occasionally it is cut with arsenic or other cocainelike powders that may themselves be highly dangerous.

 what do you THINK?

Have all segments of society been affected by crack use? If not, which segments of the U.S. population experience the greatest impact from crack use? ▪ **Why might this be the case?** ▪ **Is there a difference in the profile of a person who uses crack rather than cocaine? Explain your answer.**

Amphetamines The **amphetamines** include a large and varied group of synthetic agents that stimulate the central nervous system. Small doses of amphetamines improve alertness, lessen fatigue, and generally elevate mood. With repeated use, however, physical and psychological dependency develops. Sleep patterns are affected (insomnia); heart rate, breathing rate, and blood pressure increase; restlessness, anxiety, appetite suppression, and vision problems are common. High doses over long time periods can produce hallucinations, delusions, and disorganized behavior.

Certain types of amphetamines are used for medicinal purposes. Drugs such as Ritalin and Adderall are used to treat children with attention deficit/hyperactive disorder. However, in recent years these drugs have taken the place of caffeine on college campuses, and many students misuse them to stay awake for all-night cramming sessions (see the Health Ethics box on page 435). In fact, Ritalin is on the Drug Enforcement Administration's Top Ten list of most often stolen prescription drugs. There is a false perception that these drugs improve academic performance. According to a 2004 national survey, over 4 percent of college students had used Ritalin in the past year.

Methamphetamine An increasingly common form of amphetamine, **methamphetamine** is a potent, long-acting, addictive drug that strongly activates the brain's reward center by producing a sense of euphoria. Methamphetamine can cause brain damage that results in impaired motor skills and cognitive functions, as well as psychosis and increased risk for heart attack and stroke.

Methods of Methamphetamine Use Methamphetamine can be snorted, smoked, injected, or orally ingested. Depending on the method of use, the drug will affect the user in different ways. Users often experience tolerance immediately, making methamphetamine a highly addictive drug from the very first time it is used. When snorted, the effects can be felt in 3 to 5 minutes; if orally ingested, the user will experience effects within 15 to 20 minutes. The pleasurable effects of methamphetamine are typically an intense rush lasting only a few minutes when snorted; in contrast, smoking the drug can produce a high lasting over 8 hours.

Physical Effects of Methamphetamine As shown in Figure 14.4, in smaller doses methamphetamine increases physical activity and alertness, and decreases appetite. However, the drug's effects quickly wear off, and the user seeks more. Long-term use of methamphetamine can

amphetamines A large and varied group of synthetic agents that stimulate the central nervous system.

methamphetamine A powerfully addictive drug that strongly activates certain areas of the brain and affects the central nervous system.

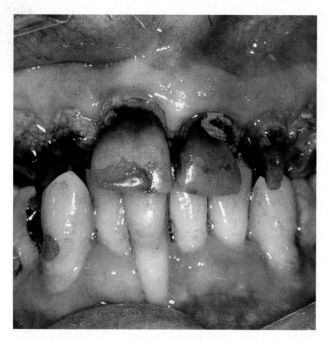

Methamphetamine users often damage their teeth beyond repair due to the toxic chemicals in the substance. This condition is referred to as "meth mouth."

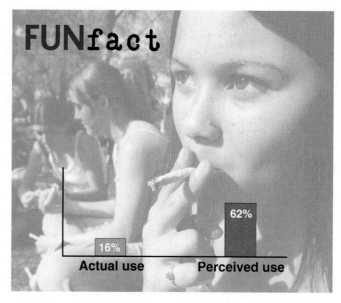

16% Actual use   62% Perceived use

FIGURE 14.5 College Students' Actual Use of Marijuana versus Perceived Use

Students have a false sense of actual marijuana use by their peers.

Source: American College Health Association, National College Health Assessment, Fall 2005, www.acha.org.

cause severe dependence, psychosis, paranoia, aggression, weight loss, and stroke. Abusers often do not sleep or eat for days, as they continually inject up to 1 gram of the drug every 2 to 3 hours. A high state of irritability and agitation has been associated with violent behavior among some users.

Abuse of methamphetamine is an increasingly serious problem, especially in more rural areas of the United States, Hawaii, and the West Coast. In 2005, 4.5 percent of high school seniors reported using methamphetamine in their lifetime. Rates among adults are difficult to determine, but it is believed that over 12 million Americans have tried meth.[11] A possible contributing factor to the increasing rate of methamphetamine use is that it is relatively easy to make. Methamphetamine is produced by "cookers" using recipes that often include common over-the-counter ingredients such as ephedrine and pseudoephedrine, found in cold and allergy medication. Many states, such as Oregon, have taken action by requiring retailers to move all cold and allergy medication behind the pharmacist's counter, so high-volume buyers can be carefully monitored. Additionally, laws have strengthened the penalties associated with manufacturing methamphetamine.

Ice is a potent form of methamphetamine that is imported primarily from Asia, particularly from South Korea and

Taiwan. It is purer and more crystalline than the version manufactured in many large U.S. cities, and is odorless when smoked. Ice is usually smoked, like crack cocaine, and its effects can last for more than 12 hours.

Like other methamphetamines, the "down" side of this drug is devastating. Prolonged use can cause fatal lung and kidney damage as well as long-lasting psychological damage. In some instances, major psychological dysfunction can persist as long as two-and-a-half years after last use.

Marijuana

Although archaeological evidence documents the use of **marijuana** ("grass," "weed," "pot") as far back as 6,000 years, the drug did not become popular in the United States until the 1960s. Marijuana receives less media attention today than it did then, but it still is the illicit drug used most frequently by far. Nearly one of every three Americans over the age of 12 has tried marijuana at least once. Some 12 million Americans have used it; more than 1 million cannot control their use. Marijuana use is also on the rise on college campuses, following the trend of increased use set by the general population.[12] However, students do not use marijuana as much as is perceived (Figure 14.5).

Physical Effects of Marijuana Marijuana is derived from either the *Cannabis sativa* or *Cannabis indica* (hemp) plant. Current American-grown marijuana is a turbocharged version of the hippie weed of the late 1960s. Developed using crossbreeding, genetic engineering, and American farming ingenuity, top-grade cannabis packs a punch very

ice A potent, inexpensive methamphetamine that has long-lasting effects.

marijuana Chopped leaves and flowers of *Cannabis indica* or *Cannabis sativa* plants (hemp); a psychoactive stimulant that intensifies reactions to environmental stimuli.

"PHARMING" PARTIES: THE NEW DRUG ABUSE VENUE

Several teens are sitting at the kitchen table listening to a girl tell about how she got OxyContin from the medicine chest at home. "It was left over," she says, "from my sister's wisdom teeth surgery." "What did you get? I'll give you some of this"—indicating a bottle of Ritalin—"for some of that painkiller." "Is this generic, or is it the good stuff?" he asks. This is not an ordinary party—it's a pharming party, a get-together arranged so teens and young adults can barter for their favorite prescription drugs. Pharming parties represent a growing trend among teenage drug abusers, and college students as well. Whereas use of illegal substances like speed, heroin, and pot has declined over the past decade, according to a report by Columbia University National Center on Addiction and Substance Abuse (CASA), abuse of prescription drugs has increased sharply. CASA says about 1 out of every 10 teens took legal medications illegally in 2003, the last year the figures were available. Among college students, the results of the 2004 *Monitoring the Future* (MTF) study found that over 7 percent of college students had used Vicodin, a prescription painkiller, without a doctor's prescription in the past year and over 4 percent had abused a stimulant such as Ritalin.

Why is prescription drug abuse growing in popularity?

Unfortunately, prescription drugs are often easier to obtain than illegal ones. Some teenagers and college students come by them legitimately (such as those who have a prescription for an amphetamine-based prescription drug) but trade them for others, like painkillers, that hold more appeal because of their potent high. Others order from shady Internet pharmacies where prescriptions are not always required. Some students may fake or exaggerate symptoms in order to persuade physicians to write prescriptions.

Studies also find that many who are abusing prescription medications are also abusing illegal drugs at the same time. According to the MTF study, students who obtained prescription painkillers from peers reported higher levels of binge drinking and marijuana abuse than nonabusers or those who received painkillers from family. This poses another set of problems, as alcohol in combination with any one of these medications can make a dangerous cocktail. If a friend or someone you know seems unusually drunk, drowsy, slurs speech, has trouble moving, or passes out, call for help immediately.

Because abuse of prescription medicines is a growing and not highly recognized problem, many do not realize the dangers. "My friend told me to save the painkillers for when I'm drinking or getting high," says a 17-year-old with a chuckle as she smokes her last cigarette. She doesn't think of herself as an addict. But she recog-

nizes the signs of addiction among her friends. "I know a lot of people who live by pills. Pills can dictate your life, I have seen it." Painkillers such as OxyContin, Percocet, Percodan, Vicodin, and others are highly addictive if taken for prolonged periods of time. OxyContin, in particular, can be a highly addictive and dangerous narcotic when abused. Users may take the pill orally, snort it, or dissolve it in a solution they can inject. The "rush" is similar to that of heroin. Chronic use can also result in increasing tolerance, and more of the drug is needed to achieve the desired effect. Occasional pharming parties can quickly spiral into an out-of-control addiction.

Should parents have to monitor the family medicine chest? What practical steps should be taken to prevent the misuse of prescription medications in the house? What steps, if any, should be taken about Internet pharmacies that allow medications to be purchased without a prescription? Why do you think prescription medications are not thought of as possible drugs of abuse?

Sources: Excerpt from C. Banta, "Trading for a High," *Time,* August 1, 2005; L. D. Johnston et al., *Monitoring the Future National Survey Results on Drug Use, 1975–2004: Volume II, College Students and Adults* (NIH Publication No. 05-5727) (Bethesda, MD: National Institute on Drug Abuse, 2005); L. Whitten, "Studies Identify Factors Surrounding Rise in Abuse of Prescription Drugs by College Students," *NIDA Notes* 20, no. 4, 2006.

similar to that of hashish. **Tetrahydrocannabinol (THC)** is the psychoactive substance in marijuana and the key to determining how powerful a high it will produce.

How potent is marijuana today? Samples of THC are taken from marijuana confiscated by law enforcement agencies to determine the average strength of the drug. Today, most marijuana contains 5 percent THC; more potent forms of the drug can contain up to 27 percent THC, but average 12 percent. Hashish has an average of 10 percent, ranging from 1 percent to 26 percent.[13]

Hashish, a potent cannabis preparation derived mainly from the thick, sticky resin of the female plant flowers,

contains high concentrations of THC. Hash oil, a substance produced by percolating a solvent such as ether through dried marijuana to extract the THC, is a tarlike liquid that may contain up to 300 mg of THC in a dose, or an average of 10 percent.[14]

tetrahydrocannabinol (THC)   The chemical name for the active ingredient in marijuana.

hashish   The sticky resin of the cannabis plant; it is high in THC.

MEDICINAL USE OF MARIJUANA: LEGAL CHALLENGES CONTINUE

For years, marijuana's legal status for medical purposes has been hotly debated nationally. Currently, 30 states and the District of Columbia have laws that recognize marijuana's medical value. Eleven states with therapeutic research program laws are nevertheless unable to give patients legal access to medical marijuana because of federal laws. Eight states have symbolic laws that recognize marijuana's medical value but fail to protect patients from arrest for possession of an illegal drug. Voters in Alaska, California, Colorado, Hawaii, Maine, Montana, Oregon, Nevada, Rhode Island, Vermont, and Washington state have chosen to legalize marijuana for medicinal use (see accompanying figure). These new state laws however, conflict with federal laws against the possession of marijuana and have led to new, yet unresolved, battles in court.

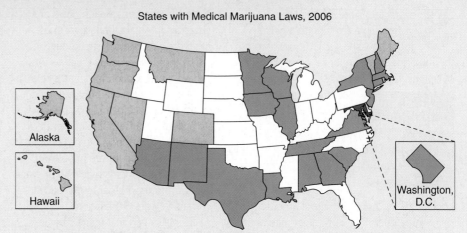

States with Medical Marijuana Laws, 2006

☐ Eleven states have laws that protect patients who possess and grow their own medical marijuana (with their doctors' recommednation or certification) from both criminal penalties and the threat of arrest.

■ Maryland protects medical marijuana patients from jail, but not from the threat of arrest.

▨ Eighteen states and the District of Columbia have laws that recognize marijuana's medical value, but they are ineffective because they rely on federal cooperation.

Source: Marijuana Policy Project, "State by State Medical Marijuana Laws: How To Remove the Threat of Arrest," 2006, www.mpp.org/atf/cf/{fc4e88df-6ace-4aa6-851c-0688a929d3c5}/2006_sbs _report.pdf.

Most of the time, marijuana is rolled into cigarettes (joints) or smoked in a pipe or water pipe (bong). Effects are generally felt within 10 to 30 minutes and usually wear off within 3 hours.

The most noticeable effect of THC is the dilation of the eyes' blood vessels, which produces the characteristic bloodshot eyes. Smokers of the drug also exhibit coughing, dry mouth and throat ("cotton mouth"), increased thirst and appetite, lowered blood pressure, and mild muscular weakness, primarily exhibited in drooping eyelids. Users can also experience severe anxiety, panic, paranoia, and psychosis.

Users may have intensified reactions to various stimuli; colors, sounds, and the speed at which things move may seem altered. High doses of hashish may produce vivid visual hallucinations.

Effects of Chronic Marijuana Use Because marijuana is illegal in most parts of the United States and has been widely used only since the 1960s, long-term studies of its effects have been difficult to conduct. Also, studies conducted in the 1960s involved marijuana with THC levels only a fraction of today's levels, so their results may not apply to the stronger forms available today.

> **Are there any negative long-term effects from marijuana use?**

Most current information about chronic marijuana use comes from countries such as Jamaica and Costa Rica, where the drug is not illegal. These studies of long-term users (for ten or more years) indicate that it causes lung damage comparable to that caused by tobacco smoking. Indeed, smoking a single joint may be as bad for the lungs as smoking three tobacco cigarettes. Inhalation of marijuana transfers carbon monoxide to the bloodstream. Because the blood has a greater affinity for carbon monoxide than it does for oxygen, this diminishes the oxygen-carrying capacity of the blood. The heart must work harder to pump the vital element to oxygen-starved tissues. Furthermore, the tar from cannabis contains higher levels of carcinogens than does tobacco smoke. Smoking marijuana results in three times more tar inhalation and retention in the respiratory tract than does tobacco use.

Other risks associated with marijuana include suppression of the immune system, blood pressure changes, and impaired memory function. Recent studies suggest that pregnant women who smoke marijuana are at a higher risk for stillbirth or miscarriage and for delivering low–birth weight babies and babies with abnormalities of the nervous system. Babies born to marijuana smokers are five times more likely to have features similar to those exhibited by children with fetal alcohol syndrome.

Debates concerning the effects of marijuana on the reproductive system have yet to be resolved. Studies conducted in the mid-1970s suggested that marijuana inhibited testosterone (and thus sperm) production in males and caused chromosomal breakage in both ova and sperm. Subsequent research in these areas is inconclusive. The question of whether the high-THC plants currently available will increase the risks associated with this drug is, as yet, unanswered.[15]

Marijuana and Medicine Although recognized as a dangerous drug by the U.S. government, marijuana has several medical purposes. It helps control the side effects (such as severe nausea and vomiting) produced by chemotherapy (chemical treatment for cancer). It improves appetite and forestalls the loss of lean muscle mass associated with AIDS-wasting syndrome (previously known as AIDS-related complex or ARC). Marijuana reduces the muscle pain and spasticity caused by diseases such as multiple sclerosis. It also temporarily relieves the eye pressure of glaucoma, although it is unclear whether it is more effective than legal glaucoma drugs.[16] Marijuana's legal status for medicinal purposes continues to be hotly debated (see the New Horizons in Health box).

Marijuana and Driving Marijuana use presents clear hazards for drivers of motor vehicles as well as others on the road. The drug substantially reduces a driver's ability to react and make quick decisions. In a study by the National Highway Traffic Safety Administration, a moderate dose of marijuana alone was shown to impair driving performance; however, the effects of even a low dose of marijuana combined with alcohol were markedly greater than for either drug alone. Studies show that approximately 6 to 11 percent of fatal accident victims test positive for THC.[17] In many of these cases, alcohol is detected as well. Perceptual and other performance deficits resulting from marijuana use may persist for some time after the high subsides. Users who attempt to drive, fly, or operate heavy machinery often fail to recognize their impairment.

 what do you THINK?

Why do you think that marijuana is the most popular illicit drug on college campuses? ■ How widespread is marijuana use on your campus?

Opiates

Among the oldest pain relievers known to humans, opiates cause drowsiness, reduce pain, and induce euphoria. A type of **narcotic,** opiates are derived from the parent drug **opium,** a dark, resinous substance made from the milky juice of the

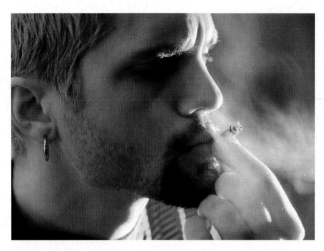

Marijuana is the most commonly used illicit drug.

opium poppy seed pod. Other opiates include morphine, codeine, heroin, and black tar heroin.

Until the early twentieth century, many patent medicines contained opiates and were advertised as cures for everything from menstrual cramps to teething pains. More powerful than opium, **morphine** (named after Morpheus, the Greek god of sleep) was widely used as a painkiller during the Civil War. **Codeine,** a less powerful analgesic (pain reliever) derived from morphine, also became popular.

As opiates became more common, physicians noted that patients tended to become dependent on them. Growing concern about addiction led to government controls of narcotic use. The Harrison Act of 1914 prohibited the production, dispensation, and sale of opiate products unless prescribed by a physician. Subsequent legislation required physicians prescribing opiates to keep careful records. Physicians are still subject to audits of their prescriptions.

Some opiates are still used today for medical purposes. Morphine is sometimes prescribed for severe pain, and codeine is found in prescription cough syrups and other painkillers. Several prescription drugs, including Percodan, Demerol, and Dilaudid, contain synthetic opiates. Although all opiate use is strictly regulated, illicit use of OxyContin, another powerful opiate, has increased dramatically in recent years.

narcotic Drugs that induce sleep and relieve pain; primarily the opiates.

opium The parent drug of the opiates; made from the seed pod resin of the opium poppy.

morphine A derivative of opium; sometimes used by medical practitioners to relieve pain.

codeine A drug derived from morphine; used in cough syrups and certain painkillers.

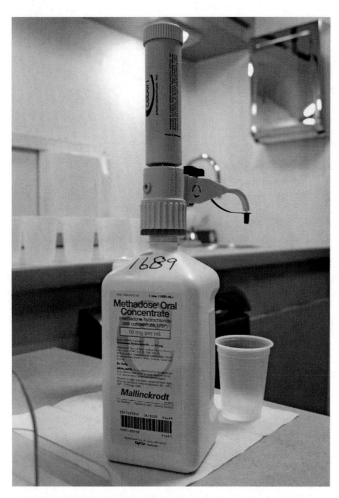

Methadone is one type of heroin treatment and allows many users to lead somewhat normal lives.

Physical Effects of Opiates

Opiates are powerful depressants of the central nervous system. In addition to relieving pain, these drugs lower heart rate, respiration, and blood pressure. Side effects include weakness, dizziness, nausea, vomiting, euphoria, decreased sex drive, visual disturbances, and lack of coordination. Of all the opiates, heroin has the greatest notoriety as an addictive drug. The following section discusses the progression of heroin addiction; addiction to any opiate follows a similar path.

Heroin Addiction

Heroin is a white powder derived from morphine. **Black tar heroin** is a sticky, dark brown, foul-smelling form of heroin that is relatively pure and

heroin An illegally manufactured derivative of morphine, usually injected into the bloodstream.

black tar heroin A dark brown, sticky form of heroin.

endorphins Opiate-like hormones that are manufactured in the human body and contribute to natural feelings of well-being.

inexpensive. Once considered a cure for morphine dependency, heroin was later discovered to be even more addictive and potent than morphine. Today, heroin has no medical use.

It is estimated that 3.7 million people have used heroin at one time in their lives. The highest number of users occurs among young adults, aged 26 or older. Heroin can be snorted, injected, or smoked; injection remains the most common route of administration. However, the contemporary version of heroin is so potent that users can get high by snorting or smoking the drug. This has attracted a more affluent group of users who may not want to inject, for reasons such as the increased risk of contracting a disease such as HIV.

Heroin is a depressant that produces drowsiness and a dreamy, mentally slow feeling. It can cause drastic mood swings, with euphoric highs followed by depressive lows. Heroin also slows respiration and urinary output and constricts the pupils of the eyes. In fact, pupil constriction is a classic sign of narcotic intoxication; hence, the stereotype of the drug user hiding behind a pair of dark sunglasses. Symptoms of tolerance and withdrawal can appear within three weeks of first use.[18]

The most common route of administration for heroin addicts is "mainlining"—intravenous injection of powdered heroin mixed in a solution. Many users describe the "rush" they feel when injecting themselves as intensely pleasurable, whereas others report unpredictable and unpleasant side effects. The temporary nature of the rush contributes to the drug's high potential for addiction—many addicts shoot up four or five times a day. Mainlining can cause veins to scar and eventually collapse. Once a vein has collapsed, it can no longer be used to introduce heroin into the bloodstream. Addicts become expert at locating new veins to use: in the feet, the legs, even the temples. When they do not want their needle tracks (scars) to show, they inject themselves under the tongue or in the groin.

The physiology of the human body could be said to encourage opiate addiction. Opiate-like substances called **endorphins** are manufactured in the body and have multiple receptor sites, particularly in the central nervous system. When endorphins attach themselves at these points, they create feelings of painless well-being. Medical researchers refer to them as "the body's own opiates." When endorphin levels are high, people feel euphoric. Long-distance runners, for example, experience "runner's high" from elevated endorphin levels. The same euphoria occurs when opiates or related chemicals are active at the endorphin receptor sites.

Treatment for Opiate Addiction

Programs to help heroin addicts, and those addicted to other opiates such as OxyContin or morphine, kick the habit have not been very successful. The rate of recidivism (tendency to return to previous behaviors) is high. Some addicts resume drug use even after years of drug-free living because the craving for the injection rush is very strong. It takes a great deal of discipline to seek alternative, nondrug highs.

Opiate addicts experience a distinct pattern of withdrawal. They begin to crave another dose four to six hours after their last dose. Symptoms of withdrawal include intense desire for the drug, yawning, a runny nose, sweating, and crying. About 12 hours after the last dose, addicts experience sleep disturbance, dilated pupils, loss of appetite, irritability, goose bumps, and muscle tremors. The most difficult time in the withdrawal process occurs 24 to 72 hours following last use. All of the preceding symptoms continue, along with nausea, abdominal cramps, restlessness, insomnia, vomiting, diarrhea, extreme anxiety, hot and cold flashes, elevated blood pressure, and rapid heartbeat and respiration. Once the peak of withdrawal has passed, all these symptoms begin to subside. Still, the recovering addict has many hurdles to jump.

Methadone maintenance is one treatment available for people addicted to heroin or other opiates. Methadone is a synthetic narcotic that blocks the effects of opiate withdrawal. It is chemically similar enough to the opiates to control the tremors, chills, vomiting, diarrhea, and severe abdominal pains of withdrawal. Methadone dosage is decreased over a period of time until the addict is weaned off the drug.

Methadone maintenance is controversial because of the drug's own potential for addiction. Critics contend that the program merely substitutes one addiction for another. Proponents argue that people on methadone maintenance are less likely to engage in criminal activities to support their habits than heroin addicts are. For this reason, many methadone maintenance programs are financed by state or federal government and are available to clients free of charge or at reduced cost.

A number of new drug therapies for opiate dependence are emerging. Naltrexone (Trexan), an opiate antagonist, has been approved as a treatment. While on naltrexone, recovering addicts do not have the compulsion to use heroin, and if they do use it, they don't get high, so there is no point in using the drug. More recently, researchers have reported promising results with Temgesic (buprenorphine), a mild, nonaddicting synthetic opiate, which, like heroin and methadone, bonds to certain receptors in the brain, blocks pain messages, and persuades the brain that its cravings for heroin have been satisfied. Addicts report that while they are taking buprenorphine, they do not crave heroin anymore.

Hallucinogens (Psychedelics)

Hallucinogens are substances that are capable of creating auditory or visual hallucinations. These types of drugs are also known as **psychedelics,** a term adapted from the Greek phrase meaning "mind manifesting." Hallucinogens are a group of drugs whose primary pharmacological effect is to alter feelings, perceptions, and thoughts in a user. The major receptor sites for most of these drugs are in the part of the brain that is responsible for filtering extraneous or irrelevant outside stimuli before allowing these signals to travel to other parts of the brain. This area, the **reticular formation,** is located in the brain stem at the upper end of the spinal cord (Figure 14.6). When a hallucinogen is present at a reticular formation site, messages become scrambled, and the user

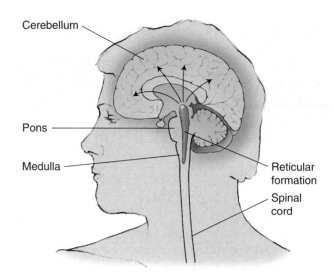

FIGURE 14.6 The Reticular Formation

may see wavy walls instead of straight ones or may smell colors and hear tastes. This mixing of sensory messages is known as **synesthesia.** In addition to synesthetic effects, users may become less inhibited or recall events long buried in the subconscious mind.

The most widely recognized hallucinogens are LSD, mescaline, psilocybin, and PCP. All are illegal and carry severe penalties for manufacture, possession, transportation, or sale.

LSD Of all the psychedelics, **lysergic acid diethylamide (LSD)** is the most notorious. First synthesized in the late 1930s by Swiss chemist Albert Hoffman, LSD resulted from experiments to derive medically useful drugs from the ergot fungus found on rye and other cereal grains. Because LSD seemed capable of unlocking the secrets of the mind,

methadone maintenance A treatment for people addicted to opiates that substitutes methadone, a synthetic narcotic, for the opiate of addiction.

hallucinogens Substances capable of creating auditory or visual distortions and heightened states.

psychedelics Drugs that distort the processing of sensory information in the brain.

reticular formation An area in the brain stem that is responsible for relaying messages to other areas in the brain.

synesthesia A drug-created effect in which sensory messages are incorrectly assigned—for example, the user hears a taste or smells a sound.

lysergic acid diethylamide (LSD) Psychedelic drug causing sensory disruptions; also called acid.

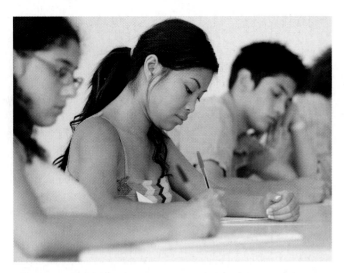

Addiction can creep up on anyone, even if they are doing well in school and other aspects of their life appear to be in order.

psychiatrists initially felt it could be beneficial to patients unable to remember suppressed traumas. From 1950 through 1968, the drug was used for such purposes.

Media attention focused on LSD in the 1960s. Young people used the drug to "turn on" and "tune out" the world that gave them the war in Vietnam, race riots, and political assassinations. In 1970, federal authorities, under intense pressure from the public, placed LSD on the list of controlled substances (Schedule I). LSD's popularity peaked in 1972, then tapered off, primarily because of users' inability to control dosages accurately.

Because of the recent wave of nostalgia for the 1960s, this dangerous psychedelic drug has been making a comeback. Known on the street as "acid," LSD is now available in virtually every state. Over 11 million Americans, most of them under age 35, have tried LSD at least once. LSD especially attracts younger users. Approximately 1.8 percent of high school seniors report having tried it at least once in the past year.[19] A national survey of college students showed that 1.2 percent had used the drug in the past year.[20]

An odorless, tasteless, white crystalline powder, LSD is most frequently dissolved in water to make a solution that can be used to manufacture the street forms of the drug. The most common form is blotter acid—small squares of blotterlike paper that have been impregnated with the liquid. The blotter is swallowed or chewed briefly. LSD also comes in tiny thin squares of gelatin called windowpane and in tablets called microdots, which are less than an eighth of an inch across (it would take ten or more to add up to the size of an aspirin tablet). Microdots and windowpane are just a

mescaline   A hallucinogenic drug derived from the peyote cactus.

peyote   A cactus with small "buttons" that, when ingested, produce hallucinogenic effects.

sideshow; blotter is the medium of choice. As with any illegal drug, purchasers run the risk of buying an impure product.

One of the most powerful drugs known to science, LSD can produce strong effects in doses as low as 20 micrograms (µg). (To give you an idea of how small a dose this is, the average postage stamp weighs approximately 60,000 µg.) The potency of the typical dose currently ranges from 20 to 80 µg, compared to 150 to 300 µg commonly used in the 1960s.

Despite its reputation as primarily a psychedelic, LSD produces a number of physical effects, including increased heart rate, elevated blood pressure and temperature, goose flesh (roughened skin), increased reflex speeds, muscle tremors and twitches, perspiration, increased salivation, chills, headaches, and mild nausea. Because the drug also stimulates uterine muscle contractions, it can lead to premature labor and miscarriage in pregnant women. Research into long-term effects has been inconclusive.

The psychological effects of LSD vary. The mindset of the user and setting in which the drug is used are influential factors. Euphoria is the common psychological state produced by the drug, but dysphoria (a sense of evil and foreboding) may also be experienced. The drug also shortens attention span, causing the mind to wander. Thoughts may be interposed and juxtaposed, so the user experiences several different thoughts simultaneously. Synesthesia occurs occasionally. Users become introspective and suppressed memories may surface, often taking on bizarre symbolism. Many more effects are possible, including decreased aggressiveness and enhanced sensory experiences.

LSD causes distortions of ordinary perceptions, such as the movement of stationary objects. "Bad trips," the most publicized risk of LSD, are commonly related to the user's mood. The person, for example, may interpret increased heart rate as a heart attack (a "bad body trip"). Often bad trips result when a user confronts a suppressed emotional experience or memory (a "bad head trip").

Although there is no evidence that LSD creates physical dependency, it may well create psychological dependence. Many LSD users become depressed for one or two days following a trip and turn to the drug to relieve this depression. The result is a cycle of LSD use to relieve post-LSD depression, which often leads to psychological addiction.

 what do you THINK?

Are people today using LSD for the same reasons it was used in the 1960s? ■ What are the perceived attractions and the real dangers of LSD use?

Mescaline   **Mescaline** is one of hundreds of chemicals derived from the **peyote** cactus, a small, buttonlike cactus that grows in the southwestern United States and Latin America. Natives of these regions have long used the dried peyote buttons for religious purposes. In fact, members of the Native American Church (a religion practiced by thousands of North American Indians) have been granted special permission to use the drug during religious ceremonies in some states.

Users normally swallow 10 to 12 dried peyote buttons. These buttons taste bitter and generally induce immediate nausea or vomiting. Longtime users claim that the nausea becomes less noticeable with frequent use.

Those who are able to keep the drug down begin to feel the effects within 30 to 90 minutes, when mescaline reaches maximum concentration in the brain. (It may persist for up to nine or ten hours.) Mescaline is a powerful hallucinogen. It is also a central nervous system stimulant.

Products sold on the street as mescaline are likely to be synthetic chemical relatives of the true drug. Street names of these products include DOM, STP, TMA, and MMDA. Any of these can be toxic in small quantities.

Psilocybin

Psilocybin **Psilocybin** and *psilocin* are the active chemicals in a group of mushrooms sometimes called "magic mushrooms." Psilocybe mushrooms, which grow throughout the world, can be cultivated from spores or harvested wild. Because many mushrooms resemble the psilocybe variety, people who use wild mushrooms for any purpose should be certain of what they are doing. Mushroom varieties can easily be misidentified, and mistakes can be fatal. Psilocybin is similar to LSD in its physical effects, which generally wear off in four to six hours.

PCP

PCP **Phencyclidine,** or **PCP,** is a synthetic substance that became a black-market drug in the early 1970s. PCP was originally developed as a dissociative anesthetic, which means that patients administered this drug could keep their eyes open, apparently remain conscious, and feel no pain during a medical procedure. Afterward, they would experience amnesia for the time the drug was in their system. Such a drug had obvious advantages as an anesthetic, but its unpredictability and drastic effects (postoperative delirium, confusion, and agitation) made doctors abandon it, and it was withdrawn from the legal market.

On the illegal market, PCP is a white, crystalline powder that users often sprinkle onto marijuana cigarettes. It is dangerous and unpredictable regardless of the method of administration. Common street names for PCP are "angel dust" for the crystalline powdered form and "peace pill" and "horse tranquilizer" for the tablet form. (It was used as a veterinary anesthetic for a time.)

The effects of PCP depend on the dosage. A dose as small as 5 mg will produce effects similar to those of strong central nervous system depressants—slurred speech, impaired coordination, reduced sensitivity to pain, and reduced heart and respiratory rate. Doses between 5 and 10 mg cause fever, salivation, nausea, vomiting, and total loss of sensitivity to pain. Doses greater than 10 mg result in a drastic drop in blood pressure, coma, muscular rigidity, violent outbursts, and possible convulsions and death.

Psychologically, PCP may produce either euphoria or dysphoria. It is also known to produce hallucinations as well as delusions and overall delirium. Some users experience a prolonged state of "nothingness." The long-term effects of PCP use are unknown.

Designer Drugs (Club Drugs)

Designer drugs are produced in chemical laboratories, often manufactured in homes, and sold illegally. These drugs are easy to produce from available raw materials. The drugs themselves were once technically legal because the law had to specify the exact chemical structure of an illicit substance. However, there is now a law in place that bans all chemical cousins of illegal drugs.

Collectively known as **club drugs,** these dangerous substances include Ecstasy, GHB, Special K, and Rohypnol. Although users may think them harmless, research has shown that club drugs can produce a range of unwanted effects, including hallucinations, paranoia, amnesia, and, in some cases, death. Some club drugs work on the same brain mechanisms as alcohol and can dangerously boost the effects of both substances. Because the drugs are odorless and tasteless, people can easily slip them into drinks. Some of them have been associated with sexual assault and for that reason are referred to as "date rape drugs" (see the Spotlight on Your Health box on the following page).

Ecstasy (methylene dioxymethylamphetamine, or MDMA), once dubbed the "LSD of the 80s," has had a resurgence of popularity on many college campuses. Almost one of every four students at some universities report having used it. Ecstasy creates feelings of openness and warmth, combined with the mind-expanding characteristics of hallucinogens. Effects begin within 30 minutes and can last for four to six hours. Young people may use Ecstasy initially to improve mood or get energized so they can keep dancing; it also increases heart rate and blood pressure and may raise body temperature to the point of kidney and/or cardiovascular failure. Chronic use appears to damage the brain's ability to think and to regulate emotion, memory, sleep, and pain. Combined with alcohol, Ecstasy can be extremely dangerous and sometimes fatal. Recent studies indicate that Ecstasy may cause long-lasting neurotoxic effects by damaging brain cells that produce serotonin, and it is unknown whether these brain cells will regenerate.[21]

Inhalants

Inhalants are chemicals that produce vapors which, when inhaled, can cause hallucinations and create intoxicating and

---

psilocybin The active chemical found in psilocybe mushrooms; it produces hallucinations.

phencyclidine (PCP) A drug, commonly called "angel dust," that causes hallucinations, delusions, and delirium.

designer drugs (club drugs) Synthetic analogs (drugs that produce similar effects) of existing illicit drugs.

Ecstasy A club drug that creates feelings of openness and warmth but also raises heart rate and blood pressure.

inhalants Products that are sniffed or inhaled in order to produce highs.

CLUB DRUGS ON CAMPUS

Among 18 to 25-year-olds surveyed in 2004, 13.8 percent reported lifetime MDMA use, 3.1 percent reported past-year MDMA use, and 0.7 percent reported past-month MDMA use.* Every era seems to have its hot drug. At one point it was Valium, then LSD, and then crack. Currently the so-called club drugs are popular on college campuses. Three of note include Rohypnol (flunitrazepam), also called "ropies" or "roofies"; GHB (gamma-hydroxybutyrate), or, as it is known on the street, "grievous bodily harm"; and Special K (ketamine).

Rohypnol is a potent tranquilizer similar in nature to Valium, but many times stronger. The drug produces a sedative effect, amnesia, muscle relaxation, and slowed psychomotor responses. Commonly known as the "date rape" drug, Rohypnol has gained notoriety as a growing problem on college campuses. The drug has been added to punch and other drinks at fraternity parties and college social gatherings, where it is reportedly given to female partiers in hopes of lowering their inhibitions and facilitating potential sexual conquests. The manufacturer changed the formula to give the drug a bright blue color that would make it easy to detect in most drinks, so would-be perpetrators are turning to blue tropical drinks and punches to disguise the drug.

Although "ropie" fervor has subsided somewhat, it continues to be a concern. See the Spotlight on Your Health box in Chapter 4 on strategies to protect yourself from being dosed with Rohypnol.

Rohypnol has been joined by a newer, liquid substance called GHB, or gamma-hydroxybutyrate. GHB is used as a muscle builder, a tranquilizer, and an aphrodisiac to increase one's sense of touch and sexual prowess. GHB is an odorless, tasteless fluid that can be made easily at home or in a chemistry lab. Like Rohypnol, GHB has been slipped into drinks without being detected, resulting in loss of memory, unconsciousness, amnesia, and even death. Other side effects of GHB include nausea, vomiting, seizures, memory loss, hallucinations, coma, and respiratory distress. During the 1980s, GHB was available in U.S. health food stores. Concerns about its use led the FDA to ban over-the-counter sales in 1990 and GHB is now a Schedule I controlled substance.

The Special K we're referring to is not the breakfast cereal, but rather ketamine, used as an anesthetic in many hospital and veterinary clinics. On the street, Special K is most often diverted in liquid form from veterinary offices or medical suppliers. Dealers dry the liquid (usually by cooking it) and grind the residue into powder. Special K causes hallucinations as it inhibits the relay of sensory input; the brain fills the

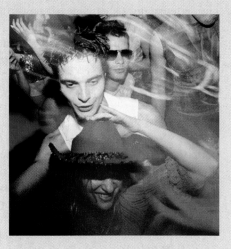

resulting void with visions, dreams, memories, and sensory distortions. The effects of Special K are not as severe as those of Ecstasy, so it has grown in popularity among people who have to go to work or school after a night of partying.

Sources: Office of National Drug Control Policy, "Rohypnol Fact Sheet," June 2004; Office of National Drug Control Policy, "Gamma-Hydroxybutyrate (GHB) Fact Sheet," June 2004; National Institute on Drug Abuse, "NIDA InfoFacts: Club Drugs," 2006, www.drugabuse.gov/infofacts/clubdrugs.html. * Substance Abuse and Mental Health Services Administration, "Results from the 2004 National Survey on Drug Use and Health: National Findings," September 2005, http://oas.samhsa.gov/nsduh/2k4nsduh/2k4Results/2k4Results.htm#toc.

euphoric effects. Not commonly recognized as drugs, inhalants are legal to purchase and universally available but dangerous when used incorrectly. They generally appeal to young people who can't afford or obtain illicit substances.

Some of these agents are organic solvents representing the chemical by-products of the distillation of petroleum products. Rubber cement, model glue, paint thinner, lighter fluid, varnish, wax, spot removers, and gasoline belong to this group. Most of these substances are sniffed by users in search of a quick, cheap high.

Because they are inhaled, the volatile chemicals in these products reach the bloodstream within seconds. An inhaled

substance is not diluted or buffered by stomach acids or other body fluids and thus is more potent than it would be if swallowed. This characteristic, along with the fact that dosages are extremely difficult to control because everyone has unique lung and breathing capacities, makes inhalants particularly dangerous.

The effects of inhalants usually last for fewer than 15 minutes. Users may experience dizziness, disorientation, impaired coordination, reduced judgment, and slowed reaction times. Signs of inhalant use include the following: unjustifiable collection of glues, paints, lacquer thinner, cleaning fluid, and ether; sniffles similar to those produced by a cold;

and a smell on the breath similar to the inhalable substance. The effects of inhalants resemble those of central nervous system depressants, and combining inhalants with alcohol produces a synergistic effect. In addition, combining these substances can cause severe liver damage that can be fatal.

An overdose of fumes from inhalants can cause unconsciousness. If the user's oxygen intake is reduced during the inhaling process, death can result within five minutes. Whether a user is a first-time or chronic user, sudden sniffing death (SSD) syndrome can be a fatal consequence. This syndrome can occur if a user inhales deeply and then participates in physical activity or is startled.

Amyl Nitrite

Amyl Nitrite Sometimes called "poppers" or "rush," **amyl nitrite** is packaged in small, cloth-covered glass capsules that can be crushed to release the active chemical. The drug is often prescribed to alleviate chest pain in heart patients because it dilates small blood vessels and reduces blood pressure. Dilation of blood vessels in the genital area is thought to enhance sensations or perceptions of orgasm. It also produces fainting, dizziness, warmth, and skin flushing.

Nitrous Oxide

Nitrous Oxide **Nitrous oxide** is sometimes used as an adjunct to dental anesthesia or minor surgical anesthesia. It is also a propellant chemical in aerosol products such as whipped toppings. Users experience a state of euphoria, floating sensations, and illusions. Effects also include pain relief and a "silly" feeling, demonstrated by laughing and giggling (hence its nickname "laughing gas"). Regulating dosages of this drug can be difficult. Sustained inhalation can lead to unconsciousness, coma, and death.

Steroids

Public awareness of **anabolic steroids** has been heightened by media stories about their use by amateur and professional athletes, especially today's professional baseball players, and other high-profile athletes. Anabolic steroids are artificial forms of the male hormone testosterone that promote muscle growth and strength. These **ergogenic drugs** are used primarily by young men who believe the drugs will increase their strength, power, bulk (weight), speed, and athletic performance.

Most steroids are obtained through the black market. It was once estimated that approximately 17 to 20 percent of college athletes used them. Now that stricter drug-testing policies have been instituted by the NCAA, reported use of anabolic steroids among intercollegiate athletes has dropped to 1.1 percent. However, a recent survey among high school students found a significant increase in the use of anabolic steroids since 1991. Few data exist on the extent of steroid abuse by adults. It has been estimated that hundreds of thousands of people aged 18 and older abuse anabolic steroids at least once a year. Among both adolescents and adults, steroid abuse is higher among males than females. However, steroid abuse is growing most rapidly among young women.[22]

Steroids are available in two forms: injectable solutions and pills. Anabolic steroids produce a state of euphoria, diminished fatigue, and increased bulk and power in both sexes. These qualities give steroids an addictive quality. When users stop, they can experience psychological withdrawal and sometimes severe depression, in some cases leading to suicide attempts. If untreated, depression associated with steroid withdrawal has been known to last for a year or more after steroid use stops.

Men and women who use steroids experience a variety of adverse effects. These drugs cause mood swings (aggression and violence), sometimes known as "'roid rage"; acne; liver tumors; elevated cholesterol levels; hypertension; kidney disease; and immune system disturbances. There is also a danger of transmitting AIDS and hepatitis (a serious liver disease) through shared needles. In women, large doses of anabolic steroids may trigger the development of masculine attributes such as lowered voice, increased facial and body hair, and male pattern baldness; they may also result in an enlarged clitoris, smaller breasts, and changes in or absence of menstruation. When taken by healthy males, anabolic steroids shut down the body's production of testosterone, causing men's breasts to grow and testicles to atrophy.

To combat the growing problem of steroid use, the U.S. Congress passed the Anabolic Steroids Control Act (ASCA) of 1990. This law makes it a crime to possess, prescribe, or distribute anabolic steroids for any use other than the treatment of specific diseases. Anabolic steroids are now classified as a Schedule III drug. Penalties for their illegal use include up to five years' imprisonment and a $250,000 fine for the first offense and up to ten years' imprisonment and a $500,000 fine for subsequent offenses.

A new and alarming trend is the use of other drugs to achieve the effects of steroids. The two most common steroid alternatives are gamma-hydroxybutyrate (GHB) and clenbuterol. GHB is a deadly, illegal drug that is a primary ingredient in many "performance-enhancing" formulas. GHB does not produce a high. It does, however, cause headaches, nausea, vomiting, diarrhea, seizures, and other central nervous system disorders, and possibly death. Clenbuterol is used in some countries for veterinary treatments but is not approved for any use—in animals or humans—in the United States.

New attention was drawn to the issue of steroids and related substances when former St. Louis Cardinals slugger Mark McGwire admitted to using a supplement containing

amyl nitrite A drug that dilates blood vessels and is properly used to relieve chest pain.

nitrous oxide The chemical name for "laughing gas," a substance properly used for surgical or dental anesthesia.

anabolic steroids Artificial forms of the hormone testosterone that promote muscle growth and strength.

ergogenic drug Substance believed to enhance athletic performance.

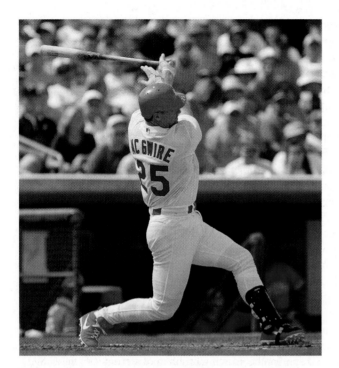

In March 2005, major league baseball players, such as Mark McGwire, were subpoenaed to testify before Congress on the use of steroids in the sport. McGwire has admitted to the use of the hormone supplement, andro, in the past.

androstenedione (andro), an adrenal hormone that is produced naturally in both men and women. Andro raises levels of the male hormone testosterone, which helps build lean muscle mass and promotes quicker recovery after injury. McGwire had done nothing illegal, as the supplement could be purchased over the counter (with sales estimated at $800 million a year) and its use was legal in baseball at that time, although banned by the NFL, NCAA, and International Olympic Committee. A recent study found that when men take 100 milligrams of andro three times daily, it increases estrogen levels by up to 80 percent, enlarges the prostate gland, and increases heart disease risk by 10 to 15 percent. Major league baseball banned its use in 2004.

Visits to the locker rooms of many sports teams would disclose large containers of other alleged muscle-building supplements, such as creatine. Although they are legal, questions remain whether enough research has been done concerning the safety of these supplements. Some experts worry that they may bring consequences similar to those of steroids, such as liver damage and heart problems. Some of these performance-enhancing supplements are discussed further in Chapter 23, Complementary and Alternative Medicine.

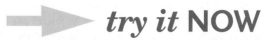

try it NOW

Drug misuse can eventually lead to addiction, and hurt your chances of achieving lifelong goals. On a piece of paper, identify one long-term goal you would like to achieve, such as becoming a lawyer. Be sure your goal is specific. Next, write down three steps you need to take to reach the goal (e.g., an internship with the district attorney, getting into the law school of your choice, passing the bar exam). Finally, think about drug misuse, its consequences, and how these factors will make your goal difficult to achieve or prevent you from reaching it at all.

Illegal Drug Use in the United States

Stories of people who have tried illegal drugs, enjoyed them, and suffered no consequences may tempt you to try them yourself. You may tell yourself it's "just this once," convincing yourself that one-time use is harmless. Given the dangers surrounding these substances, however, you should think twice. The risks associated with drug use extend beyond the personal. The decision to try any illicit substance encourages illicit drug manufacture and transport, thus contributing to the national drug problem. The financial burden of illegal drug use on the U.S. economy is staggering, with an estimated economic cost of around $180.9 billion.[23] This estimate includes costs associated with substance abuse treatment and prevention, health care, reduced job productivity and lost earnings, and social consequences such as crime and social welfare.

In addition, roughly half of all expenditures to combat crime are related to illegal drugs. The burden of these costs is absorbed primarily by the government (46 percent), followed by those who abuse drugs and members of their households (44 percent). One study found that Americans spend $64 billion on illicit drugs annually. These numbers break down as follows: $35 billion on cocaine, $10 billion each on marijuana and heroin, and $5 billion on methamphetamines. This is eight times what the federal government spends on research on HIV/AIDS, cancer, and heart disease put together.[24]

what do you THINK?

What do you believe are the moral and ethical issues surrounding drug testing? ■ Are you in favor of drug testing? ■ Should all employees be subjected to drug tests or just those in high-risk jobs? ■ Is it the employer's right to conduct drug testing at the worksite? Explain your answer.

Drugs in the Workplace

According to the National Survey on Drug Abuse and Health, 75.2 percent of all U.S. workers who use illicit drugs are employed full or part time.[25] With such a large segment of drug users employed to some degree, the cost to American businesses soars into the billions of dollars. These costs reflect reduced work performance and efficiency, lost productivity, absenteeism, and turnover. Drug-abusing workers function at about 67 percent of their capacity, costing American businesses roughly $81 billion in lost productivity alone in one year.[26]

The highest rates of illicit drug use among workers exist in the food preparation, food service, bartending, construction, and transportation and material-moving industries. Of people who work full time, those who admit to being current drug users are between the ages of 18 and 25, less educated, male, divorced or never married, white, and low paid. In addition, drug users are 2.2 times more likely to request early dismissal or time off, 2.5 times more likely to have absences of eight days or more, and 3 times more likely to be late for work.[27]

Is it legal for employers to require employees to take a drug test?

Many companies have instituted drug testing for their employees. Mandatory drug urinalysis is controversial. Critics argue that such testing violates Fourth Amendment rights of protection from unreasonable search and seizure. Proponents believe the personal inconvenience entailed in testing pales in comparison to the problems caused by drug use in the workplace. Several court decisions have affirmed the right of employers to test their employees for drug use. They contend that Fourth Amendment rights pertain only to employees of government agencies, not to those of private businesses. Most Americans apparently support drug testing for certain types of jobs.

Drug testing is expensive, with costs running as high as $100 per test. Moreover, some critics question the accuracy and reliability of the results. Both false positives and false negatives can occur. As drug testing becomes more common in the work environment, it is gaining greater acceptance by employees, who see testing as a step to improving safety and productivity.

Solutions to the Problem

Americans are alarmed by the increasing use of illegal drugs. Respondents in public opinion polls feel that the most important strategy for fighting drug abuse is educating young people. They also endorse strategies such as stricter border surveillance to reduce drug trafficking, longer prison sentences for drug dealers, increased government spending on prevention, enforcing antidrug laws, and greater cooperation between government agencies and private groups and individuals providing treatment assistance. All of these approaches will probably help up to a point, but they do not offer a total solution to the problem. Drug abuse has been a part of human behavior for thousands of years, and it is not likely to disappear in the near future. For this reason, it is necessary to educate ourselves and to develop the self-discipline necessary to avoid dangerous drug dependence.

For many years, the most popular antidrug strategies were total prohibition and "scare tactics." Both approaches proved ineffective. Prohibition of alcohol during the 1920s created more problems than it solved, as did prohibition of opiates in 1914. Outlawing other illicit drugs has neither eliminated them nor curtailed their traffic across U.S. borders.

In general, researchers in the field of drug education agree that a multimodal approach is best. Students should be taught the difference between drug use and abuse. Factual information that is free of scare tactics must be presented; lecturing and moralizing do not work. Emphasis should be placed on things that are important to young people. Telling adolescent males that girls will find them disgusting if their breath stinks of cigarettes or pot will get their attention. Likewise, lecturing on the negative effects of drug use is a much less effective deterrent than teaching young people how to negotiate the social scene. Drug Abuse Resistance Education, commonly called DARE, is one program intended to educate students but has been largely ineffective. Education efforts need to focus on achieving better outcomes for preventing drug use.

We must also study at-risk groups so we can better understand the circumstances that make them susceptible to drug use. Time, money, and effort by educators, parents, and policy makers are needed to ensure that today's youth receive the love and security essential for building productive and meaningful lives and rejecting drug use.

what do you THINK?

Do you feel the public has a social responsibility to fight drug abuse? ■ What is the cost society pays for drug use? ■ Have you ever personally known someone who has suffered because of addiction to drugs? ■ How did you respond?

TAKING charge

Summary

- The six categories of drugs are prescription drugs, OTC drugs, recreational drugs, herbal preparations, illicit drugs, and commercial preparations. Routes of administration include oral ingestion, injection (intravenous, intramuscular, and subcutaneous), inhalation, inunction, and suppositories.
- People from all walks of life use illicit drugs, although college students report higher usage rates than the general population. Drug use has declined since the mid-1980s.

- Controlled substances include cocaine and its derivatives, amphetamines, methamphetamine and ice, marijuana, opiates, hallucinogens/psychedelics, designer drugs (club drugs), inhalants, and steroids. Users tend to become addicted quickly to such drugs.
- The drug problem reaches everyone through crime and elevated health care costs. Drugs are a major problem in the workplace; workplace drug testing is one proposed solution to this problem.

Chapter Review

1. An example of what is *not* considered drug *misuse* is
   a. excessive use of and dependency on a drug.
   b. taking a friend's prescription medicine.
   c. taking medicine more than is recommended to do so.
   d. not following the instructions when taking a medicine.

2. The most common method of injection among drug abusers is
   a. intramuscular.
   b. intravenous.
   c. subcutaneous.
   d. All of the above.

3. A person who takes excessive drugs on a continuous basis, even when it is not necessary to, describes
   a. drug misuse.
   b. drug addiction.
   c. drug tolerance.
   d. drug abuse.

4. The most common method for taking drugs is
   a. injection.
   b. inhalation.
   c. orally.
   d. inunction.

5. The most widely used illegal drug in the United States is
   a. alcohol.
   b. heroin.
   c. marijuana.
   d. methamphetamine.

6. Which of the following is classified as a stimulant drug?
   a. amphetamines
   b. alcohol
   c. marijuana
   d. LSD

7. *Freebasing* is
   a. mixing cocaine with heroin.
   b. inhaling heroin fumes.
   c. injecting a drug into the veins.
   d. smoking the fumes of cocaine.

8. Drugs that depress the central nervous system are known as
   a. narcotics.
   b. sedatives.
   c. depressants.
   d. psychedelics.

9. The one illegal drug that does not appear to cause physical dependency is
   a. cocaine.
   b. heroin.
   c. marijuana.
   d. LSD.

10. The psychoactive drug mescaline is found in what plant?
    a. mushrooms
    b. peyote cactus
    c. marijuana
    d. belladona

Answers to these questions can be found on page A-1.

Questions for Discussion and Reflection

1. What is the current theory that explains how drugs work in the body? Explain this theory.
2. Do you think there is such a thing as responsible use of illicit drugs? Would you change any of the current laws governing drugs? How would you determine what is legitimate use and illegitimate use?
3. Why do you think that many people today feel that marijuana use is not dangerous? What are the arguments in favor of legalizing marijuana? What are the arguments against legalization? How common is the use of marijuana on your campus?
4. How do you and your peers feel about illicit drug use? Has your opinion changed in recent years? If so, how and why?
5. Debate the issue of workplace drug testing. Would you apply for a job that had drug testing as an interview requirement? As a continuing requirement?
6. What could you do to help a friend who is fighting a substance abuse problem? What resources on your campus could help you?
7. Why are drugs such as Rohypnol and Ecstasy of great concern these days? If someone has "consensual" sex with another person after secretly lacing his or her drink with one of these drugs, do you think it's a case of rape and should be prosecuted as such? Why or why not?
8. How do you think reports in the media about the use of stimulants and/or steroids by athletes affect the popularity of these drugs? Would you consider taking such a drug to improve your appearance or your athletic performance? Explain your answer.
9. What types of programs do you think would be effective in preventing drug abuse among high school and college students? How might programs for high school differ from those for college students?

Accessing Your Health on the Internet

The following websites explore further topics and issues related to personal health. You'll also find links to each organization's website on the Companion Website for *Access to Health,* Tenth Edition, at www.aw-bc.com/donatelle.

1. *Club Drugs.* A website designed to disseminate science-based information about club drugs. www.clubdrugs.org
2. *Join Together.* An excellent site for the most current information related to substance abuse. This site also includes information on gun violence and provides advice on organizing and taking political action. www.jointogether.org
3. *National Institute on Drug Abuse.* The home page of this U.S. government agency has information on the latest statistics and findings in drug research. www.nida.nih.gov
4. *Substance Abuse and Mental Health Services Administration (SAMHSA).* Outstanding resource for information about national surveys, ongoing research, and national drug interventions. www.samhsa.gov

Further Reading

Elster, J. (ed.). *Addiction: Entries and Exits.* New York: Russell Sage Foundation, 2000.

> *Addresses current addiction controversies from an international perspective, with authors from the United States and Norway. Topics include whether addicts have a choice in their behavior and current addiction theories.*

Goldstein, A. *Addiction: From Biology to Drug Policy.* New York: Oxford University Press, 2001.

> *This book discusses how drugs impact the brain, how each drug causes addiction, and how addictive drugs impact society. The author offers an explanation of what we know about drug addiction, how we know what we know, and what we can and cannot do about the drug problem.*

Greenburg, S. *2005 Physician's Desk Reference for Nonprescription Drugs and Dietary Supplements.* Montvale, NJ: Thomson Medical Economics, 2005.

> *Outlines proper uses, possible dangers, and effective ingredients of nonprescription medications.*

Griffith, W. H., and S. Moore. *Complete Guide to Prescription and Nonprescription Drugs, 2005.* New York: Perigee, 2004.

> *This essential guide answers every conceivable question about prescription and nonprescription drugs and contains information about dosages, side effects, precautions, interactions, and more. More than 5,000 brand name and 800 generic drugs are profiled in an easy-to-use format.*

Ray, O. S., and C. Ksir. *Drugs, Society and Human Behavior,* 11th ed. New York: McGraw-Hill. 2006.

> *This book examines drugs and behavior from the behavioral, pharmacological, historical, social, legal, and clinical perspectives.*

The National Center on Addiction and Substance Abuse. *Women Under the Influence: Alcohol Problems in Adolescents and Young Adults: Epidemiology, Neurobiology, Prevention* *and Treatment*. Baltimore: Johns Hopkins University Press, 2006.

> Women Under the Influence *is a scholarly analysis of substance abuse among American women. This lucidly written book provides a perceptive and compassionate discussion of the factors that contribute to abuse of a wide spectrum of substances and of the associated social and health consequences for women.*

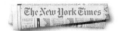

e-themes from *The New York Times*

For up-to-date articles about current health issues, visit www.aw-bc.com/donatelle, select *Access to Health,* Tenth Edition, Chapter 14, and click on "e-themes."

References

1. Substance Abuse and Mental Health Services Administration, "Substance Abuse: A National Health Challenge," October 4, 2006, www.samhsa.gov/oas/oas.html.
2. Ibid.
3. P. Kittenger and D. Herron, "Patient Power: Over-the-Counter Drugs—Brief Analysis," National Center for Policy Analysis, 2005, www.ncpa.org/pub/ba/ba524.
4. Ibid.
5. L. D. Johnston et al., *Monitoring the Future National Survey Results on Drug Use, 1975–2004: Volume II, College Students and Adults* (NIH Publication No. 05-5727) (Bethesda, MD: National Institute on Drug Abuse, 2005).
6. Ibid.
7. Ibid.
8. M. Fisherman and C. Johanson, "Cocaine," in *Pharmacological Aspects of Drug Dependence: Towards an Integrated Neurobehavior Approach, Handbook of Experimental Pharmacology,* C. Shuster and M. Kuhar, eds. (Hamburg, Germany: Springer-Verlag, 1996): 159–195.
9. Ibid.
10. U.S. Department of Health and Human Services, *Substance Abuse and Mental Health Services Administration, 2004 National Survey on Drug Abuse and Health* (Rockville, MD: Office of Applied Studies, 2005).
11. L. D. Johnston et al., *Monitoring the Future National Survey Results on Drug Use, 1975–2005: Volume I, Secondary School Students* (NIH Publication No. 06-5883) (Bethesda, MD: National Institute on Drug Abuse, 2006).
12. W. Compton et al., "Prevalence of Marijuana Use Disorders in the United States 2001–2002," *Journal of the American Medical Association* 291 (2004): 2114–2121.
13. U.S. Department of Health and Human Services, *Marijuana: Facts for Teens* (NIH Publication No. 04-4037, 2004).
14. Ibid.
15. H. C. Ashton, "Pharmacology and Effects of Cannabis: A Brief Review," *British Journal of Psychiatry* 178 (2001): 101–106.
16. American Academy of Ophthalmology, Medical Library, "The Use of Marijuana in the Treatment of Glaucoma," 2003, www.medem.com.
17. U.S. Department of Health and Human Services, National Institute on Drug Abuse, Research Report, *Marijuana Abuse* (NIH Publication No. 05-3859, 2005).
18. Office of National Drug Control Policy, "Fact Sheet: Heroin," 2002, www.whitehousedrugpolicy.gov/publications/factsht/heroin/index.html.
19. Johnston, *Monitoring the Future National Survey Results on Drug Use, 1975–2004: Volume II.*
20. Johnston, *Monitoring the Future National Survey Results on Drug Use, 1975–2005: Volume I.*
21. National Institute on Drug Abuse (NIDA), "NIDA Launches Initiative to Combat Club Drugs," *NIDA Notes* 14, no. 2 (2000).
22. National Institute on Drug Abuse (NIDA), "Anabolic Steroids" *NIDA for Teens,* 2005, http://teens.drugabuse.gov/drnida/drnida_ster1.asp.
23. National Drug Intelligence Center, "National Drug Threat Assessment, 2006: The Impact of Drugs on Society," 2006, www.usdoj.gov/ndic/pubs11/18862/impact.htm.

24. Office of National Drug Control Policy, "2002 National Drug Control Strategy" 2002, www.whitehousedrugpolicy.gov.

25. U.S. Department of Health and Human Services, *Substance Abuse and Mental Health Services Administration, 2004 National Survey on Drug Abuse and Health* (Rockville, MD: Office of Applied Studies, 2005).

26. U.S. Department of Health and Human Services, "Drugs in the Workplace: What the Employer Needs to Know," 2005, http://dwp.samhsa .gov/DrugTesting/Files_Drug_Testing/FactSheet/factsheet041906 .aspx.

27. Ibid.

15

Cardiovascular Disease

REDUCING YOUR RISK

What's the **difference** between good cholesterol and bad cholesterol?

What's the best way to eat for a **healthy** heart?

Does cardiovascular **disease** run in families?

Can **aspirin** really prevent heart disease?

Does **red wine** really prevent heart disease?

OBJECTIVES

- Discuss the incidence, prevalence, and outcomes of cardiovascular disease in America, including its impact on society.

- Describe the anatomy and physiology of the heart and circulatory system and the importance of healthy heart function.

- Review major types of heart disease, factors that contribute to their development, diagnostic and treatment options, and the importance of lifestyle for prevention.

- Discuss controllable and uncontrollable risk factors for cardiovascular disease, your own risk profile, and determine the risk factors you can and cannot control.

- Discuss methods of diagnosing and treating cardiovascular disease and the importance of being a wise health care consumer.

451

One out of every three adult men and women in the United States has some type of **cardiovascular disease (CVD),** the broad term used to describe diseases of the heart and blood vessels. To put this into perspective, deaths from CVD claim more lives each year than the next four leading causes of death combined (cancer, chronic lower respiratory diseases, accidents, and diabetes), and accounted for nearly 38 percent of all deaths in the United States in 2005.[1] Although we've made considerable advances in battling CVD, it continues to pose a serious threat to the health of all Americans, no matter their age, gender, or race (Figure 15.1). This is not a new phenomenon; since 1900 CVD has been the number-one killer in the United States in every year but one—1918, when a particularly virulent strain of influenza (flu) struck with blinding force. With this exception, CVD deaths continue to rise (Figure 15.2). It is important to note that in 2005 researchers reported that while CVD continued to be the leading cause of death among Americans in all age groups, cancer surpassed CVD as the leading cause of death for the first time for those under the age of 85 (see Chapter 16). In order to better understand the impact of CVD on individuals, families, and health care providers, consider the following:[2]

- Over 2,500 Americans die each day from CVD, or an average of one death every 35 seconds. This totals more than 1.4 million CVD-related deaths annually. Many of these fatalities are **sudden cardiac deaths,** meaning that these Americans die from abrupt, profound loss of heart function (cardiac arrest), either instantly or shortly after symptoms occur.
- Almost 152,000 Americans killed by CVD are under age 65.
- The probability at birth of eventually dying of CVD is 47 percent; of dying from cancer, 22 percent; from accidents, 3 percent; from diabetes, 2 percent; and from HIV, 0.7 percent.
- Among women, 1 in 30 deaths is from breast cancer; 1 in 2.6 is from CVD.
- An estimated 30 percent of non-Hispanic white men and 24 percent of non-Hispanic white women have CVD.
- Among non-Hispanic blacks, about 41 percent of men and 40 percent of women have CVD. The rate of high blood pressure in African Americans is among the highest in the world.
- Among Hispanic Americans, 29 percent of men and 27 percent of women have CVD. They are less likely than

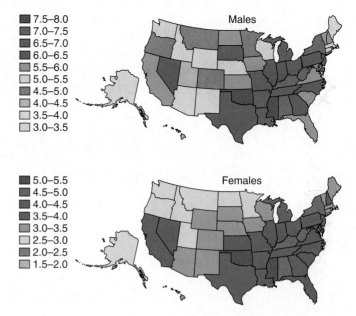

FIGURE 15.1 2001 Total Cardiovascular Disease Death Rates by State and Gender, Age Adjusted

Source: C. Murray et al., "Understanding the Coronary Heart Disease versus Total Cardiovascular Disease Mortality Paradox," *Circulation* 113 (2006): 2071–2081.

other groups to have high blood pressure but also are less likely to be aware of it and to be treated for it.
- Thirty-six percent of American Indians or Alaskan Natives will die prematurely (before age 65) from CVD.
- Adults over age 18 often have more than one risk factor for CVD. Forty-nine percent of African American adults have two or more risks; 38 percent of men and 36 percent of women have multiple risks; 26 percent of college graduates have multiple risk factors, while 53 percent of those who only have a high school diploma have two or more risk factors for CVD.
- In terms of total deaths, in every year since 1984, CVD has claimed the lives of more women than men.

Of the millions of Americans who currently live with one of the major categories of CVD, many do not know they have a serious problem.[3] In spite of major improvements in medication, surgery, and other health care procedures, the prognosis for many of these individuals is not good:[4]

- Twenty-five percent of men and 38 percent of women will die within one year after having an initial heart attack. In part because women have heart attacks at an older age than men do, women are more likely to die from heart attacks within just a few weeks.
- People who survive the acute stages of a heart attack have a chance of illness and death that is 1.5 to 15 times higher than that of the general population, depending on their sex and clinical outcomes. The risk of another heart attack, sudden death, angina pectoris, heart failure, and stroke—for both men and women—is substantial.

cardiovascular disease (CVD) Disease of the heart and blood vessels.

sudden cardiac death Death that occurs as a result of abrupt, profound loss of heart function.

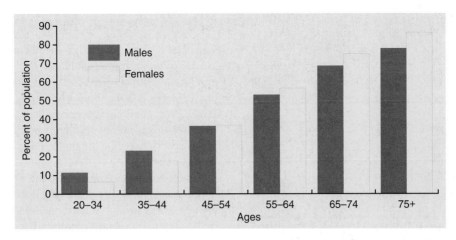

FIGURE 15.2 Prevalence of Cardiovascular Diseases in U.S. Men and Women, Aged 20 and Older

Source: National Center for Health Statistics, "Prevalence of Cardiovascular Diseases in Americans Age 20 and Older by Age and Sex, NHANES 1999–2002," 2006, www.cdc.gov.

- Within six years of a recognized heart attack, 18 percent of men and 35 percent of women will have another heart attack, 7 percent of men and 6 percent of women will experience sudden death, and about 22 percent of men and 46 percent of women will be disabled with heart failure.
- CHD will permanently disable 19 percent of the U.S. labor force.
- Although older adults are at higher risk, CVD is also one of the leading causes of death for children under the age of 15. Increasing numbers of children have congenital heart defects and strokes are a serious problem in babies under one year of age.[5] It is important to recognize that risk factors for CVD increase with age, making early prevention even more critical.

Although it is impossible to place a monetary value on human life, the economic burden of cardiovascular disease on our society is staggering—more than $403 billion estimated for 2006.[6] This figure includes the cost of physician and nursing services, hospital and nursing home services, medications, and lost productivity resulting from disability. As Americans live longer with chronic diseases, costs will continue to increase, resulting in a tremendous burden on the health care system. Although many Americans think that CVD can be cured with a bypass or other surgical procedure, in truth the effects of CVD can be long term and take a toll on patients, their families, individuals, and society. Importantly, CVD is not a uniquely American health problem (Figure 15.3, page 454).

The best defense against CVD is to prevent it from developing in the first place. How can you cut your risk? By taking steps today to reduce your risk factors. Controlling high blood pressure and reducing intake of saturated fats and cholesterol are two examples of things you can do to lower your chances of heart attack. By maintaining your weight, exercis-

ing, decreasing your intake of sodium, not smoking, and changing your lifestyle to reduce stress, you can lower your blood pressure. You can also monitor the levels of fat and cholesterol in your blood and adjust your diet to prevent arteries from becoming blocked. Having combinations of risk factors seems to increase overall risk by a factor greater than those of the combined risks. Happily, the converse is also true: reducing several risk factors can have a dramatic effect. Answer the questions in the Assess Yourself box on pages 456–457 to determine your overall coronary risk. Understanding how your cardiovascular system works will help you understand your risk and how to reduce it.

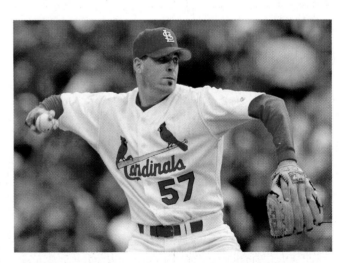

Cardiovascular disease can affect even the youngest and most fit people. Daryl Kile, a 33-year-old professional baseball player, died suddenly from atherosclerosis. It was discovered after his death that two of the main arteries in his heart were 80 to 90 percent blocked. His heart was also enlarged, weighing 20 percent more than normal.

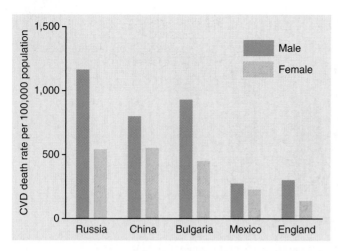

FIGURE 15.3 **Death Rates for Cardiovascular Disease, Including CHD and Stroke, for Selected Countries**

Source: American Heart Association, "International Cardiovascular Disease Statistics, 2005," www.americanheart.org.

Understanding the Cardiovascular System

The **cardiovascular system** is the network of organs and elastic tubes through which blood flows as it carries oxygen and nutrients to all parts of the body and removes waste. It includes the *heart, arteries, arterioles* (small arteries), and *capillaries* (minute blood vessels). It also includes *venules* (small veins) and *veins,* the blood vessels through which blood flows as it returns to the heart and lungs.

cardiovascular system A complex system consisting of the heart and blood vessels that transports nutrients, oxygen, hormones, metabolic wastes, and enzymes throughout the body and regulates temperature, the water levels of cells, and the acidity levels of body components.

atria The two upper chambers of the heart, which receive blood.

ventricles The two lower chambers of the heart, which pump blood through the blood vessels.

arteries Vessels that carry blood away from the heart to other regions of the body.

arterioles Branches of the arteries.

capillaries Minute blood vessels that branch out from the arterioles; their thin walls allow for the exchange of oxygen, carbon dioxide, nutrients, and waste products among body cells.

The Heart: A Mighty Machine

The heart is a muscular, four-chambered pump, roughly the size of your fist. It is a highly efficient, extremely flexible organ that contracts 100,000 times each day, pumping the equivalent of 2,000 gallons of blood to all areas of the body. In a 70-year lifetime, an average human heart beats 2.5 billion times. This number is significantly higher for those who are overweight and out of shape, requiring their heart to work harder.

Under normal circumstances, the human body contains approximately 6 quarts of blood. Blood transports nutrients, oxygen, waste products, hormones, and enzymes throughout the body. Blood also regulates body temperature, cellular water levels, and acidity levels of body components and aids in bodily defense against toxins and harmful microorganisms. An adequate blood supply is essential to health and well-being.

The heart's four chambers work together to recirculate blood constantly throughout the body (Figure 15.4). The two upper chambers of the heart, called **atria** or *auricles,* are large collecting chambers that receive blood from the rest of the body. The two lower chambers, known as **ventricles,** pump the blood out again. Small valves regulate the steady, rhythmic flow of blood between chambers and prevent inappropriate backwash. The *tricuspid valve* (located between the right atrium and the right ventricle), the *pulmonary valve* (between the right ventricle and the pulmonary artery), the *mitral valve* (between the left atrium and left ventricle), and the *aortic valve* (between the left ventricle and the aorta) permit blood to flow in only one direction.

Heart Function Heart activity depends on a complex interaction of biochemical, physical, and neurological signals. Here are the basic steps involved in heart function:

1. Deoxygenated blood enters the right atrium after having been circulated through the body.

2. From the right atrium, blood moves to the right ventricle and is pumped through the pulmonary artery to the lungs, where it receives oxygen.

3. Oxygenated blood from the lungs then returns to the left atrium of the heart.

4. Blood from the left atrium is forced into the left ventricle.

5. The left ventricle pumps blood through the aorta to all body parts.

Various types of blood vessels are required for different parts of this process. **Arteries** carry blood away from the heart; most arteries transport oxygenated blood, but the pulmonary arteries carry deoxygenated blood to the lungs, where it picks up oxygen and gives off carbon dioxide. As the arteries branch off from the heart, they divide into smaller blood vessels called **arterioles,** and then into even smaller blood vessels known as **capillaries.** Capillaries have thin walls that permit the

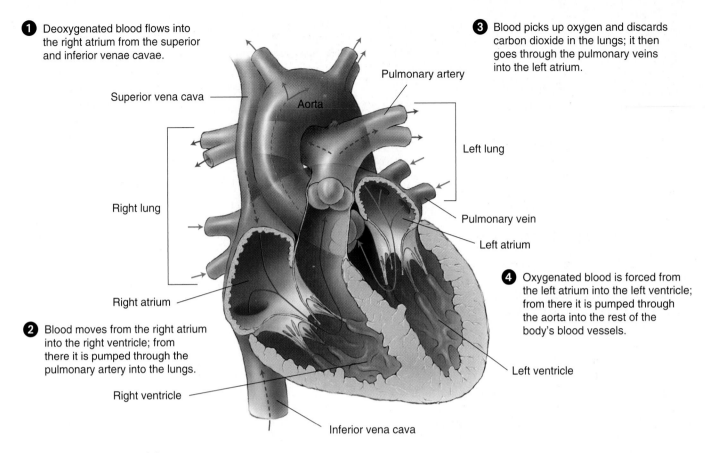

1 Deoxygenated blood flows into the right atrium from the superior and inferior venae cavae.

3 Blood picks up oxygen and discards carbon dioxide in the lungs; it then goes through the pulmonary veins into the left atrium.

Superior vena cava

Aorta

Pulmonary artery

Right lung

Left lung

Pulmonary vein

Left atrium

Right atrium

4 Oxygenated blood is forced from the left atrium into the left ventricle; from there it is pumped through the aorta into the rest of the body's blood vessels.

2 Blood moves from the right atrium into the right ventricle; from there it is pumped through the pulmonary artery into the lungs.

Right ventricle

Left ventricle

Inferior vena cava

FIGURE 15.4 Anatomy of the Heart

exchange of oxygen, carbon dioxide, nutrients, and waste products with body cells. The carbon dioxide and waste products are transported to the lungs and kidneys through **veins** and **venules** (small veins).

For the heart to function properly, the four chambers must beat in an organized manner. Your heartbeat is governed by an electrical impulse that directs the heart muscle to move when the impulse moves across it, which results in a sequential contraction of the four chambers. This signal starts in a small bundle of highly specialized cells, the **sinoatrial node (SA node),** located in the right atrium. The SA node serves as a natural pacemaker for the heart. People with a damaged SA node (either a congenital defect or one injured by disease) must often have a mechanical pacemaker implanted to ensure the smooth passage of blood through the sequential phases of the heartbeat.

The average adult heart at rest beats 70 to 80 times per minute, although a well-conditioned heart may beat only 50 to 60 times per minute to achieve the same results. When overly stressed, a heart may beat over 200 times per minute, particularly in an individual who is overweight or out of shape. A healthy heart functions more efficiently and is less likely to suffer damage from overwork.

Types of Cardiovascular Disease

There are several types of cardiovascular disease (see Figure 15.5 on page 458):

- Atherosclerosis (fatty plaque buildup in arteries)
- Coronary heart disease (CHD)
- Chest pain (angina pectoris)
- Irregular heartbeat (arrhythmia)
- Congestive heart failure (CHF)
- Congenital and rheumatic heart disease
- Stroke (cerebrovascular accident)

Prevention and treatment of these diseases range from changes in diet and lifestyle to medications and surgery.

(Text continues on page 458)

veins Vessels that carry blood back to the heart from other regions of the body.

venules Branches of the veins.

sinoatrial node (SA node) Cluster of electric-generating cells that serves as a form of natural pacemaker for the heart.

ASSESS yourself

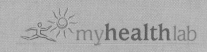

UNDERSTANDING YOUR CVD RISK

Fill out this assessment online at
www.aw-bc.com/myhealthlab or
www.aw-bc.com/donatelle.

Each of us has a unique level of risk for various diseases. Some of these risks are things you can take action to change; others are risks that you need to consider as you plan a life-long strategy for overall risk reduction. Complete each of the following questions and total your points in each section. If you score between 1 and 5 in any section, consider your risk. The higher the number, the greater your risk. If you answered "don't know" for any question, talk to your parents or other family members as soon as possible to find out if you have any unknown risks.

PART I: ASSESS YOUR FAMILY RISK FOR CVD

	Yes (1 point)	No (0 points)	Don't Know
1. Do any of your primary relatives (mother, father, grandparents, siblings) have a history of heart disease or stroke?	❑	❑	❑
2. Do any of your primary relatives (mother, father, grandparents, siblings) have diabetes?	❑	❑	❑
3. Do any of your primary relatives (mother, father, grandparents, siblings) have high blood pressure?	❑	❑	❑
4. Do any of your primary relatives (mother, father, grandparents, siblings) have a history of high cholesterol?	❑	❑	❑
5. Would you say that your family consumed a high-fat diet (lots of red meat, dairy, butter/margarine) during your time spent at home?	❑	❑	❑

Total points _____

PART II: ASSESS YOUR LIFESTYLE RISK FOR CVD

	Yes	No	Don't Know
1. Is your total cholesterol level higher than it should be?	❑	❑	❑
2. Do you have high blood pressure?	❑	❑	❑
3. Have you been diagnosed as prediabetic or diabetic?	❑	❑	❑
4. Do you smoke?	❑	❑	❑
5. Would you describe your life as being highly stressful?	❑	❑	❑

Total points _____

PART III: ASSESS YOUR ADDITIONAL RISKS FOR CVD

1. How would you best describe your current weight?
   a. Lower than what it should be for my height and weight (0 points)
   b. About what it should be for my height and weight (0 points)
   c. Higher than it should be for my height and weight (1 point)
2. How would you describe the level of exercise that you get each day?
   a. Less than what I should be exercising each day (1 point)
   b. About what I should be exercising each day (0 points)
   c. More than what I should be exercising each day (0 points)
3. How would you describe your dietary behaviors?
   a. Eating only the recommended number of calories/day (0 points)
   b. Eating less than the recommended number of calories each day (0 points)
   c. Eating more than the recommended number of calories each day (1 point)

4. Which of the following best describes your typical dietary behavior?
   a. I eat from the major food groups, trying hard to get the recommended fruits and vegetables. (0 points)
   b. I eat too much red meat and consume much saturated fat from meats and dairy products each day. (1 point)
   c. Whenever possible, I try to substitute olive oil or canola oil for other forms of dietary fat. (0 points)
5. Which of the following best describes you?
   a. I watch my sodium intake and try to reduce stress in my life. (0 points)
   b. I have a history of chlamydia infection. (1 point)
   c. I try to eat 5 to 10 milligrams of soluble fiber each day and to substitute a soy product for an animal product in my diet at least once each week. (0 points)

Total points _____

MAKE it happen!

ASSESSMENT: The Assess Yourself activity evaluates your risk of heart disease and the status of your LDL cholesterol. Based on your results and the advice of your physician, you may need to reduce your cholesterol level and risk of CVD.

MAKING A CHANGE: In order to change your behavior, you need to develop a plan. Follow the steps below and complete your Behavior Change Contract to take action.

1. Evaluate your behavior and identify patterns and specific things you are doing. What can you change now? What can you change in the near future?

2. Select one pattern of behavior that you want to change.

3. Fill out the Behavior Change Contract found at the front of your book. It should include your long-term goal for change, your short-term goals, the rewards you'll give yourself for reaching these goals, potential obstacles along the way, and strategies for overcoming these obstacles. For each goal, list the small steps and specific actions that you will take.

4. Chart your progress in a journal. At the end of a week, consider how successful you were in following your plan. What helped you be successful? What made change more difficult? What will you do differently next week?

5. Revise your plan as needed: Are the short-term goals attainable? Are the rewards satisfying?

ONE STUDENT'S PLAN: Nathan knew that his father had a history of heart disease, so he knew it was important to monitor his own risk. Using the results from his most recent checkup, he completed the self-assessment. Although his initial score for ten-year risk of heart attack (in step 1 of the assessment) was less than 10 percent, the combination of two major coronary risk factors (high systolic blood pressure and family history of CVD) with an LDL level of 140 showed in step 2 of the assessment that he needed to start making some lifestyle changes. At 6 feet in height, he weighed 220 pounds, which he discovered is close to obese according to the Body Mass Index calculations. He decided to manage his weight through exercise and improved eating habits. He also expected a modified diet would help lower his cholesterol levels.

Nathan's first step was to keep track of everything he normally ate for a week. When he analyzed his food journal, he saw that he rarely ate breakfast, which made him more likely to grab a doughnut later in the morning and eat a big lunch. He bought some whole-wheat, high-fiber cereal and skim milk and started getting up 15 minutes earlier so he had time to eat his healthy breakfast. For the days when he didn't feel like eating cold cereal, he bought some five-minute oatmeal that also had healthy fiber and nutrients and had been shown to lower LDL levels. Nathan found that he was not as tempted by the doughnuts and other unhealthy snacks during the day, and that he didn't overeat as much at lunch. He even had more energy during the day. As he started to lose weight, he felt more able to begin a moderate exercise program. All of these changes—losing weight, eating more fiber and less fat, and adding some exercise to his life—made Nathan confident that his next checkup with his doctor would show a lower LDL level and, perhaps, lower blood pressure. When Nathan is in a healthier range on these measures, he plans to buy himself a new DVD player.

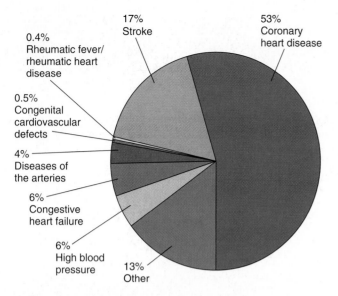

FIGURE 15.5 Percentage Breakdown of Deaths from Cardiovascular Disease in the United States

Source: American Heart Association, *Heart Disease and Stroke Statistics—2006* (Dallas, TX: American Heart Association, 2006). © 2006 American Heart Association. Reproduced with permission. www.americanheart.org.

Atherosclerosis

Arteriosclerosis is a condition that underlies many cardiovascular health problems, and is believed to be the biggest contributor to disease burden globally. **Atherosclerosis** is actually a type of arteriosclerosis and is characterized by deposits of fatty substances, cholesterol, cellular waste products, calcium, and fibrin (a clotting material in the blood) in the inner lining of the artery. **Hyperlipidemia** (an abnormally high blood lipid level) is a key factor in this process, and the resulting buildup is referred to as **plaque.**[7]

Often, atherosclerosis is called *coronary artery disease (CAD)* because of the resultant damage done to coronary arteries. According to current thinking, four factors are responsible for this damage: inflammation, elevated levels of cholesterol and triglycerides in the blood, high blood pressure, and tobacco smoke.[8]

arteriosclerosis   A general term for thickening and hardening of the arteries.

atherosclerosis (coronary artery disease)   Condition characterized by deposits of fatty substances, cholesterol, cellular waste products, calcium, and fibrin in the inner lining of an artery.

hyperlipidemia   Elevated levels of lipids in the blood.

plaque   Buildup of deposits in the arteries.

metabolic syndrome   A group of three or more characteristics, including waist circumference and blood pressure, that can cause metabolic problems that raise CVD risk.

Early Theories   Initially, it was thought that plaque developed in response to injury and tended to collect at sites of injury. Many scientists believed that the process of plaque buildup began because the protective inner lining of the artery (*endothelium*) became damaged, and fats, cholesterol, and other substances in the blood tend to aggregate in these damaged areas. High blood pressure surges, elevated cholesterol and triglyceride levels in the blood, and cigarette smoking were the main suspects in having caused this injury to artery walls. As a result of national campaigns aimed at reducing dietary fat, millions of people cut down on animal fat and dairy products. However, despite massive lifestyle changes and the use of cholesterol-lowering drugs, cardiovascular diseases continue to be the leading cause of death in the United States, Europe, and most of Asia.[9]

Inflammatory Risks   Today, scientists are beginning to look for other factors in the formation of atherosclerotic lesions. New research has led many experts to believe that atherosclerosis is an *inflammatory* disease and that inflamed vessels are more prone to plaque formation.[10] What causes this inflammation in arterial walls? Though researchers aren't sure, there is evidence that a pathogen may be at the root of it. The most likely culprits are *Chlamydia pneumoniae* (a sexually transmitted infection), *Helicobacter pylori* (which causes stomach ulcers), *herpes simplex virus* (a virus to which the majority of Americans have been exposed by age five), and *cytomegalovirus* (another herpesvirus transmitted through body fluids and infecting most Americans before the age of 40). Clearly, if findings about these viruses hold up, there will be yet another good reason to avoid unprotected sex.

During an inflammatory reaction, *C-reactive proteins (CRPs)* tend to be present at high levels. Many scientists believe the presence of these proteins may signal elevated risk for angina and heart attack. Doctors could opt to test patients using a highly sensitive assay (hs-CRP); if levels are high, action could be taken to prevent progression to a heart attack or other coronary event. In the near future, hs-CRP tests might be given as routinely as cholesterol screening tests for heart disease.

Other possible causes of inflammation include elevated low-density lipoproteins, free radicals caused by cigarette smoking, high blood pressure, diabetes mellitus, and the amino acid homocysteine (see the New Horizons in Health box on page 460).

In an effort to combat the effects of inflammation, an explosive amount of research is being published to assess the potential role of anti-inflammatory drugs, such as aspirin, ibuprofen, statins, and a new generation of "super-aspirins."[11]

Metabolic Syndrome   A group of obesity related health risk factors, **metabolic syndrome** dramatically increases the risk of heart disease and diabetes. Also known as Syndrome X or MetS, metabolic syndrome is believed to increase the risk for atherosclerotic cardiovascular disease by as much as threefold. Affecting over 26 percent of adults or

50 million people, this disease has gained increasing attention in the last 2 to 3 years worldwide.[12]

How does one develop MetS? Weight gain, particularly in the abdominal area, and insulin resistance are two of the main characteristics of metabolic syndrome. Insulin resistance is not clearly understood, but it means cells don't work properly in handling blood glucose levels. High blood pressure is also a common feature of metabolic syndrome. Today, scientists indicate that when there are three or more of the following, the diagnosis is metabolic syndrome:

- Abdominal obesity (waist measurement of more than 40 inches in men or 35 in women)
- Elevated blood fat (triglycerides greater than 150)
- Low levels of "good" high-density lipoprotein cholesterol (HDL): less than 40 in men and less than 50 in women
- Elevated blood pressure greater than 130/85
- Elevated fasting glucose greater than 100 mg/dl (a sign of insulin resistance)

For those who have an increased risk for insulin resistance, criteria for diagnosis may be a bit lower.[13]

Coronary Heart Disease

Of all the major cardiovascular diseases, coronary heart disease (CHD) is the greatest killer. In fact, this year well over 1,200,000 people will suffer a heart attack, and over 40 percent of them will die.[14] Those of you raised on a weekly dose of TV doctor programs will recognize *code blue* as the term for a **myocardial infarction (MI),** or **heart attack.** A heart attack involves an area of the heart that suffers permanent damage because its normal blood supply has been blocked. This condition is often brought on by a **coronary thrombosis,** or blood clot in the coronary artery, or through an atherosclerotic narrowing that blocks an artery. When a blood clot, or **thrombus,** becomes dislodged and moves through the circulatory system, it is called an **embolus.** When blood does not flow readily, there is a corresponding decrease in oxygen flow. If the blockage is extremely minor, an otherwise healthy heart will adapt over time by enlarging existing blood vessels and growing new ones (in a process known as *angiogenesis*) to reroute needed blood through other areas. This system, known as **collateral circulation,** is a form of self-preservation that allows an affected heart muscle to cope with the damage.

When heart blockage is more severe, however, the body is unable to adapt on its own, and outside lifesaving support is critical. The hour following a heart attack is the most crucial period—over 40 percent of heart attack victims die within this time. See the Skills for Behavior Change box on page 461 to learn what to do in case of a heart attack.

Sudden death from cardiac arrest can occur within minutes, when the heart's electrical impulses become rapid (*ventricular tachycardia*) and then chaotic (*ventricular fibrillation,* or *VF*). Portable defibrillators, CPR, and other emergency techniques can save lives.

Although young adults can also succumb to cardiac arrest, abnormalities of the heart are the most likely cause of cardiac death in this age group. Under certain conditions, various

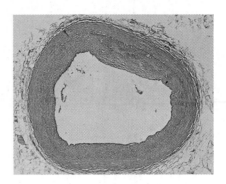

(a)

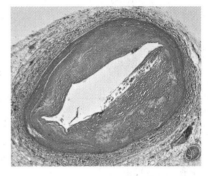

(b)

(a) Cross section of a normal coronary artery. **(b)** A coronary artery narrowed by plaque.

heart medications, other prescription drugs, or illicit drugs can lead to abnormal heart rhythms that cause cardiac arrest or death. Respiratory arrest caused by asthma, electrocution, high blood pressure, drowning, choking, and trauma are other potential causes.

 what do you THINK?

What risk factors might typical college-aged students have for plaque formation? ■ What information should new CVD prevention guidelines include if the new theories discussed in this section prove true?

myocardial infarction (MI)   Heart attack.

heart attack   A blockage of normal blood supply to an area in the heart.

coronary thrombosis   A blood clot occurring in the coronary artery.

thrombus   Blood clot attached to the wall of a blood vessel.

embolus   A blood clot that becomes dislodged from a blood vessel wall and moves through the circulatory system.

collateral circulation   Adaptation of the heart to partial damage accomplished by rerouting needed blood through unused or underused blood vessels while the damaged heart muscle heals.

Is it time to forget the cholesterol and fat in your diet altogether and focus on other risks? No. However, researchers are investigating new factors that may contribute to CVD risk as much as that juicy steak or high-fat ice cream.

Like C-reactive protein (CRP) and inflammation, researchers have discovered another substance that may signal increased risk for CVD. Recent studies indicate that *homocysteine,* an amino acid normally present in the blood, may be related to higher risk of coronary heart disease, stroke, and other vascular disease when present at high levels. In fact, it is theorized that homocysteine may work in much the same way as CRP, inflaming the inner lining of arteries and promoting fat deposits on the damaged walls and development of blood clots.

Folic acid and other B vitamins such as B_6 and B_{12} may help break down homocysteine in the body; many scientists are currently assessing the precise role of high homocysteine levels in increasing CVD risk, and the role folic acid and B vitamins might play in reducing the risk. Because conclusive evidence of risk reduction from folic acid is not available, authorities such as the American Heart Association do not recommend taking folic acid supplements to lower homocysteine levels and prevent CVD. For now, a healthy, balanced diet that includes at least five servings of fruits and vegetables a day is the best preventive action. Citrus fruit, tomatoes, vegetables, and grain products that are fortified with folic acid are good sources of the daily recommended 400 micrograms.

Sources: American Heart Association, "Homocysteine, Folic Acid, and Cardiovascular Disease,"2006, www.americanheart.org; F. Sofi et al., "Dietary Habits, Lifestyles, and Cardiovascular Risk Factors in a Clinically Healthy Italian Population," *European Journal of Clinical Nutrition* 59, no. 5 (2005) 731; J. K. Victanen et al., "Homocysteine as a Risk Factor for CVD Mortality in Men with Other CVD Risk Factors: The Kuopio Ischemic Heart Risk Factor (KIHF) Study," *Journal of Internal Medicine* 257, no. 3 (2005): 209–317.

Angina Pectoris

Atherosclerosis and other circulatory impairments often reduce the heart's blood and oxygen supply, a condition known as **ischemia.** People with ischemia often suffer from varying degrees of **angina pectoris,** or chest pain. In fact, an estimated 2.6 million men and 4.2 million women suffer mild to crushing forms of chest pain each day.[15] Many people experience short episodes of angina during physical exertion. Symptoms may range from slight indigestion to a feeling that the heart is being crushed. Generally, the more serious the oxygen deprivation, the more severe the pain. Although angina pectoris is not a heart attack, it does indicate underlying heart disease.

Currently, there are several methods of treating angina. In mild cases, rest is critical. The most common treatments for more severe cases involve using drugs that affect (1) the supply of blood to the heart muscle or (2) the heart's demand for oxygen. Pain and discomfort are often relieved with *nitroglycerin,* a drug used to relax (dilate) veins, thereby reducing the amount of blood returning to the heart and thus lessening its workload. Patients whose angina is caused by spasms of the coronary arteries are often given drugs called *calcium channel blockers,* drugs that prevent calcium atoms from passing through coronary arteries and causing heart contractions. They also appear to reduce blood pressure and slow heart rate. *Beta blockers,* the other major type of drugs used to treat angina, control potential overactivity of the heart muscle.

Arrhythmias

Over 4 million Americans experience some type of **arrhythmia,** an irregularity in heart rhythm; about 480,400 of these cases result in death.[16] A person who complains of a racing heart in the absence of exercise or anxiety may be experiencing *tachycardia,* the medical term for abnormally fast heartbeat. On the other end of the continuum is *bradycardia,* or abnormally slow heartbeat. When a heart goes into **fibrillation** of either the atrial or ventricular regions of the heart, it beats in a sporadic, quivering pattern, resulting in extreme inefficiency in moving blood through the cardiovascular system. If untreated, fibrillation may be fatal.

Not all arrhythmias are life-threatening. In many instances, excessive caffeine or nicotine consumption can trigger an arrhythmia episode. However, severe cases may require drug therapy or external electrical stimulus to prevent serious complications.

ischemia Reduced oxygen supply to a body organ or part.

angina pectoris Chest pain occurring as a result of reduced oxygen flow to the heart.

arrhythmia An irregularity in heartbeat.

fibrillation A sporadic, quivering pattern of heartbeat, resulting in extreme inefficiency in moving blood through the cardiovascular system.

SKILLS FOR behavior change

WHAT TO DO IN THE EVENT OF A HEART ATTACK

B ecause heart attacks are so frightening, we would prefer not to think about them. However, knowing how to act in an emergency could save your life or that of somebody else.

KNOW THE WARNING SIGNS OF A HEART ATTACK

- Uncomfortable pressure, fullness, squeezing, or pain in the center of the chest, lasting two minutes or longer
- Jaw pain and/or shortness of breath
- Pain spreading to the shoulders, neck, or arms
- Dizziness, fatigue, fainting, sweating, and/or nausea

Not all these warning signs occur in every heart attack. For instance, women's heart attacks tend to show up as shortness of breath, fatigue, and jaw pain, stretched

out over hours rather than minutes. If any of these symptoms do appear, however, don't wait. Get help immediately!

KNOW WHAT TO DO IN AN EMERGENCY

- Find out which hospitals in your area have 24-hour emergency cardiac care.
- Determine (in advance) the hospital or medical facility that's nearest your home and office, and tell your family and friends to call this facility in an emergency.
- Keep a list of emergency rescue service numbers next to your telephone and in your pocket, wallet, or purse. Be aware of whether your local area has a 911 emergency service.
- If you have chest or jaw discomfort that lasts more than two minutes, call the emergency rescue service. Do not drive yourself to the hospital.

BE A HEART SAVER

- If you're with someone who is showing signs of a heart attack and the warning signs last for two minutes or longer, act immediately.
- Expect a denial. It's normal for someone to deny the possibility of anything as serious as a heart attack. Don't take no for an answer, however. Insist on taking prompt action.
- Call the emergency rescue service, or get to the nearest hospital emergency room that offers 24-hour emergency cardiac care.
- Give CPR (mouth-to-mouth breathing and chest compression) if it's necessary and if you're properly trained.

Source: American Heart Association, *Heart Disease and Stroke Facts* (Dallas, TX: American Heart Association, 2006), www.americanheart.org.

Congestive Heart Failure

When the heart muscle is damaged or overworked and lacks the strength to keep blood circulating normally through the body, its chambers are often taxed to the limit. **Congestive heart failure (CHF)** affects over 5 million Americans and dramatically increases risk of premature death.[17] The heart muscle may be injured by a number of health conditions, including rheumatic fever, pneumonia, heart attack, or other cardiovascular problems. In some cases, the damage is due to radiation or chemotherapy treatments for cancer. These weakened muscles respond poorly, impairing blood flow out of the heart through the arteries. The return flow of blood through the veins begins to back up, causing congestion in body tissues. This pooling of blood enlarges the heart, makes it less efficient, and decreases the amount of blood that can be circulated. Fluid begins to accumulate in other body areas, such as the vessels in the legs, ankles, or lungs, causing swelling or difficulty in breathing.

Today, CHF is the single most frequent cause of hospitalization in the United States.[18] If untreated, congestive heart failure can be fatal. However, most cases respond well to treatment that includes *diuretics* (water pills) to relieve fluid accumulation; drugs, such as *digitalis*, that increase the

pumping action of the heart; and drugs called *vasodilators* that expand blood vessels and decrease resistance, allowing blood to flow more easily and making the heart's work easier.

Congenital and Rheumatic Heart Disease

Approximately 1 out of every 125 children is born with some form of **congenital heart disease** (disease present at birth).[19] These forms may be relatively minor, such as slight *murmurs* (low-pitched sounds caused by turbulent blood flow through the heart or problematic heart valve action) resulting from valve irregularities that some children outgrow. Other

---

congestive heart failure (CHF)   An abnormal cardiovascular condition that reflects impaired cardiac pumping and blood flow; pooling blood leads to congestion in body tissues.

congenital heart disease   Heart disease that is present at birth.

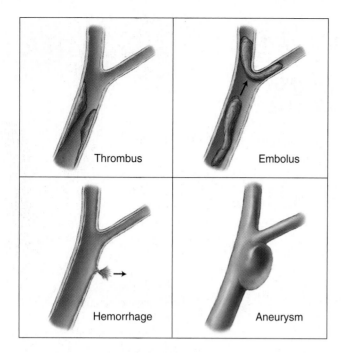

FIGURE 15.6 Common Blood Vessel Disorders

congenital problems involve serious complications in heart function that can be corrected only with surgery. Their underlying causes are unknown but may be related to hereditary factors; maternal diseases, such as rubella, that occurred during fetal development; or chemical intake (particularly alcohol) by the mother during pregnancy. Because of advances in pediatric cardiology, the prognosis for children with congenital heart defects is better than ever before.

Rheumatic heart disease can cause similar heart problems in children. It is attributed to rheumatic fever, an inflammatory disease that may affect many connective tissues of the body, especially those of the heart, joints, brain, or skin, and which is caused by an unresolved *streptococcal infection* of the throat (strep throat). In a small number of cases, this infection can lead to an immune response in which antibodies attack the heart as well as the bacteria. Many of the 82,000 annual operations on heart valves in the United States (at an average cost of $85,000 each) are related to rheumatic heart disease.[20]

rheumatic heart disease A heart disease caused by untreated streptococcal infection of the throat.

stroke A condition occurring when the brain is damaged by disrupted blood supply.

aneurysm A weakened blood vessel that may bulge under pressure and, in severe cases, burst.

transient ischemic attacks (TIAs) Brief interruptions of the blood supply to the brain that cause only temporary impairment; often an indicator of impending major stroke.

Stroke

Like heart muscle, brain cells must have a continuous adequate supply of oxygen in order to survive. A **stroke** (also called a *cerebrovascular accident*) occurs when the blood supply to the brain is interrupted. Strokes may be caused by a thrombus (a clot in a blood vessel), an embolus (a clot that has broken off from a blood vessel wall and is floating in the bloodstream), or an **aneurysm** (a weakening in a blood vessel that causes it to bulge and, in severe cases, to burst). Figure 15.6 illustrates these blood vessel disorders. When any of these events occurs, oxygen deprivation kills brain cells, which do not have the capacity to heal or regenerate. Some strokes are mild and cause only temporary dizziness or slight weakness or numbness. More serious interruptions in blood flow may cause speech impairments, memory problems, and loss of motor control.

Other strokes affect parts of the brain that regulate heart and lung function and kill within minutes. Stroke killed 157,000 Americans in 2003 and accounted for 1 in 15 deaths, surpassed only by CHD and cancer. Each year, about 700,000 people experience a new or recurrent stroke, which averages out to one person suffering a stroke every 45 seconds, and one person dying as a result every 3 minutes.[21]

About one in ten major strokes is preceded days, weeks, or months earlier by **transient ischemic attacks (TIAs),** brief interruptions of the blood supply to the brain that cause only temporary impairment. Symptoms of TIAs include dizziness, particularly at first rising in the morning, weakness, temporary paralysis or numbness in the face or other regions, temporary memory loss, blurred vision, nausea, headache, slurred speech, or other unusual physiological reactions. TIAs are often indications of an impending major stroke.

Warning signs of stroke include:

- Sudden weakness or numbness of the face, arm, or leg on one side of the body
- Sudden dimness or loss of vision, particularly in only one eye
- Loss of speech or trouble talking or understanding speech
- Sudden, severe headaches with no known cause
- Unexplained dizziness, unsteadiness, or sudden falls, especially with any of the previously listed symptoms

If you experience any of these symptoms, or if you are with someone who does, seek medical help *immediately.* The earlier treatment starts, the more effective it will be.

One of the greatest medical successes in recent years has been the decline in the fatality rate from strokes, a rate that has dropped by one-third in the United States since the 1980s and continues to fall. Improved diagnostic procedures, better surgical options, clot-busting drugs injected soon after a stroke has occurred, and acute care centers specializing in stroke treatment and rehabilitation have all been factors. Increased awareness of risk factors for stroke, especially high blood pressure, knowledge of warning signals, and an emphasis on prevention also have contributed. It is estimated that more than half of all remaining strokes could be avoided if more people followed the recommended preventive standards.

Unfortunately, those who survive a stroke do not always make a full recovery. Some 50 to 70 percent of stroke survivors regain functional independence, while 15 to 30 percent are permanently disabled and require assistance. Today, stroke is a leading cause of serious long-term disability and contributes a significant amount to Medicaid and Medicare expenses for older Americans.[22]

Reducing Your Risk for Cardiovascular Disease

What is your own risk for heart disease? Factors that increase the risk for cardiovascular problems fall into two categories: those we can control and those we cannot. Fortunately, we can take steps to minimize many risk factors.

Risks You Can Control

Avoid Tobacco As early as 1964, the Surgeon General of the United States asserted that smoking was the greatest risk factor for heart disease. Today, more than one in five deaths from CVD are directly related to smoking. The risk for cardiovascular disease is 70 percent greater for smokers than for nonsmokers. Smokers who have a heart attack are more likely to die suddenly (within one hour) than are nonsmokers. Evidence also indicates that chronic exposure to environmental tobacco smoke (ETS or secondhand smoke) increases the risk of heart disease by as much as 30 percent.[23]

How does smoking damage the heart? There are two plausible explanations. One theory is that nicotine increases heart rate, heart output, blood pressure, and oxygen use by heart muscles. Because the carbon monoxide in cigarette smoke displaces oxygen in heart tissue, the heart is forced to work harder to obtain sufficient oxygen. The other theory states that chemicals in smoke damage the lining of the coronary arteries and cause inflammation, allowing cholesterol and plaque to accumulate more easily. This additional buildup constricts the vessels, increasing blood pressure and causing the heart to work harder.

When people stop smoking, regardless of how long or how much they've smoked, their risk of heart disease declines rapidly.[24] Although the exact reasons are unknown, new findings from the Lung Health Study indicate that women have greater lung function improvements than their male counterparts after sustained smoking cessation.[25]

Cut Back on Saturated Fat and Cholesterol

How concerned should you be about the type of fat and amount of fat and cholesterol in your diet? Very concerned. According to recent evidence, cholesterol risks may be greater than ever for Americans. When dietary experts from

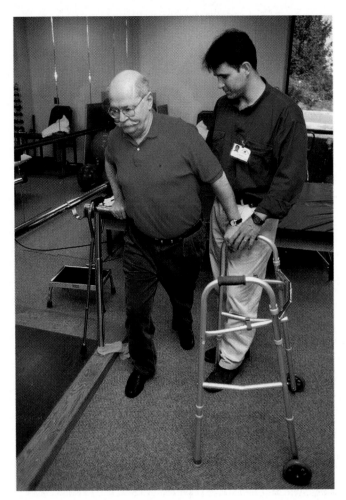

Recovery after a stroke can be a long process, often requiring therapy to improve speech and mobility.

the National Heart, Lung, and Blood Institute met to prepare the *Third Report of the National Cholesterol Education Program Expert Panel on Detection, Evaluation, and Treatment of High Blood Cholesterol in Adults,* they gave Americans a wake-up call by drastically reducing the levels of cholesterol that are considered acceptable. These guidelines not only show that cholesterol levels are out of control in the United States, but also indicate that the number of people who need cholesterol-cutting drugs may be three times what was originally thought. In fact, nearly 36 million people in the United States—one-fifth of all adults—may require medications to avoid cardiovascular problems.[26]

Why all the fuss about fats and cholesterol? Diets high in saturated fat are known to raise cholesterol levels, send the body's blood-clotting system into high gear, and make the blood more viscous in just a few hours, increasing the risk of heart attack or stroke. Studies indicate that fatty foods apparently trigger production of *factor VII,* a blood-clotting substance. Switching to a low-fat diet lowers the risk of clotting.[27]

A fatty diet also increases the amount of cholesterol in the blood, contributing to atherosclerosis. In past years,

TABLE 15.1

TABLE 15.1 — Classification of LDL, Total, and HDL Cholesterol (mg/dl) and Recommended Levels for Adults

LDL Cholesterol

<100	Optimal
100–129	Near optimal/above optimal
130–159	Borderline High
160–189	High
=190	Very high

Total Cholesterol

<200	Desirable
200–239	Borderline high
=240	High

HDL Cholesterol

<40	Low
=60	High

Triglycerides

<150	Normal
150–199	Borderline high
200–499	High
=500	Very high

Source: National Heart, Lung, and Blood Institute, *Third Report of the Expert Panel on Detection, Evaluation, and Treatment of High Blood Cholesterol in Adults* (NIH Publication No. 05-3290), 2005, www.nhlbi.nih.gov/health/public/heart/chol.wyntk.htm.

cholesterol levels between 200 to 240 milligrams per 100 milliliters of blood (mg/ml) were considered normal. Recent research indicates that levels between 180 and 200 mg/ml are more desirable and that 150 mg/ml levels would be even better to reduce CVD risks. People with multiple risk factors for CVD are advised to follow even more stringent guidelines.[28] See Table 15.1 for recommendations.

However, it isn't just the total cholesterol level that you should be concerned about. Cholesterol comes in two main

low-density lipoproteins (LDLs) Compounds that facilitate the transport of cholesterol in the blood to the body's cells, and cause the cholesterol to build up on artery walls.

high-density lipoproteins (HDLs) Compounds that facilitate the transport of cholesterol in the blood to the liver for metabolism and elimination from the body.

triglycerides The most common form of fat in the body; excess calories are converted into triglycerides and stored as body fat.

What's the difference between good cholesterol and bad cholesterol?

varieties: **low-density lipoprotein (LDL)** and **high-density lipoprotein (HDL).** Low-density lipoprotein, often referred to as "bad" cholesterol, is believed to build up on artery walls. In contrast, high-density lipoprotein, or "good" cholesterol, appears to remove cholesterol from artery walls, and transports it to the liver for metabolism and elimination from the body. In theory, if LDL levels get too high or HDL levels too low—largely because of too much saturated fat in the diet, a lack of physical exercise, high stress levels, or genetic predisposition—cholesterol will accumulate inside arteries and lead to cardiovascular problems. Scientists now believe that there are other factors that may also increase CVD risk. A component of HDL known as Lp(a) may be the most important element of the HDL makeup. Lp(a), a lipoprotein, plays an important role in plaque accumulation and increased risk for stroke and coronary events, particularly in males. The higher the Lp(a) level, the higher the risk.[29]

The goal is to manage the ratio of HDL to total cholesterol by lowering LDL levels, raising HDL, or both. Regular exercise and a healthy diet low in saturated fat continue to be the best methods for maintaining healthy ratios. However, if dietary efforts and exercise do not reduce total cholesterol or LDL, several medications are available that may help.

Triglycerides, another type of fat in the blood, also appear to promote atherosclerosis. As people get older, heavier, or both, their triglyceride and cholesterol levels tend to rise. Although some CVD patients have elevated triglyceride levels, a causal link between high triglyceride levels and CVD has yet to be established. It may be that high triglyceride levels do not directly cause atherosclerosis but, rather, are among the abnormalities that speed its development.

Current guidelines suggest that you should reduce consumption of saturated fat (which comes mostly from animal products) to less than 7 percent of your total daily caloric intake and minimize your consumption of *trans* fats (see Chapter 8), which is found in partially hydrogenated products such as margarine, many fast foods, and many packaged foods. (If the ingredients list includes "shortening," "partially hydrogenated vegetable oil," or "hydrogenated vegetable oil," the food contains *trans* fats.) By cutting your intake of saturated fats and *trans* fats, experts from the National Heart, Lung, and Blood Institute (NHLBI) believe that you can reduce your LDL levels by as much as 10 percent.[30] In addition, NHLBI experts indicate that you should consume fewer than 200 milligrams per day of cholesterol, which is found mainly in eggs and meat. Doing so may reduce LDL by as much as 5 percent.[31] For information on types of fat and how to reduce total fat in your diet, see "An Eating Plan for Healthy Americans: Our AHA Diet" on the American Heart Association's website (www.americanheart.org).

Though it is wise to cut back on saturated fat, be aware that some fat is necessary to overall health. Ironically, the consumption of too many low-fat or fat-free foods, such as salad dressings and other products, may actually contribute to the escalating problem of obesity in America. It is better to eat foods with olive oil, canola oil, and other monounsaturated fats than to consume low-fat or no-fat products. (For a complete discussion of this topic, see Chapter 8.) Of course, all fat intake should be in moderation.

Monitor Your Cholesterol Levels To get an accurate assessment of your total cholesterol and LDL and HDL levels, consider a lipoprotein analysis. This analysis should be done by a reputable health provider and requires that you not eat or drink anything for 12 hours prior to the test. The LDL level is derived using a standard formula:

LDL = total cholesterol – HDL – (triglycerides/5)

For example, if the level of total cholesterol is 200, the level of HDL 45, and the level of triglycerides 150, the LDL level would be 125 (200 – 45 – 30).

In general, LDL is more closely associated with cardiovascular risk than is total cholesterol. However, most authorities agree that looking only at LDL ignores the positive effects of HDL. Perhaps the best method of evaluating risk is to examine the ratio of HDL to total cholesterol or the percentage of HDL in total cholesterol. If the level of HDL is lower than 35, the risk increases dramatically.

Change Lifestyle to Reduce Your Risk Of the more than 100 million Americans who need to worry about their cholesterol levels, almost half, particularly those at the low-to-moderate risk levels, should be able to reach their LDL and HDL goals through lifestyle changes alone. People who are at higher risk or those for whom lifestyle modifications are not effective may need to take cholesterol-lowering drugs while they continue modifying their lifestyle. Among the most commonly prescribed drugs are statins (Lipitor, Baycol, and Pravachol are examples), which are very effective in reducing LDL levels. Folic acid and niacin drugs are often prescribed for people with low HDL and high triglyceride levels.

Maintain a Healthy Weight No question about it—body weight plays a role in CVD. Researchers are not sure whether high-fat, high-sugar, high-calorie diets are a direct risk for CVD or whether they invite risk by causing obesity, which strains the heart, forcing it to push blood through the many miles of capillaries that supply each pound of fat. A heart that has to continuously move blood through an overabundance of vessels may become damaged.

Overweight people are more likely to develop heart disease and stroke even if they have no other risk factors. If you're heavy, losing even 5 to 10 pounds can make a significant difference of as much as 5 percent LDL reduction.[32] This is especially true if you're an "apple" (thicker around your upper body and waist) rather than a "pear" (thicker around your hips and thighs). See Chapter 9 to learn how to determine if you are at a healthy weight and for more tips on weight management.

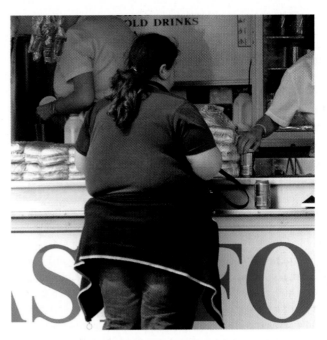

Excessive body weight increases the risk of developing CVD. Weight management should be a primary goal for CVD prevention.

What's the best way to eat for a healthy heart?

Modify Other Dietary Habits The NHLBI guidelines recommend the following dietary changes to reduce CVD risk:

- Consume 5 to 10 mg per day of soluble fiber from sources such as psyllium seeds, oat bran, fruits, vegetables, and legumes (see Chapter 8). Even this small dietary modification may result in another 5 percent drop in LDL levels.

- Consume about 2 g per day of plant sterols or sterol derivatives from substances such as Benecol or Take Control margarine. These were the first widely available sources of sterols, but there are many more choices. This amount of plant sterols has the potential to reduce LDL by another 5 percent.

Exercise Regularly According to all available evidence, inactivity is a definite risk factor for CVD.[33] The good news is that you do not have to be an exercise fanatic to reduce your risk. Even modest levels of low-intensity physical activity—walking, gardening, housework, dancing—are beneficial if done regularly and over the long term. Exercise can increase HDL, lower triglycerides, and reduce coronary risks in several ways. For more information, see Chapter 10.

Making the above modifications could reduce LDL levels by as much as 35 percent—similar to taking any of the statin drugs typically prescribed. However, despite these recommendations and the clear benefits of regular exercise, only 31.3 percent of American adults aged 18 and older engage in any regular physical activity.[34]

try it NOW

Determine your resting heart rate. You can find this out by taking your pulse. Gently press the pads of your first two fingers against the inside of your opposite wrist, just below the base of your thumb. Sit quietly, and count the number of beats that occur during a 10-second period. Multiply the number of beats by 6. Repeat the process. Now you have a baseline to monitor how your heart rate changes based on physical activity and emotions like stress or excitement.

Control Diabetes The NHLBI guidelines underscore the unique CVD risks for people with diabetes. Diabetics who have taken insulin for a number of years have a greater chance of developing CVD. In fact, CVD is the leading cause of death among diabetic patients. Because overweight people have a higher risk for diabetes, distinguishing between the effects of the two conditions is difficult. Diabetics also tend to have elevated blood fat levels, increased atherosclerosis, and a tendency toward deterioration of small blood vessels, particularly in the eyes and extremities. However, through a prescribed regimen of diet, exercise, and medication, diabetics can control much of their increased risk for CVD (see Chapter 18).

Control Your Blood Pressure Hypertension refers to sustained high blood pressure. If it cannot be attributed to any specific cause, it is known as **essential hypertension.** Approximately 90 percent of all cases of hypertension fit this category. **Secondary hypertension** refers to hypertension caused by specific factors, such as kidney disease, obesity, or tumors of the adrenal glands. In general, the higher your blood pressure, the greater your risk for CVD.

Hypertension is known as the "silent killer" because it usually has no symptoms. Its prevalence has increased by over 30 percent in the last 10 years, with data indicating that there are 65 million adults in the United States with high blood pressure. This means that more than 1 in 3 American

hypertension   Sustained elevated blood pressure.

essential hypertension   Hypertension that cannot be attributed to any known cause.

secondary hypertension   Hypertension caused by specific factors, such as kidney disease, obesity, or tumors of the adrenal glands.

systolic pressure   The upper number in the fraction that measures blood pressure, indicating pressure on the walls of the arteries when the heart contracts.

diastolic pressure   The lower number in the fraction that measures blood pressure, indicating pressure on the walls of the arteries during the relaxation phase of heart activity.

adults have blood pressure above the recommended level, and may be on medication, working to reduce risk factors—or unaware that they have a problem. Another 28 percent of American adults over the age of 18 have *prehypertension,* and are well on their way to hypertension.[35]

Blood pressure is measured in two parts and is expressed as a fraction—for example, 110/80, or 110 over 80. Both values are measured in *millimeters of mercury* (mm Hg). The first number refers to **systolic pressure,** or the pressure being applied to the walls of the arteries when the heart contracts, pumping blood to the rest of the body. The second value is **diastolic pressure,** or the pressure applied to the walls of the arteries during the heart's relaxation phase. During this phase, blood is reentering the chambers of the heart, preparing for the next heartbeat.

Normal blood pressure varies depending on weight, age, and physical condition, and for different groups of people, such as women and minorities. Systolic blood pressure tends to increase with age, while diastolic blood pressure increases until age 55 and then declines. As a rule, men have a greater risk for high blood pressure than women until age 55, when their risks become about equal. At age 75 and over, women are more likely to have high blood pressure than men.[36]

For the average person, 110 over 80 is a healthy blood pressure level. High blood pressure is usually diagnosed when systolic pressure is 140 or above. Diastolic pressure does not have to be high to indicate high blood pressure. When only systolic pressure is high, the condition is known as *isolated systolic hypertension (ISH),* the most common form of high blood pressure in older Americans.[37] Causes of high blood pressure include narrowing of the arteries and the heart beating more quickly or more forcefully than it should. However, many times the underlying cause is not known. If your blood pressure exceeds 140 over 90, you need to take steps to lower it. See Table 15.2 for a summary of blood pressure values and what they mean. If either your diastolic or systolic pressure is too high, then you would be classified as having high blood pressure.

Treatment of hypertension can involve dietary changes (reducing salt and calorie intake), weight loss (when appropriate), the use of diuretics and other medications (only when prescribed by a physician), regular exercise, and the practice of relaxation techniques and effective coping and communication skills.

Manage Stress Some scientists have noted a relationship between CVD risk and a person's stress level, behavior habits, and socioeconomic status. These factors may influence established risk factors. For example, people under stress may start smoking or smoke more than they otherwise would. A recent study funded by the National Heart, Lung, and Blood Institute found that impatience and hostility, two key components of the Type A behavior pattern, increase young adults' risk of developing high blood pressure. Other related factors, such as competitiveness, depression, and anxiety, did not appear to increase risk. The research was the first to study these factors as a group rather than individually and has clear implications for prevention.[38]

In other studies, researcher-physician Robert S. Eliot demonstrated that approximately one out of five people has an extreme cardiovascular reaction to stressful stimulation. These people experience alarm and resistance so strongly that, when under stress, their bodies produce large amounts of stress chemicals, which in turn cause tremendous changes in the cardiovascular system, including remarkable increases in blood pressure. These people are called *hot reactors.* Although their blood pressure may be normal when they are not under stress—for example, in a doctor's office—it increases dramatically in response to even small amounts of everyday tension. *Cold reactors* are those who are able to experience stress (even to live as Type As) without showing harmful cardiovascular responses. Cold reactors may internalize stress, but their self-talk and perceptions about the stressful events lead them to a nonresponse state in which their cardiovascular system remains virtually unaffected.[39]

Since Eliot's early work, research in this area has been inconclusive, although more recent studies suggest that personality does indeed play an important role in effective coping. Some research indicates that people who have an underlying predisposition toward a toxic core personality (in other words, who are chronically hostile and hateful) may be at greatest risk for a CVD event. See Chapter 3 for tips on managing your stress, whether you are a hot or cold reactor.

Risks You Cannot Control

Does cardiovascular disease run in families?

There are, unfortunately, some risk factors for CVD that we cannot prevent or control. The most important are these:

- *Heredity.* A family history of heart disease appears to increase the risk significantly. Whether the increase is due to genetics or environment is an unresolved question.
- *Age.* Seventy-five percent of all heart attacks occur in people over age 65. The rate of CVD increases with age for both sexes.
- *Gender.* Men are at greater risk for CVD until about age 60. Women under 35 have a fairly low risk unless they have high blood pressure, kidney problems, or diabetes. Oral contraceptives and smoking also increase the risk. Hormonal factors appear to reduce risk for women, although after menopause or after estrogen levels are otherwise reduced (for example, because of hysterectomy), women's LDL levels tend to go up, increasing their chances for CVD. (For more on the gender factor, see the next section.)
- *Race.* Blacks are at 45 percent greater risk for hypertension and thus at greater risk for CVD than whites. In addition, African Americans are less likely to survive a heart attack. Figure 15.7 on page 468 reveals the impact of race on CVD risk.

TABLE 15.2	Blood Pressure Classifications		
Classification	Systolic Reading (mm Hg)		Diastolic Reading (mm Hg)
Normal	<120	and	<80
Prehypertension	120–139	or	80–89
Hypertension			
Stage 1	140–159	or	90–99
Stage 2	≥160	or	≥100

Note: If systolic and diastolic readings fall into different categories, treatment is determined by the highest category. Readings are based on the average of two or more properly measured, seated readings on each of two or more health care provider visits.

Source: National Heart, Lung, and Blood Institute, *The Seventh Report of the Joint National Committee on Prevention, Detection, Evaluation, and Treatment of High Blood Pressure* (NIH Publication No. 03-5233) (Bethesda, MD: National Institutes of Health, May 2003).

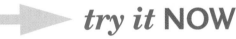

try it NOW

Early prevention and modification of risk factors for heart disease can be key to whether or not you develop CVD later in life. Right now, find out if you are prone to CVD and take steps to lower your risk. Do heart disease, high blood pressure, or high cholesterol run in your family? If so, discuss steps you can take to reduce your risk and monitor your heart health with your health care provider. Though you can't control your genetic susceptibility, you can make other positive lifestyle changes to reduce your risk now.

Women and Cardiovascular Disease

Whereas men tend to have more heart attacks and to suffer them earlier in life than do women, some interesting trends in survivability have emerged. In 2003, CVD claimed the lives of 426,800 men and a surprising 483,800 women.[40] Why do more men have heart attacks but more women die from them? Why do some studies say that women have about the same mortality rate after MI and others indicate there are vast differences, supported by actual numbers?

Although we understand the mechanisms that cause heart disease in men and women (or at least we think we do!), their experiences in the health care system, their reactions to life-threatening diseases, and a host of other technological and environmental factors may play a role in these statistics.

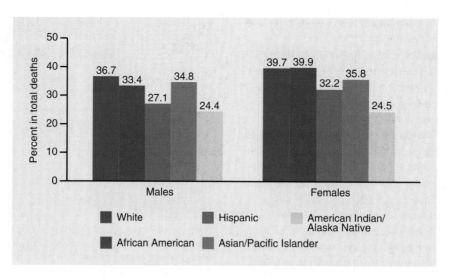

FIGURE 15.7 Deaths from Cardiovascular Disease in the United States by Age and Race, 2002

Source: American Heart Association, *Heart Disease and Stroke Statistics—2006* (Dallas, TX: American Heart Association, 2006). © 2006 American Heart Association. Reproduced with permission. www.americanheart.org.

Risk Factors for Heart Disease in Women

The Role of Estrogen Premenopausal women are unlikely candidates for heart attacks, unless they suffer from diabetes, high blood pressure, or kidney disease or have a genetic predisposition to high cholesterol levels. Family history and smoking can also increase the risk. However, once her estrogen production drops with menopause, a woman's chance of developing CVD rises rapidly. A 60-year-old woman has the same heart attack risk as a 50-year-old man. By her late seventies, a woman's heart attack risk may exceed that of a man her age. Look back to Figure 15.2 to see how CVD rates between men and women compare as we age. To date, much of this changing risk has been attributed to the aging process, but the role of estrogen and other hormones remains unclear. Early studies of various **hormone replacement therapies (HRTs)** indicated that HRT might reduce the risk of CVD by as much as 12 to 25 percent. However, subsequent findings strongly called into question what was previously believed to be the health-enhancing powers of HRT (see the Women's Health/Men's Health box on CVD and hormones on pages 470–471). Today, new evidence points to the potential benefits of estrogen to women in their fifties. Even when their total blood cholesterol levels are higher than men's, however, women may be at less risk because they typically have a higher percentage of HDL.[41]

hormone replacement therapies (HRTs) Therapies that replace estrogen in postmenopausal women.

That is only part of the story. It's true that women aged 25 and over tend to have lower cholesterol levels than men of the same age—but when they reach 45, things change. Most men's cholesterol levels become more stable, while both LDL and total cholesterol levels in women start to rise. The gap widens further beyond age 55.

Before age 45, women's total blood cholesterol levels average below 220 mg/ml. By the time she is 45 to 55, the average woman's blood cholesterol rises to between 223 and 246 mg/ml. Studies of men have shown that for every 1 percent drop in cholesterol, there is a 2 percent decrease in CVD risk.[42] If this holds true for women, prevention efforts focusing on dietary intervention and exercise may significantly help postmenopausal women.

Neglect of Heart Disease Symptoms in Women

During the past decade, research has suggested three main reasons that the signs of heart disease in women may get overlooked: (1) Physicians may be gender biased in their delivery of health care, tending to concentrate on women's reproductive organs rather than on the whole body; (2) physicians tend to view male heart disease as a more severe problem because men have traditionally had a higher incidence of the disease; and (3) women decline major procedures more often than men do. Other explanations for diagnostic and therapeutic difficulties encountered by women with heart disease include:

- Delay in diagnosing a possible heart attack
- The complexity involved in interpreting chest pain in women

- Typically less aggressive treatment of female heart attack victims
- Women's older age, on average, and greater frequency of other health problems
- The fact that women's coronary arteries are often smaller than men's, making surgical or diagnostic procedures more difficult technically
- The increased incidence of postinfarction angina and heart failure in women

In addition, symptoms of heart attack often differ for women and men, making it more difficult for women to determine whether to go to the doctor (see the Women's Health/ Men's Health box on page 472).

Gender Bias in CVD Research?

The traditional view that heart disease is primarily a male problem has carried over into research as well. A well-publicized example was a study suggesting that aspirin could help prevent heart attacks—based entirely on its effects in 22,000 male doctors. To address such concerns, the National Institutes of Health has launched a 15-year, $625 million study of 140,000 postmenopausal women (known as the Women's Health Initiative), focusing on the leading causes of death and disease. Researchers hope to determine how a healthy lifestyle and increased medical attention can help prevent women's heart disease, as well as cancer and osteoporosis. As discussed elsewhere, the study has already had important implications for women using HRT.

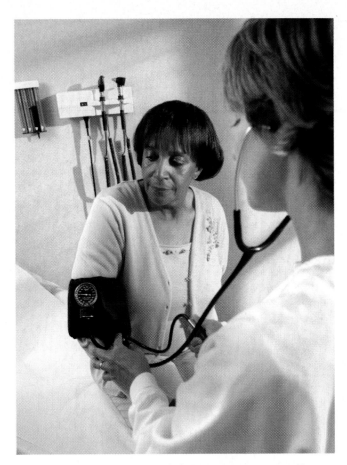

Women at risk for heart disease need to have their blood pressure and other CVD risk factors carefully monitored.

 what do you THINK?

How do men and women differ in their experiences related to CVD? ■ Why do you think women's risks were largely ignored until fairly recently? ■ What actions do you think individuals can take to help improve the situation for both men and women? ■ What actions can communities and medical practitioners take?

New Weapons Against Heart Disease

The victim of a heart attack today has many options that were not available a generation ago. Medications can strengthen heartbeat, control arrhythmias, remove fluids in case of congestive heart failure, and relieve pain. New surgical procedures are saving many lives.

Techniques of Diagnosing Heart Disease

Several techniques are used to diagnose heart disease, including electrocardiogram, angiography, and positron emission

tomography scans. An **electrocardiogram (ECG)** is a record of the electrical activity of the heart. Patients may undergo a stress test, such as walking or running on a treadmill, while their hearts are monitored. A more accurate method of testing for heart disease is **angiography** (often referred to as *cardiac catheterization*), in which a needle-thin tube called a *catheter* is threaded through heart arteries, a dye is injected, and an X ray is taken to discover which areas are blocked. A more recent and even more effective method of measuring heart activity is a **positron emission tomography (PET) scan,** which produces three-dimensional images of the heart as

electrocardiogram (ECG) A record of the electrical activity of the heart; may be measured during a stress test.

angiography A technique for examining blockages in heart arteries. A catheter is inserted into the arteries, a dye is injected, and an X ray is taken to find the blocked areas. Also called cardiac catheterization.

positron emission tomography (PET) scan Method for measuring heart activity by injecting a patient with a radioactive tracer that is scanned electronically to produce a three-dimensional image of the heart and arteries.

CVD PROTECTION OR RISK? THE HORMONE CONTROVERSY CONTINUES

For decades, the prevailing wisdom was that taking hormones during and after menopause would not only reduce hot flashes, it would protect against cardiovascular disease in women. The rate of CVD increases in women after menopause, leading experts to believe that keeping hormone levels high after menopause would control CVD risk. Although scientists didn't really know why this apparent relationship existed, they began to prescribe hormones to millions of women. The results of a major study in the mid-1990s, the Postmenopausal Estrogen/Progestin Intervention (PEPI) Trial, seemed to prove that hormone replacement therapy (HRT) lowered CVD risk by raising levels of HDL and decreasing LDL. This led to widespread promotion of HRT by professional organizations, doctors, educators, and the community at large. Other studies seemed to confirm these facts, and women moved to take HRT in unprecedented numbers—some 38 percent of all postmenopausal women in the most recent data.

Women choose to take HRT for various reasons. Although reducing CVD risk has been one of them, many women take HRT because it is the most effective treatment for menopausal symptoms such as hot flashes, night sweats, sexual dysfunction and vaginal dryness, insomnia, and hair loss. For women experiencing these problems, short-term use of HRT to get them through the years when the symptoms are most disruptive may have seemed worth any small risk. Other women took HRT because it has been shown to reduce the risk of bone fractures and osteoporosis, another major threat to older women's health.

NEW FINDINGS RAISE QUESTIONS

Recently, results from several studies provided growing evidence that the advice to take HRT to prevent CVD was not only inaccurate, it may have been deadly for some of those who followed it. In light of these studies, many woman have stopped taking HRT. Consider the following:

- The 1998 Heart and Estrogen/Progestin Replacement Study, a large-scale randomized, placebo-controlled clinical trial, showed that after four years, there was no difference in heart attack rates but higher rates of coronary death for those on HRT compared with those taking a placebo.
- The 2000 Estrogen Replacement and Atherosclerosis Trial, the first study to use angiographic images to assess the effects of HRT and estrogen replacement therapy (ERT) on women with preexisting coronary disease, showed no effect from hormone replacement.
- In 2002, investigators conducting the huge Women's Health Initiative (WHI) study stirred even more controversy. Researchers announced that women on HRT in the study were experiencing a small but unacceptable increase in heart attacks, blood clots in the lungs (pulmonary embolism) and legs (deep vein thrombosis), and stroke. Although the project was scheduled to continue until 2005, these results caused the researchers to stop it early. One version of HRT, Prempro, appeared to pose a greater risk than others.
- In 2004, a multicenter heart disease prevention study (part of WHI) found that estrogen-only therapy had no effect on coronary heart disease risk but increased the risk of stroke in postmenopausal women. The study also showed an increased risk of deep vein thrombosis, no effect on breast or colorectal cancer, and reduced risk of hip and other fractures. Like its HRT counterpart, the study was stopped early and notices sent to health care providers.

blood flows through it. During a PET scan, a patient receives an intravenous injection of a radioactive tracer at rest and during exercise. As the tracer decays, it emits positrons that are picked up by the scanner and transformed by a computer into color images of the heart. Newer single-photon emission computed tomography (SPECT) scans provide an even better view. Other tests include:

- *Radionuclide imaging* (includes tests such as thallium test, multinucleated gated angiography [MUGA scan], and acute infarct scintigraphy). These procedures involve injecting substances called radionuclides into the bloodstream. Computer-generated pictures can then show them in the heart. These tests can show how well the heart muscle is supplied with blood, how well the heart's chambers are functioning, and which part of the heart has been damaged by a heart attack.
- *Magnetic resonance imaging (MRI)*. This test uses powerful magnets to look inside the body. Computer-generated pictures can show the heart muscle and help physicians identify damage from a heart attack, diagnose congenital heart defects, and evaluate disease of larger blood vessels such as the aorta.
- *Ultrafast computed tomography (CT)*. This is an especially fast form of X ray of the heart designed to evaluate bypass grafts, diagnose ventricular function, and measure calcium deposits.
- *Digital subtraction angiography (DSA)*. This modified form of computer-aided imaging records pictures of the heart and its blood vessels.

Amidst these facts, new research continues to fuel more controversy, and cause confusion among consumers. In 2006, the estrogen controversy grew as a newer study indicated that women aged 50 to 59 could gain some protective benefit against CHD by taking estrogen at low doses.

WHAT ARE THE IMPLICATIONS FOR CONSUMERS?

Should a woman toss out her hormones based on the earlier WHI results? Generally, experts recommended that if you are overweight, with high cholesterol and/or a family history of heart disease, you may already be at increased risk for cardiovascular disease, and it may be prudent to look for alternatives. However, as the newer research demonstrates, these guidelines might be accurate for women under age 50, but for those aged 50 and older, estrogen could be protective.

How great is the risk? The accompanying table demonstrates estimates if 10,000 women took HRT for one year.

It should be noted that these increased risks are drawn from studies of HRT, as estrogen-alone studies are still being analyzed. The decision to use ERT or HRT is complex and should be made in consultation with knowledgeable health care providers and after reviewing the latest information from reputable sources. The most important thing to take away from the WHI findings is that HRT does not seem to prevent or improve cardiovascular risks, so no woman should take it solely to protect against heart attack or stroke.

If you have questions about these studies or want additional information, the references below are valuable sources of information.

Sources: K. L. Brubaker et al., "Effects of Estrogen-Alone Treatment in Postmenopausal Women," *Journal of the American Medical Association* 292, no. 6 (2004): 686–696; L. Mosca et al., "Hormone Replacement Therapy and Cardiovascular Disease," *Circulation* 104 (2001): 499; Writing Group for the Women's Health Initiative Investigators, "Risks and Benefits of Estrogen Plus Progestin in Healthy Postmenopausal Women," *Journal of the American Medical Association* 288, no. 3 (2002): 321–333; U.S. Preventive Services Task Force, "Hormone Replacement Therapy for Primary Prevention of Chronic Conditions: Recommendations and Rationale," October 2002 (Rockville, MD: Agency for Healthcare Research and Quality), www.ahrq.gov/clinic/3rduspstf/hrt/hrtrr.htm; J. Hsia et al., "Conjugated Equine Estrogens and Coronary Heart Disease: The Women's Health Initiative," *Archives of Internal Medicine* 166, no. 3 (2006): 357–365.

The number of women with	Would increase by	Would decrease by
Breast cancer	8[a]	
Heart attack	7	
Stroke	8	
Pulmonary embolism	8[b]	
Venous thrombosis	10[b]	
Colorectal cancer		6[c]
Hip fracture		5

a. Risk appears after four years of use
b. Risk is greatest in first two years of use
c. Benefit appears after three years of use

Angioplasty versus Bypass Surgery

Coronary bypass surgery has helped many patients who suffered coronary blockages or heart attacks. In coronary bypass surgery, a blood vessel is taken from another site in the patient's body (usually the *saphenous* vein in the leg or the *internal mammary artery*) and implanted to "bypass" blocked arteries and transport blood. Death rates are generally much lower at medical centers where surgical teams and intensive care teams see large numbers of patients.[43]

Another procedure, **angioplasty** (sometimes called *balloon angioplasty*), carries fewer risks and may be more effective than bypass surgery in selected cases. As in angiography, a thin catheter is threaded through blocked heart arteries. The catheter has a balloon at the tip, which is inflated to flatten fatty deposits against the arterial walls, allowing blood to flow more freely. Angioplasty patients are generally awake but sedated during the procedure. In about 30 percent of patients,

coronary bypass surgery A surgical technique whereby a blood vessel is implanted to bypass a clogged coronary artery.

angioplasty A technique in which a catheter with a balloon at the tip is inserted into a clogged artery; the balloon is inflated to flatten fatty deposits against artery walls, allowing blood to flow more freely.

As more research is done concerning diagnosis and treatment of CVD, it is clear that women sometimes experience different symptoms and benefit from different treatments than men do. For example, consider the following:

FEELING PAIN

Several studies have documented that women experience pain more acutely and frequently than men, indicating that the sexes may detect and react to pain differently. In a study of dental patients, women responded more favorably than men to a class of pain relievers known as kappa opioids, including pentazocine. This finding suggests that receptors for inhibiting pain may vary by sex. Also, women appear to be less responsive than men to non-steroidal anti-inflammatory drugs, such as ibuprofen. Women typically need slightly lower doses of aspirin and should be warned that taking 325 mg of aspirin per day may result in anticoagulation levels that exceed those of men. Surgical risks, risks from accidents that lead to excessive bleeding, and so on, may be greater for aspirin-using women.

NOTING HEART ATTACK SYMPTOMS

We are taught that the classic symptom of a heart attack is chest-crushing pain. However, this symptom is not that common in women. Women's heart attacks, by contrast, tend to show up as shortness of breath, fatigue, and jaw pain, stretched out over hours rather than minutes. Women tend to suffer their first heart attack ten years later than men; and, in part because they are older when they have these attacks, they are more likely to die.

TREATING CVD

Interestingly, drugs used to break up clots and stabilize erratic heartbeats are less effective in women than in men. Beta blockers, one common form of treatment for reducing blood pressure and migraines, take longer to metabolize in women than in men, meaning that women often have more difficulty regulating dosage and preventing side effects. Until recently, hormone replacement therapy was believed to help, but recent research has shown otherwise (see the Women's Health/Men's Health box on the hormone controversy, page 470). Recent studies have shown that angioplasty is one of the best techniques for reducing women's risk of heart attack.

---

the treated arteries become clogged again within six months. Some patients may undergo the procedure as many as three times within a five-year period. Some surgeons argue that given this high rate of recurrence, bypass may be a more effective treatment.

Today, newer forms of laser angioplasty and atherectomy, a procedure that removes plaque, are being done in several clinics. These procedures are often followed by procedures in which the affected area has a small wire mesh tube (a stent) inserted to prop open the artery cleared by angioplasty.

Research suggests that in many instances, drug treatments may be just as effective in prolonging life as invasive surgical techniques, but it is critical that doctors prescribe an aggressive drug treatment program and that patients comply with it.

Aspirin for Heart Disease: Can It Help?

Research indicates that low doses of aspirin (80 mg daily or every other day) are beneficial to heart patients due to

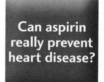

Can aspirin really prevent heart disease?

aspirin's blood-thinning properties. Higher levels do not provide significantly more protection. Aspirin has even been advised as a preventive strategy for people with no current heart disease symptoms; however, aspirin should only be taken as a preventive if under the advice of a person's own physician. Major problems associated with chronic aspirin use are gastrointestinal intolerance and a tendency for some people to have difficulty with blood clotting, and these factors may outweigh aspirin's benefits in some cases. People taking aspirin face additional risks from emergency surgery or accidental bleeding. Although the findings concerning aspirin and heart disease are still inconclusive, the research seems promising.[44] See the New Horizons in Health box on page 474 for more on promising news in reducing CVD risk.

Thrombolysis

Whenever a heart attack occurs, prompt action is vital. When a coronary artery is blocked, the heart muscle doesn't die immediately, but time determines how much damage occurs. If a victim reaches an emergency room and is diagnosed fast enough, a form of reperfusion therapy called **thrombolysis** can be performed. Thrombolysis involves injecting an agent such as TPA (tissue plasminogen activator) to dissolve the

thrombolysis Injection of an agent to dissolve clots and restore some blood flow, thereby reducing the amount of tissue that dies from ischemia.

clot and restore some blood flow, thereby reducing the amount of tissue that dies from ischemia.[45] These drugs must be administered within one to three hours after a heart attack for best results.

what do you THINK?

With all the new diagnostic procedures, treatments, and differing philosophies about various prevention and intervention techniques, how can typical health consumers ensure that they will get the best treatment? ■ Where can they go for information? ■ Why might women, members of certain minority groups, and older adults need a "health advocate" who can help them get through the system?

Cardiac Rehabilitation

Every year, nearly 1 million people survive heart attacks. Over 7 million more have unstable angina, and about 650,000 undergo bypass surgery or angioplasty. In 2003, a total of 7 million people in the United States underwent a cardiovascular operation.[46] Heart failure is the most common discharge diagnosis for hospitalized Medicare patients and the fourth most common diagnosis among all patients hospitalized in the United States. Most of these patients are eligible for cardiac rehabilitation (including exercise training and health education classes on good nutrition and CVD risk management), needing only a doctor's prescription for these services. However, many Americans do not have access to these programs. Even larger numbers are finding it difficult to afford them in light of skyrocketing costs for prescription drugs. Some patients must choose between home health care and cardiac rehabilitation; others stay away from such programs because of cost, transportation, or other factors. Perhaps the biggest deterrent is fear of having another attack due to exercise. The benefits of cardiac rehabilitation (including increased stamina and strength and faster recovery), however, far outweigh the risks when these programs are run by certified health professionals.

Personal Advocacy and Heart-Smart Behaviors

People who suspect they have cardiovascular disease are often overwhelmed and frightened. Where should they go for diagnosis? What are the best treatments? Answering these questions becomes even more difficult if they are upset, scared, or tend to listen unquestioningly to doctors' orders. If you or a loved one must face a CVD crisis, it is important to act with knowledge, strength, and assertiveness. The following suggestions will help you deal with hospitals and health care providers in the wake of a cardiac event or any major health problem (see Chapter 22 for more on being a smart consumer of health care services).

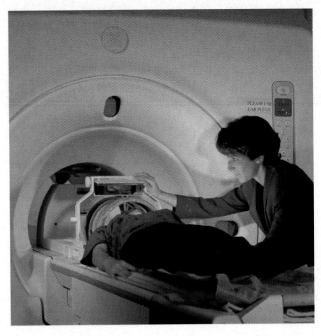

Magnetic resonance imaging is one of several methods to detect heart damage, abnormalities, or defects.

1. *Know your rights as a patient.* Ask about the risks and costs of various diagnostic tests. Some procedures, particularly angiography, may pose significant risks for people who are older, who have a history of minor strokes, or who have had chemotherapy or other treatments that could have damaged their blood vessels. Ask for test results and an explanation of any abnormalities.

2. *Find out about informed consent procedures, living wills, durable power of attorney, organ donation, and other legal issues before you become sick.* Having someone shove a clipboard in your face and ask you if life support can be terminated in case of a problem is one of the great horrors of many people's hospital experiences. Be prepared.

3. *Ask about alternative procedures.* If possible, seek a second opinion at a different health care facility (in other words, get at least two opinions from doctors who are not in the same group and who cannot read each other's diagnoses). New research indicates that doctors may not use drug treatments as aggressively as they could and that medications may be as effective as major bypass or open-heart surgeries. Ask, ask, and ask again. Remember, it is your life, and there is always the possibility that another treatment will be better for you.

4. *Remain with your loved one as a "personal advocate."* If your loved one is weak and unable to ask questions, ask the questions yourself. Inquire about new medications, tests, and other potentially risky procedures that may be undertaken during the course of treatment or recovery. If you feel your loved one is being removed from intensive care or other closely monitored areas

NEW HORIZONS in health

Just when we thought that indulging in certain dietary delights should be avoided, there is growing evidence that the antioxidant compound class known as "flavonoids," found in fruits, teas, red wine, and cocoa, may protect us from heart disease, stroke, and even diabetes. Sound too good to be true? Exciting new research indicates that the flavonoids in red wine in particular may act as an anti-inflammatory and protect us from CVD. Though the evidence supporting these claims is promising, research into these compounds and exactly how they protect against CVD is still in its infancy, and scientists warn that it is too early to come to a solid conclusion.

Does red wine really prevent heart disease?

Consider these studies:

- At an international conference on the health benefits of cocoa, researchers revealed that cocoa flavonol molecules may reduce the risk of blood clotting and improve blood flow in the brain.
- Results from over 51 epidemiological studies suggest that risk of CHD may decrease by as much as 20 percent when 0 to 2 alcoholic drinks per day are consumed.
- In a study of 329 heart disease patients, consumption of a small amount of wine or tea daily corresponded to a 24 percent decrease in CHD risk.
- Results from the Health Professionals Follow-Up Study, in which 38,077 male health professionals who were free of cardiovascular disease were observed for 12 years, suggested that drinking 1 to 2 drinks per day, 3 to 4 days per week decreased the risk of heart attack by as much as 32 percent. In the same study, it was found that light alcohol consumption can reduce the risk of stroke by 20 percent.

In spite of the promising nature of these studies, most experts warn that non-drinkers should not begin drinking to improve their health. Although the benefits of light alcohol consumption are suggested, they still do not outweigh the overall risk of alcohol consumption (see Chapter 12 for more on these risks). Likewise, don't abandon balanced nutrition for a daily candy bar. However, this research does indicate that perhaps some day scientists will discover how to isolate the beneficial compounds in these foods, and offer them in the form of preventive medications for those at risk for CVD.

Sources: C. Keen, "Specific Compound Identified Behind Aspirin-Like Effect" (presentation, Cocoa Flavonols Meeting, Lucerne, Switzerland, July 25–27, 2002); P. Lagiou et al., "Intake of Specific Flavonoid Classes and Coronary Heart Disease: A Case-Control Study in Greece," *European Journal of Clinical Nutrition* 58, no. 12 (2004): 1643–1648; P. Szmitko and V. Subodh, "Red Wine and Your Heart," *Circulation* 111 (2004): e10–e11.

prematurely, ask if the hospital is taking this action to comply with DRGs (established limits of treatment for certain conditions) and if this action is warranted. Most hospitals have waiting areas or special rooms so family members can stay close to a patient. Exercise your right to this option.

5. *Monitor the actions of health care providers.* To control costs, some hospitals are hiring nursing aides and other personnel who may lack the training that registered nurses have in handling patients with CVD. Ask about the patient-to-nurse ratio, and make sure that people monitoring you or your loved ones have appropriate credentials.

6. *Be considerate of your care provider.* One of the most stressful jobs any person can be entrusted with is care of a critically ill person. Although questions are appropriate and your emotions are running high, be as tactful and considerate as possible. Nurses often carry a disproportionate responsibility for the care of patients during critical times and are often forced to carry a higher than optimal patient load. Try to remain out of their way, ask questions as necessary, and report any irregularities in care to the supervisor.

7. *Be patient with the patient.* The pain, suffering, and fears associated with a cardiac event often cause otherwise nice people to act in not-so-nice ways. Be patient and helpful, and allow time for the person to rest. Talk with the patient about his or her feelings, concerns, and fears. Do not ignore these concerns to ease your own anxieties.

We still have much to learn about CVD and its causes, treatments, and risk factors. Staying informed is an important part of staying healthy. Good dietary habits, regular exercise, stress management, prompt attention to suspicious symptoms, and other healthy behaviors will greatly enhance your chances of remaining CVD free. Other factors that influence risk include how much emphasis our health care systems place on access to health care for all underserved populations, education about risk, and other community-based interventions. Action on both community and individual levels can help address the challenge of CVD.

TAKING charge

Summary

- Cardiovascular disease incidence and prevalence rates have changed considerably in the past 50 years. Certain segments of the population have disproportionate levels of risk.
- The cardiovascular system consists of the heart and circulatory system and is a carefully regulated, integrated network of vessels that supply the body with the nutrients and oxygen necessary to perform daily functions.
- Cardiovascular diseases include atherosclerosis (hardening of the arteries), heart attack, angina pectoris, arrhythmias, congestive heart failure, congenital and rheumatic heart disease, and stroke. These combine to be the leading cause of death in the United States today.
- Many risk factors for cardiovascular disease can be controlled, such as cigarette smoking, high blood fat and cholesterol levels, hypertension, lack of exercise, a high-fat diet, obesity, diabetes, and emotional stress. Some risk factors, such as age, gender, and heredity, cannot be controlled. Many of these factors have a compounded effect when combined. Dietary changes, exercise, weight reduction, and attention to lifestyle risks can greatly reduce susceptibility to cardiovascular disease.
- Women have a unique challenge in controlling their risk for CVD, particularly after menopause, when estrogen levels are no longer sufficient to be protective.
- New methods developed for treating heart blockages include coronary bypass surgery, angioplasty, and insertion of stents. Also, drugs such as beta blockers and calcium channel blockers can reduce high blood pressure and treat other symptoms. Research has provided important clues on how best to prevent or reduce risk of CVD today. Recognizing your own risks and acting now to reduce risk are important elements of lifelong cardiovascular health.

Chapter Review

1. The upper chambers of the heart are called the
   a. pericardium.
   b. ventricles.
   c. atrium.
   d. myocardium.

2. The function of the aorta is to
   a. return the blood from the lungs.
   b. pump the blood to the arteries in the rest of the body.
   c. pump blood to the lungs.
   d. return blood back to the heart.

3. What does cholesterol measure in the body?
   a. The formation of fatty substances called plaque which can clog the arteries.
   b. The level of triglycerides in the blood which can increase risk of coronary disease.
   c. Hypertension which leads to hardening of the arteries.
   d. None of the above.

4. Arteriosclerosis is more commonly referred to as
   a. hardening of the arteries.
   b. heart attack.
   c. high blood pressure.
   d. plaque.

5. A stroke results when
   a. a heart attack occurs.
   b. when CPR has failed to revive the stopped heart.
   c. when blood to the brain has been blocked off.
   d. when the blood pressure rises too high.

6. An irregularity in the heartbeat is called a(n)
   a. fibrillation.
   b. bradycardia.
   c. tachycardia.
   d. arrhythmia.

7. The "bad" type of cholesterol found in the bloodstream is known as
   a. high density lipoprotein.
   b. low density lipoprotein.
   c. total cholesterol.
   d. triglyceride.

8. Ken's physician informed him that he has hypertension and must work at lowering it to avoid a possible heart attack. Hypertension, in simpler terms, means
   a. high blood pressure.
   b. high cholesterol.
   c. a fast heart beat.
   d. thrombolysis.

9. Dan complained to his doctor that he was experiencing a "racing heart." The doctor informed him that he was experiencing
   a. bradycardia.
   b. tachycardia.
   c. hyperlipidemia.
   d. atherosclerosis.

10. What percentage of women will die within one year after their initial heart attack?
    a. 10 percent
    b. 25 percent
    c. 38 percent
    d. 45 percent

Answers to these questions can be found on page A-1.

Questions for Discussion and Reflection

1. Trace the path of a drop of blood from the time it enters the heart until it reaches the extremities.
2. List the different types of CVD. Compare and contrast their symptoms, risk factors, prevention, and treatment.
3. What are the major indicators that CVD poses a particularly significant risk to people of your age? To people over 65? To people from selected minority groups?
4. Discuss the role that exercise, stress management, dietary changes, checkups, and other factors can play in reducing risk for CVD. What role might chronic infections play in CVD risk?
5. Discuss why age is such an important factor in women's risk for CVD. What can be done to decrease women's risk in later life?
6. Describe some of the diagnostic and treatment alternatives for CVD. If you had a heart attack today, which treatment would you prefer? Explain why.

Accessing Your Health on the Internet

The following websites explore further topics and issues related to personal health. You'll also find links to each organization's website on the Companion Website for *Access to Health*, Tenth Edition, at www.aw-bc.com/donatelle.

1. *American Heart Association.* Home page for the leading private organization dedicated to heart health. This site provides information, statistics, and resources regarding cardiovascular care, including an opportunity to test your own risk for CVD. www.americanheart.org
2. *Johns Hopkins Cardiac Rehabilitation home page.* Information about prevention of heart disease and rehabilitation from CVD from one of the best cardiac care centers in the United States, including information about programs available to help individuals stop smoking, lose weight, lower blood pressure and blood cholesterol, and reduce emotional stress. www.jhbmc.jhu.edu/cardiology/rehab/rehab.html
3. *National Heart, Lung, and Blood Institute.* A valuable resource for information on all aspects of cardiovascular health and wellness. www.nhlbi.nih.gov
4. *Adult Congenital Heart Association.* The Adult Congenital Heart Association (ACHA) is a nonprofit organization that seeks to improve the quality of life and extend the lives of adults with congenital heart defects through education, outreach, advocacy, and promotion of research. www.achaheart.org

Further Reading

American Heart Association. *Heart Disease and Stroke Facts.* Dallas, TX: American Heart Association.

An annual overview providing facts and figures concerning cardiovascular disease in the United States. Supplement provides key statistics about current trends and future directions in treatment and prevention.

McCrum, Robert. *My Year Off: Recovering after a Stroke.* New York: Broadway Books, 1999.

The chronicle of a young man's recovery from a severe stroke.

Pashkow, F. and C. Libov. *The Women's Heart Book.* New York: Hyperion, 2001.

Gersh, B. and M. Wood, eds. *The Mayo Clinic Heart Book.* New York: William Morrow, 2000.

These two books provide an overview of heart disease in America, including risk factors, trends, and options for heart patients.

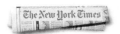

e-themes from *The New York Times*

For up-to-date articles about current health issues, visit www.aw-bc.com/donatelle, select *Access to Health,* Tenth Edition, Chapter 15, and click on "e-themes."

References

1. Report of the American Heart Association Statistics Committee and Stroke Statistics Sub-Committee, "Heart Disease and Stroke Statistics—2006 Update," *Circulation* 113 (2006): 1–118.
2. Ibid.
3. American Heart Association, *Heart Disease and Stroke Statistics* (Dallas: American Heart Association, 2006).
4. Ibid.
5. Ibid.
6. Ibid.
7. Ibid.
8. American Heart Association, *Heart Disease and Stroke Statistics,* C. Langenberg, et al., "Cardiovascular Death and the Metabolic Syndrome: The Role of Adipose Signaling Hormones and Inflammatory Markers," *Diabetes Care* 29 (2006): 1363–1369; J. de Jager et al., "Endothelial Dysfunctions and Low-Grade Inflammation Explain Much of the Excess Mortality in Individuals with Type 2 Diabetes: The Hoorn Study," *Arteriosclerosis, Thrombosis, and Vascular Biology* 26 (2006): 1086–1093; C. Meisinger et al., "Plasma Oxidized Low-Density Lipoprotein: A Strong Predictor for Acute Coronary Heart Disease Events in Apparently Healthy Middle-Aged Men in the General Population," *Circulation* 112 (2005): 651–657.
9. World Health Organization, "The World Health Report, 2006" (Geneva, Switzerland: World Health Organization, 2006); American Heart Association, *Heart Disease and Stroke Statistics.*
10. Langenberg et al., "Cardiovascular Death and the Metabolic Syndrome"; de Jager et al., "Endothelial Dysfunctions and Low-Grade Inflammation."
11. J. Berger et al., "Aspirin for the Primary Prevention of Cardiovascular Disease in Men and Women," *Journal of the American Medical Association* 295, no. 3 (2006): 306–313.
12. S. Mora et al., "Enhanced Risk Assessment in Asymptomatic Individuals with Exercise Testing and Framingham Risk Scores," *Circulation* 112, no. 11 (2005): 1566–1572; G. Hu et al., "Prevalence of the Metabolic Syndrome and Its Relation to All-Cause and Cardiovascular Mortality in Non-Diabetic European Men and Women," *Archives of Internal Medicine* 164, no. 10 (2004): 1066–76; L. Girman et al., "An Exploratory Analysis of Criteria for the Metabolic Syndrome and Its Prediction of Cardiovascular Outcomes: The Hoorn Study," *American Journal of Epidemiology* 162 no. 5 (2005): 438–447; J. Ford et al., "Risks for All-Cause Mortality, Cardiovascular Disease, and Diabetes Associated with the Metabolic Syndrome: A Summary of Evidence," *Diabetes Care* 28, no. 7 (2005): 1769–1778; J. Bertrais et al., "Sedentary Behaviors, Physical Activity, and Metabolic Syndrome in Middle-Aged French Subjects," *Obesity Research* 13, no. 6 (2005): 936–944.
13. American Heart Association, *Heart Disease and Stroke Statistics.*
14. Ibid.
15. Ibid.
16. Ibid.
17. Ibid.
18. Ibid.
19. Ibid.
20. Ibid.
21. American Heart Association, *Stroke Facts, 2006: All Americans* (Dallas: American Heart Association, 2006).
22. American Heart Association, *Heart Disease and Stroke Statistics.*
23. Ibid.
24. Ibid.
25. N. R. Anthonisen et al., for the Lung Health Study Research Group, "The Effects of a Smoking Cessation Intervention on 14.5-Year Mortality: A Randomized Controlled Trial," *Annals of Internal Medicine* 142 (2005): 223–239.
26. National Heart, Lung, and Blood Institute, *Third Report of the National Cholesterol Education Program (NCEP) Expert Panel on Detection, Evaluation, and Treatment of High Blood Cholesterol in Adults (Adult Treatment Panel III),* 2001, www.nhlbi.nih.gov/guidelines/cholesterol/index.htm.
27. B. Howard et al., "Low-Fat Diet and Risk of Cardiovascular Disease," *Journal of the American Medical Association* 295, no. 6 (2006): 655–666.
28. National Heart, Lung, and Blood Institute, "Third Report of the Expert Panel on Detection, Evaluation, and Treatment of High Blood Cholesterol in Adults."
29. S. M. Marovina et al., "NHLBI Workshop on Lipoprotein a and CVD: Recent Advances and Future Directions," 2004, www.nhlbi.nih.gov; A. Ariyo, C. Thach, and R. Tracy, "Lp(a) Lipoprotein, Vascular Disease, and Mortality in the Elderly," *New England Journal of Medicine* 349, no. 22 (2003): 2108–2115.
30. National Heart, Lung, and Blood Institute, "Third Report of the Expert Panel on Detection."
31. Ibid.
32. Ibid.
33. Report of the American Heart Association, "Heart Disease and Stroke Statistics."
34. National Center for Health Statistics, "Vital and Health Statistics," series 10 (219), February 2004.
35. American Heart Association, *Heart Disease and Stroke Statistics.*
36. Ibid.
37. National Heart, Lung, and Blood Institute, "Understanding High Blood Pressure," 2006, www.nhlbi.nih.gov/hbp/hbp/intro.htm.
38. L. L. Yan et al., "Psychosocial Factors and Risk of Hypertension," *Journal of the American Medical Association* 290, no. 16 (2003): 2138–2148.
39. R. Eliot, "Changing Behavior: A New Comprehensive and Quantitative Approach" (keynote address, Annual Meeting of the American College of Cardiology on Stress and the Heart, Jackson Hole, WY, July 3, 1987).
40. J. Hsia et al., "Conjugated Equine Estrogens and Coronary Heart Disease," *Archives of Internal Medicine* 166, no. 3 (2006): 357–365.
41. American Heart Association, *Heart Disease and Stroke Statistics.*
42. Ibid.
43. M. Eisenberg et al., "Outcomes and Cost of Coronary Artery Bypass Graft Surgery in the United States and Canada," *Archives of Internal Medicine* 165 (2005): 1506–1513.
44. Berger et al., "Aspirin for the Primary Prevention of Cardiovascular Disease in Men and Women."
45. Agency for Healthcare Policy and Research, "Cardiac Rehabilitation: Exercise, Training, Education, Counseling, and Behavioral Interventions" (Publication #96-0672) (Rockville, MD: Author, 1996).
46. Report of the American Heart Association, "Heart Disease and Stroke Statistics."

16

Cancer

REDUCING YOUR RISK

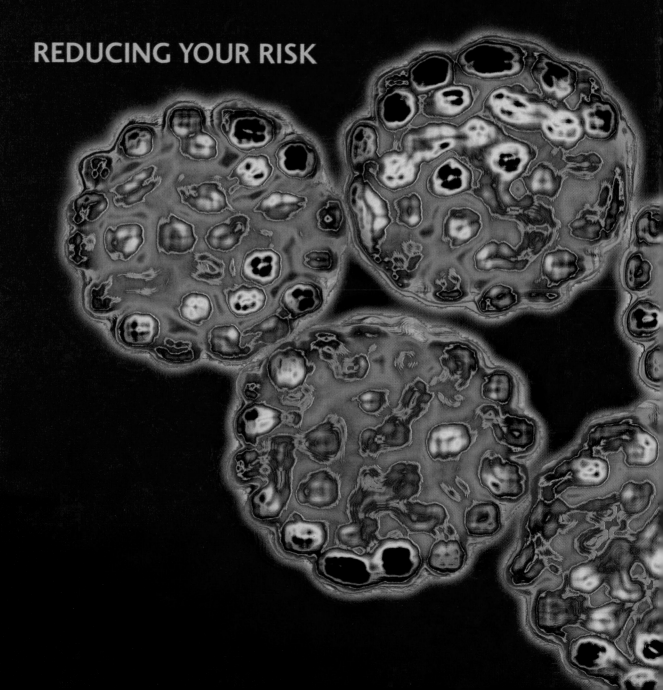

Does being **overweight** cause cancer?

If I quit **smoking** now, will I reduce my risk of lung cancer?

Is a **tanning** booth safer than the sun?

What are some ways cancer is **detected**?

What **treatment** types are the most cutting edge?

OBJECTIVES

- Understand what cancer is, how it develops, and its causes.
- Describe the different types of cancer and the risks they pose to people at different ages and stages of life.
- Explain the importance of early detection, self-exams, medical exams, and symptoms related to different types of cancer.
- Discuss ways to prevent cancer and the implications of behavioral risks.
- Discuss cancer diagnosis and treatment, including radiation therapy, chemotherapy, immunotherapy, and other common methods of detection and treatment.

As recently as 50 years ago, a diagnosis of cancer was usually a death sentence. Health professionals could only guess at the cause, and treatments were often as deadly as the disease itself. Because we had no idea how a person "got" cancer, fears about possible infection led to ostracism and bigotry aimed at people who desperately needed support, much like people with HIV were treated in the early days of the AIDS epidemic.

Fortunately, we've come a long way since then. Today we know that there are multiple causes of cancer and understand that even though you cannot "catch" cancer from another person, there are some infectious agents that increase your risk. Early detection and vast improvements in technology have dramatically improved the prognosis for most cancer patients. We also know that there are many actions we can take individually and as a society to prevent cancer. Understanding the facts about cancer, recognizing your own risk, and taking action to reduce your risk are important steps in the battle.

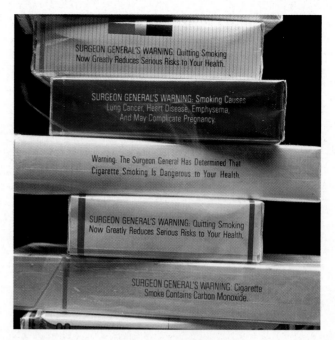

Of the several lifestyle risk factors for cancer, tobacco use is perhaps the most significant and the most preventable.

An Overview of Cancer

In 2005 a startling chronic disease statistic was revealed: Cancer became the leading cause of death for Americans under the age of 85, overtaking heart disease for the first time ever.[1] According to American Cancer Society data, 476,009 Americans under 85 died of cancer, compared with 450,637 who died of heart disease. Why did this news surprise public health experts? Cancer-related mortality rates have declined over the last decade and five-year survival rates (the relative rates for survival in persons who are living cancer free five years after diagnosis) for all cancers diagnosed between 1995 and 2001 were 65 percent, up dramatically from the 50 percent survivals in the 1970s.[2] However, though cancer-related deaths have declined over the last decade, they have not declined as quickly as deaths related to heart disease. New drug regimens, surgical techniques, and other anti–heart disease measures have been largely responsible for declines in heart disease (see Chapter 15). Although noteworthy improvements have been made in many cancer survival rates, certain cancers, such as pancreatic and liver, remain particularly resistant to treatment.

For Americans of all age groups, cancer continues to be the second leading cause of death. During 2006, approximately 564,830 Americans died of cancer, and nearly 1.4 million new cases were diagnosed. Put into perspective, this means that every day more than 1,500 Americans—one-quarter of all deaths—die of some form of cancer. Of these, one-third of the cancers were related to poor nutrition, physi-

cal inactivity, and obesity, which means they could have been prevented.

Certain other cancers are related to exposure to infectious diseases such as hepatitis B virus (HBV), human papillomavirus (HPV), HIV, *Helicobacter pylori* bacterium, and others, and could be prevented through behavioral changes, vaccines, or antibiotics.[3]

However, it is important to note that although approximately 1.4 million people will be diagnosed with cancer in a year, over 65 percent will be alive five years after diagnosis. Many will be considered "cured," meaning that they have no subsequent cancer in their bodies five years after diagnosis and can expect to live a long and productive life.[4] Some cancers that only a few decades ago presented a very poor outlook are often cured today, including acute lymphocytic leukemia in children, Hodgkin's disease, Burkitt's lymphoma, Ewing's sarcoma (a form of bone cancer), Wilms' tumor (a kidney cancer in children), testicular cancer, and osteogenic (bone) sarcoma.

What Is Cancer?

Cancer is the name given to a large group of diseases characterized by the uncontrolled growth and spread of abnormal cells.[5] Think of a healthy cell as a small computer, programmed to operate in a particular fashion. Under normal conditions, healthy cells are protected by a powerful overseer, the immune system, as they perform their daily functions of growing, replicating, and repairing body organs. When something interrupts normal cell programming, however, uncontrolled growth and abnormal cellular development result in a new growth of tissue serving no physiological function,

cancer A large group of diseases characterized by the uncontrolled growth and spread of abnormal cells.

TABLE 16.1	Probability of Developing Invasive Cancers Over Selected Age Intervals by Sex, United States 2000 to 2002*				
		Birth to 39 (%)	40 to 59 (%)	60 to 69 (%)	70 & Older (%)
All sites[†]	Male	1.43	8.57	16.46	39.61
	Female	1.99	9.06	10.54	26.72
Breast	Female	0.48	4.11	3.82	7.13
Colon and rectum	Male	0.07	0.90	1.66	4.94
	Female	0.06	0.70	1.16	4.61
Leukemia	Male	0.15	0.22	0.35	1.17
	Female	0.13	0.14	0.19	0.78
Lung and bronchus	Male	0.03	1.00	2.45	6.33
	Female	0.03	0.80	1.68	4.17
Melanoma of skin	Male	0.13	0.51	0.51	1.25
	Female	0.21	0.40	0.26	0.56
Prostate	Male	0.01	2.66	7.19	14.51

*For those free of cancer at beginning of age interval. Based on cancer cases diagnosed during 2000 to 2002.

[†]All sites exclude basal and squamous cell skin cancers and in situ cancers except urinary bladder.

Source: DevCan: Probability of Developing or Dying of Cancer Software, Version 6.0. Statistical Research and Applications Brance, National Cancer Institute, 2005, http://srab.cancer.gov/devcan; American Cancer Society, Surveillance Research, 2006.

which is called a **neoplasm.** This neoplasmic mass often forms a clumping of cells known as a **tumor.**

Not all tumors are **malignant** (cancerous); in fact, most are **benign** (noncancerous). Benign tumors are generally harmless unless they grow in such a fashion as to obstruct or crowd out normal tissues. A benign tumor of the brain, for instance, is life-threatening when it grows enough to restrict blood flow and cause a stroke. The only way to determine whether a tumor is malignant is through **biopsy,** or microscopic examination of cell development.

Benign and malignant tumors differ in several key ways. Benign tumors generally consist of ordinary-looking cells enclosed in a fibrous shell or capsule that prevents their spreading to other body areas. Malignant tumors are usually not enclosed in a protective capsule and can therefore spread to other organs. This process, known as **metastasis,** makes some forms of cancer particularly aggressive in their ability to overcome bodily defenses. By the time they are diagnosed, malignant tumors have frequently metastasized throughout the body, making treatment extremely difficult. Unlike benign tumors, which merely expand to take over a given space, malignant cells invade surrounding tissue, emitting clawlike protrusions that disturb the ribonucleic acid (RNA) and deoxyribonucleic acid (DNA) within normal cells. Disrupting these substances, which control cellular metabolism and reproduction, produces **mutant cells** that differ in form, quality, and function from normal cells.

How great is your own risk of cancer? Table 16.1 helps put this into perspective. Age and gender have a great deal to do with who gets cancer and who does not. For example, women under age 39 have a relatively low rate of breast cancer (1 in 209). However, women aged 60 and older face a dramatic increase in risk of breast cancer, at 1 in 26.[6] Assess your own cancer risk by completing the Assess Yourself box on page 482.

Disparities in Cancer Rates

Cancer strikes people of all ages, races, cultures, and socioeconomic levels, but some Americans are at greater risk. There are many demographic and socioeconomic factors

(Text continues on page 484)

neoplasm A new growth of tissue that serves no physiological function and results from uncontrolled, abnormal cellular development.

tumor A neoplasmic mass that grows more rapidly than surrounding tissue.

malignant Very dangerous or harmful; refers to a cancerous tumor.

benign Harmless; refers to a noncancerous tumor.

biopsy Microscopic examination of tissue to determine if a cancer is present.

metastasis Process by which cancer spreads from one area to different areas of the body.

mutant cells Cells that differ in form, quality, or function from normal cells.

ASSESS yourself

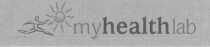

Fill out this assessment online at
www.aw-bc.com/myhealthlab or
www.aw-bc.com/donatelle.

Although you may be predisposed to some types of cancer due to genetic, biological, and/or environmental causes, there are many more that may be prevented through lifestyle changes and risk reduction strategies. If you carefully assess your risks, you can then make behavior changes that may make you less susceptible to various cancers. The following questions will give you an indication of your susceptibility. Of course, no single instrument can serve as a complete risk assessment or diagnostic guide. These questions merely serve as the basis for personal introspection and thoughtful planning about ways to reduce your risk.

Read each question and circle the number corresponding to each Yes or No. Be honest and accurate in order to get the most complete understanding of your cancer risks. Individual scores for specific questions should not be interpreted as a precise measure of relative risk, but the totals in each section give a general indication of your risk.

	Yes	No
SECTION 1: BREAST CANCER		
1. Do you check your breasts at least monthly using breast self-examination (BSE) procedures?	1	2
2. Do you look at your breasts in the mirror regularly, checking for any irregular indentations/lumps, discharge from the nipples, or other noticeable changes?	1	2
3. Has your mother, sister, or daughter been diagnosed with breast cancer?	2	1
4. Have you ever been pregnant?	1	2
5. Have you had a history of lumps or cysts in your breasts or underarm?	2	1
Total points _____		
SECTION 2: SKIN CANCER		
1. Do you spend a lot of time in the sun, either at work or at play?	2	1
2. Do you use sunscreens with an SPF rating of 15 or more when you are in the sun?	1	2
3. Do you use tanning beds or sun booths regularly to maintain a tan?	2	1
4. Do you examine your skin once a month, checking any moles or other irregularities, particularly in hard-to-see areas such as your back, genitals, neck, and under your hair?	1	2
5. Do you purchase and wear sunglasses that adequately filter out harmful sun rays?	1	2
Total points _____		
SECTION 3: CANCERS OF THE REPRODUCTIVE SYSTEM		
Men		
1. Do you examine your penis regularly for unusual bumps or growths?	1	2
2. Do you perform regular testicular self-examination?	1	2
3. Do you have a family history of prostate or testicular cancer?	2	1
4. Do you practice safer sex and wear condoms with every sexual encounter?	1	2
5. Do you avoid exposure to harmful environmental hazards such as mercury, coal tars, benzene, chromate, and vinyl chloride?	1	2
Total points _____		
Women		
1. Do you have a regularly scheduled Pap test?	1	2
2. Have you been infected with the human papillomavirus, Epstein-Barr virus, or other viruses believed to increase cancer risk?	2	1
3. Has your mother, sister, or daughter been diagnosed with breast, cervical, endometrial, or ovarian cancer (particularly at a young age)?	2	1

		Yes	No
4.	Do you practice safer sex and use condoms with every sexual encounter?	1	2
5.	Are you obese, taking estrogen, and/or consuming a diet that is very high in saturated fats?	2	1

Total points _____

SECTION 4: CANCERS IN GENERAL

		Yes	No
1.	Do you smoke cigarettes on most days of the week?	2	1
2.	Do you consume a diet that is rich in fruits and vegetables?	1	2
3.	Are you obese and/or do you lead a primarily sedentary lifestyle?	2	1
4.	Do you live in an area with high air pollution levels and/or work in a job where you are exposed to several chemicals on a regular basis?	2	1
5.	Are you careful about the amount of animal fat in your diet, substituting olive oil or canola oil for animal fat whenever possible?	1	2
6.	Do you limit your overall consumption of alcohol?	1	2
7.	Do you eat foods rich in lycopenes (such as tomatoes) and antioxidants?	1	2
8.	Are you "body aware" and alert for changes in your body?	1	2
9.	Do you have a family history of ulcers or of colorectal, stomach cancer, or other digestive system cancers?	2	1
10.	Do you avoid unnecessary exposure to radiation, cell phone emissions, and microwave emissions?	1	2

Total points _____

Analyzing Your Scores

Take a careful look at each question for which you received a "2" score. Are there any areas in which you received mostly "2s"? Did you receive total points of 6 or higher in Sections 1 through 3? Did you receive total points of 11 or higher in Section 4? If so, you have at least one identifiable risk. The higher the score, the more risks you may have. However, rather than focusing just on your score, focus on which items you might change. Review the suggestions throughout this chapter and list actions that you could take right now that might help you reduce your risk for these cancers.

MAKE it happen!

ASSESSMENT: The Assess Yourself activity above identifies certain behaviors that can contribute to increased cancer risks. If you have identified particular behaviors that may be putting you at risk, consider steps you can take to change these behaviors and improve your future health.

MAKING A CHANGE: In order to change your behavior, you need to develop a plan. Follow the steps below and complete your Behavior Change Contract to take action.

1. Evaluate your behavior, and identify patterns and specific things you are doing. What can you change now? What can you change in the near future?

2. Select one pattern of behavior that you want to change.

3. Fill out the Behavior Change Contract found at the front of your book. It should include your long-term goal for change, your short-term goals, the rewards you'll give yourself for reaching these goals, potential obstacles along the way, and strategies for overcoming these obstacles. For each goal, list the small steps and specific actions that you will take.

4. Chart your progress in a journal. At the end of a week, consider how successful you were in following your plan. What helped you be successful? What made change more difficult? What will you do differently next week?

5. Revise your plan as needed. Are the short-term goals attainable? Are the rewards satisfying?

ONE STUDENT'S PLAN: Keisha's assessment showed that, though she was taking precautions to reduce her cancer risk

(continued)

in most areas, she was not doing what she should about her breast cancer risk. Her score in this area was 8, because she did not regularly examine her breasts, her mother had been diagnosed with breast cancer two years ago, and she had never been pregnant. Keisha decided she needed to learn how to examine her breasts and to make a plan to ensure she did it every month. After studying this textbook's illustrations, she made an appointment with her gynecologist. While she was there, she asked the doctor to confirm that she was doing the examination correctly.

Next, Keisha decided that she would spend the first ten minutes of her morning once a month to do the exam and that she would give herself a reward for each month that she examined herself on schedule. On her way to campus after doing the exam, she would treat herself to a latte and a scone. After she stuck with her schedule for six months in a row, she would buy herself a new outfit. She also resolved to talk to her younger sister, who was also at risk, about the importance of the exam.

associated with health-related disparities, including income, race/ethnicity, culture, geography (urban/rural), age, sex, sexual orientation, and literacy.[7]

Poverty is widely believed to be the most important factor affecting health and longevity. People from lower socioeconomic levels tend to smoke more, be obese and sedentary, have less access to healthy fruits and vegetables, are often under- or uninsured (and therefore can access health care only when the cancer is in its later stages of development), may not be able to afford medications or uncompensated medical charges, and have difficulty communicating with their health care providers and understanding health information. Cultural factors, including ability to speak English, beliefs about the benefits and risks of treatment, beliefs about illness, and other factors may also affect the ability to access quality health care.[8] Culture can influence values and belief systems related to whether or not people seek care, take action to reduce risk, participate in preventive screenings, and comply with medical regimens.

How serious are the disparities? Consider the following:[9]

- Of all racial or ethnic groups in the United States, African Americans have the highest death rates from all cancer sites combined. Death rates for African American males are 1.4 times higher than for whites, and for females, they are 1.2 times higher.
- A person living in an affluent census tract has a five-year survival rate that is 10 percent higher than a person living in a tract below the poverty level.
- The gap between socioeconomic and ethnic groups in cancer mortality rates is greater now than it was in 1975.
- Men from poorer census counties have a 22 percent higher death rate from prostate cancer than their affluent county comparison groups.
- African Americans with stage I or stage II lung cancer are less likely to receive the recommended treatment of

surgery than whites, a disparity that accounts for much of the difference in survival.
- African Americans with cervical cancer are more likely than whites to go unstaged (that is, not to have their cancer's progression classified) and receive no treatment.
- Whites are more likely to receive aggressive treatment for colorectal cancer.

Though the above examples provide a disheartening look at the disparities that exist, reducing disparities is a major initiative of the National Institutes of Health and other professional groups. Planned actions include:

- *Advocacy.* Including media campaigns, information dissemination, lobbying and coalition formation, and action at the federal, state, and local levels, these efforts are designed to make it easier for those who are subjected to disparities to navigate the health care system. Public policies, other legislative action, and increased funding to get the word out all help disadvantaged groups have a better chance of quality care.
- *Research.* By increasing funding for research on the mechanisms of cancer initiation and factors likely to improve treatment among the poor and disadvantaged, health outcomes for cancer patients will definitely improve.
- *Education.* By broadening the base for bilingual information and educational materials, more diverse populations will be reached with key information about signs and symptoms, risk factors, and prevention strategies. In addition, providing at-risk populations with better information about navigating the health care system, accessing health care products and services, and other key information elements will result in earlier diagnosis and better prognosis for treatment.

See Figure 16.1 for some statistics that illustrate the severity of the problem of disparities in cancer death rates.

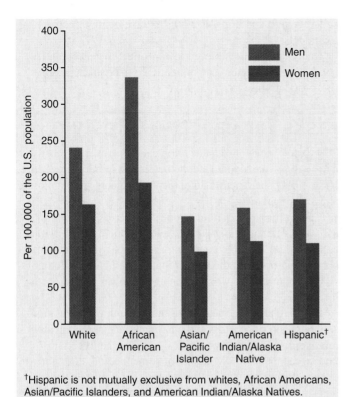

FIGURE 16.1 Cancer Death Rates, by Race and Ethnicity, United States, 1998–2002

Source: Surveillance, Epidemiology, and End Results Program, 1975–2002, Division of Cancer Control and Population Sciences, National Cancer Institute, 2005.

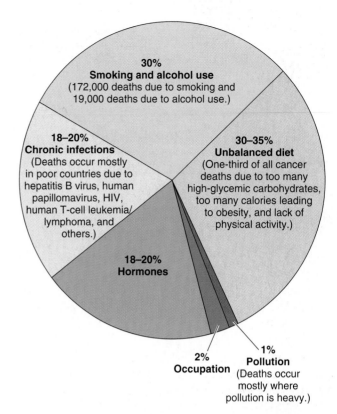

FIGURE 16.2 Factors Believed to Contribute to Global Causes of Cancer

Sources: S. Heacht et al., Public Session/Panel Discussion (Portland, OR: Linus Pauling Institute International Conference on Diet and Optimal Health, 2001); American Cancer Society, *Cancer Facts & Figures 2006* (Atlanta: American Cancer Society, 2006).

What Causes Cancer?

After decades of research, most cancer epidemiologists believe that cancers are, at least in theory, preventable, and many could be avoided by suitable choices in lifestyle and environment. Many specific causes of cancer are well documented, the most important of which are smoking, obesity, and a few organic viruses. However, wide global variations in common cancers, such as those of the breast, prostate, colon, and rectum, remain unexplained (Figure 16.2).

Most research supports the idea that cancer is caused by both *external* (chemicals, radiation, viruses, and lifestyle) and *internal* (hormones, immune conditions, and inherited mutations) factors. Causal factors may act together or in sequence to promote cancer development. We do not know why some people have malignant cells in their body and never develop cancer, while others may take ten years or more to develop the disease.

Cellular Change/Mutation Theories

One theory of cancer development proposes that cancer results from spontaneous errors that occur during cell reproduc-

tion. Perhaps cells that are overworked or aged are more likely to break down, causing genetic errors that result in mutant cells.

Another theory suggests that cancer is caused by some external agent or agents that enter a normal cell and initiate the cancerous process. It is believed that 75 to 85 percent of all deaths from cancer are related to environmental factors. These include radiation, chemicals, hormonal drugs, immunosuppressant drugs (drugs that suppress the normal activity of the immune system), and other toxins, which are considered possible **carcinogens** (cancer-causing agents); perhaps the most common carcinogen is the tar in cigarettes. The greater the dose or exposure to environmental hazards, the greater the risk of disease. People who are forced to work, live, and pass through areas that have high levels of environmental toxins may be at greater risk for several types of cancers.[10]

A third theory on the cause of cancer emerged from research on certain viruses believed to cause tumors in

carcinogens Cancer-causing agents.

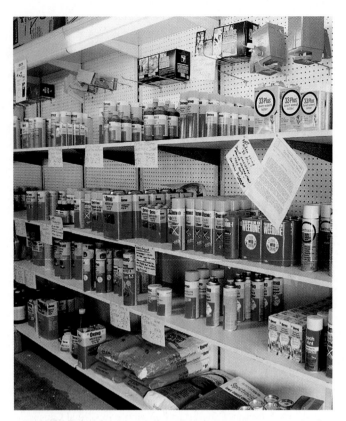

Research suggests that exposure to the chemicals found in many common products, like pesticides, may cause cancer.

animals. Scientists discovered **oncogenes,** suspected cancer-causing genes that are present on chromosomes. Although oncogenes are typically dormant, scientists theorize that certain conditions such as age, stress, and exposure to carcinogens, viruses, and radiation may activate them. Once activated, they grow and reproduce in an out-of-control manner.

Scientists are uncertain whether only people who develop cancer have oncogenes or whether we all have **protooncogenes,** genes that can become oncogenes under certain conditions. Many **oncologists** (physicians who specialize in the treatment of malignancies) believe that the oncogene theory may lead to a greater understanding of how individual

oncogenes   Suspected cancer-causing genes present on chromosomes.

protooncogenes   Genes that can become oncogenes under certain conditions.

oncologists   Physicians who specialize in the treatment of malignancies.

relative risk   A measure of the strength of the relationship between risk factors and the condition being studied, such as a particular cancer.

cells function and bring us closer to developing effective treatments.

Many factors are believed to contribute to cancer, and combining risk factors can dramatically increase a person's risk of the disease.

Risks for Cancer—Lifestyle

Anyone can develop cancer; however, most cases affect adults beginning in middle age. In fact, nearly 76 percent of cancers are diagnosed at ages 55 and over.

Cancer researchers refer to one's cancer risk when they assess risk factors. *Lifetime risk* refers to the probability that an individual, over the course of a lifetime, will develop cancer or die from it. In the United States, men have a lifetime risk of about one in two; women have a lower risk of one in three.[11]

Relative risk is a measure of the strength of the relationship between risk factors and a particular cancer. Basically, relative risk compares your risk if you engage in certain known risk behaviors with that of someone who does not engage in such behaviors. For example, if you are a male and smoke, your chances of getting lung cancer are about 23 times greater than those of a nonsmoker.[12]

Over the years, researchers have found that people who engage in certain behaviors show a higher incidence of cancer. In particular, diet, sedentary lifestyle (and resultant obesity), consumption of alcohol or cigarettes, stress, and other lifestyle factors seem to play a role. Likewise, colon and rectal cancer occur more frequently among persons with a high-fat, low-fiber diet; in those who don't eat enough fruits and vegetables; and in those who are inactive.[13] (See Chapter 8 on nutrition for information about certain dietary risks related to cancer and the role of supplements in prevention.) More research is needed to pinpoint the mechanisms that act in the body to increase the odds of cancer. For now, there is compelling evidence that certain actions are clearly associated with a greater than average risk of the disease.

Keep in mind that a high relative risk does not guarantee cause and effect. It merely indicates the likelihood of a particular risk factor being related to a particular outcome.

Smoking and Cancer Risk   Of all the potential risk factors for cancer, smoking is among the greatest. In the United States, tobacco is responsible for nearly one in five deaths annually, accounting for at least 30 percent of all cancer deaths and 87 percent of all lung cancer deaths.[14]

In the last 20 years, British and American lung cancer rates have declined however, lung cancer rates among men are still increasing in most developing countries and in Eastern Europe, where consumption of cigarettes remains high and is still increasing in some areas. Figure 16.3 demonstrates the correlation between smoking and lung cancer. See Chapter 13 for more on global trends in tobacco use.

Most authorities have believed that cigarettes cause only cancers of the lung, pancreas, bladder, and kidney, and (synergistically with alcohol) the larynx, mouth, pharynx, and esophagus. However, more recent evidence indicates that several other types of cancer are also related to tobacco. Most notably, cancers of the stomach, liver, and cervix seem to be directly related to long-term smoking.

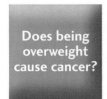

Obesity and Cancer Risk It is difficult to sort through the accumulated evidence about the role of certain nutrients, obesity, sedentary lifestyle, and related variables. Nevertheless, a body of research has emerged that points to a potential cancer link. Cancer is more common among people who are overweight, and risk increases as obesity increases. Several studies indicate a relationship between a high body mass index and death rates for cancers such as those of the esophagus, colon, rectum, liver, stomach, kidney, and pancreas. Women with a high BMI have a higher mortality rate from breast, uterine, cervical, and ovarian cancers; men with a high BMI have higher death rates from prostate and stomach cancers. In a study of over 900,000 U.S. adults, 34 percent of all cancer deaths were attributable to overweight and obesity. Numerous other studies support this link:[15]

- The relative risk of breast cancer in postmenopausal women is 50 percent higher for obese women than for nonobese women.
- The relative risk of colon cancer in men is 40 percent higher for obese men than for nonobese men.
- The relative risks of gallbladder and endometrial cancer are five times higher in obese individuals than in individuals of "healthy" weight.
- Some studies show a positive association between obesity and cancers of the kidney, pancreas, rectum, esophagus, and liver.
- Obesity is believed to alter complex interactions among diet, metabolism, physical activity, hormones, and growth factors.

Biological Factors

Early theorists believed that we inherit a genetic predisposition toward certain forms of cancer.[16] Cancers of the breast, stomach, colon, prostate, uterus, ovaries, and lung appear to run in families. For example, a woman runs a much higher risk of breast cancer if her mother or sisters (primary relatives) have had the disease, particularly at a young age. Hodgkin's disease and certain leukemias show similar familial patterns. Can we attribute these familial patterns to genetic susceptibility or to the fact that people in the same families experience similar environmental risks?

To date, the research in this area is inconclusive. It is possible that we can inherit a tendency toward a cancer-prone, weak immune system or, conversely, that we can inherit a cancer-fighting potential. But the complex interaction of hereditary predisposition, lifestyle, and environment on the

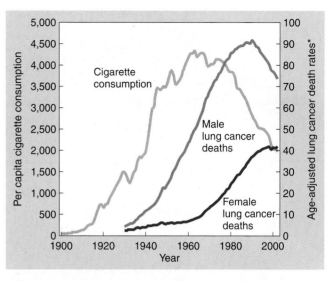

FIGURE 16.3 Tobacco Use in the United States, 1900–2002

Sources: Death Rates: U.S. Mortality Public Use Tapes, National Center for Health Statistics, 2005; Cigarette Consumption: U.S. Department of Agriculture, 1900–2002.

development of cancer makes it a challenge to determine a single cause. However, research resulting from the Human Genome Project indicates certain types of genetic predisposition to certain types of cancer. This body of research is expected to grow.

Biological sex also affects the likelihood of developing certain forms of cancer. For example, breast cancer occurs primarily among females, although men do occasionally get breast cancer. Obviously, factors other than heredity and familial relationships affect which sex develops a particular cancer. In the 1950s, for example, women rarely contracted lung cancer. But with increases in the number of women who smoke and the length of time they have smoked, lung cancer rates have soared to become the leading cause of cancer death in women. However, while gender plays a role in certain cases of cancer, other variables such as lifestyle are probably more significant.

Reproductive and Hormonal Risks for Cancer The effects of reproductive factors on breast and cervical cancer have been well documented. Late menarche, early menopause, early first childbirth, and high parity (having many children) have been shown to reduce a woman's risk of breast cancer. Pregnancy and estrogen supplementation in the form of oral contraceptives or hormone replacement therapy increase a woman's chances of breast cancer. A higher risk of endometrial cancer is also associated with hormone replacement therapy.[17]

Breast cancer is much more common in most Western countries than in developing countries. This is partly—and perhaps largely—accounted for by dietary effects (consuming a diet high in calories and fat), combined with later first childbirth, lower parity (having fewer children), shorter breast-feeding, higher obesity rates, and a longer life

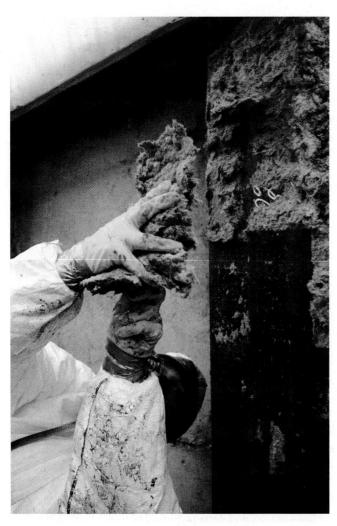

This worker is removing asbestos, a known carcinogen, from a building. What can his employer do to ensure his heath and safety?

expectancy among Western women (people do not live long enough to develop cancer).[18]

Occupational and Environmental Factors

Overall, workplace hazards account for only a small percentage of all cancers. However, various substances are known to cause cancer when exposure levels are high or prolonged. One of the most common occupational carcinogens is asbestos, a fibrous material once widely used in the construction, insulation, and automobile industries. Nickel, chromate, and chemicals such as benzene, arsenic, and vinyl chloride have been shown definitively to be carcinogens for humans. Also, people who routinely work with certain dyes and radioactive substances may have increased risks for cancer. Working with coal tars, as in the mining profession, or with inhalants, as in the auto-painting business, is hazardous. So is working with herbicides and pesticides, although the evidence is inconclusive for low-dose exposures. Several federal and state agencies are responsible for monitoring such exposures and ensuring that businesses comply with standards designed to protect workers.

Radiation: Ionizing and Nonionizing Ionizing radiation (IR)—radiation from X rays, radon, cosmic rays, and ultraviolet radiation (primarily ultraviolet B, or UVB radiation)—is the only form of radiation proven to cause human cancer. (See the section on skin cancer on page 496.) Incidents such as the Chernobyl nuclear accident in the 1980s focused attention on the potential risks of ionizing radiation. Evidence that high-dose IR causes cancer comes from studies of atomic bomb survivors, patients receiving radiotherapy, and certain occupational groups (for example, uranium miners). Virtually any part of the body can be affected by IR, but bone marrow and the thyroid are particularly susceptible. Radon exposures in homes can increase lung cancer risk, especially in cigarette smokers. To reduce the risk of harmful effects, diagnostic medical and dental X rays are set at the lowest dose levels possible.

Although nonionizing radiation produced by radio waves, cell phones, microwaves, computer screens, televisions, electric blankets, and other products has been a topic of great concern in recent years, research has not proven excess risk to date.[19]

Social and Psychological Factors

Many researchers claim that social and psychological factors play a major role in determining whether a person gets cancer. Stress has been implicated in increased susceptibility to several types of cancers. By reducing stress levels in your daily life, you may, in fact, lower your risk for disease. A number of therapists have even established preventive treatment centers where the primary focus is on "being happy" and "thinking positive thoughts." Is it possible to laugh away cancer?

Although medical personnel are skeptical of overly simplistic solutions, we cannot rule out the possibility that negative emotional states contribute to illness.[20] People who are under chronic, severe stress or who suffer from depression or other persistent emotional problems show higher rates of cancer than their healthy counterparts. Sleep disturbances, diet, or a combination of factors may weaken the body's immune system, increasing susceptibility to cancer. Although psychological factors may play a part in cancer development, lifestyle habits such as tobacco use are far more important.

Chemicals in Foods

Among the food additives suspected of causing cancer is *sodium nitrate,* a chemical used to preserve and give color to red meat. The actual carcinogen is not sodium nitrate but *nitrosamines,* substances formed when the body digests the sodium nitrates. Sodium nitrate has not been banned, primarily because it kills *Clostridium botulinum,* the bacterium that causes the highly virulent foodborne disease botulism. It

TABLE 16.2   Preventing Cancer through Diet and Lifestyle

Type of Cancer	Factors that Decrease Risk	Factors that Increase Risk
Breast	Engage in physical activity for at least 4 hours per week; consume lots of fruits and vegetables	Obesity and weight gain; alcohol consumption; hormone replacement therapy
Colorectal	Engage in regular, moderate physical activity; consume lots of fruits and vegetables	High intake of red meat; smoking; alcohol consumption; obesity
Lung	Consume at least 5 servings of fruits and vegetables daily	Tobacco use; some occupations
Oral/Throat	Consume at least 5 servings of fruits and vegetables daily; engage in regular, moderate physical activity	Tobacco use; obesity; alcohol consumption; salted foods
Prostate	Consume at least 5 servings of fruits and vegetables daily	High intake of red meat and high-fat dairy products
Stomach	Consume at least 5 servings of fruits and vegetables daily; refrigerate food	Salted foods; *Helicobacter pylori* bacteria

Here are some additional tips issued by a panel of cancer researchers:

- Avoid being underweight or overweight, and limit weight gain during adulthood to less than 11 pounds.
- If you don't get much exercise at work, take a 1-hour brisk walk or similar exercise daily, and exercise vigorously for at least 1 hour a week.
- Eat 8 or more servings a day of cereals and grains (such as rice, corn, breads, and pasta), legumes (such as peas), roots (such as beets, radishes, and carrots), tubers (such as potatoes), and plantains (including bananas).
- Limit consumption of refined sugar.
- Limit alcoholic drinks to less than 2 a day for men and 1 for women.
- Limit intake of red meat to less than 3 ounces a day, if eaten at all.
- Limit consumption of salted foods and use of cooking and table salt. Use herbs and spices to season foods.

Sources: World Cancer Research Fund, American Institute for Cancer Research, "Food, Nutrition and the Prevention of Cancer," www.wecf-uk.org; American Cancer Society, "The Complete Guide: Nutrition and Physical Activity," www.cancer.org.

should also be noted that the bacteria found in the human intestinal tract may contain more nitrates than a person could ever take in from eating cured meats or other nitrate-containing food products. Nonetheless, concern about the carcinogenic properties of nitrates has led to the introduction of meats that are nitrate-free or contain reduced levels of the substance.

Much of the concern about chemicals in foods centers on the possible harm caused by pesticide and herbicide residues. Whereas some of these chemicals cause cancer at high doses in experimental animals, the very low concentrations found in some foods are well within established government safety levels. Continued research regarding pesticide and herbicide use is essential, and scientists and consumer groups stress the importance of a balance between chemical use and the production of high-quality food products. Prevention efforts should focus on policies to protect consumers, develop low-chemical pesticides and herbicides, and reduce environmental pollution. See Table 16.2 for more information on preventing cancer through diet and lifestyle.

Infectious Diseases and Cancer

According to recent estimates, 17 percent of new cancers worldwide will be attributable to infection in 2005.[21] Infec-

tions are thought to influence cancer development in several ways, most commonly through (1) chronic inflammation, (2) suppression of the immune system, and/or (3) chronic stimulation.

HBV, HCV, and Liver Cancer Viruses such as hepatitis B (HBV) and C (HCV) are believed to stimulate cancer cells in the liver because they are chronic diseases that cause inflammation of liver tissue. This may prime the liver for cancer or make it more hospitable for cancer development. Global increases in hepatitis B and C rates and concurrent rises in liver cancer rates seem to provide evidence of such an association.

HPV and Cervical Cancer Nearly 100 percent of women with cervical cancer have evidence of human papillomavirus (HPV) infection, believed to be a major cause of cervical cancer. Fortunately, only a small percentage of HPV cases progress to cervical cancer.[22] Today, HPV can not only be controlled, but there is also a new vaccine against HPV. For more on this recent news, see Chapter 17.

Medical Factors

Some medical treatments increase a person's risk for cancer. One famous example is the prescription drug *diethylstilbestrol (DES),* widely used from 1940 to 1960 to control

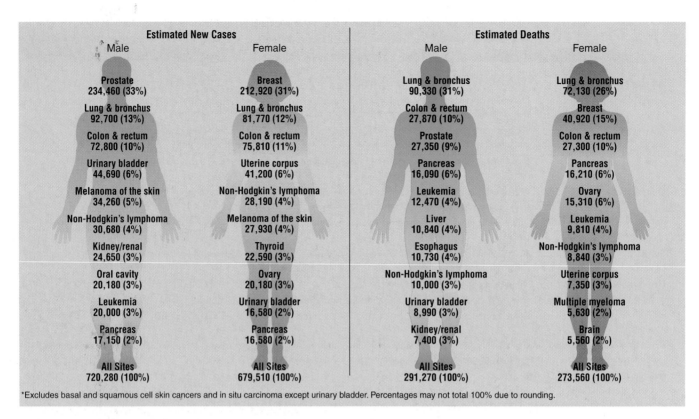

Estimated New Cases		Estimated Deaths	
Male	**Female**	**Male**	**Female**
Prostate 234,460 (33%)	Breast 212,920 (31%)	Lung & bronchus 90,330 (31%)	Lung & bronchus 72,130 (26%)
Lung & bronchus 92,700 (13%)	Lung & bronchus 81,770 (12%)	Colon & rectum 27,870 (10%)	Breast 40,920 (15%)
Colon & rectum 72,800 (10%)	Colon & rectum 75,810 (11%)	Prostate 27,350 (9%)	Colon & rectum 27,300 (10%)
Urinary bladder 44,690 (6%)	Uterine corpus 41,200 (6%)	Pancreas 16,090 (6%)	Pancreas 16,210 (6%)
Melanoma of the skin 34,260 (5%)	Non-Hodgkin's lymphoma 28,190 (4%)	Leukemia 12,470 (4%)	Ovary 15,310 (6%)
Non-Hodgkin's lymphoma 30,680 (4%)	Melanoma of the skin 27,930 (4%)	Liver 10,840 (4%)	Leukemia 9,810 (4%)
Kidney/renal 24,650 (3%)	Thyroid 22,590 (3%)	Esophagus 10,730 (4%)	Non-Hodgkin's lymphoma 8,840 (3%)
Oral cavity 20,180 (3%)	Ovary 20,180 (3%)	Non-Hodgkin's lymphoma 10,000 (3%)	Uterine corpus 7,350 (3%)
Leukemia 20,000 (3%)	Urinary bladder 16,580 (2%)	Urinary bladder 8,990 (3%)	Multiple myeloma 5,630 (2%)
Pancreas 17,150 (2%)	Pancreas 16,580 (2%)	Kidney/renal 7,400 (3%)	Brain 5,560 (2%)
All Sites 720,280 (100%)	All Sites 679,510 (100%)	All Sites 291,270 (100%)	All Sites 273,560 (100%)

*Excludes basal and squamous cell skin cancers and in situ carcinoma except urinary bladder. Percentages may not total 100% due to rounding.

FIGURE 16.4 Leading Sites of New Cancer Cases and Deaths, 2006 Estimates

Source: Reprinted by permission of the American Cancer Society, *Cancer Facts & Figures 2006* (Atlanta: American Cancer Society, 2006).

problems with bleeding during pregnancy and reduce the risk of miscarriage. Not until the 1970s did the dangers of this drug became apparent. Although DES caused few side effects in the millions of women who took it, their daughters were found to have an increased risk for cancers of the reproductive organs. Another example is the use of estrogen in treating menopausal symptoms. Estrogen use is now recognized to contribute to multiple cancer risks, and to provide fewer benefits than was originally believed. Prescriptions for estrogen therapy have declined dramatically, and many women are trying to reduce or eliminate their use of the hormone. Ironically, another medical factor is chemotherapy, which, while being used to treat one cancer, may increase the patient's risk of other forms of cancer.

Types of Cancers

As mentioned earlier, the term *cancer* refers not to a single disease, but to hundreds of different diseases. They are grouped into four broad categories based on the type of tissue from which the cancer arises.

Classifications of Cancer

- *Carcinomas.* Epithelial tissues (tissues covering body surfaces and lining most body cavities) are the most common sites for cancers. Carcinomas of the breast, lung, intes-

tines, skin, and mouth are examples. These cancers affect the outer layer of the skin and mouth as well as the mucous membranes. They metastasize through the circulatory or lymphatic system initially and form solid tumors.
- *Sarcomas.* Sarcomas occur in the mesodermal, or middle, layers of tissue—for example, in bones, muscles, and general connective tissue. They metastasize primarily via the blood in the early stages of disease. These cancers are less common but generally more virulent than carcinomas. They also form solid tumors.
- *Lymphomas.* Lymphomas develop in the lymphatic system—the infection-fighting regions of the body—and metastasize through the lymphatic system. Hodgkin's disease is an example. Lymphomas also form solid tumors.
- *Leukemias.* Cancer of the blood-forming parts of the body, particularly the bone marrow and spleen, is called leukemia. A nonsolid tumor, leukemia is characterized by an abnormal increase in the number of white blood cells.

Trained oncologists determine the seriousness and general prognosis of a particular cancer. Once laboratory results and clinical observations have been made, cancers are rated by level and stage of development. Those diagnosed as "carcinoma in situ" are localized at the point of origin and are often curable. Cancers with higher level or stage ratings have spread farther and are less likely to be cured. Figure 16.4 shows the most common sites of cancer and the number of deaths annually from each type.

Lung Cancer

Lung cancer killed an estimated 174,470 people in 2006, and it continues to be the leading cancer killer for men and women.[23] Since 1987, more women have died each year from lung cancer than from breast cancer, which over the previous 40 years had been the major cause of cancer deaths in women. As smoking rates have declined over the past 30 years, we have seen significant declines in male lung cancer, but these rates are not dropping as quickly among women. Another cause for concern is that although fewer adults are smoking, tobacco use among youth is again on the rise, and young women appear to be particularly vulnerable.

Symptoms and Treatment Symptoms of lung cancer include a persistent cough, blood-streaked sputum, chest pain, and recurrent attacks of pneumonia or bronchitis. Treatment depends on the type and stage of the cancer. Surgery, radiation therapy, and chemotherapy are all options. If the cancer is localized, surgery is usually the treatment of choice. If it has spread, surgery is combined with radiation and chemotherapy. Unfortunately, despite advances in medical technology, survival rates for lung cancer have improved only slightly over the past decade. Just 15 percent of lung cancer patients live five or more years after diagnosis. These rates improve to 50 percent with early detection, but only 16 percent of lung cancers are discovered in their early stages.[24]

Prevention Smokers, especially those who have smoked for over 20 years, and people who have been exposed to industrial substances such as arsenic and asbestos or to radiation are at the highest risk for lung cancer. The American Cancer Society estimates that 1 in 5 deaths are due to tobacco use in the United States.[25] Exposure to secondhand cigarette smoke, known as *environmental tobacco smoke* or *ETS,* increases the risk for nonsmokers. Researchers theorize that 90 percent of all lung cancers could be avoided if people did not smoke. Substantial improvements in overall prognosis have been noted in smokers who quit at the first signs of precancerous cellular changes and allowed their bronchial linings to return to normal.

> If I quit smoking now, will I reduce my risk of lung cancer?

Breast Cancer

About one out of eight women will develop breast cancer at some time in her life. Although this oft-repeated ratio has frightened many women, remember that it represents *lifetime* risk. Thus, not until the age of 80 does a woman's risk of breast cancer rise to one in eight.[26]

In 2006, approximately 212,920 women in the United States were diagnosed with invasive breast cancer for the first time. In addition, 61,980 new cases of *in situ* breast cancer, typically ductal carcinoma in situ (DCIS), a more localized cancer, were diagnosed. The increase in detection of DCIS is a direct result of earlier detection through mammography. In the same year, about 1,720 new cases of breast cancer were diagnosed in men. About 40,970 women (and 460 men) died, making breast cancer the second leading cause of cancer death for women. According to the most recent data, mortality rates went down dramatically from 1990 to 2002, with the largest decrease in younger women, under the age of 50.[27] This decline may be due to earlier diagnosis and better treatment, as numerous studies have shown that early detection increases survival and treatment options.

Detection and Symptoms The earliest signs of breast cancer are usually observable on mammograms, often before lumps can be felt. However, mammograms are not foolproof. Hence, regular breast self-examination (BSE) and careful attention to subtle body changes are important. If a mammogram detects a suspicious mass, a biopsy is performed to provide a more definitive assessment. Once breast cancer has grown to where it can be palpated, symptoms may include persistent breast changes, such as a lump in the breast or surrounding lymph nodes, thickening, dimpling, skin irritation, distortion, retraction or scaliness of the nipple, nipple discharge, or tenderness. Breast pain is commonly due to noncancerous conditions, such as fibrocystic breasts, and is not usually a first symptom. However, any time pain or tenderness persists in the breast or underarm area, it is a good idea to seek medical attention. Women who have ignored this symptom have been shocked to find out later that it was, for them, a symptom of cancer.

Risk Factors The incidence of breast cancer increases with age. Although there are many possible risk factors, those that are supported by research include:[28]

- Personal or family history of breast cancer (primary relatives such as mother, daughter, sister); the younger the relative was when diagnosed, the greater the family risk
- Biopsy-confirmed atypical hyperplasia (excessive increase in the number of cells or tissue growth)
- Long menstrual history (menstrual periods that started early and ended late in life)
- Obesity after menopause
- Recent use of oral contraceptives or postmenopausal estrogens or progestin (see the Women's Health/Men's Health box on hormones in Chapter 15)
- Never having children, or having a first child after age 30
- Consuming two or more drinks of alcohol per day
- Higher education and socioeconomic status

Risk factors that need more rigorous research before being firmly established as risks include:[29]

- Consuming a diet high in saturated fats
- Exposure to pesticides and other chemicals
- Weight gain, particularly after menopause
- Physical inactivity
- Genetic predisposition through *BRCA1* and *BRCA2* genes. (Genes appear to account for approximately 5 to 10 percent of all cases of breast cancer. Screening for these

How to Examine Your Breasts

The best time for a woman to examine her breasts is when the breasts are not tender or swollen. Women who are pregnant, breast-feeding, or have breast implants can also choose to examine their breasts regularly.

1. Lie down and place your right arm behind your head. The exam is done while lying down, not standing up, because when lying down the breast tissue spreads evenly over the chest wall and it is as thin as possible, making it much easier to feel all the breast tissue.

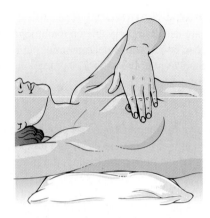

2. Use the finger pads of the three middle fingers on your left hand to feel for lumps in the right breast. Use overlapping dime-sized circular motions of the finger pads to feel the breast tissue.

3. Use three different levels of pressure to feel all the breast tissue. Light pressure is needed to feel the tissue closest to the skin; medium pressure to feel a little deeper; and firm pressure to feel the tissue closest to the chest and ribs. A firm ridge in the lower curve of each breast is normal. If you're not sure how hard to press, talk with your doctor or nurse. Use each pressure level to feel the breast tissue before moving on to the next spot.

4. Move around the breast in an up and down pattern starting at an imaginary line drawn straight down your side from the underarm and moving across the breast to the middle of the chest bone. Be sure to check the entire breast area going down until you feel only ribs and up to the neck or collar bone (clavicle).

    There is some evidence to suggest that the up and down pattern (sometimes called the vertical pattern) is the most effective pattern for covering the entire breast without missing any breast tissue.

5. Repeat the exam on your left breast, using the finger pads of the right hand.

6. While standing in front of a mirror with your hands pressing firmly down on your hips, look at your breasts for any changes of size, shape, contour, or dimpling. (The pressing down on the hips position contracts the chest wall muscles and enhances any breast changes.)

7. Examine each underarm while sitting up or standing and with your arm only slightly raised so you can easily feel in this area. (Raising your arm straight up tightens the tissue in this area and makes it difficult to examine.)

FIGURE 16.5 Breast Self-Examination

Note that the American Cancer Society recommends the use of mammography and clinical breast exam in addition to self-examination.

Source: American Cancer Society, "Breast Awareness and Self-Examination," 2006, www.cancer.org/docroot/CRI/content/CRI_2_4_3X _Can_breast_cancer_be_found_early_5.asp?sitearea=.

genes is recommended for women with a family history of breast cancer, when counseling is available.)

Although risk factors are useful indicators, they do not always predict individual susceptibility. However, because of increased awareness, better diagnostic techniques, and improved treatments, breast cancer patients have a better chance of surviving today. The five-year survival rate for people with localized breast cancer (which includes all people living five years after diagnosis, whether the patient is in remission, disease free, or under treatment) has risen from 80 percent in the 1950s to 98 percent today. These statistics vary dramatically, however, based on the stage of the cancer when it is first detected. As with most cancers, the earlier the stage, the greater the chances of a full recovery. If the cancer has spread to surrounding tissue, the five-year survival rate is 81 percent; if it has spread to distant parts of the body, the rate falls to 26 percent; and if the breast cancer has not spread at all, the survival rate approaches 100 percent.[30]

Patients who become actively involved in treatment decision making, who seek out the best oncologists with the most experience with their type of cancer, and who become knowledgeable about options and treatments often fare best. Of course, this takes time, access to health care providers, supportive family members, and attention to health-promoting lifestyles before, during, and after treatment.

Prevention International differences in breast cancer incidence correlate with variations in diet, especially fat intake, although a causal role for these dietary factors has not been firmly established. Sudden weight gain has also been implicated. Exciting new research about the *BRCA1* and *BRCA2* genes for breast cancer offers new hope for early detection.

Regular self-examination (Figure 16.5) and mammograms are the best ways to prevent and detect breast cancer early. The American Cancer Society offers guidelines for how often women should get mammograms and checkups (Table 16.3). All women, no matter their age, should be in the habit of breast self-examination every month.

Some research also shows that exercise can reduce risk, and the good news is that it does not have to be heavy

TABLE 16.3	Recommendations for the Early Detection of Cancer in Asymptomatic People
Site	**Recommendation**
Cancer-related checkup	For individuals undergoing periodic health examinations, a cancer-related checkup should include health counseling and, depending on a person's age, might include examination for cancers of the thyroid, oral cavity, skin, lymph nodes, testes, and ovaries, as well as for some nonmalignant diseases.
Breast	Women 40 and older should have an annual mammogram and an annual clinical breast exam (CBE) performed by a health care professional and should perform monthly breast self-examination (BSE). Ideally, the CBE should occur before the scheduled mammogram.
	Women aged 20–39 should have a clinical breast exam performed by a health care professional every 3 years and should perform monthly breast self-examination.
Colon and rectum	Beginning at age 50, men and women should follow one of the examination schedules below:
	■ A fecal occult blood test (FOBT) every year, or a flexible sigmoidoscopy (FSIG) every 5 years, or annual fecal occult blood test and flexible sigmoidoscopy every 5 years*
	■ A double-contrast barium enema every 5 to 10 years
	■ A colonoscopy every 10 years
Prostate	The American Cancer Society recommends that both the prostate-specific antigen (PSA) blood test and the digital rectal examination be offered annually, beginning at age 50, to men who have a life expectancy of at least 10 more years.
	Men at high risk (African American men and men with a strong family history of one or more first-degree relatives diagnosed with prostate cancer at an early age) should begin testing at age 45.
	Information should be provided to patients about what is known and what is uncertain about the benefits and limitations of early detection and treatment of prostate cancer so that they can make an informed decision.
Uterus	**Cervix:** Screening should begin approximately 3 years after a woman begins having vaginal intercourse but no later than 21 years of age. Screening should be done every year with Pap tests or every 2 years using liquid-based tests. At or after age 30, women who have had 3 normal tests in a row may get screened every 2–3 years, unless they have certain risk factors, such as HIV infection or a weak immune system.
	Endometrium: The American Cancer Society recommends that all women should be informed about the risks and symptoms of endometrial cancer and strongly encouraged to report any unexpected bleeding or spotting to their physicians. Annual screening for endometrial cancer with endometrial biopsy beginning at age 35 should be offered to women with or at risk for hereditary nonpolyposis colon cancer (HNPCC).

*Combined testing is preferred over either annual FOBT or FSIG every five years alone. People who are at moderate or high risk for colorectal cancer should talk with a doctor about a different testing schedule.

Source: American Cancer Society, *Cancer Facts & Figures 2006* (Atlanta: American Cancer Society, 2006). Reproduced with permission. www.cancer.org. © 2006, American Cancer Society, Inc.

exercise to be beneficial. Researchers speculate that exercise may protect women by altering the production of the ovarian hormones estrogen and progesterone during menstrual cycles.[31]

Treatment Today, people with breast cancer (like people with nearly any type of cancer) have many treatment options to choose from. It is important to thoroughly check out a physician's track record and his or her philosophy on the best treatment. Is the physician's recommendation consistent with that of major cancer centers in the country? Check out the doctor's credentials and the experiences of patients who have seen this doctor as well as the surgeon who will perform your biopsy and other surgical techniques. If possible, seek a facility that has a significant number of breast cancer patients, does many surgeries, is regarded as a teaching facility for new oncologists, has the "latest and greatest" in terms of technology, and is highly regarded by past patients. Often, cancer support groups can provide invaluable information and advice.

Treatments range from a lumpectomy to radical mastectomy to various combinations of radiation or chemotherapy. Figure 16.6 on page 494 reviews these options. Among nonsurgical options, promising results have been noted among women using *selective estrogen-receptor modulators (SERMs)* such as tamoxifen and raloxifene, particularly among women whose cancers appear to grow in response to estrogen. These drugs, as well as new *aromatase inhibitors*, work by blocking estrogen.[32] Remember that it is always a good idea to seek more than one opinion before making a decision.

Colon and Rectal Cancers

Colorectal cancers (cancers of the colon and rectum) continue to be the third most common cancer in both men and women, with over 148,610 cases diagnosed in 2006.[33] Although colon cancer rates have increased steadily in recent decades, many people are unaware of their risk.

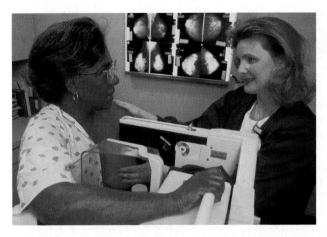

Early detection through mammography and other techniques greatly increases a woman's chance of surviving breast cancer.

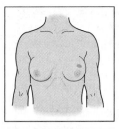

Lumpectomy
Performed when tumor is in earliest localized stages. Prognosis for recovery is better than 95%. Only tumor itself is removed. Some physicians may also remove normal tissue in surrounding area.

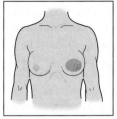

Simple mastectomy
Removal of breast and underling tissue. Prognosis for full recovery better than 80%.

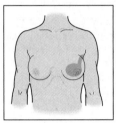

Modified radical mastectomy
Breast and lymph nodes in immediate area removed. Prognosis for full recovery dependent on level of spread.

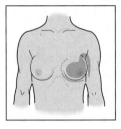

Radical mastectomy
Removal of breast, lymph nodes, pectoral muscles, all fat, and underlying tissue. Prognosis for full recovery may be as low as 60%, depending on level of spread.

Detection and Symptoms
In its early stages, colorectal cancer has no symptoms. Bleeding from the rectum, blood in the stool, and changes in bowel habits are the major warning signals. Because colorectal cancer tends to spread slowly, the prognosis is quite good if it is caught in the early stages. Early screening programs can detect precancerous polyps or early stage colorectal cancer, and aid to diagnose the disease at more treatable stages. However, in spite of major educational campaigns, many Americans fail to have the most basic screening test—the fecal occult blood test. Colonoscopy or barium enemas are recommended screening tests for at-risk populations and everybody over age 50.

Risk Factors
Anyone can get colorectal cancer, but people who are over age 50, who are obese, who have a family history of colon and rectal cancer, a personal or family history of polyps (benign growths) in the colon or rectum, or inflammatory bowel problems such as colitis run an increased risk. Other possible risk factors include diets high in fat or low in fiber, smoking, sedentary lifestyle, high alcohol consumption, and low intake of fruits and vegetables. Indeed, approximately 90 percent of all colorectal cancers are preventable.[34] Recent studies have suggested that estrogen replacement therapy and nonsteroidal anti-inflammatories such as aspirin may reduce colorectal risk.[35]

Prevention and Screening
Regular exercise, a diet with lots of fruits and plant-origin foods, a healthy weight, and moderation in alcohol consumption appear to be among the most promising prevention strategies. New research also suggests that aspirin-like drugs, postmenopausal hormones, folic acid, calcium supplements, selenium, and vitamin E may also contribute to prevention; however, more research must be conducted to conclusively determine if and how these substances reduce risk.[36]

The most commonly recommended screenings, particularly for those over age 50, include:[37]

FIGURE 16.6 Surgical Procedures for Diagnosed Breast Cancer
These surgeries are typically followed by radiation treatment and/or chemotherapy.

- *Fecal occult blood test (FOBT).* Cancers and large polyps often bleed sporadically into the intestine. The FOBT detects "hidden," or "occult," blood in a stool sample. You take samples of your own stool in the privacy of your home, place them in a preservative medium, and mail them to a lab for evaluation. This is a relatively inexpensive test (less than $20 in most cases), and it has been proven to play a significant role in early detection.
- *Digital rectal exam.* In this test, a physician inserts his or her finger into the rectum to feel for irregularities. This is often part of a routine examination, but when used alone, it is not sufficient to rule out possible problems.
- *Flexible sigmoidoscopy.* In this test, a two-foot-long, slender, flexible, hollow, lighted tube is inserted into the rectum and up into the lower region of the colon. This test requires less preparation, is safer than a colonoscopy, and is a helpful early screening exam. However, it can only detect problems in the lower colon, and any polyps or other irregularities that are found will require a colonoscopy to assess the entire bowel. The cost is $150 or more.

- *Barium enema with air contrast.* For this test, the bowel must be completely clean and a white, chalky substance known as barium sulfate is introduced into the colon and allowed to spread, while air is pumped into the colon. X rays monitor irregular outcroppings and deviations that might indicate tumor invasion. The cost is $300 to $500 or more. If abnormalities are found, a colonoscopy may still need to be performed.
- *Colonoscopy.* Like the sigmoidoscopy, this test allows for direct visual examination of the colon and rectum, but it includes a much larger portion of the colon. Polyps can be removed via the colonoscope; the cost is $1,000 or more.
- *Newer tests.* In the future, genetic-based fecal screening and other techniques may be widely available. It is currently possible to swallow a small camera and have a form of virtual examination of the colon as the camera passes through. However, this technique is more time consuming and the optics are not yet as clear and reliable as the regular colonoscopic techniques.

For many people, the preparation for any of these tests, which may include laxatives to induce bowel movements, self-enemas, fasting, and other techniques, is an obstacle that must be reduced or overcome to ensure better participation.

Treatment Treatment often consists of radiation or surgery. Chemotherapy, although not used extensively in the past, is today a possibility. A permanent *colostomy,* the creation of an abdominal opening to eliminate body wastes, is seldom required for people with colon cancer and even less frequently for those with rectum cancer.

Prostate Cancer

Cancer of the prostate is the most common cancer in American males today, excluding skin cancer, and the second leading cause of cancer death in men, after lung cancer. In 2006, about 234,460 new cases of prostate cancer were diagnosed in the United States. About 1 man in 3 will be diagnosed with prostate cancer during his lifetime, but only 1 man in 33 will die of it.[38] Put into perspective, prostate cancer accounts for about 10 percent of cancer-related deaths in men each year.

Ironically, many people do not know what the prostate is or what function it serves in the body. The prostate is a muscular, walnut-sized gland that surrounds part of the urethra, the tube that transports urine and sperm out of the body. As part of the male reproductive system, its primary function is to produce seminal fluid, the fluid that transports sperm. During an orgasm, the muscles of the prostate contract to push semen through the urethra and out through the penis. Located directly below the bladder, if the prostate becomes enlarged, either through inflammation or cancerous growth, it may block the urethra, thus disrupting flow out of the bladder, or push on the bladder and cause pain or discomfort. That is why pain and difficulty in urination are often symptoms of problems with the prostate.

Symptoms Most symptoms of prostate cancer are non-specific, that is, they mimic signs of infection or an enlarged prostate. Symptoms may include weak or interrupted urine flow; difficulty starting or stopping urination; feeling the urge to urinate frequently; pain upon urination; blood in the urine; or **referred pain** (pain that originates in one spot but is felt elsewhere) in the low back, pelvis, or thighs. It is important to note that many men are **asymptomatic** (have no symptoms) in the early stages, which is why testing and early diagnosis are becoming more important as the risks of prostate cancer rise in the general population. Most prostate cancers grow slowly and are believed to take years to develop.

New research that is particularly relevant to college-aged men has found that prostate cancer may begin with a condition called *prostatic intraepithelial neoplasia (PIN).* In this condition, there are changes in the microscopic appearance of prostate gland cells, ranging from a bit different than normal to abnormal. The important part of this is that these changes are believed to occur in men in their twenties and by the time men reach age 50, nearly 50 percent of them have these changes.[39]

Risk Factors Although the causes of prostate cancer continue to elude health professionals, there are several factors that appear to increase risk. Among the most likely are:[40]

- *Age.* Chances of developing prostate cancer increase dramatically with age. More than 70 percent of cancers are diagnosed in men over the age of 65. Usually the disease has progressed to the point of displaying symptoms in these older men, or they are more likely to be seeing a doctor for other problems and get a screening test or **prostate-specific antigen (PSA)** test.
- *Race.* African American men are 61 percent more likely to develop prostate cancer than white men and are much more likely to be diagnosed at an advanced stage. Being diagnosed at an advanced stage means that they are also more likely to die of the disease than other races. Prostate cancer is less common among Asian men and occurs at about the same rates among Hispanic men as it does among white men.
- *Nationality.* Prostate cancer is most common in North America and northwestern Europe and less common in Asia, Africa, Central America, and South America. The reasons for these differences are not well understood but may be due to the fact that men in the latter countries are less likely to be diagnosed (are less likely to receive PSA testing) or that, in some countries where AIDS is a leading

referred pain Pain caused by a condition in one place that is felt in a different place.

asymptomatic Having a disease but no symptoms.

prostate-specific antigen (PSA) An antigen found in prostate cancer patients.

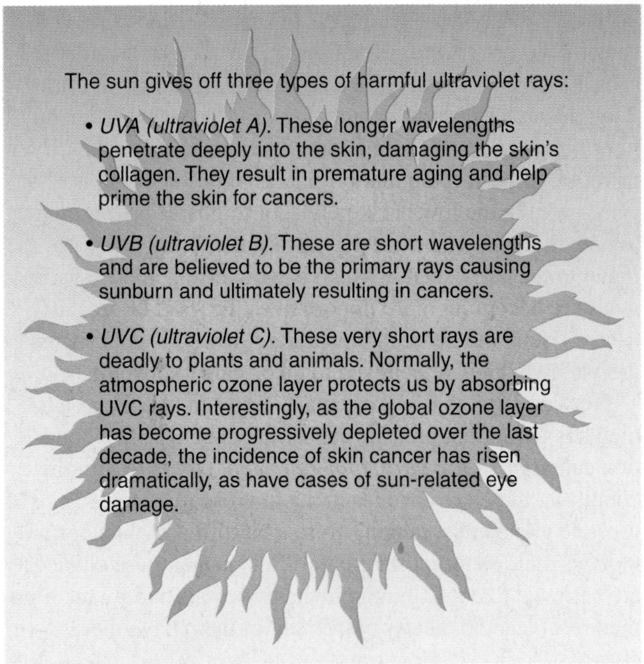

The sun gives off three types of harmful ultraviolet rays:

- *UVA (ultraviolet A)*. These longer wavelengths penetrate deeply into the skin, damaging the skin's collagen. They result in premature aging and help prime the skin for cancers.

- *UVB (ultraviolet B)*. These are short wavelengths and are believed to be the primary rays causing sunburn and ultimately resulting in cancers.

- *UVC (ultraviolet C)*. These very short rays are deadly to plants and animals. Normally, the atmospheric ozone layer protects us by absorbing UVC rays. Interestingly, as the global ozone layer has become progressively depleted over the last decade, the incidence of skin cancer has risen dramatically, as have cases of sun-related eye damage.

FIGURE 16.7 Types of Ultraviolet Rays

killer of men, men may not live long enough to develop the disease.

- *Family history.* Having a father or brother with prostate cancer more than doubles a man's risk of getting prostate cancer (interestingly, the risk is higher for men with an affected brother than it is for those with an affected father). The genes that predispose men to prostate cancer have not been clearly identified; thus, genetic tests like those for breast cancer in women are not yet available.

- *Diet.* Although diet is widely believed to be a risk factor for prostate cancer, most studies have not yet conclusively identified specific risks. The fact that men in countries where high-fat diets are consumed have higher risks of prostate cancer than men in countries with lower fat is the most compelling indicator for the role of dietary fats.

- *Physical activity and overweight/obesity.* Some studies have suggested that regular physical activity and maintaining a healthy weight may help reduce the risk of developing or dying from prostate cancer; however, this link is not clear.

- *Vasectomy.* Although there is concern among some groups that having a vasectomy, particularly before the age of 35, increases the risk of prostate cancer, most recent studies have not found this to be true. More research examining this issue is currently under way.

Prevention and Treatment A quick look at the risk factors for prostate cancer tells you that many of these factors, such as age and race, are beyond your control. However,

malignant melanoma A virulent cancer of the melanocytes (pigment-producing cells) of the skin.

there are some things that you could do that appear promising. Eating more fruits and vegetables, particularly those containing lycopenes, may lower your risk. Some studies suggest that taking 50 milligrams (400 International Units) of vitamin E and adequate amounts of selenium in your diet may reduce risk, while consuming high levels of vitamin A may increase your risks. Until more definitive proof of nutrient effectiveness in risk reduction is available, the best advice would be to follow the dietary recommendations discussed in Chapter 8. Otherwise, keeping your weight healthy, getting regular amounts of exercise, sleeping sufficient amounts, and reducing stress keeps your immune system functioning effectively and may help you resist some forms of cancer development.

Another important strategy is to get diagnostic tests on the schedule recommended by the American Cancer Society and the National Cancer Institute. Every man over the age of 40 should have an annual digital rectal prostate examination. The American Cancer Society recommends that men age 50 and over have an annual prostate-specific antigen (PSA) test (see the Women's Health/Men's Health box). African American men and those with brothers or fathers who have had prostate cancer need to be particularly attentive to getting PSA and other diagnostic tests and discussing their concerns with physicians.

Fortunately, even with so many generalized symptoms, 83 percent of all prostate cancers are detected while they are still in the local or regional stages and tend to progress slowly. The five-year survival rate in these early stages is 100 percent.

Skin Cancer: Sun Worshippers Beware

If you are one of the millions of people each year who try to get a "healthy tan," think again. In fact, that phrase isn't just an oxymoron; it stands for premature aging and wrinkling at the very least, and life-threatening illness at worst. The damage to your skin from a single bad sunburn lasts the rest of your life! Even worse, such damage is cumulative. Early signs of sun damage (photodamage) include sunburn, tanning, and increased freckling. Later, these "cute" freckles are followed by wrinkling, premature aging and age spots, cataracts and other forms of eye damage, sagging of the skin, and the most serious consequence: skin cancer. If you are an avid sunbather, compare areas such as your hands and face to areas that are almost always covered from the sun's rays, such as your buttocks or breasts. The differences that you see are almost always the result of sun exposure over time.[41]

The long-term effects of sun exposure can be devastating:[42]

- Skin cancer is the most common form of cancer in the United States today, affecting over 1 million people every year (one in five of all adults). This year 10,710 people are estimated to die of skin cancer. Of those, 7,910 will die of melanoma and 2,800 will die of other forms of skin cancer.

- **Malignant melanoma,** the deadliest form of skin cancer, is beginning to occur at a much higher rate in women

PSA TESTS: WHAT DO THE NUMBERS MEAN TO YOU?

Prostate-specific antigen (PSA) tests are blood tests that detect PSA, a substance made by the prostate gland. Although PSA is found primarily in semen, a small amount is also found in the blood; hence the test involves taking a blood sample from the arm. The blood is sent to a laboratory and, if normal, the result will be a value of 4 nanograms per milliliter (ng/ml) of blood.

If the person has prostate cancer, these values normally go above 4. In general, the greater the number, the higher your risk of actually having cancer. If the value is between 4 and 10, you may have a 25 percent chance of having prostate cancer; if greater than 10, your risk goes up proportionally. Some groups recommend that if your values are 3 or higher, you should consult with your doctor and have a more definitive test.

It is important to know that PSA tests are not perfect and many false positives (tests that show positive values but are actually negative) and false negatives (tests that show negative values when you may actually have cancer) occur. Several factors are believed to influence the reliability of these tests:

- Benign prostate hypertrophy, a non-cancerous enlargement of the prostate
- Prostatitis, inflammation of the prostate
- Ejaculation, which can cause a temporary increase in blood PSA levels (you should abstain from ejaculating for two days before the test)
- Some medications, such as finasteride (Proscar or Propecia) and dutasteride (Avodart), may falsely lower PSA values
- Herbal preparations, particularly those labeled for prostate health

There are other PSA tests (such as the percent-free PSA) that are more sensitive and provide a better indicator of your risk. If you or a loved one gets a preliminary high value and none of the above factors apply, ask the doctor for a more definitive test. In addition, doctors may choose to biopsy the tissue, do digital rectal examinations, perform ultrasound tests such as a transrectal ultrasound, or employ other more sophisticated diagnostic tools. Consult the patient information websites established by the American Cancer Society and the National Cancer Institute and ask questions, particularly if you have siblings or a father who have been diagnosed previously.

Source: American Cancer Society, *Cancer Facts & Figures 2006* (Atlanta: American Cancer Society, 2006). Reproduced with permission. www.cancer.org. © 2006, American Cancer Society, Inc.

---

under age 40. In fact, whereas relatively few people die from the highly treatable basal or squamous cell skin cancers, the highly virulent malignant melanoma has become the most frequent cancer in women aged 25 to 29 and runs second only to breast cancer in women aged 30 to 34.

- Rates of melanoma are ten times higher among whites than blacks.

What happens when you expose yourself to sunlight? Biologically, the skin responds to photodamage by increasing its thickness and the number of pigment cells (melanocytes), which produce the "tan" look. The skin's cells that ward off infection are also prone to photodamage, lowering the normal immune protection of our skin and priming it for cancer.[43] Photodamage also causes wrinkling by impairing the elastic substances (collagens) that keep skin soft and pliable.

Although sun exposure risks have been widely reported, over 60 percent of Americans aged 25 years and under report that they are "working on a tan" at some point during the year. Despite the red flag, why do people continue to tan? Recent research suggests a connection between high levels of ultraviolet light and endorphins. Those who tan in the sun or artificially may experience a short "high" for this reason, and

tanning can become a type of addiction. For more on the safety of tanning booths and other artificial tans, see the Spotlight on Your Health box on page 501.

Risk Factors Who's at risk for skin cancer? Anyone who overexposes himself or herself without adequate protection. The risk is greatest for people who fit the following categories:

- Have fair skin; blonde, red, or light brown hair; blue, green, or gray eyes
- Always burn before tanning or burn easily and peel readily
- Don't tan easily, but spend lots of time outdoors
- Have previously been treated for skin cancer or have a family history of skin cancer (if you have a family history of melanoma, see your physician for regular skin exams)
- Use no or low-SPF sunscreens

Preventing skin cancer is a matter of limiting exposure to harmful UV rays (Figure 16.7). If you do get sunburned, be careful about treating it:

- Drink more fluids than usual.
- Take aspirin or ibuprofen to reduce inflammation; apply cool compresses gently, without rubbing the area; when you shower or bathe, use a mild soap.

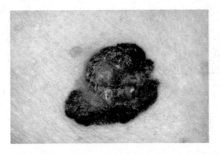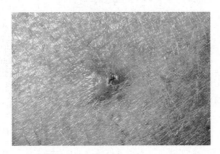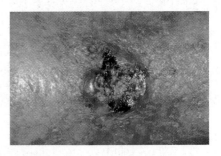

Prevention of skin cancer requires keeping a careful watch for any new pigmented growths and for changes to any moles. Melanoma symptoms, as shown in the left photo, include scalloped edges, asymmetrical shapes, discoloration, and an increase in size. Basal cell carcinoma and squamous cell carcinoma (middle and right photos, respectively) should be brought to your physician's attention but are not as deadly as melanoma.

TABLE 16.4	Safe Sun Tips

- Avoid the sun, or seek shade, from 10 AM to 2 PM, when the sun's rays are strongest. Even on a cloudy day, up to 80 percent of the sun's rays can get through.
- Apply an SPF 15 or higher sunscreen evenly to all uncovered skin before going outside. Look for a "broad-spectrum" sunscreen that protects against both UVA and UVB radiation. Check the label for the correct amount of time you should allow between applying the product and going outdoors. If the label does not specify, apply it 30 minutes before going outside. Ask a doctor before applying sunscreen to children under six months old.
- Remember to apply sunscreen to your eyelids, lips, nose, ears, neck, hands, and feet.
- If you don't have much hair, apply sunscreen to the top of your head. Better still, wear a wide-brimmed, light-colored hat to protect your head and face.
- Reapply sunscreen often. The label will tell you how often you need to reapply it. If it isn't waterproof, reapply it after taking a dip, or if you are sweating a lot.
- Wear loose-fitting, light-colored clothing.
- Use sunglasses with 99 to 100 percent UV protection to protect your eyes.
- Avoid artificial tanning methods such as sun lamps, tanning beds, tanning pills, and tanning makeup.
- Check your skin regularly for signs of skin cancer.

Sources: U.S. Food and Drug Administration, "Safer Sunning in Seven Steps," 2006, www.fda.gov/opacom/lowlit/sunsafty.html; Medline Plus, "Sun Exposure," 2006, www.nlm.nih.gov/medlineplus/sunexposure.html.

- Moisturize the skin with aquaphor petroleum jelly, plain calamine lotion, or Sarna lotion. Some forms of aloe work well, but make sure you read the ingredients on the label.
- Avoid "-caine" products such as benzocaine.
- For severe symptoms, including nausea, vomiting, chills, malaise, weakness, and blistering, stay awake and see a doctor.

See Table 16.4 for more tips on staying safe in the sun.

Detection, Symptoms, and Treatment Many people do not know what to look for when examining themselves for skin cancer. Basal and squamous cell carcinomas can be a recurrent annoyance, showing up most commonly on the face, ears, neck, arms, hands, and legs as warty bumps, colored spots, or scaly patches. Bleeding, itchiness, pain, or oozing are other symptoms that warrant attention. Surgery may be necessary to remove them, but they are seldom life-threatening.

In striking contrast is the insidious melanoma, an invasive killer that quickly spreads to regional organs and throughout the body, accounting for over 75 percent of all skin cancer deaths. Risks increase dramatically among whites after age 20.[44] Often, melanoma starts as a normal-looking mole but quickly develops abnormal characteristics. A simple *ABCD* rule outlines the warning signs of melanoma:

- *Asymmetry.* One half of the mole does not match the other half.
- *Border irregularity.* The edges are uneven, notched, or scalloped.
- *Color.* Pigmentation is not uniform. Melanomas may vary in color from tan to deeper brown, reddish black, black, or deep bluish black.
- *Diameter.* Greater than 6 millimeters (about the size of a pea).

If you notice any of these symptoms, consult a physician promptly.

Treatment of skin cancer depends on its seriousness. Surgery is performed in 90 percent of all cases. Radiation therapy, *electrodesiccation* (tissue destruction by heat), and *cryosurgery* (tissue destruction by freezing) are also common forms of treatment. For melanoma, treatment may involve surgical removal of the regional lymph nodes, radiation, or chemotherapy.

Testicular Cancer

Testicular cancer is one of the most common types of solid tumors found in young adult males, affecting nearly 8,250 young men in 2006. Those between the ages of 15 and 35 are at greatest risk. There has been a steady increase in tumor

How to Examine your Testicles

The best time to perform a testicular self-examination is after a warm shower or bath, when the testicles descend and the scrotal skin is relaxed.

1. Use a mirror to examine the scrotum for any visible swelling.

2. Using both hands, place the index and middle fingers of each hand on the underside of the testicle and the thumbs on top. Gently roll the testicle between the thumbs and fingers.

3. Identify the epididymis, the structure behind the testicle that carries sperm, so that you don't mistake it for a lump.

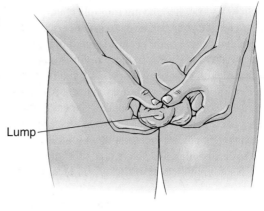

Lump

FIGURE 16.8 Testicular Self-Examination

frequency over the past several years in this age group.[45] Although the cause of testicular cancer is unknown, several risk factors have been identified. Males with undescended testicles appear to be at greatest risk, and some studies indicate a genetic influence.

In general, testicular tumors first appear as a painless enlargement of the testis or thickening in testicular tissue. Because this enlargement is often painless, it is extremely important that all young males practice regular testicular self-examination (Figure 16.8).

One of the most remarkable testicular cancer stories is the survival of Tour de France champion Lance Armstrong. Struck by an invasive form of testicular cancer that had spread to several parts of his body, including his brain, Armstrong's indomitable spirit set a wonderful example of hope for thousands of young men afflicted with the disease. He survived through a combination of superior medical care, exercise, and dietary and lifestyle changes, as well as a spiritual journey. The Lance Armstrong Foundation receives millions of dollars from sales of yellow wristbands carrying the words "LiveStrong" and now worn by millions of Americans.

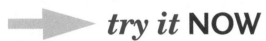

try it NOW

The survival rate of breast and testicular cancer patients greatly increases with early detection. Make a commitment to perform a breast or testicular self-exam monthly (see pages 492 and this page for instructions). Knowing your body and detecting abnormalities is one way you can take an active role in cancer prevention.

Ovarian Cancer

Ovarian cancer is the fifth leading cause of cancer death for women, diagnosed in almost 20,180 of them in 2006 and killing 15,310.[46] Ovarian cancer causes more deaths than any other cancer of the reproductive system because its insidious, often silent, course means women tend not to discover it until the cancer is at an advanced stage.

Symptoms The most common symptom is enlargement of the abdomen (or a feeling of bloating) in women over age 40. Abnormal vaginal bleeding or discharge is rarely a symptom until the disease is advanced. Other symptoms include vague digestive disturbances (stomach discomfort, gas, pressure, distention), fatigue, pain during intercourse, unexplained weight loss, unexplained changes in bowel or bladder habits, urinary frequency, and incontinence.[47] Women who have these symptoms in the absence of other problems will often be diagnosed with stomach irritability or other digestive problems. If symptoms persist, women must insist on further evaluation, including a thorough pelvic examination and other relevant tests.

Risk Factors The exact causes of ovarian cancer are not known. However, studies show that the following factors may increase chances of developing the disease:[48]

- *Family history.* First-degree relatives (mother, daughter, sister) of a woman who has had ovarian cancer are at increased risk. A family history of breast or colon cancer is also associated with increased risk.
- *Childbearing.* Women who have never been pregnant are more likely to develop ovarian cancer than those who have had a child, and the more children a woman has had, the less risk she faces.
- *Cancer history.* Women who have had breast or colon cancer have a greater chance of developing ovarian cancer than women who have not had either cancer.
- *Fertility drugs.* Drugs that cause a woman to ovulate may slightly increase her chance of developing ovarian cancer.
- *Talc.* Some studies suggest that women who have used talcum powder in their genital area for many years may have increased risk.
- *Genetic predisposition.* Mutation of the *BRCA1* and *BRCA2* genes (already linked to breast cancer) may increase risk. Another genetic syndrome, hereditary non-polyposis colon cancer, has also been linked to increased risk of developing ovarian cancer. Also, white women and women of Jewish descent are at higher risk.

Prevention Research shows that the use of birth control pills, adherence to a low-fat diet, having multiple children, or breast-feeding can reduce your risk of ovarian cancer. So, should you go out and get pregnant or start taking birth control pills to reduce risk? No. However, these results, particularly when combined with cardiovascular risks and other health information, provide yet another reason to eat plenty of vegetables and cut down on your fat intake. General prevention strategies like focusing on diet, exercise, sleep, stress management, and weight control are good ideas for this and any of the cancers discussed in this chapter, as substantiated by recent research studying the role of lifestyle in breast and ovarian cancer.[49]

To protect yourself, thorough annual pelvic examinations are important. Pap tests, although useful in detecting cervical cancer, do not reveal ovarian cancer. Women over the age of 40 should have a cancer-related checkup every year. Transvaginal ultrasound and a tumor marker, *CA125,* may assist in diagnosis but are not recommended for routine screening.[50] If you have any symptoms of ovarian cancer and they persist, see your doctor promptly.

Cervical and Endometrial (Uterine) Cancer

In 2006, an estimated 9,710 new cases of cervical cancer and 41,200 cases of endometrial cancer were diagnosed in the United States. Most uterine cancers develop in the body of the uterus, usually in the endometrium (lining). The rest develop in the cervix, located at the base of the uterus. The overall incidence of early-stage uterine cancer—cervical cancer—has increased slightly in recent years in women under the age of 50.[51] In contrast, invasive, later-stage forms of the disease appear to be decreasing. This may be due to more regular screenings of younger women using the **Pap test,** a procedure in which cells taken from the cervical region are examined for abnormal cellular activity. Although these tests are very effective for detecting early stage cervical cancer, they are less effective for detecting cancers of the uterine lining and not effective at all for detecting cancers of the fallopian tubes or ovaries.[52]

Risk factors for cervical cancer include early age at first intercourse, multiple sex partners, cigarette smoking, and certain sexually transmitted infections, including the human papillomavirus (the cause of genital warts) and the herpesvirus. For endometrial cancer, risk factors include age, endometrial hyperplasia, estrogen replacement therapy, being overweight, diabetes and high blood pressure, a history of other cancers,

Pap test A procedure in which cells taken from the cervical region are examined for abnormal cellular activity.

race (white women are at higher risk), and treatment with tamoxifen for breast cancer. (Doctors emphasize that the benefits of tamoxifen far outweigh its possible risks, and close monitoring for endometrial cancer is an important part of tamoxifen treatment.) Other risk factors also related to estrogen include having few or no children and entering menopause late in life.[53]

Early warning signs of uterine cancer include bleeding outside the normal menstrual period or after menopause or persistent unusual vaginal discharge. These symptoms should be checked by a physician immediately.[54]

Pancreatic Cancer

The incidence of cancer of the pancreas, known as a "silent" disease, has increased substantially during the last 25 years to 33,730 cases in 2006. Chronic inflammation of the pancreas (pancreatitis), obesity, physical inactivity, diabetes, cirrhosis, and a high-fat diet may contribute to its development. Smokers have double the risk of nonsmokers.[55]

Unfortunately, pancreatic cancer is one of the worst cancers to get. Only 4 percent of patients live more than five years after diagnosis, usually because the disease is well advanced by the time there are any symptoms.

Leukemia

Leukemia is a cancer of the blood-forming tissues that leads to proliferation of millions of immature white blood cells. These abnormal cells crowd out normal white blood cells (which fight infection), platelets (which control hemorrhaging), and red blood cells (which carry oxygen to body cells). As a result, symptoms such as fatigue, paleness, weight loss, easy bruising, repeated infections, nosebleeds, and other forms of hemorrhaging occur. In children, these symptoms can appear suddenly.[56]

Leukemia can be acute or chronic in nature and can strike both sexes and all age groups. It currently affects over 35,000 Americans.[57] Chronic leukemia can develop over several months and have few symptoms. The five-year survival rate for patients with chronic lymphocytic leukemia, one of the most common types, has risen to 74 percent.

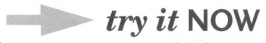 *try it* NOW

There are many actions you can take right away to improve your lifestyle and prevent your risk of developing cancer. Take advantage of the salad bar in your dining hall, and load up on greens, or request veggies like steamed broccoli or sautéed spinach. Don't forget the sunscreen: make applying a sunscreen with SPF 15 (at least) part of your daily routine, and stay in the shade from noon to 2 PM (when the sun is strongest).

ARTIFICIAL TANS: SACRIFICING HEALTH FOR BEAUTY?

In a recent study of American attitudes about tanning conducted by the American Academy of Dermatology, 26 percent of young people under age 25 had used a tanning bed in the past year. Of that 26 percent, more than half were young women.*

Men and women of all ages, shapes, and sizes are searching for an easy way to get that "summery, outdoorsy look" before or instead of spending time in the sun. Are any of the sun substitutes a safe alternative?

TANNING BOOTHS AND BEDS

Is a tanning booth safer than the sun?

On an average day, more than 1.3 million Americans visit a tanning salon, including teenagers and young adults. Researchers using data from the *National Longitudinal Study of Adolescent Health* report that over 25 percent of white female adolescents and 11 percent of males used tanning booths at least three times in the last year. Factors associated with indoor tanning include being female, residence in the Midwest or South, rural school location, increased age, use of tobacco and alcohol, and increased levels of discretionary cash for personal spending. Adolescents who tanned easily were more likely to visit tanning booths, while women who reported higher levels of physical activity were less likely to use them.

Most tanning salon patrons incorrectly believe that tanning booths are safer than sitting in the sun. However, the truth is that there is no such thing as a safe tan from *any* source! Essentially, a tan is the skin's response to an injury and every time you tan, you accumulate injury and increase your risk for disfiguring forms of skin cancer, premature aging, eye problems, unsightly skin spots, wrinkles and leathery skin, and possible death from melanoma.

To make matters worse, the industry is difficult to monitor and regulate due to the many salons that are springing up across the country. Dermatologists cite additional factors that make tanning in a salon as bad as—or even worse than—sitting in the sun:

- Tanning facilities sometimes fail to enforce regulations, such as insuring that customers wear eye protection and that overexposure does not occur.
- Some tanning facilities do not calibrate the UVA output of their tanning bulbs or insure sufficient rotation of newer and older bulbs, which can lead to more or less exposure than you paid for.
- Tanning facility patrons often try for a total body tan. The buttocks and genitalia are particularly sensitive to UV radiation and are prone to develop skin cancer.
- Another concern is hygiene. Don't assume that those little colored water sprayers used to "clean" the inside of the beds are sufficient to kill organisms. Any time you come in contact with body secretions from others, you run the risk of an infectious disease. The busier the facility, the more likely you are to come into contact with germs that could make you ill.

SPRAY-ON TANS

Some companies offer a sunless option that involves spraying customers in a tanning booth with the color additive dihydroxyacetone (DHA). DHA interacts with the dead surface cells in the outermost layer of the skin to darken skin color. DHA has been approved by the FDA for use in coloring the skin since 1977, and has typically been used in lotions and creams. Its use is restricted to external application, which means that it shouldn't be sprayed in or on the mouth, eyes, or nose because the risks, if any, are unknown. If you choose to use DHA spray at home or in tanning booths, be sure to cover these areas. Remember that the spray is a dye and does

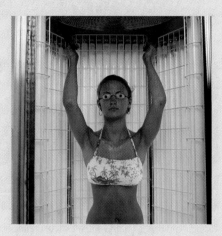

not increase your protection from the damaging rays of the sun.

TANNING PILLS

Although there are no tanning pills approved by the FDA, some companies market pills that contain the color additive canthaxanthin. When large amounts of canthaxanthin are ingested, the substance can turn the skin a range of colors, from orange to brown. However, canthaxanthin is only approved for use as a color additive in foods and oral medications, and only in small amounts. Tanning pills have been associated with health problems, including an eye disorder called canthaxanthin retinopathy, which is the formation of yellow deposits on the eye's retina. According to the American Academy of Dermatology, canthaxanthin has also been reported to cause liver injury and a severe itching condition called urticaria.

Sources: C. A. Demko et al., "Teenagers in the UV Tanning Booth?" *Archives of Pediatric and Adolescent Medicine* 157, no. 9 (2003): 854–860; University of Alabama at Birmingham, "'Dear Doctor' Column: Tanning Beds," 2002, www.health.uab.edu; University of Alabama at Birmingham, "'Dear Doctor' Column: Tanning (Sunless)," 2004, www.health.uab.edu; Food and Drug Administration (FDA), "Protect the Skin You're In!" *The FDA and You* 3 (2004), www.fda .gov/cdrh/fdaandyou/issue 03.html. * S. Danoff-Borg and C. E. Mosher, "Predictors of Tanning Salon Use: Behavioral Alternatives for Enhancing Appearance, Relaxing and Socializing," *Journal of Health Psychology* 11, no. 3 (2006): 511–518.

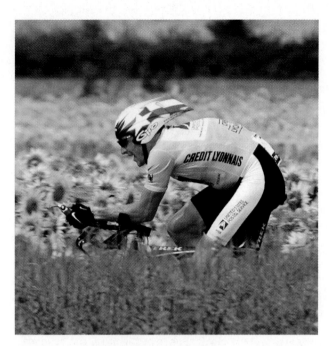

Lance Armstrong's battle with testicular cancer brought attention to a disease that strikes men who may consider themselves "too young" to be at risk for cancer.

Facing Cancer

Based on current rates, about 83 million—or one in three of us now living—will eventually develop cancer. Despite these gloomy predictions, recent advancements in the diagnosis and treatment of many forms of cancer have reduced some of the fear and mystery that once surrounded this disease.

Detecting Cancer

What are some ways cancer is detected?

The earlier cancer is diagnosed, the better the prospect for survival. Make a realistic assessment of your own risk factors and avoid the ones that you can control. Do you have a family history of cancer? If so, what types? Make sure you know which symptoms to watch for, and follow the recommendations for self-exams and medical checkups in

magnetic resonance imaging (MRI) A device that uses magnetic fields, radio waves, and computers to generate an image of internal tissues of the body for diagnostic purposes without the use of radiation.

computerized axial tomography (CAT) scan A scan by a machine that uses radiation to view internal organs not normally visible in X rays.

radiotherapy The use of radiation to kill cancerous cells.

chemotherapy The use of drugs to kill cancerous cells.

Table 16.3. Avoid known carcinogens—such as tobacco—and other environmental hazards. Eat a nutritious diet. Heeding the suggestions for primary prevention can significantly decrease your own risk for cancer.

Several high-tech tools to detect cancer have been developed:

- In **magnetic resonance imaging (MRI),** a huge electromagnet detects hidden tumors by mapping the vibrations of the various atoms in the body on a computer screen. The **computerized axial tomography (CAT) scan** uses X rays to examine parts of the body. In both of these painless, noninvasive procedures, cross-sectioned pictures can reveal a tumor's shape and location more accurately than can conventional X rays.
- *Prostatic ultrasound* (a rectal probe using ultrasonic waves to produce an image of the prostate) is being investigated as a means to increase the early detection of prostate cancer. Prostatic ultrasound has been combined with the PSA blood test.

Most of the sites that pose the highest risk for cancer have screening tests available for early detection. Other common forms of cancer have readily identifiable symptoms. Health care reforms that provided coverage for regular checkups and preventive services would help many poor and middle-class Americans seek medical care early, when the chances of a cure are best.

Table 16.5 lists seven warning signals of cancer. If you notice any of these signals, and they don't appear to be related to anything else, see a doctor immediately. For example, difficulty swallowing may be due to a cold or flu. However, if you are otherwise symptomless and the difficulty continues, consult your physician. Make sure you receive all appropriate diagnostic tests.

New Hope in Cancer Treatments

Although cancer treatments have changed dramatically over the past 20 years, surgery, in which the tumor and surrounding tissue are removed, is still common. Today, treatments such as **radiotherapy** (the use of radiation) or **chemotherapy** (the use of drugs) to kill cancerous cells are also used.

Radiation works by destroying malignant cells or stopping cell growth. It is most effective in treating localized cancer masses. Unfortunately, in the process of destroying malignant cells, radiotherapy also destroys some healthy cells. It may also increase the risk for other types of cancers. Despite these drawbacks, radiation continues to be one of the most common and effective forms of treatment.

When cancer has spread throughout the body, it is necessary to use some form of chemotherapy. Currently, over 50 different anticancer drugs are in use, some of which have excellent records of success. Ongoing research promises to result in new drugs that are less toxic to normal cells and more potent against tumor cells.

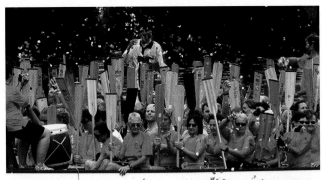

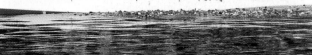

Cancer survivors can lead long and healthy lives. Some, such as these breast cancer survivors, take part in a variety of activities to raise money for cancer research and treatment and to increase public awareness about prevention.

Whether used alone or in combination, radiotherapy and chemotherapy have side effects, including extreme nausea, nutritional deficiencies, hair loss, and general fatigue. Long-term damage to the cardiovascular system and other body systems can be significant. It is important to discuss these matters fully with doctors when making treatment plans.

Substances found in nature, such as taxol (originally found in Pacific yew trees), are now being synthesized in laboratories and tested on a variety of cancers. Other compounds, including those derived from sea urchins, are rich in resources for anticancer drugs.

What treatment types are the most cutting edge?

Today, researchers are targeting cancer as a genetic disease that is brought on by some form of mutation, either inherited or acquired. Promising treatments focus on stopping the cycle of these mutant cells, targeting toxins through monoclonal antibodies, and rousing the immune system to be more effective. Others include the following:[58]

- **Immunotherapy** enhances the body's own disease-fighting systems to help control cancer. Interferon (a naturally occurring body protein that protects healthy cells and kills cancer cells), interleukin-2 (a growth factor that stimulates cells of the immune system to find cancer), and other biological response modifiers are under study.
- One of the most exciting new approaches for spurring the immune system to ward off cancer is the use of *cancer-fighting vaccines*. Cancer vaccines alert the body's immune defenses; but, instead of warning of germs, they provide indicators of good cells that have gone bad. Consequently, rather than preventing disease, they help people who are already ill. These vaccines may be the next generation of cancer treatment.
- Research on the effectiveness of *gene therapy* has moved into early clinical trials. Scientists have found hopeful signs of a virus carrying genetic information that makes the cells it infects susceptible to an antiviral drug. Scientists also are looking at ways to transfer genes that increase the patient's immune response to the cancerous tumor or that confer drug resistance to the bone marrow so that higher doses of chemotherapeutic drugs can be given.
- In other studies, researchers are testing compounds that may stop tumors from forming new blood vessels, a process known as *angiogenesis*. By inhibiting angiogenesis, scientists hope to inhibit the flow of nutrient- and oxygen-rich blood to the cancerous tumors and slow their growth.
- In recent years, scientists have identified various steps in what is termed the *cancer pathway*. These include oncogene actions, hormone receptors, growth factors, metastasis, and angiogenesis. Preliminary studies are under way to design compounds (*rational drug design*) aimed at specific molecules along the cancer pathway with the intent of inhibiting actions at these various steps.
- A powerful enzyme inhibitor, *TIMP-2*, shows promise for slowing the metastasis of tumor cells. A metastasis suppressor gene, *NM23*, has also been identified.
- *Neoadjuvant chemotherapy* (using chemotherapy to shrink the tumor and then removing it surgically) has been tried against various types of cancers.
- *Stem cell research* is another promising avenue for potential treatment, although controversy around the use of stem cells continues to slow research (see Chapter 19).

In addition, psychosocial and behavioral research has become increasingly important as health professionals learn more about lifestyle factors that influence risk and survivability. Health care practitioners have become more aware of the psychological needs of patients and families and have begun to tailor treatment programs to meet their diverse needs.

Participation in clinical trials has provided a new source of hope for many undergoing cancer treatment. Clinical trials

immunotherapy A process that stimulates the body's own immune system to combat cancer cells.

are people-based studies of new drugs or procedures. Because of the many unknown variables, deciding whether to participate in a clinical trial can be a difficult decision. Despite the risks, which should be carefully considered, thousands have benefited from treatments that would otherwise be unavailable to them.

Talking with Your Doctor about Cancer

Any time cancer is suspected, people react with anxiety, fear, and anger. Emotional distress is sometimes so intense that they are unable to make critical health care decisions. If you find it difficult to know what to ask your doctor during a routine exam, imagine how hard it would be to discuss life-or-death options for yourself or a loved one. Before you arrive at the doctor's office, prepare a list of important questions to discuss. Remember, your health care provider should be your partner and help you make the best decisions for you.

If the diagnosis is cancer, here are some suggestions for questions to ask:

- What kind of cancer do I have? What stage is it in? Based on my age and stage, what prognosis do I have?
- What are my treatment choices? Which do you recommend? Why?
- What are the benefits of each kind of treatment?
- What are the short- and long-term risks and possible side effects for each treatment?
- Would a clinical trial be appropriate for me?

If surgery is recommended, ask:

- What kind of operation will it be, and how long will it take? What form of anesthesia will be used? How many similar procedures has this surgeon done in the past month? What is his or her success rate?
- How will I feel after surgery? If I have pain, how will you help me?
- Where will the scars be? What will they look like? Will they cause disability?
- Will I have any activity limitations after surgery? What kind of physical therapy, if any, will I need? When will I get back to normal activities?

If radiation is recommended, ask:

- Why do you think this treatment is better than my other options?
- How long will I need to have treatments, and what will the side effects be in the short and long term? What body organs or systems may be damaged?
- What can I do to take care of myself during therapy? Are there services available to help me?
- What is the long-term prognosis for people of my age with my type of cancer who are using this treatment?

If chemotherapy is recommended, ask:

- Why do you think this treatment is better than my other options?
- Which drug combinations pose the fewest risks and most benefits?
- What will be the short- and long-term side effects on my body?

Before beginning any form of cancer therapy, it is imperative to be a vigilant and vocal consumer. Read and seek information from cancer support groups. Check the skills of your surgeon, your radiation therapist, and your doctor in terms of clinical experience and interpersonal interactions.

Cancer Survivors: Life After Cancer

Heightened public awareness and an improved prognosis have made the cancer experience less threatening and isolating than it once was. In fact, assistance for the cancer patient is more readily available than ever before. Cancer support groups, cancer information workshops, and low-cost medical consultation are just a few of the forms of assistance now offered in many communities. Groups have successfully lobbied the U.S. Congress to increase cancer research dollars. As a result, government funding has increased substantially over the past decade. The battle for funds continues. Increasing efforts in cancer research, improvements in diagnostic equipment, and advances in treatment provide hope for the future.

TAKING charge

Summary

- Cancer is a group of diseases characterized by uncontrolled growth and spread of abnormal cells. These cells may create tumors. Benign (noncancerous) tumors grow in size but do not spread; malignant (cancerous) tumors spread to other parts of the body.
- Several causes of cancer have been identified. Lifestyle factors include smoking and obesity. Biological factors include

inherited genes and gender. Occupational and environmental hazards are carcinogens present in people's home or work environments. Chemicals in foods that may act as carcinogens include preservatives and pesticides. Infectious diseases that may lead to cancer include herpes, mononucleosis, and human papillomavirus (which causes genital warts). Medical factors include certain drug therapies given for other conditions that may elevate the chance of cancer. Combined risk refers to a combination of the above factors, which tends to compound the risk for cancer.

- There are many different types of cancer, each of which poses different risks, depending on a number of factors. Common forms include lung, breast, colon and rectum, prostate, skin, testicular, ovarian, uterine, and pancreatic cancers, as well as leukemia.
- Early diagnosis improves survival rate. Self-exams for breast, testicular, and skin cancer and knowledge of the seven warning signals of cancer aid early diagnosis.
- New types of cancer treatments include various combinations of radiotherapy, chemotherapy, and immunotherapy.

Chapter Review

1. When cancer cells have *metastasized*
   a. they have grown into a malignant tumor.
   b. they have spread to other parts of the body, including vital organs.
   c. the cancer is retreating and cancer cells are dying off.
   d. None of the above.

2. A cancerous neoplasm is
   a. a biopsy.
   b. benign.
   c. a tumor.
   d. malignant.

3. Who is at a higher risk for developing skin cancer?
   a. People who have fair skin.
   b. People who freckle and burn more when in the sun.
   c. People who have a history of bad sunburn as a child.
   d. All of the above.

4. "If you are male and smoke, your chances of getting lung cancer are 23 times greater as compared to a nonsmoker." This statement refers to a statistical risk known as
   a. relative risk.
   b. comparable risk.
   c. cancer risk.
   d. genetic predisposition.

5. The greatest number of cancer deaths for both men and women combined are from
   a. colon/rectal cancer.
   b. pancreatic cancer.
   c. lung cancer.
   d. stomach cancer.

6. The leading type of cancer in men is
   a. lung.
   b. bladder.
   c. oral.
   d. prostate.

7. The leading type of cancer in women is
   a. ovarian.
   b. uterine.
   c. breast.
   d. thyroid.

8. One of the best ways to reduce a person's risk of developing cancer is to
   a. quit smoking now if currently smoking.
   b. eat a very healthy diet with more antioxidant-type fruits and vegetables.
   c. have frequent screening and testing if high risk for a certain cancer type.
   d. All of the above.

9. The type of cancer usually found in the connective tissues of the body, such as bones and muscles, is
   a. sarcoma.
   b. leukemia.
   c. carcinoma.
   d. lymphoma.

10. The more serious and life-threatening type of skin cancer is
    a. basal cell cancer.
    b. squamous cell cancer.
    c. melanoma cancer.
    d. lymphoma cancer.

Answers to these questions can be found on page A-1.

Questions for Discussion and Reflection

1. What is cancer? How does it spread? What is the difference between a benign and a malignant tumor?
2. List the likely causes of cancer. Do any of them put you at greater risk? What can you do to reduce this risk? What risk factors do you share with family members? Friends?
3. What are the symptoms of lung, breast, prostate, and testicular cancer? What can you do to reduce your risk of developing these cancers or increase your chances of surviving them?
4. What are the differences between carcinomas, sarcomas, lymphomas, and leukemia? Which is the most common? Least common?
5. Why are breast and testicular self-exams important for women and men? What could be the consequences of not doing these exams regularly?
6. Discuss the seven warning signals of cancer. What could indicate that you have cancer instead of a minor illness? How soon should you seek treatment for any of the suspicious symptoms?

Accessing Your Health on the Internet

The following websites explore further topics and issues related to personal health. You'll also find links to each organization's website on the Companion Website for *Access to Health,* Tenth Edition, at www.aw-bc.com/donatelle.

1. *American Cancer Society.* Resources from the leading private organization dedicated to cancer prevention. This site provides information, statistics, and resources regarding cancer. www.cancer.org
2. *National Cancer Institute.* Check here for valuable information on clinical trials and the Physician Data Query (PDQ), a comprehensive database of cancer treatment information. www.cancer.gov
3. *National Women's Health Information Center (NWHIC).* Provides a wealth of information about cancer in women. Cosponsored by the National Cancer Institute. www.4woman.gov
4. *Oncolink.* Sponsored by the University of Pennsylvania Cancer Center, this site seeks to educate cancer patients and their families by offering information on support services, cancer causes, screening, prevention, and common questions. www.oncolink.com

Further Reading

American Cancer Institute Journal, published monthly.

Focuses on current cancer risk factors, prevention, and treatment research.

American Cancer Society. *Cancer Facts & Figures.* Atlanta, GA: American Cancer Society, published annually.

A summary of major facts relating to cancer. Provides information on incidence, prevalence, symptomology, prevention, and treatment. Available through local divisions of the American Cancer Society. Contains up-to-date information about the disease, medical options, and emotional support.

American Cancer Society. *A Breast Cancer Journey: Your Personal Guidebook,* 2nd ed. Atlanta, Georgia: American Cancer Society, 2004.

Contains up-to-date information on treatments, medicines, reconstructive surgery, and complementary and alternative options. Also includes information for caregivers, family, and friends.

Armstrong, L. *It's Not About the Bike: My Journey Back to Life.* New York: Penguin, 2000.

Lance Armstrong's incredible description of his triumph over testicular cancer and his Tour de France victories. A book full of inspiration for young men with this disease, their families, and anyone facing cancer.

Nutrition and Cancer Journal, published monthly.

Focuses on etiological aspects of various dietary factors and research on risks for cancer development. Also includes current research on dietary factors and cancer prevention.

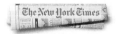

e-themes from *The New York Times*

For up-to-date articles about current health issues, visit www.aw-bc.com/donatelle, select *Access to Health,* Tenth Edition, Chapter 16, and click on "e-themes."

References

1. A. Jemel et al., "Cancer Statistics," *CA: A Journal for Cancer Clinicians* 55 (2005): 10–30.
2. American Cancer Society, *Cancer Facts & Figures 2006* (Atlanta: American Cancer Society, 2006).
3. Ibid.
4. Ibid.
5. Ibid.
6. Ibid.
7. N. Kreiger, "Defining and Investigating Social Disparities in Cancer: Critical Issues," *Cancer Causes and Control* 16, no. 1 (2005): 10552–10564.
8. C. Brach, I. Fraser, and K. Paez, "Crossing the Language Chasm," *Health Affairs* 24, no. 2 (2005): 424–434.
9. American Cancer Society, *Cancer Facts & Figures 2006.*
10. Ibid.
11. Ibid.
12. Ibid.
13. D. Goodarz et al., "Causes of Cancer in the World: Comparative Risk Assessment of Nine Behavioral and Environmental Risk Factors," *The Lancet* 366, no. 9499 (2005): 1784–1793; R. Prentice et al., "Low Fat Dietary Patterns and Risk of Invasive Breast Cancer," *Journal of the American Medical Association* 295, no. 6 (2006): 629–642.
14. American Cancer Society, *Cancer Facts & Figures 2006.*
15. K. Rapp et al., "Obesity and Incidence of Cancer: A Large Cohort Study of over 145,000 Adults in Austria," *British Journal of Cancer* 93 (2005): 1062–1067; S. Freedland, "Obesity and Prostate Cancer: A Growing Problem," *Clinical Cancer Research* 11, no. 19 (2005): 6763–6766; R. MacInnis et al., "Body Size and Composition and Colon Cancer Risk in Women," *International Cancer Journal* 118, no. 6 (2005): 1496–1500; C. Samanic et al., "Relation of Body Mass Index to Cancer Risk in 362,552 Swedish Men," *Cancer Causes and Control* 17, no. 7 (2005): 10552–10600; M. McCullough et al., "Risk Factors for Fatal Breast Cancer in African American Women and White Women in a Large U.S. Prospective Cohort," *American Journal of Epidemiology* 162, no. 8 (2005): 734–742; P. Soliman et al., "Risk Factors for Young Premenopausal Women with Endometrial Cancer," *Obstetrics and Gynecology* 105 (2005): 575–580.
16. R. Eeles et al., *Genetic Predisposition to Cancer,* 2nd ed. (New York: Oxford University Press, 2004).
17. P. Soliman et al., "Risk Factors for Young Premenopausal Women with Endometrial Cancer."
18. B. Binkumar and A. Mathew, "Dietary Fat and Risk of Breast Cancer," *World Journal of Surgical Oncology* 3, no. 45 (2005): 1477.
19. A. Swerdlow et al., "Mobile Phone Use and Risk of Acoustic Neuroma," *British Journal of Cancer* 93, no. 7 (2005): 842–848.
20. M. Bennett et al., "Humor and Laughter May Influence Health: Complementary Therapies and Humor in a Clinical Population," *Evidence-Based Complementary and Alternative Medicine* 3, no. 2 (2006): 187–190.
21. P. Pisani, *Estimates of Number of Cancer Cases throughout the World Attributable to Infectious Disease* (Lyon, France: International Agency for Research on Cancer, 2004).
22. B. W. Stewart and P. Kleihues, eds., "Cancers of the Female Reproductive Tract," *World Cancer Report* (Lyon, France: IARC Press, 2003).
23. American Cancer Society, *Cancer Facts & Figures 2006.*
24. Ibid.
25. Ibid.
26. Ibid.
27. Ibid.
28. Ibid.
29. Ibid.
30. Ibid.
31. M. Holmes et al., "Physical Activity Might Improve Survival in Women with Breast Cancer," *Journal of the American Medical Association* 527 (2005).
32. National Breast Cancer Organization, "Hormonal Therapy," 2006, www.y-me.org.
33. American Cancer Society, *Cancer Facts & Figures, 2006.*
34. Ibid.
35. P. A. Janne and R. J. Mayer, "Chemoprevention of Colorectal Cancer," *New England Journal of Medicine* 342 (2000): 1960–1968; Writing Group—WHI, "Risks and Benefits of Estrogen Plus Progesterone on the Health of Postmenopausal Women," *Journal of the American Medical Association* 288, no. 3 (July 17, 2002).
36. American Cancer Society, *Cancer Facts & Figures 2006.*
37. L. Seeff et al., "Screening for Colorectal Cancer in the United States," *Journal of Family Practice* 51 (2002): 761–766.
38. Ibid.
39. Ibid.
40. Ibid.
41. University of Wisconsin Health Service, "Sunburn: Prevention/Treatment," 2002, www.uhs.wisc.edu/ex/selfcare/resource/sunburn.php.
42. American Cancer Society, *Cancer Facts & Figures 2006.*
43. University of Wisconsin Health Service, "Sunburn: Prevention/Treatment."
44. American Cancer Society, *Cancer Facts & Figures 2006.*
45. Ibid.
46. Ibid.
47. Ibid.
48. National Cancer Institute, "Ovarian Cancer and You," 2006, www.cancer.gov/cancerinfo/pdq/screening/ovarian/patient.
49. G. C. Zografos, M. Panou, and N. Panou, "Common Risk Factors of Breast and Ovarian Cancer: Recent Review," *International Journal of Gynecological Cancer* 14, no. 5 (2004): 721–740; C. T. Berkelman, "Risk Factors and Risk Reduction of Breast and Ovarian Cancer," *Current Opinion in Obstetrics and Gynecology* 15, no. 1 (2003): 63–68.
50. American Cancer Society, *Cancer Facts & Figures 2006.*
51. Ibid.
52. Ibid.
53. National Cancer Institute, "Endometrial Cancer Overview," 2006, www.cancer.gov.
54. American Cancer Society, *Cancer Facts & Figures 2006.*
55. Ibid.
56. Ibid.
57. Ibid.
58. Ibid.

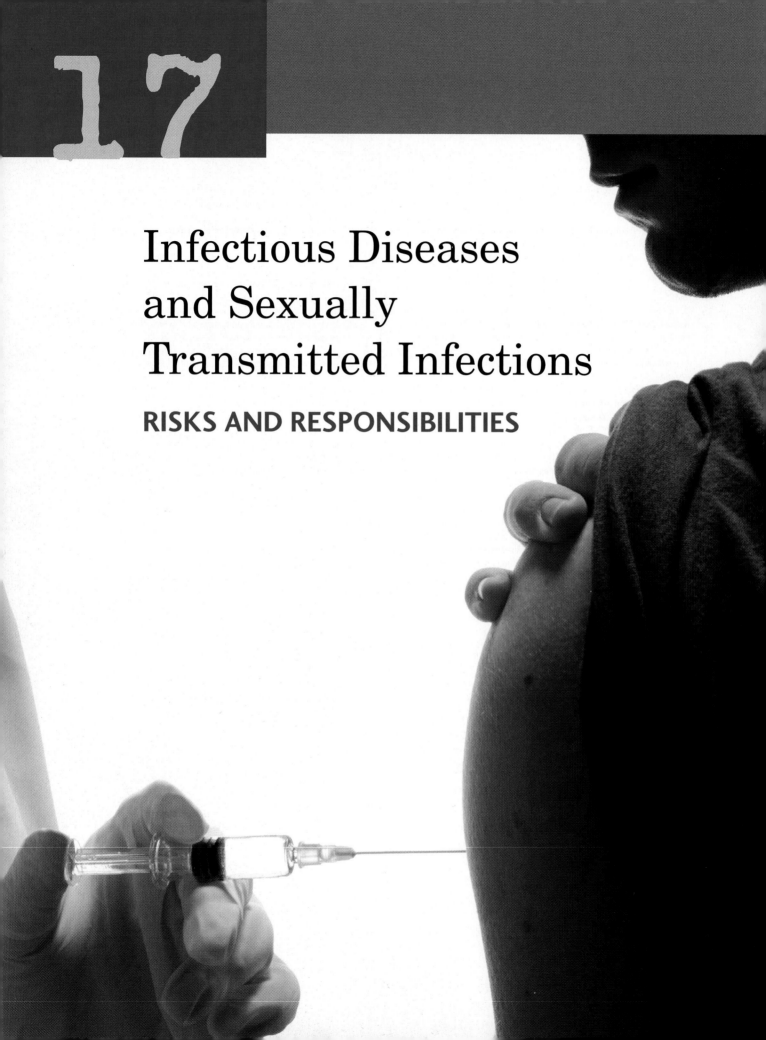

17

Infectious Diseases and Sexually Transmitted Infections

RISKS AND RESPONSIBILITIES

Will **vitamin C** cure my cold?

How does my body **fight** an infection?

Can I get a sexually transmitted **infection** from "outercourse"?

How is herpes **transmitted**?

How worried about **bird flu** should I be?

OBJECTIVES

■ Understand the risk factors for infectious diseases, and how your immune system works to protect you, and what factors may make it less effective.

■ Discuss the most common pathogens infecting humans today and the typical diseases caused by each.

■ Explain the major emerging and resurgent diseases affecting humans today; discuss why they are increasing in incidence and what actions are being taken to reduce risks.

■ Discuss the various sexually transmitted infections, their means of transmission, and actions that can be taken to prevent their spread.

■ Discuss human immunodeficiency virus (HIV) and acquired immunodeficiency syndrome (AIDS) trends in infection and treatment, and the impact on special populations and

very moment of every day, you are in contact with microscopic organisms that have the ability to make you ill or even kill you. These disease-causing agents, known as **pathogens,** are found in air and food and on nearly every object or person with whom you come in contact. Although new varieties of pathogens arise all the time, many have existed for as long as there has been life on this planet. Fossil evidence shows that infections afflicted the earliest human beings. At times, infectious diseases wiped out whole groups of people through **epidemics** such as the Black Death, or bubonic plague, that killed up to one-third of the population of Europe and Asia in the 1300s. A **pandemic,** or global epidemic, of influenza killed more than 20 million people in 1918, while strains of tuberculosis and cholera continue to cause premature death among populations throughout the world.

In spite of our best efforts to eradicate them, these diseases are a continuing menace to all of us. Although vaccines, pasteurization, improvements in sanitation, and other public health measures have slowed or stopped the spread of many diseases, some infections that were once held in check by antibiotics have begun to resurge, or emerge, in new and more deadly resistant forms. If we are unable to limit the emergence and spread of resistance, some diseases may simply become untreatable and deadly once again, much as they were in the *preantibiotic* era.

The news isn't all bad, however. Our immune systems are remarkably adept at protecting us. *Endogenous microorganisms* are those that live in peaceful coexistence with their human host most of the time. For people in good health and whose immune systems are functioning properly, endogenous organisms are usually harmless. However, in sick people or those with weakened immune systems, these normally harmless pathogenic organisms can cause serious health problems.

Exogenous microorganisms are organisms that do not normally inhabit the body. When they do, however, they are apt to produce an infection and/or illness. The more easily these pathogens can gain a foothold in the body and sustain themselves, the more **virulent** (aggressive) they may be in causing disease. If your immune system is strong, you will often be able to fight off even the most virulent attacker. Several factors influence your susceptibility to disease.

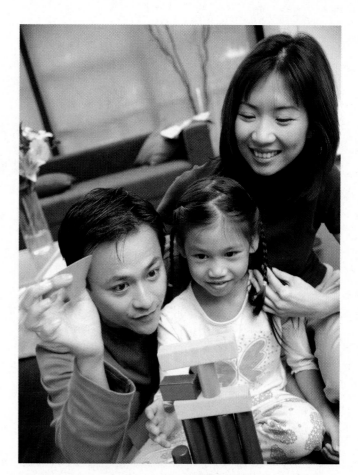

Genetic factors are one of the greatest indicators of our disease risk. A child might inherit certain immune traits that will make her more or less prone to disease.

Assessing Your Disease Risks

Most diseases are **multifactorial diseases**—that is, they are caused by the interaction of several factors from inside and outside the person. For a disease to occur, the host must be *susceptible,* meaning that the immune system must be in a weakened condition; an agent capable of *transmitting* a disease must be present; and the *environment* must be *hospitable* to the pathogen in terms of temperature, light, moisture, and other requirements. Other risk factors may increase or decrease susceptibility. Figure 17.1 summarizes the body's defenses against invasion.

Risk Factors You Can't Control

Unfortunately, some risk factors are beyond our control. This section discusses some of the most common risks.

Heredity Perhaps the single greatest factor influencing disease risk is genetics. Being born into a family in which heart disease, cancer, or other illnesses are prevalent increases a person's risk. Still other diseases are caused by

pathogens   Disease-causing agents.

epidemic   Disease outbreak that affects many people in a community or region at the same time.

pandemic   Global epidemic of a disease.

virulent   Strong enough to overcome host resistance and cause disease.

multifactorial disease   Disease caused by interactions of several factors.

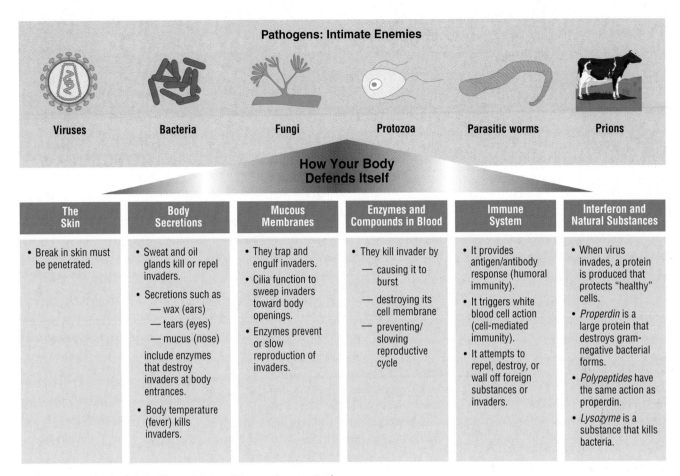

How Your Body Defends Itself

The Skin	Body Secretions	Mucous Membranes	Enzymes and Compounds in Blood	Immune System	Interferon and Natural Substances
• Break in skin must be penetrated.	• Sweat and oil glands kill or repel invaders. • Secretions such as — wax (ears) — tears (eyes) — mucus (nose) include enzymes that destroy invaders at body entrances. • Body temperature (fever) kills invaders.	• They trap and engulf invaders. • Cilia function to sweep invaders toward body openings. • Enzymes prevent or slow reproduction of invaders.	• They kill invader by — causing it to burst — destroying its cell membrane — preventing/ slowing reproductive cycle	• It provides antigen/antibody response (humoral immunity). • It triggers white blood cell action (cell-mediated immunity). • It attempts to repel, destroy, or wall off foreign substances or invaders.	• When virus invades, a protein is produced that protects "healthy" cells. • *Properdin* is a large protein that destroys gram-negative bacterial forms. • *Polypeptides* have the same action as properdin. • *Lysozyme* is a substance that kills bacteria.

FIGURE 17.1 The Body's Defenses Against Disease-Causing Pathogens

direct chromosomal inheritance. For example, **sickle-cell anemia,** an inherited blood disease that primarily affects African Americans, may be transmitted to the fetus if both parents carry the sickle-cell trait. It is often unclear whether hereditary diseases occur as a result of inherited chromosomal traits or inherited insufficiencies in the immune system. Some believe that we may even inherit immune system quality, so that some people are naturally "tougher" than others and more resilient to disease and infection.

Aging After age 40, we become more vulnerable to most of the chronic diseases. As we age, our immune system responds less efficiently to invading organisms, increasing the risk for infection and illness. The same flu that produces an afternoon of nausea and diarrhea in a younger person may cause days of illness or even death in an older person. The very young are also at risk for many diseases, particularly if they are not vaccinated against them.

Environmental Conditions Unsanitary conditions and the presence of drugs, chemicals, and hazardous pollutants and wastes in food and water probably have a great effect on our immune systems. A growing body of research points to changes in the environment (like global warming) and natural disasters as a significant contributor to increasing

numbers of infectious diseases.[1] It is well documented that poor environmental conditions can weaken **immunological competence**—the body's ability to defend itself against pathogens.

Organism Resistance Some organisms, such as the foodborne organism **botulism,** are particularly virulent, and even tiny amounts may make the most hardy of us ill. Other organisms have mutated and are resistant to the body's defenses as well as other conventional treatments designed to protect against them. Still other, newer pathogens pose unique challenges for our immune systems—ones that our bodily defenses are ill-adapted to fight. See the New Horizons in Health box on page 512 for more on problems due to organism resistance to antibiotics.

sickle-cell anemia Genetic disease commonly found among African Americans; results in organ damage and premature death.

immunological competence Ability of the immune system to defend the body from pathogens.

botulism A resistant foodborne organism that is extremely virulent.

ANTIBIOTIC RESISTANCE: WHAT DOESN'T KILL THEM MAKES THEM STRONGER

Imagine a world where people die from common colds, diarrhea, ear infections, and superficial cuts and infections. Though this sounds like the stuff of science fiction or bioterrorism run amok, the facts indicate that such a scenario is not that outrageous. In fact, according to the World Health Organization, "People of the world may only have a decade or two to make use of many of the medicines presently available to stop infectious diseases before antimicrobial resistance begins to be a major threat to health." Today, antibiotic resistance has been called one of the world's most pressing health issues, threatening the lives of millions. Either we develop entirely new classes of antibiotics at a previously unheard-of rate, or we face the truth about the dwindling effectiveness of penicillin and other antibiotics. As pharmaceutical companies shift their emphasis from developing a new arsenal of weapons to fight microbial threats to developing more profitable drugs that treat chronic conditions, the state of our health is in serious jeopardy.

RESISTANT INFECTIONS

Drug-resistant infectious agents—those that are not killed or inhibited by antimicrobial compounds—are on the rise globally. A key factor in their development is the ability to genetically adapt quickly to new environmental conditions. Tuberculosis, gonorrhea, malaria, and childhood ear infections are just a few of the diseases that have become difficult, if not impossible, to treat due to the emergence of drug-resistant pathogens. At particular risk are those in hospitals, where every year 2 million patients in the United States get drug-resistant infections, and over 90,000 die. The Institute of Medicine, part of the National Academy of Sciences, has estimated that the annual cost of treating antibiotic-resistant infections in the United States may be as high as $30 billion. How serious is the problem? Consider the following facts:

- Strains of *Staphylococcus aureus* resistant to most antibiotics are endemic in many hospitals today. In some cities 31 percent of staph infections are resistant, and in nursing homes as many as 71 percent of staph infections defy traditional antibiotic regimens.
- *Streptococcus pneumoniae* causes thousands of cases of meningitis and pneumonia and 7 million cases of ear infections in the United States each year. Currently, about 30 percent of these cases are resistant to penicillin, the primary drug for treatment. Many penicillin-resistant strains are also resistant to other antibiotics.
- An estimated 300 million to 500 million people worldwide are infected with parasites that cause malaria, and an estimated 700,000 to 2.7 million people die each year from the disease. Re-

sistance to chloroquine, once a widely used and highly effective treatment, is now found in most regions of the world, with other treatments losing their effectiveness at alarming rates.

- Strains of multidrug-resistant tuberculosis have emerged over the last decade.
- Diarrheal diseases cause almost 3 million deaths per year—mostly in developing countries where resistant forms of *Campylobacter, Shigella, Escherichia coli, Vibrio cholerae,* and *Salmonella* food poisoning have emerged. In some areas, as much as 50 percent of the *Campylobacter* cases are resistant to Cipro, the most effective treatment. A potentially deadly "superbug" known as *Salmonella enterica typhimurium,* resistant to most antibiotics, has appeared in Europe, Canada, and the United States.
- Resistant fungal diseases such as *Pneumocystis carinii* pneumonia are on the rise internationally.
- Viral resistance to HIV treatment means that many drugs quickly lose their effectiveness in treating HIV.

In the battle between drugs and bugs, the bugs are clearly scoring some big wins.

WHY IS ANTIMICROBIAL RESISTANCE GROWING?

Although the actual mechanisms are complex, antibiotics typically wipe out certain bacteria that are susceptible to them. However, when used improperly, the antibiotics

Risk Factors You Can Control

The good news is that we all have some degree of personal control over many risk factors for disease, because lifestyle behaviors play a huge role in our immune system's resilience. Too much stress, inadequate nutrition, a low level of physical fitness, lack of sleep, misuse or abuse of legal and illegal substances, poor personal hygiene, high-risk behaviors, and other variables significantly increase the risk for a number of diseases. Those we have the most control over, via lifestyle decisions and behaviors, are noted on the following list with an asterisk (*):

- Personal habits: smoking, alcohol use, sleep, exercise, stress levels, drug use/abuse*
- Dosage, virulence, and where the disease-causing agent enters the body
- Age at time of infection
- Preexisting level of immunity*
- Health and vigor of immune system response*
- Genetic factors controlling immune response
- Nutritional status of host*
- Comorbidities: the number of battles your immune system is fighting at the same time*

kill only the weak bacteria and leave the strongest versions to thrive and replicate. Because bacteria can swap genes with one another under the right conditions, hardy drug-resistant germs can share their resistance mechanisms with other germs. Eventually, an entire colony of resistant bugs grows and passes on its resistance traits to new generations of bacteria.

Resistance commonly stems from incorrect use of antibiotics. For example, patients may begin an antibiotic regimen, start to feel better, and stop taking the drug to save money by using the drug another time. The surviving bacteria then build immunity to the drugs used to treat them. Also, doctors have overused antibiotics; the CDC estimates that one-third of the 150 million prescriptions written each year are unnecessary, resulting in bacterial strains that are tougher than the drugs used to fight them.

Whereas patient noncompliance and doctor overuse are believed to be the most significant contributors to our epidemic of resistant bacteria, other factors are also contributors.

- Overuse of antibiotics in food production has contributed to increased drug resistance. About 70 percent of antibiotic production today is used to treat sick animals and encourage growth in livestock and poultry. Although research is only in its infancy, many believe that ingesting meats and animal products that are rich in antibiotics may actually contribute to antibiotic resistance in humans.
- Another area of concern is the American obsession with cleanliness. One need only look at the antibacterial soaps, cleaning products, and other products on the shelves to know that personal and home cleaning products are the rage. Just how much these soaps and other products contribute to overall resistance is also in question; as with antibiotics, the germs these products do not kill may become stronger than before.

REDUCING THE RISK OF ANTIMICROBIAL RESISTANCE

What can be done to slow the growth of resistant organisms? Individual and community actions include the following:

- Enact policies that severely restrict the use of antibiotics, growth hormones, and other products in our food supply.
- Buy foods and products that are antibiotic free.
- Motivate people to take medications as prescribed and to finish all medications: kill the bugs the first time, all the time.
- Encourage doctors to prescribe antibiotics only when absolutely necessary and to educate patients about their use.
- Encourage consumers not to pressure doctors to give them antibiotics for their ailments.
- Educate consumers about the fact that germs are not inherently bad and that

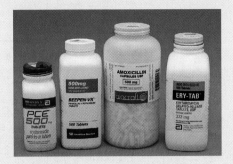

exposure to many of them helps our immune systems develop arsenals capable of fighting pathogens.
- Educate people that washing their hands with a good flow of water and regular soap for a bit longer time than normal is better than using antibacterial soaps.
- Encourage pharmaceutical companies to develop, test, and market new classes of antibiotics to keep up with growing resistance.

Sources: National Institute of Allergy and Infectious Diseases, "Fact Sheet: Antimicrobial Resistance," 2004, www.niaid.nih.gov/factsheets/antimicro.htm; National Center for Infectious Diseases, "Malaria Fact Sheet," 2004, www.cdc.gov/malaria/facts.htm; World Health Organization, "Anti-Microbial Resistance," www.who.int; Centers for Disease Control and Prevention, "About Antibiotic Resistance," 2006, www.cdc.gov/drugresistance/community/antibiotic-resistance.htm; M. S. Smolinski et al., *Special Report: Microbial Threats to Health* (Washington DC: National Academies Press, 2003)

- Environmental surroundings, such as temperature, humidity, and sanitary conditions*
- Psychological factors (motivation, emotional status, and so on)*

❓ *what do you* THINK?

If you were to list your own risk factors for infectious diseases, what would they be? ■ What actions can you take to reduce your risks? ■ Are your risks greater today than before you entered college? ■ Why or why not?

Types of Pathogens and Routes of Transmission

Pathogens can enter the body in several ways (Table 17.1 on page 514). They may be transmitted by *direct contact* between infected persons, such as during sexual relations, kissing, or touching, or by *indirect contact*, such as by touching an object the infected person has had contact with. The hands are probably the greatest source of infectious disease transmission. For example, you may touch the handle of a drinking fountain that was just touched by someone whose

TABLE 17.1 Routes of Disease Transmission

Mode of Transmission	Aspects of Transmission
Contact	Either *direct* (e.g., skin or sexual contact) or *indirect* (e.g., infected blood or body fluid)
Food- or waterborne	Eating or coming in contact with contaminated food or water or products passed through them
Airborne	Inhalation; droplet spread as through sneezing, coughing, or talking
Vectorborne	Vector-transmitted via secretions, biting, egg-laying, as done by mosquitoes, ticks, snails, avians, etc; depends on how infectious the organism is
Perinatal	Similar to contact infection; happens in the uterus or as the baby passes through the birth canal

hands were contaminated by a recent sneeze or failure to wash after using the toilet. You may also **autoinoculate** yourself, or transmit a pathogen from one part of your body to another. For example, you may touch a cold sore on your lip that is teeming with viral herpes, then transmit the virus to your eye when you scratch your itchy eyelid.

Pathogens are also transmitted by *airborne contact*—you can breathe in air that carries a particular pathogen—or by *foodborne infection* if you eat something contaminated by microorganisms. Recent episodes of food poisoning from *Salmonella* bacteria in certain foods and *Escherichia coli* (*E. coli*) bacteria in undercooked beef have raised concerns about the safety of the U.S. food supply. As a direct result of these concerns, food labels caution consumers to cook meats thoroughly, wash utensils, and take other food-handling precautions.

autoinoculate Transmit a pathogen from one part of your own body to another part.

interspecies transmission Transmission of disease from humans to animals or from animals to humans.

bacteria Single-celled organisms that may cause disease.

toxins Poisonous substances produced by certain microorganisms that cause various diseases.

staphylococci Round, gram-positive bacteria, usually found in clusters.

epidermis The outermost layer of the skin.

toxic shock syndrome (TSS) A potentially life-threatening bacterial infection that is most common in menstruating women who use tampons.

Your best friend may be the source of *animal-borne pathogens*. Dogs, cats, livestock, and wild animals can spread numerous diseases through their bites or feces or by carrying infected insects into living areas and transmitting diseases either directly or indirectly. Although **interspecies transmission** of diseases (the passing of diseases from humans to animals and vice versa) is rare, it does occur. *Waterborne diseases* are transmitted directly from drinking water and indirectly from foods washed or sprayed with contaminated water. These pathogens can also invade your body if you wade or swim in contaminated streams, lakes, and reservoirs. Pathogens may also transmit *insectborne diseases* via mosquitoes, ticks, and other hosts that spread disease through sucking or biting. Mothers may transmit diseases *perinatally* to an infant in the womb or as the baby passes through the vagina during birth.

We can categorize pathogens into six major types: bacteria, viruses, fungi, protozoa, parasitic worms, and prions. Each has a particular route of transmission and characteristic elements that make it unique. Some are particularly virulent and can successfully invade a host and sustain themselves in a potentially hostile environment. Others are weak and die before they even penetrate the body because of the far-reaching body defense system. In the following pages we discuss each of these categories and give an overview of diseases they cause that have a significant impact on public health.

Bacteria

Bacteria are single-celled organisms that are plantlike in nature but lack chlorophyll (the pigment that gives plants their green coloring). There are three major types of bacteria: cocci, bacilli, and spirilla. Each type is distinguished by its shape, size, and other unique characteristics.

Although there are several thousand species of bacteria, just over 100 cause disease in humans. In many cases, it is not the bacteria themselves that cause disease but rather the poisonous substances, called **toxins,** that they produce. The following are the most common bacterial infections.

Staphylococcal Infections

Staphylococci are normally present on our skin at all times and usually cause few problems; but when there is a cut or break in the **epidermis,** or outer layer of the skin, staphylococci may enter and cause a localized infection. If you have ever suffered from acne, boils, styes (infections of the eyelids), or infected wounds, you have probably had a staph infection.

At least one staph-caused disorder, **toxic shock syndrome (TSS),** is potentially fatal. Although most cases of TSS have occurred in menstruating women, the disease was first reported in 1978 in a group of children and continues to appear in people of either gender recovering from wounds, surgery, or other injury.

If you are a menstruating woman, you can reduce the likelihood of TSS by taking the following precautions: (1) avoid superabsorbent tampons except during the heaviest menstrual flow; (2) change tampons at least every four hours; and (3) use pads at night instead of tampons. Men and women can prevent TSS by making sure that cuts and wounds remain clean and by seeking medical attention if there are signs of skin infection such as redness, swelling, or abnormal drainage near the wound.[2] Call your doctor immediately if you experience any of the following symptoms: high fever, headache, vomiting, diarrhea and chills, stomach pains, or shocklike symptoms such as faintness, rapid pulse, pallor (which can be caused by a drop in blood pressure), or a sunburnlike rash, particularly on fingers and toes.

Streptococcal Infections At least five types of the **streptococcus** microorganism—groups A, B, C, D, and G—are known to cause bacterial infections. Most strep infections are caused by the group A variety, including streptococcal pharyngitis ("strep throat") and scarlet fever, which is often preceded by a sore throat.[3] Most of these infections respond readily to antibiotics. However, resistant forms of streptococcal infections are emerging and pose threats for the future.

Another variety of strep is group B streptococcus (GBS), which can cause illness in newborn babies, pregnant women, the elderly, and adults with other illnesses or compromised immune systems. GBS can cause life-threatening blood infections (sepsis), pneumonia, bladder infections, womb infections, and stillbirth. Twenty percent of those with GBS die. This has caused increasing concern among health professionals.[4]

A third type of strep, *necrotizing fasciitis ("flesh-eating strep"),* is the stuff of science fiction. This organism caused hysteria in the United States in 1994 as hospital patients fell prey to this illness that slowly invaded and killed tissue in healing wounds. This form of strep is treatable, but suddenly becomes the victor in the delicate war between antibiotics and microbes. Today, newer antibiotics can treat it.[5]

Meningitis **Meningitis** is an infection of the *meninges,* the membranes that surround the brain and spinal cord. Meningitis can cause acute inflammation of the brain, and can be caused by a virus (less severe) or bacteria (fatal). Some forms of bacterial meningitis are contagious and can be spread through contact with saliva, nasal discharge, feces, or respiratory and throat secretions. *Pneumococcal meningitis* is the most dangerous type of bacterial meningitis, with a fatality rate of 20 percent. Approximately 6,000 cases of pneumococcal meningitis are reported in the United States each year. Symptoms may include nausea and vomiting, confusion and disorientation, drowsiness, and poor appetite.

College students living in dormitories have a higher risk of contracting *meningococcal meningitis,* a virulent form of meningitis that has risen dramatically on college campuses in recent years.[6] The signs of meningitis are sudden fever, severe headache, and a stiff neck, particularly having difficulty touching your chin to your chest.

Persons who are suspected of having meningitis should receive immediate, aggressive medical treatment. The infec-

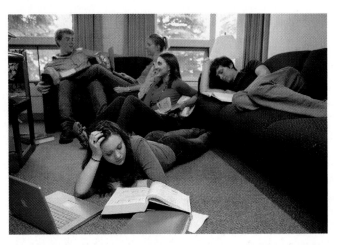

Close quarters, such as college dorms, are prime breeding grounds for some contagious diseases, like meningitis.

tion can progress quickly and early treatment is critical to the outcome.

Pneumonia In the early twentieth century, **pneumonia** was a leading cause of death in the United States. This disease is characterized by chronic cough, chest pain, chills, high fever, fluid accumulation, and eventual respiratory failure. One of the most common forms of pneumonia is due to bacterial infection and responds readily to antibiotic treatment in the early stages. Other forms are caused by viruses, chemicals, or other substances in the lungs and are more difficult to treat. Although medical advances have reduced the overall incidence and severity of pneumonia, it continues to be a major threat in the United States and worldwide. Vulnerable populations include older adults and those already suffering from other illnesses such as AIDS.

Legionnaire's Disease This bacterial disorder gained widespread publicity in 1976, when several Legionnaires at an American Legion convention in Philadelphia contracted it and died before the invading organism was isolated and effective treatment devised. Symptoms mimic the flu, but within a few days can become severe and require hospitalization. Although one of the lesser known diseases, its waterborne nature has led to several recent outbreaks around the world, particularly on cruise ships.[7] In people whose resistance is lowered, particularly the elderly, delayed identification can have serious consequences.

streptococcus A round bacterium, usually found in chain formation.

meningitis An infection of the meninges, the membranes that surround the brain and spinal cord.

pneumonia Bacterially caused disease of the lungs.

Tuberculosis A major killer in the United States in the early twentieth century, **tuberculosis (TB),** or "consumption" or "white death" as it was once known, was largely controlled in the United States by 1950 due to improved sanitation, isolation of infected persons, and treatment with drugs such as *rifampin* or *isoniazid*. Although many health professionals assumed that TB had been conquered, that appears not to be the case. During the past 20 years, several factors have led to an epidemic rise in the disease: deteriorating social conditions, including overcrowding and poor sanitation; failure to isolate active cases of TB; a weakening of public health infrastructure, which has led to less funding for screening; and migration of TB to the United States through international travel. In 2005, there were over 14,093 active cases of TB in the United States. Foreign-born individuals have a higher risk than Americans.[8] In the United States between 1998 and 2003, the top five countries of origin for foreign-born persons with TB were Mexico, the Philippines, Vietnam, India, and China.[9] Newer strains of multiple-drug-resistant tuberculosis make this epidemic potentially more devastating than previous outbreaks.

The World Health Organization (WHO) ranks tuberculosis among the most serious health threats in the world. It is estimated that one-third of the world's inhabitants (over 2 billion humans) carry the TB bacterium, *Mycobacterium tuberculosis,* and infection is spreading at the rate of 1 person per second. An estimated 15 million people live with active TB, and 2 million people die from it each year.[10]

Tuberculosis is caused by bacterial infiltration of the respiratory system that results in a chronic inflammatory reaction in the lungs. Airborne transmission via the respiratory tract is the primary and most efficient mode of transmitting TB. People with active cases can transmit the disease while talking, coughing, sneezing, or singing. Fortunately, it is fairly difficult to catch, and prolonged exposure, rather than single exposure, is the typical mode of infection. A rare mode of transmission is by infected urine, especially for young children using the same toilet facilities. People residing in overcrowded prisons and homeless shelters with poor ventilation (which means that people continuously inhale the same contaminated air) are at higher risk. The poor, especially children and the chronically ill, seem to be among those at greatest risk. As the HIV/AIDS epidemic has evolved, persons with compromised immune systems are also at high risk for TB infection.

Many people infected with TB are contagious without actually showing any symptoms themselves. Symptoms include persistent coughing, weight loss, fever, and spitting up blood. If you or someone you know has these symptoms, check with a doctor. A simple skin test can indicate infection, to be followed by chest X rays and other confirmatory tests. Treatments are effective for most nonresistant cases. Treatment includes rest, careful infection-control procedures, and drugs to combat the infection.

Periodontal Diseases Disorders of the tissue around the teeth, called **periodontal diseases,** affect three out of four adults over age 35. Improper tooth care, including lack of flossing and poor brushing habits, and the failure to obtain regular professional dental care lead to increased bacterial growth, caries (tooth decay), and gum infections. If left untreated, permanent tooth loss may result.

Rickettsia-Caused Diseases Once believed to be closely related to viruses, **rickettsia** are now considered a small form of bacteria. They produce toxins and multiply within small blood vessels, causing vascular blockage and tissue death.

Rickettsia require an insect vector (carrier) for transmission to humans. Two common forms of human rickettsial disease are Rocky Mountain spotted fever (RMSF), carried by a tick, and typhus, carried by a louse, flea, or tick. These diseases produce similar symptoms, including high fever, weakness, rash, and coma, and both can be life-threatening. You do not actually have to be bitten by a vector to contract these diseases. Because the insects harbor the developing rickettsia in their intestinal tracts, insect excrement deposited on the skin and entering the body through abrasions and scratches may be a common source of infection.[11]

what do you THINK?

Why do you think we are experiencing global increases in diseases such as tuberculosis today? ■ Should we be concerned about diseases in other countries? ■ Do we have an obligation to help the world's population in its struggle against these diseases? ■ What policies, programs, and services might help?

Viruses

Viruses are the smallest known pathogens, 100 to 200 times smaller than bacteria. Because of their tiny size, they are visible only under an electron microscope and were not identified until the twentieth century.[12]

Hundreds of viruses infect almost every single type of living organism. Over 150 viruses are known to cause diseases in humans, although their role in the development of various cancers and chronic diseases remains unclear. In fact, we still have much to learn about viruses, one of the most unusual microorganisms that infect humans.

tuberculosis (TB) A disease caused by bacterial infiltration of the respiratory system.

periodontal diseases Diseases of the tissue around the teeth.

rickettsia A small form of bacteria that live inside other living cells.

viruses Minute parasitic microbes that live inside another cell.

Essentially, a virus consists of a protein structure that contains either *ribonucleic acid (RNA)* or *deoxyribonucleic acid (DNA)*. Incapable of carrying out the normal cell functions of respiration and metabolism, a virus cannot reproduce on its own and can exist only in a parasitic relationship with the cell it invades. In fact, some scientists question whether viruses should even be considered living organisms.

When viruses attach themselves to host cells, they inject their own RNA or DNA, causing the host cells to begin reproducing new viruses. Once they take control of a cell, these new viruses overrun it until, filled to capacity, the cell bursts, putting thousands of new viruses into circulation to begin the process of cell invasion and reproduction all over again.

Because viruses cannot reproduce outside living cells, they are especially difficult to culture in a laboratory, making their detection and study extremely time consuming. Viral diseases can be difficult to treat because many viruses can withstand heat, formaldehyde, and large doses of radiation with little effect on their structure. In addition, some viruses may have **incubation periods** (the length of time required to develop fully and therefore cause symptoms in their hosts) that are measured in years rather than hours or days. Termed **slow-acting viruses,** these viruses infect the host and remain in a semidormant state for years, causing a slowly developing illness. HIV is the most recent deadly example of a slow-acting virus.

Drug treatment for viral infections is also limited. Drugs powerful enough to kill viruses generally kill the host cells, too, although some medications block stages in viral reproduction without damaging the host cells.

When exposed to certain viruses, the body produces a protein substance known as **interferon.** Interferon does not destroy the invading microorganisms but sets up a protective mechanism to aid healthy cells in their struggle against the invaders. Although interferon research is promising, it should be noted that not all viruses stimulate interferon production.

The Common Cold

In everyday life, perhaps no ailment is as bothersome as the common cold, with its irritating symptoms of runny nose, itchy eyes, and generally uncomfortable sensations. Colds are responsible for more days lost from work and more uncomfortable days spent at work than any other ailment.

Caused by any number of viruses (some experts claim there may be over 100 different viruses responsible), colds are **endemic** (always present to some degree) among people throughout the world. Current research indicates that otherwise healthy people carry cold viruses in their noses and throats most of the time. These viruses are held in check until the host's resistance is lowered. In the true sense of the word, it is possible to "catch" a cold—from the airborne droplets of another person's sneeze or from skin-to-skin or mucous membrane contact—though recent studies indicate that the hands are the greatest avenue for transmitting colds and other viruses. Obviously, then, covering your nose and mouth with a tissue, handkerchief, or even the crook of your elbow when sneezing is better than using your bare hand, particularly if

you next use your hand to touch food, shake your friend's hand, or open a door.

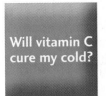

Will vitamin C cure my cold?

Although numerous theories exist concerning how to "cure" the common cold, including taking megadoses of vitamin C, little hard evidence supports any of them. The best rule of thumb is to keep your resistance level high. Sound nutrition, adequate rest, stress reduction, and regular exercise appear to be the best bets in fighting off infection. Avoid people with newly developed colds (colds appear to be most contagious during the first 24 hours of onset). If you contract a cold, bed rest, plenty of fluids, and aspirin to relieve pain and discomfort are the tried-and-true remedies for adults. Children should not be given aspirin for colds or the flu because this could lead to development of *Reye's syndrome,* a potentially fatal disease. Several nonaspirin over-the-counter preparations are effective for alleviating certain symptoms.

Influenza In otherwise healthy people, **influenza,** or flu, is usually not life-threatening. Symptoms, including aches and pains, nausea, diarrhea, fever, and coldlike ailments, generally pass quickly. (Figure 17.2 on page 518 compares cold and flu symptoms.) However, in combination with other disorders, such as respiratory or heart disease, or among people over age 65 or under age 5, the flu can be very serious. Five to 20 percent of Americans get the flu each year, and of these, 200,000 people will need hospitalization and 36,000 will die.[13]

To date, three major varieties of flu virus have been discovered, with many different strains existing within each variety. The A form of the virus is generally the most virulent, followed by the B and C varieties. See the New Horizons in Health box on page 519 for information on avian flu. If you contract one form of influenza you may develop immunity to it, but you will not necessarily be immune to other forms of the disease. Little can be done to treat flu patients once the infection has become established.

Today, vaccines provide significant protection for vulnerable populations and these individuals receive the highest priority for annual flu shots. Some vaccines have proven effective against certain strains of flu virus, but they are

incubation period The time between exposure to a disease and the appearance of symptoms.

slow-acting viruses Viruses having long incubation periods and causing slowly progressive symptoms.

interferon A protein substance produced by the body that aids the immune system by protecting healthy cells.

endemic Describing a disease that is always present to some degree.

influenza A common viral disease of the respiratory tract.

SYMPTOMS	COLD	FLU
Fever	Rare	Characteristically high (102–104°F); lasts 3–4 days
Headache	Rare	Prominent
General aches/pain	Slight	Usual; often severe
Fatigue, weakness	Quite mild	Can last up to 2–3 weeks
Extreme exhaustion	Never	Early and prominent
Stuffy nose	Common	Sometimes
Sneezing	Usual	Sometimes
Sore throat	Common	Sometimes
Chest discomfort, cough	Mild to moderate; hacking cough	Common; can become severe
Nausea, vomiting	Not common	Sometimes
COMPLICATIONS	Sinus congestion, sinus infection, or earache	Bronchitis, pneumonia; can be life-threatening
PREVENTION	None; avoid contact with infected persons; wash hands; cover mouth when sneezing	Annual vaccination; amantadine or rimantadine (antiviral drugs)
TREATMENT	Palliative, temporary	Amantadine or rimantadine within 24–48 hours of symptoms

FIGURE 17.2 Is It a Cold or the Flu?

Source: Adapted from National Institute of Allergy and Infectious Diseases, "Is It a Cold or the Flu?" 2000.

totally ineffective against others. In spite of minor risks, it is recommended that people over age 65, pregnant women, people with heart or lung disease, and those with certain other illnesses be vaccinated. Because flu shots take two to three weeks to become effective, you should get these shots in the fall, before the flu season begins. An inhaled vaccine called FluMist is also available for healthy, nonpregnant adults up to age 49. Because the vaccine contains a weakened version of the live virus, people who receive the vaccine may pose a risk to anyone with a weakened immune system who is around them.

Infectious Mononucleosis Initial symptoms of **mononucleosis,** or "mono," include sore throat, fever, headache, nausea, chills, and pervasive weakness or fatigue. As the disease progresses, lymph nodes may enlarge and

jaundice, and spleen enlargement, aching joints, and body rashes may occur.

Theories on the transmission and treatment of mononucleosis are highly controversial. Caused by the *Epstein-Barr virus,* mononucleosis is readily detected through a *monospot test,* a blood test that measures the percentage of specific forms of white blood cells. Because many viruses are caused by transmission of body fluids, it was once believed that young people passed the disease on by kissing (hence its nickname "the kissing disease"). Although this is still considered a possible cause, mononucleosis is not believed to be highly contagious. It does not appear to be easily contracted through normal, everyday personal contact. Multiple cases among family members are rare, as are cases between intimate partners.

Treatment of mononucleosis is often a lengthy process that involves bed rest, balanced nutrition, and medications. Gradually, the body develops immunity to the disease and the person returns to normal activity.

Hepatitis One of the most highly publicized viral diseases is **hepatitis,** a virally caused inflammation of the liver. Hepatitis symptoms include fever, headache, nausea, loss of appetite, skin rashes, pain in the upper right abdomen, dark yellow (with brownish tinge) urine, and the possibility

mononucleosis A viral disease that causes pervasive fatigue and other long-lasting symptoms.

hepatitis A virally caused disease in which the liver becomes inflamed, producing symptoms such as fever, headache, and possibly jaundice.

A NEW PANDEMIC? AVIAN INFLUENZA

As the flu season of 2005–2006 approached, headlines warning of a massive flu pandemic, and images of chickens and other birds going to slaughter across Asia and Europe, began to emerge. The media flurry was sparked by concern in the international community over a strain of avian (bird) influenza called H5N1. This newly emerging virulent flu strain had appeared in bird populations throughout Asia, including domestic birds such as chickens and ducks, as early as 1997. Why all the concern now? Scientists have noted that recently, bird flu has appeared in regions of the world previously unaffected. As of this book's publication, bird flu has spread to many regions of the world, with human cases reported in Asia, Africa, China, Europe, and Russia. Though it spreads primarily through domestic and wild birds, cases have been documented in pigs, house cats, and other small mammals.

How worried about bird flu should I be?

THE THREAT TO HUMAN HEALTH

Many scientists suggest that this virus is virulent enough to surpass the lethality of the influenza epidemic of 1918 that swept the global community, causing millions of deaths. In a 2005 World Health Organization (WHO) meeting devoted to the H5N1 bird flu strain, public health officials warned that a worldwide bird flu pandemic could easily kill millions of people and cost the global economy more than $800 billion.

Why does bird flu pose such a severe threat to humans? The H5N1 strain is so new and unique that human beings have no natural immunity to it. With the common flu virus, our immune system is able to recognize the antigens and develop antibodies to fight back. H5N1 is considered so virulent because it is so different from other flu antigens. Though the virus has yet to mutate into a form highly infectious to humans, outbreaks in rural areas of the world (where people often live in close proximity to poultry) would provide avian flu with an ideal environment to jump to humans.

PREVENTING A PANDEMIC

WHO officials warn that the world is not prepared to fight a flu pandemic. The current spread of H5N1 throughout global bird populations has seemed to spur international governments into action, although progress is slow. People in poorer countries may rely heavily on poultry for their livelihood, which makes destroying infected birds economically difficult, and many cases may go unreported. Many countries are preparing strategic action plans to develop early warning systems, prevent the spread of disease, and develop vaccines. However, developing countries are of great concern, as they do not have the necessary resources to enact such preparations. African nations and rural areas of Asia could be devastated by a pandemic.

Research studies are under way to develop a vaccine, but no vaccine is ready for production currently and producing and distributing enough vaccine for an epidemic is yet another challenge. Despite this, there are some promising treatments, and tips for prevention.

- Antiviral medications, such as Tamiflu, can reduce the severity and duration of illness. Countries worldwide, and the WHO, are building a stockpile of these medications, and developing plans for rapid distribution should an outbreak occur.
- To date, researchers do not believe the virus can be transmitted via cooked poultry, but precaution should be used when eating poultry or eggs in countries experiencing outbreaks. Foods should be properly cooked and handled during food preparation. Exposure can occur

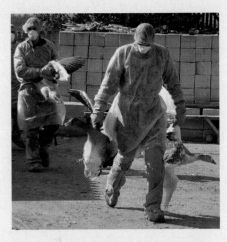

during preparation of raw poultry for cooking.
- Wash your hands (see the Try it Now on page 525 for tips on proper handwashing). This is one of the best defenses against infection. If you cannot wash your hands with soap and water, use an alcohol-based hand sanitizer.

WHEN WILL THE PANDEMIC HIT?

Scientists can't be sure but it has undoubtedly already taken many years for the current strain of avian flu to evolve into this virulent, deadly version. A pandemic will occur only when:

- A newer and more highly contagious subtype of the virus emerges
- The new subtype can readily infect humans, and be sustainable in humans

To date, H5N1 has infected over 100 people worldwide and killed 50 percent of them. The stage is set for the pandemic to strike, so government intervention that is effective and a drug regimen that is equally effective and available are of utmost importance.

Sources: World Health Organization, "Avian Influenza: Frequently Asked Questions," 2006, www.who.int/csr/disease/avian_influenza/avian_faqs/en/print.html; Centers for Disease Control and Prevention, "Avian Influenza: Current Situation," 2006, www.cdc.gov/flu/avian/outbreaks/current.htm.

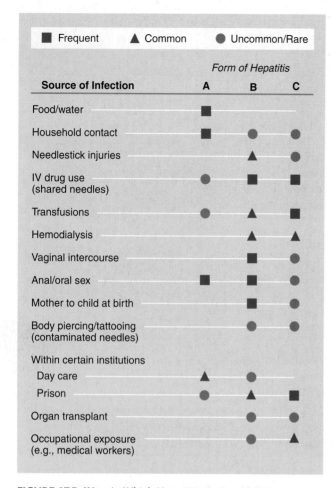

Source of Infection	Form of Hepatitis		
	A	B	C
Food/water	■		
Household contact	■	●	●
Needlestick injuries		▲	●
IV drug use (shared needles)	●	■	■
Transfusions	●	▲	■
Hemodialysis		▲	▲
Vaginal intercourse		■	●
Anal/oral sex	■	■	●
Mother to child at birth		■	●
Body piercing/tattooing (contaminated needles)		●	●
Within certain institutions			
Day care	▲	●	
Prison	●	▲	■
Organ transplant		●	●
Occupational exposure (e.g., medical workers)		●	▲

■ Frequent   ▲ Common   ● Uncommon/Rare

FIGURE 17.3 Ways in Which Hepatitis A, B, and C Are Contracted

Source: American Liver Foundation, "Getting Hip to Hep: What You Should Know about Hepatitis A, B, and C," 2006, www.liverfoundation.org (75 Maiden Lane, Suite 603, New York, NY 10038, 1-800-GO-LIVER).

of jaundice (yellowing of the whites of the eyes and the skin). In some regions of the United States and among certain segments of the population, hepatitis has reached epidemic proportions. Internationally, viral hepatitis is one of the most frequently reported diseases and a major contributor to acute and chronic liver disease, accounting for high morbidity and mortality. Currently, there are seven known forms of hepatitis, with hepatitis A, B, and C having the highest rates of incidence (see Figure 17.3). In the United States, hepatitis continues to be a major threat in spite of a safe blood supply and massive efforts at education about hand washing (hepatitis A) and safer sex (hepatitis B and C). Treatment of all the forms of viral hepatitis is somewhat limited. A proper diet, bed rest, and antibiotics that combat bacterial invaders, which may cause additional problems, are recommended.

Hepatitis A (HAV). HAV is contracted from eating food or drinking water contaminated with human excrement. Today, largely due to vaccinations, rates of HAV have dropped, but there are still over 50,000 new infections in the United States each year, typically through something in the household,

sexual contact, day care attendance, or international travel.[14] Infected food handlers, people who ingest seafood from contaminated water, and those who use contaminated needles are also at risk. Fortunately, individuals infected with hepatitis A do not become chronic carriers.

Hepatitis B (HBV). One out of every 20 people in the United States will be infected with HBV in their lifetime. It is spread primarily via body fluids being shared through unprotected sex. However, it is also contracted via sharing needles when injecting drugs, through needlesticks on the job, or, in the case of a newborn baby, from an infected mother. Although 30 percent of those who are infected have no symptoms, symptoms can include jaundice, fatigue, abdominal pain, loss of appetite, nausea and vomiting, and joint pain.

HBV infection has been on the decline, largely due to a vaccine for HBV that has been available since 1982 and is now available on most college campuses for a modest cost.[15] This means that HBV is one of the only vaccine-preventable sexually transmitted infections in society today. However, because the vaccine can be costly, and is not widely available globally, over 350 million people worldwide are chronic carriers.[16] A combination series vaccine for HAV and HBV is also an option. If you work in a day care or health care facility, or plan to travel to regions of the world where HAV or HBV are prevalent, you should discuss the risk with your physician.

Hepatitis C (HCV). This disease was spread primarily through blood transfusions or organ transplants prior to mass screenings that began in 1992. Since then, the more common means of transmission has been when blood or body fluids from an infected person follow a variety of routes to enter the body of a person who is not infected. HCV infections are on an epidemic rise in many regions of the world today. Currently, it is estimated that there are 25,000 new cases of hepatitis C in the United States each year, with over 3 million people chronically infected.[17] Over 85 percent of those infected develop chronic infections; if the infection is left untreated, the person may develop cirrhosis of the liver, liver cancer, or liver failure. Liver failure due to chronic hepatitis C is the leading cause of liver transplants in the United States.[18]

Symptoms of HCV are similar to those of HBV, with jaundice, fatigue, abdominal pain, loss of appetite, and nausea occurring frequently. Dark urine is a hallmark symptom. The prognosis for a cure is bleak compared with other forms of hepatitis. About 75 to 85 percent of those infected develop chronic HCV and 70 percent of those who become chronic carriers also develop chronic liver disease.[19]

Although there is no vaccine for HCV, one is currently being tested and may be available shortly.[20]

Reducing Your Risk of Contracting HBV and HCV Follow these strategies:

■ Use latex condoms correctly every time you have sex. (Note: The efficacy of latex condoms in preventing infection with HBV is unknown, but their proper use may reduce transmission.)

- Don't share personal care items that might have blood on them, such as razors or toothbrushes.
- If you are pregnant, get a blood test for HBV; infants born to HBV-infected mothers should be given HBIG (hepatitis B immunoglobulin) and vaccine within 12 hours of birth.
- Do not inject drugs, and never share needles.
- Consider the risks of tattoos and body piercings. Only go to reputable artists or piercers who follow established sterilization and infection control protocols.
- If you have had HBV or are HCV positive, do not donate blood, organs, or tissues.
- If you are a health care or public safety worker, get vaccinated and follow routine barrier precautions.

Mumps

In 1968, a vaccine became available for mumps, a common viral disorder among children, and the disease seemed to be largely under control, with reported cases declining from 80 per 100,000 people in 1968 to less than 2 per 100,000 people in 1984. Since then, mumps rates have risen, and a recent epidemic of mumps infected thousands of people mainly in Iowa and the Central United States. No one knows how this outbreak started, but it is suspected that many do not receive their second mumps vaccination, making them particularly susceptible.

Approximately one-half of all mumps infections are not apparent because they produce only minor symptoms. Many cases are never reported, so the actual incidence may be higher than indicated.

Typically, there is an incubation period of 16 to 18 days, followed by symptoms caused by the lodging of the virus in the glands of the neck. The most common symptom is the swelling of the parotid (salivary) glands; however, about one-third of all infected people never have this symptom. One of the greatest dangers associated with mumps is the potential for sterility in men who contract the disease in young adulthood. Some victims suffer hearing loss.

Chickenpox (HVZV) and Shingles

Caused by the *herpes varicella zoster* virus (HVZV), chickenpox produces characteristic symptoms of fever and fatigue 13 to 17 days after exposure, followed by skin eruptions that itch, blister, and produce a clear fluid. The virus is present in these blisters for approximately one week. Symptoms are generally mild, and immunity to subsequent infection appears to be lifelong. (Some children experience more serious side effects, such as scarring, high fever, and other complications.) Although a vaccine for chickenpox is available, and all children should receive it, many parents incorrectly assume that the vaccine is not necessary. The failure to vaccinate means that many children still contract the disease.

For a small segment of the population, however, the virus may become reactivated. This disease, known as *shingles,* affects over 5 percent of the population each year. More than half the sufferers are over age 50.

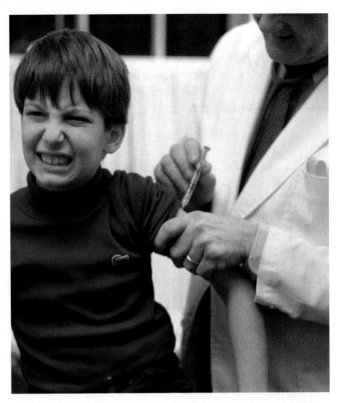

Following the recommended immunization schedule is an easy and effective way to protect a child from serious illnesses, while also helping to eradicate life-threatening disease.

Measles

Technically referred to as *rubeola,* **measles** is a viral disorder that often affects young children. Symptoms, appearing about ten days after exposure, include an itchy rash and a high fever. **Rubella (German measles)** is a milder viral infection that is believed to be transmitted by inhalation, after which it multiplies in the upper respiratory tract and passes into the bloodstream. It causes a rash, especially on the upper extremities. It is not generally a serious health threat and usually runs its course in three to four days. The major exceptions to this rule are among newborns and pregnant women. Rubella can damage a fetus, particularly during the first trimester, creating a condition known as congenital rubella, in which the infant may be born blind, deaf, retarded, or with heart defects. Immunization has reduced the incidence of both measles and rubella. Infections in children not immunized against measles can lead to fever-induced problems such as rheumatic heart disease, kidney damage, and neurological disorders.

> **measles** A viral disease that produces symptoms including an itchy rash and a high fever.
>
> **rubella (German measles)** A milder form of measles that causes a rash and mild fever in children and may cause damage to a fetus or a newborn baby.

Rabies The **rabies** virus infects many warm-blooded animals. Bats are believed to be **asymptomatic** (symptom-free) carriers. Their urine, which they spray when flying, contains the virus, and even the air of densely populated bat caves may be infectious. In most other hosts, the disease is extremely virulent and usually fatal. A characteristic behavior of rabid animals is the frenzied biting of other animals and people. Not only does this behavior cause injury, but it also spreads the virus through the infected animal's saliva. The most obvious symptoms of the disease are extreme activity in the cerebral region of the brain, rage, increased salivation, spasms in the pharynx (throat) muscles, extreme drive to find water, and the inability to swallow.

The incubation period for rabies is usually one to three months, although it may range from one week to one year. The disease may be fatal if not treated immediately with the rabies vaccine. Anyone bitten by an animal that might carry rabies should seek immediate medical attention and try to bring the animal along for testing.

Other Pathogens

Fungi Hundreds of species of **fungi,** multi- or unicellular primitive plants, inhabit our environment. Many fungi are useful, providing such foodstuffs as edible mushrooms and some cheeses. But some species of fungi can produce infections. Candidiasis (a vaginal yeast infection), athlete's foot, toenail fungus, ringworm, and jock itch are examples of fungal diseases. Keeping the affected area clean and dry plus treatment with appropriate medications will generally bring prompt relief.

Protozoa **Protozoa** are microscopic single-celled organisms that are generally associated with tropical diseases such as African sleeping sickness and malaria. Although these pathogens are prevalent in nonindustrialized countries, they are largely controlled in the United States. A common water-borne protozoan disease in many regions of the country is giardiasis. Persons who drink or are exposed to the *Giardia* pathogen may suffer intestinal pain and discomfort weeks after infection. Protection of water supplies is the key to prevention.

Parasitic Worms **Parasitic worms** are the largest of the pathogens. Ranging in size from the relatively small pinworms typically found in children to the large tapeworms found in all warm-blooded animals, most parasitic worms are more a nuisance than a threat. Of special note today are the worm infestations associated with eating raw fish in Japanese sushi restaurants. Cooking fish and other foods to temperatures sufficient to kill the worms and their eggs can prevent this.

Prions A **prion,** or unconventional virus, is a self-replicating, protein-based agent that can infect humans and other animals. Believed to be the underlying cause of spongiform diseases such as "mad cow disease," this agent systematically destroys brain cells. We will say more about prion-based diseases in the Emerging and Resurgent Diseases section later in this chapter.

Your Body's Defenses: Keeping You Well

Although all the pathogens just described pose a threat if they take hold in your body, the chances that they will do so are actually quite small. First, they must overcome a number of effective barriers, many of which were established in your body before you were even born. Table 17.2 details how you can keep your body in top shape to defend against invaders.

Physical and Chemical Defenses: Your Body Responds

Perhaps our single most critical early defense system is the skin. Layered to provide an intricate web of barriers, the skin allows few pathogens to enter. **Enzymes,** complex proteins manufactured by the body that appear in body secretions such as sweat, provide additional protection, destroying microorganisms on skin surfaces by producing inhospitable pH levels. Normal body pH is 7.0, but enzymatic or biochemical changes may cause the body chemistry to become more acidic (pH of less than 7.0) or more alkaline (pH of more than 7.0). In either case, microorganisms that flourish at a selected pH will be weakened or destroyed as these changes occur. Only when cracks or breaks occur in the skin can pathogens gain easy access to the body.

The linings of the body provide yet another protection. Mucous membranes in the respiratory tract and other linings of the body trap and engulf invading organisms. Cilia,

---

rabies A viral disease of the central nervous system; often transmitted through animal bites.

asymptomatic Without symptoms, or symptom free.

fungi A group of plants that lack chlorophyll and do not produce flowers or seeds; several microscopic varieties are pathogenic.

protozoa Microscopic single-celled organisms.

parasitic worms The largest of the pathogens, most of which are more a nuisance than a threat.

prion A recently identified pathogen that infects humans and animals; a self-replicating protein-based agent that systematically destroys brain cells.

enzymes Organic substances that facilitate chemical reactions, some of which cause bodily changes and destruction of microorganisms.

TABLE 17.2	Keeping Defenses Healthy
■ Limit exposure to germs	Limit contact with those who are getting colds or have symptoms. Wash your hands and avoid touching hands to eyes and mouth. Avoid antibacterial soaps, which contribute to germ resistance.
■ Exercise regularly	Exercising raises core body temperature, which kills many invaders.
■ Get enough sleep	Refresh your body regularly. Take time out and time off. Experience your spiritual side.
■ Eat healthy foods	Follow established guidelines, consuming adequate amounts of water, protein, carbohydrates, fats, vitamins, and minerals. Moderation in using supplements is recommended.
■ Don't overuse antibiotics	"Use it and lose it" is a phrase that aptly describes what has happened as antibiotics are used over and over again and bacteria adapt to become more resistant to them. Many antibiotics are used inappropriately because patients demand them.
■ Manage stress	Use strategies such as exercise and relaxation techniques to lower stress levels in your life.

Source: Adapted from T. Mitchell, "Make Your Immnue System Invincible," *USA Weekend,* January 7–9, 2000. Reprinted by permission of T. L. Mitchell, *USA Weekend* Health Editor.

hairlike projections in the lungs and respiratory tract, sweep invaders toward body openings, where they are expelled. Tears, nasal secretions, earwax, and other secretions found at body entrances contain enzymes designed to destroy or neutralize pathogens.

Finally, any organism that manages to breach these initial lines of defense faces a formidable specialized network of defenses thrown up by the immune system (Figure 17.4 on page 524).

The Immune System: Your Body Fights Back

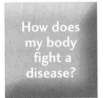
How does my body fight a disease?

Immunity is a condition of being able to resist a particular disease by counteracting the substance that produces the disease. Any substance capable of triggering an immune response is called an **antigen.** An antigen can be a virus, a bacterium, a fungus, a parasite, or a tissue or cell from another individual. When invaded by an antigen, the body responds by forming substances called **antibodies** that are matched to that specific antigen much as a key is matched to a lock. Antibodies belong to a mass of large molecules known as *immunoglobulins,* a group of nine chemically distinct protein substances, each of which plays a role in neutralizing, setting up for destruction, or actually destroying antigens.

Once an antigen breaches the body's initial defenses, the body begins a process of antigen analysis. It considers the size and shape of the invader, verifies that the antigen is not part of the body itself, and then produces a specific antibody to destroy or weaken the antigen. This process, which is much more complex than described here, is part of a system called the humoral immune response. Humoral immunity is the body's major defense against many bacteria and bacterial toxins.

Cell-mediated immunity is characterized by the formation of a population of *lymphocytes* (specialized white blood cells) that can attack and destroy the foreign invader. These lym-

phocytes constitute the body's main defense against viruses, fungi, parasites, and some bacteria, and are found in the blood, lymph nodes, bone marrow, and certain glands. Other key players in this immune response are known as macrophages (a type of phagocytic, or cell-eating, white blood cell).

Two forms of lymphocytes in particular, the **B lymphocytes (B cells)** and **T lymphocytes (T cells),** are involved in the immune response. They are named according to the area of the body in which they develop: most B cells are manufactured in the soft tissue of the hollow shafts of the long bones. T cells, in contrast, develop and multiply in the thymus, a multilobed organ that lies behind the breastbone.

T cells assist the immune system in several ways. *Regulatory T cells* help direct the activities of the immune system and assist other cells, particularly B cells, to produce antibodies. Dubbed "helper T's," these cells are essential for activating B cells, other T cells, and macrophages. Another form of T cell, known as *killer T cells* or "cytotoxic T's," directly attacks infected or malignant cells. Killer T's enable the body to rid itself of cells that have been infected by viruses or transformed by cancer; they are also responsible for the rejection of tissue and organ grafts. The third type of T cells, *suppressor T cells,* turns off or suppresses the activity

antigen Substance capable of triggering an immune response.

antibodies Substances produced by the body that are individually matched to specific antigens.

B lymphocytes (B cells) Specialized white blood cells that are manufactured in the soft tissue of the hollow shafts of the long bones, and are part of the immune response system.

T lymphocytes (T cells) Specialized white blood cells that are manufactured in the thymus, a multilobed organ that lies behind the breastbone. There are several types of T cells that aid in the immune response.

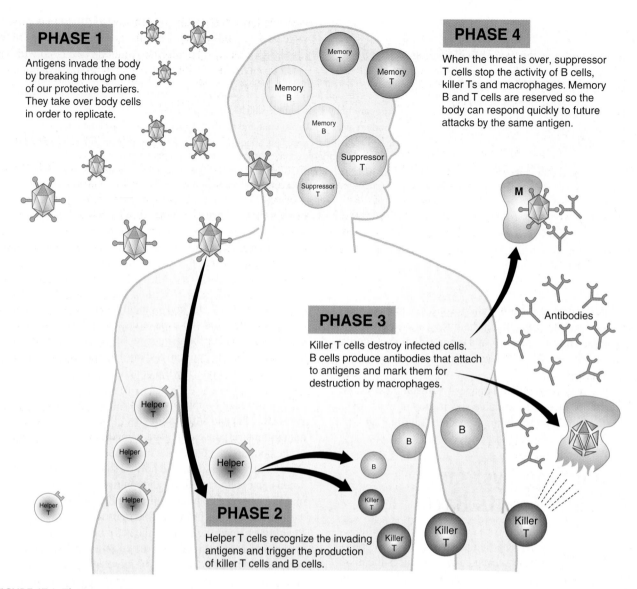

PHASE 1

Antigens invade the body by breaking through one of our protective barriers. They take over body cells in order to replicate.

PHASE 4

When the threat is over, suppressor T cells stop the activity of B cells, killer Ts and macrophages. Memory B and T cells are reserved so the body can respond quickly to future attacks by the same antigen.

Memory T
Memory T
Memory B
Memory B
Suppressor T
Suppressor T

M

Antibodies

PHASE 3

Killer T cells destroy infected cells. B cells produce antibodies that attach to antigens and mark them for destruction by macrophages.

Helper T
Helper T
Helper T
Helper T
Helper T

B
B
B
Killer T
Killer T
Killer T
Killer T

PHASE 2

Helper T cells recognize the invading antigens and trigger the production of killer T cells and B cells.

FIGURE 17.4 **The Immune Response**

of B cells, killer T's, and macrophages. Suppressor T cells circulate in the bloodstream and lymphatic system, neutralizing or destroying antigens, enhancing the effects of the immune response, and helping to return the activated immune system to normal levels.

After a successful attack on a pathogen, some of the attacker T and B cells are preserved as *memory T* and *B cells,* enabling the body to quickly recognize and respond to subsequent attacks by the same kind of organism at a later time. Thus macrophages, T and B cells, and antibodies are the key factors in mounting an immune response.

Once people have survived certain infectious diseases, they become immune to those diseases, meaning that in all probability they will not develop them again. Upon subsequent attack by the disease-causing microorganisms, their memory T and B cells are quickly activated to come to their defense.

Autoimmune Diseases Although white blood cells and the antigen–antibody response generally work in our favor by neutralizing or destroying harmful antigens, the body sometimes makes a mistake and targets its own tissue as the enemy, builds up antibodies against that tissue, and attempts to destroy it. This is known as *autoimmune* disease (*auto* means "self"). Common autoimmune disorders are rheumatoid arthritis, lupus erythematosus, and myasthenia gravis, and are discussed further in Chapter 18.

In some cases, the antigen–antibody response completely fails to function. The result is a form of *immunodeficiency syndrome.* Perhaps the most dramatic case of this syndrome was the "bubble boy," a youngster who died in 1984 after living his short life inside a sealed-off environment designed to protect him from all antigens. A much more common immune system disorder is *acquired immunodeficiency syndrome (AIDS),* which we will discuss later in this chapter (page 538).

Fever

If an infection is localized, pus formation, redness, swelling, and irritation often occur. These symptoms indicate that the invading organisms are being fought systemically. Another indication is the development of a *fever,* or a rise in body temperature above the norm of 98.6°F. Fever frequently results from toxins secreted by pathogens that interfere with the control of body temperature. Although extremely elevated temperature is often harmful to the body, fever is believed to act as a form of protection. Raising body temperature by even one or two degrees provides an environment that destroys some disease-causing organisms. A fever also stimulates the body to produce more white blood cells, which destroy more invaders.

Pain

Although we do not usually think of pain as a defense mechanism, it is a response to injury, and it plays a valuable role in the body's response to invasion. Pain may be either direct, caused by the stimulation of nerve endings in an affected area, or referred, meaning it is present in one place although the source is elsewhere. An example of **referred pain** is the pain in the arm or jaw often experienced by someone having a heart attack. Most pain responses are accompanied by inflammation. Pain tends to be the earliest sign that an injury has occurred and often causes the person to slow down or stop the activity that was aggravating the injury, thereby protecting against further damage. Because it is often one of the first warnings of disease, persistent pain should not be overlooked or masked with short-term pain relievers.

Vaccines: Bolstering Your Immunity

Recall that once people have been exposed to a specific pathogen, subsequent attacks will activate their memory T and B cells, giving them immunity. This is the principle on which **vaccination** is based.

A vaccine consists of killed or attenuated (weakened) versions of a disease-causing microorganism or an antigen that is similar to but less dangerous than the disease antigen. It is administered to stimulate the person's immune system to produce antibodies against future attacks—without actually causing the disease (or by causing a very minor case of the disease). Vaccines are given orally or by injection, and this form of artificial immunity is termed **acquired active immunity,** in contrast to **naturally acquired active immunity** (which is obtained by exposure to antigens in the normal course of daily life) or *naturally acquired passive immunity* (as occurs when a mother passes immunity to her fetus via their shared blood supply or to an infant via breast milk).

Depending on the virulence of the organism, vaccines containing live, attenuated, or dead organisms are given for a variety of diseases. In some instances, if a person is already weakened by other health problems, vaccination may provoke an actual mild case of the disease, so the decision for an ill person to receive the vaccine should be discussed with that person's physician. Childhood vaccinations are key, but so are adult vaccinations. Figure 17.5 on page 526 shows the recommended schedule for adult vaccinations.

Active and Passive Immunity

If you are exposed to an organism, either during daily life or through vaccination, you will eventually develop an active acquired immunity to that organism. Your body will produce its own antibodies, and, in most cases, you will not have to worry about subsequent exposures to that disease.

In some cases, however, the risks associated with contracting a disease are so severe that a person may not be able to wait the days or weeks that the body needs to produce antibodies. Also, in the event that resistance is terribly weakened as a result of cancer chemotherapy or other reasons, the body may be unable to produce its own antibodies. In this case, antibodies formed in another person or animal (called the donor) are often given. Termed **passive immunity,** this type of immunity is often short-lived but provides the necessary boost to get a person through a potentially critical period. Antibodies utilized for passive immunity are taken from *gamma globulins,* proteins synthesized from a donor's blood. A mother also confers passive immunity on her newborn baby through breast-feeding.

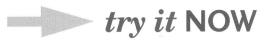

try it NOW

Wash your hands to prevent infection. How can you clean your hands properly? Wet your hands with warm water and lather up with soap; scrub your hands for about 20 seconds—try counting to 20 or saying the alphabet. Rinse well and dry your hands. Start following this basic procedure today whenever you use the bathroom, eat or prepare food, blow your nose, cough, or sneeze.

---

referred pain   Pain that is present at one location, although the source of pain is elsewhere.

vaccination   Inoculation with killed or weakened pathogens or similar, less dangerous antigens in order to prevent or lessen the effects of some disease.

acquired active immunity   Immunity developed in response to a prior disease or vaccination to prevent disease.

naturally acquired active immunity   Immunity obtained by exposure to an antigen in the normal course of life.

passive immunity   Antibodies formed in another person or animal, and then given to someone with a weakened immune system such as when a mother passes immunity to her fetus.

	Age group		
Vaccine	19–49 years	50–64 years	≥ 65 years
Tetanus, diphtheria (Td)	1-dose booster every 10 years		
Measles, mumps, rubella (MMR)	1 or 2 doses	1 dose	
Varicella	2 doses (0, 4–8 weeks)	2 doses (0, 4–8 weeks)	
— — —Vaccines below broken line are for selected populations — — —			
Influenza	1 dose annually	1 dose annually	
Pneumococcal (polysaccharide)	1–2 doses		1 dose
Hepatitis A	2 doses (0, 6–12 mos, or 0, 6–18 months)		
Hepatitis B	3 doses (0, 1–2, 4–6 months)		
Meningococcal	1 or more doses		

For all persons in this category who meet the age requirements and who lack evidence of immunity (e.g., lack documentation of vaccination or have no evidence of prior infection)

Recommended if some other risk factor is present (e.g., based on medical, occupational, lifestyle, or other indications)

FIGURE 17.5 Recommended Adult Immunization Schedule, by Vaccine and Age Group, 2006

Note that there are important explanations and additions to these recommendations that should be consulted by checking the latest schedule (available on the Centers for Disease Control and Prevention website).

Source: Centers for Disease Control and Prevention, "Recommended Adult Immunization Schedule, October 2005–September 2006," 2006, www.cdc.gov/nip/recs/adult-schedule.htm.

Emerging and Resurgent Diseases

Although our immune systems are remarkably adept at responding to challenges, they are threatened by an army of microbes that is so diverse, virulent, and insidious that the invaders appear to be gaining ground. Within the past decade, rates for infectious diseases have rapidly increased, particularly for reemerging diseases such as tuberculosis. This can be attributed to a combination of overpopulation, inadequate health care systems, increasing poverty, extreme environmental degradation, and drug resistance.[21] As international travel increases (over 1 million people per day cross international boundaries), with germs transported from remote regions to huge urban centers within hours, the likelihood of infection by microbes previously unknown on U.S. soil increases. Table 17.3 identifies major contributors to the emergence and resurgence of infectious diseases.

Tiny Microbes: Lethal Threats

Today's arsenal of antibiotics appears to be increasingly ineffective, with penicillin-resistant strains of diseases on the rise as microbes are able to outlast and outsmart even the best of our antibiotic weapons. Old scourges are back, and new ones are emerging.

"Mad Cow Disease" The American cattle industry is under new scrutiny, with confirmed U.S. cases of *bovine spongiform encephalopathy* (BSE, or "mad cow disease") detected in 2003, and two more in 2005 and 2006. Evidence indicates that there is a relationship between ongoing outbreaks in Europe of BSE and a disease in humans known as *new variant Creutzfeldt-Jakob disease* (NvCJD).[22] Both disorders are invariably fatal brain diseases with unusually long incubation periods measured in years, and both are caused by unconventional transmittable agents known as prions.

BSE is thought to be transmitted when cows are fed a protein-based substance (slaughterhouse leftovers from sheep, poultry, and cows) to help them put on weight and grow faster. Failure to treat this protein by-product sufficiently to kill the BSE organism allowed it to infect the cows. The disease is believed to be transmitted to humans through the meat of these slaughtered cows. The resultant variant of BSE in humans, NvCJD, is characterized by progressively worsening neurological damage and death.

As scientists continue to investigate the presence of BSE in U.S. cattle, the USDA has cut back on its testing of beef cattle. Why? USDA officials say that there is a very low risk to humans, amidst bans on U.S. beef from countries around the world. To date, there have been no known human infections from U.S. beef. People living in the United States who have developed the disease are believed to have been infected during international travel.

A related prion-caused disease similar to BSE, *chronic wasting disease,* has been found in deer. Studies are under way to investigate the implications of this disease for human health.

Contributing Factors	Possible Solutions
Hardier bugs: tiny size, adaptability, resistant strains, misuse of antibiotics	Increased pharmaceutical efforts, new drug development, selective use of new drugs; improved vaccination rates; funding of new research
Failure to prioritize public health initiatives on national level	Increased government funding; improved efforts aimed at prevention and intervention (Less than 1 percent of the federal budget goes to prevention programs.)
Explosive population growth: resource degradation, overcrowding, land use atrocities, increased urbanization	Population control, wise use of natural resources, environmental controls, reduced deforestation, and increased pollution prevention efforts
International travel	Education or risk reduction; restrictions related to unvaccinated populations; improved air quality and venting on commercial airlines
Human behaviors, particularly intravenous (IV) drug use and risky sexual behavior	Education about risky behaviors; incentives for improved behaviors; increased personal motivation
Vector management failures: widespread overuse/misuse of pesticides and antimicrobial agents that hasten resistance	Management of pesticide use; focus on pollution prevention; regulation; enforcement of laws
Food and water contamination; globalization of food supply and centralized processing	Control of population growth; animal controls; food controls; improved environmental legislation; food safety; pollution prevention
Complacency and apathy	Education—develop "we" mentality rather than "me" mentality
Poverty	Government support; international aid for vaccination programs, early diagnosis, and treatment; care for disadvantaged
War and mass refugee migration, famine, disasters	Government intervention; international aid
Aging of population	Support for prevention/intervention against controllable age-related health problems
Irrigation, deforestation, and reforestation projects that alter habitats of disease-carrying insects and animals	Improved techniques for conservation; responsible use of resources; policies and programs that protect environment
Increased human contact with tropical rainforests and other wilderness habitats that are reservoirs for insects and animals that harbor unknown infectious agents	Increased regulation to reduce human impact; more research to improve interactions between humans and environment

Sources: Author; information from Centers for Disease Control and Prevention, "Emerging Infectious Diseases: A Strategy for the 21st Century," 2006, www.cdc.gov/ncidod/emergplan.

Dengue and Dengue Hemorrhagic Fever

Transmitted by mosquitoes, **dengue** viruses are the most widespread mosquito-borne viruses in the world. Today, 2.5 billion people are at risk for dengue.[23] Dengue symptoms include flulike nausea, aches, and chronic fatigue and weakness. Each year, it is estimated that more than 100 million people are infected, and over 8,000 die.[24] A more serious form of the disease, **dengue hemorrhagic fever,** can kill children in 6 to 12 hours, as the virus causes capillaries to leak and spill fluid and blood into surrounding tissue. Dengue is on the rise in the United States, largely due to increased international travel.

West Nile Virus
Until 1999, few Americans had heard of *West Nile virus (WNV),* which like dengue is spread by the bite of an infected mosquito. Today, only Alaska and Hawaii remain disease free, and during 2006 over 3,800 cases of WNV were reported, with 119 deaths nationwide.

Most people who become infected with West Nile virus will have either mild symptoms or none at all. Rarely, West Nile virus infection can result in severe and sometimes fatal illness. Symptoms include fever, headache, and body aches, often with skin rash and swollen lymph glands, and a form of encephalitis (inflammation of the brain). There is no vaccine or specific treatment for WNV, but avoiding mosquito bites is the best way to prevent WNV. Strategies to prevent mosquito bites include using a bug repellent with DEET (diethyl tolumide) and wearing long-sleeved clothing and long pants when outdoors; staying indoors during dawn, dusk, and other peak mosquito feeding times; and removing any standing water sources around the home.

dengue   A disease transmitted by mosquitoes; causes flulike symptoms.

dengue hemorrhagic fever   A more serious form of dengue.

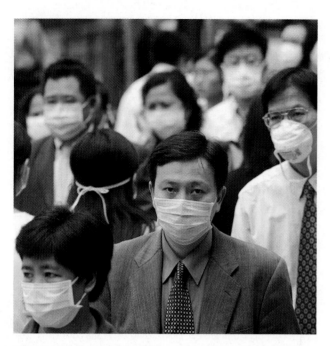

Emerging diseases such as SARS can cause communities to take widespread precautions to prevent transmission.

Ebola Hemorrhagic Fever (Ebola HF)
Ebola HF is a severe, often fatal, disease in humans and nonhuman primates (monkeys, gorillas, and chimpanzees). Although much about Ebola is unknown, researchers believe that the virus is zoonotic (animal-borne) and normally occurs in animal hosts that are native to the African continent.[25] The virus is spread via direct contact with blood and/or secretions and may be aerosol disseminated (airborne). With an incubation period of 2 to 21 days, the course of the disease is quick and characterized by fever, headache, joint and muscle aches, sore throat, and weakness, followed by diarrhea, vomiting, and stomach pain. A rash, red eyes, hiccups, and internal and external bleeding often occur in later phases.[26] Although there have been no known cases of human transmission in the United States, several outbreaks have occurred in various regions of Africa. Fortunately, Ebola is not as prevalent worldwide as dengue fever.

Severe Acute Respiratory Syndrome (SARS)
SARS is a viral respiratory illness that first emerged in Asia in 2003 and eventually infected over 8,000 people worldwide, with 774 deaths. SARS is caused by a coronavirus and is thought to be spread by close personal contact with those infected, though research on other methods of transmission is ongoing. Symptoms of SARS include high fever, body aches, headache, diarrhea, and a cough. Eventually, this cough can progress to a pneumonia-like upper respiratory illness.[27]

Escherichia coli O157:H7
E. coli O157:H7, as it is commonly referred to, is one of over 170 types of *E. coli* bacteria that can infect humans. Though most *E. coli* organisms are harmless and live in the intestines of healthy animals and humans, *E. coli* O157:H7 produces a lethal toxin and can cause severe illness or death.

E. coli O157:H7 can live in the intestines of healthy cattle and then contaminate food products at slaughterhouses. Eating ground beef that is rare or undercooked is a common way of becoming infected (see Chapter 8 for more information on safe food-handling practices). Drinking unpasteurized milk or juice and drinking or swimming in sewage-contaminated water or public pools can also cause infection via ingestion of feces that contain *E. coli*.

A symptom of infection is nonbloody diarrhea, usually two to eight days after exposure; however, asymptomatic cases have been noted. Children and older adults are particularly vulnerable to such serious side effects as kidney failure, as are persons whose immune systems have been weakened by other diseases.

Although *E. coli* organisms continue to pose threats to public health, strengthened regulations on the cooking of meat and regulation of chlorine levels in pools have helped. However, the 2006 *E. coli* outbreak linked to contaminated spinach has caused the USDA and others in the agriculture industry to review regulations and consider new safety measures.

Cholera
Cholera, an infectious disease transmitted through fecal contamination of food or water supplies, has been rare in the United States for most of a century. Recent epidemic outbreaks in the Western hemisphere (over 900,000 cases), however, have started to affect the United States. One theory of how cholera is introduced into distant regions of the world is that ships from endemic areas release contaminated bilge water into port towns, contaminating local shellfish.[28] Efforts to control cholera may be increasingly difficult as international travel and trade increase.

Listeriosis
Foods that are improperly cooked or that don't require cooking (such as luncheon meats) are particularly susceptible to carrying listeriosis, and it has proved fatal in many cases in recent years. Early symptoms begin with mild or low fever and progress to headache and inflammation of the brain. Those who are immunocompromised and pregnant women are at greatest risk. New regulations that require strict monitoring of food-processing plants should help reduce the risk of listeria infection.

Malaria
In the 1960s, after massive international efforts, malaria, a vectorborne disease transmitted by the *Anopheles* mosquito, seemed to be on the decline. However, today there has been a major resurgence of malaria outbreaks, particularly in Africa, Asia, and Latin America. Currently, the malaria prevention effort is focused on personal protection against bites rather than elimination of mosquitoes.

Bioterrorism: The New Global Threat

The idea of using infectious microorganisms as weapons is not new. In fact, during the English wars with American Indians, blankets impregnated with scabs from smallpox patients were traded to Native Americans in hopes of causing disease.[29]

The threat of delivering a lethal load of anthrax or other deadly microorganisms in the warheads of missiles or by a single person is a topic of much discussion among today's world leaders, particularly after the instances of anthrax being delivered via the mail following the September 11, 2001, terrorist attacks. For more on biological threats, see the New Horizons in Health box on bioterrorism in Chapter 4.

Sexually Transmitted Infections

Sexually transmitted infections (STIs) have been with us since our earliest recorded days on Earth. Today, there are more than 20 known types of STIs. Once referred to as "venereal diseases" and then "sexually transmitted diseases," the most current terminology is more reflective of the number and types of these communicable diseases. More virulent strains and more antibiotic-resistant forms spell trouble for at-risk populations in the days ahead.

STIs affect men and women of all backgrounds and socioeconomic levels. In the United States alone, an estimated 15.3 million new cases of STIs are reported each year. Additional facts to note include the following:

- More than 65 million people are currently living with an incurable STI.[30]
- Two-thirds of all STIs occur in people 25 years of age or younger.[31]
- One in four new STI infections occurs in teenagers.[32]
- One in five Americans has genital herpes, with 500,000 new cases each year.[33]

STIs disproportionately affect women, minorities, and infants. In addition, STIs are most prevalent in teens and young adults.[34] In 2003, approximately 53 percent of high school students had engaged in sexual intercourse. Of these 53 percent, 14 percent had four or more sex partners and 37 percent did not use a condom in their most recent sexual encounter.[35]

Early symptoms of an STI are often mild and unrecognizable (Figure 17.6). Left untreated, some of these infections can have grave consequences, such as sterility, blindness, central nervous system destruction, disfigurement, and even death. Infants born to mothers carrying the organisms for these infections are at risk for a variety of health problems.

As with many communicable diseases, much of the pain, suffering, and anguish associated with STIs can be eliminated

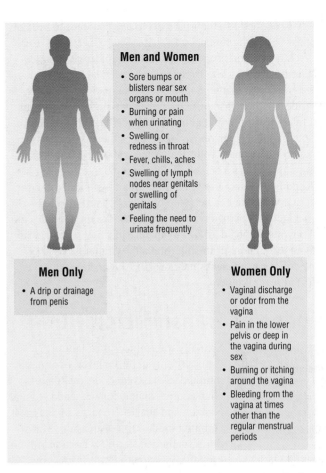

FIGURE 17.6 Signs or Symptoms of Sexually Transmitted Infections (STIs)
In their early stages, many STIs may be asymptomatic or have such mild symptoms that they are easy to overlook.

through education, responsible action, simple preventive strategies, and prompt treatment. STIs can happen to anyone, but they won't if you take appropriate precautions when you decide to engage in a sexual relationship.

Possible Causes: What's Your Risk?

Several reasons have been proposed to explain the present high rates of STIs. The first relates to the moral and social stigma associated with these infections. Shame and embarrassment often keep infected people from seeking treatment. Unfortunately, these people usually continue to be sexually active, thereby infecting unsuspecting partners. People who are uncomfortable discussing sexual issues may also be less

sexually transmitted infections (STIs) Infectious diseases transmitted via some form of intimate, usually sexual, contact.

likely to use and ask their partners to use condoms to protect against STIs and pregnancy.

Another reason proposed for the STI epidemic is our casual attitude about sex. Bombarded by media hype that glamorizes easy sex, many people take sexual partners without considering the consequences. Others are pressured into sexual relationships they don't really want. Generally, the more sexual partners a person has, the greater the risk for contracting an STI. Evaluate your own attitude about STIs by completing the Assess Yourself box on page 532.

Ignorance—about the infections, their symptoms, and the fact that someone can be symptom free but still infected—is also a factor. A person who is infected but asymptomatic can unknowingly spread an STI to an unsuspecting partner, who may in turn ignore or misinterpret any symptoms. By the time either partner seeks medical help, he or she may have infected several others.

Modes of Transmission

| Can I get a sexually transmitted infection from "outercourse"? |

Sexually transmitted infections are generally spread through some form of intimate sexual contact. Sexual intercourse, oral–genital contact, hand–genital contact, and anal intercourse are the most common modes of transmission. More rarely, pathogens for STIs are transmitted mouth to mouth or through contact with fluids from body sores. Although each STI is a different infection caused by a different pathogen, all STI pathogens prefer dark, moist places, especially the mucous membranes lining the reproductive organs. Most of them are susceptible to light, excess heat, cold, and dryness, and many die quickly on exposure to air. (The toilet seat is not a likely breeding ground for most bacterial or viral STIs!) Although most STIs are passed on by sexual contact, other kinds of close contact, such as sleeping on sheets used by someone who has pubic lice, may also infect you.

Like other communicable infections, STIs have both pathogen-specific incubation periods and periods of time during which transmission is most likely, called periods of communicability.

Chlamydia

Chlamydia, a disease that often presents no symptoms, tops the list of the most commonly reported infections in the

---

chlamydia   Bacterially caused STI of the urogenital tract.

conjunctivitis   Serious inflammation of the eye caused by any number of pathogens or irritants; can be caused by STIs such as chlamydia.

pelvic inflammatory disease (PID)   Term used to describe various infections of the female reproductive tract.

United States. Chlamydia infects about 2.8 million people annually in the United States, the majority of them women.[36] Public health officials believe that the actual number of cases is probably higher because these figures represent only those cases reported. College students account for over 10 percent of infections, and these numbers seem to be increasing yearly.

In males, early symptoms may include painful and difficult urination, frequent urination, and a watery, puslike discharge from the penis. Symptoms in females may include a yellowish discharge, spotting between periods, and occasional spotting after intercourse. However, many chlamydia victims display no symptoms and therefore do not seek help until the disease has done secondary damage. Females are especially likely to be asymptomatic; over 70 percent do not realize they have the disease until secondary damage occurs.

The secondary damage resulting from chlamydia is serious in both genders. Men can suffer injury to the prostate gland, seminal vesicles, and bulbourethral glands, as well as arthritis-like symptoms and damage to the blood vessels and heart. In women, chlamydia-related inflammation can injure the cervix or uterine tubes, causing sterility, and damage the inner pelvic structure, leading to pelvic inflammatory disease (PID). If an infected woman becomes pregnant, she has a high risk for miscarriage and stillbirth. Chlamydia may also be responsible for one type of **conjunctivitis,** an eye infection that affects not only adults but also infants, who can contract the disease from an infected mother during delivery. Untreated conjunctivitis can cause blindness.

If detected early, chlamydia is easily treatable with antibiotics such as tetracycline, doxycycline, or erythromycin. In most cases, treatment is successfully completed in two to three weeks. Unfortunately, chlamydia tests are not a routine part of many health clinics' testing procedures. Usually a person must specifically request a chlamydia check.

Pelvic Inflammatory Disease

Pelvic inflammatory disease (PID) is a term used to describe a number of infections of the uterus, uterine tubes, and ovaries. Although PID often results from an untreated sexually transmitted infection, especially chlamydia or gonorrhea, it is not actually an STI. Several nonsexual factors increase the risk of PID, particularly excessive vaginal douching, cigarette smoking, and substance abuse.

Symptoms of PID vary but generally include lower abdominal pain, fever, unusual vaginal discharge, painful intercourse, painful urination, and irregular menstrual bleeding. Major consequences of untreated PID are infertility, ectopic pregnancy, chronic pelvic pain, and recurrent upper genital infections. Risk factors include young age at first sexual intercourse, multiple sex partners, high frequency of sexual intercourse, and change of sexual partners within the past 30 days. Regular gynecological examinations and early treatment for STI symptoms reduce risk.

Gonorrhea

Gonorrhea is one of the most common STIs in the United States, surpassed only by chlamydia in number of cases. The Centers for Disease Control (CDC) estimates that there are over 700,000 cases per year, plus numbers that go unreported.[37] Health economists estimate that the annual cost of gonorrhea and its complications is over $1.1 billion.[38] Caused by the bacterial pathogen *Neisseria gonorrhoeae,* this infection primarily infects the linings of the urethra, genital tract, pharynx, and rectum. It may spread to the eyes or other body regions via the hands or body fluids, typically during vaginal, oral, or anal sex. Most victims are males between the ages of 20 and 24, with sexually active females between the ages of 15 and 19 also at high risk.[39]

In males, a typical symptom is a white, milky discharge from the penis accompanied by painful, burning urination two to nine days after contact. This is usually enough to send most men to the physician for treatment. However, about 20 percent of all males with gonorrhea are asymptomatic.

In females, the situation is just the opposite: only 20 percent experience any discharge, and few develop a burning sensation upon urinating until much later in the course of the infection (if ever). The organism can remain in the woman's vagina, cervix, uterus, or uterine tubes for long periods with no apparent symptoms other than an occasional slight fever. Thus a woman can be unaware that she has been infected and that she is infecting her sexual partners.

If the infection is detected early, an antibiotic regimen is generally effective within a short period of time. If the infection goes undetected in a woman, it can spread throughout the urogenital tract to the uterine tubes and ovaries, causing sterility, or, at the very least, severe inflammation and PID. The bacteria can also spread up the reproductive tract or, more rarely, through the blood and infect the joints, heart valves, or brain. If an infected woman becomes pregnant, the infection can cause conjunctivitis in her infant. To prevent this, physicians routinely administer silver nitrate or penicillin preparations to the eyes of newborn babies.

In a man, untreated gonorrhea may spread to the prostate, testicles, urinary tract, kidney, and bladder. Blockage of the ductus deferentia due to scar tissue formation may cause sterility. In some cases, the penis develops a painful curvature during erection.

Syphilis

Syphilis is also caused by a bacterial organism, the spirochete known as *Treponema pallidum.* Because it is extremely delicate and dies readily upon exposure to air, dryness, or cold, the organism is generally transferred only through direct sexual contact. Typically, this means contact between sexual organs during intercourse; but, in rare instances, the organism enters the body through a break in the skin, through deep kissing in which body fluids are exchanged, or through some other transmission of body fluids.

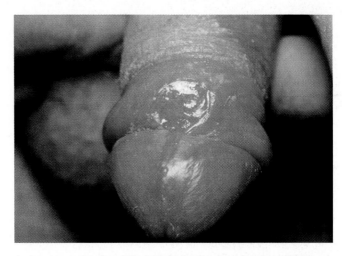

A chancre on the site of the initial infection is a symptom of primary syphilis.

Syphilis is called the "great imitator" because its symptoms resemble those of several other infections. Left untreated, syphilis generally progresses through several distinct stages. It should be noted, however, that some people experience no symptoms at all.

Primary Syphilis The first stage of syphilis, particularly for males, is often characterized by the development of a **chancre** (pronounced "shank-er"), a sore located most frequently at the site of initial infection (see photo above). Although painless, the dime-sized chancre is oozing with bacteria, ready to infect an unsuspecting partner. Usually it appears three to four weeks after contact.

In males, the site of the chancre tends to be the penis or scrotum because this is where the organism first enters the body. But, if the infection was contracted through oral sex, the sore can appear in the mouth, throat, or other first contact area. In females, the site of infection is often internal, on the vaginal wall or high on the cervix. Because the chancre is not readily apparent in females, the likelihood of detection is not great. In both males and females, the chancre will completely disappear in three to six weeks.

Secondary Syphilis A month to a year after the chancre disappears, secondary symptoms may appear, including a rash or white patches on the skin or on the mucous

(Text continues on page 534)

gonorrhea   Second most common STD in the United States; if untreated, may cause sterility.

syphilis   One of the most widespread STIs; characterized by distinct phases and potentially serious results.

chancre   Sore often found at the site of syphilis infection.

ASSESS yourself

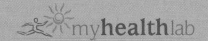

STI ATTITUDE AND BELIEF SCALE

**Fill out this assessment online at
www.aw-bc.com/myhealthlab or
www.aw-bc.com/donatelle.**

The following quiz will help you evaluate whether your beliefs and attitudes about STIs lead you to behaviors that increase your risk of infection. Indicate that you believe the following items are true or false by checking the box under True or False. Then consult the answer key that follows.

	True	False
1. You can usually tell whether someone is infected with an STI, especially HIV infection.	❑	❑
2. Chances are that if you haven't caught an STI by now, you probably have a natural immunity and won't get infected in the future.	❑	❑
3. A person who is successfully treated for an STI needn't worry about getting it again.	❑	❑
4. So long as you keep yourself fit and healthy, you needn't worry about STIs.	❑	❑
5. The best way for sexually active people to protect themselves from STIs is to practice safer sex.	❑	❑
6. The only way to catch an STI is to have sex with someone who has one.	❑	❑
7. Talking about STIs with a partner is so embarrassing that it's better not to raise the subject and instead hope the other person will.	❑	❑
8. STIs are mostly a problem for people who have numerous sex partners.	❑	❑
9. You don't need to worry about contracting an STI so long as you wash yourself thoroughly with soap and hot water immediately after sex.	❑	❑
10. You don't need to worry about AIDS if no one you know has ever come down with it.	❑	❑
11. When it comes to STIs, it's all in the cards. Either you're lucky or you're not.	❑	❑
12. The time to worry about STIs is when you come down with one.	❑	❑
13. As long as you avoid risky sexual practices, such as anal intercourse, you're pretty safe from STIs.	❑	❑
14. The time to talk about safer sex is before any sexual contact occurs.	❑	❑
15. A person needn't be concerned about an STI if the symptoms clear up on their own in a few weeks.	❑	❑

Scoring Key

1. *False.* While some STIs have telltale signs, such as the appearance of sores or blisters on the genitals or disagreeable genital odors, others do not. Several STIs, such as chlamydia, gonorrhea (especially in women), internal genital warts, and even HIV infection in its early stages, cause few if any obvious signs or symptoms. You often cannot tell whether your partner is infected with an STI. Many of the nicest-looking and most well-groomed people carry STIs, often unknowingly. The only way to know whether a person is infected with HIV is by an HIV-antibody test.

2. *False.* If you practice unprotected sex and have not contracted an STI to this point, count your blessings. The thing about good luck is that it eventually runs out.

3. *False.* Sorry. Successful treatment does not render immunity against reinfection. You still need to take precautions to avoid reinfection, even if you have had an STI in the past and were successfully treated. If you answered true to this item, you're not alone. About one in five college students polled in a recent survey of more than 5,500 college

students across Canada believed that a person who gets an STI cannot get it again.

4. *False.* Even people in prime physical condition can be felled by the tiniest of microbes that cause STIs. Physical fitness is no protection against these microscopic invaders.

5. *True.* If you are sexually active, practicing safer sex is the best protection against contracting an STI.

6. *False.* STIs can also be transmitted through nonsexual means, such as by sharing contaminated needles or, in some cases, through contact with disease-causing organisms on towels and bedsheets or even toilet seats.

7. *False.* Because of the social stigma attached to STIs, it's understandable that you may feel embarrassed about raising the subject with your partner. But don't let embarrassment prevent you from taking steps to protect your own and your partner's welfare.

8. *False.* Though it stands to reason that people who are sexually active with numerous partners have a greater chance that one of their sexual partners will carry an STI, all it

takes is one infected partner to pass along an STI to you, even if he or she is the only partner you've had or even if the two of you had sex only once. STIs are a potential problem for anyone who is sexually active.

9. *False.* Though washing your genitals immediately after sex may have some limited protective value, it is no substitute for practicing safer sex.

10. *False.* You can never know whether you may be the first among your friends and acquaintances to become infected. Moreover, symptoms of HIV infection may not appear for years after initial infection with the virus, so you may have sexual contacts with people who are infected but don't know it and who are capable of passing along the virus to you. You in turn may then pass it along to others, whether or not you are aware of any symptoms.

11. *False.* Nonsense. While luck may play a part in determining whether you have sexual contact with an infected partner, you can significantly reduce your risk of contracting an STI.

12. *False.* The time to start thinking about STIs (thinking helps, but worrying only makes you more anxious than you need be) is now, not after you have contracted an infection. Some STIs, like herpes and AIDS, cannot be cured. The only real protection you have against them is prevention.

13. *False.* Any sexual contact between the genitals, or between the genitals and the anus, or between the mouth and genitals, is risky if one of the partners is infected with an STI.

14. *True.* Unfortunately, too many couples wait until they have commenced sexual relations to have "a talk." By then it may already be too late to prevent the transmission of an STI. The time to talk is before any intimate sexual contact occurs.

15. *False.* Several STIs, notably syphilis, HIV infection, and herpes, may produce initial symptoms that clear up in a few weeks. But whereas the early symptoms may subside, the infection is still at work within the body and requires medical attention. Also, as noted previously, the infected person is capable of passing along the infection to others, regardless of whether noticeable symptoms were ever present.

Interpreting Your Score

First, add up the number of items you got right. The higher your score, the lower your risk. The lower your score, the greater your risk. A score of 13 correct or better may indicate that your attitudes toward STIs would probably decrease your risk of contracting them. Yet even one wrong response on this test may increase your risk of contracting an STI. You should also recognize that attitudes have little effect on behavior unless they are carried into action. Knowledge alone isn't sufficient to protect yourself from STIs. You need to ask yourself how you are going to put knowledge into action by changing your behavior to reduce your chances of contracting an STI.

Source: From J. S. Nevid with F. Gotfried, *Choices: Sex in the Age of STDs,* 10–13. © Copyright 1995 by Allyn & Bacon. Reprinted by permission.

MAKE it happen!

ASSESSMENT: The Assess Yourself activity gave you the chance to consider your beliefs and attitudes about STIs, and possible risks you may be facing. Now that you have considered these results, you can begin to change behaviors that may be putting you at risk.

MAKING A CHANGE: In order to change your behavior, you need to develop a plan. Follow these steps below and complete your Behavior Change Contract to take action.

1. Evaluate your behavior and identify patterns and specific things you are doing. What can you change now? What can you change in the near future?

2. Select one pattern of behavior that you want to change.

3. Fill out the Behavior Change Contract found at the front of your book. It should include your long-term goal for change, your short-term goals, the rewards you'll give yourself for reaching these goals, potential obstacles along the way, and strategies for overcoming these obstacles. For each goal, list the small steps and specific actions that you will take.

4. Chart your progress in a journal. At the end of a week, consider how successful you were in following your plan. What helped you be successful? What made change more difficult? What will you do differently next week?

(continued)

5. Revise your plan as needed: Are the short-term goals attainable? Are the rewards satisfying?

ONE STUDENT'S PLAN: Carlos had never thought that he was at risk for an STI. He only dated one woman at a time, and he had never had an STI himself. After he reviewed his answers to the self-assessment, however, he saw that there were several ways in which he was putting himself at risk.

He had thought that he would be able to tell whether someone was infected with an STI but question 1's answer described how, especially among women, there are few if any obvious signs or symptoms of some STIs. Carlos also believed that he was not at risk because he dated only one woman at a time, but the answer to question 8 pointed out that a person can pass on an STI that he or she contracted from a previous sex partner. Carlos decided it was time to take responsibility for his sexual activity. He had been on three dates with Sherry and felt things were progressing toward a

more intimate stage; he wanted to be sure that they discussed STIs before they put themselves at risk.

Carlos was nervous when he thought about talking to Sherry, so he wrote out a few ideas of ways to bring up the subject. This made him more confident that he would be able to talk honestly with Sherry. He also made sure that he had a supply of condoms, so there wouldn't be any reason not to practice safer sex. During their next date, Carlos asked Sherry if they could have a serious conversation about the next step. When he told her that he wanted to talk about STIs, she told him that she was relieved that he had brought up the subject. She knew that she was healthy and hadn't been sure how to find out his status. Carlos was relieved that Sherry was as concerned about the issue as he was, and they were both glad that embarrassment had not prevented them from having this conversation.

---

membranes of the mouth, throat, or genitals. Hair loss may occur, lymph nodes may enlarge, and the victim may develop a slight fever or headache. In rare cases, sores develop around the mouth or genitals. As during the active chancre phase, these sores contain infectious bacteria, and contact with them can spread the infection. In a few cases, there may be arthritic pain in the joints. Because symptoms vary so much and appear so much later than the sexual contact that caused them, the victim seldom connects the two. The infection thus often goes undetected even at this second stage. Symptoms may persist for a few weeks or months and then disappear, leaving the person thinking that all is well.

Latent Syphilis After the secondary stage, the syphilis spirochetes begin to invade body organs. After this period, the infection is rarely transmitted to others, except during pregnancy, when it can be passed to the fetus. The child will then be born with *congenital syphilis,* which can cause death or severe birth defects such as blindness, deafness, or disfigurement. Because in most cases the fetus does not become infected until after the first trimester, treatment of the mother during this time will usually prevent infection of the fetus. One way that some states protect against congenital syphilis

is by requiring prospective marriage partners to be tested for syphilis prior to obtaining a marriage license.

Late Syphilis Years after syphilis has entered the body, its effects become all too evident. Late-stage syphilis indications include heart damage, central nervous system damage, blindness, deafness, paralysis, premature senility, and, ultimately, dementia.

Treatment for Syphilis Because the organism is bacterial, it is treated with antibiotics, usually penicillin, benzathine penicillin G, or doxycycline. The major obstacles to treatment are misdiagnosis of this "imitator" infection and lack of access to health care.

Pubic Lice

Pubic lice, often called "crabs," are small parasites that are usually transmitted during sexual contact. More annoying than dangerous, they move easily from partner to partner during sex. They have an affinity for pubic hair, attaching themselves to the base of these hairs, where they deposit their eggs (nits). One to two weeks later, these nits develop into adults that lay eggs and migrate to other body parts, thus perpetuating the cycle.

Treatment includes washing clothing, furniture, and linens that may harbor the eggs. It usually takes two to three weeks to kill all larval forms. Although sexual contact is the most common mode of transmission, you can "catch" pubic lice

pubic lice (crabs) Parasites that can inhabit various body areas, especially the genitals.

from lying on sheets that an infected person has slept on. Sleeping in hotel and dormitory rooms in which sheets are not washed regularly or sitting on toilet seats where the nits or larvae have been dropped and lie in wait for a new carrier increases your risk.

Genital Warts (Human Papillomavirus)

Genital warts (also known as venereal warts or condylomas) are caused by a small group of viruses known as **human papillomavirus (HPV).** A person becomes infected when HPV penetrates the skin and mucous membranes of the genitals or anus through sexual contact. HPV is among the most common forms of STI, infecting over 5.5 million Americans each year. The virus appears to be relatively easy to catch. The typical incubation period is from six to eight weeks after contact. Many people have no symptoms, particularly if the warts are located inside the reproductive tract. Others may develop a series of itchy bumps on the genitals, ranging in size from small pinheads to large cauliflower-like growths. On dry skin (such as the shaft of the penis), the warts are commonly small, hard, and yellowish gray, resembling warts that appear on other parts of the body.

Genital warts are of two different types: (1) *full-blown genital warts* that are noticeable as tiny bumps or growths, and (2) the much more prevalent *flat warts* that are not usually visible to the naked eye. In females, these flat warts are often first detected by a doctor during a routine Pap test. Abnormal Pap results may prompt the physician to perform a procedure in which a vinegar-like solution is applied to the insides of the vaginal walls and cervix to bleach potential warts. The area is then viewed through a special magnifying instrument known as a colposcope. A photographic procedure known as a cerviscope can also detect genital warts. During a cerviscope, vinegar is applied to the vaginal and cervical areas, and an image of the area is projected onto a screen for a specialist to diagnose. This technique is relatively inexpensive and is believed to be five times more sensitive than standard colposcopy. An even newer method is the *DNA probe,* a technique that identifies the genetic makeup of possible warts.

Whereas women must see a physician for a diagnosis, a male can check for suspicious lesions by wrapping his penis in vinegar-soaked gauze or cloth, waiting for five minutes, and then checking for white bleached areas indicative of flat warts. However, genital warts of the rectum must be diagnosed by a physician.

Risks of Genital Warts

Genital warts pose a significant risk for cervical cancer. Genital warts may lead to *dysplasia,* or changes in cells that may lead to a precancerous condition. Exactly how HPV infection leads to cervical cancer is uncertain. It is known that within five years after infection, 30 percent of all HPV cases will progress to the precancerous stage. Of those cases that become precancerous

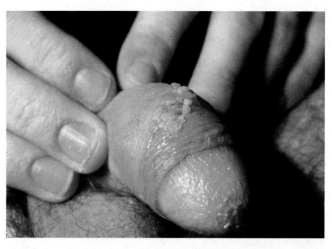

Genital warts are caused by the human papillomavirus and can be either full-blown or flat.

and are left untreated, 70 percent will eventually result in actual cervical cancer. In addition, genital warts may pose a threat to a pregnant woman's unborn fetus if the fetus is exposed to the virus during birth. Cesarean deliveries may be considered in serious cases.

New research has also implicated HPV as a possible risk factor for coronary artery disease. It is hypothesized that HPV causes an inflammatory response in the artery walls, which makes cholesterol and plaque build up. (See Chapter 15.)

Treatment for Genital Warts Treatment for genital warts may take several forms:

1. Warts may be painted with a medication called *podophyllin* during a visit to the doctor's office. The podophyllin is washed off after about four hours, and a few days later the warts begin to dry up and fall off. Sometimes more than one trip to the doctor is necessary. This procedure is relatively painless, but there are potential side effects. Because podophyllin may be absorbed through the skin, pregnant women should not use it. Some patients may experience skin reactions.

2. Warts may be removed by *cryosurgery,* a procedure in which an instrument treated with liquid nitrogen is held to the affected area, freezing the tissue. Within a few days, the warts fall off.

3. Depending on size and location, some warts are removed by *simple excision.*

genital warts Warts that appear in the genital area or the anus; caused by the human papillomavirus (HPV).

human papillomavirus (HPV) A small group of viruses that cause genital warts.

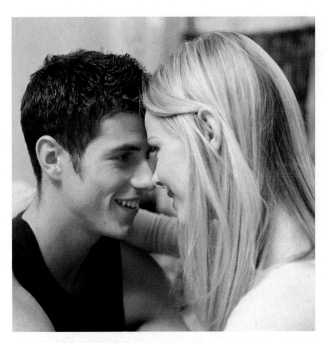

You can't tell if someone has an STI just by looking at them. Being open and honest with your partners, and expecting the same, is an important part of prevention.

4. For larger warts, *laser surgery* is often used. This is a major procedure that usually requires general anesthesia.

5. Creams containing *5-fluorouracil* (an anticancer drug) are being used to prevent further precancerous cell development.

6. For external warts, injections of *interferon* are sometimes given to keep the virus from spreading to healthy tissue.

New Hope for Prevention: HPV Vaccination

In June 2006 a new vaccine was approved by the FDA to prevent HPV. The vaccine protects against the four types of HPV that lead to 70 percent of cervical cancers and 90 percent of genital warts. The vaccine is meant primarily for women aged 9 to 26, and is administered via a series of shots over a 6-month period.[40]

Candidiasis (Moniliasis)

Unlike many STIs, which are caused by pathogens that come from outside the body, the yeastlike fungus caused by the *Candida albicans* organism normally inhabits the vaginal

---

candidiasis (yeast infection, moniliasis) Yeastlike fungal disease often triggered sexually.

vaginitis Set of symptoms characterized by vaginal itching, swelling, and burning.

trichomoniasis Protozoan infection characterized by foamy, yellowish discharge and unpleasant odor.

---

tract in most women. Only under certain conditions, in which the normal chemical balance of the vagina is disturbed, will these organisms multiply to abnormal quantities and begin to cause problems.

Symptoms of **candidiasis** include severe vaginal itching and burning of the vagina and vulva. A white, cheesy discharge and swelling of the vulva may also occur. These symptoms are often collectively called **vaginitis,** which means an inflammation of the vagina. When this microbe infects the mouth, whitish patches form, and the condition is referred to as *thrush*. This monilial infection also occurs in males and is easily transmitted between sexual partners.

Antifungal drugs applied on the surface or by suppository usually cure it in just a few days. For approximately one out of ten women, however, nothing seems to work, and the infection returns again and again. Symptoms can be aggravated by contact of the vagina with scented soaps, douches, perfumed toilet paper, chlorinated water, and spermicides. Tight-fitting jeans and pantyhose can provide the combination of moisture and irritant the organism thrives on.

Trichomoniasis

Unlike many STIs, **trichomoniasis** is caused by a protozoan. Although as many as half of the men and women in the United States may carry this organism, most remain free of symptoms until their bodily defenses are weakened. Both men and women may transmit the infection, but women are the more likely candidates for infection. Symptoms include a foamy, yellowish, unpleasant-smelling discharge accompanied by a burning sensation, itching, and painful urination. These symptoms are most likely to occur during or shortly after menstruation, but they can appear at any time or be absent altogether.

Although usually transmitted by sexual contact, the "trich" organism can also be spread by toilet seats, wet towels, or other items that have discharged fluids on them. You can also contract trichomoniasis by sitting naked on the locker room bench at your local health spa or gym. Treatment includes oral metronidazole, usually given to both sexual partners to avoid the possible "ping-pong" effect of repeated cross-infection so typical of STIs.

General Urinary Tract Infections (UTIs)

Although *general urinary tract infections (UTIs)* can be caused by various factors, particularly the insertion of catheters and other devices during hospitalization, some forms are sexually transmitted. Any time invading organisms enter the genital area, they can travel up the urethra and enter the bladder. Similarly, organisms normally living in the rectum, urethra, or bladder may travel to the sexual organs and eventually be transmitted to another person.

You can also get a UTI through autoinoculation, often during the simple task of wiping yourself after defecating. Wiping from the anus forward can transmit organisms found in feces to the vaginal opening or the urethra. Contact between the hands and the urethra and between the urethra and other objects are also common means of autoinoculation. Women, with their shorter urethras, are more likely to contract UTIs. Handwashing with soap and water prior to sexual intimacy, foreplay, and so on, is recommended.

Treatment depends on the nature and type of pathogen. Visiting with your doctor and obtaining medications from a pharmacy is the best course of action.

Herpes

Herpes is a general term for a family of infections characterized by sores or eruptions on the skin. Caused by herpesviruses, the herpes family of diseases is not transmitted

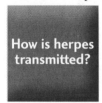
How is herpes transmitted?

exclusively by sexual contact. Kissing or sharing eating utensils can also exchange saliva and transmit the infection. Herpes infections range from mildly uncomfortable to extremely serious. **Genital herpes** is an infection caused by the herpes simplex virus (HSV), and affects over 45 million Americans aged 12 and older.[41]

There are two types of herpes simplex virus (HSV). Both herpes simplex types 1 and 2 can infect any area of the body, producing lesions (sores) in and around the vaginal area, on the penis, around the anal opening, buttocks, or thighs, and around the mouth. For example, you may have a type 1 infection on your lip and transmit the HSV-1 organism to your partner's genitals during oral sex. Practically speaking, the resulting symptoms would be virtually the same as if you had transmitted the type 2 virus. Occasionally, sores appear on other parts of the body. HSV remains in certain nerve cells for life and can flare up, or cause symptoms, when the body's ability to maintain itself is weakened.[42]

The *prodromal* (precursor) phase of the infection is characterized by a burning sensation and redness at the site of infection. During this time prescription medicines such as acyclovir and over-the-counter medications such as Abreva will often keep the disease from spreading. However, this phase of the disease is quickly followed by the second phase, in which a blister filled with a clear fluid containing the virus forms. If you pick at this blister or otherwise touch the site and spread this fluid with fingers, lipstick, lip balm, or other products, you can autoinoculate other body parts. Particularly dangerous is the possibility of spreading the infection to your eyes, for a herpes lesion on the eye can cause blindness.

Over a period of days, the unsightly blister will crust over, dry up, and disappear, and the virus will travel to the base of an affected nerve supplying the area and become dormant. Only when the victim becomes overly stressed, when diet and sleep are inadequate, when the immune system is overworked, or when excessive exposure to sunlight or other stressors occurs will the virus become reactivated (at the same site every time) and begin the blistering cycle all over again. These sores cast off (shed) viruses that can be highly infectious.

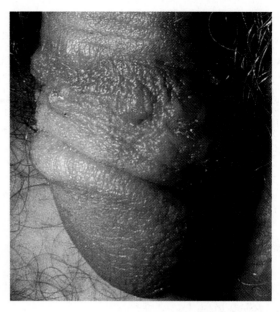
Genital herpes is a highly contagious and incurable STI. It is characterized by recurring cycles of painful blisters on the genitalia.

However, it is important to note that a herpes site can shed the virus even when no overt sore is present, particularly during the interval between the earliest symptoms and blistering. People may get genital herpes by having sexual contact with others who don't know they are infected or who are having outbreaks of herpes without any sores. A person with genital herpes can also infect a sexual partner during oral sex. The virus is spread only rarely, if at all, by touching objects such as a toilet seat or hot tub seat.[43]

Genital herpes is especially serious in pregnant women because the baby can be infected as it passes through the vagina during birth. Many physicians recommend cesarean deliveries for infected women. Additionally, women with a history of genital herpes appear to have a greater risk of developing cervical cancer.

Although there is no cure for herpes at present, certain drugs can reduce symptoms. Unfortunately, they seem to work only if the infection is confirmed during the first few hours after contact. As you may guess, this is rather rare. The effectiveness of other treatments, such as L-lysine, is largely unsubstantiated. Newer over-the-counter medications seem to be moderately effective in reducing the severity of symptoms. Although lip balms and cold-sore medications may provide temporary anesthetic relief, remember that rubbing anything on a herpes blister can spread herpes-laden fluids to other body parts. Table 17.4 on page 538 details how you can prevent contracting herpes.

genital herpes STI caused by the herpes simplex virus.

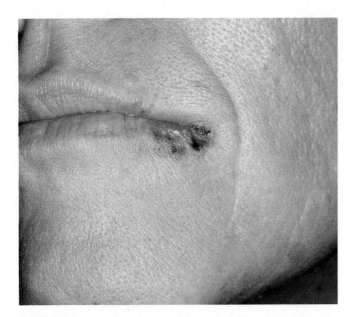

Oral herpes, caused by the same virus as genital herpes, is extremely contagious, and can cause painful sores and blisters around the mouth.

HIV/AIDS

Acquired immunodeficiency syndrome (AIDS) is a significant global health threat. Since 1981, when AIDS was first recognized, over 60 million people in the world have become infected with **human immunodeficiency virus (HIV),** the virus that causes AIDS. Today, an estimated 38.6 billion people are living with HIV or AIDS and an estimated 4.1 million new cases were diagnosed worldwide in 2005.[44] Women are becoming increasingly affected by the virus, accounting for approximately 50 percent of cases.[45] In the United States, as of 2002, over 859,000 men, women, and children with AIDS have been reported to the Centers for Disease Control and Prevention (CDC), and at least 501,669 have died.[46] The CDC estimates that at least 40,000 new infections occur each year in the United States. See the Health in a Diverse World box for more on the global impact of HIV/AIDS.

The Onset of AIDS

Researchers believe that the AIDS virus may actually have been present in the United States since the early 1950s, although medical and government officials did not note problems related to the disease until the spring of 1981. Suddenly, federal officials began to receive an increasing number of

acquired immunodeficiency syndrome (AIDS)
Extremely virulent sexually transmitted disease that renders the immune system inoperative.

human immunodeficiency virus (HIV)   The slow-acting virus that causes AIDS.

requests for an experimental drug used to treat a rare disease called *Pneumocystis carinii pneumonia (PCP)*. Caused by a protozoan, PCP appeared to be affecting significant numbers of previously healthy young men in New York and California.

At about the same time, increasing numbers of men in California were being diagnosed with a rare form of cancer known as *Kaposi's sarcoma*. These two groups of patients—those with PCP and those with Kaposi's sarcoma—tended to share many characteristics. They were typically white and homosexual, came from similar geographical regions, used specific types of drugs, and had generalized lymphadenopathy (chronic swelling of the lymph nodes) and general malfunctioning of the immune system. Because of the last problem, many of these people developed several diseases at the same time, making diagnosis of one underlying cause extremely difficult.

For many months, epidemiologists investigated possible causes of this disease, including the types of drugs used by many gay men and the water supplies in their communities. In 1984, two researchers, Robert C. Gallo at the National Cancer Institute in the United States and Luc Montagnier at the Pasteur Institute in Paris, independently isolated the retrovirus (a type of slow-acting virus) that causes AIDS. Initially called the human T cell lymphotropic virus type III (HTLV-III) by most American researchers, this pathogen is today generally referred to as the human immunodeficiency virus (HIV).

THE STAGGERING TOLL OF HIV/AIDS IN THE GLOBAL COMMUNITY

Although the rates of HIV/AIDS may be slowing in the United States, the disease has had an increasingly devastating impact on other regions of the world. Here are some facts about this global epidemic.

- Sub-Saharan Africa remains the most affected region in the world. Two-thirds of all people living with HIV are in sub-Saharan Africa, where 24.5 million people were living with HIV in 2005.
- Growing epidemics are under way in Eastern Europe and Central Asia, where

220,000 people were newly infected with HIV in 2005.

- Worldwide, less than one in five people at risk of becoming infected with HIV have access to basic prevention services. Across the world, only one in eight people who want to be tested are currently able to do so.
- Each day, 1,800 children worldwide become infected with HIV, the vast majority of them newborns. In 2005, 9 percent of pregnant women in low- and middle-income countries were of-

fered services to prevent transmission to their newborns.

- According to the latest UNAIDS/WHO "3 by 5" progress report, approximately 1.3 million people living with HIV are receiving ARV therapy in low-and middle-income countries—this means that 20 percent of those in need of treatment are now receiving it.

Source: The Body, The Complete HIV/AIDS Resource, "Global Facts and Figures," 2006, www.thebody.com/unaids/global_facts.html.

Although during the early days of the epidemic it appeared that HIV infected only homosexuals, it quickly became apparent that the disease was not confined to groups of people, but rather was related to high-risk behaviors such as unprotected sexual intercourse and sharing needles.

A Shifting Epidemic

Initially, people with HIV were diagnosed as having AIDS only when they developed blood infections, the cancer known as Kaposi's sarcoma, or any of 21 other indicator diseases, most of which were common in male AIDS patients. The CDC has expanded the indicator list to include pulmonary tuberculosis, recurrent pneumonia, and invasive cervical cancer. Perhaps the most significant new indicator is a drop in the level of the body's master immune cells, called CD4s, to 200 per cubic millimeter (one-fifth the level in a healthy person).

AIDS cases have been reported state by state throughout the United States since the early 1980s as a means of tracking the disease. Though the numbers of actual reported cases have always been suspect, improved reporting and surveillance methods have helped increase accuracy. Today, the CDC recommends that all states report HIV infections as well as AIDS. Because of medical advances in treatment and increasing numbers of HIV-infected persons who do not progress to AIDS, it is believed that AIDS incidence statistics may not provide a true picture of the epidemic, the long-term costs of treating HIV-infected individuals, and other key information. HIV incidence data also provide a better picture of infection trends. Currently, most states mandate that those who test positive for the HIV antibody be reported. Although

there is significant pressure to mandate reporting in all states, there is controversy over implementing such a mandate. Many believe that if we require reporting of HIV-positive tests, many people will refuse to be tested even if they suspect they are infected.

what do you THINK?

Do you favor mandatory reporting of HIV and AIDS cases? ■ If you knew that your name and vital statistics would be "on file" if you tested positive for HIV, would you be less likely to take the HIV test to begin with? ■ On the other hand, do people who carry this contagious fatal disease have a responsibility to inform the general public and the health professionals who will provide their care? ■ Explain your answer.

Women and AIDS

HIV is an equal-opportunity pathogen that can attack anyone who engages in high-risk behaviors. This is true regardless of race, gender, sexual orientation, or socioeconomic status. Consider the following facts:[47]

- By 2005, women accounted for over 27 percent of newly reported AIDS cases in the United States.
- American women most at risk are ethnic minorities and the economically disadvantaged.
- Among sexually active heterosexual teenagers, college students, and health care workers, nearly 60 percent of HIV cases are women.

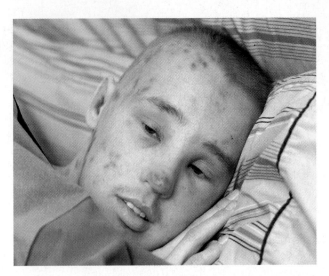

The effects of HIV/AIDS can be seen here in the form of Kaposi's sarcoma and AIDS-wasting syndrome.

■ Women of color are disproportionately affected by HIV. Although African American and Hispanic females comprise less than 25 percent of all U.S. women, together they account for 79 percent of AIDS cases among women in the United States.
■ AIDS is one of the top ten causes of death for people aged 15 to 64 in the United States.

Compounding the problems of women with HIV are serious deficiencies in our health and social service systems, including inadequate treatment for female addicts and lack of access to child care, health care, and social services for families headed by single women. Women with HIV/AIDS are also the major source of infection in infants. Virtually all new HIV infections among children in the United States are attributable to perinatal transmission of HIV.[48]

Special Concerns of Women with HIV/AIDS

Women often have an even more difficult time protecting themselves from infection and taking care of themselves if they become ill. Irrefutable evidence indicates that HIV/AIDS disproportionately affects women as they are four to ten times more likely than men to contract HIV through unprotected sexual intercourse with an infected partner. This discrepancy can be traced to both biological and socioeconomic factors.
Biological factors include:

■ HIV can enter through mucous membrane surfaces of the genital tract; the vagina has a greater exposed mucous membrane area than does the urethra of the penis.
■ The vaginal area is more likely to incur microtears during sexual intercourse, which facilitates entry of HIV.
■ During intercourse, a woman is exposed to more semen than is the male to vaginal fluids.
■ Semen is more likely to enter the vagina with force, whereas vaginal fluids do not enter the penis with force.

■ Women who have STIs are more likely to be asymptomatic and therefore unaware they have a disease; STIs increase the risk of HIV transmission.

Socioeconomic factors include:

■ Women have been underrepresented in clinical trials for HIV treatment and prevention.
■ Women are more vulnerable to sexual abuse from their male partners and are more likely to be involved in nonconsensual sex or sex without condoms.
■ Women are more likely to be economically dependent on men.
■ Women may be less likely to seek medical treatment because of caregiving burdens, transportation problems, and lack of money.
■ In the United States, HIV-positive women are likely to be younger and less educated than HIV-positive men.
■ Cultural norms place women in a relatively passive role in taking responsibility for protection during sexual intercourse and in general sexual decision making, particularly in third world countries.

Efforts must be initiated to help women take control of their sexual health and participate actively in sexual decisions made with their partners. In addition, women often carry the responsibility of caring for their children or for others who may be infected with HIV or suffering from AIDS. If the mother's role as caretaker must be abandoned due to illness, family members often suffer. As more and more women become infected with HIV, national efforts aimed at prevention, intervention, and treatment will undoubtedly increase.

 what do you THINK?

■ Why do you think HIV/AIDS is increasing among women and minority groups in America? ■ Why are some women particularly vulnerable to diseases such as AIDS? ■ What actions can we take as a nation to reduce the spread of HIV/AIDS among women and minority groups? ■ Should Americans be concerned about the global HIV/AIDS epidemic? Why or why not?

How HIV Is Transmitted

HIV typically enters one person's body when another person's infected body fluids (semen, vaginal secretions, blood, etc.) gain entry through a breach in body defenses. Mucous membranes of the genital organs and the anus provide the easiest route of entry. If there is a break in the mucous membranes (as can occur during sexual intercourse, particularly anal intercourse), the virus enters and begins to multiply.

After initial infection, HIV multiplies rapidly, invading the bloodstream and cerebrospinal fluid. It progressively destroys helper T cells (recall that these cells call the rest of the immune response to action), weakening the body's resistance to disease. The virus also changes the genetic structure of the cells it attacks. In response to this invasion, the body quickly begins to produce antibodies.

Despite some myths, HIV is not a highly contagious virus. Studies of people living in households with an AIDS patient have turned up no documented cases of HIV infection due to casual contact. Other investigations provide overwhelming evidence that insect bites do not transmit HIV.

Engaging in High-Risk Behaviors

AIDS is not a disease of gay people or minority groups. If you engage in high-risk behaviors, you increase your risk for the disease. If you do not practice these behaviors, your risk is minimal. It is as simple as that.

Unfortunately, this message has not gotten through to many Americans. They assume that because they are heterosexual, do not inject illegal drugs, and do not have sex with sex workers, they are not at risk. They couldn't be more wrong. Anyone who engages in unprotected sex is at risk, especially sex with a partner who has engaged in other high-risk behaviors. Sex with multiple partners is the greatest threat.

You can't determine the presence of HIV by looking at a person; you can't tell by questioning unless the person has been tested recently, is HIV negative, *and* is giving an honest answer. So what should you do?

Of course, the simplest answer is abstinence. If you don't exchange body fluids, you won't get the disease. As a second line of defense, if you decide to be intimate, the next best option is to use a condom. However, in spite of all the educational campaigns, surveys consistently indicate that most college students throw caution to the wind if they think they "know" someone—they have unprotected sex. Even when they do not know the individual involved well, most of them have unprotected sex.

Why do so many of us act so irresponsibly when the outcome is so deadly? The answer is probably a combination of ignorance, denial that it could be you who is HIV positive, a certain degree of apathy, and a bit of very real fear. People who are afraid often avoid testing. If they have symptoms, they may still avoid testing out of fear that they may be diagnosed positive and not have any real options for a cure.

Recognize the risk factors, and remember, if you do not engage in activities that are known to spread the virus, your chances of becoming infected are extremely small. The following activities are high-risk behaviors.

Unprotected Sexual Intercourse

The greatest risk factor is the exchange of HIV-infected body fluids during vaginal or anal intercourse. Substantial research indicates that blood, semen, and vaginal secretions are the major fluids of concern. However, even though these risks are well documented, millions of Americans report inconsistent safer sex practices, particularly when drugs or alcohol affect rational thinking.

Although the virus was found in one person's saliva (out of 71 people in a study population), most health officials state

TABLE 17.5	Tattoo and Piercing Safety

A look around any college campus reveals many examples of the widespread trend of body piercing and tattooing, also referred to as "body art." There are many health risks to consider though, ranging from serious infection to scarring. If you opt for tattooing or body piercing, remember the following points:

- Look for clean, well-lit work areas, and ask about sterilization procedures.
- Immediately before piercing or tattooing, the body area should be carefully sterilized. The artist should put on new latex gloves and touch nothing else while working.
- Packaged, sterilized needles should be used only once and then discarded. A piercing gun should not be used because it cannot be sterilized properly.
- Leftover tattoo ink should be discarded after each procedure. Do not allow the artist to reuse ink that has been used for other customers.
- Only jewelry made of noncorrosive metal, such as surgical stainless steel, niobium, or solid 14-karat gold, is safe for new piercing.
- If any signs of pus, swelling, redness, or discoloration persist, remove the piercing object and contact a physician.

Source: Center for Food Safety and Applied Nutrition, "Tattoos and Permanent Makeup," Office of Cosmetics Fact Sheet, U.S. Food and Drug Administration, 2004, www.cfsan.fda.gov/~dms/cos-204.html.

that saliva is not a high-risk body fluid unless blood is present; saliva is a less significant risk than other shared body fluids. The fact that the virus has been found in saliva does provide a good rationale for caution when engaging in deep, wet kissing.

Injecting Drugs

A significant percentage of AIDS cases in the United States result from sharing or using HIV-contaminated needles and syringes. Though users of illegal drugs are commonly considered the only members of this category, others may also share needles—for example, people with diabetes who inject insulin or athletes who inject steroids. People who share needles and also engage in sexual activities with members of high-risk groups, such as those who exchange sex for drugs, increase their risks dramatically. Tattooing and piercing is another risk (see Table 17.5).

Receiving a Blood Transfusion Prior to 1985

Prior to 1985, a small group of people had become infected after receiving blood transfusions or infected organ transplants. Today, because of massive screening efforts, the risk of receiving HIV-infected blood is almost nonexistent.

Mother-to-Infant (Perinatal) Transmission

Approximately one in three of the children who have contracted AIDS received the virus from their infected mothers while in the womb or while passing through the vaginal tract during delivery.

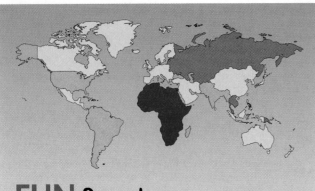

FUNfact

There are 38.6 million people living with HIV in the world today. How many people is that? Enough to fill the Super-Dome in New Orleans over 5,200 times.

FIGURE 17.7 A Global View of HIV Infection

Source: UNAIDS, "A Global View of HIV Infection," 2006, www.unaids.org.

Breast-feeding likely poses little risk. Initially, public health officials also included breast milk in the list of high-risk fluids because a few infants apparently contracted HIV while breast-feeding. Subsequent research has indicated that HIV could have been transmitted by bleeding nipples as well as by actual consumption of breast milk and other fluids.

Symptoms of HIV Disease

A person may go for months or years after infection by HIV before any significant symptoms appear. The incubation time varies greatly from person to person. Children have shorter incubation periods than adults. Newborns and infants are particularly vulnerable to AIDS because human beings do not become fully immunocompetent (that is, their immune system is not fully developed) until they are 6 to 15 months old. Research suggests that some very young children have shown the adult progression of AIDS.[49]

For adults who receive no medical treatment, it takes an average of eight to ten years for the virus to cause the slow, degenerative changes in the immune system that are characteristic of AIDS. During this time, the person may experience a large number of opportunistic infections (infections that gain a foothold when the immune system is not functioning effec-

ELISA Blood test that detects the presence of antibodies to the HIV virus.

Western blot A more accurate test than ELISA to confirm the presence of HIV antibodies.

tively). Colds, sore throats, fever, tiredness, nausea, night sweats, and other generally nonlife-threatening conditions commonly appear and are described as pre-AIDS symptoms.

Testing for HIV Antibodies

Once antibodies have formed in reaction to HIV, a blood test known as the **ELISA** test may detect their presence. If sufficient antibodies are present, the ELISA results will be positive. When a person who previously tested *negative* (no HIV antibodies present) has a subsequent test that is *positive,* seroconversion is said to have occurred. In such a situation, the person would typically take another ELISA test, followed by a more expensive, precise test known as the **Western blot,** to confirm the presence of HIV antibodies.

Although the ELISA is viewed as quite accurate, it is a conservative test in that it errs on the side of caution, meaning it produces a large number of *false-positive results.* It was deliberately designed to do this because it was intended as a test for screening the nation's blood supply. There have also been instances of *false-negative results.* Some health professionals believe that there are chronic carriers of HIV who, for unknown reasons, continually show false-negative results on both the ELISA and Western blot tests. This, of course, raises serious concerns about risks for these people's sexual partners.

It should be noted that these tests are not AIDS tests per se. Rather, they detect antibodies for the disease, indicating the presence of HIV in the person's system. Whether the person will develop AIDS depends to some extent on the strength of the immune system. Although we have made remarkable progress in prolonging the relatively symptom-free periods between infection, HIV-positive status, and progression to symptomatic AIDS, it is important to note that a cure does not yet exist. The vast majority of all infected people eventually develop some form of the disease.

As testing for HIV antibodies has improved, scientists have explored various ways of making it easier for individuals to be tested. Health officials distinguish between reported and actual cases of HIV infection because it is believed that many HIV-positive people avoid being tested. One reason is fear of knowing the truth. Another is the fear of discrimination from employers, insurance companies, and medical staff if a positive test result becomes known to others. (Although it is illegal to discriminate against a person who is HIV positive or has AIDS, discrimination is not always an overt act that is easily punished. Subtle acts of discrimination and harassment continue to be reported.) Early detection and reporting are important, because immediate treatment for someone in the early stages of HIV disease is critical.

New Hope and Treatments

New drugs and new drug combinations have slowed the progression from HIV to AIDS and have prolonged life expectancies for most AIDS patients. Though these new therapies

SKILLS FOR behavior change

STAYING SAFE IN AN UNSAFE SEXUAL WORLD

HIV transmission depends on specific behaviors; this is true of other STIs as well. The following will help you protect yourself and reduce your risk.

- Avoid casual sexual partners. Ideally, have sex only if you are in a long-term, mutually monogamous relationship with someone who is equally committed to the relationship and whose HIV status is negative.

- Avoid unprotected sexual activity involving the exchange of blood, semen, or vaginal secretions with people whose present or past behaviors put them at risk for infection. Postpone sexual involvement until you are assured that he or she is not infected.

- All sexually active adults who are not in a lifelong monogamous relationship should practice safer sex by using latex condoms. Remember, however, that condoms still do not provide 100 percent safety.

- Never share injecting needles with anyone for any reason.

- Never share any devices through which the exchange of blood could occur, including needles, razors, tattoo instruments, body-piercing instruments, and any other sharp objects.

- Avoid injury to body tissue during sexual activity. HIV can enter the bloodstream through microscopic tears in anal or vaginal tissues.

- Avoid unprotected oral sex or any sexual activity in which semen, blood, or vaginal secretions could penetrate mucous membranes through breaks in the membrane. Always use a condom or a dental dam during oral sex.

- Avoid using drugs that may dull your senses and affect your ability to take responsible precautions with potential sex partners.

- Wash your hands before and after sexual encounters. Urinate after sexual relations and, if possible, wash your genitals.

- Although total abstinence is the only absolute means of preventing the sexual transmission of HIV, abstinence can be a difficult choice to make. If you have any doubt about the potential risks of having sex, consider other means of intimacy, at least until you can assure your safety. Try massage, dry kissing, hugging, holding and touching, and masturbation (alone or with a partner).

- Be sure medical professionals take appropriate precautions to prevent potential transmission, including washing their hands and wearing gloves and masks. All equipment used for treatment should be properly sterilized.

- If you are worried about your own HIV status, have yourself tested. Don't risk infecting others.

- If you are a woman and HIV positive, you should take the steps necessary to ensure that you do not become pregnant.

- If you suspect that you may be infected or if you test positive for HIV antibodies, do not donate blood, semen, or body organs.

At no time in your life is it more important to communicate openly than when you are considering an intimate relationship. Ask questions, so you can make an informed decision about whether to get involved. Remember that you can't tell if someone has an STI. Anyone who has ever had sex with anyone else or has injected drugs is at risk, and they may not even know it. The following will help you to communicate about potential risks.

- Remember that you have a responsibility to your partner to disclose your own status. You also have a responsibility to

yourself to stay healthy. Ask about your partner's HIV status. Suggest going through the testing together as a means of sharing something important.

- Be direct, honest, and determined in talking about sex before you become involved. Do not act silly or evasive. Get to the point, ask clear questions, and do not be put off in receiving a response. A person who does not care enough to talk about sex probably does not care enough to take responsibility for his or her actions.

- Discuss the issues without sounding defensive or accusatory. Develop a personal comfort level with the subject prior to raising the issue with your partner. Be prepared with complete information, and articulate your feelings clearly. Reassure your partner that your reasons for desiring abstinence or safer sex arise from respect and not distrust.

- Encourage your partner to be honest and to share feelings. This will not happen overnight. If you have never had a serious conversation with this person before you get into an intimate situation, you cannot expect honesty and openness when the lights go out.

- Analyze your own beliefs and values ahead of time. Know where you will draw the line on certain actions, and be very clear with your partner about what you expect. If you believe that using a condom is necessary, make sure you communicate this.

- Decide what you will do if your partner does not agree with you. Anticipate potential objections or excuses, and prepare your responses accordingly.

- Discuss the significance of monogamy in your partner's relationships. Decide early how important this relationship is to you and how much you are willing to work at arriving at an acceptable compromise on lifestyle.

offer the promise of extended life for many, they may have inadvertently led to a recent increase in risky behaviors and a rise in cases of infection. Although AIDS fell from the top ten to the fourteenth leading cause of death in 1997 and has remained at that ranking, many experts fear that we are taking steps backward. Advocates for AIDS patients believe the medications still cost too much money and cause too many side effects.

Current treatments combine selected drugs, especially protease inhibitors and reverse transcriptase inhibitors. *Protease inhibitors* (for example, amprenavir, ritonavir, and saquinavir) resemble pieces of the protein chain that the HIV protease normally cuts. They block the HIV protease enzyme from cutting the protein chains needed to produce new viruses. Other drugs, including the nucleoside analogs (such as AZT, ddI, ddC, d4T, and 3TC), inhibit the HIV enzyme *reverse transcriptase* before the virus has invaded the cell. Protease inhibitors act to prevent the production of the virus in chronically infected cells that HIV has already invaded. In effect, the older drugs work by preventing the virus from infecting new cells, and the protease inhibitors work by preventing infected cells from reproducing new HIVs.

Although protease inhibitors show promise, they have proved difficult to manufacture, and some have failed while others are successful. Side effects vary from person to person, and getting the right dose is critical for effectiveness. All of the protease drugs seem to work best in combination with other therapies. These combination treatments are still quite experimental, and no combination has proved to be absolute for all people as yet. Also, as with other antiviral treatments, resistance to the drugs can develop. Individuals who already show resistance to AZT may not be able to use a protease-AZT combination. This can pose a problem for many people who have been taking the common drugs who then find their options for combination therapy limited.

Although these drugs provide new hope and longer survival rates for people living with HIV, it is important to maintain caution. We are still a long way from a cure. Apathy and carelessness may abound if too much confidence is placed in these treatments. Newer drugs that held much promise are becoming less effective as HIV develops resistance to them. Costs of taking multiple drugs are prohibitive and side effects common. There is no cure. Furthermore, the number of people becoming HIV-infected each year has stabilized and even increased in some communities, meaning that we are still a long way from beating this disease. In fact, while AIDS death rates in America dropped nearly 66 percent during the 1995–1998 period, we are now seeing modest increases in the death rate, as drug regimens lose effectiveness and rates of infection rise.[50]

Preventing HIV Infection

Although scientists have been working on a variety of HIV vaccines, none are currently available. The only way to prevent HIV infection is to avoid risky behaviors. HIV infection and AIDS are not uncontrollable conditions. You can reduce your risk by the choices you make in sexual behaviors and

by taking responsibility for your own health and the health of your loved ones. The Skills for Behavior Change box on page 543 presents ways to reduce your risk for contracting HIV and other STIs.

Because the status of your immune system is an important factor in your susceptibility to any of the STIs, it is important that you do everything possible to protect yourself. Adequate nutrition, sleep, stress management, vaccinations, and other preventive maintenance strategies can do a great deal to ensure your long-term health.

Where to Go for Help If you are concerned about your own risk or the risk of a close friend, arrange a confidential meeting with the health educator or other health professional at your college health service. He or she will provide you with the information that you need to decide whether you should be tested for HIV antibodies. If the student health service is not an option for you, seek assistance through your local public health department or community STI clinic. Local physicians, counselors, professors, and other responsible people can help you discover the answers you are looking for.

TAKING charge

Summary

- The major uncontrollable risk factors for contracting infectious diseases are heredity, age, environmental conditions, and organism resistance. Major controllable risk factors include stress, nutrition, fitness level, sleep, hygiene, avoidance of high-risk behaviors, and drug use.
- The major pathogens are bacteria, viruses, fungi, protozoa, prions, and parasitic worms. Bacterial infections include

staphylococcal infections, streptococcal infections, meningitis, pneumonia, Legionnaire's disease, tuberculosis, periodontal diseases, and rickettsia. Major viral infections include the common cold, influenza, infectious mononucleosis, hepatitis, mumps, chickenpox and shingles, dengue fever, Ebola, severe acute respiratory syndrome (SARS), West Nile virus, measles, and rabies.

- Your body uses a number of defense systems to keep pathogens from invading. The skin is our major protection, helped by enzymes. The immune system creates antibodies to destroy antigens. In addition, fever and pain play a role in defending the body. Vaccines bolster the body's immune system against specific diseases.
- Emerging and resurgent diseases pose significant threats for future generations. Many factors contribute to these risks. Possible solutions focus on a public health approach to prevention.
- Sexually transmitted infections are spread through intercourse, oral sex, anal sex, hand–genital contact, and sometimes mouth-to-mouth contact. Major STIs include chlamydia, pelvic inflammatory disease (PID), gonorrhea, syphilis, pubic lice, genital warts, candidiasis, trichomonia-sis, and herpes. Sexual transmission may also be involved in some general urinary tract infections.
- Acquired immunodeficiency syndrome (AIDS) is caused by the human immunodeficiency virus (HIV). HIV is not confined to certain high-risk groups. Globally, HIV/AIDS has become a major threat to the world's population. Anyone can get HIV by engaging in high-risk sexual activities that include exchange of body fluids, by having received a blood transfusion or organ transplant before 1985, by injecting drugs, or by having sex with anyone who engages in any of these high-risk activities. Women appear to be particularly susceptible to infection. You can cut your risk for AIDS significantly by deciding not to engage in risky sexual activities.

Chapter Review

1. Which of the following pathogens requires a living host to grow and multiply?
   a. bacteria
   b. fungi
   c. viruses
   d. parasitic worms

2. Which of the following substances in the antibody system is considered to be the scavenger cells that devour foreign cells in the body?
   a. antigens
   b. lymphocytes
   c. macrophages
   d. None of the above.

3. An example of a passive immunity one would receive is
   a. inoculation with a vaccine containing weakened antigens.
   b. when the body makes its own antibodies to a pathogen.
   c. the antibody-containing part of the vaccine that came from someone else.
   d. None of the above.

4. One of the best ways to prevent contagious viruses from spreading is to
   a. frequently wash your hands.
   b. replace worn toothbrushes often.
   c. eat a healthy diet.
   d. All of the above.

5. The population that makes up approximately 50 percent of new sexually transmitted infections in the United States is
   a. pre-teens.
   b. teenage to college-aged young adults.
   c. married couples.
   d. senior citizens.

6. If infected, which STI will remain in the human body for life, regardless of treatment?
   a. chlamydia
   b. gonorrhea
   c. syphilis
   d. herpes

7. Pelvic inflammatory disease (PID) is
   a. a sexually transmitted infection.
   b. a type of urinary tract infection.
   c. an infection of a woman's fallopian tubes or uterus.
   d. a disease that both men and women can get.

8. The most widespread sexually transmitted bacterium is
   a. gonorrhea.
   b. chlamydia.
   c. syphilis.
   d. chancroid.

9. Jennifer touched her viral herpes sore on her lip and then touched her eye. She ended up with the herpesvirus in her eye as well. This is an example of
   a. acquired immunity.
   b. passive spread.
   c. autoinoculation.
   d. self vaccination.

10. Which of the following is *not* a true statement about the HIV/AIDs virus?
    a. You can tell if a potential sex partner has the virus by looking at them.
    b. The virus can be spread either through semen or vaginal fluids.
    c. You cannot get HIV from a public restroom toilet seat.
    d. Unprotected anal sex increases risk of exposure to the HIV virus.

Answers to these questions can be found on page A-1.

Questions for Discussion and Reflection

1. What are the major controllable risk factors for contracting infectious diseases? Using this knowledge, how would you change your current lifestyle to prevent such infection?

2. What is a pathogen? What are the similarities and differences between pathogens and antigens? Discuss uncontrollable and controllable risk factors that can threaten your health. What can you do to limit the effects of either type of risk factor?

3. What are the six types of pathogens? What are the various means by which they can be transmitted? How have social conditions among the poor and homeless increased the risks for certain diseases, such as tuberculosis, influenza, and hepatitis? Why are these conditions a challenge to the efforts of public health officials?

4. What is the difference between active and passive immunity? How do they compare to natural and acquired immunity? Explain why it is important to wash your hands often when you have a cold.

5. Identify possible reasons for the spread of emerging and resurgent diseases. Indicate public policies and programs that might reduce this trend.

6. Identify five sexually transmitted infections. What are their symptoms? How do they develop? What are their potential long-term effects?

7. Why are women more susceptible to HIV infection than men? What implication does this have for prevention, treatment, and research?

8. Should Americans be concerned about soaring HIV/AIDS rates elsewhere in the world? Explain your answer.

Accessing Your Health on the Internet

The following websites explore further topics and issues related to personal health. You'll also find links to each organization's website on the Companion Website for Access to Health, Tenth Edition, at www.aw-bc.com/donatelle.

1. *Centers for Disease Control and Prevention (CDC).* Home page for the government agency dedicated to disease intervention and prevention, with links to all the latest data and publications put out by the CDC, including the *Morbidity and Mortality Weekly Report (MMWR), HIV/AIDS Surveillance Report,* and the *Journal of Emerging Infectious Diseases,* and access to the CDC research database, Wonder. www.cdc.gov

2. *National Center for Infectious Disease.* Up-to-date perspectives on infectious diseases of significance to the global community. www.cdc.gov/ncidod

3. *The New England Journal of Medicine Online.* Online version of a weekly journal reporting the results of important medical research worldwide; includes articles from current and past publications. http://content.nejm.org

4. *World Health Organization.* Access to the latest information on world health issues; direct access to publications and fact sheets, with keywords to find topics of interest. www.who.int

Further Reading

Champeau, D. and R. Donatelle. *AIDS and STIs: A Global Perspective.* Boston: Pearson Custom Publishing, 2000.

> *An overview of issues, trends, and ethics surrounding the global pandemic of HIV/AIDS and sexually transmitted infections.*

Chin, J., ed. *Control of Communicable Diseases Manual,* 17th ed. Washington, DC: American Public Health Association, 2003.

> *Outstanding pocket reference for information on infectious diseases. Updated every three to five years to cover emerging diseases.*

Klatt, E. *Pathology of AIDS: Version 17.* Gainesville, FL: Florida State University Press, 2006.

> *Overview of AIDS risks, prevention, and control as well as pathological development and historical basis.*

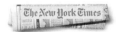

e-themes from *The New York Times*

For up-to-date articles about current health issues, visit www.aw-bc.com/donatelle, select *Access to Health,* Tenth Edition, Chapter 17, and click on "e-themes."

References

1. P. Wilkinson, "Infectious Diseases: Preparing for the Future," 2006, www.foresight.gov.uk.
2. Centers for Disease Control and Prevention, "Toxic Shock Syndrome," 2006, www.cdc.gov/ncidod/dbmd/diseaseinfo/toxishock_t.htm.
3. Centers for Disease Control and Prevention, "Group A Streptococcal Disease (GAS)," 2005, www.cdc.gov/ncidod.
4. Centers for Disease Control and Prevention, "Bacterial and Mycotic Diseases," 2005, www.cdc.gov/groupbstrep/gbs/gen_public_adult.htm.
5. New York State Department of Health, "Streptococcal Infections," 2004, www.health.state.ny.us/nysdoh/communicable_diseases/en/gas.htm.
6. J. Tully et al., "Students May Have Higher Risk for Meningococcal Disease Than Other Adolescents," *British Medical Journal* 332 (2006): 1136–1142.
7. Centers for Disease Control and Prevention, "Cruise Ships Associated with Legionnaire's Disease," *Morbidity and Mortality Weekly Report* 54, no. 45 (2005): 1153–1155.
8. R. Pratt et al., "Trends in Tuberculosis—U.S.," *Journal of the American Medical Association* 295, no. 19 (2005): 2243–2245.
9. Ibid.
10. Kaiser Family Foundation, "Global Health Report," 2006, www.globalhealthreporting.org/tb.asp.
11. Centers for Disease Control and Prevention, "Rocky Mountain Spotted Fever: Questions and Answers," 2005, www.cdc.gov/ncidod/dvrd/rmsf/.
12. G. Tortora, B. Funke, and C. Case, *Microbiology: An Introduction,* 9th ed. (San Francisco: Benjamin Cummings, 2007).
13. Centers for Disease Control and Prevention, "Key Facts about Influenza and the Influenza Vaccine," 2006, www.cdc.gov/flu/keyfacts.htm.
14. National Center for Infectious Diseases, "Disease Burden from Hepatitis A, B, and C in the United States," 2006, www.cdc.gov/ncidod/diseases/hepatitis/resource/dz_burden02.htm.
15. URO Today, "Hepatitis B," 2006, www.urotoday.com/browse_categories/hepatitis-b/1220/.
16. Ibid.
17. National Center for Infectious Diseases, "Disease Burden from Hepatitis A, B, and C in the United States."
18. Ibid.
19. National Center for Infectious Diseases, "Viral Hepatitis C Fact Sheet," 2004, www.cdc.gov/ncidod/diseases/hepatitis/c/fact.htm.
20. National Immunization Program, "Viral Hepatitis Vaccines," 2004, www.cdc.gov/nip/vaccine/hep/default.htm.
21. J. Ritterman, "Preventing Microbial Resistance: The Next Step," *The Permanent Journal* 10, no. 3 (2006): 22–24.
22. National Center for Infectious Diseases, "BSE and CJD Information and Resources," 2003, www.cdc.gov/ncidod/dvrd/vcjd/index.htm.
23. Centers for Disease Control and Prevention, "Dengue Fever," 2005, www.cdc.gov/ncidod/dvbid/dengue/index.htm.
24. Ibid.
25. Centers for Disease Control and Prevention, "Diseases—Ebola Hemorrhagic Fever," 2004, www.cdc.gov/ncidod/dvrd/spb/mnpages/dispages/ebola.htm.
26. Ibid.
27. Centers for Disease Control and Prevention, "Fact Sheet: Basic Information about SARS," 2005, www.cdc.gov.
28. K .E Nelson and C. F Williams, *Infectious Disease Epidemiology Theory and Practice,* 2nd ed. (Boston: Jones and Bartlett, 2007), 325.
29. R. Fenner, *The History of Smallpox and Its Spread Around the World* (Geneva, Switzerland: World Health Organization, 1988).
30. National Institute of Allergy and Infectious Diseases, "Profile Fiscal Year 2003. Sexually Transmitted Infections," 2004, www.niaid.nih.gov/facts/profile_fy2003/PDF/SSAR_SEXUALLY.pdf.
31. Centers for Disease Control and Prevention, "STDs Today," 2006, www.cdc.gov/std/default.htm.
32. National Centers for Chronic Disease Prevention and Health Promotion, "Healthy Youth, Sexual Behaviors," 2004, www.cdc.gov/HealthyYouth/sexualbehaviors/index.htm.
33. Centers for Disease Control and Prevention, "STDs Today."
34. Ibid.
35. National Centers for Chronic Disease Prevention and Health Promotion, "Healthy Youth, Sexual Behaviors."
36. National Center for HIV, STD, and TB Prevention, "Chlamydia Fact Sheet," 2006, www.cdc.gov/std/Chlamydia/STDFact-Chlamydia.htm.
37. National Center for HIV, STD, and TB Prevention, "Gonorrhea Fact Sheet," 2004, www.cdc.gov/std/Gonorrhea/STDFact-Gonorrhea.htm.
38. Ibid.
39. A. Evans and P. Brachman, *Bacterial Infections of Humans: Epidemiology and Control,* 3rd ed. (New York: Plenum, 1998).
40. Centers for Disease Control and Prevention, "Sexually Transmitted Diseases: HPV Vaccine Questions and Answers," 2006, www.cdc.gov.
41. National Center for HIV, STD, and TB Prevention, "Genital Herpes Fact Sheet," 2006, www.cdc.gov/std/herpes/STDFact-Herpes.htm.
42. Ibid.
43. Ibid.
44. UNAIDS, "2006 Report of the Global AIDS Epidemic," www.data.unaids.org/pub/globalreport/2006/2006_GR_CH02_en.pdf.
45. Ibid.
46. Centers for Disease Control and Prevention, "HIV/AIDS Surveillance," 2005, www.cdc.gov.
47. National Institute of Allergy and Infectious Diseases, "HIV and Women Fact Sheets," 2006, www.niaid.nih.gov.
48. Ibid.
49. National Institute of Allergy and Infectious Diseases, "HIV Infection in Infants and Children," 2006, www.niaid.nih.gov.
50. R. Conviser, "Changing Care Costs for HIV/AIDS," 2002, http://hab.hrsa.gov/reports/changingcost/sld001.htm.

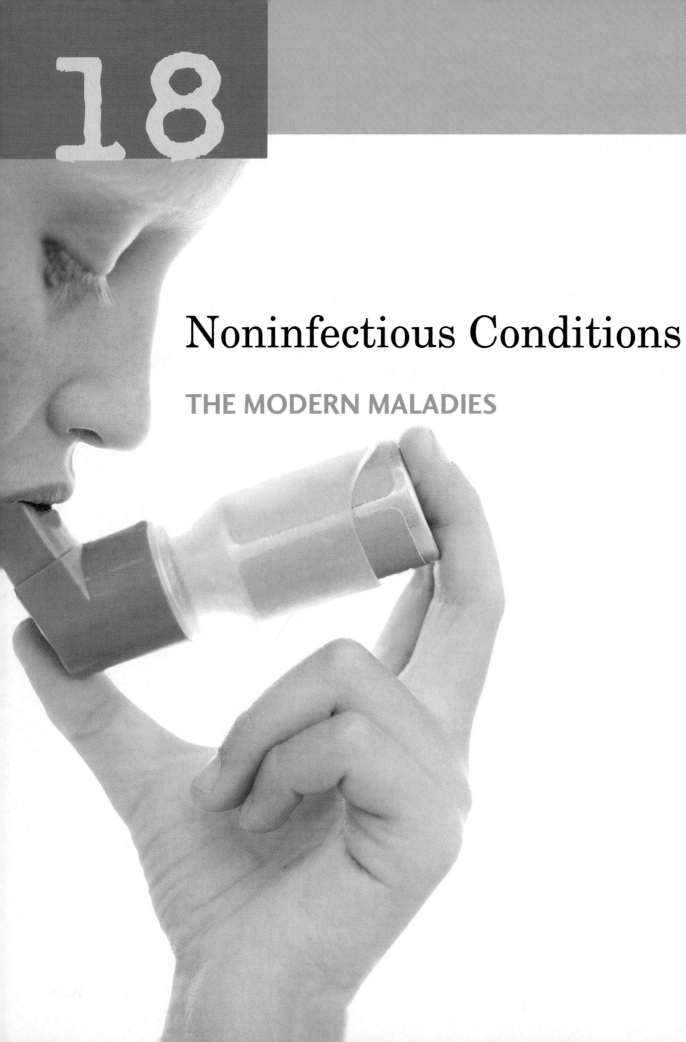

18

Noninfectious Conditions

THE MODERN MALADIES

What causes **asthma**?

What can I do to reduce my **risk** for diabetes?

How can I prevent migraine **headaches**?

Is lactose intolerance an **allergic** reaction to dairy products?

Is my heavy backpack causing my **back pain**?

OBJECTIVES

- Discuss key chronic respiratory diseases, including bronchitis, asthma, and emphysema, and respiratory complications associated with allergies and sleep apnea.
- Explain common neurological disorders, including headaches and seizure disorders.
- Describe common gender-related disorders, including risk factors, symptoms, and methods to control or prevent them.
- Understand diabetes and how it develops, and other digestion-related disorders.
- Discuss the effects of varied musculoskeletal diseases, including arthritis and other bone and joint problems.

Typically, when we think of the major ailments and diseases affecting Americans today, we think of "killer" diseases such as cancer and heart disease. Clearly, these diseases make up the major portion of life-threatening diseases, accounting for nearly two-thirds of all deaths. Yet although they do not capture much media attention, other forms of chronic disease can also cause substantial pain, suffering, and disability. Fortunately, most of them can be prevented or their symptoms relieved.

Generally, noninfectious conditions are not transmitted by a pathogen or by any form of personal contact. They often develop over a long period of time and cause progressive damage to human tissues. Although these conditions normally do not result in death, they do lead to illness and suffering for many people. Lifestyle and personal health habits are often implicated as underlying causes; however, a number of "newer" maladies seem to defy conventional wisdom about causation. For those known maladies and **idiopathic** (of unknown cause) disorders, education, reasonable changes in lifestyle, pharmacological agents, and public health efforts aimed at research, prevention, and control can minimize their effects. In this chapter, we will discuss common noninfectious conditions and the factors that contribute to them.

Chronic Lower Respiratory Disease

Chronic lower respiratory disease is the term used to describe conditions affecting the lower respiratory system, the

---

idiopathic   Of unknown cause.

chronic lower respiratory disease   Term used to describe all conditions affecting the lower respiratory system.

dyspnea   Shortness of breath, usually associated with disease of the heart or lungs.

chronic obstructive pulmonary diseases (COPDs)   A collection of chronic lung diseases including asthma, emphysema, and chronic bronchitis.

bronchitis   Inflammation of the lining of the bronchial tubes.

acute bronchitis   A form of bronchitis most often caused by viruses.

chronic bronchitis   A serious respiratory disorder in which the bronchial tubes become so inflamed and swollen that respiratory function is impaired.

emphysema   A respiratory disease in which the alveoli become distended or ruptured and are no longer functional.

alveoli   Tiny air sacs of the lungs where gas exchange occurs (oxygen enters the body and carbon dioxide is removed).

---

fourth leading cause of death in America today.[1] Chronic lower respiratory diseases are marked by airflow obstruction that is irreversible, and symptoms such as a chronic, productive cough, **dyspnea** (a form of uncomfortable breathlessness) with even mild exertion, and wheezing.[2]

Chronic Obstructive Pulmonary Diseases

Chronic obstructive pulmonary diseases (COPDs) include bronchitis and emphysema, and are largely preventable. In fact, between 80 and 90 percent of persons with COPD have a history of smoking.[3] In addition to smokers, those who have been exposed to dust, fumes, or gases that irritate the lungs over time or in one big dose (such as the policemen and firemen responding to the 9/11 terrorist attack on the World Trade Center) may be particularly vulnerable. Breathing difficulty can make it hard for individuals to perform activities of daily living (ADLs), which we learned about in Chapter 1.

Bronchitis   **Bronchitis** is inflammation of the lining of the bronchial tubes (*bronchi*), often occurring right after some type of lung infection, such as a cold. When the bronchi become inflamed or infected, less air is able to flow from the lungs, and heavy mucus begins to form. Although mucus is normal and necessary, when it is the dreaded yellow-gray or green color and it is coughed up in unusual amounts, one may have bronchitis. Other symptoms include a tight, sore sensation in the chest, a sore throat, difficulty catching breath, and tiredness. Although infections are common triggers for bronchitis, you may find that certain household cleaners and cigarette smoke trigger an attack. Usually, **acute bronchitis** is the most common form of bronchitis and symptoms often begin to go away in a week or two.

When the symptoms of bronchitis last for at least three months of the year in two consecutive years, you probably have the more serious form, **chronic bronchitis.** In some cases, this chronic inflammation and irritation of the lungs may lead to other chronic respiratory problems, such as asthma or emphysema. According to the most recent statistics, over 9 million Americans suffer from chronic bronchitis.[4]

Emphysema   If you have ever heard someone gasping for air for no apparent reason or watched someone hooked up to an oxygen tank and struggling to breathe while climbing a flight of stairs, you have probably witnessed an emphysemic episode. **Emphysema** involves the gradual destruction of the **alveoli** (tiny air sacs through which gas exchange occurs) of the lungs. Over 3.5 million Americans suffer from emphysema.[5] As the alveoli are destroyed, the affected person finds it more and more difficult to exhale. The victim struggles to take in a fresh supply of air before the air held in the lungs has been expended. Over time the chest cavity gradually expands, producing a barrel-shaped chest.

The cause of emphysema is uncertain. There is, however, a strong relationship between emphysema and long-term cigarette smoking and exposure to air pollution. Victims of emphysema often suffer discomfort for many years. In fact, studies show that lung function decline begins early in life, and noticeable symptoms, like "smoker's cough," appear once the damage has begun.[6] What most of us take for granted—the easy, rhythmic flow of air in and out of the lungs—becomes a continuous struggle for people with emphysema. Inadequate oxygen supply, combined with the stress of overexertion on the heart, eventually takes its toll on the cardiovascular system and leads to premature death.

Asthma

Asthma is a long-term, chronic inflammatory disorder that blocks airflow in and out of the lungs. Asthma causes tiny airways in the lung to overreact with spasms in response to certain triggers. Although most asthma attacks are mild and non–life-threatening, they can trigger bronchospasms (contractions of the bronchial tubes in the lungs) that are so severe that without rapid treatment, death may occur.

The good news is that asthma is a treatable condition, and it can be managed. All asthma attacks give a warning. Learning to recognize the warning signs and responding to them early can help prevent attacks or keep them from getting worse.[7] Warning signs can include increased shortness of breath or wheezing, disturbed sleep caused by shortness of breath, cough, chest tightness or pain, increased need to use bronchodilators (medications that open up airways by relaxing the surrounding muscles), and a fall in peak flow rates (as measured by a simple device that allows monitoring of lung function).

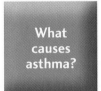

What causes asthma?

A number of factors can trigger an asthma attack or increase your risk of having one. These include living in a large urban area; exposure to secondhand smoke, occupational chemicals, pollen, molds, dust, or pet dander; having one or both parents with asthma, respiratory infections in childhood, low birth weight, obesity, and gastroesophageal reflux disease.[8] In some individuals, stress, exercise, certain medications, cold air, and sulfites are also potential triggers.

Asthma can occur at any age but is most likely to appear in children between infancy and age 5 and in adults before age 40. In childhood, asthma strikes more boys than girls; in adulthood, it afflicts more women than men. Also, the asthma rate is 50 percent higher among African Americans than whites, and four times as many African Americans die of asthma as do whites.[9] If you are younger than 30, your asthma is probably triggered by some type of allergy. Over age 30, attacks are often triggered by environmental irritants.

In the last decade, asthma rates have risen dramatically, particularly among inner-city children. Consider these points regarding its spread:[10]

- Asthma is the only chronic disease, besides AIDS and tuberculosis, with an increasing death rate. Each day 14 Americans die from asthma, an annual total of 5,000.

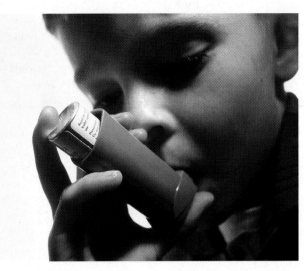

The marked increase of asthma and other respiratory problems among young children worries health officials.

- Asthma has become the most common chronic disease of childhood, accounting for one-fourth of all school absences and affecting more than one child in 20. Adolescent asthma can be unpredictable and difficult to control.
- Asthma affects over 17 million Americans, including 7 to 10 million children; 15 percent of all students aged 5 to 19 have it.
- The annual direct costs of asthma are over $15 billion. Among adults, asthma is the fourth leading cause of work absence, resulting in over 10 million lost workdays per year.
- The number of asthma sufferers has increased by more than 65 percent since the 1980s; one in ten new cases is diagnosed in people over age 65.
- The World Health Organization estimates that between 100 and 150 million people worldwide have asthma, and this number is rising.

What causes asthma? Most experts point to a potential allergenic cause, whereas others look to environmental, infectious, and familial links to explain the increase.

People with asthma fall into one of two distinctly different types. *Nonallergic* or *intrinsic asthma* may have allergic triggers, but any unpleasant event or stimulant may trigger an attack. In contrast, the most common form of asthma, known as *allergic* or *extrinsic (slow onset) asthma,* is associated with allergic triggers. This type tends to run in families and develop in childhood. Often, by adulthood, a person has few episodes, or the disorder completely goes away. A common form of extrinsic asthma is *exercise-induced asthma (EIA),* which may or may not have an allergic connection. Some

asthma   A chronic respiratory disease characterized by attacks of wheezing, shortness of breath, and coughing spasms.

Although asthma rates continue to increase around the world, there is much that individuals and communities can do to reduce risk.

- Work with local leaders to reduce air pollution in your community. Investigate regulations on the burning of household and yard trash, field burning, wood-burning stoves, and secondhand smoke from cigarettes—all known triggers for asthma attacks—and work to revise them as necessary.
- Purchase a good air filter for your home, and clean furnace filters regularly. Clean your house often, using a high-suction vacuum rather than a broom to reduce dust particles suspended in the air.
- Wash pillows regularly to avoid pesky mites and other debris inside the pillows. Use pillow protectors and mat-

tress protectors, which keep dust mites and other critters out of your face and trapped inside the pillow or mattress. Don't purchase used mattresses, which may be teeming with mites.

- Avoid having cats or dogs that are known for high dander production in the home. If you're a pet lover but animal dander bothers you, try a nonshedding breed such as a poodle. Keep all pets off your bed, and wash them and their bedding weekly. Vacuum their hair regularly.
- Have asthma medications handy, and know where they are kept in case of an emergency.
- Keep your home clean and pest free; cockroaches and other vermin have enzymes in their saliva or particles on their bodies that may trigger allergic reactions.
- Keep mold concentrations low by using antimold cleaners or by running a de-

humidifier to keep moisture levels down.

- Avoid mowing the lawn or excessive outdoor exposure to pollen during high-pollen times. Local news stations often provide pollen warnings. If you must be outdoors, wear a pollen mask.
- Exercise regularly to keep your lungs functioning well.
- Avoid cigarette, cigar, and pipe smoke.
- If you have a fireplace or wood-burning stove, check it regularly to make sure that it is not spewing smoke and particulate matter.
- Let people close to you know that you are asthmatic, and educate them about what to do if you have an asthma attack. Understanding and knowledge are powerful tools for health consumers. Make sure your loved ones have access to information.

---

athletes have no allergies, yet live with asthma. Cold, dry air is believed to exacerbate EIA (make it more intense); thus, keeping the lungs moist and warming up prior to working out may help. The warm, moist air around a swimming pool is one of the best environments for people with asthma.

Relaxation techniques appear to help some asthma sufferers. Drugs may be necessary for serious cases. Determining whether a specific allergen provokes asthma attacks, taking steps to reduce exposure, avoiding triggers such as certain types of exercise or stress, and finding the most effective medications are big steps in asthma prevention and control. Numerous new drugs are available that cause fewer side effects than older medications. Finding a doctor who specializes in asthma treatment and stays up-to-date on possible options is critical. Today the focus is on disease management

and controlling triggers. The Skills for Behavior Change box identifies important preventive measures.

Allergy-Induced Respiratory Problems

An **allergy** occurs as part of the body's attempt to defend itself against a specific *antigen* or *allergen* by producing specific *antibodies*. When foreign pathogens such as bacteria or viruses invade the body, it responds by producing antibodies to destroy these invading antigens. Under normal conditions, the production of antibodies is a positive element in the body's defense system. However, for unknown reasons, in some people the body overreacts by developing an overly elaborate protective mechanism against relatively harmless substances. The resulting *hypersensitivity reaction* to specific allergens or antigens in the environment is fairly common, as anyone who has awakened with a runny nose or itchy eyes will testify. Most commonly, these hypersensitivity, or allergic, responses occur as a reaction to environmental antigens such as molds, animal dander (hair and dead skin), pollen, ragweed, or dust. Once

allergy Hypersensitive reaction to a specific antigen or allergen in the environment in which the body produces excessive antibodies to that antigen or allergen.

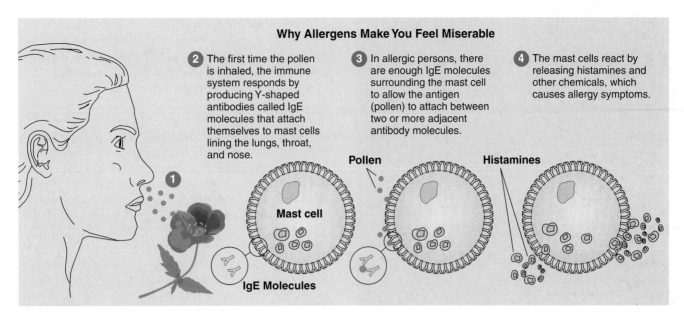

Why Allergens Make You Feel Miserable

2 The first time the pollen is inhaled, the immune system responds by producing Y-shaped antibodies called IgE molecules that attach themselves to mast cells lining the lungs, throat, and nose.

3 In allergic persons, there are enough IgE molecules surrounding the mast cell to allow the antigen (pollen) to attach between two or more adjacent antibody molecules.

4 The mast cells react by releasing histamines and other chemicals, which causes allergy symptoms.

Pollen

Histamines

Mast cell

IgE Molecules

FIGURE 18.1 **Steps of an Allergic Response**

excessive antibodies to these antigens are produced, they trigger the release of **histamines,** chemical substances that dilate blood vessels, increase mucous secretions, cause tissues to swell, and produce other allergy-like symptoms, particularly in the respiratory system (Figure 18.1).

Over 60 million Americans have asthma or allergies.[11] Although many people think of allergies as childhood diseases, in reality allergies tend to become progressively worse with time and with increased exposure to allergens. In these circumstances, allergic responses become chronic in nature, and treatment becomes difficult. Many people take allergy shots to reduce the severity of their symptoms, with some success. In most cases, once the offending antigen has disappeared, allergy-prone people suffer few symptoms.

Hay Fever

Perhaps the best example of an allergy-induced respiratory problem is **hay fever.** Usually considered a seasonally related disease (most prevalent when ragweed and flowers are blooming), hay fever is common throughout the world. Hay fever attacks, which are characterized by sneezing and itchy, watery eyes and nose, make countless people miserable. The disorder appears to run in families, and research indicates that lifestyle is not as great a factor in developing hay fever as it is in other chronic diseases. Instead, an overzealous immune system and exposure to environmental allergens including pet dander, dust, pollen from various plants, and other substances appear to be the critical factors that determine vulnerability. For people who are unable to get away from the cause of their hay fever response, medical assistance in the form of injections or antihistamines may provide the only relief. Over 18 million adults and 6 million children have a diagnosis of hay fever.[12]

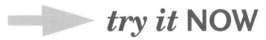 *try it* NOW

For those who have allergies or asthma, dust in the home can be your worst enemy. If you or someone you live with has allergies, take these steps today to control dust. Keep pillows, cushions, and mattresses in zippered covers. Wash bedding weekly in hot water, and wipe surfaces with a damp rag weekly to keep dust to a minimum.

Sleep-Related Disorders

In Chapter 2, we learned about the importance of sleep, and sleep problems such as insomnia and sleep apnea. Insomnia is characterized by the inability to fall asleep or stay asleep. Sleep apnea is one of the growing numbers of disorders responsible for insomnia-like sleep patterns.

histamines Chemical substances that dilate blood vessels, increase mucous secretions, and produce other symptoms of allergies.

hay fever A chronic respiratory disorder that is most prevalent when ragweed and flowers bloom.

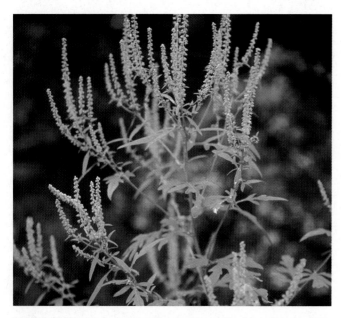

Hay fever, often seasonal and triggered by pollen from plants such as ragweed (pictured above), is one of the most common forms of allergies.

Sleep Apnea

As we learned in Chapter 2, **sleep apnea** is a serious, potentially life-threatening condition that involves brief interruptions in breathing. This disorder may be as pervasive as diabetes in the United States and is believed to affect more than 18 million adults, particularly those who are overweight.

There are two major types of sleep apnea: central and obstructive. *Central sleep apnea* occurs when the brain fails to tell the breathing muscles to initiate breathing. Abuse of alcohol and other medications can cause this condition. The more common form, *obstructive sleep apnea,* occurs when air cannot move in and out of a person's nose or mouth, even though the body tries to breathe.

It is a common misperception that breathing always stops entirely during the apnea phases of sleep. Often, breathing continues and the chest rises and falls, but the level of air that is exchanged is minimal. When the body doesn't get enough oxygen, the heart races, blood pressure goes up, body chemistry may change, and a host of other subtle and not-so-subtle events occur. Most importantly, as oxygen saturation levels in the blood fall, the body's autonomic nervous system moves to protect you and signals your body to breathe, often with a sudden gasp of breath. This response may wake a person, causing sufferers to rarely reach deep sleep, and wake up feeling tired and unwell. This is often one of the first symptoms of a person with sleep apnea.

sleep apnea Disorder in which a person has numerous episodes of breathing stoppage during a night's sleep.

What causes sleep apnea? Typically, obstructive apnea occurs when a person's throat muscles and tongue relax during sleep and block the airways.[13] People who are overweight or obese often have more tissue to flap or sag, making their risk of apnea greater; however, not all people with sleep apnea are obese.

Why should we be concerned? Chronic high blood pressure, irregular heartbeats, heart attack, and stroke are among the more serious risks. Chronic fatigue, inattentiveness when driving, and general feelings of tiredness and depression may also be of concern. Some people have early-morning headaches. People with untreated sleep apnea are three times more likely to have automobile accidents than people who do not suffer from it.[14]

If diagnosed, there are several options available for treatment, the most common of which is a *continuous positive airway pressure* (CPAP) device, which consists of an airflow device, long tube, and mask. Persons with sleep apnea wear this mask during sleep, and air is forced into the nose to keep the airway open. Snoring and sleep disturbances generally stop with the use of this machine. There are also surgical, laser, and other techniques for treating sleep apnea, but the results of these treatments are mixed. In people who have weight problems, losing weight often reduces the number and severity of apnea events; however, since many apnea patients have a hereditary predisposition to loose skin in the throat area without being obese, weight loss does not always solve the problem.

❓ *what do you* THINK?

Which of the respiratory diseases described in this section do you or your family have problems with? ■ How many of your college friends have these COPDs? ■ What difficulties do they have in controlling their diseases? ■ Why do you think the incidence of COPDs, as a group, is increasing? ■ What actions can you or the people in your community take to reduce risks and problems from these diseases?

Neurological Disorders

Headaches

If you think you are alone when you get a headache, think again (Figure 18.2). Over 50 million people see their doctors for headaches each year, and many more just silently put up with the pain or pop pain relievers to blunt the symptoms. Over 80 percent of women and 65 percent of men experience them on a regular basis.[15]

It is small comfort to know that headaches are usually not the sign of a serious disease or underlying condition and will go away fairly quickly. Over 90 percent of all headaches are of three major types: *tension headaches, migraines,* and *cluster headaches.*

Tension Headaches

These are the most common type of headache and produce what is usually a mild to moderate level of diffuse pain in the head. They occur randomly, and as the name implies, stress and muscular tension in the jaw, neck, or other body areas cause this type of headache; however, newer thinking is that this headache is due to chemical and neuronal imbalances in the brain or other, as yet unknown, causes. Possible triggers for this imbalance include red wine, lack of sleep, fasting or extreme dieting, menstruation, or certain food additives or preservatives. If you suffer from this type of headache, the best thing to do might be to take over-the-counter pain medications such as aspirin, get more sleep, and record when you seem to have symptoms. If stress is a trigger, try to relax with a hot bath, relaxing music, hot compresses, massage, or other relaxation techniques. If you seem to get these headaches after eating certain foods or with other triggers, avoid them. The good news is that these types of headaches are often short lived. If they occur frequently or in combination with migraine symptoms, consult your doctor.

Migraine Headaches

More than 29 million Americans—three times more women than men—suffer from **migraines,** a type of headache that often has severe, debilitating symptoms. One of four households has a migraine sufferer.[16] Whereas all headaches can be painful, migraines can be disabling. Symptoms vary greatly by individual, and attacks can last anywhere from 4 to 72 hours, with distinct phases of symptoms. Usually migraine incidence peaks in young adulthood, the prime years for college students, aged 20 to 45.[17] Migraines are often hereditary. If both parents have them, there is a 75 percent chance their children will have them; if only one parent has them, there is a 50 percent chance their children will have them. If any of your relatives have them, there is a 20 percent risk for you.[18] In about 15 percent of cases, migraines are preceded by a sensory warning sign known as an *aura,* such as flashes of light, flickering vision, blind spots, tingling in arms or legs, or a sensation of odor or taste. Sometimes nausea, vomiting, and extreme sensitivity to light and sound are present.[19] Symptoms of migraines include pain behind or around one eye and usually on the same side of the head. Pain may be excruciating and can last for hours or days. In some people, there is sinus pain, neck pain, or an aura without headache.

How can I prevent migraine headaches?

Patients report that migraines can be triggered by emotional stress, weather, certain foods, lack of sleep, and a litany of other causes. When tested under laboratory settings, however, much of this evidence is inconclusive. What is known is that migraines occur when blood vessels dilate in the membrane that surrounds the brain. Historically, treatments have centered on reversing or preventing this dilation, with the most common treatment derived from

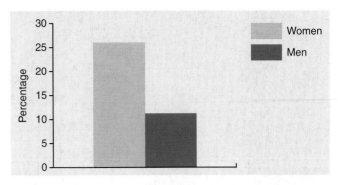

FIGURE 18.2 Prevalence of U.S. Adults with Migraine or Severe Headache During the Last Three Months, by Sex, Aged 18–44

Source: National Health Interview Survey, "Prevalence of U.S Adults with Migraine or Severe Headache During the Last Three Months," 2005, www.cdc.gov/nchs/nhis.htm.

the rye fungus *ergot.* Today, fast-acting ergot compounds are available by nasal spray, vastly increasing the speed of relief. However, ergot drugs have many side effects, the least of which may be that they are habit forming, causing users to wake up with "rebound" headaches each morning after use, prompting the user to take more medication.[20]

Critics of the blood vessel dilation theory question why only blood vessels of the head dilate in these situations. Furthermore, why aren't people who take hot baths or those who exercise more prone to migraine attacks? They suggest that migraines originate in the cortex of the brain, where certain pain sensors are stimulated.

When true migraines occur, relaxation is only minimally effective as a treatment. Often, strong pain-relieving drugs prescribed by a physician are necessary. Imitrex, a drug tailor-made for migraines, works for about 80 percent of those who try it. However, Imitrex is expensive and its side effects make it inappropriate for anyone with uncontrolled high blood pressure or heart disease. Recently, treatment with lidocaine has shown promising results, and newer drugs called triptans, such as Zomig, Amerge, and Maxalt, are now available. Consult your doctor to learn more about the newest drugs available to treat migraines.

Cluster Headaches

Fortunately, cluster headaches are among the more rare forms of headache, affecting less than 1 percent of people, usually men.[21] Although cluster headaches are less common than migraines, the pain can be worse. Usually these headaches cause stabbing pain on one side of the head, behind the eye, or in one defined spot. They can last for weeks and disappear quickly but, most commonly, last for

migraine A condition characterized by localized headaches that possibly result from alternating dilation and constriction of blood vessels.

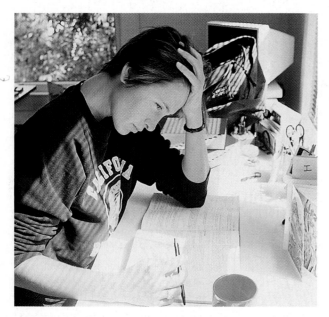

Tension headaches are triggered by many factors, including lack of sleep, stress, and strain on head and neck muscles.

30 to 45 minutes.[22] Oxygen therapy, drugs, and even surgery have been used to treat severe cases.

Secondary Headaches Secondary headaches arise as a result of some other underlying, usually organic, condition. Hypertension, blocked sinuses, allergies, low blood sugar, diseases of the spine, the common cold, poorly fitted dentures, problems with eyesight, and other types of pain or injury can trigger this condition. Relaxation and pain relievers such as aspirin are of little help in treating secondary headaches. Rather, medications or other therapies to relieve the underlying organic cause of the headache must be included in the treatment regimen.

Seizure Disorders

The word **epilepsy** derives from the Greek *epilepsia,* meaning "seizure." Reports of epilepsy appeared in Greek medical records as early as 300 BC. Ancient peoples interpreted seizures as invasions of the body by evil spirits or as punishments by the gods. Although much of the mystery surrounding epileptic seizures has been solved in recent years, the stigma and lack of understanding remain. Over 2 million people in the United States suffer from some form of seizure-related disorder, and between 5 and 10 percent of the population will experience at least one seizure in their lives.

epilepsy A neurological disorder caused by abnormal electrical brain activity; can be accompanied by altered consciousness or convulsions.

Each year, over 180,000 people in the United States will have a seizure for the first time.[23]

These disorders are generally caused by abnormal electrical activity in the brain and are characterized by loss of control of muscular activity and unconsciousness. Symptoms vary widely from person to person and can range from temporary confusion to major seizing.

Epilepsy is most common in childhood and after age 65 but can occur at any time. Typically, seizures fall into one of two categories. When they seem related to abnormal activity in just one region of the brain, they are classified as partial. When they involve all or most parts of the brain, they are generalized. Common seizure disorders include:[24]

- *Narcolepsy.* A condition in which the individual falls asleep at unpredictable times
- *Grand mal,* or *major motor, seizure.* These seizures are often preceded by the perception of a shrill cry or a seizure aura (body sensations such as ringing in the ears or a specific smell or taste). Convulsions and loss of consciousness generally occur and may last from 30 seconds to several minutes or more. Keeping track of the length of time elapsed is one aspect of first aid.
- *Petit mal,* or *minor, seizure.* These seizures involve no convulsions. Rather, a minor loss of consciousness occurs, which may even go unnoticed. Minor twitching of muscles may take place, usually for a shorter time than grand mal convulsions.
- *Psychomotor seizure.* These seizures involve both mental processes and muscular activity. Symptoms include mental confusion and a listless state characterized by activities such as lip smacking, chewing, and repetitive movements.
- *Jacksonian,* or *focal, seizure.* This is a progressive seizure that often begins in one part of the body, such as the fingers, and moves to other parts, such as the hand or arm. Usually only one side of the body is affected.

About half of all cases of seizure disorder are of unknown origin. Stroke and head injury or trauma are possible causes; other causes include congenital abnormalities, injury or illness resulting in inflammation of the brain or spinal column, drug or chemical poisoning, tumors, nutritional deficiency, and heredity.

In most cases, people afflicted with seizure disorders can lead normal, seizure-free lives when under medical supervision. Public ignorance about these disorders is one of the most serious obstacles confronting them. Improvements in medication and surgical interventions to reduce some causes of seizures are among the most promising treatments today.

Providing First Aid for Seizures There are several things you can do to help people during and after seizures.

1. *Note the length of the attack.* Seizures in which a person remains unconscious for long periods of time should be monitored closely. If medical help arrives, be sure to tell the medical personnel how long the person has been unconscious.

DISPARITIES IN DISEASE TRENDS

I n a review of the leading causes of death in the United States, clear gender, racial, and ethnic differences exist. African Americans, Hispanic Americans, Asian Americans, and white Americans display vastly different risk profiles. These differences are found not only among life-threatening disorders such as cardiovascular disease and cancer, but in many chronic conditions as well. Consider the following:

- Prevalence rates of asthma are consistently higher for blacks than for whites by approximately 50 percent. Among Hispanic Americans, death rates due to asthma are approximately 50 percent higher than among non-Hispanics.
- Females report approximately 50 percent more chronic bronchitis than males, and whites are 50 percent more likely to develop the condition than are blacks.
- Osteoarthritis is more common among males under age 45 than among their female counterparts. However, over the age of 54, osteoarthritis is more common among women than men.
- No significant racial differences in morbidity for rheumatoid arthritis are apparent; however, several American Indian tribes show a high prevalence of the disease, including the Yakima of Central Washington and the Mille-Lac Band of Chippewa in Minnesota.
- Older Americans and minority populations suffer disproportionately high rates of diabetes and diabetes-related complications.
- Fibromyalgia and chronic fatigue are much more common among females.
- Parkinson's disease rates are higher among men than among women and more common in whites than in blacks.

Sources: B. Hamann, *Disease: Identification, Prevention and Control* (New York: McGraw-Hill, 2007); National Center for Health Statistics, *Health: United States, 2005,* 2006, www.cdc.gov/nchs.

---

2. *Remove obstacles that could harm the victim.* Because seizure victims may lose motor control during a convulsion, they inadvertently thrash around. To reduce the chances of serious injury, clear away any objects that could pose a threat.

3. *Loosen clothing, and turn the victim's head to the side.* This procedure will ensure adequate ventilation and allow fluids or vomit to drain from the mouth.

4. *Do not force objects into the victim's mouth.* Although seizure victims may bite their tongues, causing possible damage, they will not swallow them. If the victim's mouth is clamped shut, forcing objects into the mouth may break teeth or cause more harm than doing nothing.

5. *Get help.* After you have completed steps 1 through 4, get help or send someone for help. This is particularly important if the victim does not regain consciousness within a few minutes.

6. *Reassure the victim.* In too many instances, the seizure victim regains consciousness only to face a crowd of staring people. When administering first aid, try to dissuade curious bystanders from hanging around. Calmly reassure the victim that everything is okay.

7. *Allow the person to rest.* After a seizure, many people will be exhausted. Allow them to sleep if possible.

what do you THINK?

Do you suffer from recurrent headaches or other neurological problems? ■ What might cause your problems? ■ What actions could you take to reduce your risks and symptoms?

Parkinson's Disease

Over 1.5 million Americans are believed to have **Parkinson's disease,** a chronic, slowly progressive neurological condition that typically strikes after age 50. Rates of Parkinson's have quadrupled in the past 30 years and may increase even more dramatically as growing numbers of baby boomers pass age 60. Nearly 60,000 new cases are diagnosed each year. Fifteen percent of the people diagnosed are under age 50.[25]

The hallmark of Parkinson's disease, and the symptom most commonly associated with it, is a tremor, or "shaking

---

Parkinson's disease A chronic, progressive neurological condition that causes tremors and other symptoms.

palsy." Tremors can become so severe that the simplest tasks, such as eating or brushing one's teeth, become difficult or impossible. Additional symptoms may include:

- Tremor of the hand when in a relaxed position or when under stress
- Rigid or stiff muscles
- Slowness in movement and a delay in initiating movements
- Poor balance
- Difficulty in walking, shuffling steps, and inability to take next steps
- Slurred speech, slowness in thought, and small, cramped handwriting

Although many theories exist concerning the causes of this disease, most are only speculative. The most common factors being studied include:[26]

- Familial predisposition, particularly for younger patients (about 15 to 20 percent of those who have Parkinson's have a close relative with it). However, newer research indicates that heredity is probably not as great a factor as was previously believed.
- Acceleration of age-related changes
- Exposure to environmental toxins such as pesticides
- Past illnesses/disorders
- Trauma

Parkinson's is progressive and incurable. However, new drug therapies, including levodopa, dopamine antagonists, and MAOIs, work to keep symptoms under control, possibly for years. Surgical options such as brain tissue transplants and the use of fetal tissue stem cells, or genetically engineered cell transplants have also provided promising results.

Multiple Sclerosis

Multiple sclerosis (MS) is a degenerative neurological disease in which the myelin, a fatty material that surrounds our nerves and facilitates transmission of nerve impulses, breaks down and causes nerve malfunction, or short-circuiting. As the myelin degenerates, it scars, often in multiple places. Typically, MS appears between ages 16 and 60 and is characterized by periods of relapse (when symptoms flare up) and remission (when symptoms are not present). MS affects over 500,000 Americans.[27]

multiple sclerosis (MS) A degenerative neurological disease in which myelin, an insulator of nerves, breaks down.

fibrocystic breast condition A common, noncancerous condition in which a woman's breasts contain fibrous or fluid-filled cysts.

endometriosis Abnormal development of endometrial tissue outside the uterus, resulting in serious side effects.

Symptoms of MS vary considerably from one person to the next. Some experience mild problems of episodic numbness, dizziness, fatigue, changes in gait, and temporary vision loss. Others face more severe symptoms, including loss of bladder control and severe muscle weakness, necessitating a wheelchair for mobility. Most MS patients lead fairly normal lives and have few disease flare-ups.

Though several hypotheses address possible causes of MS, none has been proved conclusively. Allergies, viral exposure to an unknown pathogen, and environmental factors all have been considered possible causes.

Those who have been diagnosed with MS should practice commonsense strategies for preventing flare-ups. As with most neurological problems, risk reduction includes practicing a healthy lifestyle—particularly getting adequate sleep, eating a well-balanced diet, and controlling stress.[28] Temperature extremes, including exposure to cold, damp weather or to excessive heat and humidity, can make symptoms flare.

Gender-Related Disorders

Fibrocystic Breast Condition

A common, noncancerous problem among women in the United States is **fibrocystic breast condition.** Symptoms range in severity from one small, palpable lump to large masses of irregular tissue found in both breasts. The underlying causes of the condition are unknown. Although some experts relate it to hormonal changes that occur during the normal menstrual cycle, many women report that the condition neither worsens nor improves during their cycles. In fact, in most cases, the condition appears to run in families and to become progressively worse with age, irrespective of pregnancy or other hormonal disruptions. Although most cyst formations consist of fibrous tissue, some are filled with fluid. Treatment often involves removing fluid from the affected area or surgically removing the cyst itself.

Does fibrocystic breast condition predispose a woman to breast cancer? Experts believe that the risks for breast cancer among women with certain types of fibrocystic disease may be slightly higher than among the general populace, but it is likely that other factors, discussed in detail in Chapter 16, present much greater risks.

Endometriosis

Endometriosis is characterized by abnormal growth and development of endometrial tissue (the tissue lining the uterus) in regions of the body other than the uterus. It is most likely to appear between the ages of 20 and 40.

Symptoms of endometriosis include severe cramping during and between menstrual cycles, irregular periods, unusually heavy or light menstrual flow, abdominal bloating, fatigue, painful bowel movements with periods, painful

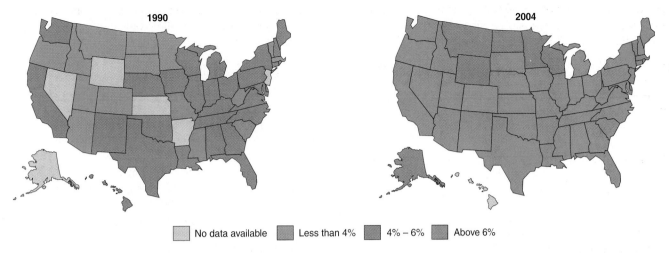

FIGURE 18.3 Percentage of Adults with Diagnosed Diabetes*

*Includes women with gestational diabetes

Source: Centers for Disease Control and Prevention, "Diabetes Prevalence, 2004," 2006, www.cdc.gov/diabetes/statistics/prev/state/index.htm.

intercourse, constipation, diarrhea, infertility, and low back pain. Among the most widely accepted theories concerning the causes of endometriosis are the transmission of endometrial tissue to other regions of the body during surgery or through the birthing process; the movement of menstrual fluid backward through the uterine tubes during menstruation; and abnormal cell migration through body-fluid movement. Women with cycles shorter than 27 days or flows lasting over a week are at increased risk. The more aerobic exercise a woman engages in and the earlier she starts it, the less likely she is to develop endometriosis.

Treatment for endometriosis ranges from bed rest and stress reduction to **hysterectomy** (the removal of the uterus) and/or the removal of one or both ovaries and the uterine tubes. More conservative treatments that involve dilation and curettage, surgically scraping endometrial tissue off the uterine tubes and other reproductive organs, and combinations of hormone therapy have become more acceptable. Hormonal treatments include gonadotropin-releasing hormone (GnRH) analogs, various synthetic progesterone-like drugs (Provera), and oral contraceptives.

Diabetes: Disabling, Deadly, and on the Rise

Diabetes is a serious, widespread, and costly chronic disease, affecting not just the 21 million Americans who must live with it, but also their families and communities. Between 1980 and 2002, diagnosed diabetes increased over 50 percent among U.S. adults, giving it the dubious distinction of being the fastest growing chronic disease in American history, which continues to rise unchecked today (Figure 18.3).[29] A recent study by the Centers for Disease Control indicated that diabetes seems to be increasing even more dramatically among younger adults—it is up by almost 70 percent among those in their thirties.[30]

In 2005, 1.5 million people aged 20 and over were diagnosed with diabetes and 225,000 die each year of related complications, making diabetes the sixth leading cause of death in America today.[31] Diabetes has its greatest impact on the elderly and certain racial and ethnic groups. One in five adults over age 65 has diabetes. Among adults aged 20 and older, African Americans are twice as likely as whites to have diabetes, and American Indians and Alaska Natives are 2.6 times more likely to develop it.[32] Overall diabetes rates are projected to double by 2050.

What causes this serious disease? In healthy people, the *pancreas,* a powerful enzyme-producing organ, produces the hormone **insulin** in sufficient quantities to allow the body to use or store glucose (blood sugar). When the pancreas fails to produce enough insulin to regulate sugar metabolism or when the body fails to use insulin effectively, a disease known as **diabetes mellitus** occurs (Figure 18.4 on page 560). Diabetics exhibit **hyperglycemia,** or elevated blood sugar levels, and high glucose levels in their urine. Other symptoms include excessive thirst, frequent urination, hunger, tendency to tire easily, wounds that heal slowly, numbness or tingling in the extremities, changes in vision, skin eruptions, and, in

hysterectomy   Surgical removal of the uterus.

insulin   A hormone produced by the pancreas; required by the body for the metabolism of carbohydrates.

diabetes mellitus   A disease in which the pancreas fails to produce enough insulin or the body fails to use insulin effectively.

hyperglycemia   Elevated blood sugar levels.

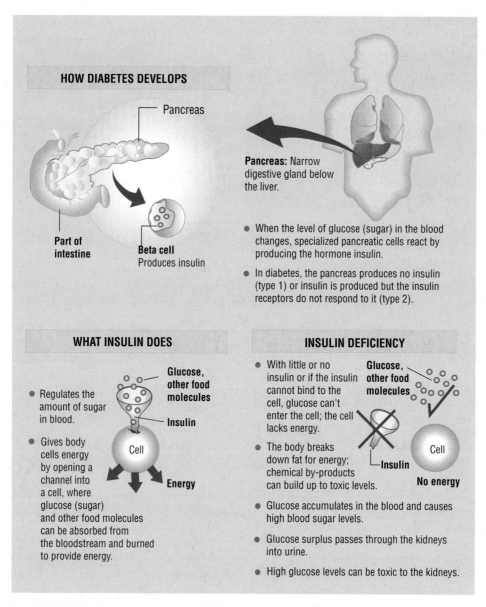

FIGURE 18.4 Diabetes: What It Is and How It Develops

Sources: Adaptation based on *Oregonian*, September 5, 2000, A6; *FDA Consumer* magazine; J. Mordis and W. Manis, *The Healing Handbook for Persons with Diabetes*, 3rd ed., 2000, www.umassmed.edu/diabeteshandbook; L. Urdang, ed., *The Bantam Medical Dictionary*, 3rd ed. (New York: Bantam, 2000); American Medical Association, *American Medical Association Family Medical Guide*, 4th ed. (New York: Wiley, 2004); research by Jutta Scheibe.

women, a tendency toward vaginal yeast infections. Of the 21 million people in the United States today who have diabetes, nearly 6 million are unaware of their condition.

How does a person become diabetic? The more serious form, known as *type 1 diabetes* (formerly known as insulin-dependent, or juvenile, diabetes), is an autoimmune disease in which the immune system destroys the insulin-making beta cells and most often appears during childhood or adolescence.[33] Type 1 diabetics typically must depend on insulin injections or oral medications for the rest of their lives because insulin is not present in their bodies.

In *type 2 diabetes* (formerly known as noninsulin-dependent, or adult-onset, diabetes), insulin production is deficient or the body is unable to utilize available insulin. Type 2 diabetes accounts for 90 to 95 percent of all diabetes cases and most often appears after age 40.[34] However, type 2 diabetes is now being diagnosed at younger ages, even among children and teens. This form of diabetes is typically linked to obesity and physical inactivity, both of which can be modified to control diabetes and improve health. If people with type 2 diabetes change their lifestyle, they may be able to avoid oral medications or insulin indefinitely.

A third type of diabetes, called *gestational diabetes,* can develop in a woman during pregnancy and affects 2 to 5 percent of all pregnant women. The condition usually disappears after childbirth, but it does leave the woman at greater risk of

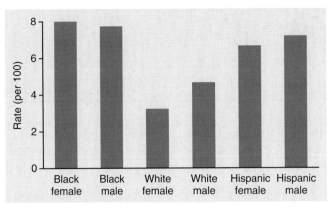

FIGURE 18.5 Age-Adjusted Prevalence of Diagnosed Diabetes, by Race/Ethnicity and Sex, 2004

Source: Centers for Disease Control and Prevention, "Diabetes Surveillance System," 2005, www.cdc.gov/diabetes/statistics/prev/national/fig2004.htm.

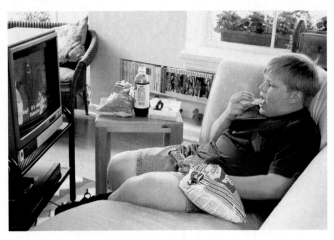

Unhealthy eating habits and a sedentary lifestyle can lead to type 2 diabetes even among children.

developing type 2 diabetes at some point. Other, less common, forms of diabetes can result from genetic syndromes, surgery, drugs, malnutrition, infections, and other illnesses.[35]

Understanding Risk Factors

What can I do to reduce my risk for diabetes?

Diabetes tends to run in families.[36] Being overweight, coupled with inactivity, dramatically increases the risk of type 2 diabetes. Older persons and mothers of babies weighing over 9 pounds at birth also run an increased risk. Approximately 80 percent of all type 2 patients are overweight at the time of diagnosis. Weight loss, better nutrition, control of blood glucose levels, and regular exercise are important factors in lowering blood sugar and improving the efficiency of cellular use of insulin. These improvements can help to prevent overwork of the pancreas and the development of diabetes. In fact, recent findings show that modest, consistent physical activity and a healthy diet can cut a person's risk of type 2 diabetes by a significant amount.[37] For unknown reasons, African Americans, Hispanics, and American Indians have the highest rates of type 2 diabetes in the world—much higher than that of whites.[38] (See Figure 18.5 for a comparison of rates.)

People who develop diabetes today have a much better prognosis than they would have had just 20 years ago. Recognize your own risk for this disease and take steps to reduce it. The Assess Yourself box on page 562 will help you determine if you are at risk for diabetes.

Controlling Diabetes

Most physicians attempt to control type 1 and later stages of type 2 diabetes with a variety of insulin-related drugs. Most of these drugs are taken orally, although self-administered hypodermic injections are prescribed when other treatments are inadequate. Recent breakthroughs in individual monitoring and implantable insulin monitors and insulin infusion pumps that regulate

insulin intake "on demand" have provided many diabetics with the opportunity to lead normal lives.

Newer forms of insulin that last longer in the body and have fewer side effects are now available. An insulin inhaler is now available, freeing patients from the painful necessity of insulin injections. All of these treatments come at a price. On average, health care costs for diabetics are $10,000 to $20,000 higher per year than for healthy patients. The direct and indirect costs of treating diabetes in the United States total $132 billion per year.[39] However, the full burden of diabetes is hard to measure: death records often do not reflect the role of diabetes in a person's death, and the costs related to undiagnosed diabetes are unknown.

Some people find that they can manage their diabetes effectively by eating foods that are rich in complex carbohydrates, low in sodium, and high in fiber; by losing weight; and by getting regular exercise. Developing a routine for monitoring and controlling this disease can be stressful, particularly in the beginning. Some reports even suggest that people with diabetes may be at a greater-than-average risk for clinical depression. Attention to psychosocial needs is often an important aspect of diabetic health.

Preventing Complications

Depending on the type and severity of the disease, diabetes can cause many complications and increase the severity of other existing conditions. If diabetes rates can be reduced, the real impact may be seen in reductions in diabetes complications and prevention of diabetes-related diseases. Consider the following problems that diabetes causes or contributes to and actions that may help reduce their burden:[40]

■ *Eye disease and blindness.* Each year, 12,000 to 24,000 people become blind because of diabetic eye disease. In fact, it is the leading cause of new blindness in America today. Non-Hispanic blacks are nearly 50 percent more likely to develop diabetes-related eye disease than non-Hispanic whites.

ASSESS *yourself*

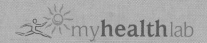

ARE YOU AT RISK FOR DIABETES?

Fill out this assessment online at
www.aw-bc.com/myhealthlab or
www.aw-bc.com/donatelle.

Certain characteristics place people at greater risk for diabetes. Nevertheless, many people remain unaware of the symptoms of diabetes until after the disease has begun to progress. If you answer yes to three or more of the following questions, you should consider seeking medical advice. Talk to health professionals at your student health center, or make an appointment with your family physician.

	Yes	No
1. Do you have a history of diabetes in your family?	❑	❑
2. Do any of your primary relatives (mother, father, sister, brother, grandparents) have diabetes?	❑	❑
3. Are you overweight or obese?	❑	❑
4. Are you typically sedentary (seldom, if ever, engage in vigorous aerobic exercise)?	❑	❑
5. Have you noticed an increase in your craving for water or other beverages?	❑	❑
6. Have you noticed that you have to urinate more frequently than you used to during a typical day?	❑	❑
7. Have you noticed any tingling or numbness in your hands and feet, which might indicate circulatory problems?	❑	❑
8. Do you often feel a gnawing hunger during the day, even though you usually eat regular meals?	❑	❑
9. Have you noticed that you are losing weight but don't seem to be doing anything in particular to make this happen?	❑	❑
10. Are you often so tired that you find it difficult to stay awake to study, watch television, or engage in other activities?	❑	❑
11. Have you noticed that you have skin irritations more frequently and that minor infections don't heal as quickly as they used to?	❑	❑
12. Have you noticed any unusual changes in your vision (blurring, difficulty in focusing, etc.)?	❑	❑
13. Have you noticed unusual pain or swelling in your joints?	❑	❑
14. Do you often feel weak or nauseated if you wait too long to eat a meal?	❑	❑
15. If you are a woman, have you had several vaginal (yeast) infections during the past year?	❑	❑

- *Kidney disease.* In 2005, 44,400 people with diabetes developed kidney failure; each year over 100,000 are in treatment for this condition. Better control of blood pressure and blood glucose levels could reduce diabetes-related kidney failure by about 50 percent.
- *Amputations.* Over 60 percent of nontraumatic amputations of lower limbs are due to diabetes. Foot care programs that include regular examinations and patient education could prevent up to 85 percent of these amputations.

- *Cardiovascular disease.* Heart disease and stroke cause about 65 percent of deaths among people with diabetes. More than 70 percent of diabetics have hypertension.
- *Pregnancy complications.* Poorly controlled diabetes can cause major birth defects in 5 to 10 percent of all pregnancies and causes 15 to 20 percent of all spontaneous abortions.
- *Flu- and pneumonia-related deaths.* Each year, 10,000 to 30,000 people with diabetes die of complications from flu

MAKE it happen!

ASSESSMENT: The Assess Yourself box asks you to evaluate whether you are at risk for diabetes. Now that you have considered your results, you may need to take steps to further understand and address your risks.

MAKING A CHANGE: In order to change your behavior, you need to develop a plan. Follow the steps below and complete your Behavior Change Contract to take action.

1. Evaluate your behavior and identify patterns and specific things you are doing. What can you change now? What can you change in the near future?

2. Select one pattern of behavior that you want to change.

3. Fill out the Behavior Change Contract found at the front of your book. It should include your long-term goal for change, your short-term goals, the rewards you'll give yourself for reaching these goals, potential obstacles along the way, and strategies for overcoming these obstacles. For each goal, list the small steps and specific actions that you will take.

4. Chart your progress in a journal. At the end of a week, consider how successful you were in following your plan. What helped you be successful? What made change more difficult? What will you do differently next week?

5. Revise your plan as needed: Are the short-term goals attainable? Are the rewards satisfying?

ONE STUDENT'S PLAN: When Jamie answered the questions in the self-assessment, he found that he had three "yes" answers. He was overweight (which he knew from calculating his body mass index), he was typically sedentary, since he didn't have a regular exercise program, and he felt like he was always hungry, even though he had regular meals. He decided to check into his family's medical history to further consider his risk for diabetes.

When Jamie spoke to his mother, he was surprised to find out that both his father and his grandmother had diabetes. Even more surprising, his 12-year-old brother had recently been diagnosed as being at risk.

Jamie immediately made an appointment at his student health center and soon was tested. His results were borderline normal, but he was advised to make changes to prevent developing diabetes. Among the changes were reducing his weight, eating more fiber, and starting a regular exercise program. Jamie talked to his roommates about his results, and they helped him come up with some ideas to make these changes. His first step was to ride his bicycle to campus every day, instead of driving. This gave him some physical activity that didn't take too much extra time from his day. Jamie also knew that he needed to improve his diet, by cutting down on junk food and looking for ways to include more fiber in his meals. He decided to start bringing snacks of carrots or apples with him to school. This would help him eat a balanced diet and keep him from buying candy from the vending machines. He also made sure to pay attention to his various options when he ate at the dining hall and to try to steer clear of the high-fat entrees and desserts.

Jamie's blood sugar will be retested in two months. If the level has come down to closer to the normal range, he will reward himself with tickets to see his favorite baseball team play its cross-town rivals.

---

or pneumonia. They are roughly three times more likely to die of these complications than people without diabetes, yet only 55 percent of people with diabetes get an annual flu shot.

New Choices in Care for Diabetics
In January 2006 the FDA approved the use of an inhalable form of insulin called Exubera. This will eliminate complications for those who find injecting difficult due to pain or infection. The inhaler should not be used by those who smoke or suffer from a COPD.

There are also new options for those who must prick their fingers to check blood glucose levels. One is a device that looks like a watch and can noninvasively check blood glucose by detecting changes on the skin's surface.

Digestion-Related Disorders

Lactose Intolerance

Is lactose intolerance an allergic reaction to dairy?

As many as 50 million Americans are unable to eat dairy products such as milk, cheese, or ice cream. They suffer from **lactose intolerance,** meaning that they have lost the ability to produce the digestive enzyme lactase, which is necessary for the body to convert milk sugar (lactose) into glucose. That cold glass of milk becomes a source of stomach cramping, diarrhea, nausea, gas, and related symptoms. (See Chapter 8 for a discussion of other things we eat that may cause intolerance.) Once diagnosed, it can be treated by introducing low-lactose or lactose-free foods into the diet. Through trial and error, individuals usually find that they can tolerate one type of low-lactose food better than others. Some people purchase special products that supply the missing lactase, enabling them to eat dairy foods without serious side effects. It should be noted, however, that these products do not work for everyone; someone who is lactose intolerant may need to experiment before settling into a diet that works. Furthermore, many people who think they are lactose intolerant actually are not. If you suspect that you are lactose intolerant, diagnostic tests can provide conclusive evidence.

Colitis and Irritable Bowel Syndrome

Ulcerative colitis is a disease of the large intestine in which the mucous membranes of the intestinal walls become inflamed. Victims with severe cases may have as many as 20 bouts of bloody diarrhea a day. Colitis can also produce severe stomach cramps, weight loss, nausea, sweating, and fever. Although some experts believe that colitis occurs more frequently in people with high stress levels, this theory is controversial. Hypersensitivity reactions, particularly to milk and certain foods, have also been considered a possible cause. Treatment focuses on relieving the symptoms. Increasing fiber intake and taking anti-inflammatory drugs, steroids, and other medications to reduce inflammation and soothe irritated intestinal walls can relieve symptoms.

Irritable bowel syndrome (IBS) is a condition characterized by nausea, pain, gas, diarrhea attacks, or cramps occurring after eating certain foods or during unusual stress. IBS symptoms commonly begin in early adulthood. Symptoms may vary from week to week and can fade for long periods of time, only to return.

The cause is unknown, but researchers suspect that people with IBS have digestive systems that are overly sensitive to what they eat and drink, to stress, and to certain hormonal changes. They may also be more sensitive to pain signals from the stomach. Stress management, relaxation techniques, regular activity, and diet can control IBS in the vast majority of cases. Some sufferers benefit from anticholinergic drugs, which relax the intestinal muscle, or from antidepressant drugs and psychological counseling. Medical advice should be sought whenever such conditions persist.

Diverticulosis

Diverticulosis occurs when the walls of the intestine weaken for undetermined reasons and small pea-sized bulges develop. These bulges often fill with feces and, over time, become irritated and infected, causing pain and discomfort. If this irritation persists, bleeding and chronic obstruction may occur, either of which can be life-threatening.

Although diverticulosis may appear in any part of the intestinal wall, it most commonly occurs in the small intestine. Often the person affected may be unaware that the problem exists. However, in some cases, a person may actually have an attack similar to the pain of appendicitis except that the pain is on the left side of the body instead of the right, where the appendix is located. Although diverticulosis most frequently occurs during and after middle age, it can appear at any age. If you have persistent discomfort in the lower abdominal region, seek medical attention at once.

Peptic Ulcers

An ulcer is a lesion or wound that forms in body tissue as a result of some form of irritant. A **peptic ulcer** is a chronic ulcer that occurs in the lining of the stomach or the section of the small intestine known as the *duodenum.* The lining of these organs becomes irritated, the protective covering of mucus is reduced, and the gastric acid begins to digest the dying tissue, just as it would a piece of food. Typically, this irritation causes pain that disappears when the person eats but returns about an hour later.

For many years, doctors believed that peptic ulcers were caused by eating spicy foods and acid-reducing drugs were the accepted treatment. However, research now indicates that

---

lactose intolerance   Inability to produce lactase, an enzyme needed to convert milk sugar into glucose.

ulcerative colitis   An inflammatory disorder that affects the mucous membranes of the large intestine, producing bloody diarrhea.

irritable bowel syndrome (IBS)   Nausea, pain, gas, or diarrhea caused by certain foods or stress.

diverticulosis   A condition in which bulges form in the walls of the intestine; results in irritation and infection of the intestine.

peptic ulcer   Damage to the stomach or intestinal lining, usually caused by digestive juices.

a common bacterium, *Helicobacter pylori (H-pylori)*, causes most ulcers. This means that antibiotics can effectively treat this disorder, which affects over 4 million Americans every year, and significantly reduce the risk of recurrence. In addition to antibiotic treatment, people with ulcers should also avoid high-fat foods, alcohol, and substances such as aspirin that may irritate organ linings or cause increased secretion of stomach acids and thereby exacerbate this condition. In extreme cases, surgery is necessary to relieve persistent symptoms.

Gallbladder Disease

Also known as *cholecystitis*, **gallbladder disease** occurs when the gallbladder has been repeatedly irritated by chemicals, infection, or overuse, thus reducing its ability to release bile used for the digestion of fats. One of the characteristic symptoms of gallbladder disease is acute pain in the upper right portion of the abdomen after eating fatty foods. This pain, which can last for several hours, may feel like a heart attack or an ulcer and is often accompanied by nausea.

Who gets gallbladder disease? The old adage about the "five Fs" of risk factors frequently holds true. Anyone who is "female, fat, fair, forty, and flatulent" (prone to passing gas) appears to be at increased risk. However, people who don't fit this picture also get the disease.

Current treatment of gallbladder disease usually involves medication to reduce irritation, restriction of fat consumption, and surgery to remove the gallstones.

Gastroesophageal Reflux Disease

Gastroesophageal Reflux Disease (GERD), commonly referred to as heartburn or acid reflux, affects 5 to 7 percent of the U.S. population. Heartburn is caused by the backflow of stomach acid into the esophagus, and is often associated with discomfort or a burning sensation behind your breastbone. Symptoms usually occur after a meal and can range from mild to more severe. If you suffer from severe heartburn, talk to your doctor. The symptoms may be nothing more than a mild annoyance now, but the disease can progress to a precancerous condition in your esophagus due to the damage caused by stomach acid. For more on acid reflux, see Table 18.1.

Musculoskeletal Diseases

Most of us will encounter chronic musculoskeletal disease during our lifetime. Some form of arthritis will afflict half of those over 65; low back pain hits 85 percent of us at some point. Arthritis and musculoskeletal diseases are the most common causes of physical disability in the United States.[41]

TABLE 18.1	Acid Reflux: Symptoms, Complications, Prevention
Symptoms	A backflow of stomach acid into the esophagus. Characterized by coughing, choking, heartburn, or vomiting.
Complications	Interrupts sleep; bleeding of the stomach or esophagus; ulcers; cancer of the esophagus
Risk factors	Risk factors include age, diet, alcohol use, obesity, pregnancy, smoking.
Prevention	Avoid foods that are acidic, spicy, tomato based, fried or fatty, or caffeinated. Consult your doctor about medication options.

Arthritis: Many Types, Many Problems

Called "the nation's primary crippler," **arthritis** strikes one in seven Americans, or over 38 million people. Symptoms range from the occasional tendinitis of the weekend athlete to the horrific pain of rheumatoid arthritis. There are over 100 types of arthritis diagnosed today, accounting for over 30 million lost workdays annually. The cost to the U.S. economy is over $86 billion per year in lost wages and productivity and untold amounts in hospital and nursing home services, prescriptions, and over-the-counter pain relief.[42]

Osteoarthritis (OA), also known as degenerative joint disease, is a progressive deterioration of bones and joints that has been associated with the "wear-and-tear" theory of aging. More recent research indicates that as joints are used, they release enzymes that digest cartilage, while other cells in the cartilage try to repair the damage. When the enzymatic breakdown overpowers cellular repair, the cartilage is destroyed. Bones rub directly against each other, causing the pain, swelling, and limited movement characteristic of arthritis. Weather extremes, excessive strain, and injury often lead to osteoarthritis flare-ups, but a specific precipitating event does not seem to be necessary. Obesity, joint trauma, and repetitive joint usage all increase the risk and thus are important targets for prevention.

gallbladder disease A disease caused by repeated irritation of the gallbladder, which leads to the formation of gallstones.

arthritis Painful inflammatory disease of the joints.

osteoarthritis (OA) Progressive deterioration of bones and joints that has been associated with the "wear-and-tear" theory of aging.

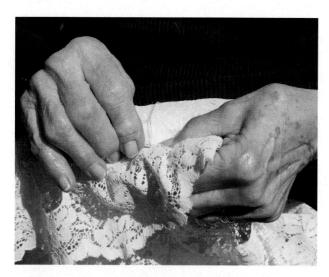

Arthritis can make simple tasks both painful and difficult to accomplish.

Although age and injury are undoubtedly factors in osteoarthritis, heredity, abnormal use of the joint, diet, abnormalities in joint structure, and impaired blood supply to the joint may also contribute. Osteoarthritis of the hands seems to have a particularly strong genetic component. Over 80 percent of those with OA report an activity limitation; OA of the knee can be as disabling as any cardiovascular disease short of stroke.[43] When joints become so distorted that they impair activity, surgical intervention is often necessary. Joint replacement and bone fusion are common surgical repair techniques. For most people, anti-inflammatory drugs and pain relievers such as aspirin and cortisone-related agents ease discomfort. In some sufferers, applications of heat, mild exercise, and massage may also relieve the pain. Today 20.7 million Americans have osteoarthritis, the majority of them women.[44]

Rheumatoid arthritis is an autoimmune disease involving chronic inflammation that can appear at any age, but it most commonly appears between ages 20 and 45; it affects over 2.1 million Americans. It is three times more common among women than among men during early adulthood but equally common among men and women in the over-70 age group. Symptoms include stiffness, pain, redness, and swelling of multiple joints, often including the hands and wrists, and can be gradually progressive or sporadic, with occasional unexplained remissions. Other symptoms include loss of appetite, fever, loss of energy, anemia, and generalized aches.[45]

Rheumatoid arthritis typically attacks the synovial membrane, which produces the lubricating fluids for the joints. Advanced rheumatoid arthritis often involves destruction of the bony ends of joints. The remedy for this condition is typically bone fusion, which leaves the joint immobile. In some instances, joint replacement may be a viable alternative.

Although the cause of rheumatoid arthritis is unknown, some theorists believe it is caused by some form of invading microorganism that takes over the joint. Toxic chemicals and stress have also been mentioned as possible causes. Genetic predisposition is a strong predictor of risk, and a genetic marker called *HLA-DR4* has been identified.[46]

Regardless of the cause, treatment of rheumatoid arthritis is similar to that for osteoarthritis treatments, emphasizing pain relief and improved functional mobility of the patient. In some instances, immunosuppressant drugs can reduce the inflammatory response.

Fibromyalgia

Fibromyalgia is a chronic, painful, rheumatoid-like disorder that affects 5 to 6 percent of the general population with bouts of muscle pain and extreme fatigue. Persons with fibromyalgia experience an array of other symptoms, including headaches, dizziness, numbness and tingling, itching, fluid retention, chronic joint pain, abdominal or pelvic pain, and even occasional diarrhea. Fibromyalgia usually is diagnosed in women in their thirties and forties. Suspected causes have ranged from sleep disturbances, stress, emotional distress, and viruses to autoimmune disorders; however, none has been proved in clinical trials. Because of fibromyalgia's multiple symptoms, it is usually diagnosed only after myriad tests have ruled out other disorders. The American College of Rheumatology identifies these major diagnostic criteria:[47]

- History of widespread pain of at least three months' duration in the axial skeleton as well as in all four quadrants of the body
- Pain in at least 11 of 18 paired tender points on digital palpation of about 4 kilograms of pressure

Treatments vary based on the severity of symptoms. Typically, adequate rest, stress management, relaxation techniques, dietary supplements and selected herbal remedies, and pain medications are prescribed. Patients are advised to avoid extreme temperatures, which can exacerbate symptoms.

Systemic Lupus Erythematosus

Systemic lupus erythematosus (SLE, or lupus) is an autoimmune disease in which antibodies destroy or injure organs such as the kidneys, brain, and heart. The symptoms include sensitivity to sunlight, arthritis, kidney problems, anemia, aching muscles and joints, and multiple infections; they range from mild to severe and may disappear for periods of time. A butterfly-shaped rash covering the bridge of the nose and both cheeks is common. The disease affects 1 in 700 Caucasians

rheumatoid arthritis   A serious inflammatory joint disease.

fibromyalgia   A chronic, rheumatoid-like disorder that can be highly painful and difficult to diagnose.

systemic lupus erythematosus (SLE, or lupus)   A disease in which the immune system attacks the body, producing antibodies that destroy or injure organs such as the kidneys, brain, and heart.

but 1 in 250 African Americans; 90 percent of all victims are females who show initial symptoms between the ages of 18 and 45. Extensive research has not yet found a cure for this sometimes fatal disease, although new studies suggest that there may be a genetic predisposition to it.

Scleroderma

Scleroderma (hardening of the skin) is a disease characterized by an increasing fibrous growth of connective tissue underlying the skin and body organs. These areas may form hard skin patches or a more generalized "ever-tightening case of steel," making movement difficult. Scleroderma may cause swelling of the hands, face, or feet. Symptoms range from minor discomfort to severe pain. In some instances, scleroderma is life-threatening.

Raynaud's Syndrome

For most of us, a few minutes in the cold causes only minor discomfort. For people suffering from **Raynaud's syndrome,** fingers and toes go numb, then turn white, then deep purple; as fingers and toes warm, they throb. Raynaud's is caused by exaggerated constriction of small arteries in the extremities that shunts blood away from them and toward the vital organs. It is believed that Raynaud's affects 5 to 10 percent of the population, with women accounting for the majority of sufferers. The cause is unknown. Treatment for Raynaud's consists of controlling body temperature by wearing warm gloves and boots, avoiding drugs that may alter blood flow (like nicotine), taking drugs to regulate blood flow, and surgery to improve circulation or repair damaged areas.

Low Back Pain

Approximately 85 percent of all Americans will experience low back pain (LBP) at some point. Some of these episodes result from muscular damage and are short-lived and acute; others may involve dislocations, fractures, or other problems with spinal vertebrae or discs, resulting in chronic pain or requiring surgery. Low back pain is epidemic throughout the world and the major cause of disability for people aged 20 to 45 in the United States, who suffer more frequently and severely from this problem than older people do.[48] See the Spotlight on Your Health box on page 568 for more on students with LBP.

LBP causes more lost work time in the United States than any other illness except upper respiratory infections. Back injuries are the most frequently mentioned complaints in injury-related lawsuits and result in high medical and rehabilitation bills, costing businesses and industries in the United States over $90 billion annually in direct and indirect costs.[49] As a result, employers throughout the country have become increasingly interested in preventing these injuries.

Risk Factors for Low Back Pain Health experts believe that the following factors contribute to LBP:

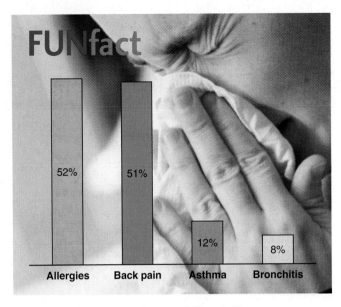

FIGURE 18.6 College Students and Chronic Illness
Do you think chronic diseases and health problems are only a concern for older Americans? Think again. College students are affected by chronic health issues, too.

Source: American College Health Association, American College Health Association-National College Health Assessment Web Summary, 2006, www.acha.org/projects_programs/ncha_sampledata.cfm.2006.

- *Age.* People between the ages of 20 and 45 run the greatest risk of LBP. At age 50, the condition becomes less common. After age 65, the incidence again rises, apparently because of bone and joint deterioration.
- *Body type.* Many studies have indicated that people who are very tall, or those with a high BMI, or lanky body type run an increased risk of LBP. However, much of this research is controversial.
- *Posture.* Poor posture may be one of the greatest contributors to LBP. If you routinely slouch, particularly during daily tasks, you run an increased risk.
- *Strength and fitness.* People with LBP tend to have less overall trunk strength than do other people. Weak abdominal muscles and back muscles also increase risk. In addition, one's total level of fitness and conditioning is a factor. The more fit you are, the better.
- *Psychological factors.* Numerous psychological factors appear to increase risk for LBP. Depression, apathy, inattentiveness, boredom, emotional upsets, drug abuse, and family and financial problems all heighten risk.

scleroderma A disease in which fibrous growth of connective tissue underlying the skin and body organs hardens and makes movement difficult.

Raynaud's syndrome A disease in which exposure to cold temperatures produces exaggerated constriction of the small arteries in the extremities, causing fingers and toes to go numb, turn white, and then turn deep purple.

COLLEGE STUDENTS AND LOWER BACK PAIN: OH, MY ACHING BACKPACK?

Are you wondering why over 52 percent of your college student peers suffer from problems with their backs? To answer this question, look no further than the typical student lugging around a backpack. What's inside this bulging portable office? Computers, books, bottled water, purses, iPods, Blackberries, headphones, cell phones, and a change of shoes or a T-shirt. The list may go on, or vary for some, but lugging such an assortment around each day can do some damage to your back.

> **Is my heavy backpack causing my back pain?**

Whereas hikers have long recognized the importance of internal frames and heavy-duty hip straps to displace the weight of heavy packs, most college students carry less supportive (and cheaper) daypacks with only a shoulder strap to carry as much as 30 to 40 pounds of weight. Over time, this weight can wreak havoc on even the most fit and healthy backs and shoulders. Older students are not alone; studies show that elementary school children are trying to emulate their older student models by carrying heavy backpacks in ever-increasing numbers—sometimes in amounts that are 10 to 15 percent of their total body weight. Because such repetitive strain on the back

can result in a lifetime of pain and disability, prevention is imperative. If you must carry a pack all day, consider the following:

- Opt for the lightest pack available and make sure that it has a heavy-duty hip strap, so that you are not carrying the bulk of the weight around your back and shoulders. Adjust the strap so that the weight is primarily on the hips.
- If you can afford a small internal-frame pack, invest in your back and buy one. There are many excellent packs available from mountain supply companies.
- Use and carry the lightest computer possible. Though big screens are nice, they add weight. Remember that a portable computer is meant to be portable. Those bigger varieties often are designed for business travelers who may use packs with wheels.
- Keep extras to a minimum when loading your pack each day. Xerox chapters of books you might want to read, rather than carrying a 5-pound book with you; carry a smaller note pad; store files on a jump drive and upload to a campus computer to do work.
- Limit the amount of personal non-essential items you carry each day. Wallets, makeup, hair products, etc., should be cut to a minimum.
- When lifting your pack to put it on your back, make sure you are standing with

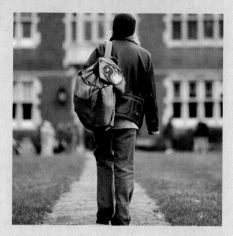

both feet on the ground, knees slightly flexed, and with your back straight. Common twisting of the back while swinging up the load can cause back injuries.
- Pack heavy items as close to the back, and the bottom, as possible.
- Once you're ready to go, weigh the pack. If it's over 15 pounds, reassess what is necessary and ditch some of the rest.

Sources: L. Hestbaek et al., "The Course of Low Back Pain from Adolesence to Adulthood: Eight-Year Follow-Up of 9,600 Twins", *Spine* 31, no. 4 (2006): 468–472; C. Hsin-Yu et al., "Gender-Age Environmental Associates of Middle-School Students' Low Back Pain," *IOS Press* 26, no. 1 (2006): 19–28, http://isopress.metapress.com/(wkwo3xaprfwq0a4525crreuv)/app/home/contribution.asp?

- *Occupational risk.* Type of work and work conditions greatly affect risk. For example, truck drivers, who must endure the bumps and jolts of the road while in a sitting position, frequently suffer from back pain.

Preventing Back Pain and Injury
What can you do to protect yourself from possible back injury? Almost 90 percent of all back problems occur in the lumbar region of the spine (lower back). You can avoid many problems by consciously maintaining good posture. Other preventive hints include the following:

- Purchase a supportive mattress, and avoid sleeping on your stomach.

- Avoid high-heeled shoes, which tilt the pelvis forward. Shoes should have good arch support.
- Control your weight.
- Lift objects with your legs, not your back.
- Buy a chair with good lumbar support for doing your work.
- Move your car seat forward so your knees are elevated slightly.
- Warm up before exercising.
- Exercise regularly—in particular, do exercises that strengthen the abdominal muscles and stretch the back muscles.

I t seems logical that we should allocate research dollars to health problems based on the number of people affected and the risk for death and disability associated with a particular disease. However, that is not necessarily how money is distributed. Disability rankings are based on complex formulas and calculations in which numbers of persons affected, age, degree of functional capacity lost, and death are factored together to assess the level of disability that a condition represents in a population. For example, if many people die or are disabled at a very young age from a particular condition, it would be ranked as more severe than if it killed only older people, due to accounting for years of potential life lost.

Consider the expenditures and disability rankings for the conditions shown below. Although heart disease exacts the greatest human toll, its funding for research, prevention, and intervention does not fully reflect the significance of its impact.

Do you notice any other large discrepancies between societal impact and level of federal funding for battling a disease? Does the ranking or funding for any disease

Disease Areas	NIH Funding in 2007: Millions of Dollars for Research (Estimates)	Disability Ranking
HIV/AIDS	2,888	15
Heart disease	2,103	1
Diabetes	1,053	8
Breast cancer	690	14
Prostate cancer	373	19
Schizophrenia	352	10
Stroke	338	4
Lung cancer	285	6
Asthma	295	17
Parkinson's disease	222	21
Multiple sclerosis	108	25

surprise you? If so, why? What factors might influence the amount of funding allocated for fighting a given disease or disability? What factors should influence funding priorities? Does the guideline of providing major research funding mainly for conditions that afflict numerous individuals disadvantage any groups of people? Explain your answer.

Source: National Institutes of Health, "Estimates of Funding for Various Diseases, Conditions, Research Areas," 2006, www.nih.gov/news/fundingresearchareas.htm.

Other Maladies

During the past 20 years, several afflictions have surfaced that seem to be products of our times. Some of these health problems relate to specific groups of people, some are due to technological advances, and others are still a mystery.

Chronic Fatigue Syndrome

Fatigue is a subjective condition in which people feel tired before they begin activities, lack the energy to accomplish tasks that require sustained effort and attention, or become abnormally exhausted after normal activities. All of us experience fatigue occasionally. Since the late 1980s, several U.S. clinics have noted a characteristic set of symptoms including chronic fatigue, headaches, fever, sore throat, enlarged lymph nodes, depression, poor memory, general weakness, nausea,

and symptoms remarkably similar to those of mononucleosis. Researchers initially believed these symptoms were caused by the same virus as mononucleosis, the Epstein-Barr virus. At first the disease was called *chronic Epstein-Barr disease,* or "yuppie flu," because the pattern of symptoms appeared most commonly in baby boomers. Some cases were so severe that patients required hospitalization. Since those initial studies, however, researchers have all but ruled out the Epstein-Barr virus. Despite extensive testing, no viral cause has been found to date.

Today, in the absence of a known pathogen, many researchers believe that the illness, now commonly referred to as **chronic fatigue syndrome (CFS),** may have strong

chronic fatigue syndrome (CFS) A condition of unknown cause characterized by extreme fatigue that is not caused by other illness.

psychosocial roots. Our heightened awareness of health makes some of us scrutinize our bodies so carefully that the slightest deviation becomes amplified. The more we focus on the body and on our perception of health, the worse we feel. In addition, the growing number of people who suffer from depression seem to be good candidates for chronic fatigue syndrome. Experts worry, however, that too many scientists approach CFS as something that is "in the person's head" and that such an attitude may prevent them from doing the serious research needed to find a cure.

The diagnosis of chronic fatigue syndrome depends on two major criteria and eight or more minor criteria. The major criteria are debilitating fatigue that persists for at least six months and the absence of other illnesses that could cause the symptoms. Minor criteria include headaches, fever, sore throat, painful lymph nodes, weakness, fatigue after exercise, sleep problems, and rapid onset of these symptoms. Because the cause is not apparent, treatment of CFS focuses on improved nutrition, rest, counseling for depression, judicious exercise, and development of a strong support network.

> **repetitive stress injury (RSI)**   An injury to nerves, soft tissue, or joints due to the physical stress of repeated motions.
>
> **carpal tunnel syndrome**   A common occupational injury in which the median nerve in the wrist becomes irritated, causing numbness, tingling, and pain in the fingers and hands.

Repetitive Stress Injuries

It's the end of the term, and you have finished the last of several papers. After hours of nonstop typing, your hands are numb and you feel an intense, burning pain that makes the thought of typing one more word almost unbearable. If you are like one of the thousands of students and workers who every year must stop doing a particular task due to pain, you may be suffering from a **repetitive stress injury (RSI).** These are injuries to nerves, soft tissue, or joints that result from the physical stress of repeated motions.

Although no good mechanism of reporting exists for students suffering from RSIs, the U.S. Bureau of Labor Statistics estimates that 25 percent of all injuries in the labor force that result in lost work time are due to repetitive motion or stress injuries. RSIs cost employers over $22 billion a year in workers' compensation and an additional $85 billion in related costs, such as absenteeism.

One of the most common RSIs is **carpal tunnel syndrome,** a product of both the information age and the age of technology in general. Hours spent typing at the computer, flipping groceries through computerized scanners, or other jobs "made simpler" by technology can irritate the median nerve in the wrist, causing numbness, tingling, and pain in the fingers and hands. Although carpal tunnel syndrome risk can be reduced by proper placement of the keyboard, mouse, wrist pads, and other techniques, RSIs are often overlooked until significant damage has been done. Better education and ergonomic workplace designs can eliminate many injuries of this nature.

TAKING charge

Summary

- Chronic lung diseases include allergies, hay fever, asthma, emphysema, and chronic bronchitis. Allergies are part of the body's natural defense system. Chronic obstructive pulmonary diseases (COPDs) are the fourth leading cause of death in the United States. Sleep apnea is another breathing-related malady increasing in prevalence.
- Neurological conditions include headaches and seizure disorders. Headaches may be caused by a variety of factors, the most common of which are tension, dilation and/or contraction of blood vessels in the brain, chemical influences on muscles and vessels that cause inflammation and pain, and underlying physiological and psychological disorders. The most common types of headache are tension, migraine, and cluster. Other neurological disorders include Parkinson's disease and multiple sclerosis.

- Several modern maladies affect only women. Fibrocystic breast condition is a common, noncancerous buildup of irregular tissue. Endometriosis is the buildup of endometrial tissue in regions of the body other than the uterus.
- Diabetes develops when the pancreas fails to produce enough insulin to regulate sugar metabolism. Its increase in prevalence is related to increases in obesity and other factors. Other conditions, such as colitis, irritable bowel syndrome, gallbladder disease, and peptic ulcers, are the direct result of functional problems in various digestion-related organs or systems. Pathogens, problems in enzyme or hormone production, anxiety or stress, functional abnormalities, and other problems are possible causes.
- Musculoskeletal diseases such as arthritis, fibromyalgia, systemic lupus erythematosus, scleroderma, Raynaud's

syndrome, and lower back pain cause significant pain and disability in millions of people. Age, occupation, gender, posture, abdominal strength, and psychological factors contribute to the development of lower back problems.

■ Chronic fatigue syndrome (CFS) and repetitive stress injuries (such as carpal tunnel syndrome) have emerged as major chronic maladies. CFS is associated with depression. Repetitive stress injuries are preventable by proper equipment placement and usage.

Chapter Review

1. Diseases and unknown disorders of the human body that appear to have no explanation are referred to as
   a. homeopathic.
   b. mysterious.
   c. idiopathic.
   d. psychotic.

2. Diabetes mellitus does not allow the body to
   a. metabolize sugars.
   b. produce insulin.
   c. respond to saturated fats in the diet.
   d. All of the above.

3. Typically, older people develop type 2 diabetes. Today, however, many more _____ are developing type 2 diabetes.
   a. babies
   b. children and teenagers
   c. college-aged young adults
   d. pregnant women

4. The gradual destruction of the alveoli in a smoker's lung usually causes the respiratory condition
   a. dyspnea.
   b. bronchitis.
   c. emphysema.
   d. asthma.

5. School-aged children miss school for this condition more than any other illness.
   a. bronchitis
   b. coughs and colds
   c. attention deficit disorder
   d. asthma

6. Julie has found that she cannot seem to handle a glass of milk without suffering from cramps and diarrhea. The same symptoms happen when she consumes cheese or ice cream. What condition is she likely to be suffering from?
   a. irritable bowel syndrome
   b. colitis
   c. lactose intolerance
   d. diabetes

7. Which of the following conditions is the leading cause of employee sick time and lost productivity in the United States?
   a. low back pain
   b. upper respiratory infections
   c. asthma
   d. on the job injuries

8. One of the most common forms of repetitive stress injury (RSI) is
   a. low back pain from overexertion.
   b. carpal tunnel of the wrist or hand.
   c. arthritis from bending the knees too often.
   d. headaches caused by neck tension.

9. Margaret experiences attacks of wheezing, difficulty in breathing, shortness of breath, and coughing spasms on occasion. What chronic respiratory disorder is she likely suffering from?
   a. sleep apnea
   b. bronchitis
   c. asthma
   d. chronic obstructive pulmonary disease

10. Type 1 diabetes is a form of
    a. adult-onset diabetes.
    b. insulin-dependent diabetes.
    c. narcolepsy.
    d. type 2 diabetes.

Answers to these questions can be found on page A-1.

Questions for Discussion and Reflection

1. What are some of the major noninfectious chronic diseases affecting Americans today? Do you think there is a pattern in the types of diseases that we get? What are the common risk factors?
2. List the common respiratory diseases affecting Americans. Which of these diseases has a genetic basis? An environmental basis? An individual basis? What, if anything, is being done to prevent, treat, or control each of these conditions?
3. Compare and contrast the different types of headaches, including their symptoms and treatments.
4. What are the medical risks of fibrocystic breast condition and endometriosis? How can they be treated?
5. Describe the risk factors for diabetes and its symptoms and treatment. What is the difference between type 1 diabetes and type 2 diabetes?
6. Compare the symptoms of colitis, diverticulosis, peptic ulcers, and gallbladder disease. How can you tell whether your stomach is reacting to final exams or telling you that you have a serious medical condition?
7. What are the major disorders of the musculoskeletal system? Why do you think there aren't any cures? Describe the difference between osteoarthritis and rheumatoid arthritis.
8. Chronic fatigue syndrome (CFS) is often associated with depression. Experts argue about whether depression precedes CFS or CFS causes depression. What do you think?

Accessing Your Health on the Internet

The following websites explore further topics and issues related to personal health. You'll also find links to each organization's website on the Companion Website for *Access to Health*, Tenth Edition, at www.aw-bc.com/donatelle.

1. *American Academy of Allergy, Asthma, and Immunology.* Provides an overview of asthma information, particularly as it applies to children with allergies. Offers interactive quizzes to test your knowledge as well as an "ask the expert" section. www.aaai.org
2. *American Diabetes Association.* Excellent resource for diabetes information. www.diabetes.org
3. *American Lung Association.* Includes the latest in asthma news, including a free monthly newsletter, *The Breathe Easy/Asthma Digest.* www.lungusa.org
4. *National Center for Chronic Disease Prevention and Health Promotion (NCCDPHP).* Access to a wide range of information from this CDC-linked organization dedicated to chronic diseases and health promotion. www.cdc.gov/nccdphp
5. *National Institute of Neurological Disorders and Stroke.* Many of the modern maladies result in chronic pain. This site provides up-to-date information to help you cope with pain-related difficulties. www.ninds.nih.gov

Further Reading

National Center for Health Statistics. *Monthly Vital Statistics Report* and *Advance Data from Vital and Health Statistics.* Hyattsville, MD: Public Health Service.

Detailed government reports, usually published monthly, concerning mortality and morbidity data for the United States, including changes occurring in the rates of particular diseases and in health practices so patterns and trends can be analyzed.

Public Health Services, Centers for Disease Control. *Chronic Disease News and Notes.* Washington, DC: U.S. Department of Health and Human Services.

Quarterly publication focusing on relevant chronic disease topics and issues.

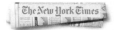

e-themes from *The New York Times*

For up-to-date articles about current health issues, visit www.aw-bc.com/donatelle, select *Access to Health*, Tenth Edition, Chapter 18, and click on "e-themes."

References

1. National Center for Health Statistics, "Health, United States, 2005," 2006, www.cdc.gov/nchs/hus.htm.
2. American Lung Association, "Results from the National Health Interview Survey, 1998–2004," 2006, www.lungusa.org; American Lung Association Epidemiology and Statistics Unit, "Trends in Chronic Bronchitis and Emphysema Morbidity and Mortality," 2005, www.lungusa.org.
3. Ibid.
4. Ibid.
5. Ibid.
6. B. Sean et al., "Early Emphysematous Changes in Asymptomatic Smokers: Detection with 3HE Imaging Radiology," *Radiology* 239 (2006): 875–883.
7. MayoClinic.com, "Asthma Signs and Symptoms," 2004, www.mayoclinic.com/invoke.cfm?id=DS00021.
8. R. Cohn et al., "National Prevalence and Exposure Risk of Cockroach Allergies in U.S. Households," *Environmental Health Perspectives* 114, no. 4 (2006): 522–526.
9. American Lung Association, "Asthma Trends," 2006, www.lungusa.org.
10. Ibid.
11. Asthma and Allergy Foundation of America, "Allergy Facts," 2006, www.aafa.org.
12. National Center for Health Statistics, "FASTSATS: Allergies and Hay Fever," 2006, www.cdc.gov/nchs/fastats/allergies.htm.
13. National Sleep Foundation, "Sleep Apnea," 2006, www.sleepfoundation.org/publications/sleepap.cfm; American Sleep Apnea Association, "Information about Sleep Apnea," 2006, www.sleepapnea.org/geninfo.html.
14. Ibid.
15. National Headache Foundation, "Headache Topic Sheets," 2006, www.headaches.org.
16. Ibid.
17. Ibid.
18. Ibid.
19. Ibid.
20. Ibid.
21. MayoClinic.com, "Cluster Headache," 2005, www.mayoclinic.com/invoke.cfm?id=DS00487.
22. National Headache Foundation, *Cluster Headache*, 2006, www.headache.org/consumer.
23. Epilepsy Foundation, "About Epilepsy," 2006, www.epilepsyfoundation.org/answerplace/ABOUTepilepsy.cfm.
24. Ibid.
25. National Parkinson Foundation, "Parkinson Primer," 2006, www.parkinson.org.
26. Ibid.
27. Multiple Sclerosis Foundation, "Frequently Asked Questions," 2006, www.msfacts.org/info_faq.php.
28. Ibid.
29. Centers for Disease Control and Prevention, "National Diabetes Fact Sheet," 2006, www.cdc.gov/diabetes/statistics.
30. Ibid.
31. Ibid.
32. Ibid.
33. Ibid.
34. Ibid.
35. American Diabetes Association, "Statistics," 2006, www.diabetes.org/diabetesstatistics.jsp.
36. H. Brekke et al., "Long-Term Effects of Lifestyle Intervention in Type 2 Diabetes Relatives," *Diabetes Research and Clinical Practice* 70 (2005): 225–234.
37. L. Azadbakaht et al., "Beneficial Effects of Dietary Approaches to Stop Hypertension Eating Plan on Features of the Metabolic Syndrome," *Diabetes Care* 29 (2006): 954–955.
38. Centers for Disease Control and Prevention, "National Diabetes Fact Sheet."
39. American Diabetes Association, "Statistics."
40. American Diabetes Association, "Complications of Diabetes in the United States," 2006, www.diabetes.org.
41. E. Hills, "Mechanical Low Back Pain," 2006, www.emedicine.com/pmr/topic13.htm.
42. Centers for Disease Control and Prevention, "Direct and Indirect Costs of Arthritis and Other Rheumatic Conditions in the U.S." *Morbidity and Mortality Weekly Report* 53 (2004): 388–389.
43. Arthritis Foundation, "Osteoarthritis," 2006, www.arthritis.org/conditions/DiseaseCenter/oa.asp.
44. Ibid.
45. Ibid.
46. Ibid.
47. R. Brownson, P. Remington, and J. Davis, eds., *Chronic Disease Epidemiology and Control* (Washington, DC: American Public Health Association, 1998), 389.
48. National Institute of Neurological Disorders and Stroke, Low Back Pain Fact Sheet, 2006, www.ninds.nin.gov/disorders/backpain/detail_backpain.htm.
49. X. Luo et al., "Care and Indemnity Costs Across a Natural History of Disability in Outpatient Low Back Pain," *Spine* 29, no. 1 (2004): 79–86.

19

Healthy Aging

A LIFELONG PROCESS

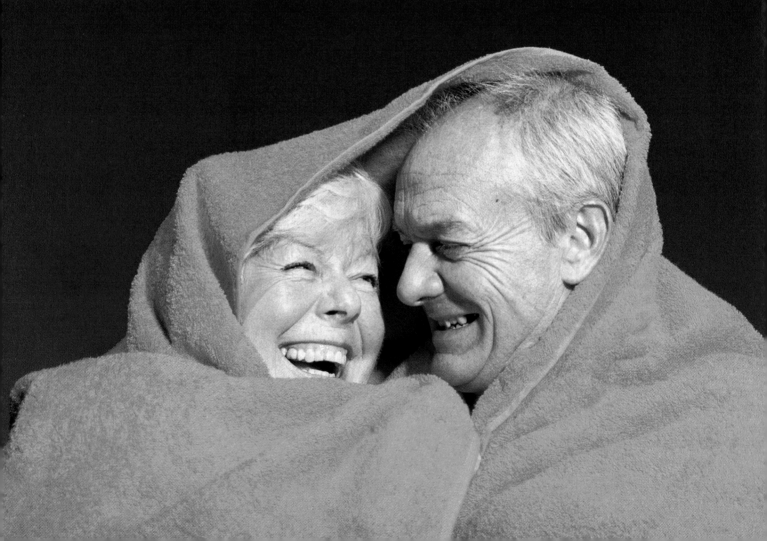

Is it really possible to "age **gracefully**"?

Can the **government** meet the needs of our aging population?

What types of physical **changes** can I expect as I grow older?

Is there a cure for **Alzheimer's** yet?

What makes **stem cells** different from other types of cells?

OBJECTIVES

- Define aging, and explain the related concepts of biological, psychological, social, legal, and functional age.
- Explain how the growing population of older adults will impact society, including considerations of economics, health care, living arrangements, and ethical and moral issues.
- Discuss the biological and psychosocial theories of aging, and examine how knowledge of these theories may have an impact on your own aging process.
- Summarize major physiological changes that occur as a result of the aging process.
- Discuss unique health challenges faced by older adults, such as alcohol abuse, use of prescription medication and over-the-counter drugs, osteoporosis, urinary incontinence, depression, and Alzheimer's disease.
- Discuss strategies for healthy aging that can begin during young adulthood.

Grow old along with me!
The best is yet to be,
The last of life, for which the first was made . . .

—Robert Browning, *Rabbi Ben Ezra*

I n a society that seems to worship youth, researchers have begun to offer good—even revolutionary—news about the aging process: growing old doesn't have to mean a slow slide to disability, loneliness, and declining physical and mental health. Health promotion, disease prevention, and wellness-oriented activities can prolong vigor and productivity, even among those who haven't always led model lifestyles or made healthful habits a priority. In fact, getting older can mean getting better in many ways—particularly socially, psychologically, and intellectually.

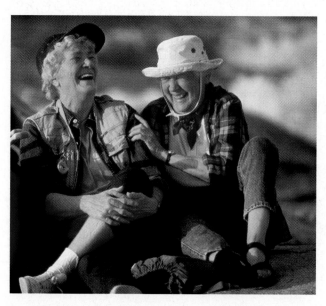

For many, the secret to aging well is to stay active and enjoy the company of good friends.

Growing Old: Life Passages

Every moment of every day, we are involved in a steady aging process. Everything in the universe—animals, plants, mountains, rivers, planets, even atoms—changes over time. This process is commonly referred to as aging. Aging is something that we cannot avoid, despite the perennial human quest for a fountain of youth. Since you can't stop the clock, why not resolve to have a positive aging experience by improving your understanding of this process, taking steps to maximize your potential, and developing strengths you can draw upon over a lifetime?

The manner in which you view aging (either as a natural part of living or an inevitable decline toward disease and death) is a crucial factor in how successfully you will adapt to life's transitions. If you view these transitions as periods of growth, as changes that will lead to improved mental, emotional, spiritual, and physical phases in your development as a human being, your journey through even the most difficult times will be easier. No doubt you have encountered vigorous 80-year-olds who wake up every morning looking forward to whatever challenges the day may bring. Such persons are socially active, have a zest for life, and seem much younger than their chronological ages. In contrast, you have probably met 50-year-olds who lack energy and enthusiasm, who seem resigned to tread water for the rest of their lives. These

people often appear much older than their chronological age. In short, people experience the aging process in different ways. Explore your own notions about aging with the Assess Yourself box on page 578.

Aging has traditionally been described as the patterns of life changes that occur in members of all species as they grow older. Some believe that it begins at the moment of conception. Others contend that it starts at birth. Still others believe that true aging does not begin until we reach our forties.

Typically, experts and laypersons alike have used chronological age to assign a person to a particular life cycle stage. However, people of different chronological ages view age very differently. To the 4-year-old, a college freshman seems quite old. To the 20-year-old, parents in their forties are over the hill. Views of aging are also colored by occupation. For example, most professional athletes are considering other careers by the time they reach 40, while writers, musicians, and even college professors may work well into their seventies and eighties. Perhaps we need to reexamine our traditional definitions of aging.

Redefining Aging

The study of individual and collective aging processes, known as **gerontology,** explores the reasons for aging and the ways in which people cope with and adapt to this process. Gerontologists have identified several age-related characteristics that define where a person is in terms of biological, psychological, social, legal, and functional life-stage development:[1]

■ *Biological age* refers to the relative age or condition of the person's organs and body systems. Research shows that healthy lifestyle behaviors such as being active, eating a healthy diet, and not smoking are the most influential factors on how your body ages.[2]

aging The patterns of life changes that occur in members of all species as they grow older.

gerontology The study of individual and collective aging processes.

- *Psychological age* refers to a person's adaptive capacities, such as coping abilities and intelligence, and to the person's awareness of his or her individual capabilities, self-efficacy, and general ability to adapt to new situations. Research documents that older adults maintain a positive attitude and do successfully cope with the physical and cognitive changes associated with aging.[3] Even if chronic illness renders someone physically handicapped, the person may have tremendous psychological reserves and remain alert and fully capable of making decisions.
- *Social age* refers to a person's habits and roles relative to society's expectations. People in a particular life stage often share similar tastes in music and television shows, for example.
- *Legal age* is probably the most common definition of age in the United States. Based on chronological years, legal age is used as a factor in determining voting rights, driving privileges, drinking age, eligibility for Social Security payments, and a host of other rights and obligations.
- *Functional age* refers to the ways—heart rate, hearing, etc.—in which people compare to others of a similar age. It is difficult to separate functional aging from many of the other types of aging, particularly chronological and biological aging.

What Is Successful Aging?

As people pass through critical periods in their lives, gerontologists discuss whether they are aging "successfully." Those who are successful usually develop positive coping skills that carry over into other areas of their lives. They have realistic, achievable goals that bring them pleasure and they tend to think confidently and independently. In short, successful agers are more prepared to "experience" life. Those who are less successful in these rites of passage either develop a sense of learned helplessness and lose confidence in their ability to succeed or learn to compensate for their failures in other ways (Figure 19.1).

Today, it is easier to find positive examples of aging than at any other time in our history. Many of today's "elderly" individuals lead active, productive lives. For instance, 49,000 Americans aged 65 and older are currently enrolled in college, and 14 percent are employed. By the year 2030, one quarter of those over 65 will have an undergraduate degree.[4]

Typically, people who have aged successfully have the following characteristics:

- In general, they have managed to avoid serious, debilitating diseases and disability.
- They function well physically, live independently, and engage in most normal activities of daily living.
- They have maintained cognitive function and are actively engaged in mentally challenging and stimulating activities.
- They are actively engaged in social and productive pursuits.
- They are resilient and able to cope reasonably well with physical, social, and emotional changes.
- They believe that they have a sense of control over circumstances in their lives.[5]

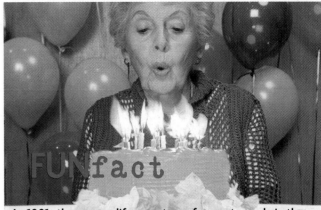

In 1901, the average life expectancy for most people in the United States was 40 years old. Flash forward 105 years, and many can expect to live an average of 77.85 years, an increase of 38 percent since the turn of the twentieth century.

FIGURE 19.1 Looking Back: Changes in Average Life Expectancy between 1901 and 2006

Although the process of aging has often been viewed with dread due to physical changes that inevitably occur, only in the past decade have we begun to fully appreciate the gains and positive aspects of normal adult development throughout the life span. According to gerontologist Dr. Karen Hooker, older adults as a population display much more differentiation in personalities, coping styles, and "possible selves" than any other age group. She states that "successful aging and development as individuals can be viewed as dynamic processes of adaptation between the self and the environment. Throughout our lives we make choices and respond to changes in vastly different ways. Each person is born with certain traits that stay reasonably stable throughout life, but character is deeply affected by personal action constructs that change with time and life history."[6] Thus, aging is not a static process, but one in which each of us changes and becomes someone uniquely fashioned by our life's story.

Gerontologists have devised several categories for specific age-related characteristics. People aged 65 to 74 are viewed as the **young-old**; those aged 75 to 84 are the **middle-old** group; those 85 and over are classified as the **old-old**.

Is it really possible to "age gracefully"?

However, the question is not how many years someone has lived, but how much life the person has packed into those years. This quality-of-life index, combined with the chronological process, appears to be the best indicator of the

young-old People aged 65 to 74.

middle-old People aged 75 to 84.

old-old People aged 85 and over.

ASSESS yourself

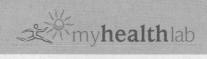

WHERE DO YOU WANT TO BE?

Fill out this assessment online at
www.aw-bc.com/MyHealthLab or
www.aw-bc.com/donatelle.

When we are young, aging is the furthest thing from our minds. However, thinking about aging and what we expect from life are important elements of a satisfying adult develop- ment process. Take a few minutes to answer the following questions. Your answers may tell you a great deal about yourself.

1. At this point in your life, what do you value most?
2. What do you think will be most important to you when you reach your forties? Fifties? Sixties? What similarities and differences do you notice, and what causes these similarities and differences?
3. Do you think your parents are happy with the way their lives have turned out? If they could change anything, what do you think they might do differently?
4. What about your own direction thus far in life is similar to that of your parents? What have you done differently? Are the similarities and differences good? Why or why not?
5. What do you think are the keys to a happy and satisfying life?
6. What do you want to accomplish by the time you are 40? By the time you are 50? By the time you are 60?
7. Have you ever thought of retirement? Describe your retirement.
8. Describe the "you" that you would like to be at the age of 70. How is that person similar to or different from the "you" of today? What actions will you need to take to be that person in the future?

MAKE it happen!

ASSESSMENT: The Assess Yourself activity above encouraged you to consider some of the deepest questions in life: What are your values? How do you want your life to compare with that of your parents? How would you like to be described at age 70? Now that you have considered your an- swers, perhaps there are actions you can take that will help you create the life you want.

MAKING A CHANGE: In order to change your behavior, you need to develop a plan. Follow the steps below and complete your Behavior Change Contract to take action:

1. Evaluate your behavior and identify patterns and specific things you are doing. What can you change now? What can you change in the near future?

2. Select one pattern of behavior that you want to change.

3. Fill out the Behavior Change Contract found at the front of your book. It should include your long-term goal for change, your short-term goals, the rewards you'll give yourself for reaching these goals, potential obstacles along the way, and strategies for overcoming these ob- stacles. For each goal, list the small steps and specific actions that you will take.

4. Chart your progress in a journal. At the end of a week, consider how successful you were in following your plan. What helped you be successful? What made change more difficult? What will you do differently next week?

5. Revise your plan as needed: Are the short-term goals attainable? Are the rewards satisfying?

ONE STUDENT'S PLAN: When Eric answered the Assess Yourself questions, he realized he had not thought deeply about where he wanted to be at various stages in his life. In particular, he wanted to take more time to look at his parents' lives and careers, as well as those of older adults around him in the community. He set a goal of asking his parents and grandparents some of these same questions about their goals and lives to see where he might agree and disagree with them and how he might develop his own val- ues and priorities. As he began thinking more seriously about the types of careers that he thought might be fulfilling, he arranged to meet with adults who had gone into professions that he was considering. He also decided to take a philoso- phy class as one of his electives in the next year, in which he could actually get school credit for thinking about these big questions.

---

phenomenon of "aging gracefully." Most experts agree that the best way to experience a productive, full, and satisfying old age is to lead a productive, full, and satisfying life prior to old age. Essentially, older people are the product of their life- long experiences and behaviors.

Older Adults: A Growing Population

There are 36.3 million people aged 65 or older in the United States, over 13 percent of the total population. The number of older Americans has increased more than tenfold since 1900, when there were only 3 million people aged 65 or older (4 percent of the total population). The number of those 65 and over is projected to hit 71.5 million by 2030, almost 20 percent of the U.S. population (Figure 19.2).[7] Other nations report a similar trend. The World Health Organization predicts that, worldwide by 2050, there will be more people over the age of 60 than those under 60 for the first time in human history (see the Health in a Diverse World box on page 581).[8] Within the United States, the population of those over 65 will increase substantially over the next two decades, due to the aging "baby boomer" generation. Researchers at the Administration on Aging predict that this will have a major impact on housing, health care, and social services for the elderly.[9]

What will this growth of the over-65 population mean to the American economy, health care system, and social structure? Leaders must take a proactive stance in developing programs and services to promote health and prevent premature disease and disability. In Utah, state officials are targeting 40-year-olds through their Healthy Aging program, encouraging regular checkups, exercise, healthy eating habits, and overall improved health behaviors. More health plans are considering ways to motivate clients to take more initiative and to work harder at health improvements that will save insurers money in the long run. Instead of focusing on negative aspects of aging, more health and social service leaders are focusing on "successful aging—what it means and what it will take to ensure that each of us can achieve it." By enhancing collective understanding of the aging process and the role of current behaviors in developing lifetime habits to inoculate us against the stresses and strains of living, we will improve our chances of achieving our "possible selves."

Health Issues for an Aging Society

Can the government meet the needs of our aging population?

The concerns of government officials over the impending growth in the older population center around meeting this population's financial and medical needs. No doubt you have heard discussions on the potential bankruptcy of the Social Security system and the large increases in out-of-pocket costs for people on Medicare. According to the latest statistics, life expectancy for a person born in 2006 is 77.9 years, about 30 years longer than for a child born in 1900.[10]

With fewer people contributing to the system and greater numbers drawing on it, the likelihood of problems arising is

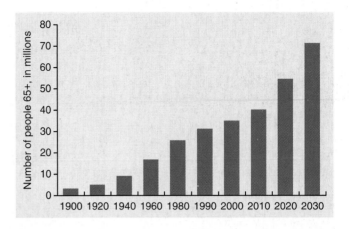

FIGURE 19.2 Number of Americans Aged 65 and Older (in Millions)

Source: Administration on Aging, "A Profile of Older Americans: 2005," 2005, www.aoa.gov/prof/Statistics/profile/2005/2005profile.pdf.

great. Where will these older people live? How will they pay for their medical costs, and how long will they need to work to support themselves? These and other questions pose many challenges for all of us.

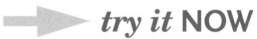

try it NOW

Estimate your life expectancy. How long you live has to do with a lot more than just good genes. Healthy behaviors, which you have control over, have a direct impact on whether or not you'll live to see 100. Visit this life expectancy calculator website to see how long you'll live: www.livingto100.com/lifecalc.html?accept.php.

Health Care Costs

Today, older Americans average $3,899 per year in out-of-pocket medical expenses, an increase of 46 percent since 1993.[11] As people live longer, the chances of developing a costly chronic disease increase, and as technology improves, chronic illnesses that once were quickly fatal may now be treated successfully for years. Projected future costs are staggering. Health care expenditures rise with age, and 77 million baby boomers are now in middle age. Compared with people ages 18 to 44, people ages 45 to 64 are nearly three times more likely to be disabled, six times more likely to have high blood pressure, and 15 times more likely to die of cancer. Meeting the nation's long-term care needs will become even more challenging as the population ages and more people require assistance with living. By the year 2020, 12 million older Americans will need long-term care, and most will be cared for at home. Whereas the majority of the elderly are cared for by family and friends, a study by the U.S. Department of Health and Human Services indicates that those who reach the age of 65 will have a 40 percent chance of entering a nursing home.[12]

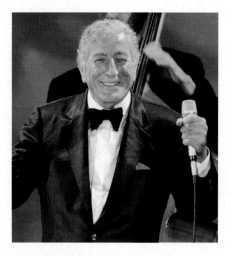
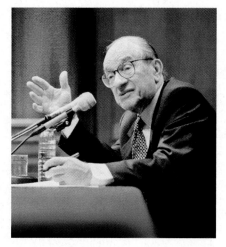
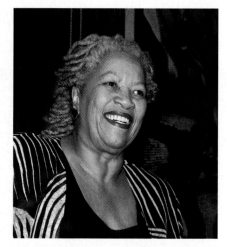

Singer Tony Bennett, economist Alan Greenspan, and author Toni Morrison are examples of people who stay active and vigorous in their professions well into their seventies and eighties.

Another large group of Americans falls into the category of "uninsured" or "underinsured"—those having only small levels of insurance, usually insufficient for their needs. It is important to note here that the highest percentage of uninsured Americans today (22 percent) occurs in the 15- to 44-year-old age group; another 13 percent are in the 45- to 64-year-old age group. Recent stock market downturns and company failures that wiped out retirement savings may make it even more difficult for older Americans to afford health insurance in the next decade. For more on health insurance, see Chapter 22.

Major questions loom: Will working Americans be willing to pay an increased share of the health care costs for people on fixed incomes who cannot pay for themselves? If not, what will become of older Americans? Perhaps most important, who will ultimately pay?

Housing and Living Arrangements

Contrary to popular opinion, most older people (over 95 percent) never live in a nursing home. Many continue to live with a spouse; others live alone or make other arrangements such as living with relatives or friends (Figure 19.3 on page 582). Community living, assisted living, skilled nursing care, and other options are new possibilities for those who have financial means or who have purchased some form of long-term-care insurance. However, housing problems for the low-income elderly remain. Who will provide the necessary social services, and who will pay the bill? Will the family of the future be forced to coexist with several generations under one roof?

Ethical and Moral Considerations

Difficult ethical questions arise when we consider the implications of an increasing population of older adults for an already overburdened health care system. Given the shortage of donor organs, will we be forced to decide whether a 50-year-old should receive a heart transplant instead of a 75-year-old? The debate over stem cell research asks us to balance scientific achievements with questions of morality (see the Health Ethics box on page 583). Is the prolongation of life at all costs a moral imperative, or will future generations be forced to devise a set of criteria for deciding who will be helped and who will not? Understanding the process of aging and knowing what actions you can take to prolong your own healthy years are part of our collective responsibility.

what do you THINK?

What do you think people over 65 would do if they suddenly didn't have Medicare? ■ Why are the aging of the population and the impending difficulties with health care costs and access important to all of us?

Theories on Aging
Biological Theories

Explanations for the biological causes of aging include the following:

■ *The wear-and-tear theory* states that, like everything else in the universe, the human body wears out. Inherent in this theory is the idea that the more you abuse your body, the faster it will wear out. Fortunately, today's older adults can achieve high levels of fitness without having to be marathoners. Strength training, walking, gardening, yoga, tai chi, and other activities allow even the most out of shape to improve. You don't have to feel pain to realize healthy gains.

AGING: THE WORLD'S OLDEST COUNTRIES

The growth of older populations around the world results from major achievements—reliable birth control that has decreased fertility rates, improvements in medical care and sanitation that have reduced infant and maternal mortality and infectious and parasitic diseases, and improvements in nutrition and education. Every month, the net increase in the world's population aged 60 and over is more than 1 million; 70 percent of this increase occurs in developing countries and 30 percent in industrialized countries. Between 2005 and 2050, the world population over age 60 is projected to more than double, to 22 percent, hitting 2 billion people. Nearly two-thirds of this growth will be in less developed nations, such as Malaysia and Colombia, where the growth of the older population is projected to triple in size by the year 2030. Almost half of today's older adults live in just four nations: China, India, Russia, and the United States. (The chart shows countries with the highest percentages of people over 60.) China, in particular, will continue to experience a boom in its aging population, with 349 million people aged 65 and older by the year 2050.

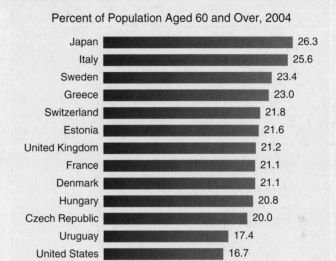

Percent of Population Aged 60 and Over, 2004

Country	Percent
Japan	26.3
Italy	25.6
Sweden	23.4
Greece	23.0
Switzerland	21.8
Estonia	21.6
United Kingdom	21.2
France	21.1
Denmark	21.1
Hungary	20.8
Czech Republic	20.0
Uruguay	17.4
United States	16.7

Source: United Nations Population Division, "World Population Prospects Population Database," 2005, http://esa.un.orgunpp.

Sources: United Nations, "World Population Prospects: 2004 Revision," 2005, www.un.org/esa/population/publications/wpp2004_volume 3.htm; U.S. Bureau of the Census, *Global Aging: Comparative Indicators and Future Trends* (Washington, DC: Government Printing Office, 1991); U.S. Bureau of the Census, International Programs Center, "International Database," 1998; United Nations Population Division, "World Population Prospects Population Database," 2005, http://esa.un.org/unpp.

- *The cellular theory* states that at birth we have only a certain number of usable cells, which are genetically programmed to divide or reproduce a limited number of times. Once these cells reach the end of their reproductive cycle, they die, and the organs they make up begin to deteriorate. The rate of deterioration varies from person to person, and its impact depends on the system involved.

- *The autoimmune theory* attributes aging to the decline of the body's immunological system. Studies indicate that as we age, our immune systems become less effective in fighting disease. Eventually, bodies that are subjected to too much stress, lack of sleep, and so on, show signs of disease and infirmity, especially if these factors are coupled with poor nutrition. In some instances, the immune system appears to lose control and turn its protective mechanisms inward, actually attacking the person's own body. Although autoimmune disorders occur in all age groups, some gerontologists believe that they increase in frequency and severity with age.

- *The genetic mutation theory* proposes that the number of cells exhibiting unusual or different characteristics increases with age. Proponents of this theory believe that aging is related to the amount of mutational damage within the genes. The greater the mutation, the greater the chance that cells will not function properly, leading to eventual dysfunction of body organs and systems.

Psychosocial Impacts on Aging

Numerous psychological and sociological factors also influence the manner in which people age. Psychologists Erik Erikson and Robert Peck have formulated theories of

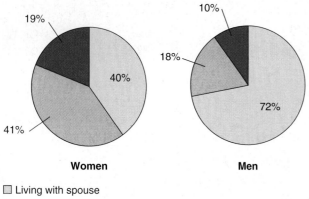

FIGURE 19.3 Living Arrangements of Americans Aged 65 and Older

☐ Living with spouse
☐ Living alone
■ Other

Source: Administration on Aging, "A Profile of Older Americans: 2005," 2005, www.aoa.gov/prof/Statistics/profile/2005/2005profile.pdf.

personality development that emphasize adaptation and adjustment. In his developmental model, Erikson states that people must progress through eight critical stages during a lifetime. If a person does not receive the proper stimulus or develop effective methods of coping with life's turmoil from infancy onward, problems are likely to develop later in life. According to this theory, maladjustments in old age are often a result of problems encountered in earlier stages of a person's life.

Peck argues that during middle and old age, people face a series of increasingly stressful tasks. Those who are poorly adjusted psychologically or who have not developed appropriate coping skills are likely to undergo a painful aging process.

A new group of "postive psychology" theorists believe that an optimistic attitude, having strong social networks, and remaining both mentally and physically engaged may have significant effects on healthy aging.

Changes in the Body and Mind
Typical Physical Changes

Although the physiological consequences of aging can differ in severity and timing, certain standard changes occur as a result of the aging process.

osteoporosis A degenerative bone disorder characterized by increasingly porous bones.

urinary incontinence Inability to control urination.

What types of physical changes can I expect as I grow older?

The Skin As a normal consequence of aging, the skin becomes thinner and loses elasticity, particularly in the outer surfaces. Fat deposits, which add to the soft lines and shape of the skin, diminish. Starting at about age 30, lines develop on the forehead as a result of sun exposure and facial expressions such as smiling and frowning. These lines become more pronounced, with added "crow's feet" around the eyes, during the forties. During a person's fifties and sixties, the skin begins to sag and lose color, leading to pallor in the seventies. Body fat in underlying layers of skin continues to be redistributed away from the limbs and extremities into the trunk region of the body. Age spots become more numerous because of excessive pigment accumulation under the skin, particularly in those with heavy sun exposure.

Bones and Joints Throughout the life span, bones are continually changing because of the accumulation and loss of minerals. By the third or fourth decade of life, mineral loss from bones becomes more prevalent than mineral accumulation, resulting in a weakening and porosity (diminishing density) of bony tissue. This loss of minerals (particularly calcium) occurs in both sexes, although it is much more common in females. Loss of calcium can contribute to **osteoporosis,** a disease characterized by low bone density and structural deterioration of bone tissue. These porous, fragile bones are susceptible to fracture.[13] (See the Spotlight on Your Health box on page 585.)

Another bone condition that afflicts almost 21 million Americans is osteoarthritis, a progressive breakdown of joint cartilage that becomes more common with age and is the leading cause of disability in the United States.[14] For information on osteoarthritis and other forms of arthritis, see Chapter 18.

The Head With age, features of the head enlarge and become more noticeable. Increased cartilage and fatty tissue cause the nose to grow a half inch wider and another half inch longer. Earlobes get fatter and longer, while overall head circumference increases one quarter of an inch per decade, even though the brain itself shrinks, because the skull becomes thicker with age.

The Urinary Tract At age 70, the kidneys can filter waste from the blood only half as fast as they could at age 30. The need to urinate more frequently occurs because the bladder's capacity declines from 2 cups of urine at age 30 to 1 cup at age 70.

One problem sometimes associated with aging is **urinary incontinence,** which ranges from passing a few drops of urine while laughing or sneezing to having no control over urination. Approximately 35 percent of older women and 22 percent of older men have some degree of urinary incontinence.[15] Incontinence can pose major social, physical, and emotional problems. Embarrassment and fear of wetting oneself may cause an older person to become isolated and avoid

HEALTH ETHICS
conflict and controversy

THE DEBATE OVER STEM CELLS

Stem cells are unique—and controversial. Stem cells are body cells with two important characteristics: (1) they are unspecialized (meaning their specific function is yet to be determined) and capable of renewing themselves by dividing repeatedly, and (2) they can be induced to become specialized cells that perform specific functions, such as muscle cells that make the heart beat or nerve cells that enable the brain to function.

What makes stem cells different from other types of cells?

These qualities have led many scientists to believe that stem cells have the potential to cure debilitating health problems such as Alzheimer's, heart disease, diabetes, Parkinson's, and glaucoma. These conditions all involve the destruction of certain crucial cells—in the case of type 1 diabetes, the pancreatic cells that secrete insulin. In the laboratory, researchers are working to coax stem cells to develop into these pancreatic cells. The plan is to transplant the new cells into diabetic patients, where they could replace the patients' damaged cells and produce insulin. If successful, this approach could prevent the destructive complications of the disease and free diabetics from the painful burden of injecting insulin for the rest of their lives. Other therapies under investigation involve growing new cells to replace those ravaged by spinal injuries, heart attacks, muscular dystrophy, and vision and hearing loss.

The controversy over stem cells arises from their origins. Generally, stem cells are derived from eggs that were fertilized in vitro. Typically these are "extra" embryos created during fertility treatments at clinics but not used for implantation. Only four to five days old, embryonic stem cells are pluripotent (capable of developing into many different cell types).

Embryonic stem cell research has provoked fierce debate. Opponents believe that an embryo is a human being and we have no right to create life and then destroy it, even for humanitarian purposes. Advocates counter that the eggs from which these embryos developed were given freely by donors and would otherwise be discarded.

Are adult stem cells a solution to this ethical dilemma? An adult stem cell is an undifferentiated cell, found in body tissues, that can specialize to replace certain types of cells. For example, human bone marrow contains at least two kinds of adult stem cells. One kind gives rise to the various types of blood cells, while the other can differentiate into bone, cartilage, fat, or fibrous connective tissue. Other tissues that may contain adult stem cells include the brain, liver, skeletal muscles, and blood vessels. Whereas research indicates that adult stem cells may be more versatile than previously thought, many scientists believe that embryonic stem cells, with their unlimited potential, are far more promising medically.

In the United States, embryonic stem cell research is limited by law. Federal funding—a major source of support for universities and labs—is restricted to experiments on only 71 stem cell lines (a stem cell line refers to a set of pluripotent, embryonic stem cells that have grown in the laboratory for at least six months). Some scientists worry that this pool is too small to develop valid medical therapies. Opponents believe that even this compromise allows unethical practices to continue. California has established a research initiative that would ban human reproductive cloning but permit embryonic stem cell research for therapeutic purposes.

As debate rages in the United States, embryonic stem cell research is moving forward in other countries. For example, the United Kingdom has licensed a British university to clone stem cells for diabetes research, and South Korean scientists have developed better laboratory techniques for deriving new stem cell lines.

Do you feel that embryonic stem cell research is ethical? Explain your answer. Would you feel differently if you or a loved one suffered from a disease that might respond to stem cell therapy?

Sources: F. Yates et al., "New Breakthrough in Nuclear Transfer," International Society for Stem Cell Research, June 9, 2005, www.isscr.org/public/breakthrough.htm; National Institutes of Health, Stem Cell Information, "Stem Cell Basics," revised August 12, 2005, http://stemcells.nih.gov/info/basics/; M. Waldholz and A. Regalado, "Biggest Struggles in Stem-Cell Fight May Be in the Lab," *The Wall Street Journal,* August 12, 2004: A1, A6; International Society for Stem Cell Research, "The Ethics of Embryonic Stem Cell Research," updated February 2, 2005, www.isscr.org/public/ethics.htm; Associated Press, "U.K. Grants First Cloning License to Develop Research Stem Cells," *The Wall Street Journal,* August 12, 2004: D3.

social functions. Caregivers may become frustrated with incontinent patients. Prolonged wetness and the inability to properly care for oneself can lead to irritation, infections, and other problems.

Incontinence is not an inevitable part of aging, but there are a host of causes, including obesity, diabetes, difficult childbirth, and prostate problems. Some cases are caused by medications, highly treatable neurological problems that affect the central nervous system, infections of the pelvic muscles, weakness in the pelvic wall, or other problems. When the problem is treated, the incontinence usually vanishes.[16]

The Heart and Lungs Resting heart rate stays about the same over the course of a person's life, but the stroke volume (the amount of blood the muscle pushes out per beat) diminishes as heart muscle deteriorates. Vital capacity, or the

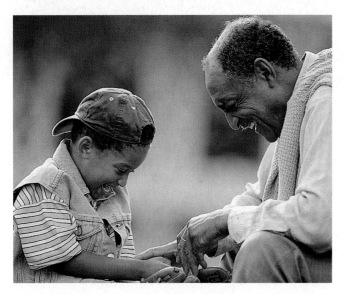

Learning to cope with challenges and changes early in life develops attitudes and skills that contribute to a full and satisfying old age.

amount of air that moves when you inhale and exhale at maximum effort, also declines with age. Exercise can do a great deal to preserve heart and lung function.

Eyesight
By age 30, the lens of the eye begins to harden, causing problems by the early forties. The lens begins to yellow and loses transparency, while the pupil of the eye shrinks, allowing less light to penetrate. Activities such as reading become more difficult, particularly in dim light. By age 60, depth perception declines and farsightedness often develops. A need for reading glasses usually develops in the forties, and this evolves into a need for bifocals or trifocals. In addition to these normal changes, some elderly people develop an eye disease such as cataracts, glaucoma, or macular degeneration.

By age 80, more than half of all Americans either have **cataracts** (clouding of the lens) or have had cataract surgery.[17] Normally, the lens is a transparent structure inside the eye that focuses incoming light and images. Over time, the lens can darken or become clouded by clumps of protein, blurring images and impairing night vision. Smoking, high blood pressure, diabetes, and extensive exposure to sunlight increase the risk of developing cataracts. Fortunately, surgical removal of of cataracts is common and comes with a high

cataracts Clouding of the lens that interrupts the focusing of light on the retina, resulting in blurred vision or eventual blindness.

glaucoma Elevation of pressure within the eyeball, leading to hardening of the eyeball, impaired vision, and possible blindness.

macular degeneration Disease that breaks down the macula, the light-sensitive part of the retina responsible for sharp, direct vision.

success rate; 90 percent of people who undergo cataract surgery enjoy better vision afterward.[18]

Glaucoma (elevated pressure within the eyeball) affects about 2.2 million adult Americans.[19] Inside the front of the eye, there is a space called the anterior chamber. Normally, a clear fluid flows freely in and out of this chamber to nourish nearby tissues. If for some reason the fluid cannot drain from the anterior chamber, pressure can build up inside the eyeball and eventually damage the optic nerve that carries visual information to the brain. Glaucoma is usually painless, and many people don't realize they have it until they have already lost some vision permanently. Risk factors include nearsightedness, age (most cases develop after age 60), and a family history of the disease. For unknown reasons, Mexican Americans and African Americans have a higher risk. If you are in a high-risk group, make sure you have your eyes thoroughly examined every two years. There is no cure for glaucoma, but medicated eyedrops can lower the pressure and control the disease. The earlier the treatment begins, the better. Surgery may also help.[20]

Approximately 1.8 million Americans over age 40 have advanced **macular degeneration,** and it is the leading cause of vision loss in those aged 60 and over.[21] This condition breaks down the macula, the part of the retina responsible for the sharp, direct vision needed to read, watch television, or drive. Macular degeneration can cause permanent blindness in the central vision plane. The exact causes of age-related macular degeneration are unknown; however, smoking, high blood pressure, farsightedness, obesity, and a family history of the condition tend to increase the risk. Although many researchers and eye specialists believe that certain nutrients such as zinc, antioxidants such as vitamins A, C, and E, and lutein may reduce risks, these theories have not been proven in clinical trials. Efforts to treat macular degeneration are under way, but progress to date has been slow.

Hearing
The ability to hear high-frequency consonants (for example, *s, t,* and *z*) diminishes with age. Much of the actual hearing loss lies in the ability to distinguish extreme ranges of sound rather than normal conversational tones.

Sexual Changes
As men age, they experience notable alterations in sexual function. Whereas the degree and rate of change vary greatly from person to person, changes that generally occur in men include:

- Slowed ability to obtain an erection
- Diminished ability to maintain an erection
- Increased length of the refractory period between orgasms
- A decline in angle of the erection
- Shortened duration of orgasm

Women also experience several changes:

- Menopause usually occurs between the ages of 45 and 55. Women may experience hot flashes, mood swings, weight gain, development of facial hair, or other hormone-related symptoms.

OSTEOPOROSIS: PREVENTING AN AGE-OLD PROBLEM

When you hear that someone has osteoporosis, the image that may come to mind is a slumped-over woman with a characteristic "dowager's hump" in the upper back; however, this is a relatively rare, extreme version of the disease. Although many people consider osteoporosis a disease only of older women, osteoporosis can occur at any age and it can pose a problem for men, too. Osteoporosis is progressive and occurs over many years. Without proper prevention in the form of diet, weight-bearing exercise, and overall fitness (see Chapter 10), each of us risks developing this condition. As awareness increases, millions of Americans are requesting bone density tests to determine just how far gone their bones and joints may really be.

EPIDEMIOLOGY

Prevalence data indicate the following:

- The hips, wrists, and spine are most vulnerable to the ravages of osteoporosis.
- In the United States, osteoporosis affects over 44 million Americans, 68 percent of whom are women.
- Each year osteoporosis causes 1.5 million fractures: 300,000 at the hip, 700,000 in the vertebrae, 250,000 in the wrists, and more than 300,000 at other sites.
- One out of every two women and one in four men over age 50 will have an osteoporosis-related fracture sometime in life.
- More than 2 million American men have osteoporosis and millions more are at risk. Each year, 80,000 men suffer a hip fracture, and one-third of them die within a year.

RISK FACTORS

A number of factors may predispose a person to developing osteoporosis. Risk factors that we cannot control include:

- *Gender.* Chances of developing osteoporosis are greater if you are a woman.

Women have less bone tissue and lose bone more rapidly than men because of the hormonal changes resulting from menopause.
- *Age.* The older you are, the greater your risk of osteoporosis. Your bones become less dense and weaker as you age.
- *Body size.* Small, thin-boned women are at greatest risk.
- *Ethnicity.* Caucasian and Asian women are at highest risk; African American and Latina women have a lower but still significant risk.
- *Family history.* Susceptibility to fracture may be, in part, hereditary. People whose parents have a history of fractures also seem to have reduced bone mass.

The following risk factors can be modified by our choices in lifestyle behaviors, medication, and diet:

- Levels of sex hormones—abnormal absence of menstrual periods (amenorrhea), low estrogen levels (menopause), and low testosterone levels in men may signal potential problems.
- Being very thin—women who are underweight produce less estrogen. Patients with severe anorexia can develop osteoporosis as early as their twenties.
- A lifetime diet low in calcium and vitamin D.
- Use of certain medications, such as glucocorticoids or some anticonvulsants.
- An inactive lifestyle or extended bed rest.
- Cigarette smoking.
- Excessive consumption of alcohol.

PREVENTION

Increased calcium and vitamin D intake and consistent weight-bearing exercise can help all of us reduce our risk of osteoporosis.

Many studies indicate that if you don't consume enough calcium, you will be at increased risk for osteoporosis. Calcium requirements change over the course of a

lifetime, with greater needs during childhood and adolescence when the skeleton is growing and during pregnancy and breast-feeding. Postmenopausal women and older men also need more, and medications may deplete calcium reserves as well. Be sure to take vitamin D, which helps the body absorb and utilize calcium more efficiently.

Like muscle, bone is living tissue that responds to exercise by becoming stronger. The best exercise for the bones is weight-bearing exercise that forces you to work against gravity. Examples include walking, hiking, jogging, weight training, tennis, and dancing.

Research conducted by Dr. Christine M. Snow, director of Oregon State University's bone research lab and internationally known exercise scientist, has shed interesting light on the importance of exercise for residents of nursing homes. Residents were given modest exercises to do while wearing weighted vests. They improved not only bone density, but also balance and strength, which together can reduce the risk of falling and fracturing bones. In addition, residents were able to walk faster, which made them less likely to fall if they lost balance. In studies of young gymnasts, Snow has found that bone density can be increased through various types of exercise. She emphasizes that it is vitally important to begin exercising early in life to ensure bone health in later years.

Sources: Osteoporosis and Related Bone Diseases—National Resource Center, "What People with Anorexia Nervosa Need to Know About Osteoporosis," revised October 2002, www.osteo.org/newfile.asp?doc=r803i&doctitle =What+People+with+Anorexia+Nervosa+Need +to+Know+About+Osteoporosis&doctype =HTML+Fact+Sheet; Osteoporosis and Related Bone Diseases—National Resource Center, "Fast Facts," December 2002, www.osteo.org/ osteo.html.

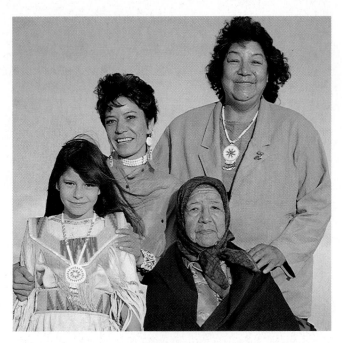

In most cases, you need look no further than your family tree to get an idea of the effects that aging will have on you.

- The walls of the vagina become less elastic and the epithelium thins, possibly making intercourse painful.
- Vaginal secretions, particularly during sexual activity, diminish.
- The breasts become less firm. Loss of fat in various areas leads to fewer curves, with a decrease in the soft lines of body contours.

Though these physiological changes may sound somewhat discouraging, the fact is that sex is an essential component to the lives of those aged 45 and over, and many people remain sexually active throughout their entire adult lives.[22] Indeed, a landmark study by the National Council on Aging refuted long-held beliefs that sexual desire decreases as we age. Results indicated that nearly half of Americans over age 60 engage in sexual activity at least once a month, and 4 out of 10 would like to have sex more frequently than they currently do.[23] With the advent of drugs designed to treat sexual dysfunction, such as Viagra, many older adults may get their wish.

Body Comfort Because of the loss of body fat, thinning epithelium, and diminished glandular activity, older adults experience greater difficulty regulating body temperature. This limits their ability to withstand extreme cold or heat, increasing the risks of hypothermia, heatstroke, and heat exhaustion. Thinning skin also makes older adults more vulnerable to bed sores and other skin ulcers.

ageism Discrimination based on age.

Typical Mental Changes

Intelligence Recent research demonstrates that many of our previous beliefs about the intelligence of older adults were based on inappropriate testing procedures. Given an appropriate length of time, older people learn and develop skills in a similar manner to younger people. Researchers have also determined that what many older adults lack in speed of learning they make up for in practical knowledge—that is, the "wisdom of age."

Memory Have you ever wondered why your grandfather seems unable to remember what he did last weekend but can vividly describe an event that occurred 40 years ago? This phenomenon is not unusual. Research indicates that although short-term memory may fluctuate on a daily basis, the ability to remember events from past decades seems to remain largely unchanged.

Adaptability Although it is widely believed that people become more like one another as they age, nothing could be further from the truth. Having lived through a multitude of experiences and faced diverse joys, sorrows, and obstacles, the typical older person has developed unique methods of coping with life. These unique adaptive variations make for interesting differences in how they confront the many changes brought on by the aging process. As a group, the elderly are extremely heterogeneous. They flex and adapt and "make do" in ways that younger adults may not be able to duplicate. Labeling this highly flexible and resilient group as rigid or unmovable is inaccurate and misleading.

Depression Most adults continue to lead healthy, fulfilling lives. However, some older people do suffer from mental and emotional disturbances. Some research indicates that depression may be the most common psychological problem facing older adults. However, the rate of major depression is actually lower among older people than among younger adults.

Regardless of age, people who have a poor perception of their health, have multiple chronic illnesses, take a lot of medications, abuse alcohol and other drugs, lack social support, and do not exercise face more challenges that require many emotional strengths to surmount. Strong coping skills and support systems will often lessen the duration and severity of the depression. However, those who are ill-equipped to deal with life's changes or who lack close ties may consider suicide a means of solving their problems.

Senility: Getting Rid of Ageist Attitudes
Discrimination against people based on age is known as **ageism.**

Over the years, older adults have often suffered from ageist attitudes. People who were chronologically old were often labeled "senile" whenever they displayed memory failure, errors in judgment, disorientation, or erratic behavior.

Today scientists recognize that these same symptoms can occur at any age and for various reasons, including disease (such as vitamin B deficiency) or the use of over-the-counter and prescription drugs. When the underlying problems are corrected, the memory loss and disorientation also improve. Currently, the term **senility** is seldom used except to describe a very small group of organic disorders.

Alzheimer's Disease Progressive brain impairments that interfere with memory and normal intellectual functioning are known as **dementias**. Although there are many types of dementia, one of the most common forms is **Alzheimer's disease (AD).** Attacking over 4.5 million Americans and killing over 100,000 of them every year, this disease is one of the most painful and devastating conditions that families can endure.[24] It kills its victims twice: first through a slow loss of personhood (memory loss, disorientation, personality changes, and eventual loss of the ability to function independently), and then through the deterioration of body systems as they gradually succumb to the powerful impact of neurological problems.

The number of Americans with Alzheimer's has more than doubled since 1980, and by 2050, it is projected that the number of individuals with the disease could reach 11 to 16 million. The average lifetime cost of care for a person with Alzheimer's is a staggering $174,000, much of which is paid by family members. With the U.S. population gradually aging, the number of people afflicted and the economic burden are certain to increase.[25] Patients with Alzheimer's live for an average of 8 years after diagnosis, though the disease can last for up to 20 years.[26] Although most people associate the disease with the aged, Alzheimer's has been diagnosed in people in their late forties. In fact, about 5 percent of all cases occur before age 65.

Contrary to what many people think, Alzheimer's is not a new disease. Named after Alois Alzheimer, a German neuropathologist who recorded it as early as 1906, Alzheimer's refers to a degenerative disease of the brain in which nerve cells stop communicating with one another. Ordinarily, brain cells communicate by releasing chemicals that allow the cells to receive and transmit messages for various types of behavior. In Alzheimer's patients, the brain doesn't produce enough of these chemicals, cells can't communicate, and eventually the cells die.

This degeneration occurs in the sections of the brain that affect memory, speech, and personality, leaving the parts that control other bodily functions, such as heartbeat and breathing, functioning at near normal levels. Thus, the mind begins to go while the body lives on. It all happens in a slow, progressive manner, and it may take 20 years before symptoms are noticed. This can exact a heavy toll on families, especially once the disease progresses to later stages; the average cost of nursing care is between $40,000 and $70,000 each year.[27]

Alzheimer's is generally detected first by families, who note changes, particularly memory lapses and personality changes, in their loved ones. Medical tests rule out under-lying causes, and certain neurological tests help confirm the diagnosis.

Alzheimer's disease characteristically progresses in three stages. During the *first stage,* symptoms include forgetfulness, memory loss, impaired judgment, increasing inability to handle routine tasks, disorientation, lack of interest in one's surroundings, and depression. These symptoms accelerate in the *second stage,* which also includes agitation and restlessness (especially at night), loss of sensory perceptions, muscle twitching, and repetitive actions. Many patients become depressed, combative, and aggressive. In the *final stage,* disorientation is often complete. The person becomes completely dependent on others for eating, dressing, and other activities. Identity loss and speech problems are common. Eventually, control of bodily functions may be lost.

Researchers are investigating a number of possible causes of the disease, including genetic predisposition, malfunction of the immune system, a slow-acting virus, chromosomal or genetic defects, chronic inflammation, uncontrolled hypertension, and neurotransmitter imbalance. Preliminary research indicates that a defect in the chromosomes may be the most likely cause, partly because virtually everyone with Down's syndrome eventually develops Alzheimer's.

Is there a cure for Alzheimer's yet?

There is no treatment that can stop the progression of Alzheimer's disease, but there are some medications such as tacrine, donepezil, or galantamine that can prevent some symptoms from progressing for a short period of time. A newer drug, memantine, has been approved by the FDA to treat more severe AD, but, like the others, its effects are limited. These medicines do treat some behavioral symptoms associated with AD such as sleeplessness, depression, anxiety, agitation, and wandering. Treating these symptoms often makes patients more comfortable and can make things easier for caregivers as well.[28]

Some researchers are looking at anti-inflammatory drugs, theorizing that Alzheimer's may develop in response to an inflammatory ailment. Others are focusing on stimulating the brains of Alzheimer's-prone individuals, believing that as people learn, more connections between cells are formed that may offset those that are lost.

Much attention has also focused on the family, as the family is often another victim when Alzheimer's occurs. Having to decide between tending to a loved one at home or

---

senility A term associated with judgment and orientation problems and the loss of memory occurring in a small percentage of the elderly.

dementias Progressive brain impairments that interfere with memory and normal intellectual functioning.

Alzheimer's disease (AD) A chronic condition involving changes in nerve fibers of the brain that results in mental deterioration.

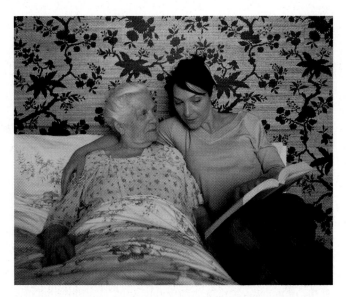

Caring for loved ones who may be too infirm to perform life's daily tasks any longer can be a very emotional experience for family members.

seeking the assistance of a long-term-care facility can be heartbreaking. Caring for Alzheimer's patients is a challenge for even the most dedicated family members. And even the best preparation for the final days of a loved one with this disease does not make the process easy. Knowing what the options are and being able to recognize the differences between normal physiological aging and the ravages of certain diseases can make it easier to cope with age-related problems, for both older patients and their families.

Health Challenges of Older Adults

Some health problems common in older adults are brought on by failing health, others by society or a perceived loss of control over life's events—watching loved ones die, facing health problems, and confronting an uncertain economy on a fixed income. Developing life skills and a network of social support during earlier years can significantly reduce problems in old age.

Alcohol Use and Abuse

Early studies reported that 2 to 10 percent of older Americans were alcoholics, but the exact percentages are controversial today. However, a person who is prone to alcoholism during the younger and middle years is more likely to continue during later years. The older alcoholic is probably no more common in American society than the young alcoholic, despite the stereotype of the old, lost soul, hiding his or her sorrows in a bottle. Often, when people think they see a drunken older person, they are really seeing a confused individual who has taken too many different prescription medications and is experiencing a form of drug interaction.

Men tend to have a higher risk for alcoholism at all ages. Alcohol abuse is five times more common among older men than among older women. Yet as many as half of all older men and an even higher proportion of older women don't drink at all. Those who do drink do so less than younger persons, consuming only five to six drinks weekly.

If the more recent studies are accurate, the reason there aren't many heavy drinkers among older adults may be that very heavy drinkers tend either to die of alcoholic complications before they reach old age or to reform their drinking habits. Some older people reduce their consumption because they find they cannot process alcohol as readily as they did when they were younger or because they are afraid of combining it with the prescription drugs they must take. If the older reports are accurate, alcoholism among the elderly may be disguised by a tendency among health professionals and family members to associate forgetfulness, incontinence, poor grooming, dementia-like reactions, injuries, and so on with old age rather than with an alcohol problem. It is important to note that most older adults who consume alcohol are neither alcoholics nor people who drink to cope with their losses. Most drinking among older people is social and may, in fact, be much less of a problem than previously thought.

Prescription Drug Use

It is extremely rare for older people to use illicit drugs, but some do overuse and grow dependent on prescription drugs. Some take more than six prescription drugs a day. Reported numbers of drugs taken are substantially higher for residents of health care institutions, because drugs that many of us purchase over the counter, such as aspirin, are counted in the total numbers.

Anyone who combines different drugs runs the risk of dangerous drug interactions. The risks of adverse effects are even greater for people with impaired circulation and declining kidney and liver function. Older people displaying symptoms of these drug-induced effects, which may include bizarre behavior patterns or disorientation, are all too often misdiagnosed as senile rather than examined for underlying causes and treated.

Currently there is no one system that tracks all of a patient's prescriptions. Pharmacists may not know about other drugs, vitamins, or herbal supplements that a patient is taking and thus may not warn of possible drug interactions. Illness or physiological abnormalities may affect the way drugs are metabolized, contributing to dose irregularities and other problems. To avoid drug interactions and other problems, older adults should use the same pharmacy consistently, ask questions about medicines and dosages, and read the directions carefully.

Over-the-Counter Remedies

A substantial segment of the over-60 population avoids professional medical treatment, viewing it as only a last resort. This is becoming increasingly true as Medicare coverage becomes less adequate and older adults are forced to pay larger medical bills out of their own resources. The poor are particularly prone to turn to folk medicine and over-the-counter (OTC) preparations as cheaper, less intimidating alternatives. Aspirin and laxatives head the list of commonly used OTC medications.

Strategies for Healthy Aging

As you know from reading this book, you can do many things to prolong your life and improve the quality of your life. To provide for healthy older years, make each of the following part of your younger years.

Develop and Maintain Healthy Relationships

Social bonds lend vigor and energy to life. Be willing to give to others, and seek variety in your relationships rather than befriending only people who agree with you. By experiencing diverse people and interacting with different points of view, we gain a new perspective on life.

Enrich the Spiritual Side of Life

Although we often take this for granted, cultivating a relationship with nature, the environment, a higher being, and yourself is a key factor in personal growth and development. Take time for thought and quiet contemplation, and enjoy the sunsets, sounds, and energy of life. These moments spent in time prioritized for "you" will leave you invigorated and fresh—better able to cope with the ups and downs of life. If you don't take time for yourself now, it just may be that you won't have time in the later years.

Improve Fitness

If you're basically sedentary, just about any moderate-intensity exercise that gets your heart beating faster and increases strength and/or flexibility will maximize your physical health and functional years. The research presented in Chapter 10 shows that there is hope even for the most die-hard couch potato.

One of the inevitable physical changes that the body undergoes is **sarcopenia,** age-associated loss of muscle mass. The less muscle you have, the less energy you will burn even while resting. The lower your metabolic rate, the more likely you will gain weight. With regular strength training, you can increase your muscle mass, boost your metabolism, strengthen your bones, lower the risk of osteoporosis, and, in general, feel better and function more efficiently. The Skills for Behavior Change box on page 590 provides tips for exercise.

So, get moving and keep moving, no matter what the activity is. And remember, it is never too late to start. Even if you're in your sixties or seventies, exercise can increase life expectancy by improving circulation, reducing blood pressure, and reducing overall health risks. A lifetime of exercise and movement will pay dividends in later years.

Eat for Health

Although other chapters in this text provide detailed information about nutrition and weight control, certain nutrients are especially essential to healthy aging:

- *Calcium.* Bone loss tends to increase in women, particularly in the hip region, shortly before menopause. During perimenopause and menopause, this bone loss accelerates rapidly, with an average of about 3 percent skeletal mass lost per year over a five-year period. The result is an increased risk for fracture and disability. Few women actually consume daily the 1,000 milligrams of calcium recommended during the younger years or the 1,500 milligrams recommended during and after menopause.
- *Vitamin D.* Vitamin D is necessary for adequate calcium absorption, yet as people age, particularly in their fifties and sixties, they do not absorb vitamin D from foods as readily as they did in their younger years. If vitamin D is unavailable, calcium levels are also likely to be lower.
- *Protein.* As older adults become more concerned about cholesterol and fatty foods, and as their budgets shrink, one nutrient that often takes the "hit" is protein. It costs more, takes longer to cook, and often has that "fat" stigma associated with animal products. Many older people cut back on protein to a point that is below the recommended daily amount. Large numbers of women in particular cut back so far that they get less than half of the daily amount necessary. Because protein is necessary for muscle mass, protein insufficiencies can spell trouble.

Other nutrients, including vitamin E, folic acid (folate), iron, potassium, and vitamin B_{12} (cobalamin), are important to the aging process, and most of these are readily available in any diet that follows food pyramid recommendations.

Caring for Older Adults

Older women far outnumber older men in American society, and the discrepancy increases with age. Because women live seven years longer than men on average, older women are more likely to be living alone. Further, they are more likely to experience poverty, and to have multiple chronic health problems, a situation referred to as **comorbidity.** Consequently,

sarcopenia Age-related loss of muscle mass.

comorbidity The presence of a number of diseases at the same time.

SKILLS FOR behavior change

AGING AND EXERCISE

Whether you're 20, 50, or 80 years old, you can exercise and improve your health. Exercising has even helped 90-year-olds living in nursing homes grow stronger and more independent.

Staying physically active is a key to good health well into later years. Yet only about one in four older adults exercises regularly. Many think they are too old or too frail, but nothing could be further from the truth. Physical activity of any kind—from heavy-duty exercises such as jogging or bicycling to easier efforts like walking—is good for you. Vigorous exercise can help strengthen your heart and lungs. Taking a brisk walk regularly will lower your risk of health problems like heart disease and depression. Climbing stairs, calisthenics, and housework will increase strength, stamina, and self-confidence. Weight lifting or strength training is a good way to slow down muscle and bone loss. Your daily activities will become easier as you feel better.

You can exercise at home alone, with a buddy, or as part of a group. Talk to your doctor before you begin, especially if you are over 40 or have a medical problem. Move at your own speed, and don't take on too much at first. A class is a good idea if you haven't exercised for a long time or are just beginning. A qualified teacher will make sure you are doing the exercise in the right way.

Set a goal of 30 minutes of moderate activity every day. You don't have to exercise for 30 minutes all at once. Short bursts of activity, like taking the stairs instead of the elevator or walking instead of driving, can add up to 30 minutes of exercise a day. Raking leaves, playing actively with children or pets, gardening, and even doing household chores can count toward your daily total.

Include a mix of stretching, strength training, and aerobic or endurance exercise in your exercise plan. People who are weak or frail should start slowly. Begin with stretching and strength training; add aerobic exercises later. Aerobic exercises are safer and easier once you feel balanced and your muscles are stronger.

Stretching improves flexibility, eases movement, and lowers the risk of injury and muscle strain. It also increases blood flow and gets your body ready for exercise. A warm-up and cool-down period of 5 to 15 minutes should be done slowly and carefully, before and after all types of exercise. In addition to being relaxing, stretching can loosen muscles in the arms, shoulders, back, chest, stomach, buttocks, thighs, and calves.

Strength training (also called resistance training or weight lifting) builds muscle and bone, both of which decline with age. Lifting weights or working out with machines or an elastic band will strengthen the upper and lower body. It is very important to have an expert teach you how to work with weights; otherwise you could get hurt. With help, older adults can work their way up to many of the same weight-lifting routines as younger adults. Once you know what to do, you can do simple strength-training exercises at home. Try using household items, such as soup cans or milk jugs filled with water or sand, as weights. Strength training does not have to take a lot of time; 30 to 40 minutes at least two or three times each week are all that's needed. Try not to exercise the same muscles two days in a row.

Aerobic exercises (also called endurance exercises) strengthen the heart and improve overall fitness by increasing the body's ability to use oxygen. Swimming, walking, and dancing are "low-impact" aerobic activities. They avoid the muscle and joint pounding of more "high-impact" exercises like jogging and jumping rope. Aerobic exercises raise the number of heartbeats each minute (heart rate). Try to

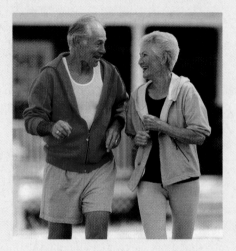

get your heart rate to a certain level and keep it there for 20 minutes or more. If you have not exercised in a while, start slowly. As you get stronger, try to increase your heart rate. Aerobics should be done for 20 to 40 minutes at least three times each week.

Before starting any aerobics program, check with your doctor and ask about your target heart rate. Some blood pressure medicines, for example, can affect how you calculate target heart rate.

Not sure where to start? Local gyms, universities, or hospitals can help you find a teacher or program that works for you. You can also check with local churches or synagogues, senior and civic centers, parks, recreation associations, YMCAs, YWCAs, and even local shopping malls for exercise and wellness programs. Many community centers also offer programs for older people who are worried about special health problems like heart disease or falling. Look for books and tapes at your local library.

Source: Adapted from the National Institute on Aging, "Don't Take It Easy—Exercise!" (Gaithersburg, MD: National Institute on Aging), www.medaccess.com/seniors/agepg/ap41.htm.

more older women than men are likely to need assistance from children, other relatives, friends, and neighbors.

Women have usually been the primary caregivers for older Americans, often for their ailing husbands. Research also indicates that women spend more hours than men (38 hours versus 27 hours per week) in caregiving activities and perform a wider range of activities. Regardless of the time spent, caregiving is a difficult and stressful experience for both women and men. **Respite care,** or care that is given by someone who relieves the primary caregiver, should be available to ease the burden. As the population ages and more older adults require care, it will become even more important to support caregivers' health and well-being.

 what do you THINK?

Why are women often the primary caregivers for aging spouses and other family members? ■ What problems can such caregiving cause? ■ How can caregivers learn to cope with the stresses and strains of their situation?

respite care The care provided by substitute caregivers to relieve the principal caregiver from his or her continuous responsibility.

TAKING charge

Summary

- Aging can be defined in terms of biological age, referring to a person's physical condition; psychological age, referring to a person's coping abilities and intelligence; social age, referring to a person's habits and roles relative to society's expectations; legal age, based on chronological years; or functional age, relative to how other people function at varied ages.
- The growing numbers of older adults (aged 65 and older) will have an important impact on society in terms of the economy, health care, housing, and ethical considerations.
- Two broad groups of theories—biological and psychosocial—purport to explain the physiological and psychological changes that occur with aging. The biological theories include the wear-and-tear theory, the cellular theory, the autoimmune theory, and the genetic mutation theory. Psychosocial theories center on adaptation and adjustments related to self-development.

- Aging changes the body and mind in many ways. Physical changes occur in the skin, bones and joints, head, urinary tract, heart and lungs, senses, sexual functioning, and temperature regulation. Major physical concerns are osteoporosis, urinary incontinence, and changes in eyesight and hearing. Most older people maintain a high level of intelligence and memory. Potential mental problems include depression and Alzheimer's disease.
- Special challenges for older adults include alcohol abuse, prescription drug and OTC interactions, questions about vitamin and mineral supplementation, and issues regarding caregiving.
- Lifestyle choices we make today will affect health status later in life. Choosing to exercise, eat a healthy diet, and foster lasting relationships will contribute to healthy aging. Decisions about caring for older adults and stresses related to caregiving are ongoing concerns as the U.S. population ages.

Chapter Review

1. The fastest growing segment of the U.S. population today is
   a. young children.
   b. teenagers.
   c. baby boomers.
   d. seniors 65 and older.

2. One of the best ways to age healthfully is to
   a. consume megadosages of vitamins.
   b. eat more carbohydrates and protein instead of saturated fats.
   c. exercise more, particularly aerobic exercise.
   d. have a glass of wine everyday.

3. One of the more common nutritional disorders in older adults is
   a. anorexia.
   b. binge eating disorder.
   c. eating less fiber.
   d. overweight and obesity.

4. Which of the following mental capacities of elderly people diminishes with age?
   a. reaction time
   b. understanding
   c. vocabulary
   d. verbal intelligence

5. A person's psychological age typically refers to that individual's
   a. habits and roles relative to society's expectations.
   b. chronological legal age.
   c. adaptive and coping abilities.
   d. comparable age to other people of the same age.

6. The biological theory of aging that supports the concept that body cells reproduce only so many times throughout life, thus limiting the body's ability to repair itself is known as the
   a. the wear-and-tear theory.
   b. cellular theory.
   c. autoimmune theory.
   d. genetic mutation theory.

7. Discrimination against individuals based on age is known as
   a. senility.
   b. Alzheimer's disease.
   c. dementia.
   d. ageism.

8. Alzheimer's disease degenerates the brain's capacity to control
   a. heartbeat and breathing.
   b. memory and speech.
   c. both A and B
   d. none of the above

9. The study of individual and collective aging processes is called
   a. ageism.
   b. gerontology.
   c. thanatology.
   d. none of the above

10. Which definition of age is used to determine eligibility for Social Security payments?
    a. legal
    b. social
    c. biological
    d. functional

Answers to these questions can be found on page A-1.

Questions for Discussion and Reflection

1. Discuss the various definitions of aging. At what age would you place your parents for each category?
2. As the older population grows, how will it affect your life? Would you be willing to pay higher taxes to support government social programs for older adults? For example, do you believe that Social Security should continue its yearly increases in payments, which are pegged to inflation? Why or why not?

3. Which of the biological theories of aging do you think is most correct? Why?
4. List the major physiological changes that occur with aging. Which of these, if any, can you change?
5. Explain the major health challenges that older people may face. What advice would you give to your grandparents before they took a prescription or OTC drug?
6. Discuss actions you can start taking now to help ensure a healthier aging process.

Accessing Your Health on the Internet

The following websites explore further topics and issues related to personal health. You'll also find links to each organization's website on the Companion Website for *Access to Health*, Tenth Edition, at www.aw-bc.com/donatelle.

1. *Administration on Aging.* A link to the U.S. Department of Health and Human Services agency dedicated to addressing the health needs of older Americans. www.aoa.gov
2. *Alzheimer's Association.* Archives of media releases and position statements, fact sheets on Alzheimer's disease, medical and research updates, and a brochure on how to recognize the ten warning signs of Alzheimer's. www.alz.org

3. *Healthy Aging.* The official site of the healthy aging campaign, a national ongoing program designed to broaden awareness of the positive aspects of aging and to provide information and inspiration for adults, aged 50 and over, to improve their physical, mental, social, and financial fitness. www.healthyaging.net
4. *Social Security Online.* Provides information about Social Security benefits and entitlements. Also offers links to related sites. www.ssa.gov

Further Reading

Gaby, A. R. *Preventing and Reversing Osteoporosis: Every Woman's Essential Guide.* Roseville, CA: Prima Publishing, 1995.

> Excellent reference text focusing on osteoporosis risk factors and what you can do to reduce risks.

The Johns Hopkins Medical Letter—Health After 50. www.hopkinsafter50.com.

> Monthly newsletter providing comprehensive, accurate overviews of health topics relevant to older adults.

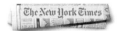

e-themes from *The New York Times*

For up-to-date articles about current health issues, visit www.aw-bc.com/donatelle, select *Access to Health,* Tenth Edition, Chapter 19, and click on "e-themes."

References

1. J. C. Cavanaugh and F. Blanchard-Fields, *Adult Development and Aging* (Belmont, CA: Wadsworth, 2006).
2. Centers for Disease Control and Prevention, "Healthy Aging," 2006, www.cdc.gov/aginginfo.htm.
3. Ibid.
4. W. He et al., "65+ in the United States: 2005," 2006,www.census .gov/prod/2006pubs/p23-209.
5. M. Lachman, "Aging Under Control?" *Psychological Science Agenda* 19, no. 1 (2005): 1–3.
6. K. Hooker, "Possible Selves and Health Behavior in Later Life," *Personality and Social Psychology Bulletin* 31, no. 5 (2005): 610–620.
7. Administration on Aging, "A Profile of Older Americans: 2005," www.aoa.gov/prof/Statistics/profile/2005/2005profile.pdf.
8. United Nations, "World Population Prospects: The 2004 Revision," 2005, www.un.org/esa/population/publications/WPP2004 _volume3.htm.
9. Administration on Aging, "A Profile of Older Americans: 2005."
10. M. Minino et al., "Deaths: Preliminary Data for 2004," 2004, www.cdc.gov/nchs/products/pubd/hestats/prelimdeaths04/preliminary deaths04.htm; National Center for Health Statistics, "FASTSTATS: Life Expectancy at Birth," 2006, www.cdc.gov/nchs.fastats/ lifexpec.htm.
11. Administration on Aging, "A Profile of Older Americans 2003: Health and Health Care," updated July 16, 2006, www.aoa.gov/ prof/Statistics/profile/2003/14.asp.
12. U.S. Department of Health and Human Services, "What Is Long-Term Care?" March 31, 2005, http://medicare.gov/longtermcare/ static/home.asp.
13. Osteoporosis and Related Bone Diseases—National Resource Center, "Osteoporosis Overview," revised January 2003, www.osteo.org/ newfile.asp?doc=osteo&doctitle=Osteoporosis+Overview& doctype=HTML+Fact+Sheet.
14. Mayo Clinic Staff, "Ostearthritis: Overview," 2005, www.mayo clinic.com/invoke.cfm?objectid=2B275878-8417-41E5-AB4FA4B6646DD7F6.
15. National Kidney and Urologic Diseases Information Clearinghouse, "Kidney and Urologic Disease Statistics for the United States" (NIH Publication No. 04-3895), February 2004, www.kidney.niddk.nih .gov/kudiseases/pubs/kustats/index.htm#up.
16. Ibid.
17. National Eye Institute, "Health Information: What Is a Cataract?" April 2006, www.nei/nih.gov/health/cataract/cataract_facts.asp#5a.
18. National Eye Institute, "Health Information: Is Cataract Surgery Effective?" April 2006, www.nei/nih.gov/health/cataract/ cataract_facts.asp#4d.
19. National Eye Institute, "Health Information: "Can Glaucoma Be Treated?" August 2006, www.nei/nih.gov/health/glaucoma/ glaucoma_facts.asp#4a.
20. Ibid.
21. National Eye Institute, "Vision Loss from Eye Diseases," 2005 www.nei.nih.gov.
22. Philadelphia Corporation for Aging, "Health Matters," no. 14, August 2004, www.pcaphl.org/healthmatters/agingsexuality.pdf.
23. X. P. Fisher and L. Fisher, "Sexuality at Midlife and Beyond," 2005, http://assets.aarp.org/rgcenter/general2004_sexuality.pdf.
24. Alzheimer's Association, "Fact Sheet," 2006, www.alz.org/ Resources/FactSheets/FSAlzheimerStats.pdf.
25. Ibid.
26. Ibid.
27. Ibid.
28. National Institute on Aging, "Alzheimer's Information: Treatment," 2006, www.nia.nih.gov/alzheimers/alzheimersinformation/treatment.

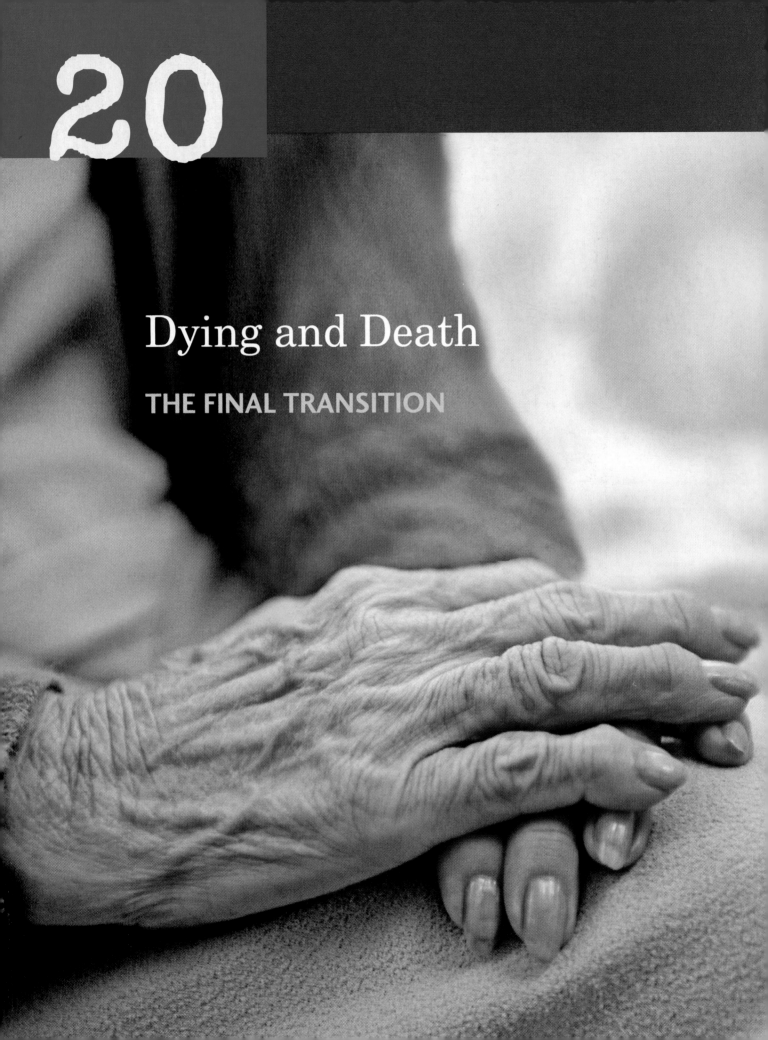

20

Dying and Death

THE FINAL TRANSITION

Does everyone experience death and **grief** in the same way?

Why should I create a **living will**?

Is physician assisted suicide **legal** in the United States?

What types of **arrangements** need to be made when a loved one dies?

How can I help a **friend** who has just experienced a loss?

OBJECTIVES

- Define death, and analyze why people deny death in Western culture.
- Discuss the stages of the grieving process and strategies for coping more effectively with death.
- Explain the ethical concerns that arise from the concepts of the right to die and rational suicide.
- Review the decisions that need to be made when someone is dying or has died, including hospice care, funeral arrangements, wills, and organ donations.

Death eventually comes to everyone, but if you live life to the fullest and learn as much about end-of-life issues as you can, you will be better able to accept the inevitable. Distractions and denial may postpone the reality of death, but they cannot eliminate it. The acceptance of death helps shape attitudes about the importance of life.

Throughout history, humans have attempted to determine the nature and meaning of death. This quest continues today. Although we will touch on moral and philosophical questions about death in this chapter, we will not explore such issues in depth. Rather, our primary focus is to present dying and death as normal components of life and to discuss how we can cope with these events.

Confrontations with death elicit different feelings depending on many factors, including age, religious beliefs, family orientation, health, personal experience with death, and the circumstances of the death itself. To cope effectively with dying, we must address the individual needs of those involved. We will identify some of these needs and offer information and suggestions that have been helpful to many people as they face this final transition. See the Assess Yourself box on page 598 to evaluate your personal level of anxiety about death.

Understanding Death

Large-scale and impersonal death seems to surround us. Often sensationalized by the news media, it is regularly woven into our entertainment. In the context of this routine exposure, it seems paradoxical that Western society in the twenty-first century has been characterized as "death-denying." Why is it that we wish to deny, or even postpone, death? Let's begin by investigating what death means, at least in medical terms (Figure 20.1).

Defining Death

Dying is the process of decline in body functions resulting in the death of an organism. **Death** can be defined as the "final and irreversible cessation of the vital functions" and also refers to a state in which these functions are "incapable of being restored."[1] This definition has become more significant as medical and scientific advances make it increasingly possible to postpone death.

---

dying The process of decline in body functions, resulting in the death of an organism.

death The permanent ending of all vital functions.

brain death The irreversible cessation of all functions of the entire brainstem.

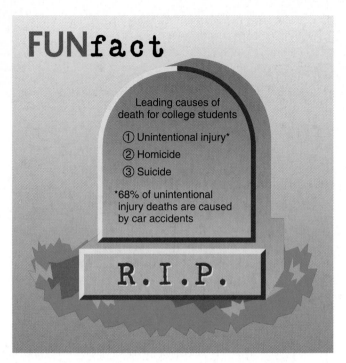

FIGURE 20.1 Top Three Causes of Death for Adults Aged 18–24

Source: National Center for Health Statistics (NCHS), National Vital Statistics System, "10 Leading Causes of Death, Ages 18–24, United States," 2003, http://webapp.cdc.gov/cgi-bin/broker.exe.

Legal and ethical issues related to death and dying led to the Uniform Determination of Death Act in 1981. This act, which has been adopted by several states, reads as follows: "An individual who has sustained either (1) irreversible cessation of circulatory and respiratory functions, or (2) irreversible cessation of all functions of the entire brain, including the brainstem, is dead. A determination of death must be made in accordance with accepted medical standards."[2]

The concept of **brain death,** defined as the irreversible cessation of all functions of the entire brainstem, has gained increasing credence. (The brainstem is a relay site for sensory and motor pathways and contains structures responsible for mediating such critical body functions as respiration, heart rate, and general levels of alertness.) As defined by the Ad Hoc Committee of the Harvard Medical School, brain death occurs when the following criteria are met:[3]

- Unreceptivity and unresponsiveness—that is, no response even to painful stimuli
- No movement during a continuous hour of observation by a physician, and no breathing after three minutes off a respirator
- No reflexes, including brainstem reflexes; fixed and dilated pupils
- A "flat" electroencephalogram (EEG, which measures electrical activity of the brain) for at least 10 minutes
- All of these tests repeated at least 24 hours later with no change

- Certainty that hypothermia (extreme loss of body heat) or depression of the central nervous system caused by use of drugs such as barbiturates are not responsible for these conditions

The Harvard report provides useful guidelines; however, the definition of *death* and all its ramifications continues to concern us.

what do you THINK?

Why is there so much concern over the definition of death? ■ How does modern technology complicate the understanding of when death occurs?

Denying Death

Attitudes toward death tend to fall on a continuum. At one end of the continuum, death is viewed as the mortal enemy of humankind. Both medical science and religion have promoted this idea of death. At the other end of the continuum, death is accepted and even welcomed. For people whose attitudes fall at this end, death is a passage to a better state of being. Most of us, however, perceive ourselves to be in the middle of this continuum. From this perspective, death is a bewildering mystery that elicits fear and apprehension while profoundly influencing attitudes, beliefs, and actions throughout life.

In the United States, a high level of discomfort is associated with death and dying. As a result, we may avoid speaking about death in an effort to limit our own discomfort. Those who deny death tend to:

- Avoid people who are grieving after the death of a loved one so they won't have to talk about it
- Fail to validate a dying person's frightening situation by talking to the person as if nothing were wrong
- Substitute euphemisms for the word death (for example, "passing away," "no longer with us," or "going to a better place")
- Give false reassurances to people who are dying by saying things like "everything is going to be okay"
- Shut off conversation about death by silencing people who are trying to talk about it
- Avoid touching people who are dying

Death denial has long been the predominant coping mechanism used by our society, but we must keep in mind that social attitudes change over time. It is therefore important to understand the climate in which these perceptions developed and took hold.

Major changes in attitudes toward death accompanied the Industrial Revolution. An emphasis on autonomy and rejection of magic meant that, as a culture, Americans had to be independent and autonomous. Yet American rituals centered on connections to other people. Recent years have shown a greater effort on the part of the American public to mourn openly, as indicated by roadside crosses and memorials

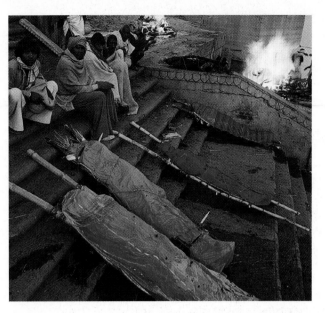

There is no single way to mourn. Each culture has its own unique ways of saying goodbye to the deceased.

placed at the sites of violent or unexpected deaths. Although these are fairly new additions to the American landscape, these memorials have long been popular in other parts of the world, particularly in predominantly Catholic countries.[4]

The attitudes we develop about death are influenced by many factors, including modern technology, personal experience and beliefs, the environment, age, access to health care, and many other factors. The complex social environment we live in has added new experiences and sometimes confusion to the complexity of our own personal beliefs about death.

what do you THINK?

"The art of living well and the art of dying well are one." What do you think this quote from the Greek philosopher Epicurus means? ■ Do you agree?

The Process of Dying

Dying is a complex process that includes physical, intellectual, social, spiritual, and emotional dimensions. Now that we have examined the physical indicators of death, we must consider the emotional aspects of dying and "social death."

Coping Emotionally with Death

Science and medicine have enabled us to understand changes associated with growth, development, aging, and social roles throughout the life span, but they have not fully explained the

(Text continues on page 600)

ASSESS yourself

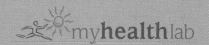

DEATH-RELATED ANXIETY SCALE

Fill out this assessment online at www.aw-bc.com/myhealthlab or www.aw-bc.com/donatelle.

How anxious or accepting are you about the prospect of your death? Indicate how well each statement describes your attitude.

		Not True at All	Mainly Not True	Not Sure	Somewhat True	Very True
1.	I tend not to be very brave in crisis situations.	0	1	2	3	4
2.	I am an unusually anxious person.	0	1	2	3	4
3.	I am something of a hypochondriac and am perhaps obsessively worried about infections.	0	1	2	3	4
4.	I have never had a semimystical, spiritual, out-of-the-body, near-death, or "peak" experience.	0	1	2	3	4
5.	I tend to be unusually frightened in planes at takeoff and landing.	0	1	2	3	4
6.	I do not have a particular religion or philosophy that helps me to face dying.	0	1	2	3	4
7.	I do not believe in any form of survival of the soul after death.	0	1	2	3	4
8.	Personally, I would give a lot to be immortal in this body.	0	1	2	3	4
9.	I am very much a city person and not really close to nature.	0	1	2	3	4
10.	Anxiety about death spoils the quality of my life.	0	1	2	3	4
11.	I am superstitious that preparing for dying might hasten my death.	0	1	2	3	4
12.	I don't like the way some of my relatives died and fear that my death could be like theirs.	0	1	2	3	4
13.	My actual experience of friends dying has been undilutedly negative.	0	1	2	3	4
14.	I would feel easier being with a dying relative if he or she had not been told he or she was dying.	0	1	2	3	4
15.	I have fears of dying alone without friends around me.	0	1	2	3	4
16.	I have fears of dying slowly.	0	1	2	3	4
17.	I have fears of dying suddenly.	0	1	2	3	4
18.	I have fears of dying before my time or while my children are still young.	0	1	2	3	4
19.	I have fears of dying before fulfilling my potential and fully using my talents.	0	1	2	3	4
20.	I have fears of dying without adequately having expressed my love to those I am close to.	0	1	2	3	4
21.	I have fears of dying before having really experienced much joie de vivre.	0	1	2	3	4
22.	I have fears of what may or may not happen after death.	0	1	2	3	4

	Not True at All	Mainly Not True	Not Sure	Somewhat True	Very True
23. I have fears of what could happen to my family after my death.	0	1	2	3	4
24. I have fears of dying in a hospital or an institution.	0	1	2	3	4
25. I have fears of those caring for me feeling overwhelmed by the strain of it.	0	1	2	3	4
26. I have fears of not getting help with euthanasia when the time comes.	0	1	2	3	4
27. I have fears of being given unofficial and unwanted euthanasia.	0	1	2	3	4
28. I have fears of getting insufficient pain control while dying.	0	1	2	3	4
29. I have fears of being overmedicated and unconscious while dying.	0	1	2	3	4
30. I have fears of being declared dead when not really dead or being buried alive.	0	1	2	3	4
31. I have fears of getting confused at death or not being able to follow my spiritual practices.	0	1	2	3	4
32. I have fears of what may happen to my body after death.	0	1	2	3	4
33. I have fears of an Alzheimer's-type mental degeneration near death.	0	1	2	3	4
34. Overall I would say that I am unusually anxious about death and dying.	0	1	2	3	4

Total points _____

Interpreting Your Scores

If you are extremely anxious (scoring 65 or more), you might consider counseling or therapy; if you are unusually anxious (scoring between 40 and 64), you might want to find a method of meditation, philosophy, or spiritual practice to help experience, explore, and accept your feelings about death. Average anxiety is a score under 40. Continue to have a thoughtful and open ability to consider your own death in time.

MAKE it happen!

ASSESSMENT: The Assess Yourself activity above encouraged you to explore your death-related anxiety. How anxious are you? Do you want to reduce your fears and increase your acceptance of this inevitable part of life?

MAKING A CHANGE: In order to change your behavior, you need to develop a plan. Follow the steps below and complete your Behavior Change Contract to take action.

1. Evaluate your behavior and identify patterns and specific things you are doing. What can you change now? What can you change in the near future?

2. Select one pattern of behavior that you want to change.

3. Fill out the Behavior Change Contract found at the front of your book. It should include your long-term goal for change, your short-term goals, the rewards you'll give yourself for reaching these goals, potential obstacles along the way, and strategies for overcoming these obstacles. For each goal, list the small steps and specific actions that you will take.

4. Chart your progress in a journal. At the end of a week, consider how successful you were in following your plan.

(continued)

What helped you be successful? What made change more difficult? What will you do differently next week?

5. Revise your plan as needed: Are the short-term goals attainable? Are the rewards satisfying?

ONE STUDENT'S PLAN: Peter's score of 60 points on the self-assessment indicated that he was unusually anxious about death. The experience of his grandmother's death had been a very difficult one. He was only 6 years old at the time of her death, and no one in his family discussed it with him. He visited her once in the hospital and witnessed an argument between his parents and her doctors over the steps that should be taken to prolong her life.

Peter decided that one way to feel more in control and less anxious about death would be to learn about advance directives. He went to a low-cost legal clinic near campus and asked for information. There, he was given a sample directive to discuss with his parents and his physician. It listed various medical procedures of which he could indicate the ones he did and did not want taken.

Peter also decided to fill out an organ donation card. He wanted to be sure his parents knew what he wanted done after his death, and he believed that donating any needed body parts was a worthy and fulfilling decision.

---

nature of death. This may partially explain why the transition from life to death evokes so much mystery and emotion. Although emotional reactions to dying vary, many people share similar experiences during this process.

> **Does everyone experience death and grief in the same way?**

Tasks, stages, and *phases* are all terms that have been used in models that have been developed to understand the process of dying. The late Elisabeth Kübler-Ross is perhaps the most well known of writers on the topic, but researchers such as Charles Corr have continued to expand on her great work. Research leading to a better understanding of the process of dying will continue as new psychological perspectives are explored.

Kübler-Ross and the Stages of Dying

Much of our knowledge about reactions to dying stems from the work of Elisabeth Kübler-Ross, a pioneer in **thanatology**, the study of death and dying. In 1969, Kübler-Ross published *On Death and Dying*, a sensitive analysis of the reactions of terminally ill patients. This pioneering work encouraged the development of death education as a discipline and prompted efforts to improve the care of dying patients. Kübler-Ross identified five psychological stages (Figure 20.2) that terminally ill patients often experience as they approach death:[5]

1. *Denial.* ("Not me, there must be a mistake.") This is usually the first stage, experienced as a sensation of shock and disbelief. A person intellectually accepts the impending death but rejects it emotionally. The patient is too confused and stunned to comprehend "not being" and thus rejects the idea.

2. *Anger.* ("Why me?") Anger is another common reaction to the realization of imminent death. The person becomes angry at having to face death when others are healthy. The dying person perceives the situation as "unfair" or "senseless" and may be hostile to friends, family, physicians, or the world in general.

3. *Bargaining.* ("If I'm allowed to live, I promise …") This stage generally occurs at about the middle of the progression. The dying person may resolve to be a better person in return for an extension of life or may secretly pray for a short reprieve from death in order to experience a special event, such as a family wedding or birth.

4. *Depression.* ("It's really going to happen to me, and I can't do anything about it.") Depression eventually sets in as vitality diminishes and the person begins to experience symptoms with increasing frequency. The person's deteriorating condition becomes impossible for him or her to deny, and feelings of doom and tremendous loss may become unbearably pervasive. Feelings of worthlessness and guilt are also common because the dying person may feel responsible for the emotional suffering of loved ones and the arduous efforts of caregivers.

5. *Acceptance.* ("I'm ready.") This is often the final stage. The patient stops battling with emotions and becomes tired and weak. The need to sleep increases, and wakeful periods become shorter and less frequent. With acceptance, the person does not "give up" and become sullen or resentfully resigned to death, but rather becomes passive. According to one dying person, the acceptance stage is "almost void of feelings…as if the pain had gone, the struggle is over, and there comes a time for the final rest

thanatology The study of death and dying.

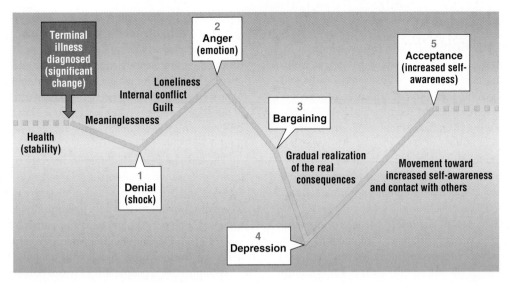

FIGURE 20.2 Kübler-Ross's Stages of Dying

before the long journey."[6] As he or she lets go, the dying person may no longer welcome visitors and may not wish to engage in conversation. Death usually occurs quietly and painlessly while the victim is unconscious.

The health care profession immediately embraced Kübler-Ross's "stage theory" and applied it in clinical settings. However, subsequent research has indicated that the experiences of dying and grieving people do not fit easily into specific stages. Some people never go through this process and instead remain emotionally calm; others may pass back and forth between the stages. Even if it is not accurate in all its particulars, however, Kübler-Ross's theory offers valuable insights for those dealing with the process of dying.

Corr's Coping Approach Since Kübler-Ross's work, others have developed alternative models for understanding the ways in which we cope with death and other significant losses. Charles Corr believes that there are unique challenges and responses for the dying person and those who love that person.[7] He suggests four dimensions of coping with loss: *physical*—doing everything possible to make ourselves comfortable and minimize pain; *psychological*—living to the fullest, focusing on life accomplishments, and seeking satisfaction in daily activities; *social*—nurturing relationships, keeping loved ones involved, and sharing emotions; and *spiritual*—identifying what matters in life and reaffirming meaningful experiences.

 what do you THINK?

Do you agree with Elisabeth Kübler-Ross's stages of dying, or do you think the stages should be expanded to include Corr's model? ■ Do you think it is important to help a person get through all the stages that Kübler-Ross has identified? Why or why not?

Social Death

The need for recognition and appreciation within a social group is nearly universal. Denying a person normal social interaction is **social death,** a seemingly irreversible situation in which a person is not treated like an active member of society. Dramatic examples of social death include the exile of nonconformists from their native countries or the excommunication of dissident members of religious groups. Numerous studies indicate that people who are dying are treated differently too. The following common behaviors contribute to the social death that often isolates people who are terminally ill:[8]

■ The dying person is referred to as if he or she were already dead.

■ The dying person may be inadvertently excluded from conversations.

■ Dying patients are often moved to terminal wards and given minimal care.

■ Bereaved family members are avoided, often for extended periods, because friends and neighbors are afraid of feeling uncomfortable in the presence of grief.

■ Medical personnel may make degrading comments about patients in their presence.

This decrease in meaningful social interaction often strips dying and bereaved people of their identity as valued members of society at a time when belonging is critical. Some dying people choose not to speak of their inevitable fate in an attempt to make others feel more comfortable and thus preserve vital relationships.

social death A seemingly irreversible situation in which a person is not treated like an active member of society.

Coping with Loss

The losses resulting from the death of a loved one are extremely difficult to cope with. The dying person, as well as close family and friends, frequently suffers emotionally and physically from the impending loss of critical relationships and roles. Words used to describe feelings and behavior related to losses resulting from death include *bereavement, grief, grief work*, and *mourning*. These terms are related but not identical in meaning. Understanding them will help in comprehending the emotional processes associated with loss and the cultural constraints that often inhibit normal coping behavior (Figure 20.3).

Bereavement is generally defined as the loss or deprivation experienced by a survivor when a loved one dies. Because relationships vary in type and intensity, reactions to losses also vary. The death of a parent, spouse, sibling, child, friend, or pet will result in different kinds of feelings. In the lives of the bereaved or of close survivors, the loss of loved ones leaves "holes." We can think of bereavement as the awareness of these holes. Time and courage are necessary to fill these spaces.

A special case of bereavement occurs in old age. Loss is an intrinsic part of growing old. The longer we live, the more losses we are likely to experience. These losses include physical, social, and emotional losses as our bodies deteriorate and more and more of our loved ones die. The theory of *bereavement overload* has been proposed to explain the effects of multiple losses and the accumulation of sorrow in the lives of some older adults. This theory suggests that the gloomy outlook, disturbing behavior patterns, and apparent apathy that characterize some people may be related more to bereavement overload than to intrinsic physiological degeneration in old age.[9]

Grief is a state of mental distress that occurs in reaction to significant loss, including one's own impending death, the death of a loved one, or a quasi-death experience (to be discussed later in this chapter). Grief reactions include any adjustments needed for one to "make it through the day" and may include changes in patterns of eating, sleeping, working, and even thinking.

When a person experiences a loss that cannot be openly acknowledged, publicly mourned, or socially supported, coping may be much more difficult. This type of grief is referred to as **disenfranchised grief.**[10] It may occur among those who miscarry during pregnancy, are developmentally disabled, or are close friends rather than relatives of the deceased. It may also include relationships that are not socially approved, such as those between extramarital lovers or gay and lesbian couples. When society does not assign significance to a high-grief death, grieving becomes even more difficult for the bereaved.

The term *mourning* is often incorrectly equated with the term *grief*. As we have noted, *grief* refers to a wide variety of feelings and actions that occur in response to bereavement. **Mourning,** in contrast, refers to culturally prescribed and accepted time periods and behavior patterns for the expression of grief. Depending on a person's relationship with the deceased, various other rituals may continue for up to a year.

In some cases, people are so overwhelmed by grief that they do not return to normal daily living. Support and counseling should be sought when this occurs. Doctors, nurses, psychologists, psychiatrists, and clergy can be helpful in solving problems associated with the loss of a loved one.

Symptoms of grief vary in severity and duration, depending on the situation and the individual. However, the bereaved person can benefit from emotional and social support from family, friends, clergy, employers, and traditional support organizations, including the medical community and the funeral industry. The larger and stronger the support system, the easier readjustment is likely to be. See the Skills for Behavior Change box on page 604 to learn about how you can best help a grieving friend.

Religion provides comfort to many dying and grieving people. Although some people question the existence of an afterlife, others gain support from religious beliefs that provide a purpose and meaning to life. By accepting dying as a part of the continuum of life, many people are able to make necessary readjustments after the death of a loved one. This holistic concept, which accepts dying as a part of the total life experience, is shared by both believers and nonbelievers.

What Is "Normal" Grief?

This is a difficult question to answer. Grief responses vary widely from person to person, but a classic acute grief syndrome often includes the following symptoms:

- Periodic waves of physical distress lasting 20 minutes to an hour
- A feeling of tightness in the throat
- Choking and shortness of breath
- A frequent need to sigh
- A feeling of emptiness in the abdomen
- A sensation of muscular weakness
- Intense anxiety that is described as actually painful

Other common symptoms of grief include insomnia, memory lapses, loss of appetite, difficulty concentrating, a tendency to engage in repetitive or purposeless behavior, an "observer" sensation or feeling of unreality, difficulty in

---

bereavement The loss or deprivation experienced by a survivor when a loved one dies.

grief The state of mental distress that occurs in reaction to significant loss, including one's own impending death, the death of a loved one, or a quasi-death experience.

disenfranchised grief Grief concerning a loss that cannot be openly acknowledged, publicly mourned, or socially supported.

mourning The culturally prescribed behavior patterns for the expression of grief.

making decisions, lack of organization, excessive speech, social withdrawal or hostility, guilt feelings, and preoccupation with the image of the deceased. Susceptibility to disease increases with grief and may even be life-threatening in severe and enduring cases.

A bereaved person may suffer emotional pain and may exhibit a variety of grief responses for many months after the death. The rate of the healing process depends on the amount and quality of grief work that a person does. **Grief work** is the process of integrating the reality of the loss into everyday life and learning to feel better. Often, the bereaved person must deliberately and systematically work at reducing denial and coping with the pain that results from memories of the deceased. This process takes time and requires emotional effort and all people do not grieve in the same way.

Worden's Model of Grieving Tasks

William Worden, a researcher into the death process, developed a more active grieving model that defined four tasks necessary for the individual to complete (Figure 20.3).[11] He explained that each person reacts differently to loss but, in general, the work of bereavement entails the following developmental tasks:

1. *Accept the reality of the loss.* At first, people may react to the death of their loved one with numbness, shock, and denial. This task requires acknowledging and realizing that the person is dead. This task takes time because it involves an intellectual acceptance as well as an emotional one. Traditional rituals, such as the funeral, help many bereaved people move toward acceptance.

2. *Work through the pain of grief.* It is necessary to acknowledge and work through the pain associated with loss, or it will manifest itself through other symptoms or behaviors. Not everyone will experience the same intensity of pain or feel it in the same way. One of the aims of grief counseling is to help facilitate people through this difficult second task so they don't carry the intense pain with them throughout their life.

3. *Adjust to an environment in which the deceased is missing.* Adjusting to a new environment means different things to different people depending on what the relationship was with the deceased. The bereaved may feel lonely and uncertain about a new identity without the person who has died. This loss confronts them with the challenge of adjusting to their own sense of self.

4. *Emotionally relocate the deceased and move on with life.* Individuals never lose memories of a significant relationship, yet eventually grieving individuals need to look forward and continue with their lives. They may need help in letting go of the emotional energy that used to be invested in the person who has died, and they may need help in finding an appropriate place for the deceased

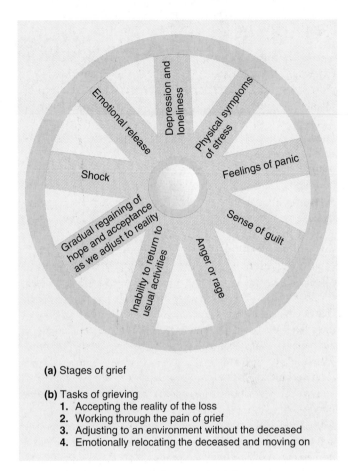

(a) Stages of grief

(b) Tasks of grieving
1. Accepting the reality of the loss
2. Working through the pain of grief
3. Adjusting to an environment without the deceased
4. Emotionally relocating the deceased and moving on

FIGURE 20.3 The Stages and Tasks of Grief

(a) People react differently to losses, but most eventually adapt. Generally, the stronger the social support system, the smoother the progression through the stages of grief. (b) Worden's developmental tasks associated with grief are another way to understand the grieving process.

in their emotional lives. Completing the necessary grief work enables them to focus less on the loss and to connect with other people by investing new energy in ongoing relationships.

In summary, models of the grief process can be viewed as "generalized maps," in that each theory is an attempt by an investigator to understand and guide grieving individuals through their pain. However, humans are unique and cannot be forced into particular patterns of behavior. Each individual will travel through grief at his or her own speed using an appropriate route.

grief work The process of accepting the reality of a person's death and coping with memories of the deceased.

SKILLS FOR behavior change

TALKING TO FRIENDS WHEN SOMEONE DIES

It's always hard to know just what to say and how to say it when talking with a grieving friend or relative. Sometimes, even though we mean well, our actions can hurt more than help. Here are some do's and don'ts.

How can I help a friend who has just experienced a loss?

DO'S

- Let your genuine concern and caring show; say you are sorry about their loss and about their pain.
- Be available to listen, run errands, help with the children, or whatever else seems needed at the time.
- Allow them to express as much grief as they are feeling at the moment and are willing to share.
- Encourage them to be patient with themselves and not worry about things they should be doing.
- Allow them to talk about the person who has died as much and as often as they want to.

- Talk about the special, endearing qualities of the person who has died.
- Reassure them that they did everything they could, that the medical care given was the best, or whatever else you know to be true and positive about the care given.

DON'TS

- Let your own sense of helplessness keep you from reaching out to a bereaved person.
- Avoid them because you are uncomfortable (this adds pain to an already intolerably painful experience).
- Say you know how they feel (unless you've suffered a similar loss, you probably don't).
- Say "you ought to be feeling better by now" or anything else that implies judgment about their feelings or what they should be doing.
- Change the subject when they mention the person who has died.
- Avoid mentioning the name of the person who has died out of fear of reminding them of their pain.

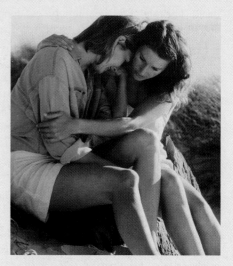

- Make any comments which in any way suggest that the care given to the deceased at home, in the hospital, or wherever was inadequate. (Bereaved people are already plagued by feelings of doubt and guilt.)

Source: Interior Alzheimer's Society, "Do's and Don'ts of Helping Bereaved People," August 24, 2006, www.alzheimer-society.ca.

? *what do you* THINK?

If you have experienced a death among your family or friends, how did you grieve? ■ Did you accomplish Worden's tasks? ■ Does the model match your experience?

When an Infant or Child Dies

At the beginning of the twentieth century, children under the age of 15 made up 34 percent of the U.S. population but accounted for 53 percent of total deaths. Today, children continue to benefit from advances in medicine and social policy that have reduced mortality rates by more than 90 percent since 1900.[12] Children are highly valued in our society, and their deaths are considered major tragedies. No matter what the cause of death—miscarriage, fatal birth defects, childhood illness, accident, suicide, homicide, natural disaster, neglect, or war injuries—the grief experienced when a child dies may be overwhelming.

The death of a child is terribly painful for the whole family. However, for several reasons, the siblings of the deceased child have a particularly hard time with grief work. Bereaved children usually have limited experience with death and therefore have not yet learned how to deal with major loss. Children may feel uncomfortable talking about death, and they may also receive less social support and sympathy than their parents do. Because so much attention and energy are devoted to the deceased child, the surviving children may feel emotionally abandoned by their parents.

A Child's Response to Death

In the past, children were thought to be miniature adults and were expected to behave as adults. It is now understood that children and adults react to death quite differently. Often, when children suffer a loss, they will react in ways that seem "normal" to the adult observer. However, children often do not show their feelings as openly as adults do. Although their actions may not reveal what they are truly feeling, children tend to experience more prolonged mourning periods. They typically grapple with these questions: (1) Did I cause the death to happen? (2) Is it going to happen to me? (3) Who is going to take care of me?[13] A child's grieving period may be less stressful when adults are open and honest and include the child in the funeral process as much as possible.

Quasi-Death Experiences

Many cultures provide social and emotional support for the bereaved in the aftermath of death. Typically, however, little support is offered when people face many other significant losses in life. Losses that in many ways resemble death and that may involve a heavy burden of grief include a child running away from home, an abduction or kidnapping, a divorce, a move to a distant place, a move to a nursing home, the loss of a romance or intimate friendship, retirement, job termination, finishing a "terminal" academic degree, or ending an athletic career.

These **quasi-death experiences** resemble death in that they involve separation, termination, loss, and a change in identity or self-perception.[14] If grief results from these losses, the pattern of the grief response will probably follow the same course as responses to death. Factors that may complicate the grieving process associated with quasi-death include uncomfortable contact with the object of loss (for example, an ex-spouse) and a lack of adequate social and institutional support.

Living with Grief

The reality of death and loss touches everyone. Coping with death is vital to your mental health. The National Mental Health Association offers these suggestions for living with grief and coping effectively with your pain.[15]

- *Seek out caring people.* Find relatives and friends who can understand your feelings of loss. Join support groups with others who are experiencing similar losses.
- *Express your feelings.* Tell others how you are feeling; it will help you to work through the grieving process.
- *Take care of your health.* Maintain regular contact with your family physician and be sure to eat well and get plenty of rest. Be aware of the danger of developing a dependence on medication or alcohol to deal with your grief.
- *Accept that life is for the living.* It takes effort to begin to live again in the present and not dwell on the past.
- *Postpone major life changes.* Try to hold off on making any major changes, such as moving, remarrying, changing jobs, or having another child. You should give yourself time to adjust to your loss.
- *Be patient.* It can take months or even years to absorb a major loss and accept your changed life.
- *Seek outside help when necessary.* If your grief seems like it is too much to bear, seek professional assistance to help work through your grief. It's a sign of strength, not weakness, to seek help.

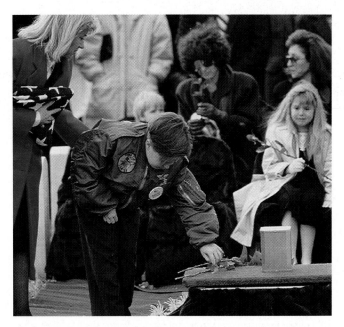

A significant loss can be particularly difficult for children.

Life-and-Death Decision Making

Many complex—and often expensive—life-and-death decisions must be made during a highly distressing period in people's lives. These emotion-laden decisions are compounded by the stresses of dying and bereavement. We will not attempt to present definitive answers to moral and philosophical questions about death; instead, we offer these topics for your consideration. We hope that this discussion of the needs of the dying person and the bereaved will help you negotiate these difficult decisions in the future.

The Right to Die

Few people would object to a proposal for the right to a dignified death. Going beyond that concept, however, many people today believe that they should be allowed to die if their condition is terminal and their existence depends on mechanical life-support devices or artificial feeding or hydration systems. Artificial life-support techniques that may be legally refused by competent patients in some states include:

- Electrical or mechanical heart resuscitation
- Mechanical respiration by machine
- Nasogastric tube feedings

quasi-death experience A loss or experience that resembles death, in that it involves separation, termination, significant loss, a change of personal identity, and grief.

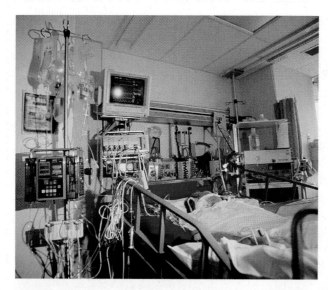

Sophisticated life-support technology allows a patient's life to be prolonged even in cases of terminal illness or mortal injury. It has also raised legal and moral questions for patients, their families, and health care professionals.

- Intravenous nutrition
- Gastrostomy (tube feeding directly into the stomach)
- Medications to treat life-threatening infections

Why should I create a living will? As long as a person is conscious and competent, he or she has the legal right to refuse treatment, even if this decision will hasten death. However, when a person is in a coma or otherwise incapable of speaking on his or her own behalf, medical personnel and administrative policy will dictate treatment. This issue has evolved into a battle involving personal freedom, legal rulings, health care administration policy, and physician responsibility. The living will and other advance directives were developed to assist in solving conflicts among these people and agencies.

Even young, apparently healthy people need a living will. Consider Terri Schiavo, who collapsed at age 26 from heart failure which led to irreversible brain damage. Schiavo, unable to survive without life support, never left any written guidelines about her wishes should she become incapacitated. After a 15-year legal battle between her parents, who wanted her to be kept alive, and her husband, who felt she should be allowed to die, the courts sided with her husband and she was removed from life support.

In other instances, there have been cases in which the wishes of people who had signed a living will (or other directive) indicating their desire not to receive artificial life support were not honored by their physician or medical institution. This problem can be avoided by choosing both a physician and a hospital that will carry out the directives of the living will. Taking this

rational suicide The decision to kill oneself rather than endure constant pain and slow decay.

precaution and discussing your personal philosophy and wishes with your family should eliminate anxiety about how you will be treated at the end of your life (Figure 20.4).

Many legal experts suggest that you take the following steps to ensure that your wishes are carried out:

1. *Be specific.* Rather than signing an advance directive (that only speaks in generalities), complete a directive that permits you to make specific choices about a variety of procedures, including cardiopulmonary resuscitation (CPR); dialysis; being placed on a ventilator; receiving food, water, or medication through tubes; receiving pain medication; and organ donation. It is also essential to attach that document to a completed copy of the standard advance directive for your state.

2. *Get an agent.* Even the most detailed directive cannot possibly anticipate every situation that may arise. You may want to also appoint a family member or friend to act as your agent, or *proxy*, by making out a form known as either a *durable power of attorney for health care* or a *health care proxy.*

3. *Discuss your wishes.* Discuss your preferences in detail with your proxy and your doctor. Your doctor or proxy may misinterpret or ignore your wishes. Going over the situations described in the form will give them a clear idea of just how much you are willing to endure to preserve your life.

4. *Deliver the directive.* Distribute several copies, not only to your doctor and your agent, but also to your lawyer and to immediate family members or a close friend. Your doctor should include this copy in your medical records. Keep the original in a place where your proxy can easily find it. Make sure someone knows to bring a copy to the hospital in the event you are hospitalized.[16]

Rational Suicide

We have discussed suicide in earlier chapters as a consequence of depression or other factors. The concept of **rational suicide** as an alternative to an extended dying process, however, deserves mention here. Rational suicide is a result of a reasoned, coherent process in which a person chooses death as a preferable alternative to unbearable pain.

Although exact numbers are not known, medical ethicists, experts in rational suicide, and specialists in forensic medicine (the study of legal issues in medicine) estimate that every year thousands of terminally ill people decide to kill themselves rather than endure constant pain and slow decay. To these people, the prospect of an undignified death is unacceptable.

Do we have a right to die? If so, is this an unlimited right, or does it apply only in certain conditions? If terminally ill patients are allowed to commit suicide legally, what other groups will demand this option? Should the courts be involved in private decisions? Should any organization be allowed to distribute information that may encourage suicide? Should loved ones or medical caregivers be allowed to assist

This directive is made this _____ day of _____ (month) _____ (year).
I, _____ being of sound mind, willfully and voluntarily make known my desire

(a) ☐ **That my life shall not be artificially prolonged** and

(b) ☐ **That my life shall be ended with the aid of a physician under circumstances set forth below, and do hereby declare:**
(You must initial (a) or (b), or both.)

1. If at any time I should have a terminal condition or illness certified to be terminal by two physicians, and they determine that my death will occur within six months,

   (a) ☐ **I direct that life-sustaining procedures be withheld or withdrawn** and

   (b) ☐ **I direct that my physician administer aid-in-dying in a humane and dignified manner.** (You must initial (a) or (b), or both.)

   (c) ☐ **I have attached Special Instructions on a separate page to the directive.** (Initial if you have attached a separate page.)

   The action taken under this paragraph shall be at the time of my own choosing if I am competent.

2. In the absence of my ability to give directions regarding the termination of my life, it is my intention that this directive shall be honored by my family, agent (described in paragraph 4), and physician(s) as the final expression of my legal right to

   (a) ☐ **Refuse medical or surgical treatment,** and

   (b) ☐ **To choose to die in a humane and dignified manner.** (You must initial (a) or (b), or both and you must initial one box below.)

   ☐ If I am unable to give directions, I *do not* want my attorney-in-fact to request aid-in-dying.

   ☐ If I am unable to give directions, I *do* want my attorney-in-fact to ask my physician for aid-in-dying.

3. I understand that a terminal condition is one in which I am not likely to live for more than six months.

4. a. I, _____
   do hereby designate and appoint _____
   as my attorney-in-fact (agent) to make health-care decisions for me if I am in a coma or otherwise unable to decide for myself as authorized in this document. For the purpose of this document, "health-care decision" means consent, refusal of consent, or withdrawal of consent to any care, treatment, service, or procedure to maintain, diagnose, or treat an individual's physical or mental condition, or to administer aid-in-dying.

   b. By this document I intend to create a Durable Power of Attorney for Health Care under The Oregon Death With Dignity Act and ORS Section 126.407. This power of attorney shall not be affected by my subsequent incapacity, except by revocation.

   c. Subject to any limitations in this document, I hereby grant to my agent full power and authority to make health-care decisions for me to the same extent that I could make these decisions for myself if I had the capacity to do so. In exercising this authority, my agent shall make health-care decisions that are consistent with my desires as stated in this document or otherwise made known to my agent, including, but not limited to, my desires concerning obtaining, refusing, or withdrawing life-prolonging care, treatment, services, and procedures, and administration of aid-in-dying.

5. This directive shall have no force or effect seven years from the date filled in above, unless I am competent to act on my own behalf and then it shall remain valid until my competency is restored.

6. I recognize that a physician's judgment is not always certain, and that medical science continues to make progress in extending life, but in spite of these facts, I nevertheless wish aid-in-dying rather than letting my terminal condition take its natural course.

7. My family has been informed of my request to die, their opinions have been taken into consideration, but the final decision remains mine, so long as I am competent.

8. The exact time of my death will be determined by me and my physician with my desire or my attorney-in-fact's instructions paramount.

I have given full consideration and understand the full import of this directive, and I am emotionally and mentally competent to make this directive. I accept the moral and legal responsibility for receiving aid-in-dying.

This directive will not be valid unless it is signed by two qualified witnesses who are present when you sign or acknowledge your signature. The witnesses must not be related to you by blood, marriage, or adoption; they must not be entitled to any part of your estate; and they must not include a physician or other person responsible for, or employed by anyone responsible for, your health care. If you have attached any additional pages to this form, you must date and sign each of the additional pages at the same time you date and sign this power of attorney.

Signed: _____

_____
City, County, and State of Residence

This document must be witnessed by two qualified adult witnesses. None of the following may be used as witnesses: (1) a health-care provider who is involved in any way with the treatment of the declarant, (2) an employee of a health-care provider who is involved in any way with the treatment of the declarant, (3) the operator of a community care facility where the declarant resides, (4) an employee of an operator of a community care facility who is involved in any way with the treatment of the declarant.

FIGURE 20.4 Directive to Physicians

An example of a directive that can be used to specify end-of-life treatments.

Source: The Oregon Death with Dignity Act, Oregon Revised Statute, Chapter 97 (1990).

HEALTH ETHICS
conflict and controversy

IS PHYSICIAN-ASSISTED SUICIDE ETHICAL?

Physician-assisted suicide (PAS) has caused a furor in the media and debate within the medical and legal professions. Consider the reasoning that follows as you develop your own position on this issue.

ARGUMENTS IN FAVOR OF PAS

Those who believe that PAS is ethically justified offer the following reasons:

1. *Respect for autonomy.* Decisions about time and circumstances of death are very personal. Competent persons should have the right to choose death.
2. *Justice.* Justice requires that we "treat like cases alike." Competent terminally ill patients are allowed to hasten death by refusing treatment; but for some patients, cutting off treatment will not suffice to hasten death—their only real option is suicide. Justice requires that we should allow assisted death for these patients.
3. *Compassion.* Suffering means more than pain; other physical and psychological burdens accompany some forms of terminal illness. It is not always possible to relieve suffering. Thus PAS may be a compassionate response to unbearable suffering.
4. *Individual liberty versus state interest.* Though society has a strong interest in preserving life, that interest lessens when a person is terminally ill and has a strong desire to end life. A complete prohibition on assisted death exces-

sively limits personal liberty. Therefore PAS should be allowed in certain cases.

5. *Openness of discussion.* Some would argue that assisted death already occurs, albeit in secret. For example, morphine drips ostensibly for pain relief may be a covert form of assisted death or euthanasia. The fact that PAS is illegal prevents open discussion of the issue and fosters secrecy in administering it. Legalization would promote open discussion.

ARGUMENTS AGAINST PAS

Those who believe that PAS should remain illegal present these arguments:

1. *Sanctity of life.* There are strong religious and secular traditions against taking human life. Assisted suicide is morally wrong because it contradicts these beliefs.
2. *Passive versus active distinction.* There is an important difference between passively "letting die" and actively "killing." Refusing treatment or withholding treatment is equivalent to letting die (a passive measure) and therefore justifiable, whereas PAS is equivalent to killing (an active measure) and is not justifiable.
3. *Potential for abuse.* Certain groups of people, lacking access to care and support, may be pushed into assisted death. Furthermore, assisted death may become a cost-containment strategy. Burdened family members and health care providers may unscrupulously en-

courage the option of assisted death in certain cases. To protect against these abuses, PAS should remain illegal.

4. *Professional integrity.* The historical ethical traditions of medicine strongly oppose taking life. For instance, the Hippocratic oath states, "I will not administer poison to anyone where asked" and "Be of benefit, or at least do no harm." Furthermore, major professional groups (such as the American Medical Association and the American Geriatrics Society) oppose assisted death because linking PAS to the practice of medicine could harm the public's image of the profession.
5. *Fallibility of the profession.* Physicians will make mistakes. For instance, there may be uncertainty in diagnosis and prognosis, errors in diagnosis and treatment of depression, or inadequate treatment of pain. Thus the state has an obligation to protect lives from these inevitable mistakes.

What are your feelings about PAS? Under what circumstances might you consider it an acceptable option? Under what circumstances should it not be an option? Where should the line be drawn?

Source: Excerpted from C. H. Braddock and M. R. Tonelli, "Physician-Assisted Suicide," *Ethics in Medicine,* February 22, 1999, http://eduserv .hscer.washington.edu/bioethics/topics/pas .html.

---

the person who wants to die by providing the means? Read the Health Ethics box to explore answers to these questions.

Euthanasia is often referred to as "mercy killing." The

active euthanasia   "Mercy killing," in which a person or organization knowingly acts to hasten the death of a terminally ill person.

passive euthanasia   The intentional withholding of treatment that would prolong life.

term **active euthanasia** has been given to ending the life of a person (or animal) that is suffering greatly and has no chance of recovery. An example might be a physician-prescribed lethal injection. **Passive euthanasia** refers to the intentional withholding of treatment that would prolong life. Deciding not to place a person with massive brain trauma on life support is an example of passive euthanasia.

Dr. Jack Kevorkian, a physician in Michigan, started a one-person campaign to force the medical profession to change its position regarding physician-assisted death. Kevorkian has assisted many terminally ill patients in dying and escaped conviction for several years. Kevorkian has argued that the present situations in our society demand a shift in the thinking and practices that medicine has had throughout most of human history. He believes that acceptance of euthanasia, specifically physician-assisted death, is one of those changes. However, the courts determined that Kevorkian's methods had gone too far; he was convicted of murder and sentenced to prison, where he remains.

Kevorkian's actions have focused attention on the issue, causing many to discuss the merits of physician-assisted suicide. According to public opinion polls, most Americans believe that suicide is morally wrong but are divided on whether physician-assisted suicide is morally acceptable. Roughly 70 percent of Americans believe doctors should be allowed to help end an incurably ill patient's life painlessly at the patient's request.[17]

Legalization of assisted suicide has been debated in many states across the nation. Currently, 38 states have enacted statutes explicitly prohibiting assisted suicide; 4 states are undecided (meaning there are no statutes or case law specifically prohibiting assisted suicide); and Oregon is the only state that allows physician-assisted suicide under certain circumstances outlined in Oregon's Death with Dignity Act.[18]

| **Is physician-assisted suicide legal in the United States?** |

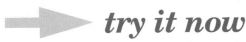

try it now

You can never be too young to consider completing an advance directive. Right now, go to www.uslivingwillregistry.com/forms.shtm, select the state you live in, and print out your state's "advance directive for health care" form. Read through the form, and think about the health care decisions you would make to complete the form.

Making Final Arrangements

Caring for dying people and dealing with the practical and legal questions surrounding death can be difficult and painful. The problems of the dying person and the bereaved loved ones involve a wide variety of psychological, legal, social, spiritual, economic, and interpersonal issues.

Hospice Care: Positive Alternatives

Since the mid-1970s, **hospice** programs have grown from a mere handful to more than 2,500, available in nearly every community. Improving the quality of care at the end of life is a top priority of the American Medical Association.

The primary goals of the hospice program are to relieve

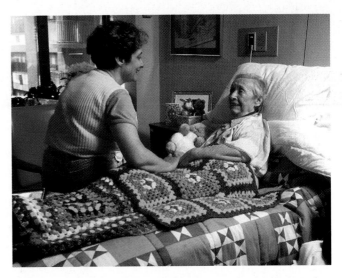

A hospice program provides support services to family members, ensures your dying loved one is comfortable, and allows family and friends to be involved in your loved one's care.

the dying person's pain, offer emotional support to the dying person and loved ones, and restore a sense of control to the dying person, family, and friends. Although home care with maximum involvement by loved ones is emphasized, hospice programs are directed by cooperating physicians, coordinated by specially trained nurses, and fortified with the services of counselors, clergy, and trained volunteers. Hospital inpatient beds are available if necessary. Hospice programs usually include the following characteristics:

1. The patient and family constitute the unit of care because the physical, psychological, social, and spiritual problems of dying confront the family as well as the patient.

2. Emphasis is placed on controlling symptoms, primarily the alleviation of pain. Curative treatments are curtailed as requested by the patient, but sound judgment must be applied to avoid a feeling of abandonment.

3. There is overall medical direction of the program, with all health care being provided under the direction of a qualified physician.

4. Services are provided by an interdisciplinary team because no one person can provide all the needed care.

5. Coverage is provided 24 hours a day, seven days a week, with emphasis on the availability of medical and nursing skills.

6. Carefully selected and extensively trained volunteers are an integral part of the health care team, augmenting staff service but not replacing it.

7. Care of the family extends through the bereavement period.

hospice A concept of care for terminally ill patients designed to maximize quality of life.

SKILLS FOR behavior change

PREPARING TO SUPPORT A DYING PERSON

Whether we have months to prepare for death or it comes suddenly, most people have difficulty knowing what to do. We push death from our consciousness, which leads to problems before and after the moment of death comes for loved ones. Although you can never be fully prepared for the loss of a loved one, you can learn skills that will help you through the trauma of loss. The following suggestions will help, particularly if you have time to prepare.

1. *Follow the wishes of the patient.* Make sure that a copy of his or her advance directive is available and accepted as the wishes of the patient. Most people, particularly in hospice, want a natural death. Think of comfort, not cure. Whenever possible, talk to the patient and allow choices to be made about the dying process. For example, if the patient wants to stay at home but being in a hospital bed would be easier for caregivers, talk this out with the patient.

2. *Help with comfort and rest.* Don't be afraid to ask for medications to help the patient deal with pain, sleeplessness, or anxiety.

3. *Prepare a list of people to call near the time of death, including family, friends, and religious support.* Talk about who the patient wants present, if anyone. Make a list of people to notify once death occurs. Keep a list of home health nurses, hospice staff, and physicians nearby so they can be contacted quickly.

4. *Call for professional help if any of the following occur:*
   - The patient experiences extreme pain or discomfort
   - The patient has difficulty breathing. Oxygen can calm the person and make the last hours more comfortable.
   - The patient has trouble urinating or passing stool. Usually the urine will be dark and in small quantity. Medications can help ease discomfort.
   - Your emotions are getting the best of you. Thoughts of impending loss can prevent you from being supportive.

5. *Touch is often comforting for the dying person.* Give back, hand, or foot rubs; apply skin lotion. Do not stand back and avoid contact. Help the patient adjust his or her position in bed if at all possible. Usually an extra sheet placed under the patient and the help of a second person will make this easier.

6. *Make the person as physically comfortable as possible.* Moisten the eyes and lips with warm, damp cloths. Apply warm or cool compresses if the person wants them.

7. *Know what to expect.* Be ready to say goodbye. Talk to the person. In some cases soft, relaxing music may be comforting. During the last moments of life, the body begins to slow down, breathing rates slow, sometimes there are long pauses between breaths. Sometimes the person will appear to wake up but will be unable to speak or recognize you. Usually this means patients are in or near coma state, and they may progress to longer and longer periods of sleep. The skin may be cool, especially around the feet and hands, and may become blue- or gray-tinged. In the last stages as death nears, the person may become incontinent or lose bowel control. Finally, the chest will stop rising, the eyes may appear glassy, and there is no more pulse.

8. *Prepare for the activities that will occur after death.* You may choose to assist with preparing the body for transport to the funeral home or other facility, or you may prefer to let others take over. Try to think about this in advance and make decisions based on your own wishes and needs.

---

8. Patients are accepted on the basis of their health needs, not their ability to pay.

Despite the growing number of people considering the hospice option, many people prefer to go to a hospital to die. Others choose to die at home, without the intervention of medical staff or life-prolonging equipment. Each dying person and his or her family should decide as early as possible what type of terminal care is most desirable and feasible. This will allow time for necessary emotional, physical, and financial preparations. Hospice care may also help the survivors cope better with the death experience. See the Skills for Behavior Change box above for information on how to prepare yourself if you expect to be with a dying person.

Making Funeral Arrangements

Anthropological evidence indicates that all cultures throughout history have developed some sort of funeral ritual. For this reason, social scientists agree that funerals assist survivors of the deceased in coping with their loss.

What types of arrangements need to be made when a loved one dies?

In the United States, with its diversity of religious, regional, and ethnic customs, funeral patterns vary. (See the Health in a Diverse World box for information on the practices of several religious traditions.) In some faiths, prior to body disposal, the deceased may be displayed to formalize last respects and increase social sup-

HEALTH IN A diverse world

FUNERAL AND MOURNING CUSTOMS AROUND THE WORLD

Traditions associated with death vary around the world, reflecting differing cultures and religious practices. However, every culture recognizes death as a significant rite of passage. The following is a global sampling of funeral customs.

BUDDHISM

In several Japanese Buddhist traditions, a funeral ceremony resembles a Christian ceremony, with a eulogy and prayers at a funeral home. Cambodian, Thai, and Sri Lankan traditions may have up to three ceremonies. In the first, which is held two days after the death, monks conduct a ceremony at the home of the bereaved. In the second, two to five days after the death, monks hold a service at a funeral home, and the third, seven days after burial or cremation, is a monk-led ceremony at a temple or the home of the bereaved. This last ceremony, called a "merit transference," seeks to generate good energy for the deceased in his or her new incarnation. There is always an open casket, with the sight of the body reminding guests of the impermanence of life.

GREEK ORTHODOX CHURCH

Mourners bow in front of the open casket and kiss an icon or cross placed on the chest of the deceased. The traditional words said to the bereaved are "May you have an abundant life" and "May their memory be eternal." At the graveside, there is a five-minute prayer ceremony and each person present places one flower on the casket. A memorial service is held on the Sunday closest to the fortieth day after the death.

HINDUISM

The body remains at the home until it is taken to the place of cremation, usually 24 hours after death. It is customary to wear white at the funeral. The major officiants at the service are Hindu priests or senior male members of the family. At the cremation, a last food offering is symbolically made to the deceased and then the body is cremated. An additional ceremony at home, performed 10 days after death for the Brahmin caste and 30 days after death for other castes, liberates the soul of the deceased for its ascent to heaven.

ISLAM

Mourners wash the body of the deceased, perfume it, and wrap it in white cloth. Mourners face Mecca and recite prayers, and then a silent procession carries the body to its burial place. All the mourners participate in filling the grave with soil.

JUDAISM

A Jewish funeral is a time of intense mourning and public grieving. Traditional Jewish law forbids cremation. Flowers are never appropriate for Orthodox or Conservative funerals but are sometimes appropriate for Reform funerals. There is never an open casket, and the officiants are a rabbi (who delivers a eulogy), a cantor (who sings), and family members or friends (who may also deliver a eulogy or memorial). At a traditional service, there is a slow procession to the grave itself with several pauses along the way. After prayers have been recited, each person puts one spade of earth into the grave.

The family sits in mourning for seven days after the funeral, called the shiva period. To symbolize the mourners' lack of interest in their comfort or how they appear to others, mirrors are covered, slippers or socks are worn, and men refrain from shaving. A special memorial candle may be burned for seven days.

AMERICAN INDIAN RELIGIONS

Funeral and mourning rituals are linked to the belief that death is the beginning of a journey into the next world. Strict rules govern the behavior of the living relatives so as to ensure the deceased a good start on this journey. Some Potawatomi, for instance, set a place for the deceased at a funeral feast so the spirit can partake of the food. Among the Yuchi, personal items may be placed in an adult male's coffin, reflecting the belief that needs in the next life are not significantly different from needs in this one.

Although American Indian beliefs assert that death is not a termination of life, the bereaved still mourn the absence of the one who has died. Many tribes restrict what bereaved relatives can eat, for example. This represents a sacrifice by the living for those who have moved on.

SOCIETY OF FRIENDS (QUAKERS)

There are two types of Quaker funerals. An unprogrammed meeting is held in the traditional manner of Friends on the basis of silence. Worshippers sit and wait for divine guidance; if so moved, they speak to the group. Programmed meetings are planned in advance and usually include singing, prayers, Bible reading, silent worship, and a sermon.

HMONG

A typical Hmong funeral lasts three days. The funeral is the most important part of Hmong culture and must be done properly to ensure a prosperous afterlife for the deceased. Family members prepare the body for burial and adorn it with objects to protect its soul from evil spirits as it journeys to the other world. They provide the soul with food, wine, clothing and money. The Hmong will also sacrifice a rooster to accompany the soul on its journey. Musicians play a pipe and set of drums to guide the soul in the direction of its ancestors.

Sources: Excerpted from *How to Be a Perfect Stranger: The Essential Religious Etiquette Handbook* © 2003 SkyLight Paths Publishing. Edited by S. M. Matlins and A. J. Magida. Permission granted by SkyLight Paths Publishing. P.O. Box 237, Woodstock, VT 05091, www .skylightpaths.com; Selected Independent Funeral Homes, *Funeral Service Practices by Religion*, 2006, www.selectedfuneralhomes .org/information/guides/religions.html.

port of the bereaved. This part of the funeral ritual is referred to as a **wake** or **viewing.** The body of the deceased is usually embalmed prior to viewing to retard decomposition and minimize offensive odors. The funeral service may be held in a church, in a funeral chapel, or at the burial site. Some people choose to replace the funeral service with a simple memorial service held within a few days of the burial. Social interaction associated with funeral and memorial services is valuable in helping survivors cope with their losses.

Common methods of body disposal include burial in the ground, entombment above ground in a mausoleum, cremation, and anatomical donation. Expenses involved in body disposal vary according to the method chosen and the available options. It should be noted that if burial is selected, an additional charge may be assessed for a burial vault. Burial vaults—concrete or metal containers that hold the casket—are required by most cemeteries to limit settling of the gravesite as the casket disintegrates and collapses. Choosing the actual container for the remains is only one of many tasks that must be dealt with when a person dies. There are many other decisions concerning the funeral ritual that can also be difficult for survivors.

Pressures on Survivors

Funeral practices in the United States today are extremely varied. A great number of decisions have to be made, usually within 24 hours. These decisions relate to the method and details of body disposal, the type of memorial service, display of the body, the site of burial or body disposition, the cost of funeral options, organ donation decisions, ordering floral displays, contacting friends and relatives, planning for the arrival of guests, choosing markers, gathering and submitting obituary information to newspapers, printing memorial folders, and many other details. Even though funeral directors are available to facilitate decision making, the bereaved may experience undue stress, especially in the event of a sudden death.

In our society, people who make their own funeral arrangements can save their loved ones from having to deal with unnecessary problems. Even making the decision regarding the method of body disposal can greatly reduce the stress on survivors.

Wills

The issue of inheritance is controversial in some families and

---

National Kidney Foundation
Please detach and give this portion of the card to my family

This is to inform you that, should the occasion ever arise, I would like to be an organ and tissue donor. Please see that my wishes are carried out by informing the attending medical personnel that I have indicated my wishes to become a donor.
Thank you.

_____
Signature   Date

For further information write or call:
National Kidney Foundation
30 East 33rd Street, New York, NY 10016
(800) 622-9010

- -
Uniform Donor Card

Of _____
(print or type name of donor)

In the hope that I may help others, I hereby make this anatomical gift, if medically acceptable, to take effect upon my death. The words and marks below indicate my wishes.
I give: ☐ any needed organs or parts
☐ only the following organs or parts

_____
(specify the organ(s), tissue(s) or part(s))

for the purposes of transplantation, therapy, medical research or education;
☐ my body for anatomical study if needed.
Limitations or special wishes, if any: _____

FIGURE 20.5 Organ Donor Card

Source: Reprinted with permission from "Uniform Donor Card." © National Kidney Foundation.

---

should be resolved before the person dies to reduce both conflict and needless expense. Unfortunately, many people are so intimidated by the thought of making a will that they never do so and die **intestate** (without a will). This is tragic, especially because the procedure for establishing a legal will is relatively simple and inexpensive. In addition, if you don't make a will before you die, the courts (as directed by state laws) will make a will for you. Legal issues, rather than your wishes, will preside. Settling an estate also takes longer when a person dies without a will.

In some cases, other types of wills may substitute for the traditional legal will. One alternative is the **holographic will,** written in the handwriting of the **testator** (person who leaves a will) and unwitnessed. Be very cautious concerning alternatives to legally written and witnessed wills because they are not honored in all states. For example, holographic wills are contestable in court. Think of the parents who never approved of the fact that their child lived with someone outside

---

wake or **viewing**   Displaying of the deceased to formalize last respects and increase social support of the bereaved.

intestate   Dying without a will.

holographic will   A will written in the testator's own handwriting and unwitnessed.

testator   A person who leaves a will or testament at death.

marriage: they could successfully challenge a holographic will in court.

Organ Donation

Another decision concerns organ donation. Organ transplant techniques have become so refined, and the demand for transplant tissues and organs has become so great, that many people are being encouraged to donate these "gifts of life" upon death. Uniform donor cards are available through the National Kidney Foundation, donor information is printed on the backs of driver's licenses, and many hospitals include the opportunity for organ donor registration in their admission procedures (Figure 20.5). Although some people are opposed to organ transplants and tissue donation, many others experience personal fulfillment from knowing that their organs may extend and improve someone else's life after their own deaths.

TAKING charge

Summary

- *Death* can be defined biologically in terms of brain death and/or the final cessation of vital functions. Denial of death results in limited communication about death, which can lead to further denial.

- Death is a multifaceted process, and individuals may experience emotional stages of dying including denial, anger, bargaining, depression, and acceptance, as noted by Kübler-Ross. Social death results when a person is no longer treated as living. Grief is the state of distress felt after loss. Worden proposes developmental tasks associated with grieving.

People differ in their responses to grief. Children need to be helped through the process of grieving.

- The right to die by rational suicide involves ethical, moral, and legal issues.

- Practical and legal issues surround dying and death. Choices of care for the terminally ill include hospice care. After death, funeral arrangements must be made almost immediately, adding to pressures on survivors. As many decisions as possible should be made in advance of death through wills and organ donation cards.

Chapter Review

1. Death of all functions of the entire human brain is referred to as
   a. brain death.
   b. cellular death.
   c. functional death.
   d. spiritual death.

2. What stage of the Kübler-Ross 'Response-to-Dying' model is the individual in when rage and resentment is expressed toward imminent death?
   a. denial
   b. anger
   c. bargaining
   d. acceptance

3. What stage of the Kübler-Ross 'Response-to-Dying' model is the individual in when there is a promise to perform good works of mercy in exchange for recovery?
   a. denial
   b. depression
   c. bargaining
   d. acceptance

4. An example of an advanced directive would include a
   a. health care proxy.
   b. do not resuscitate order.
   c. living will.
   d. All of the above.

5. When a person dies *intestate*, this means that
   a. the body can be shipped across state boundaries.
   b. burial cannot take place without some authorization.
   c. the person died without a will.
   d. the court will decide upon the funeral arrangements.

6. A body that has been incinerated after death is referred to as
   a. burial.
   b. cremation.
   c. burned to death in a fire.
   d. None of the above.

7. Mary experienced a miscarriage late in her first trimester of pregnancy. Since there was no memorial service or social support for Mary during this time of loss, she experienced which type of grief?
   a. acute grief
   b. chronic grief
   c. social grief
   d. disenfranchised grief

8. The study of death and dying is called
   a. thanatology.
   b. ageism.
   c. bereavement therapy.
   d. gerontology.

9. A physician-prescribed lethal injection to a dying patient is referred to as
   a. rational suicide.
   b. passive euthanasia.
   c. active euthanasia.
   d. right to die directive.

10. A culturally prescribed and accepted period of grief to someone who has died is known as
    a. bereavement.
    b. grief.
    c. coping with loss.
    d. mourning.

Answers to these questions can be found on page A-1.

Questions for Discussion and Reflection

1. Discuss why so many of us deny death. How could death become a more acceptable topic to discuss?
2. What are the stages that Kübler-Ross believed that terminally ill patients experience? Do you agree with the five-stage theory? Explain why or why not.
3. Define *social death* and *quasi-death experiences*.
4. Discuss coping with grief, and how to help children deal with death.
5. Identify at least one development—legal, medical, or social—that has occurred in the past five years that has affected the way we view death.
6. Debate whether rational suicide should be legalized for the terminally ill. What restrictions would you include in such a law?
7. Compare and contrast the hospital experience with hospice care. What must one consider before arranging for hospice care?
8. Discuss the legal matters surrounding death, including wills, physician directives, organ donations, and funeral arrangements.

Accessing Your Health on the Internet

The following websites explore further topics and issues related to personal health. You'll also find links to each organization's website on the Companion Website for *Access to Health,* Tenth Edition, at www.aw-bc.com/donatelle.

1. *Beyond Indigo.* This site addresses all aspects of grief and loss, including terminal illness, legal issues, and funeral planning. www.beyondindigo.com
2. *Funerals: A Consumer Guide.* This site guides the consumer through the thinking process of planning for a funeral, including preplanning, types of funerals, costs, choosing a casket, burial, and many other aspects of funeral preparation. www.ftc.gov/bcp/conline/pubs/services/funeral.htm
3. *GriefNet.org.* Resources to help people deal with the loss of loved ones, including memorial pages and e-mail support groups. www.griefnet.org
4. *Hospice Foundation.* Information about hospice care, including resources for finding a hospice, and other information to help aid in the illness, death, and grieving process. www.hospicefoundation.org
5. *Loss, Grief, and Bereavement.* This site from the National Cancer Institute covers a variety of topics related to loss, grief, and bereavement. Among the contents is a summary written by cancer experts. www.nci.nih.gov/cancertopics/pdq/supportivecare/bereavement/patient

Further Reading

Humphrey, D. and M. Clement. *Freedom to Die: People, Politics, and the Right-to-Die Movement.* Torrance, CA: Griffin, 2000.

> *Describes the history of the right-to-die movement and all sides of the debate.*

Jacobs Altman, L. *Death: An Introduction to Medical–Ethical Dilemmas.* Berkeley Heights, NJ: Enslow, 2000.

> *A multifaceted exploration of death that gives the reader much to consider.*

Mims, C. A. *When We Die: The Science, Culture, and Rituals of Death.* Torrance, CA: Griffin, 2000.

> *A look at how society views and portrays death in science and culture.*

Muth, A. S. (ed.). *Death and Dying Sourcebook: Basic Consumer Health Information for the Layperson About End-of-Life Care and Related Ethical and Legal Issues.* Detroit, MI: Omnigraphics, 2000.

> *Provides up-to-date information on the issues of nursing care, living wills, pain management, and counseling.*

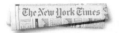

e-themes from *The New York Times*

For up-to-date articles about current health issues, visit www.aw-bc.com/donatelle, select *Access to Health,* Tenth Edition, Chapter 20, and click on "e-themes."

References

1. *The New Shorter Oxford English Dictionary* (Oxford, UK: Oxford University Press, 1993).
2. President's Commission on the Uniform Determination of Death, *Defining Death: Medical, Ethical and Legal Issues in the Determination of Death* (Washington, DC: US Government Printing Office, 1981).
3. Ad Hoc Committee of the Harvard Medical School to Examine the Definition of Brain Death, "A Definition of Irreversible Coma," *Journal of the American Medical Association* 205 (1968): 377.
4. *Religion and Ethics News Weekly,* "Belief and Practice: Roadside Crosses," February 25, 2005, www.pbs.org/wnet/religionandethics/week826/belief.html.
5. E. Kübler-Ross, and D. Kessler, *On Grief and Grieving: Finding the Meaning of Grief Through the Five Stages of Loss* (New York, NY: Scribner, 2005).
6. E. Kübler-Ross, *On Death and Dying* (New York: Macmillan, 1969), 113.
7. C. Corr, C. Nabe, and D. Corr, *Death and Dying, Life and Living,* 5th ed. (Belmont, CA: Wadsworth Publishing Company, 2005).
8. R. J. Kastenbaum, *Death, Society, and Human Experience,* 9th ed. (Boston: Allyn & Bacon, 2006).
9. Ibid.
10. K. J. Doka (ed.), *Disenfranchised Grief: New Directions, Challenges and Strategies for Practice* (Champaign, IL: Research Press, 2002).
11. J. W. Worden, *Grief Counseling and Grief Therapy: A Handbook for the Mental Health Practitioner,* 4th ed. (New York: Springer, 2004).
12. Federal Interagency Forum on Child and Family Statistics, "America's Children in Brief: Key National Indicators of Well-Being," 2006, www.childstats.gov/americaschildren/index.asp.
13. J. W. Worden, *Children and Grief: When a Parent Dies* (New York, NY: Guilford Press, 2001).
14. J. B. Kamerman, *Death in the Midst of Life* (Englewood Cliffs, NJ: Prentice Hall, 1988), 71.
15. National Mental Health Association, "Coping with Loss: Bereavement and Grief," 2005, www.nmha.org/infoctr.factsheets/42.cfm.
16. American Bar Association, "ABA Commission on Law and Aging," 2005, www.abanet.org/aging/toolkit/home.html.
17. Public Agenda, "Supreme Court Upholds Oregon Assisted Suicide Law," 2006, www.publicagenda.org.
18. Oregon Department of Human Services, "Oregon's Death with Dignity Act," 2004, www.dhs.state.or.us/publichealth/chs/pas/pas.cfm.

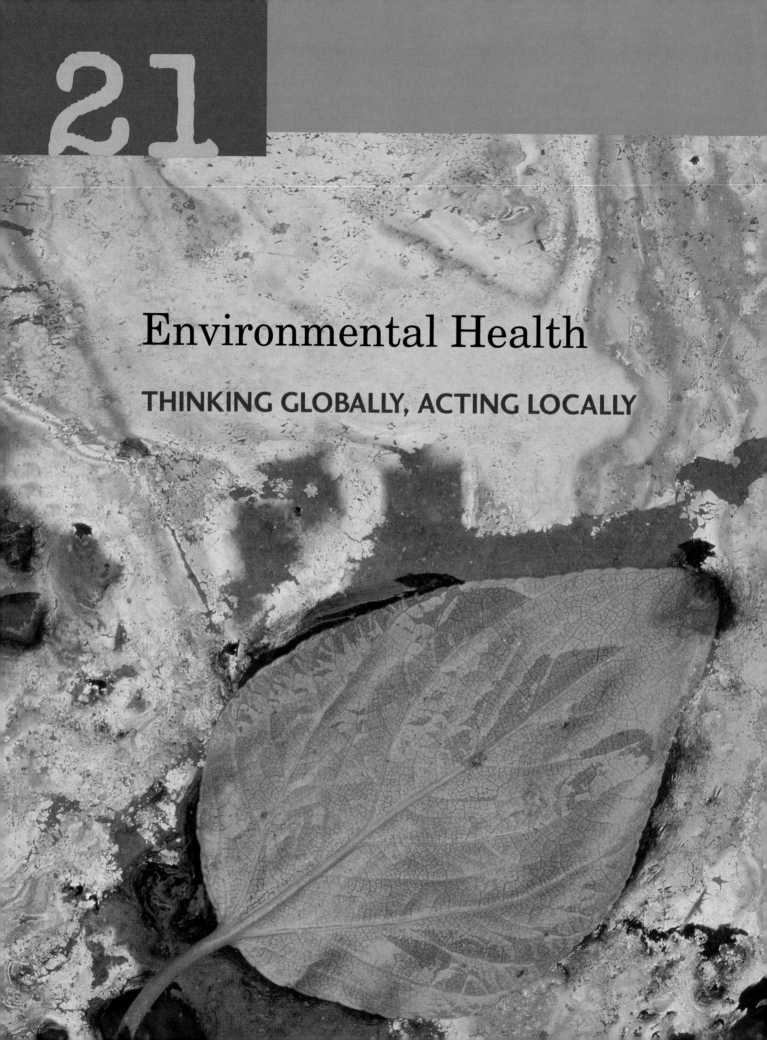

21

Environmental Health

THINKING GLOBALLY, ACTING LOCALLY

What has our **government** done to protect the ozone layer?

What is a **Superfund** site?

Can talking on my **cell phone** cause cancer?

Are there any **benefits** to using nuclear power?

What can I do to make a **positive** impact on the environment?

OBJECTIVES

- Explain the environmental impact associated with the current global population and it's projected growth.
- Discuss major causes of air pollution, and the global consequences of the accumulation of greenhouse gases and ozone depletion.
- Identify sources of water pollution and chemical contaminants often found in water.
- Describe the physiological consequences of noise pollution.
- Distinguish between municipal solid waste and hazardous waste.
- Discuss the health concerns associated with ionizing and nonionizing radiation.

617

H uman health, well-being, and the survival of all living things depend on the health and integrity of the planet on which we live. Today the natural world is under siege from the pressures of a burgeoning population that consumes massive amounts of natural resources to survive. Consequently, many citizens are interested in the health effects of environmental concerns such as global warming; depletion of the ozone layer; air, water, and solid waste pollution; deforestation; human population control; and the impact of too many people on dwindling natural resources.

In response to public and political concerns, there has been a surge in federal and state regulations along with a multibillion-dollar national infrastructure—but doubt remains as to the effectiveness of that infrastructure in reducing environmental health risks.[1] In addition, during the recent economic downturn, politicians dismantled some environmental gains by reducing regulations, easing compliance deadlines, weakening protections for endangered species, and undermining other environmental programs labeled by some in Congress as "antibusiness."[2] Today, while the federal government has decided not to participate in several international policy and planning groups designed to protect the global environment, environmental problems continue to escalate. National and international groups continue to promote an agenda based on sustainable development, or efforts to ensure that the level of productivity and activity undertaken in one generation does not compromise the environmental integrity or needed resources of the next generation.[3] In such a period of environmental pressures, an informed citizenry with a strong commitment to be responsible for the planet is essential to the survival of Earth and all living things. This chapter reviews major global environmental issues that affect us today and will continue to affect generations to come.

Overpopulation

Anthropologist Margaret Mead wrote, "Every human society is faced with not one population problem but two: how to beget and rear enough children and how not to beget and rear too many."[4] This statement has never been more important; current population growth is over 1 percent each year and the United Nations projects the present total of 6.5 billion will grow to 9.4 billion by 2050 and to 11.5 billion by 2150 (Figure 21.1).[5] Though our population is expanding, Earth's resources are not. Population experts believe that many areas of the world are already struggling with "demographic fatigue" and the most critical environmental challenge today is to slow the population growth of the world.[6]

The global population explosion is not distributed equally, with vast differences in growth rates between most developing and industrialized nations. Nearly 99 percent of all population increases take place in poor countries, while population size is static or declining in wealthy countries. Nations that

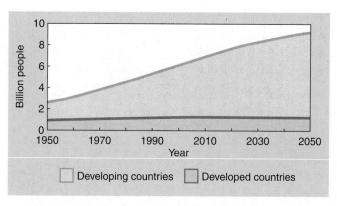

FIGURE 21.1 World Population Growth, 1950–2050 (Projected)

Source: United Nations World Population Division, Population Prospects, 2004 Revision, www.un.org/popin/wdtrends.htm.

can least afford a high birth rate in terms of economic, social, health, and nutritional needs are the ones with the most rapidly expanding populations. Overpopulation threats are most evident in Latin America, Africa, and parts of Asia—areas where poverty, devastating infectious diseases such as HIV, and problems with food and water are already prevalent.

The country projected to have the largest increase in population is India, which could add another 600 million people by the year 2050 and surpass China as the most populous country in the world. Put into perspective, the U.S. population is 300 million.[7]

The Effect of Overpopulation on the Environment

Why should we be concerned? Whether you live in an area of heavy population growth or not, the drain on the environment that results from exponential population growth is staggering. Many argue that at the current rate, we are already exceeding our capacity to provide food and clean water, and dispose of human waste. Today, 14 cities have megacity status with populations over 10 million, and by 2015, at current rates, there will be 26 megacities on Earth.[8]

Overpopulation and heavy consumption are the main factors in many of our environmental issues today. There is already heavy pressure on the capacity of natural resources to support human life and world health.[9] However, too much pressure on our planet's resources threatens ecosystems, and disturbs the careful balance between all ecosystems on our planet.

Recognizing that population control will be essential in the decades ahead, many countries have already enacted strict population control measures or have encouraged their citizens to limit the size of their families. The concept of *zero population growth (ZPG)* was introduced in the 1960s. Proponents of ZPG believe that each couple should produce only two offspring. When the parents die, these two children are their replacements, allowing the population to stabilize. By 2000,

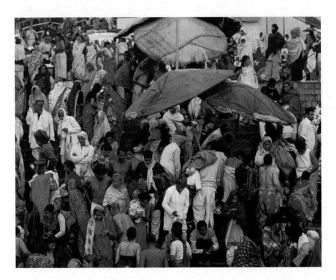

As populations increase, countries' resources become overloaded. In many parts of the world, governments struggle to meet the needs of the increasing numbers of citizens.

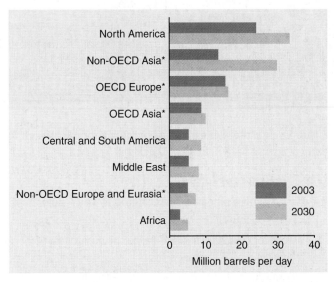

FIGURE 21.2 World Oil Consumption by Region and Country Group, 2003 and 2030

* OECD is the Organization for Economic Cooperation and Development.

Source: Energy Information Administration, International Energy Annual (May–July 2005), www.eia.doe.gov/iea.

Italy, Spain, Portugal, Greece, and Sweden were among the first to achieve zero population growth.[10] Germany, Russia, Ukraine, Hungary, and Bulgaria had actually achieved negative population growth.[11]

Working Toward Zero Population Growth

Ironically, while other nations, many of which consume far fewer natural resources and contribute far less to environmental decline, have worked hard to achieve zero or negative population growth, the United States is the only major industrialized nation to continue to have significant population growth. In 2005, the rate of U.S. growth was nearly 1 percent, far greater than that of Canada, England, or other world leaders.[12] Why does the American population continue to grow at a time when other nations are downsizing? There are many reasons for this growth, including religious beliefs that do not endorse birth control, immigration, government programs that promote family growth by giving tax breaks and other incentives for families, American values that revere the family unit, and economics that support a family consumer system. Unless the United States takes action to reduce population growth and diminish our heavy consumption patterns, we will continue to be part of the problem instead of part of the solution.

We can also do our part by recognizing that the United States consumes far more energy and raw materials per person than any other nation on Earth. Many of these resources come from other countries, and our consumption is depleting the resource balance of those countries. (See Figure 21.2 for a comparison of U.S. oil consumption with that of selected other countries.)

One simple course of action would be to control our own reproductivity. Globally, certain nations have made great strides toward achieving zero population growth. For

example, in 1970, the worldwide total fertility rate peaked at an estimated 5 births per woman; at present it is 2.7 births. However, though that may sound good, even as rates go down in many regions of the world, the sheer magnitude of the population means that the actual number of births continues to rise at an unprecedented rate. We have a long way to go before global population levels out or begins to decline.

The continued preference for large families in many developing nations is related to several factors: high infant mortality rates; the traditional view of children as "social security" (working from a young age to assist families in daily survival and supporting parents when they grow too old to work); the low educational and economic status of women that often leaves women powerless with respect to reproductive choices; and the traditional desire for sons, which keeps parents of several daughters reproducing until they have male offspring.

Education may be the single biggest contributor to zero population growth. As education levels of women increase and women achieve equality in pay and job status, fertility rates decline. However, U.S. funding for this kind of education and family planning has declined dramatically in the last four years as highly controversial "abstinence only" messages have been promoted as the only allowable interventions in many regions of the world. Most public health professionals, particularly those in the fields of research and prevention, support a much more ecological approach to population planning. They believe that a vast array of social, cultural, biological, psychological, economic, and other factors contributes to population growth and unwanted pregnancies and that simple solutions such as abstinence programs are destined to fail.

(Text continues on page 622)

ASSESS *yourself*

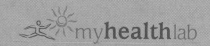

WHAT CAN I DO TO PRESERVE THE ENVIRONMENT?

Fill out this assessment online at
www.aw-bc.com/MyHealthLab or
www.aw-bc.com/donatelle.

Environmental problems often seem too big for one person to make a difference. Each day, though, there are things you can do that contribute to the health of the planet.

MAKING A DIFFERENCE

For each statement, indicate how commonly you follow the described behavior.

	Always	Usually	Sometimes	Never
1. Whenever I can, I try to walk or ride my bicycle rather than take a car.	1	2	3	4
2. I try to carpool with others to school or work.	1	2	3	4
3. ! have my car tuned up and inspected every year.	1	2	3	4
4. When I have the oil in my car changed, I make sure the oil goes into a recycling bin, not on the ground or into a floor drain.	1	2	3	4
5. I try to save fuel by not using the air conditioner except in extreme conditions.	1	2	3	4
6. I turn off the lights when a room is not being used.	1	2	3	4
7. I take a shower rather than a bath.	1	2	3	4
8. I have water-saving devices installed on my shower, toilet, and sinks.	1	2	3	4
9. I make sure faucets and toilets do not leak.	1	2	3	4
10. I use my bath towels more than once before putting them in the wash.	1	2	3	4
11. I wear my clothes more than once between washings when possible.	1	2	3	4
12. I make sure that the washing machine is full before I wash a load of clothes.	1	2	3	4
13. I try to purchase biodegradable soaps and detergents.	1	2	3	4
14. I try to use biodegradable trash bags.	1	2	3	4
15. At home, I use dishes and silverware rather than Styrofoam or plastic.	1	2	3	4
16. When I buy prepackaged foods, I choose the ones with the least packaging.	1	2	3	4
17. I try not to subscribe to newspapers and magazines when I can view them online.	1	2	3	4
18. I try not to use a hair dryer.	1	2	3	4
19. I recycle plastic bags that I get when I bring something home from the store.	1	2	3	4
20. I don't run water continuously when washing the dishes, shaving, or brushing my teeth.	1	2	3	4
21. I prefer to use unbleached or recycled paper.	1	2	3	4
22. I use both sides of printer paper and other paper when possible.	1	2	3	4

	Always	Usually	Sometimes	Never
23. If I have items I do not want to use anymore, I donate them to charity so someone else can use them.	1	2	3	4
24. I try not to buy drinks in cans with plastic rings attached to them.	1	2	3	4
25. I try not to buy bottled water in small plastic containers.	1	2	3	4
26. I clean up after myself while enjoying the outdoors (picnicking, camping, etc.).	1	2	3	4
27. I volunteer for cleanup days in the community in which I live.	1	2	3	4
28. I consider candidates' positions on environmental issues before casting my vote.	1	2	3	4

For Further Thought

Review your scores. Are your responses mostly 1s and 2s? If not, what actions can you take to become more environmentally responsible? Are there ways to help the environment on this list that you had not thought of before? Are there behaviors not on the list that you are already doing?

MAKE it happen!

ASSESSMENT: The Assess Yourself activity gave you the chance to look at your behavior and consider ways of saving water, reducing waste, and protecting the planet in other ways. Now that you have considered these results, you can begin to take steps to become more environmentally responsible.

MAKING A CHANGE: In order to change your behavior, you need to develop a plan. Follow the steps below and complete your Behavior Change Contract to take action.

1. Evaluate your behavior and identify patterns and specific things you are doing. What can you change now? What can you change in the near future?

2. Select one pattern of behavior that you want to change.

3. Fill out the Behavior Change Contract found at the front of your book. It should include your long-term goal for change, your short-term goals, the rewards you'll give yourself for reaching these goals, potential obstacles along the way, and strategies for overcoming these obstacles. For each goal, list the small steps and specific actions that you will take.

4. Chart your progress in a journal. At the end of a week, consider how successful you were in following your plan. What helped you be successful? What made change more difficult? What will you do differently next week?

5. Revise your plan as needed: Are the short-term goals attainable? Are the rewards satisfying?

ONE STUDENT'S PLAN: Marta saw that she was already doing a number of the items recommended in the self-assessment. However, she had not considered several of the ideas regarding excess packaging of her food, drinks, and so on, although she knew that extra plastic wraps and other excess packaging contribute to the need for more landfills and other environmental problems. She decided that for a week she would try to pay more attention to the packaging of her favorite foods and to buy large sizes whenever possible instead of individually packed products. This meant spending more time in the grocery store to be sure she found items with the least packaging (although she also didn't have to make as many trips to the store that week). The next week, Marta looked at how many plastic bottles she used for her water each day. She bought a durable, dishwasher-safe plastic bottle and started filling it with water each day before she left the house. After a week she was happy to discover that her garbage was not full of plastic water bottles, and she had actually saved herself some money.

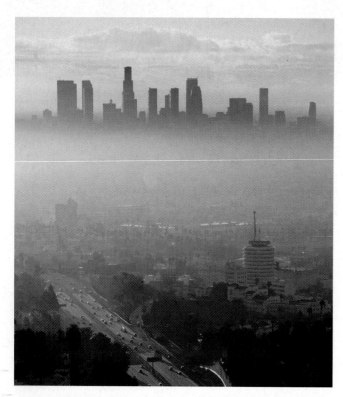

Smog and other forms of air pollution have a detrimental effect on our health and the environment.

Policies that encourage low birth rates in society and educate citizens about the consequences of unchecked population growth may be effective. In countries such as the United States, policies that encourage zero population rates or provide incentives to young parents through tax breaks for reduced family size may be a viable option.

Air Pollution

Although we often assume that the air we breathe is safe, the daily impact of a growing population makes clean air more difficult to find. Concern about air quality prompted Congress to pass the Clean Air Act in 1970 and to amend it in 1977 and again in 1990. The goal was to develop standards for six of the most widespread air pollutants that seriously affect health: sulfur dioxide, particulates, carbon monoxide, ozone,

---

sulfur dioxide A yellowish brown gaseous by-product of the burning of fossil fuels.

particulates Nongaseous air pollutants.

carbon monoxide An odorless, colorless gas that originates primarily from motor vehicle emissions.

ozone A gas formed when nitrogen dioxide interacts with hydrogen chloride.

nitrogen dioxide An amber-colored gas found in smog; can cause eye and respiratory irritations.

---

nitrogen dioxide, and lead. The Air Quality Index is the best way for the public to assess the daily quality of the air we breathe (see the New Horizons in Health box).

Sources of Air Pollution

Sulfur Dioxide A yellowish brown gas, **sulfur dioxide** is a by-product of burning fossil fuels. Electricity-generating stations, smelters, refineries, and industrial boilers are the main sources. In humans, sulfur dioxide aggravates symptoms of heart and lung disease, obstructs breathing passages, and increases the incidence of respiratory diseases such as colds, asthma, bronchitis, and emphysema. It is toxic to plants, destroys some paint pigments, corrodes metals, impairs visibility, and is a precursor to acid deposition (acid rain), which we discuss later in this chapter.

Particulates **Particulates** are tiny solid particles or liquid droplets that are suspended in the air. Cigarette smoke releases particulates. They are also by-products of industrial processes and the internal combustion engine. Particulates irritate the lungs and can carry heavy metals and carcinogenic agents deep into the lungs. When combined with sulfur dioxide, they exacerbate respiratory diseases. Particulates can also corrode metals and obscure visibility. Numerous scientific studies have found significant links between exposure to air particulate concentrations at or below current standards and adverse health effects, including premature death.[13]

Carbon Monoxide An odorless, colorless gas, **carbon monoxide** originates primarily from motor vehicle emissions. Carbon monoxide interferes with the blood's ability to absorb and carry oxygen and can impair thinking, slow reflexes, and cause drowsiness, unconsciousness, and death. Home monitors are available to test for carbon monoxide.

Ozone Ground-level **ozone** is a form of oxygen that is produced when nitrogen dioxide reacts with hydrogen chloride. These gases release oxygen, which is altered by sunlight to produce ozone. In the lower atmosphere, ozone irritates the mucous membranes of the respiratory system, causing coughing and choking. It can impair lung function, reduce resistance to colds and pneumonia, and aggravate heart disease, asthma, bronchitis, and pneumonia. One of the irritants found in smog, this ozone corrodes rubber and paint and can kill vegetation. The natural ozone found in the upper atmosphere (sometimes called "good" ozone), however, serves as a protective shield against heat and radiation from the sun. We will discuss this atmospheric ozone layer later in the chapter.

Nitrogen Dioxide Coal-powered electrical utility boilers and motor vehicles emit **nitrogen dioxide,** an amber-colored gas. High concentrations of it can be fatal, while lower concentrations increase susceptibility to colds and flu, bronchitis, and pneumonia. Nitrogen dioxide is also toxic to plant life and causes a brown discoloration of the atmosphere. It is a precursor of ozone and, along with sulfur dioxide, of acid rain.

WHAT IS THE AQI?

Air quality affects how we live and breathe. Like the weather, it can change from day to day or even hour to hour. The U.S. Environmental Protection Agency (EPA) and other groups are working to make information about outdoor air quality as available to the public as a weather report. A key tool in this effort is the Air Quality Index, or AQI.

A measure of daily air quality, the AQI tells you how clean or polluted your air is and what associated health concerns you should be aware of. The AQI focuses on health effects that can happen within a few hours or days after breathing polluted air. It reflects national air quality standards for five major air pollutants regulated by the Clean Air Act: ground-level ozone, particulate matter, carbon monoxide, sulfur dioxide, and nitrogen dioxide.

HOW DOES THE AQI WORK?

Think of the AQI as a yardstick that runs from 0 to 500. The higher the AQI value, the greater the level of air pollution and associated health risks. An AQI value of 100 generally corresponds to the national air quality standard for the pollutant, which is the level the EPA has set to protect public health. AQI values below 100 are generally considered satisfactory. When AQI values rise above 100, air quality is considered unhealthy—at first for certain groups of people, then for everyone.

UNDERSTANDING THE AQI

As shown in the accompanying table, the EPA has divided the AQI scale into six categories and color codes.

- *Good.* Air quality is satisfactory for all groups.
- *Moderate.* Air quality is acceptable except for a very small group of individuals. For example, people who are unusually sensitive to ozone may experience respiratory symptoms.
- *Unhealthy for sensitive groups.* The general public is not likely to be affected, but certain individuals may experience health effects. For example, children and adults who are active outdoors and people with respiratory disease are at greater risk from exposure to ozone, while people with heart disease are at greater risk from carbon monoxide.
- *Unhealthy.* At this point the general public may begin to notice symptoms.
- *Very unhealthy.* This may trigger a health alert, meaning everyone may experience serious health effects.
- *Hazardous.* The entire population is likely to be affected, and a warning of emergency conditions will be triggered.

Source: U.S. Environmental Protection Agency, "Air Quality Index (AQI)," 2006, www.epa.gov/airnow/aqi.html.

AQI Range	Air Quality Condition/ Level of Health Concern	Color
0–50	Good	Green
51–100	Moderate	Yellow
101–150	Unhealthy for sensitive groups	Orange
151–200	Unhealthy	Red
201–300	Very unhealthy	Purple
301–500	Hazardous	Maroon

Lead **Lead** is a metal pollutant found in paint, batteries, drinking water, pipes, dishes with lead-based glazes, dirt, soldered cans, and some candies made in Mexico. It affects the circulatory, reproductive, urinary, and nervous systems and can accumulate in bone and other tissues. Lead is particularly detrimental to children and fetuses. It can cause birth defects, behavioral abnormalities, and cognitive impairment.

The elimination of lead from gasoline and auto exhaust in the 1970s was one of the great public health accomplishments of all time. However, although stricter standards prevail, an estimated 300,000 children in the United States still have unsafe blood lead levels.[14]

Hydrocarbons Although not listed as one of the six major air pollutants in the Clean Air Act, hydrocarbons encompass a wide variety of chemical pollutants in the air. Sometimes known as *volatile organic compounds (VOCs),* **hydrocarbons** are chemical compounds containing different combinations of carbon and hydrogen. The principal source is the internal combustion engine. Most automobile engines emit hundreds of different hydrocarbon compounds. By themselves, hydrocarbons seem to cause few problems, but when they combine with sunlight and other pollutants, they form such poisons as formaldehyde, ketones, and peroxyacetylnitrate (PAN), all of which are respiratory irritants.

lead A metal found in the exhaust of motor vehicles powered by fuel containing lead and in emissions from lead smelters and processing plants.

hydrocarbons Chemical compounds that contain carbon and hydrogen.

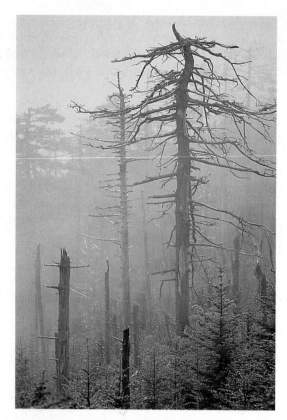

Acid deposition has many harmful effects on the environment. Because its toxins seep into groundwater and enter the food chain, it also poses health hazards to humans.

Hydrocarbon combinations such as benzene and benzo[a]-pyrene are carcinogenic. In addition, hydrocarbons play a major part in the formation of smog.

Photochemical Smog

Photochemical smog is a brown, hazy mix of particulates and gases that forms when oxygen-containing compounds of nitrogen and hydrocarbons react in the presence of sunlight. It is sometimes called *ozone pollution* because ozone is created when vehicle exhaust reacts with sunlight. In most cases, smog forms in areas that experience a **temperature inversion,** a weather condition in which a cool layer of air is trapped under a layer of warmer air, preventing the air from circulating. When gases such as hydrocarbons and nitrogen oxides are released

photochemical smog The brownish-yellow haze resulting from the combination of hydrocarbons and nitrogen oxides.

temperature inversion A weather condition occurring when a layer of cool air is trapped under a layer of warmer air.

acid deposition The acidification process that occurs when pollutants are deposited in precipitation, directly on the land, or by clouds.

into the cool air layer, they remain suspended until winds remove the warmer air layer. Sunlight filtering through the air causes chemical changes in the hydrocarbons and nitrogen oxides, which results in smog. (Smog is a combined term derived from "smoke" and "fog.") Smog is more likely to be produced in valley regions blocked by hills or mountains—for example, Los Angeles, Denver, and Tokyo.

The most noticeable adverse effects of smog are difficulty breathing, burning eyes, headaches, and nausea. Long-term exposure poses serious health risks, particularly for children, older adults, pregnant women, and people with chronic respiratory disorders such as asthma and emphysema.

what do you THINK?

Should automakers be responsible for developing cars with low emissions? ■ As a motorist, how can you help eliminate carbon monoxide emissions?

Acid Deposition and Acid Rain

Acid deposition is a broad term that encompasses the acidification process that occurs when rain, sleet, snow, clouds, and fog hold acid particles. In most scientific circles, it is replacing the term *acid rain*. Acid deposition refers to precipitation that has fallen through acidic air pollutants, particularly those containing sulfur dioxides and nitrogen dioxides. When introduced into lakes and ponds, this precipitation gradually acidifies the water. When the acid content of the water reaches a certain level, plant and animal life cannot survive. Ironically, acidified lakes and ponds become a crystal-clear deep blue, giving the illusion of beauty and health.

Acidic pollutants can be deposited in three ways:[15]

- *Wet deposition.* Pollutants are deposited in rain and snow (what is commonly termed acid rain or acid precipitation). This is the major acid deposition found in most of the Northern Hemisphere.
- *Dry deposition.* Gases and particles are deposited directly onto the land. This is the most common form of acid deposition in much of Europe.
- *Cloud deposition.* Clouds can provide a significant input of acidic pollutants over high ground.

Sources of Acid Deposition More than 95 percent of acid deposition originates in human actions, chiefly the burning of fossil fuels. The greatest sources of acid deposition in the United States are coal-fired power plants, ore smelters, oil refineries, and steel mills.

When these and other industries burn fuels, the sulfur and nitrogen in the emissions combine with oxygen and sunlight in the air to become sulfur dioxide and nitrogen oxides (precursors of sulfuric acid and nitric acids, respectively). Small acid particles are then carried by the wind and combine with moisture to produce acidic rain or snow. Rain is more acidic in the summertime because of higher concentrations of sunlight. The ability of a lake to cleanse itself and neutralize its acidity depends on several factors, the most critical of which is the buffering ability of the underlying bedrock.

Effects of Acid Deposition
In addition to damaging lakes and ponds, every year acid deposition destroys millions of trees in Europe and North America. Scientists have concluded that much of the world's forestlands are now experiencing damaging levels of sulfur deposition.[16]

Doctors believe that acid deposition aggravates and may even cause bronchitis, asthma, and other respiratory problems. People with emphysema and those with a history of heart disease may also suffer from exposure. It may also be hazardous to a pregnant woman's unborn child.

Acidic deposition can cause metals such as aluminum, cadmium, lead, and mercury to **leach** (dissolve and filter) out of the soil. If these metals make their way into water or food supplies (particularly fish), they can cause cancer in humans who consume them. Acid deposition also damages crops; laboratory experiments show that it can reduce seed yield by up to 23 percent. Actual crop losses are being reported with increasing frequency. A final consequence is the destruction of public monuments and structures, with billions of dollars in projected building damage each year.[17]

Indoor Air Pollution

In the last several years, a growing body of scientific evidence has indicated that the air within homes and other buildings can be more polluted than the outdoor air in even the most industrialized cities. Research indicates that some of the most vulnerable people are the young, older adults, and those who are sick.

Most indoor air pollution comes from sources that release gases or particles into the air. Inadequate ventilation, particularly in heavily insulated buildings with airtight windows, may increase pollution by not allowing in outside air.

Table 21.1 on page 626 describes major sources of indoor air pollution and possible health effects from these pollutants. However, the relative dose of any given chemical and the degree of its toxicity are key variables in determining risk. Some sources, such as building materials, furnishings, and household products such as air fresheners, release pollutants continuously. Others release pollutants intermittently. Health effects may develop over years of exposure or occur in response to toxic levels of pollutants. Several factors affect risk, including age, preexisting medical conditions, individual sensitivity, room temperature and humidity, and functioning of the liver, immune, and respiratory systems.[18]

Prevention of indoor air pollution should focus on three main areas: source control (eliminating or reducing individual contaminants), ventilation improvements (increasing the amount of outdoor air coming indoors), and air cleaners (removing particulates from the air).[19]

How serious is the problem? Indoor air can be 10 to 40 times more hazardous than outdoor air. There are 20 to 100 potentially dangerous chemical compounds in the average American home. Indoor air pollution comes primarily from these sources:

woodstoves, furnaces, passive cigarette smoke exposure (see Chapter 13), asbestos, formaldehyde, radon, and household chemicals. An emerging source of indoor air pollution is mold (see the New Horizons in Health box on page 627). It is not yet clear how widespread the effects of mold are.

Home Heating
Woodstoves emit significant levels of particulates and carbon monoxide in addition to other pollutants, such as sulfur dioxide. If you rely on wood for heating, make sure that your stove is properly installed, vented, and maintained. Burning properly seasoned wood reduces particulates.

People who rely on oil- or gas-fired furnaces also need to make sure that these appliances are properly installed, ventilated, and maintained. Inadequate cleaning and maintenance can allow deadly carbon monoxide to build up in the home.

Asbestos
Asbestos is a mineral that was commonly used in insulating materials in buildings constructed before 1970. When bonded to other materials, asbestos is relatively harmless, but if its tiny fibers become loosened and airborne, they can embed themselves in the lungs. Their presence leads to cancer of the lungs, stomach, and chest lining, and a fatal lung disease called mesothelioma.

Formaldehyde
Formaldehyde is a colorless, strong-smelling gas present in some carpets, draperies, furniture, particleboard, plywood, wood paneling, countertops, and many adhesives. It is released into the air in a process called *outgassing*. Outgassing is highest in new products, but the process can continue for many years.

Exposure to formaldehyde can cause respiratory problems, dizziness, fatigue, nausea, and rashes. Long-term exposure can lead to central nervous system disorders and cancer.

Ask about the formaldehyde content of products you purchase, and avoid those that contain this gas. Some houseplants, such as philodendrons and spider plants, help clean formaldehyde from the air. If you experience symptoms of formaldehyde exposure, have your home tested by a city, county, or state health agency.

Radon
Radon, an odorless, colorless gas, is the natural by-product of the decay of uranium and radium in the soil. Radon penetrates homes through cracks, pipes, sump pits, and other openings in the foundation. An estimated 15,000

---

leach   To dissolve and filter through soil.

asbestos   A substance that separates into stringy fibers and lodges in the lungs, where it can cause various diseases.

formaldehyde   A colorless, strong-smelling gas released through outgassing; causes respiratory and other health problems.

radon   A naturally occurring radioactive gas resulting from the decay of certain radioactive elements.

TABLE 21.1   Health Effects of Indoor Air Pollution

Type of Pollutant	Sources	Health Effects
Radon	Uranium in the soil or rock on which homes are built; well water also can be a source	Lung cancer from exposure in air, other health risks from swallowing in water
Environmental tobacco smoke	Smoke that comes from burning end of cigarette, pipe, or cigar	Complex mixture of more than 4,000 compounds, over 40 of which cause cancer
Biological contaminants (molds, mildew, viruses, animal dander and cat saliva, dust mites, cockroaches, and pollen)	Improper ventilation and moisture buildup, lack of cleanliness/sanitation, contaminated heating systems, household pets, rodents, insects, damp carpets, etc.	Allergic reactions, including hypersensitivity, rhinitis, asthma, infectious illnesses, sneezing, watering eyes, coughing, shortness of breath, dizziness, lethargy, fever, digestive problems
Combustion products	Unvented kerosene heaters, woodstoves, fireplaces, gas stoves	Carbon monoxide causes headaches, dizziness, weakness, nausea, confusion and disorientation, chest pain, death. Nitrogen dioxide causes irritation of nose and eyes, respiratory distress. Particles cause lung damage and irritation.
Household chemicals (see partial list below)	Paints, varnishes, cleaning products, solvents, degreasers, hobby products, etc.	Variable symptoms dependent on exposure level, including eye and respiratory tract problems, headaches, dizziness, visual disorders, and memory impairment
• Benzene	Paint, new carpet, new drapes, upholstery, fast-drying glues, caulks	Headaches, eye/skin irritation, fatigue, cancer
• Formaldehyde	Tobacco smoke, plywood, cabinets, furniture, particleboard, new carpet and drapes, wallpaper, ceiling tile, paneling	Headaches, eye/skin irritation, drowsiness, fatigue, respiratory problems, memory loss, depression, gynecological problems, cancer
• Chloroform	Paint, new drapes, new carpet, upholstery	Headaches, asthma attacks, dizziness, eye/skin irritations
• Toluene	All paper products, most finished wood products	Headaches, eye/skin irritation, sinus problems, dizziness, cancer
• Hydrocarbons	Tobacco smoke, gas burners and furnaces	Headaches, fatigue, nausea, dizziness, breathing difficulty
• Ammonia	Tobacco smoke, cleaning supplies, animal urine	Eye/skin irritation, headaches, nosebleeds, sinus problems
• Trichloroethylene	Paints, glues, caulking, vinyl coatings, wallpaper	Headaches, eye/skin irritation, upper respiratory irritation

Source: U.S. Environmental Protection Agency, "Indoor Air Pollution: An Introduction for Health Professionals," 2006, www.epa.gov/iaq/pubs/hpguide.html#intro.

to 22,000 lung cancer deaths per year have been attributed to radon, making it second only to smoking as a cause of lung cancer.[20]

The EPA estimates that 1 in 15 American homes has an elevated radon level.[21] A home-testing kit from a hardware store will enable you to test your home yourself. "Alpha track" detectors are commonly used for this type of short-term testing. They must remain in your home for 2 to 90 days, depending on the device.

Household Chemicals   Use cleansers and other cleaning products in a well-ventilated room, and be conservative in their use. Those caustic chemicals that zap mildew and grease also pose a major risk to water and the environment. Avoid buildup. Regular cleanings will reduce the need to use potentially harmful substances. Cut down on dry cleaning, as the chemicals used by many cleaners can cause cancer. If your newly cleaned clothes smell of dry-cleaning chemicals, return them to the cleaner or hang them in the open air until the smell is gone. Avoid household air freshener products containing the carcinogenic agent *dichlorobenzene*.

Indoor air pollution is also a concern in the classroom and workplace. Studies show that one in five U.S. schools has indoor air quality problems, and one in four has ventilation problems.[22] Poor air quality in classrooms may lead to drowsiness, headaches, and lack of concentration. It may also affect physical growth and development. Children with asthma are particularly at risk. Many people who work indoors complain of maladies that lessen or vanish when they leave the building. **Sick building syndrome (SBS)** is said to

sick building syndrome (SBS)   Problem that exists when 80 percent of a building's occupants report maladies that tend to lessen or vanish when they leave the building.

ARE ENVIRONMENTAL MOLDS MAKING YOU ILL?

If you've heard tales of people getting sick from living in homes or working in buildings with molds growing in the walls or attics, you are not alone. What are molds, and why all the concern? Molds are actually fungi that can be found both indoors and outdoors in most regions of the country. There are literally thousands of different mold types; and, for the most part, we live with them in peaceful coexistence. Molds produce tiny spores to reproduce, and the spores waft through the indoor and outdoor air continually. When they land on a damp spot indoors, they may begin growing and digesting whatever they are growing on, including wood, paper, carpet, and food.

However, some people are sensitive to molds, and exposure may lead to nasal stuffiness, running nose and eyes, itchy skin, or much more serious consequences. For those who are really sensitive, living in a home where mold is in the walls or under the carpets may lead to fever, headache, shortness of breath, nausea, light-headedness, or severe respiratory problems. Some people have experienced extreme autoimmune-like symptoms.

In general, the best way to prevent problems is to avoid areas that are likely to have molds, such as compost piles, cut grass, and wooded areas. Antique shops, greenhouses, saunas, flower shops, lake or beach houses, attics, and basements are all likely mold growth areas.

If you have mold in your home, you should clean it up and fix sources of dampness that may be contributing to them. Use a solution of bleach and water or purchase antimold products designed to kill growth in showers and other areas of the home. If you suspect mold-related problems in your workplace or school, contact your local health department to schedule an inspection.

Specific recommendations for reducing mold exposure include:

- Keep the humidity level in your home between 40 and 60 percent.
- Use an air conditioner or a dehumidifier during humid months.
- Be sure your home has adequate ventilation, including exhaust fans in the kitchen or bath. If there are no fans, open windows.
- Add mold inhibitors to paints before application.
- Clean bathrooms with mold-killing products.
- Do not carpet bathrooms and basements.
- Wash rugs in entryways and other areas where moisture can accumulate.
- Get rid of mattresses and other furniture that may have been exposed to moisture during moving or through bed-wetting or other situations where slow drying may occur.
- Dry clothing thoroughly before folding and putting in drawers or hanging in dark closets.

Source: National Center for Environmental Health, "Molds in the Environment," 2006, www.cdc.gov/nceh/airpollution/mold/moldfacts .htm.

---

exist when 80 percent of a building's occupants report problems. Poor ventilation is a primary cause of sick building syndrome. Other causes include faulty furnaces that emit carbon monoxide, nitrogen dioxide, and sulfur dioxide; biological air pollutants such as dander, molds, and dust; VOCs from products such as hairspray, cleaners, and adhesives; and heavy metals such as lead, particularly in older buildings. Symptoms include eye irritation, sore throat, queasiness, and worsened asthma.[23]

Ozone Layer Depletion

What has our government done to protect the ozone layer?

As mentioned earlier, the *ozone* layer forms a protective layer in the Earth's stratosphere—the highest level of the Earth's atmosphere, which is located 12 to 30 miles above the Earth's surface. The ozone layer in the stratosphere protects our planet and its inhabitants from ultraviolet B (UVB) radiation, a primary cause of skin cancer. UVB radiation may also damage DNA and weaken immune systems in both humans and animals. Thus, the ozone layer is crucial to life on the planet's surface.

In the 1970s, scientists began to warn of a breakdown in the Earth's ozone layer. Instruments developed to test atmospheric contents indicated that chemicals called **chlorofluorocarbons (CFCs),** were contributing to its rapid depletion.

At first believed to be miracle chemicals, chlorofluorocarbons were used as refrigerants (Freon), as aerosol propellants in hairsprays and deodorants, as cleaning solvents, and in medical sterilizers, rigid foam insulation, and Styrofoam. But, along with halons (found in many fire extinguishers), methyl chloroform, and carbon tetrachloride (a cleaning solvent), CFCs were eventually found to be a major cause of ozone depletion. When released into the air through spraying or outgassing, CFCs migrate upward toward the ozone layer, where

chlorofluorocarbons (CFCs) Chemicals that contribute to the depletion of the ozone layer.

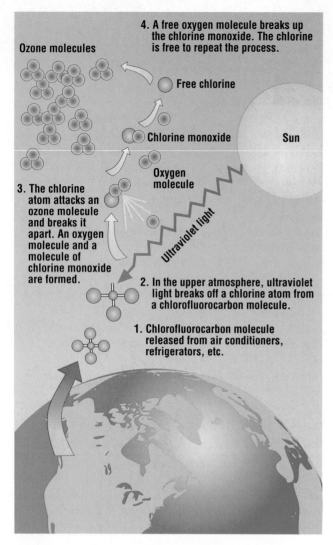

4. A free oxygen molecule breaks up the chlorine monoxide. The chlorine is free to repeat the process.

Ozone molecules

Free chlorine

Chlorine monoxide

Sun

Oxygen molecule

3. The chlorine atom attacks an ozone molecule and breaks it apart. An oxygen molecule and a molecule of chlorine monoxide are formed.

Ultraviolet light

2. In the upper atmosphere, ultraviolet light breaks off a chlorine atom from a chlorofluorocarbon molecule.

1. Chlorofluorocarbon molecule released from air conditioners, refrigerators, etc.

FIGURE 21.3 How the Ozone Layer Is Being Depleted

they decompose and release chlorine atoms. These atoms cause ozone molecules to break apart (Figure 21.3).

The U.S. government banned the use of aerosol sprays containing CFCs in the 1970s. The discovery of an "ozone hole" over Antarctica led to the 1987 Montreal Protocol, a treaty whereby the United States and other nations agreed to further reduce the use of CFCs and other ozone-depleting chemicals. The treaty was amended in 1995 to ban CFC production in developed countries. Today, over 160 countries have signed the treaty, as the international community strives to preserve the ozone layer.[24]

Although the ban on CFCs is believed to be responsible for slowing the depletion of the ozone layer, CFC replacements (including the greenhouse gases termed hydrofluorocarbons and perfluorocarbons) appear to be equally damaging. A United Nations treaty signed in Kyoto in 1997 attempted to

---

greenhouse gases Gases that contribute to global warming by trapping heat near the Earth's surface.

---

control these newer greenhouse gases. Unfortunately, the United States has so far refused to sign the treaty, amid much controversy. As the greatest producer of greenhouse gases, the United States would have been required to reduce emissions by 33 percent.

Global Warming

More than 100 years ago, scientists theorized that carbon dioxide emissions from fossil fuel burning would create a buildup of greenhouse gases in the Earth's atmosphere that could have a warming effect on the planet's surface. The century-old predictions now seem to be coming true, with alarming results. According to the National Academy of Sciences, the Earth's surface temperature has risen 1 degree Fahrenheit in the past century, with accelerated warming in the past two decades, and there is new and strong evidence that most of the warming over the last 50 years is due to human activities.[25,26]

With average global temperatures higher today than at any time since global temperatures were first recorded, the change in atmospheric temperature may be taking a heavy toll on human beings and crops. Climate researchers predicted in 1975 that the buildup of greenhouse gases would produce life-threatening natural phenomena, including drought in the midwestern United States, more frequent and severe forest fires, flooding in India and Bangladesh, extended heat waves over large areas of the Earth, and massive hurricanes in the southeastern United States, such as Hurricane Katrina. Recently, the planet has experienced all of these phenomena, and all experts agree that unless major changes are made, in less than a decade the damage to Earth will be irreversible.

Greenhouse gases include carbon dioxide, CFCs, ground-level ozone, nitrous oxide, and methane. They become part of a gaseous layer that encircles the Earth, allowing solar heat to pass through and then trapping it close to the Earth's surface. The most predominant is carbon dioxide, which accounts for 49 percent of all greenhouse gases. The United States is the greatest producer of greenhouse gases, responsible for over 22 percent of all output.

Rapid deforestation of the tropical rain forests of Central and South America, Africa, and Southeast Asia also contributes to the rapid rise in greenhouse gases. Trees take in carbon dioxide, transform it, store the carbon for food, and then release oxygen into the air. As we lose forests at the rate of hundreds of acres per hour, we lose the capacity to dissipate carbon dioxide.

Reducing Air Pollution

Air pollution problems are rooted in our energy, transportation, and industrial practices. We must develop comprehensive national strategies to address the problem of air pollution in order to clean the air for the future. We must support policies that encourage the use of renewable resources such as solar, wind, and water power as the providers of most of the world's energy.

GOING GREEN: TAKING ACTION FOR GREEN CAMPUSES

Rather than just feeling hopeless and depressed after viewing movies that portray a gloomy forecast of future environmental crisis, such as *An Inconvenient Truth,* students across the country are leading the charge to reduce energy consumption and preserve our natural environment. Hundreds of campuses are "going green" and taking positive steps to get their campuses involved in efforts to reduce global warming and other threats to health. From serving organic foods in the cafeterias and establishing compost programs for school dormitories and cafeterias to urging schools to switch to energy-efficient bulbs and recycled paper, many campuses are making an effort, and claim energy savings of 7 to 20 percent.

How can you make a difference? It isn't hard. For example, consider the amount of trash generated by paper coffee cups every single day. It's just paper though, right? Wrong. These cups can't be recycled due to a waxy film inside the cup. The simple task of bringing your own reusable cup to the coffee shop could save tons of waste each day on campuses across the country. You can also take action at a higher level and urge your college's decision makers to make some changes. Once university administrators realize the potential for saving money that could be better used elsewhere, they often enthusiastically support these programs, even when initial costs are large. Follow the lead of these green campus initiatives:

- Harvard University converted campus buses to biodiesel to reduce fuel costs and emissions.
- The student body at Northland College in Ashland, Wisconsin, voted to pay an extra $40 per year per student to purchase a wind turbine to create electricity and hybrid vehicles for campus trips.
- At Humboldt State University in California, students wrote an educational film called "Green Eye for the Conventional Gal," in which environmentalists teach ordinary students how to live a more sustainable life by eating, dressing, and using energy in a more responsible fashion (visit http://steelbluepanic.com/greeneye).
- The University of California at Berkeley's Green Campus interns created and facilitated a one-credit class, "Energy 101," in which students learn to conduct energy audits of spots on campus and report back on ways to save energy.
- Western Washington University has taken aggressive measures to use renewable electricity on campus.

Students interested in getting involved in their own green campus activities or starting their own green campus initiatives should check out websites focused on green campuses or campus climate challenge, and become involved. Each action, however small, can make a difference.

Source: Alliance to Save Energy, "Promoting Energy Efficiency World Wide", 2006, http://ase.org/content/article/detail/2497.

Most experts agree that shifting away from automobiles as the primary source of transportation is the only way to reduce air pollution significantly. Many cities have taken steps in this direction by setting high parking fees, imposing bans on city driving, and establishing high road-usage tolls. Community governments should be encouraged to provide convenient, inexpensive, and easily accessible public transportation.

Although stricter laws on carbon emissions from cars and trucks and development of new hybrid cars that operate on electricity and gas are promising, we have a long way to go to reduce fossil fuel consumption. One promising initiative is "bicycle power," with bicycles gaining popularity worldwide. Currently, China leads the world in bicycle use, followed by India. In Germany, bicycle use has increased by 50 percent, and England has a plan to quadruple bicycle use by the year 2012.[27]

Hybrid Cars Hybrid cars, capable of significantly lower emissions and less reliance on fossil fuels, have gained popularity in the United States and abroad. Improved technology, tax incentives, and other initiatives have made these a more realistic alternative to traditional cars. Newer versions of electric cars, flex-fuel cars, and low-emission diesel vehicles provide some hope for future air pollution control.

Water Pollution

Seventy-five percent of the Earth is covered with water in the form of oceans, seas, lakes, rivers, streams, and wetlands. Beneath the landmass are reservoirs of groundwater. We draw our drinking water from either this underground source or from surface freshwater. However, just 1 percent of our entire water supply is available for human use—the rest is too salty, too polluted, or locked away in polar ice caps.[28] Considering that this water must meet the world's agricultural, manufacturing, community, personal, and sanitation needs, it is no wonder that clean water is a precious commodity. Table 21.2 on page 630 shows how much water might be saved daily through simple conservation actions.

We cannot take the safety of our water supply for granted. Local and state governments, public water systems, and the

TABLE 21.2	Daily per Capita Water Use (in Gallons) in Single-Family Homes	
Type of Use	With Water-Conserving Devices	Without Water-Conserving Devices
Showers	10.0	12.6
Washing machines	10.6	15.1
Toilets	9.3	20.1
Dishwashers	1.0	1.0
Baths	1.2	1.2
Leaks	5.0	10.0
Faucets	10.8	11.1
Other domestic use	1.5	1.5
Total	49.4	72.6
Total savings: 23.3 gallons per day		

Source: Adapted from "1999 Residential Water Use Summary," by permission. Copyright © 2002, American Water Works Association.

EPA spend billions of dollars per year to protect and maintain water quality.[29] The status of our water supply reflects the pollution level of our communities and, ultimately, of the whole Earth.

How serious is our shortage of safe water for global populations? According to a 2004 World Health Organization/ UNICEF report, the world faces a silent emergency of a shortage of clean water for almost half the world's population. More than 2.6 billion people, about 40 percent of those on the planet, have no access to basic sanitation or adequate toilet facilities. More than a billion have no access to clean water, and over 4,000 children die every day from illnesses caused by contaminated water and lack of sanitation. By 2015, over 800 million people will have no safe water.[30]

Water Contamination

Many factors can contribute to water contamination. Microorganisms can flourish if water temperature and oxygen levels become hospitable to their growth, and these microbes can cause disease. Waterborne diseases such as hepatitis A, cholera, amoebic dysentery, and giardiasis can cause severe

point source pollutants Pollutants that enter waterways at a specific point.

nonpoint source pollutants Pollutants that run off or seep into waterways from broad areas of land.

leachate Liquid consisting of soluble chemicals that come from garbage and industrial waste that seeps into the water supply from landfills and dumps.

illness and death. Just because water looks clean doesn't mean it is, so never drink from a running stream or a lake without purifying water first.

In addition to microbial contamination, water can become polluted by toxic chemicals such as pesticides, herbicides, fertilizers, and a host of other chemicals. These substances end up in our sewers, our water supplies, and our general environment. The potential health hazards of mixing these thousands of chemicals together can barely be imagined.

Any substance that gets into the soil can potentially enter the water supply. Industrial pollutants, acid deposition, and pesticides eventually work their way into the soil, then into groundwater. Underground storage tanks for gasoline may leak. Oil spills contaminate coastal waterways and spill into local rivers, along with hazardous farming and industrial wastes.

A recent survey by a group of U.S. Geological Survey researchers discovered the presence of low levels of many chemical compounds—including prescription and nonprescription drugs, hormones, and wastewater compounds—in a network of 139 targeted streams across the United States. Steroids, nonprescription drugs, and insect repellent were among the most frequently detected groups of chemicals.[31]

Sources of Water Contamination The U.S. Congress has coined two terms, *point source* and *nonpoint source,* to describe the two general sources of water pollution. **Point source pollutants** enter a waterway at a specific point through a pipe, ditch, culvert, or other conduit. The two major sources of this type of pollution are sewage treatment plants and industrial facilities.

Nonpoint source pollutants—commonly known as *runoff* and *sedimentation*—run off or seep into waterways from broad areas of land rather than through a discrete conduit. It is estimated that 99 percent of the sediment in our waterways, 98 percent of the bacterial contaminants, 84 percent of the phosphorus, and 82 percent of the nitrogen come from nonpoint sources.[32] Nonpoint pollution results from a variety of human land use practices. It includes soil erosion and sedimentation, construction wastes, pesticide and fertilizer runoff, urban street runoff, wastes from engineering projects, acidic mine drainage, leakage from septic tanks, and sewage sludge.[33] (See Figure 21.4.)

Septic Systems Bacteria from human waste can leach into the water supply from improperly installed septic systems. Toxic chemicals that are dumped into septic systems can also enter groundwater.

Landfills Landfills and dumps generate a liquid called **leachate,** a mixture of soluble chemicals from household garbage, office waste, biological waste, and industrial waste. If a landfill has not been properly lined, leachate trickles through its layers of garbage and eventually gets into the water supply as acid or evaporates into the atmosphere as methane gas.

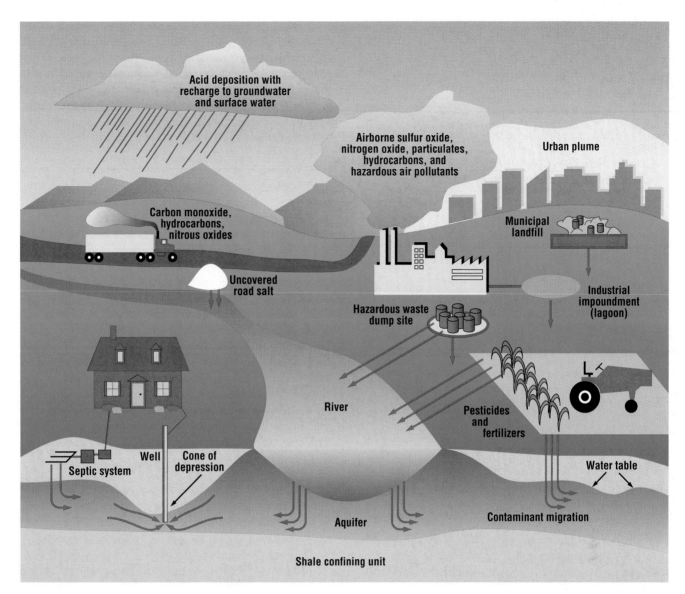

FIGURE 21.4 Sources of Groundwater Contamination

Gasoline and Petroleum Products In the United States, there are thousands of underground storage tanks for gasoline and petroleum products, most of which are located at gasoline filling stations. Most of these tanks were installed 25 to 30 years ago. They were made of fabricated steel that was unprotected from corrosion. Over time, pinpoint holes develop in the steel, and the petroleum products leak into groundwater. The most common way to detect the presence of petroleum products in water is to test for benzene, a component of oil and gasoline. Benzene is highly toxic and associated with the development of cancer. Although efforts at cleanup have been steady, many of these tanks still pose a threat.

Chemical Contaminants *Organic solvents* are chemicals designed to dissolve grease and oil. These extremely toxic substances, such as carbon tetrachloride, tetrachloroethylene, and trichloroethylene (TCE), are used to clean clothing, painting equipment, plastics, and metal parts.

Many household products, such as stain and spot removers, degreasers, drain cleaners, septic system cleaners, and paint removers, also contain these toxic chemicals.

Organic solvents work their way into the water supply in different ways. Consumers often dump leftover products into the toilet or into street drains. Industries pour leftovers into large barrels, which are then buried. After a while, the chemicals eat their way out of the barrels and leach into groundwater.

One related group of toxic substances contains chlorinated hydrocarbons. The most notorious of these substances are the **polychlorinated biphenyls (PCBs),** their cousins the *polybromated biphenyls (PBBs),* and the *dioxins.*

polychlorinated biphenyls (PCBs) Toxic chemicals that were once used as insulating materials in high-voltage electrical equipment.

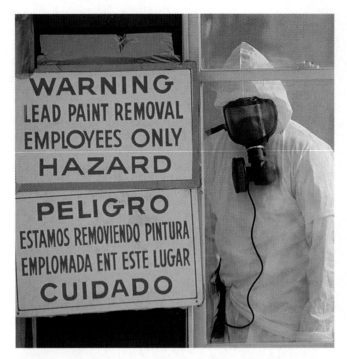

Although an expensive and cumbersome project, deleading a house is now one of the most important considerations of prospective homeowners, especially those with children.

PCBs Fire resistant and stable at high temperatures, PCBs were used for many years as insulating materials in high-voltage electrical equipment such as transformers. PCBs bioaccumulate, meaning that the body does not excrete them but rather stores them in fatty tissues and the liver. PCBs are associated with birth defects, and exposure to them is known to cause cancer. The manufacture of PCBs was discontinued in the United States in 1977, but approximately 500 million pounds of them have been dumped into landfills and waterways, where they continue to pose an environmental threat.[34] Western European countries phased out the use of many of these chemicals in the 1970s; however, elevated levels can still be detected at the mouths of major rivers, and some countries continue to produce them. PCBs bind to dust particles in the air, are deposited on plants, and end up in the food supply.[35]

Dioxins Chlorinated hydrocarbons found in herbicides (chemicals that are used to kill vegetation) and produced during certain industrial processes are called **dioxins.** Dioxins have the ability to bioaccumulate and are much more toxic than PCBs.

dioxins Highly toxic chlorinated hydrocarbons contained in herbicides and produced during certain industrial processes.

pesticides Chemicals that kill pests.

The long-term effects of bioaccumulation of these toxic substances include possible damage to the immune system and increased risk of infections and cancer. Exposure to high concentrations of PCBs or dioxins for a short period of time can also have severe consequences, including nausea, vomiting, diarrhea, painful rashes and sores, and chloracne, an ailment in which the skin develops hard, black, painful pimples that may never go away.

Pesticides Chemicals that are designed to kill insects, rodents, plants, and fungi are **pesticides.** Americans use more than 1.2 billion pounds of pesticides each year, but only 10 percent actually reach the targeted organisms. The remaining 1.1 billion pounds of pesticides settle on the land and in our air and water. Many pesticides, such as DDT, that are banned in the United States are shipped abroad. Mexico, a major crop producer for the American market, continues to use DDT.

Pesticides are volatile and evaporate readily, often being dispersed by winds over a large area or carried to the sea. This is particularly true in tropical regions, where many farmers use pesticides heavily and the climate promotes rapid release of pesticides into the atmosphere.

Pesticide residues cling to fresh fruits and vegetables and can accumulate in the body when people eat these items. Potential hazards associated with exposure to pesticides include birth defects, liver and kidney damage, and nervous system disorders.[36]

Lead The EPA has issued new standards to reduce dramatically the levels of lead in U.S. drinking water. These standards are already in place in many municipalities and will eventually reduce lead exposure for approximately 130 million people. The new rules stipulate that tap water lead values must not exceed 15 parts per billion (the previous standard allowed an average lead level of 50 parts per billion). When water suppliers identify problem areas, they will have to lower the water's acidity with chemical treatment (because acidity increases water's ability to leach lead from the pipes through which it passes), or they will have to replace old lead plumbing in the service lines.

If lead does exist in your home's water, you can reduce your risk by running tap water for several minutes before taking a drink or cooking with it. This flushes out water that has been standing overnight in lead-contaminated lines. Although leaded paints and ceramic glazes formerly posed health risks, particularly for small children who put painted toys in their mouths, the use of lead in such products has been effectively reduced in recent years.

what do you THINK?

Who should bear the financial responsibility for cleaning up hazardous waste leaks? ▪ What can you do to avoid contributing to water contamination?

Noise Pollution

Loud noise has become commonplace. We are often painfully aware of construction crews in our streets, jet airplanes roaring overhead, stereos blaring next door, and trucks rumbling down nearby freeways. Our bodies show definite physiological responses to noise, and it can become a source of physical and mental distress. Short-term exposure to loud noise reduces productivity, concentration levels, and attention spans and may affect mental and emotional health. Symptoms of noise-related distress include disturbed sleep patterns, headaches, and tension. Physically, our bodies respond to noise in a variety of ways. Blood pressure increases, blood vessels in the brain dilate, and vessels in other parts of the body constrict. The pupils of the eye dilate. Cholesterol levels in the blood rise, and some endocrine glands secrete additional stimulating hormones, such as adrenaline, into the bloodstream.

Hearing can be damaged by varying lengths of exposure to sound, which is measured in decibels (Table 21.3). If the duration of allowable daily exposure to different decibel levels is exceeded, hearing loss will result.

Unfortunately, despite increasing awareness that noise pollution is more than just a nuisance, noise control programs at federal, state, and local levels have received low budgetary priority in the United States. According to the National Institute for Occupational Safety and Health, 30 million Americans are exposed to hazardous noise at work, and 10 million suffer from permanent hearing loss.[37]

Clearly, to protect your hearing, you must take it upon yourself to avoid exposure to excessive noise. Playing stereos in your car and home at reasonable levels, keeping the volume down on your iPod, wearing ear plugs when you use power equipment, and establishing barriers such as closed windows between you and noise will help keep your hearing intact.

Land Pollution

Solid Waste

Each day, every person in the United States generates about 4 pounds of **municipal solid waste**—containers and packaging, discarded food, yard debris, and refuse from residential, commercial, institutional, and industrial sources. Approximately 73 percent of this waste is buried in landfills. Cities throughout the country are in danger of exhausting their landfill space.

As communities run out of landfill space, it is becoming more common to haul garbage out to sea to dump it or ship it to landfills in developing countries. Figure 21.5 on page 634 shows the composition of our trash and what happens to our garbage after disposal. Although experts believe that up to 90 percent of our trash is recyclable, only 26 percent of it is currently recycled. In today's throwaway society, we need to

TABLE 21.3	Noise Levels of Various Activities (in Decibels)

Decibels (db) measure the volume of sounds. Here are the decibel levels of some common sounds.

Type of Sound	Noise Level (db)
Carrier deck jet operation	150
Jet takeoff from 200 feet	140
Rock concert	120 (painful)
Auto horn (3 feet)	110 (extremely loud)
Motorcycle	100
Garbage truck	100
Pneumatic drill	90
Lawnmower	90
Heavy traffic	80
Alarm clock	80
Shouting, arguing	80 (very loud)
Vacuum cleaner	75 (loud)
Freight train from 50 feet	70
Freeway traffic	65
Normal conversation	60
Light auto traffic	50 (moderate)
Library	40
Soft whisper	30 (faint)

become aware of the amount of waste we generate every day and to look for ways to recycle, reuse, and—most desirable of all—reduce what we use (Figure 21.6 on page 634).

 *try it* NOW

Put a stop to junk mail! Tired of all those credit card offers and unwanted catalogs flooding your mailbox? Take a second to send a postcard or letter to Mail Preference Service, Direct Marketing Association, PO Box 643, Carmel, NY 15012-0643. Include your complete name, address, and zip code, and a request to "activate the preference service." You can also call 1-888-5 OPT OUT to put an end to unwanted mail.

municipal solid waste Solid wastes such as durable goods, nondurable goods, containers and packaging, food waste, yard waste, and miscellaneous wastes from residential, commercial, institutional, and industrial sources.

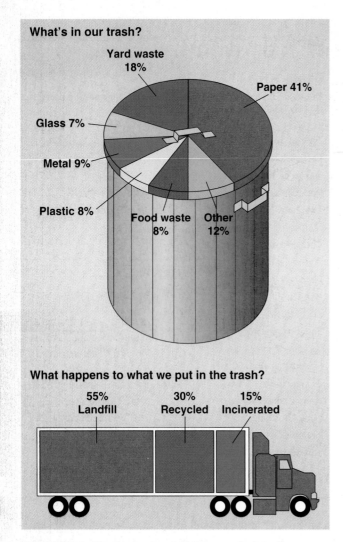

What's in our trash?

Yard waste 18%

Paper 41%

Glass 7%

Metal 9%

Plastic 8%

Food waste 8%

Other 12%

What happens to what we put in the trash?

| 55% Landfill | 30% Recycled | 15% Incinerated |

FIGURE 21.5 **The Composition and Disposal of Trash**

Hazardous Waste

The community of Love Canal, New York, has come to symbolize **hazardous waste** dump sites. The Hooker Chemical Company used Love Canal as a chemical dump site from 1947 to 1952. The area was later filled in by land developers and built up with homes and schools. In 1976, homeowners began noticing strange seepage in their basements and strong chemical odors. Babies were born with abnormal hearts and kidneys, two sets of teeth, mental handicaps, epilepsy, liver disease, and abnormal rectal bleeding. The rate of cancer and miscarriages was far above normal. The New York State Department of Health investigated and found high concentra-

hazardous waste Waste that, due to its toxic properties, poses a hazard to humans or to the environment.

Superfund Fund established under the Comprehensive Environmental Response Compensation and Liability Act to be used for cleaning up toxic waste dumps.

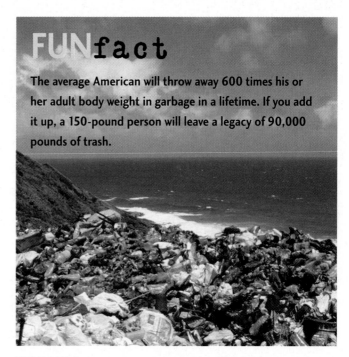

FIGURE 21.6 **Are We Leaving a Legacy of Trash?**

tions of PCBs in the storm sewers near the old canal, but it took the department another two years to order the evacuation of Love Canal homes. Over 900 families were evacuated, and the state purchased their homes. Finally, in 1978, the expensive process of cleaning up the waste dump began, and continued for years.

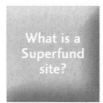

What is a Superfund site?

In 1980, the Comprehensive Environmental Response Compensation and Liability Act (**Superfund**) was enacted to provide funds for cleaning up chemical dump sites that endanger public health and land. This fund is financed through taxes on the chemical and petroleum industries (87 percent) and through general federal tax revenues (13 percent). Cost estimates for cleanup covering the years 1990 through 2020 range from $106 billion to $500 billion. Billions continue to be spent annually.[38]

To date, 32,500 potentially hazardous waste sites have been identified across the nation. After investigation, 1,498 sites were listed on the National Priorities List (NPL) as requiring action.[39] As of the end of 2004, cleanup work had been completed at 926 of the sites. Funding for projects has been scaled back due to competing economic priorities, making the cleanup difficult to complete.

The large number of U.S. hazardous waste dump sites indicates the severity of our toxic chemical problem. American manufacturers generate more than 1 ton of chemical waste per person per year (approximately 275 million tons). The Agency for Toxic Substances and Disease Registry (ATSDR) and the EPA evaluate and rank the chemicals that are considered hazardous substances (Table 21.4 on page 636).

SKILLS FOR behavior change

TAKING ACTION FOR THE ENVIRONMENT

Here are several ways to help preserve and protect the environment.

What can I do to make a positive impact on the environment?

- Listen carefully to what political candidates say about the environment. Vote for those who prioritize environmental issues and actively promote preservation, protection, and sustainable development.
- Consider state and federal initiatives on issues such as logging, fishing industries, preservation of parks, oil and natural gas drilling, protection of the food supply, restrictions on industrial polluters, solid waste disposal, and water quality.
- Become an environmentally oriented consumer. Buy products with less packaging, foods that are produced with minimal or sustainable energy, organic foods or foods with fewer chemicals and pesticides. Buy locally grown or produced foods whenever possible.

- Do not use caustic cleansers, chemicals that remove film in your shower, or dyes and fragrances in your laundry products. Use soap and water to clean surfaces, not disposable cleaning cloths and spray-on shower cleaners. All these chemicals are flushed down the drain and into the local water supply.
- Let your legislators know how you feel about environmental issues and that you will vote according to their record on the issues. When writing to any public official, keep the letter simple and to the point; avoid inflammatory statements and attacks; state the facts, cite reputable sources, and indicate what you want changed; and say it in one page or less. Proofread the letter for accuracy.
- If you buy a product with excessive packaging, call the toll-free number on the package and let the manufacturer know about your concerns.
- Educate yourself and others. Organize a discussion group of friends to read books and articles or discuss speakers

focused on environmental issues. Request environmental speakers in your class or at campus events.
- Stop buying plastic bottles of water and other beverages. Plastics are among the fastest growing sources of pollution in America. Purchase a hard plastic, wide-mouth water bottle and fill it from a filtered source. Reuse the bottle, and wash it frequently.
- Get active in community groups that deal with environmental issues. Volunteer for commissions, boards, and other groups involved in decision making. Participate in cleanup days and recycling drives. Parks, land use, animal control, zoning, public transit, street cleanup, and trash collection are a few of the many issues that have environmental components.
- Run for student government. Help your school become more involved in environmental issues. Seek practicum or internship credits for working for environmental causes. Take coursework in environmental health or science.

The EPA and the states have undertaken an aggressive program to manage hazardous wastes by monitoring their generation, transportation, storage, treatment, and final disposal. To ensure that hazardous wastes being generated today do not become complex and expensive cleanup problems tomorrow, the following steps are being taken:[40]

- Many wastes are now banned from land disposal or are being treated to reduce their toxicity before they become part of land disposal sites.
- The EPA has developed protective requirements for land disposal facilities, such as double liners, detection systems for substances that may leach into groundwater, and groundwater monitoring systems.
- Hazardous waste handlers must now clean up contamination resulting from past waste management practices as well as from current activities.
- The EPA is exploring economic incentives to encourage ingenuity in waste minimization practices and recycling.

 what do you THINK?

What items do you currently recycle? ■ What are some of the reasons you do not recycle? ■ What might encourage you to recycle more than you do? ■ What concerns would you have about living near a landfill or hazardous waste disposal site?

Radiation

A substance is said to be radioactive when it emits high-energy particles from the nuclei of its atoms. There are three types of radiation: alpha particles, beta particles, and gamma rays. *Alpha particles* are relatively massive and are not capable of penetrating human skin. They pose health hazards only when inhaled or ingested. *Beta particles* can penetrate the

TABLE 21.4	Top 20 Hazardous Substances: ATSDR/EPA Priority List

1. Arsenic
2. Lead
3. Mercury
4. Vinyl chloride
5. Polychlorinated biphenyls (PCBs)
6. Benzene
7. Cadmium
8. Polycyclic aromatic hydrocarbons
9. Benzo[*a*]pyrene
10. Benzo[*b*]fluoranthene
11. Chloroform
12. DDT, P'P'-
13. Aroclor 1254
14. Aroclor 1260
15. Trichloroethylene
16. Dibenz[*a,h*]anthracene
17. Chromium, Hexavalent
18. Dieldrin
19. Phosphorus, white
20. Chlordane

Source: Agency for Toxic Substances and Disease Registry, "Top 20 Hazardous Substances," 2003, www.atsdr.cdc.gov/cxcx3.html.

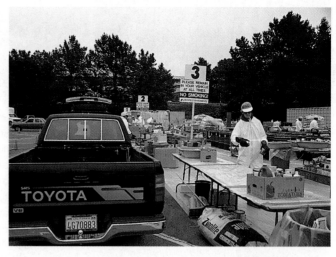

Many communities now provide special programs in which their residents can drop off any kind of hazardous waste for safe disposal.

skin slightly and are harmful if ingested or inhaled. *Gamma rays* are the most dangerous because they can pass straight through the skin, causing serious damage to organs and other vital structures.

Ionizing Radiation

Exposure to ionizing radiation is an inescapable part of life on this planet. **Ionizing radiation** is caused by the release of particles and electromagnetic rays from atomic nuclei during the normal process of disintegration. Some naturally occurring elements, such as uranium, emit radiation. Radiation can wreak havoc on human cells, leading to mutations, cancer, miscarriages, and other problems.

Reactions to radiation differ from person to person. Exposure is measured in **radiation absorbed doses,** or **RADs** (also called *roentgens*). Recommended maximum "safe" dosages range from 0.5 to 5 RADs per year. Approximately 50 percent of the radiation to which we are exposed comes from natural sources, such as building materials. Another

ionizing radiation Radiation produced by photons having high enough energy to ionize atoms.

radiation absorbed doses (RADs) Units that measure exposure to radioactivity.

45 percent comes from medical and dental X rays. The remaining 5 percent comes from computer display screens, microwave ovens, television sets, luminous watch dials, and radar screens and waves. Most of us are exposed to far less radiation than the "safe" maximum dosage per year.

Radiation can cause damage at dosages as low as 100 to 200 RADs. At this level, signs of radiation sickness include nausea, diarrhea, fatigue, anemia, sore throat, and hair loss, but death is unlikely. At 350 to 500 RADs, these symptoms become more severe, and death may result because the radiation hinders bone marrow production of the white blood cells we need to protect us from disease. Dosages above 600 to 700 RADs are invariably fatal. The effects of long-term exposure to relatively low levels of radiation are unknown. Some scientists believe that such exposure can cause lung cancer, leukemia, skin cancer, bone cancer, and skeletal deformities.

Researchers are also investigating the effects of exposure to the radio frequency waves generated by cell phones (see the New Horizons in Health box).

Electric and Magnetic Fields: Emerging Risks?

If you believe what you hear on TV or read in the papers, electric and magnetic fields (EMFs) generated by electric power delivery systems are responsible for risks for cancer (particularly among children), reproductive dysfunction, birth defects, neurological disorders, Alzheimer's disease, and other ailments. Does research support these claims about EMFs? Though many believe that the threat is legitimate, others point to major discrepancies and inconsistencies in the research. In spite of many questions, fears have increased, and there is probably more potential for exploitation of consumers than real hazard to health from this nonionizing form of exposure.

WIRELESS WORRIES: CELL PHONES AND RISKS TO HEALTH

In less than a decade, cell phones have become a household staple, with the number of subscribers skyrocketing from 16 million in 1994 to over 110 million today and still rising by 1 million per month. Although cell phones have become commonplace, their use continues to spur controversy, particularly regarding questions of potential health risk. Although the cell phone industry assures consumers that phones are safe, a former industry research director, Dr. George Carlo, argues that past studies have not provided conclusive evidence of safety and we do not know the effects of cell phone usage on future generations. He observed, "This is the first generation that has put relatively high-powered transmitters against the head, hour after hour, day after day." Depending on how close the cell phone antenna is to the head, as much as 60 percent of the microwave radiation may actually penetrate the area around the head, some of it reaching an inch to an inch-and-a-half into the brain.

Can talking on my cell phone cause cancer?

Are increases in the prevalence of brain tumors and other neurological conditions in the last decade related to cell phone use? At high power levels, radiofrequency energy, which is the energy used in cell phones, can rapidly heat biological tissue and cause damage, such as burns. However, cell phones operate at power levels well below the level at which such heating occurs. Many countries, including the United States and most of Europe, use standards set by the FCC for radiofrequency energy based on research by several scientific groups. These groups identified a whole-body *specific absorption rate (SAR)* value for exposure to radiofrequency energy. Four watts per kilogram was identified as a threshold level of exposure at which harmful biological effects may occur. The FCC requires wireless phones to comply with a safety limit of 1.6 watts per kilogram. To find the SAR for your phone, see this website: www.fda.gov/cellphones/qa.html.

The Food and Drug Administration, the World Health Organization, and other major health agencies agree that the research to date has not shown radiofrequency energy emitted from cell phones to be harmful. However, they also point to the need for more research and caution that because cell phones have only been widely used for less than a decade and no long-term studies have been done, there is not enough information to say they are risk free. Three large case-control studies and one large cohort study have compared cell phone use among brain cancer patients and individuals free of brain cancer. Key findings from these studies indicate that:

- Brain cancer patients did not report more cellular phone use overall than controls. In fact, most of the studies showed a lower risk of brain cancer among cell phone users, for unclear reasons.
- None of the studies showed a clear link between the side of the head on which the cancer occurred and the side on which the phone was used.
- There was no correlation between brain tumor risk and dose of exposure, as assessed by duration of use, date since first subscription, age at first subscription, or type of cellular phone used.

However, these studies are not conclusive, and preliminary results from smaller, well-designed studies have continued to raise questions. A recent Swedish study found higher risk of a benign brain tumor among adults who had used analog cell phones (which produce higher exposure levels than their digital counterparts) for at least ten years. At the moment, the biggest risk from cell phones appears to come from using them while driving, with a corresponding increase in crashes showing that nearly 80 percent of crashes involved

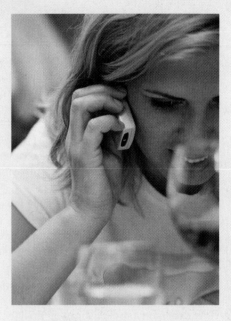

driver inattention within three seconds of the event. The most common distraction? Cell phone use. However, if you prefer to err on the side of caution, follow these hints to lower your risk:

- Limit cell phone usage. Use land-based phones whenever possible. Avoid talking on cell phones, even hands-free phones, while driving. This not only lowers your exposure, it also lowers your risk of accidents.
- Send a text message or e-mail rather than talking on the phone; this keeps the phone further from your head.
- Check the SAR level of your phone. Purchase one with a lower level if yours is near the FCC limit.

Sources: S. Grund, "Cell Phones: Do They Cause Cancer?" Medline Plus, 2004 update, www.nlm.nih.gov/medlineplus/ency/article/007151.htm; S. Lönn et al., "Mobile Phone Use and the Risk of Acoustic Neuroma," *Epidemiology* 15, no. 6 (2004): 653–659; Food and Drug Administration, "Cell Phone Facts: Consumer Information on Wireless Phones," 2004, www.fda.gov/cellphones/qa.html; American Cancer Society, "Cellular Phones," 2006, www.cancer.org; National Highway Safety Administration, "The 100-Car Naturalistic Driving Study," www.iii.org/media/hottopics/insurance/cellphones.

Nuclear Power Plants

Nuclear power plants account for less than 1 percent of the total radiation to which we are exposed. Other producers of radioactive waste include medical facilities that use radioactive materials as treatment and diagnostic tools and nuclear weapons production facilities.

> **Are there any benefits to using nuclear power?**

Proponents of nuclear energy believe that it is a safe and efficient way to generate electricity. Initial costs of building nuclear power plants are high, but actual power generation is relatively inexpensive. A 1,000-megawatt reactor produces enough energy for 650,000 homes and saves 420 million gallons of fossil fuels each year. In some areas where nuclear power plants were decommissioned, electricity bills tripled when power companies turned to hydroelectric or fossil fuel sources to generate electricity.

Nuclear reactors also discharge fewer carbon oxides into the air than fossil fuel–powered generators. Advocates believe that conversion to nuclear power could help slow the global warming trend. Over the past 15 years, carbon emissions were reduced by 298 million tons, or 5 percent.

All these advantages of nuclear energy must be weighed against the disadvantages. First, disposal of nuclear wastes is extremely problematic. Additionally, a reactor core meltdown could pose serious threats to a plant's immediate environment and to the world in general.

A **nuclear meltdown** occurs when the temperature in the core of a nuclear reactor increases enough to melt both the nuclear fuel and the containment vessel that holds it. Most modern facilities seal their reactors and containment vessels in concrete buildings with pools of cold water on the bottom. If a meltdown occurs, the building and the pool are supposed to prevent the escape of radioactivity.

One serious nuclear accident in particular contributed to a steep decline in public support for nuclear energy. The 1986 reactor core fire and explosion at the Chernobyl nuclear power plant in Russia killed 48 people and hospitalized another 200. In just 4.5 seconds, the temperature in the reactor rose to 120 times normal, causing the explosion. Officials evacuated towns and villages near the plant. Some medical workers estimate that the eventual death toll from radiation-induced cancers related to the Chernobyl incident topped 100,000.

Radioactive fallout from the Chernobyl disaster spread over most of the Northern Hemisphere. Milk, meat, and vegetables in Scandinavian countries were contaminated with radioactive iodine and cesium and were declared unfit for human consumption. Thousands of reindeer in Lapland were contaminated and had to be destroyed. In Great Britain, thousands of sheep had to be destroyed, and three years later sheep in the northern regions of the country were still found to be contaminated. Direct costs of the disaster totaled more than $13 billion, including lost agricultural output and the cost of replacing the power plant. Nuclear accidents continue to pose risks to human health, even in well-controlled settings.

> **nuclear meltdown** An accident that results when the temperature in the core of a nuclear reactor increases enough to melt the nuclear fuel and the containment vessel housing it.

 ***what do you* THINK?**

How much exposure do you have to ionizing and nonionizing radiation in a year? ▪ What measures could you take to reduce your exposure? ▪ Do you feel the advantages outweigh the disadvantages of nuclear power? Explain why or why not.

TAKING charge

Summary

- Population growth is the single largest factor affecting the demands made on the environment. Demand for more food, products, and energy—as well as sites to dispose of waste, particularly in the industrialized world—places great strain on the Earth's resources.
- The primary constituents of air pollution are sulfur dioxide, particulate matter, carbon monoxide, nitrogen dioxide, ozone, lead, and hydrocarbons. Air pollution takes the forms of photochemical smog and acid deposition, among others.

Indoor air pollution is caused primarily by woodstove smoke, furnace emissions, asbestos, tobacco smoke, formaldehyde, radon, and household chemicals. Pollution is depleting the Earth's protective ozone layer, contributing to global warming.

- Water pollution can be caused by either point (direct entry through a pipeline, ditch, etc.) or nonpoint (runoff or seepage from a broad area of land) sources. Major contributors to water pollution include dioxins, pesticides, and lead.

- Noise pollution affects our hearing and produces other symptoms such as reduced productivity, reduced concentration, headaches, and tension.
- Solid waste pollution includes household trash, plastics, glass, metal products, and paper; limited landfill space creates problems. Hazardous waste is toxic; its improper disposal creates health hazards for those in surrounding communities.

- Ionizing radiation results from the natural erosion of atomic nuclei. Nonionizing radiation is caused by the electromagnetic fields around power lines and household appliances, among other sources. The disposal and storage of radioactive wastes from nuclear power plants and weapons production pose serious potential problems for public health.

Chapter Review

1. A difference between acute and chronic health effects is that chronic effects
   a. are caused by a single severe reaction to a chemical.
   b. usually develop from repeated exposures to a harmful substance.
   c. are minor reactions caused by a single exposure to a chemical.
   d. None of the above.

2. What has global warming been doing to our planet Earth?
   a. It has caused an increase in the Earth's surface temperatures by 10 degrees.
   b. It is causing the polar ice caps to melt and may one day cause flooding in low-lying areas.
   c. It is only occurring on the North American continent.
   d. It is creating greater air pollution concerns.

3. The indoor pollutant used in home construction that can cause headaches, stinging eyes, and burning lungs is
   a. asbestos insulation.
   b. lead paint.
   c. formaldehyde foam.
   d. All of the above.

4. The clear and odorless gas that is considered radioactive and could become cancerous if it seeps into a home and is breathed is
   a. carbon monoxide.
   b. radon.
   c. hydrogen sulfide.
   d. natural gas.

5. Intensity (exposure) to sound is measured in
   a. foot candles.
   b. noise volume.
   c. hertz.
   d. decibels.

6. What is meant by the *sick building syndrome*?
   a. Buildings can get diseased like humans.
   b. New airtight buildings don't allow for adequate air circulation and this can cause illness in those who work or live in them.
   c. Older buildings are more likely to leach harmful indoor pollutants to people inside.
   d. None of the above.

7. A simple way that one can contribute to improving the global environment is to
   a. choose simply packaged items.
   b. turn off electric appliances and light fixtures when not needed.
   c. turn off the tap when shaving or brushing your teeth.
   d. All of the above.

8. The phenomenon that creates a barrier to protect us from the sun's harmful ultraviolet radiation rays is
   a. photochemical smog.
   b. the ozone layer.
   c. gray air smog.
   d. the greenhouse effect.

9. An example of a nonpoint source of water pollution would be
   a. runoff of dirty water into the sewer system.
   b. a pipe carrying raw sewage dumping into a lake.
   c. the municipal sewer treatment plant.
   d. None of the above.

10. The natural source in the environment that ionizing radiation comes from is
    a. electromagnetic rays.
    b. alpha particles that penetrate the human skin.
    c. beta particles.
    d. gamma rays.

Answers to these questions can be found on page A-1.

Questions for Discussion and Reflection

1. How are the rapidly increasing global population and consumption of resources related? Is population control the best solution? Why or why not?
2. What are the primary sources of air pollution? What can be done to reduce air pollution?
3. What causes poor indoor air quality? How does indoor air pollution affect schoolchildren?
4. What are the causes and consequences of global warming?
5. What are point and nonpoint sources of water pollution? What can be done to reduce or prevent water pollution?
6. What are the physiological consequences of noise pollution? What can you do to lessen your exposure to noise pollution?
7. Why do you think so little recycling occurs in the United States?
8. Would you feel comfortable living near a nuclear power plant? Do you think nuclear power will be an important source of energy in the future? Why or why not?

Accessing Your Health on the Internet

The following websites explore further topics and issues related to personal health. You'll also find links to each organization's website on the Companion Website for *Access to Health*, Tenth Edition, at www.aw-bc.com/donatelle.

1. *American Cancer Society - Environmental Cancer Risks.* Provides a searchable database of information about specific cancers and environmental risks, as well as a risk assessment and information about carcinogens. www.cancer .org/docroot/ped/ped_1_1.asp?sitearea=ped&level=1
2. *Data Online for Population, Health, and Nutrition (DOLPHN) Database.* DOLPHN provides demographic and health trend data relevant to the U.S. Agency for International Development. Subjects include child survival, family planning, access to clean water, and many other subjects. http://dolphn.aimglobalhealth.org
3. *Environmental Protection Agency (EPA).* A source for up-to-date statistics and background information about major risks to health from environmental hazards. www.epa.gov
4. *National Center for Environmental Health (NCEH).* A section of the Centers for Disease Control and Prevention, with information on a wide variety of environmental health issues, including a series of helpful fact sheets. www.cdc .gov/nceh
5. *National Environmental Health Association (NEHA).* This organization provides educational resources and opportunities for environmental health professionals. The NEHA website lists conferences, training, and publications and offers informational position papers. http://neha.org/
6. *Environmental Literacy Council.* This website is an excellent source of information about environmental issues in general, ranging in coverage from how the ozone layer works and why depletion is an issue to why the rain forests are an important ecosystem. www.enviroliteracy.org

Further Reading

Easton, T. *Taking Sides: Clashing Views on Environmental Issues,* 12th ed. New York: McGraw-Hill, 2007.

> Overview of key environmental issues laid out in debate style. Designed to stimulate thoughtful discussion about key issues.

Kennedy, R. F. *Crimes Against Nature: How George W. Bush and His Corporate Pals Are Plundering the Country and Hijacking Our Democracy.* New York: HarperCollins, 2004.

Michaels, P. *Meltdown: The Predictable Distortion of Global Warming by Scientists, Politicians, and the Media.* Washington, DC: Cato Institute, 2004.

> *These two books offer sharply contrasting perspectives on the environment and public policy and will provoke debate and discussion. The factual basis of the assertions made in both books should be compared to commentary and statistics available from objective sources in the scientific community.*

Speth, J. G. *Red Sky at Morning: America and the Crisis of the Global Environment.* New Haven, CT: Yale University Press, 2004.

> Overview of major environmental threats to health and projections for the future.

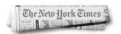

e-themes from *The New York Times*

For up-to-date articles about current health issues, visit www.aw-bc.com/donatelle, select *Access to Health,* Tenth Edition, Chapter 21, and click on "e-themes."

References

1. K. Hilgencamp, *Environmental Health: Ecological Perspectives* (Boston: Jones and Bartlett, 2006).
2. Ibid.
3. A. Yassi et al., *Basic Environmental Health* (New York: Oxford University Press, 2001), 14.
4. R. Caplan, *Our Earth, Ourselves* (New York: Bantam, 1990), 247.
5. World Resources Institute, "July 2006 Monthly Update: World Population Growth—Past, Present and Future," 2006, http://earthtrends.wri.org/updates/node/61.
6. Hilgencamp, *Environmental Health: Ecological Perspectives.*
7. U.S. Census Bureau, "U.S. and World Population Clocks," 2005, www.census.gov/main/www.popclock.html.
8. World Resources Institute, "July 2006 Monthly Update: World Population Growth."
9. G. Moore, *Living with the Earth: Concepts in Environmental Science,* 2nd ed. (Boca Raton, FL: CRC Press, 2002), 62.
10. A. Nadakavukaren, *Our Global Environment: A Health Perspective,* 6th ed. (Long Grove, IL: Waveland Press, 2005).
11. Ibid.
12. Population Reference Bureau, "2005 World Population Data Sheet," www.prb.org.
13. L. Levi et al., "Effects of New Smoking Regulations," *Annals of Oncology* 17 (2006): 1335–1339; R. Borland et al., "Support for and Reported Compliance with Smoke-Free Restaurants and Bars," *Tobacco Control* 10, Suppl (2006): iii34–iii41; M. Org et al., "Cardiovascular Health and Economic Effects of Smoke-Free Workplaces," *American Journal of Medicine* 117, no. 1 (2004): 32–38.
14. Childstats.gov, "America's Children in Brief: Key National Indicators of Well-Being—Lead in the Blood of Children," 2005, www.childstats.gov/americaschildren/2005spec2.asp.
15. Environment Agency, "Acid Rain," 2004, www.environmentagency.gov.uk/yourenv/eff/pollution/acid_rain.
16. S. Hayward, "Index of Environmental Indicators—2006," 2006, www.pacificresearch.org/Pub/Sab/Enviro/06_Enviroindex/06enviroindex.
17. U.S. Environmental Protection Agency, "Effects of Acid Rain," 2005, www.epa.gov/acidrain.
18. Ibid.
19. Ibid.
20. National Cancer Institute, "Radon and Cancer: Questions and Answers," 2004, http://cis.nci.nih.gov/fact3_52.htm.
21. U.S. Environmental Protection Agency, "The Inside Story: A Guide to Indoor Air Quality," 2002, www.epa.gov/iaq/pubs/insidest.html.
22. Ibid.
23. N. Carpenter, "'Sick' Buildings Can Be Root of Work-Related Maladies," *Boston Business Journal* 20 (2000): 36–37.
24. U.S. Environmental Protection Agency, *Questions and Answers on Ozone Depletion* (Washington, DC: Stratospheric Protection Division, 1998).
25. U.S. Environmental Protection Agency, "Global Warming—Climate," 2002, http://yosemite.epa.gov/oar/globalwarming.nsf/content/climate.html.
26. Ibid.
27. J. Abramovitz, *Taking a Stand: Cultivating a New Relationship with the World's Forests* (Washington, DC: Worldwatch Institute, 1998).
28. World Health Organization, "World in Danger of Missing Sanitation Target; Drinking Waters Target also at Risk," 2006, www.who.int/mediacenter/news/releases/2006/pr47/en/index.html.
29. U.S. Geological Survey, "New Reports on Our Nation's Water Quality," 2004, http://water.usgs.gov/pubs/fs/2004/3045.
30. World Health Organization, "World in Danger of Missing Sanitation Target."
31. U.S. Geological Survey, "National Reconnaissance of Pharmaceuticals in U.S. Streams," 2006, www.toxics.usgs.gov/highlights/impact.html.
32. U.S. Environmental Protection Agency, "National Management Measure to Control Non-Point Source Pollution from Urban Areas" (Publication No. EPA 841-B-05-004) (Washington, DC: Environmental Protection Agency, 2005).
33. Ibid.
34. Moore, *Living with the Earth.*
35. Ibid.
36. D. Barr et al., "Concentrations of Dialkyl Phosphate Metabolites of Organophosphorous Pesticides in the U.S. Population," *Population and Environmental Health Perspectives* 112, no. 2 (2004): 186–200.
37. National Institute for Occupational Safety and Health, "Work-Related Hearing Loss," 2006, www.cdc.gov/niosh/topics/noise/abouthlp/workerhl.html.
38. U.S. Environmental Protection Agency, "Superfund National Accomplishments Summary, Fiscal Year 2004," 2004, www.epa.gov/superfund/action/process/numbers04.htm.
39. Ibid.
40. Ibid.

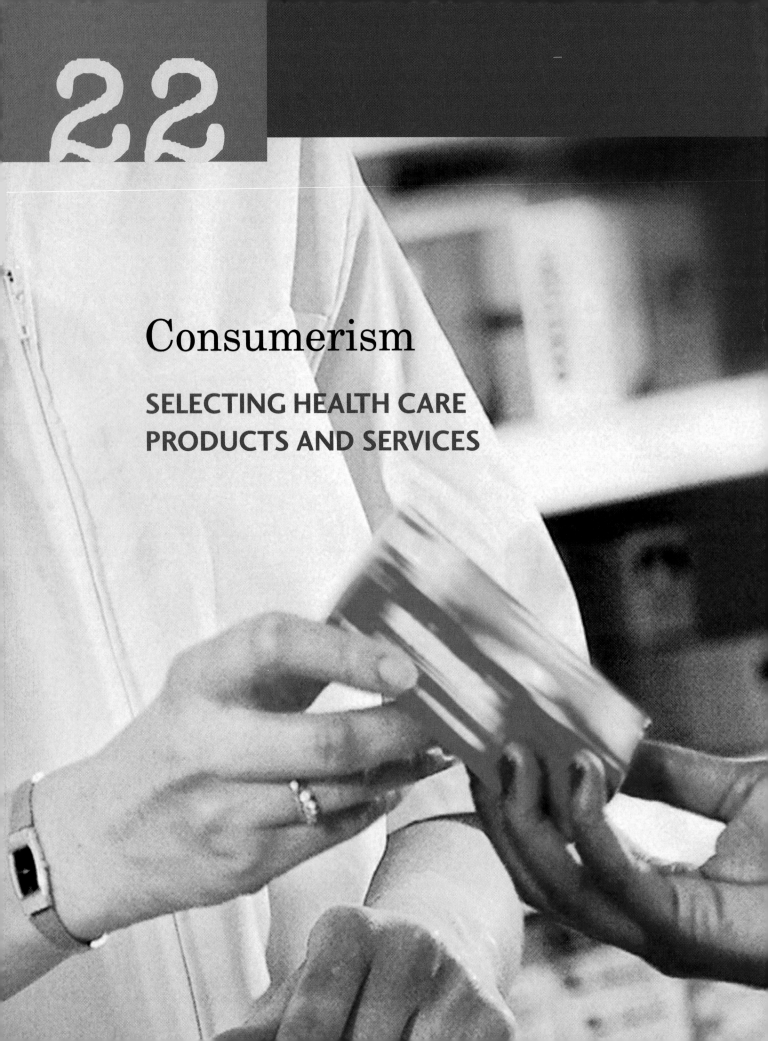

22

Consumerism

SELECTING HEALTH CARE PRODUCTS AND SERVICES

How do I know if I'm **sick** enough to see a health care provider?

Are **generic** medications the same as brand-name drugs?

Can I count on my **university** health care plan to cover my medical needs?

What types of things should I **think** about when choosing health insurance?

If I get sick, how can I ensure I receive the best **care** for my condition?

OBJECTIVES

- Explain the importance of responsible consumerism and how to encourage consumers to take action.
- Discuss why self-diagnosis, self-help, and self-care are becoming increasingly important in our quest for health and well-being.
- Explain the choices available to Americans who seek health care through allopathic avenues, as well as factors that should be considered in making decisions about health care.
- Describe the U.S. health care system in terms of types of medical practice, types of insurance, and the changing structure of the system and issues with cost, quality, and access to services.
- Understand the role health insurers play in providing health care.

There are many reasons to be an informed health care consumer. Most important, you have only one body—if you don't treat it with care, you will pay a major price in terms of financial costs and health consequences. Doing everything you can to prevent illness, stay healthy, and recover rapidly when you do get sick will enhance every other part of your life.

Here is yet another reason to be an active health consumer: as a citizen or resident of the United States, you have no constitutional right to health care. Our society generally treats health care as a private-consumption good or service to be bought and sold rather than as a social good to which everyone is entitled.

Therefore, to obtain high-quality health care at an affordable cost, you need to be both informed and assertive. However, as you may already know, medical and health care services are much harder to evaluate for need, availability, cost, and quality than are, say, clothes or vegetables. In addition, you may seek health care services in circumstances of physical or emotional distress when your decision-making powers are compromised and you find yourself very vulnerable.

This chapter will help you make better decisions about your health and health care. Our health care system is a maze of health care providers, payers (insurance, government, and individuals), and products, and many of us find it hard to thread our way through it. Health care is the fifth largest industry in our country, accounting for over 10 percent of our workforce, and many different companies aggressively market health products and services to the public. Increasingly, health care organizations are "for-profit" businesses, sold and traded on the stock market, and making a profit is the goal. Both medical professionals and consumers report that they feel overwhelmed, confused, and frustrated by the multitude of choices, seemingly divergent interests, and lack of coordination in our system.

Responsible Consumerism: Choices and Challenges

Perhaps the single greatest difficulty that we face as health consumers is the sheer magnitude of choices. If you try to select a general practitioner from the telephone book, you have to thumb through dozens of pages of specialists. When you want to purchase cough syrup, you are confronted with hundreds of options, each claiming to do more for you than the brand next to it. Even trained pharmacists find it impossible to keep up with the explosion of new drugs and health-related products.

Because there are so many profit-seekers competing for a share of the lucrative health market and because misinforma-

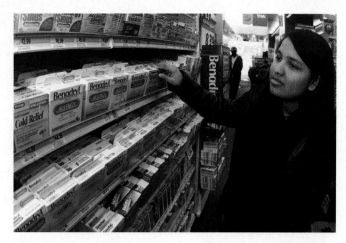

With so many options for everything—from choosing cold medicine to choosing a physician—what's a consumer to do?

tion is so common, wise health consumers use every means at their disposal to ensure that they are acting responsibly and economically. Answer the questions in the Assess Yourself box on page 646 to see how you might become a better health care consumer.

Attracting Consumers' Dollars

Today's marketing specialists identify a target audience for a given product and go after it with an arsenal of gimmicks, subtle persuaders, and sophisticated strategies. Different techniques are used to attract new customers, maintain existing customers, and encourage former consumers of the product to come back. Advertisements may present a product as a status symbol or play on inner fears and insecurities, causing you to wonder whether your deodorant is working, your breath is bad, or your skin is greasy.

Whatever your desires or fears, countless products and services are available to meet them. Although some marketing tactics are obvious, others are subtle and difficult to discern. Perfume advertisements that depict passionate embraces and automobile ads that feature expensive sports cars with beautiful young men and women are common. The implied message is that if you purchase a given perfume, your love life will improve, and if you buy that flashy car, attractive people will flock to you.

Many other marketing strategies revolve around "trendy" news items. A good example is the current fascination with the use of herbs to treat the common cold and wearable magnets to treat arthritis and painful joints. Increasingly, these advertising techniques are used for medical products as aggressively as they are for other items.

Putting *Cure* into Perspective

People often fall victim to false health claims because they mistakenly believe that a product or provider has helped them. Frequently this belief arises from two conditions: spontaneous remission and the placebo effect.

Spontaneous Remission It is said that if you treat a cold, it will disappear in a week, but if you leave it alone, it will last seven days. A **spontaneous remission** from an ailment refers to the disappearance of symptoms without any apparent cause or treatment. Many illnesses, like the common cold and even back strain, are self-limiting and will improve in time, with or without treatment. Other illnesses, such as multiple sclerosis and some cancers, are characterized by alternating periods of severe symptoms and sudden remissions. People experiencing spontaneous remissions can easily attribute their "cure" to a treatment that in fact had no real effect.

Placebo Effect The **placebo effect** is an apparent cure or improved state of health brought about by a substance, product, or procedure that has no generally recognized therapeutic value. It is not uncommon for patients to report improvements based on what they expect, desire, or were told would happen after taking simple sugar pills that they believed were powerful drugs. About 10 percent of the population is thought to be exceptionally susceptible to the power of suggestion and may be easy targets for aggressive marketing of products that are really placebos. Although the placebo effect is generally harmless, it does account for the expenditure of millions of dollars on health products and services every year. Megadoses of vitamin C have never been proven to treat cancer, nor do mud baths smooth wrinkled skin. People who use placebos when medical treatment is needed increase their risk for health problems. However, those who use low-cost, no-risk placebos and find relief, even for just a short time, should not be criticized.

Taking Responsibility for Your Health Care

As the health care industry has become more sophisticated about seeking your business, so must you become more sophisticated about purchasing its products and services. Learn how, when, and where to enter the massive technological maze that is our health care system without incurring unnecessary risk and expense. Acting responsibly in times of illness can be difficult, but the person best able to act on your behalf is you.

If you are not feeling well, you must first decide whether you really need to seek medical advice. Only a decade ago, as many as 70 percent of all trips to the doctor and nearly half of all hospital stays were believed to be unnecessary and potentially harmful.[1] These figures have been reduced considerably, however, with the advent of managed care, which carries with it a degree of out-of-pocket shared costs. Theoretically, patients who have to pay for a portion of their care will not seek care unnecessarily. As we will discuss later in this chapter, managed care involves a number of measures designed to keep people out of hospitals and emergency rooms, which are typically the most expensive form of non-emergency health care.[2]

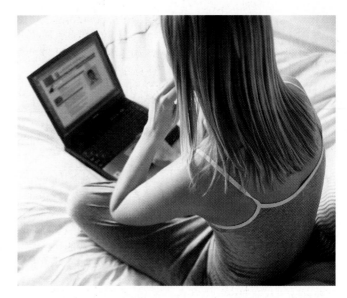

Deciding when to contact a physician can be difficult. Most people first try to diagnose and treat their condition themselves.

Yet critics of managed care point to cost savings as a part of the problem with quality and access. Not seeking treatment, whether due to high costs or limited coverage, or trying to medicate yourself when more rigorous methods of treatment are needed, is dangerous. Being knowledgeable about the benefits and limits of self-care is critical for responsible consumerism.

Self-Help or Self-Care

A recent concept in health consumerism proposes that the patient is the primary health care provider or first line of defense in health. We can practice behaviors that promote health, prevent disease, and minimize reliance on the formal medical system. We can also interpret basic changes in our own physical and emotional health and treat minor afflictions without seeking professional help. Self-care consists of knowing your body, paying attention to its signals, and taking appropriate action to improve your health and stop the progression of illness or injury.

Common forms of self-care include the following:

- Diagnosing symptoms or conditions that occur frequently but may not need physician visits (for example, colds, minor abrasions)
- Performing breast and testicular self-examinations (monthly)

spontaneous remission The disappearance of symptoms without any apparent cause or treatment.

placebo effect An apparent cure or improved state of health brought about by a substance or product that has no medicinal value.

ASSESS yourself

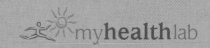

BEING A BETTER HEALTH CARE CONSUMER

Fill out this assessment online at www.aw-bc.com/MyHealthLab or www.aw-bc.com/donatelle.

Answer the following questions, and determine what you might do to become a better health care consumer.

1. Do you have a physician?
2. Do you have health insurance?
3. Have you determined which health care services are available free or at a reduced cost in your area? If so, what are they?
4. When you receive a prescription, do you ask the pharmacist if a generic brand could be substituted?
5. Do you ask the pharmacist for potential side effects before or after the prescription is filled, including possible food and drug interactions?
6. Do you take medication as directed?
7. Do you report any unusual side effects to your doctor?
8. When you receive a diagnosis, do you seek more information about the diagnosis and treatment?
9. If surgery or an invasive type of treatment is indicated by your doctor, do you seek a second opinion?
10. Where do you find most health information?
11. How do you know this source of information is a reliable and credible source?
12. When you purchase an over-the-counter (OTC) medication, do you read the label?
13. What attracts you most to a new product? (check all that apply)

    _____ price

    _____ promises of a new lifestyle

    _____ appears to meet a need

    _____ positive testimonials

    _____ savings or coupons

    _____ spokesperson

    _____ testing for product safety

14. How much of a role do you think advertising plays in your decision to purchase a new product?

- Learning first aid for common, uncomplicated injuries and conditions
- Checking blood pressure, pulse, and temperature
- Using home pregnancy and ovulation kits and HIV test kits
- Monitoring cervical mucus for natural family planning
- Doing periodic checks for blood cholesterol
- Using home stool test kits for blood and early colon cancer detection
- Learning from reliable self-help books, tapes, software, websites, and videos
- Benefiting from relaxation techniques, including meditation, nutrition, rest, and exercise

When to Seek Help

How do I know if I'm sick enough to see a health care provider?

Effective self-care also means understanding when to seek professional medical attention rather than treating a condition yourself. Deciding which conditions warrant professional advice is not always easy. Generally, you should consult a physician if you experience *any* of the following:

- A serious accident or injury
- Sudden or severe chest pains causing breathing difficulties

MAKE it happen!

ASSESSMENT: The Assess Yourself activity asks you to look at your behavior as a health care consumer. Once you have considered your responses, you may want to change or improve certain behaviors in order to get the best treatment from your health care provider and the heath care system.

MAKING A CHANGE: In order to change your behavior, you need to develop a plan. Follow the steps below and complete your Behavior Change Contract to take action.

1. Evaluate your behavior and identify patterns and specific things you are doing. What can you change now? What can you change in the near future?

2. Select one pattern of behavior that you want to change.

3. Fill out the Behavior Change Contract found at the front of your book. It should include your long-term goal for change, your short-term goals, the rewards you'll give yourself for reaching these goals, potential obstacles along the way, and strategies for overcoming these obstacles. For each goal, list the small steps and specific actions that you will take.

4. Chart your progress in a journal. At the end of a week, consider how successful you were in following your plan. What helped you be successful? What made change more difficult? What will you do differently next week?

5. Revise your plan as needed: Are the short-term goals attainable? Are the rewards satisfying?

ONE STUDENT'S PLAN: When Theo reviewed his answers in the self-assessment, it was clear to him that he needed to pay more attention to the medication he took for his asthma. Although he was supposed to take the same dose every day, when he was feeling healthy he would take only half of the prescribed dosage in order to save money. Theo also wasn't sure what side effects were considered normal with his medication and had not mentioned any of them to his doctor, Dr. Higuchi. He also had recently started taking an herbal supplement that his roommate had recommended to help his weightlifting, but he hadn't mentioned the supplement to his doctor either.

Theo's first step was to make an appointment with Dr. Higuchi to discuss some of his questions and concerns about his medication. He made a list ahead of time of what he wanted to talk about to be sure he didn't forget any of his questions. He also started keeping track of the side effects he was experiencing, so he could give the doctor a clear picture of his health. Finally, he made a note of the name and ingredients of the supplement and decided not to take it until he could ask about any potential interaction it might have with his asthma medication.

Theo's meeting with Dr. Higuchi went well. When Theo explained that he was trying to save money by using less of the medication than prescribed, Dr. Higuchi found a generic equivalent that cost much less. He reminded Theo about the importance of taking the correct dose and explained that some of the side effects that he reported were caused by the variation in the amount of medication he was taking. He also told Theo that the herbal supplement would make the asthma medication much less effective, an interaction not disclosed on the supplement's label. Theo agreed that now he could afford to take the medication exactly as prescribed and scheduled a follow-up appointment in six months to report on any further concerns he might have.

- Trauma to the head or spine accompanied by persistent headache, blurred vision, loss of consciousness, vomiting, convulsions, or paralysis
- Sudden high fever or recurring high temperature (over 102°F for children and 103°F for adults) and/or sweats
- Tingling sensation in the arm accompanied by slurred speech or impaired thought processes
- Adverse reactions to a drug or insect bite (shortness of breath, severe swelling, dizziness)
- Unexplained bleeding or loss of body fluid from any body opening
- Unexplained sudden weight loss
- Persistent or recurrent diarrhea or vomiting

- Blue-colored lips, eyelids, or nail beds
- Any lump, swelling, thickness, or sore that does not subside or that grows for over a month
- Any marked change or pain in bowel or bladder habits
- Yellowing of the skin or the whites of the eyes
- Any symptom that is unusual and recurs over time
- Pregnancy

With the vast array of home diagnostic devices currently available, it seems relatively easy for most people to take care of themselves. But some caution is in order here: although many of these devices are valuable for making an initial diagnosis, home health tests are no substitute for regular, complete examinations by a trained practitioner.

SKILLS FOR behavior change

BEING PROACTIVE IN YOUR OWN HEALTH CARE

Throughout this book, we have emphasized the importance of healthy preventive behaviors. Sometimes, however, you will still become ill. At such times, it is important that you continue to be actively involved in your care. The more you know about your own body and the factors that can affect your health, the better you will be at communicating with health care providers. It also helps you make informed decisions and recognize when a certain treatment may not be right for you. The following points can help:

> **If I get sick, how can I ensure I receive the best care for my condition?**

- Know your own and your family's medical history.
- Be knowledgeable about your condition—causes, physiological effects, possible treatments, prognosis. Don't rely on the doctor for this information. Do some research.
- Bring a friend or relative along for medical visits to help you review what the doctor says. If you go alone, take notes.
- Ask the practitioner to explain the problem and possible treatments, tests, and drugs in a clear and understandable way. If you don't understand something, ask for clarification.
- If the doctor prescribes any medications, ask whether you can take generic equivalents that cost less.

- Ask for a written summary of the results of your visit and any lab tests.
- If you have any doubt about the doctor's recommended treatment, seek a second opinion.
- If you need to take a prescription medication for an extended time, ask for the maximum number of doses allowed by your plan if you have a small pharmacy copayment.

After seeing a health care professional, consider these ideas:

- Write down an accurate account of what happened and what was said. Be sure to include the names of the doctor and all other people involved in your care, the date, and the place.
- Shop around drugstores for the best prices in the same way that you would when shopping for clothes.
- When filling prescriptions, ask to see the pharmacist's package inserts that list medical considerations concerning the medicines. Request detailed information about potential drug and food interactions.
- Write clear instructions on the label to avoid risk to others who may take the drug in error.

In addition to following the practical steps listed above, being proactively involved in your health care also means that you should be aware of your rights as a patient. Your rights include the following:

1. The right of informed consent means that before receiving any care, you should be fully informed of what is being planned, the risks and potential benefits, and possible alternative forms of treatment, including the option of no treatment. Your consent must be voluntary and without any form of coercion. It is critical that you read any consent forms carefully and amend them as necessary before signing.
2. You are entitled to know whether the treatment you are receiving is standard or experimental. In experimental conditions, you have the legal and ethical right to know if the study is one in which some people receive treatment while others do not in order to compare the results, and if any drug is being used in the research project for a purpose not approved by the Food and Drug Administration (FDA).
3. You have the right to privacy, which includes the source of payment for treatment and care. It also includes protecting your right to make personal decisions concerning all reproductive matters.
4. You have the right to receive care. You also have the legal right to refuse treatment at any time and to cease treatment at any time.
5. You are entitled to access all your medical records and to have those records remain confidential.
6. You have the right to seek the opinions of other health care professionals regarding your condition.

The Skills for Behavior Change box offers valuable information about taking an active role in your own health care.

Assessing Health Professionals

Suppose you decide that you do need medical help. You must then identify what type of help you need and where to obtain it. Selecting a professional may seem simple, yet many people have no idea how to assess the qualifications of a health care provider.

Knowledge of both traditional medical specialties and alternative, or complementary, medical treatment is critical to making an intelligent selection. In addition, numerous studies document the importance of good communication skills: the most satisfied patients are those who feel that their physician explains diagnosis and treatment options thoroughly and involves them in decisions regarding their own care.[3]

When selecting from a network of providers, make sure you understand your coverage options and consider the following questions about prospective health care providers:

- What professional educational training have they had? What license or board certification do they hold? Note that there is a difference between "board eligible" and "board certified." *Board certified* indicates that they have passed the national board examination for their specialty (such as pediatrics) and have been certified as competent in that specialty. In contrast, *board eligible* merely means that they are eligible to take the specialty board's exam but have not necessarily passed it.

- Are they affiliated with an accredited medical facility or institution? The Joint Commission on Accreditation of Healthcare Organizations (JCAHO) requires these institutions to verify all education, licensing, and training claims of their affiliated practitioners. What other doctors are in their group, and who will assist in your treatment?

- Are they open to complementary or alternative strategies? Would they refer you for different treatment modalities if appropriate?

- Do they indicate clearly how long a given treatment may last, what side effects you might expect, and what problems you should watch for?

- Are their diagnoses, treatments, and general statements consistent with established scientific theory and practice?

- Who will be responsible for your care when the doctor is on vacation or off call?

- Do they listen to you, respect you as an individual, and give you time to ask questions? Do they return your calls, and are they available to answer questions?

When a doctor orders a test, treatment, or medication, you might ask questions like these:

- How often has the doctor performed this test, surgery, or procedure and with what proportion of successful outcome?

- What are the side effects, and can these side effects be treated or reduced?

- Does this procedure require an overnight stay at a hospital, or can it be performed in a doctor's office?

- Why has this test been ordered? What is the doctor trying to find or exclude?

Asking the right questions at the right time may save you personal suffering and expense. Many patients find that writing their questions down before an appointment helps them get answers to all their questions. You should not accept a defensive or hostile response; asking questions is your right as a patient.

A recent survey found that nearly two-thirds of Americans are confident that the medical information given to them by their doctor is accurate, while the remaining third opt for a second opinion on important issues or do independent research.[4]

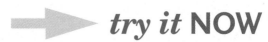

try it NOW

Make an appointment with your health care provider. When was the last time you had a regular checkup? Usually when we are healthy, we rarely have a regular physical. Prevention is key to good health, however. Make an appointment today with your health care provider for a preventive-care exam.

Choices in Health Products: Prescription and Over-the-Counter Drugs

Recall from Chapter 14 that prescription drugs can be obtained only with a written prescription from a physician, while over-the-counter drugs can be purchased without a prescription. Just as making wise decisions about providers is an important aspect of responsible health care, so is making wise decisions about medications. Consider the benefits, risks, and possible interactions related to a given drug.

Prescription Drugs

In about two-thirds of doctor visits, the physician administers or prescribes at least one medication. In fact, prescription drug use has risen by 25 percent over the past decade.[5] Even though these drugs are administered under medical supervision, the wise consumer still takes precautions. Hazards and complications arising from the use of prescription drugs are common. Responsible decision making requires the consumer to acquire basic drug knowledge.

Types of Prescription Drugs
Prescription drugs can be divided into dozens of categories. We discuss some of the most common here. Others are explored in the chapters on birth control, infectious and sexually transmitted diseases, cancer, and cardiovascular disease.

Antibiotics are drugs used to fight bacterial infection. Bacterial infections continue to be the most common serious diseases in the United States and throughout the world. The vast majority of these can be cured with antibiotic treatment. There are currently close to 100 different antibiotic drugs used to kill or stop bacterial growth. Some, called broad-spectrum antibiotics, are designed to control disease caused

antibiotics   Prescription drugs designed to fight bacterial infection.

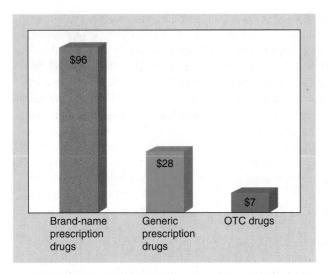

FIGURE 22.1 The Average Price of Drugs
The cost of brand-name drugs is high now and may continue to rise. Ask your doctor about generic and OTC options.

by a number of bacterial species. Other hazards of antibiotic overuse are discussed in Chapter 17.

Central nervous system depressants are sedative or hypnotic medications commonly used to treat anxiety. The two main types of drugs in this group are benzodiazepines, which include drugs such as Valium, Ativan, and Xanax, and barbiturates (examples include Amytal and Seconal). The benzodiazepines are the most widely used drug in this category, most commonly prescribed for tension, muscular strain, sleep problems, and anxiety panic attacks, and in treatment of alcohol withdrawal. They differ widely in their mechanism of action, absorption rate, and metabolism, but all produce similar intoxication and withdrawal symptoms. Benzodiazepine sleeping pills have largely replaced barbiturates, which were used medically in the past for relieving tension and inducing relaxation and sleep.

All sedative or hypnotic drugs can produce physical and psychological dependence in several weeks. A complication specific to sedatives is cross-tolerance, which occurs when users develop tolerance for one sedative or become depen-

central nervous system depressants   Sedative or hypnotic medications commonly used to treat anxiety.

antidepressants   Prescription drugs used to treat clinically diagnosed depression.

amphetamines   Prescription stimulants not commonly used today because of the dangers associated with them.

rebound effects   Severe withdrawal effects experienced by users of stimulants, including depression, nausea, and violent behavior.

generic drugs   Drugs marketed by chemical name rather than brand name.

dent on it and develop tolerance for others as well. Withdrawal from sedative or hypnotic drugs may range from mild discomfort to severe symptoms, depending on the degree of dependence. A major public health issue is whether or not persons using benzodiazepines have an increased risk of cognitive decline and dementia. Ongoing research is investigating this possible link.[6]

Antidepressants are medications typically used to treat major depression, although occasionally they are used to treat other forms of depression that may be resistant to conventional therapy. There are several groups of antidepressant medications approved for use in the United States. Prozac, Zoloft, and Paxil are well-known examples. Antidepressants are among the three most commonly prescribed classes of drugs. Over the past decade, the use of antidepressant drugs in the United States has increased by 48 percent overall and by 124 percent in children.[7] For more on antidepressants, see Chapter 2.

Amphetamines are stimulants that are prescribed less commonly now than in the past. Like many psychoactive drugs, they are purchased both legally and illegally. Amphetamines suppress appetite and elevate respiration, blood pressure, and pulse rate. Ritalin and Cylert are prescription amphetamines that are used to treat attention deficit hyperactivity disorder in children, and Pondimin is used to treat obesity.

Tolerance to these powerful stimulants develops rapidly, and the user trying to cut down or quit may experience unpleasant **rebound effects.** These severe withdrawal symptoms, peculiar to stimulants, include depression, irritability, violent behavior, headaches, nausea, and deep fatigue.

Are generic medications the same as brand-name drugs?

Generic Drugs Generic drugs,
medications sold under a chemical name rather than a brand name, have gained popularity in recent years. They contain the same active ingredients as brand-name drugs, but their price is often less than half that of the brand-name medications (Figure 22.1). If your doctor prescribes a drug, always ask if a generic equivalent exists and if it would be safe and effective for you to try.

Be aware, though, that there is some controversy about the effectiveness of generic drugs because substitutions are often made in minor ingredients that can affect the way the drug is absorbed, causing discomfort or even an allergic reaction in some users. Always note any reactions you have to medications and tell your doctor. Also, not all drugs are available as generics.

Over-the-Counter Drugs

Over-the-counter (OTC) drugs are nonprescription substances we use in the course of self-diagnosis and self-medication. More than one-third of the time people treat their own health problems with OTC medications. Self-care for many of us results from eagerness to save money and time on an office visit to the physician. We therefore diagnose our own illnesses and go to the nearest discount pharmacy to stock up on the latest and best-advertised cure for what we think ails us.

In fact, American consumers spend billions of dollars yearly on OTC preparations for relief of everything from runny noses to ingrown toenails. There are 40,000 OTC drugs and more than 300,000 brand names for those drugs. Most of these products are manufactured from a basic group of 1,000 chemicals. The many different OTC drugs available to us are produced by combining as few as two and as many as ten substances.

How Prescription Drugs Become OTC Drugs

The U.S. Food and Drug Administration (FDA) regularly reviews prescription drugs to evaluate how suitable they would be as OTC products. (See the Health Ethics box on page 652.) Typically, these are drugs for conditions that consumers can diagnose readily and manage themselves and for which clear, understandable directions can be included. For a drug to be switched from prescription to OTC status, it must meet the following criteria:

1. The drug has been marketed as a prescription medication for at least three years.

2. The use of the drug has been relatively high during the time it was available as a prescription drug.

3. Adverse drug reactions are not alarming, potential adverse effects are printed on the drug label, and the frequency of side effects has not increased during the time it was available to the public.

Since this policy has been in effect, the FDA has switched hundreds of drugs from prescription to OTC status. Some examples are the analgesic/anti-inflammatory medicines ibuprofen (Advil, Nuprin) and naproxen sodium (Aleve), the antihistamine Benadryl, the vaginal antifungal Gyne-Lotrimin, the bronchodilator Bronkaid Mist, the hydrocortisone Cortaid, and the allergy reliever Claritin. Many more prescription drugs are currently being considered for OTC status.

Types of OTC Drugs The FDA has categorized 26 types of OTC preparations. Those most commonly used are analgesics, cold/cough/allergy and asthma relievers, stimulants, sleeping aids and relaxants, and dieting aids.

Analgesics We spend more than $2 billion annually on **analgesics** (pain relievers), the largest sales category of OTC drugs in the United States. Although these pain relievers come in several forms, aspirin, acetaminophen (Tylenol, Pamprin, Panadol), and ibuprofen-like drugs such as naproxen (Aleve) and ketoprofen (Orudis) are the most common.

Most pain relievers work at receptor sites by interrupting pain signals. Some are categorized as NSAIDs (nonsteroidal anti-inflammatory drugs), which are also called **prosta-** **glandin inhibitors.** Prostaglandins are chemicals that resemble hormones and are released by the body in response to pain. (Scientists believe that the additional pain caused by the release of prostaglandins signals the body to begin the healing process.) Prostaglandin inhibitors restrain the release of prostaglandins, thereby reducing the pain. Common NSAIDs include ibuprofen (including Motrin), naproxen sodium (such as Anaprox), and aspirin.

In addition to relieving pain, NSAIDs reduce fevers by increasing the flow of blood to the skin surface, which causes sweating, thereby cooling the body. Aspirin in particular has long been used to reduce the inflammation and swelling associated with arthritis. Recently it has been discovered that aspirin's anticoagulant (interference with blood clotting) effects make it useful for reducing the risk of heart attack and stroke.

Possible side effects for many NSAIDS include allergic reactions, ringing in the ears, stomach bleeding, and ulcers. Combining NSAIDs with alcohol can compound the gastric irritant properties in the medications. As with all drugs, read the labels. Some analgesic labels caution against driving or operating heavy machinery when using the drug, and most warn that analgesics should not be taken with alcohol.

In addition, research has linked aspirin to a potentially fatal condition called Reye's syndrome. Children, teenagers, and young adults (up to age 19) who are treated with aspirin while recovering from the flu or chicken pox are at risk for developing the syndrome. Aspirin substitutes are recommended for people in these age groups.

Acetaminophen is an aspirin substitute found in Tylenol and related medications. Like aspirin, acetaminophen is an effective analgesic and antipyretic (fever-reducing drug). It does not, however, relieve inflamed or swollen joints. The side effects associated with acetaminophen are generally minimal, though overdose can cause liver damage.

Several analgesics are available as prescription or OTC drugs. Generally, the OTC drugs (for example, Nuprin, Advil, and Aleve) are milder versions of the prescription varieties. Aleve's main distinction is its lasting effect: while other analgesics must be taken every 4 to 6 hours, once every 8 to 12 hours is sufficient for Aleve.

Cold, Cough, Allergy, and Asthma Relievers The operative word in this category is *reliever*. Most of these medications are designed to alleviate the uncomfortable symptoms associated with maladies of the upper respiratory tract, but no drugs exist to cure the actual diseases. The drugs available provide only temporary relief until the sufferer's immune system prevails over the disease. Aspirin or acetaminophen is used in some cold preparations, as are several other ingredients. Both aspirin and acetaminophen are on the

---

analgesics Pain relievers.

prostaglandin inhibitors Drugs that inhibit the production and release of prostaglandins associated with arthritis or menstrual pain.

HEALTH ETHICS
conflict and controversy

IMPROVING THE SAFETY OF PRESCRIPTION DRUGS

In 1993, the Food and Drug Administration (FDA) changed its policies to speed the approval process of new drugs. These changes were made for humanitarian reasons, in response to activists seeking rapid approval of experimental drugs that offered at least a ray of hope to AIDS patients who otherwise faced certain death. The "accelerated development/review" process was seen as a way to offer drugs that might be a significant improvement over existing treatments, or that could benefit those with life-threatening illnesses for which no treatment currently exists.

Hundreds of new drugs have been approved for OTC status since then. Of that number, a handful have been withdrawn after reports of deaths and severe side effects, risks that do not outweigh the overall benefit the drug may offer. Examples of drugs that have been placed on the pharmacy shelves as a result of the FDA's more lenient approach, but have yielded detrimental or fatal results, include the COX-2 inhibitor (prescription analgesic) Bextra and the irritable bowel syndrome medication Lotronex. Bextra is a widely used drug for treating arthritis pain. In 2004, results of a large-scale study unveiled a series of cardiovascular risks associated with the medication, including heart attack and stroke, and an increased risk for a serious and potentially fatal skin reaction. In April 2005, the FDA requested that the manufacturer of Bextra (Pfizer) remove this drug from

the market. Lotronex, a drug for treating irritable bowel syndrome in women, was approved despite warnings. It has now been linked to five deaths, the removal of one patient's colon, and other bowel surgeries. Lotronex was pulled from the market voluntarily by the manufacturer after only 10 months.

In response to these events and others, the Food and Drug Administration has launched a new drug safety initiative. As part of this initiative, the Drug Safety Oversight Board will be established in order to oversee drug safety issues, consult with medical experts and consumer groups, and provide new information on medication risks and benefits to consumers and health care providers. Also at the core of current changes to the FDA, long considered by public health officials the most reliable entity for providing early warning that a product may be dangerous, will be new and improved communication channels to the general public on drug safety information.

New communication channels include:

- *The Drug Watch Web Page.* This page will include emerging information, for both previously and newly approved drugs, about possible serious side effects or other safety risks, and how risks can be avoided. The agency will enhance access to this information and call for assistance in prioritizing and further evaluating potential adverse health concerns.

- *Healthcare Professional Information Sheets.* These are one-page information sheets for health care professionals for all drugs on the FDA's Drug Watch and all drugs with Medication Guides (FDA-approved patient labeling). They contain the most important new information for safe use, including known and potential safety issues based on reports of adverse events, new information that may affect prescribing of the drug, and the approved indications and benefits of the drug.

- *Patient Information Sheets.* These are one-page information sheets for patients in a consumer-friendly format for all products on Drug Watch. Information will include new safety information as well as basic information about how to use the drug.

What standards should the FDA use to determine whether or not a drug is safe? How might consumers benefit from a rapid drug approval process? How much time do you believe is a safe amount of time for a drug trial?

Sources: U.S. Food and Drug Administration, "The FDA Speeds Medical Treatment for Serious Diseases," March/April 2006, www.fda.gov/cder; U.S. Food and Drug Administration, "Accelerated Development Review," 2006, www.fda.gov/cder/handbook; United States Department of Health and Human Services, news release, "Reforms Will Improve Oversight and Openness at FDA," February 15, 2005, www.fda.gov/cder/drugsafety.htm.

Generally Recognized as Safe (GRAS) A list of drugs generally recognized as safe, which seldom cause side effects when used properly.

Generally Recognized as Effective (GRAE) A list of drugs generally recognized as effective, which work for their intended purpose when used properly.

government's lists of medications that are **Generally Recognized as Safe (GRAS)** and **Generally Recognized as Effective (GRAE).** Table 22.1 describes the basic types of OTC cough, cold, and allergy relievers.

Sleeping Aids and Relaxants A study by the World Health Organization, conducted in 15 health centers around the globe, found that 27 percent of patients reported difficulties with sleeping.[8] Many people routinely treat their insomnia with OTC sleep aids (such as Nytol, Sleep-Eze, and Sominex) that are advertised as providing a "safe and restful" sleep. These drugs are used to induce the drowsy feelings that precede sleep. The principal ingredient in OTC sleeping aids is an antihistamine called pyrilamine maleate. Chronic reliance on sleeping aids may lead to addiction; people used to using these products may eventually find it impossible to sleep without them.

Dieting Aids In the United States, there is a $200 million market for dieting aids. Some of these drugs (such as Acutrim and Dexatrim) are advertised as "appetite suppressants." The FDA has pulled several appetite suppressants off the market because their active ingredient was phenylpropanolamine (PPA), which is a **sympathomimetic** (affecting the sympathetic nervous system). This causes reactions similar to those experienced when angry or excited, such as dry mouth and lack of appetite. PPA has been linked to increased risk of stroke.[9] More recently, the FDA also prohibited the sale of ephedra, a naturally occurring substance often billed as a dietaid, or sports and energy-enhancement drug. Ephedra use has been linked to heart attack, stroke, and death.[10]

Estimates show that, when taken as recommended, even the best OTC dieting aids significantly reduce appetite in less than 30 percent of users, and tolerance occurs in only one to three days of use. Manufacturers of appetite suppressants often include a written 1,200-calorie diet to complement their drug. However, most people who limit themselves to 1,200 calories per day will lose weight—without any help from appetite suppressants. Clearly, these products have no value in treating obesity.

Some people rely on **laxatives** and **diuretics** ("water pills") to lose weight. Frequent use of laxatives disrupts the body's natural elimination patterns and may cause constipation or even *obstipation* (inability to have a bowel movement). The use of laxatives to produce weight loss has generally unspectacular results and robs the body of needed fluids, salts, and minerals. Abuse of laxatives is associated with eating disorders (Chapter 9).

Taking diuretics to lose weight is also dangerous. Not only will the user gain the weight back upon drinking fluids, but diuretic use may contribute to dangerous chemical imbalances. The potassium and sodium eliminated by diuretics play important roles in maintaining electrolyte balance. Depletion of these vital minerals may cause weakness, dizziness, fatigue, and sometimes death. (See Table 22.2 on page 654 for side effects of other OTC drugs.)

Rules for Proper OTC Drug Use
Despite a common belief that OTC products are safe and effective, indiscriminate use and abuse can occur with these drugs as with all others. For example, people who frequently drop medication into their eyes to "get the red out" or pop antacids after every meal are likely to become dependent. Many people also experience adverse side effects because they ignore warning labels or simply do not read them. The FDA has

TABLE 22.1	Types of Over-the-Counter Cold, Cough, and Allergy Relievers

- *Expectorants.* These drugs loosen phlegm, which allows the user to cough it up and clear congested respiratory passages. GRAS and GRAE reviewers question the effectiveness of many expectorants. When combined with other medications, particularly among those used by frail or very ill individuals, safety issues may arise.
- *Antitussives.* These OTC drugs calm or curtail the cough reflex. They are most effective when the cough is dry (does not produce phlegm). Oral codeine, dextromethorphan, and diphenhydramine are the most common antitussives that are on both the GRAE and GRAS lists.
- *Antihistamines.* These central nervous system depressants dry runny noses, clear postnasal drip, clear sinus congestion, and reduce tears.
- *Decongestants.* These remedies reduce nasal stuffiness due to colds.
- *Anticholinergics.* These substances often are added to cold preparations to reduce nasal secretions and tears. None of the preparations tested was found to be GRAE or GRAS. Some cold compounds contain alcohol in concentrations that may exceed 40 percent.

developed a standard label that appears on most OTC products (Figure 22.2 on page 655). It provides directions for use, warnings, and other useful information. (Diet supplements, which are regulated as food products, have their own type of label that includes a Supplement Facts panel.)

OTC medications are far more powerful than ever before, and the science behind them is stronger as well. Most of us are self-medicators at one time or another. We find it easier to function, for example, if the headache and stuffiness of the common cold do not interfere with our studies or work. Most of us can use OTC products safely with adequate precautions, but for some people, OTCs can be as toxic as the most dangerous chemicals. Therefore, before you use any type of medication, do your homework. Observe the following rules when taking nonprescription drugs:

1. Always know what you are taking. Identify the active ingredients in the product.

2. Know the effects. Be sure you know both the desired and potentially undesired effects of each active ingredient.

sympathomimetics Drugs found in appetite suppressants that affect the sympathetic nervous system.

laxatives Medications used to soften stool and relieve constipation.

diuretics Drugs that increase the excretion of urine from the body.

TABLE 22.2 Some Side Effects of OTC Drugs

Drug	Possible Hazards
Acetaminophen	■ Bloody urine, painful urination, skin rash, bleeding and bruising, yellowing of the eyes or skin (even for normal doses)
	■ Difficulty in diagnosing overdose because reaction may be delayed up to a week
	■ Liver damage from chronic low-level use
Antacids	■ Reduced mineral absorption from food
	■ Possible concealment of ulcer
	■ Reduction of effectiveness for anticlotting medications
	■ Prevention of certain antibiotics' functioning (for antacids that contain aluminum)
	■ Worsening of high blood pressure (for antacids that contain sodium)
	■ Aggravation of kidney problems
Aspirin	■ Stomach upset and vomiting, stomach bleeding, worsening of ulcers
	■ Enhancement of the action of anticlotting medications
	■ Potentiation of hearing damage from loud noise
	■ Severe allergic reaction
	■ Association with Reye's syndrome in children and teenagers
	■ Prolonged bleeding time (when combined with alcohol)
Cold medications	■ Loss of consciousness (if taken with prescription tranquilizers)
Diet pills, caffeine, decongestants	■ Organ damage or death from cerebral hemorrhage
Ibuprofen	■ Allergic reaction in some people with aspirin allergy
	■ Fluid retention or edema
	■ Liver damage similar to that from acetaminophen
	■ Enhancement of action of anticlotting medications
	■ Digestive disturbances (half as often as with aspirin)
Laxatives	■ Reduced absorption of minerals from food
	■ Creation of dependency
Naproxen sodium	■ Potential digestive tract bleeding
	■ Possible stomach cramps or ulcers
Toothache medications	■ Destruction of the still-healthy part of a damaged tooth (for medications that contain clove oil)

3. Read the warnings and cautions.

4. Don't use anything for longer than one or two weeks. If your symptoms persist, consult a doctor.

5. Be particularly cautious if you are also taking prescription drugs.

6. If you have questions, ask your pharmacist.

7. *If you don't need it, don't take it!*

Drug Interactions Sharing medications, using outdated prescriptions, taking higher doses than recommended,

polydrug use   Use of multiple medications or illicit drugs simultaneously.

synergism   Interaction of two or more drugs that produces more profound effects than would be expected if the drugs were taken separately.

or using medications as a substitute for dealing with personal problems may result in serious health consequences. But so may **polydrug use:** taking several medications or illegal drugs simultaneously may result in very dangerous problems associated with drug interactions. The most hazardous interactions are synergism, antagonism, inhibition, and intolerance. Hazardous interactions may also occur between drugs and foods and beverages. Talk with your doctor about possible interactions before taking any medicines.

Synergism, also known as *potentiation,* is an interaction of two or more drugs in which the effects of the individual drugs are multiplied beyond what would normally be expected if they were taken alone—rather like saying 1 + 1 = 6. A synergistic interaction is most likely to occur when *central nervous system depressants* are combined. Included in this category are alcohol, opiates (morphine, heroin), antihistamines (cold remedies), sedative hypnotics (Quaalude), minor tranquilizers (Valium, Librium, and Xanax), and barbiturates. The worst possible combination is alcohol and barbiturates

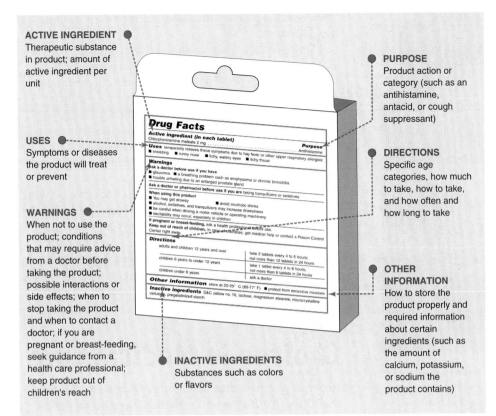

ACTIVE INGREDIENT ●
Therapeutic substance in product; amount of active ingredient per unit

USES ●
Symptoms or diseases the product will treat or prevent

WARNINGS ●
When not to use the product; conditions that may require advice from a doctor before taking the product; possible interactions or side effects; when to stop taking the product and when to contact a doctor; if you are pregnant or breast-feeding, seek guidance from a health care professional; keep product out of children's reach

INACTIVE INGREDIENTS ●
Substances such as colors or flavors

PURPOSE ●
Product action or category (such as an antihistamine, antacid, or cough suppressant)

DIRECTIONS ●
Specific age categories, how much to take, how to take, and how often and how long to take

OTHER INFORMATION ●
How to store the product properly and required information about certain ingredients (such as the amount of calcium, potassium, or sodium the product contains)

Label text:
Drug Facts
Active ingredient (in each tablet)
Chlorpheniramine maleate 2 mg .... Purpose .... Antihistamine
Uses temporarily relieves these symptoms due to hay fever or other upper respiratory allergies:
■ sneezing ■ runny nose ■ itchy, watery eyes ■ itchy throat
Warnings
Ask a doctor before use if you have
■ glaucoma ■ a breathing problem such as emphysema or chronic bronchitis
■ trouble urinating due to an enlarged prostate gland
Ask a doctor or pharmacist before use if you are taking tranquilizers or sedatives
When using this product
■ You may get drowsy ■ avoid alcoholic drinks
■ alcohol, sedatives, and tranquilizers may increase drowsiness
■ be careful when driving a motor vehicle or operating machinery
■ excitability may occur, especially in children
If pregnant or breast-feeding, ask a health professional before use.
Keep out of reach of children. In case of overdose, get medical help or contact a Poison Control Center right away.
Directions
adults and children 12 years and over | take 2 tablets every 4 to 6 hours; not more than 12 tablets in 24 hours
children 6 years to under 12 years | take 1 tablet every 4 to 6 hours; not more than 6 tablets in 24 hours
children under 6 years | ask a doctor
Other information store at 20-25° C (68-77° F) ■ protect from excessive moisture
Inactive ingredients D&C yellow no. 10, lactose, magnesium stearate, microcrystalline cellulose, pregelatinized starch

FIGURE 22.2 The Over-the-Counter Medicine Label

Source: Consumer Healthcare Products Association, "The New Over-the-Counter Medicine Label," 2002. Reprinted by permission.

(sleeping preparations such as Seconal and phenobarbital) because combining these depressants slows down the brain centers that normally control vital functions. Respiration, heart rate, and blood pressure can drop to the point of inducing coma and even death.

Prescription and OTC drugs carry labels warning the user not to combine the drug with certain other drugs or with alcohol. Because the dangers associated with synergism are so great, you should always verify any possible drug interactions before using a prescribed or OTC drug. Pharmacists, physicians, drug information centers, or community drug education centers can answer your questions. Even if one of the drugs in question is an illegal substance, you should still attempt to determine the dangers involved in combining it with other drugs. Health care professionals are legally bound to maintain confidentiality even when they know that a client is using illegal substances.

Antagonism, although not usually as serious as synergism, can produce unwanted and unpleasant effects. In an antagonistic reaction, drugs work at the same receptor site so that one drug blocks the action of the other. The "blocking" drug occupies the receptor site and prevents the other drug from attaching, thus altering its absorption and action.

With **inhibition,** the effects of one drug are eliminated or reduced by the presence of another drug at the receptor site. One common inhibitory reaction occurs between antacid tablets and aspirin. The antacid inhibits the absorption of aspirin, making it less effective as a pain reliever. Other

inhibitory reactions occur between alcohol and contraceptive pills and between antibiotics and contraceptive pills. Both alcohol and antibiotics may make birth control pills less effective.

Intolerance occurs when drugs combine in the body to produce extremely uncomfortable reactions. The drug Antabuse, used to help alcoholics give up alcohol, works by producing this type of interaction. It binds liver enzymes (the chemicals the liver produces to break down alcohol), making it impossible for the body to metabolize alcohol. As a result, an Antabuse user who drinks alcohol experiences nausea, vomiting, and, occasionally, fever.

Cross-tolerance occurs when a person develops a physiological tolerance to one drug and shows a similar tolerance to selected other drugs as a result. Taking one medication may

antagonism A type of interaction in which two or more drugs work at the same receptor site.

inhibition A type of interaction in which the effects of one drug are eliminated or reduced by the presence of another drug at the receptor site.

intolerance A type of interaction in which two or more drugs produce extremely uncomfortable symptoms.

cross-tolerance Development of a tolerance to one drug that reduces the effects of another, similar drug.

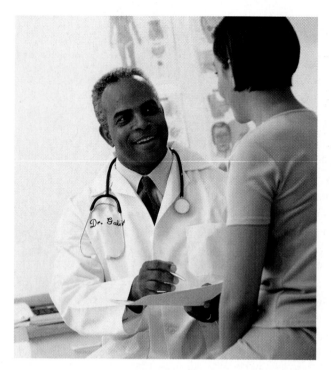

It is important to have an open and honest relationship with your health care provider. Asking questions and providing accurate information will help you make the best decisions about your medical treatment.

actually increase the body's tolerance to another. For example, cross-tolerance can develop between alcohol and barbiturates, two depressant drugs.

 what do you THINK?

What are some situations in which students misuse drugs? ■ Other than alcohol, which drugs (prescription or OTC) do students tend to abuse while they are at college?

Women and Medications

Women menstruate, can become pregnant, and go through menopause. These normal conditions all affect how women's bodies react to medication. On average, women take more prescription and nonprescription medications than do men. For these reasons, women should be especially concerned

---

allopathic medicine Conventional, Western medical practice; in theory, based on scientifically validated methods and procedures.

primary care practitioner A medical practitioner who treats routine ailments, advises on preventive care, gives general medical advice, and makes appropriate referrals when necessary.

---

about which substances they take and about how and when they take them.

Many women use oral contraceptives, commonly known as "the pill." Failure to take the pill each day can result in pregnancy, yet 25 percent of women on the pill miss or skip days. Women may also become pregnant accidentally because some medicines—such as penicillin, some sleeping pills, tuberculosis drugs, and anxiety medicines—can keep oral contraceptives from working. When a woman is prescribed a new medication, she should inform her health care provider if she is on the pill.

A woman should also inform her physician if she is taking any medication while pregnant or breast-feeding. Medications taken during these times may be passed to her fetus or baby, and some can severely affect the developmental process, resulting in physical or mental impairments or even death. The physician may be able to prescribe a different drug or a different way to take the medication that will not affect the fetus or baby.

Choices in Medical Care

How can you choose the best health care provider for your needs? Familiarize yourself with the various health professions and subspecialties (see the list in Table 22.3). These professionals all subscribe to allopathic medical procedures. Most people believe that **allopathic medicine,** or traditional Western medical practice, is based on scientifically validated methods, but be aware that not all allopathic treatments have undergone the extensive clinical trials and long-term studies of outcomes that are necessary to conclusively prove effectiveness in different populations. Even when studies appear to support the health benefits of a particular treatment or product, other studies with equal or better scientific validity often refute these claims. Also, what is recommended treatment today may change dramatically in the future as new technology and medical advances replace older practices. Like other professionals, medical doctors are only as good as their training, continuing knowledge acquisition, and resources allow them to be. A "consumer beware" attitude is always prudent, especially when making critical health care decisions.

Conventional Western (Allopathic) Medicine

Selecting a **primary care practitioner**—a medical practitioner whom you can visit for routine ailments, preventive care, general medical advice, and appropriate referrals—is not an easy task. The primary care practitioner for most people is a family practitioner, an internist, a pediatrician, or an obstetrician-gynecologist. Many people routinely see nurse practitioners or physician assistants who work for an individual doctor or a medical group, and others use nontraditional providers as their primary source of care.

Active participation in your own treatment is the only sensible course in a health care environment that encourages

TABLE 22.3 Allopathic/Traditional Medical Professionals

Allergist	A specialist who diagnoses and treats allergies
Anesthesiologist	A specialist who administers drugs during surgical procedures to reduce pain or induce unconsciousness
Cardiologist	A specialist in the diagnosis and treatment of heart and blood vessel disorders
Dermatologist	A specialist in the diagnosis and treatment of skin disorders
Dietitian	A specialist in the field of diet and human nutrition
Endocrinologist	A specialist in the diagnosis and treatment of glandular disorders
Family practitioner	A physician who offers routine medical service for a variety of ailments
Gastroenterologist	A specialist who diagnoses and treats disorders of the stomach and intestinal tract
Hematologist	A specialist who diagnoses and treats blood-related disorders
Internist	A specialist who diagnoses and treats disorders of the internal organs
Neurologist	A specialist who diagnoses and treats diseases of the brain, nervous system, and spinal cord
Nurse practitioner	Nurse specialist with additional training in a specific area, such as OB-Gyn
Obstetrician-gynecologist (OB-Gyn)	A specialist who diagnoses and treats problems of the female reproductive system
Oncologist	A specialist who diagnoses and treats cancerous growths and tumors
Orthopedist and orthopedic surgeon	Specialists who diagnose, treat, and/or provide surgical care for bone and joint injuries and problems
Otolaryngologist	A specialist who treats ear, nose, and throat disorders
Pediatrician	A physician who treats childhood diseases
Physical therapist	A specialist who rehabilitates people after impairment due to injury or disease
Plastic surgeon	A specialist who provides corrective surgery for irregularities of body or facial contours
Podiatrist	A specialist who diagnoses and treats disorders of the feet
Pulmonary specialist	A specialist who diagnoses and treats disorders of the respiratory system
Radiologist	A specialist in the diagnosis of disease by using X rays and other imaging techniques
Rheumatologist	A specialist who diagnoses and treats medical conditions of joints and surrounding tissues
Urologist	A specialist who diagnoses and treats disorders of the urinary tract

"defensive medicine." In a recent survey, 91 percent of U.S. physicians admitted they sometimes order unnecessary medical tests because they are concerned about being sued for malpractice. Approximately 50 percent of physicians have ordered unnecessary invasive procedures such as tissue biopsies, and 41 percent have prescribed unneeded drugs such as antibiotics.[11] Unnecessary drugs and procedures do not improve health outcomes, and in some cases they may even create new health problems.

Informed consent refers to your right to have explained to you—in nontechnical language you can understand—all possible side effects, benefits, and consequences of a procedure, as well as available alternatives to it. It also means that you have the right to refuse a treatment and to seek a second or even third opinion from unbiased, noninvolved providers.[12]

 what do you THINK?

Have you ever opted for a treatment other than what was recommended by your allopathic medical provider? ▪ What was the response? ▪ Did your health insurer cooperate fully and pay the bill?

Other Allopathic Specialties

Although Table 22.3 provides an overview of common sources of health care, it is by no means all-inclusive. Other specialists include **osteopaths,** general practitioners who receive training similar to a medical doctor's but who place special emphasis on the skeletal and muscular systems. Their treatments may involve manipulation of the muscles and joints. Osteopaths receive the degree of doctor of osteopathy (DO) rather than doctor of medicine (MD).

Much confusion exists about the roles of ophthalmologists and optometrists. An **ophthalmologist** holds a medical

osteopath General practitioner who receives training similar to a medical doctor's but with an emphasis on the skeletal and muscular systems, often using spinal manipulation as part of treatment.

ophthalmologist Physician who specializes in the medical and surgical care of the eyes, including prescriptions for glasses.

degree and can perform surgery and prescribe medications. An **optometrist** typically evaluates visual problems and fits glasses but is not a trained physician. If you have an eye infection, glaucoma, or other eye condition needing diagnosis and treatment, you need to see an ophthalmologist.

Dentists are specialists who diagnose and treat diseases of the teeth, gums, and oral cavity. They attend dental school for four years and receive the title of doctor of dental surgery (DDS) or doctor of medical dentistry (DMD). They must also pass both state and national board examinations before receiving their licenses to practice. The field of dentistry includes many specialties. For example, **orthodontists** specialize in the alignment of teeth. **Oral surgeons** perform surgical procedures to correct problems of the mouth, face, and jaw.

Nurses are highly trained and strictly regulated health practitioners who provide a wide range of services for patients and their families, including educating and counseling patients, disseminating community health and disease prevention information, and administering medications. They may choose from several training options. There are over 2.4 million licensed registered nurses (RNs) in the United States who have completed either a four-year program leading to a bachelor of science in nursing (BSN) degree or a two-year associate degree program. More than half a million lower-level licensed practical or vocational nurses (LPN or LVN) have completed a one- to two-year training program, which may be community college based or hospital based.

Nurse practitioners (NPs) are professional nurses having advanced training obtained through either a master's degree program or a specialized nurse practitioner program. Nurse

practitioners have the training and authority to conduct diagnostic tests and prescribe medications (in some states). They work in a variety of settings, particularly in HMOs (health maintenance organizations), clinics, and student health centers. Nurses may also earn the clinical doctor of nursing degree (ND) or doctor of nursing science (DNS and DNSc), or a research-based PhD in nursing.

More than 30,000 **physician assistants** (PAs) currently practice in the United States. Most of these are in office-based practices, including school health centers, but approximately 40 percent practice in areas where physicians are in short supply. Studies have shown that this relatively new class of midlevel practitioners may competently care for the majority of patients seeking primary care. All physician assistants must work under the supervision of a licensed physician, and they are legally permitted to prescribe drugs in 47 states.[13]

Health Care Organizations, Programs, and Facilities

Today, managed care is the dominant health payer system in the United States. Because of this, many people are restricted in their choice of a health care provider. Selective contracting between insurers or employers and health providers has limited the freedom of choice that some Americans previously enjoyed under a fee-for-service system. Two critical decisions to make are (1) choosing an insurance carrier or type of plan, and then (2) choosing from among the health care providers who participate in that plan. This section lists the most common choices.

Types of Medical Practices

In the highly competitive market for patients, many health care providers have found it essential to combine resources into a **group practice,** which can be single specialty or multispecialty. Physicians share offices, equipment, utility bills, and staff costs. Besides sharing costs, they may also share profits. Proponents of group practice maintain that it provides better coordination of care, reduces unnecessary duplication of equipment, and improves the quality of health care through peer review. Critics argue that group practice may limit competition and patients' access to services.

Solo practitioners are medical providers who practice independently of other practitioners. It is difficult for solo practitioners to survive in today's high-cost, high-technology health care market. They often have little time away from their offices and have to trade on-call hours with other doctors. For these reasons, there are far fewer solo practices today than in the past. Most solo practitioners are doctors who established their practices years ago, have a specialty that's in high demand, or work in a rural or underserved area.

---

optometrist   Eye specialist whose practice is limited to prescribing and fitting lenses.

dentist   Specialist who diagnoses and treats diseases of the teeth, gums, and oral cavity.

orthodontist   Dentist who specializes in the alignment of teeth.

oral surgeon   Dentist who performs surgical procedures to correct problems of the mouth, jaw, and face.

nurse   Health practitioner who provides many services for patients and who may work in a variety of settings.

nurse practitioner (NP)   Professional nurse with advanced training obtained through either a master's degree program or a specialized nurse practitioner program.

physician assistant   A midlevel practitioner trained to handle most standard cases of care.

group practice   A group of physicians who combine resources, sharing offices, equipment, and staff costs, to render care to patients.

solo practitioner   Physician who renders care to patients independently of other practitioners.

Integrated Health Care Organizations

Both hospitals and clinics provide a range of health care services, including emergency treatment, diagnostic tests, and inpatient and outpatient (ambulatory) care. Your selection of a hospital or clinic will depend on your particular needs, income, and insurance coverage, plus the availability of services in your community. As the number of hospitals has decreased in recent years due to an oversupply of hospital beds, a decreasing reliance on inpatient care, and an increase in competition, the number of hospital-based outpatient clinics has grown. These integrated health care organizations range from groups of loosely affiliated health service organizations and hospitals to HMOs that control their own very tightly joined hospitals, clinics, pharmacies, and even home health agencies.

There are several ways to classify hospitals: by profit status (nonprofit or for-profit); ownership (private, city, county, state, federal); specialty (children's, maternity, chronic care, psychiatric, general acute); teaching status (teaching-affiliated or not); size; and whether they are part of a chain of hospitals.

Nonprofit (voluntary) hospitals have traditionally been run by religious or other humanitarian groups. Earnings have generally been reinvested in the hospital to improve health care. These hospitals have often cared for patients whether the patients could pay or not.

The number of **for-profit (proprietary) hospitals** has multiplied over the past two decades. Today they constitute over 20 percent of nongovernmental acute-care hospitals. For-profit hospitals, which do not receive tax breaks, are not compelled to operate as a charity and typically provide fewer free services to the community than do nonprofit hospitals. Historically, some for-profit hospitals quickly transferred indigent (poor) or uninsured patients to public hospitals (those that are not heavily supported by taxes) or to nonprofit hospitals. This practice, known as *patient dumping,* was prohibited by federal law in 1986. Today, all hospital emergency rooms are required to perform a screening exam on all patients, regardless of their ability to pay. Legally, patients must be determined to be "medically stable" before they can be discharged from the emergency room or transferred to another facility, although consumer groups allege that some hospitals continue to dump less-profitable patients.[14]

More treatments and services, including surgery, are delivered on an **outpatient (ambulatory) care** basis (care that does not involve an overnight stay) by hospitals, traditional clinics, student health clinics, and nontraditional clinical centers. One type of ambulatory facility that is becoming common is the *surgicenter*—a place where minor, low-risk procedures such as vasectomies, tubal ligations, tissue biopsies, cosmetic surgery, abortions, and minor eye operations are performed.[15] To reduce the distance patients have to travel, many hospitals locate satellite clinics in cities' outlying areas, sometimes in shopping centers. A few hospitals have designated their satellites as freestanding emergency

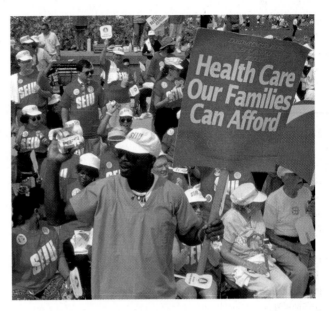

Increasing health care costs have mobilized people to take political action. Debate continues over the proper role of government, the insurance industry, and other parties.

centers, or surgicenters, that function like hospital emergency rooms for uncomplicated immediate-care cases but have lower operating costs. Some consumers refer to these as "doc-in-the-box" centers.

Many hospitals and group practices are affiliated with freestanding imaging and diagnostic laboratory centers through direct ownership or other profit-sharing arrangements. Significant debate surrounds this practice. Critics argue that when doctors own the diagnostic and laboratory services to which they refer patients, they may order an excessive number of tests. Today, such practices amount to "conflict of interest situations" and are largely prohibited by antikickback legislation.

Once located within hospitals, most health clinics today are likely to be independent facilities run by medical practitioners. Other health clinics are run by county health departments; these offer low-cost diagnosis and treatment for financially needy patients. Some 1,500 college campuses also have student health centers that, along with county, city, or community clinics, supply low-cost family planning, tests, and services related to vaccinations, sexually transmitted infections, and gynecological services.

Consumers who consider using a hospital or clinic should scrutinize the facility's accreditation. Accredited hospitals

nonprofit (voluntary) hospitals Hospitals run by religious or other humanitarian groups that reinvest their earnings in the hospital to improve health care.

for-profit (proprietary) hospitals Hospitals that provide a return on earnings to the investors who own them.

outpatient (ambulatory) care Treatment that does not involve an overnight stay in a hospital.

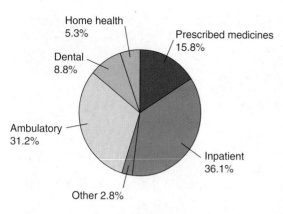

Home health
5.3%

Prescribed medicines
15.8%

Dental
8.8%

Ambulatory
31.2%

Inpatient
36.1%

Other 2.8%

Total = $596 billion

FIGURE 22.3 Where Do We Spend Our Health Care Dollars?

Source: G. L. Olin and S. R. Machlin, "Health Care Expenses in the Community Population, 1999," *Medical Expenditure Panel Survey* (MEPS Chartbook No. 11) (Rockville, MD: Agency for Healthcare Research and Quality, 2003).

have met rigorous standards set by the Joint Commission on Accreditation of Healthcare Organizations (JCAHO). If you choose an institution that has this accreditation, you have a greater likelihood of quality care.

People can also obtain information regarding prior provider malpractice insurance or sanctions from state licensure boards and the National Practitioner Data Bank. It is the responsibility of all health care consumers to report concerns about health care providers to local or state medical societies or licensing agencies for investigation. Report concerns about billing-related fraud or abuse directly to the Health Care Finance Administration (HCFA).

For more tips on how to evaluate hospitals and health care providers, see the Spotlight on Your Health box.

 what do you THINK?

Do you assume that your physicians and health care centers are licensed, certified, and accredited? ■ Have you ever checked on a doctor's or health care facility's credentials? ■ If so, what did you decide?

Issues Facing Today's Health Care System

Many Americans believe that our health care system needs fundamental reform. What are the problems that have brought us to this point? Cost, access, malpractice, restricted choices in providers and treatments, unnecessary procedures, complicated and cumbersome insurance rules, and dramatic ranges in quality are among the issues of concern. One of the most frequently voiced criticisms concerns lack of access to adequate health insurance, as many Americans have had

increasing difficulty obtaining comprehensive coverage from their employers. Until recently, insurance benefits were often lost when employees changed jobs, causing many people to remain in undesirable jobs in order to avoid losing health benefits. This phenomenon, known as *job lock,* led the federal government to pass legislation mandating the "portability" of health insurance benefits from one job to the next, thereby guaranteeing coverage during the transition. Today, individuals who leave their jobs have the option of continuing their group health insurance benefits under the Consolidated Omnibus Budget Reconciliation Act (COBRA). COBRA gives former employees, retirees, spouses, and dependents the right to continue their insurance temporarily at group rates. COBRA beneficiaries pay for their benefits but usually have better coverage than they could receive as individuals.

Over 90 million people in the United States suffer from chronic health conditions that should be at least monitored by medical practitioners.[16] Their access to care is largely determined by whether they have health insurance. Catastrophic or chronic illness among only 10 percent of the population accounts for 75 percent of all health expenditures.[17] Because we cannot perfectly predict who will fall into that 10 percent, every American is potentially vulnerable to the high cost and devastating effects of such illnesses.

Cost

Both per capita and as a percentage of gross domestic product (GDP), we spend more on health care than any other nation. Yet, unlike the rest of the industrialized world, we do not provide access for our entire population. Already, we spend over $2 trillion annually on health care, well over $5,035 for every man, woman, and child. This translates into 16.2 percent of our GDP. Does this sound like a lot? Consider that health care expenditures are projected to grow by 7.2 percent each year until they reach $4 trillion annually by 2015—nearly 20 percent of our GDP.[18]

Why do health care costs continue to spiral upward? There are many factors involved: excess administrative costs; duplication of services; an aging population; growing rates of obesity, inactivity, and related health problems; demand for new diagnostic and treatment technologies; an emphasis on crisis-oriented care instead of prevention; and inappropriate utilization of services by consumers are some of them.

Our system has more than 2,000 health insurance companies, each with different coverage structures and administrative requirements. This lack of uniformity prevents our system from achieving the *economies of scale* (bulk purchasing at a reduced cost) and administrative efficiency realized in countries where there is a single-payer delivery system. According to the Health Insurance Association of America (HIAA), commercial insurance companies commonly experience administrative costs greater than 10 percent of the total health care insurance premium, whereas the administrative cost of the government's Medicare program is less than 4 percent. Administrative expenses in the private sector contribute to the high cost of health care and force companies to require

SPOTLIGHT on your health

Suppose that you decide to buy a car. No doubt you would do some research first and compare information on various models and dealers to obtain the best vehicle for your needs.

Now suppose that you are told you need surgery. Wouldn't you like to be able to do the same kind of research on hospitals and surgeons, so you could identify the best health care providers for your case? Below are some of the most helpful sources.

THE LEAPFROG GROUP
www.leapfroggroup.org

A nationwide coalition of more than 150 public and private organizations, the Leapfrog Group focuses on identifying problems in the U.S. hospital system that can lead to medical errors, and devising solutions.

Leapfrog issues hospitals a quality rating based on CPOE (computerized physician/provider order entry) implementation and other safety practices. Its website posts the results of its hospital safety survey and ranks hospitals around the country. Note that hospital participation in the program is voluntary, and many hospitals do not participate at present.

HEALTHGRADES
www.healthgrades.com

This company provides quality reports on physicians as well as hospitals, nursing homes, and other health care facilities. In its hospital ratings, the website incorporates data from nearly 5,000 hospitals on surgery volume (how many procedures of this type are performed at that particular hospital) and patient outcomes (complication and mortality rates). Ratings of physicians detail the doctor's specialty, training, board certification, and whether there have been any governmental disciplinary actions taken against him or her.

HEALTHSCOPE
www.healthscope.org

Operated by the nonprofit coalition Pacific Business Group on Health, this website rates hospitals, medical groups, and health plans in California. Hospital ratings are based on patient questionnaires, mortality reports, patient discharge records, and quality assessments from the Leapfrog Group. Hospital participation is voluntary.

HEALTHFINDER
www.myhealthfinder.com

Sponsored by the Niagara Health Quality Coalition, this site provides quality assessments of hospitals, health insurance plans, and long-term care facilities in New York state. Hospital ratings are based on information from patients, the Joint Commission on Accreditation of Health Care Organizations, HealthGrades, and various reports. Ratings include data on surgery volume and mortality rates for coronary bypass surgery.

PENNSYLVANIA HEALTH CARE COST CONTAINMENT COUNCIL
www.phc4.org

This independent state agency seeks to lower health care costs by stimulating competition in the health care market. It collects, analyzes, and makes available to the public information on the cost and quality of health care in Pennsylvania. Hospital ratings include data such as patients' length of stay in the hospital, readmission for any reason, readmission for complications or infections, rate of transfer to acute care, mortality rates, and average hospital charges.

---

employees to share more of the costs, cut back on benefits, and drop some benefits altogether. These costs are largely passed on to consumers in the form of higher prices for goods and services. See Figure 22.3 for a breakdown of how health care dollars are spent.

The declining availability of health insurance coverage means more Americans are uninsured or underinsured. These people are unable to access preventive care and seek care only in the event of an emergency or crisis. Because emergency care is extraordinarily expensive, they often are unable to pay, and the cost is absorbed by those who *can* pay—the insured or taxpayers. This process is known as *cost shifting*.

Access

Access to health care is determined by numerous factors, including the supply of providers and facilities, proximity to care, ability to maneuver in the system, health status, and insurance coverage. Although there are approximately 700,000 physicians in the United States, many Americans lack adequate access to health services because of insurance barriers or maldistribution of providers. There is an oversupply of higher-paid specialists and a shortage of lower-paid primary care physicians (family practitioners, pediatricians, internists, OB-Gyns, geriatricians). Inner cities and some rural areas face constant shortages of physicians.

Managed care health plans determine access on the basis of participating providers, health plan benefits, and administrative rules. Often this means that consumers do not have the freedom to choose specialists, facilities, or treatment options beyond those contracted with the health plan and recommended by their primary care provider (also known as *gatekeeper*). In the United States, consumer demand has led to an expansion of benefits to include such nonallopathic therapies as chiropractic and acupuncture (see Chapter 23). However, many nonallopathic treatments remain unavailable, even to a limited degree, through current health plans.

Quality and Malpractice

The U.S. health care system employs several mechanisms for ensuring quality services: education, licensure, certification/registration, accreditation, peer review, and, as a last resort, the legal system of malpractice litigation. Some of these mechanisms are mandatory before a professional or organization may provide care, whereas others are purely voluntary. (Be aware that licensure, although state mandated for some practitioners and facilities, is only a minimum guarantee of quality.) Insurance companies and government payers may also require a higher level of quality by linking payment to whether a practitioner is board certified or a facility is accredited by the appropriate agency. In addition, most insurance plans now require prior authorization and/or second opinions not only to reduce costs, but also to improve quality of care.

Consumer, provider, and advocacy groups focus on the great variation in quality as a major problem in our health care system. A newer form of quality measurement uses "outcome" as the primary indicator for measuring health care quality at the individual level. Outcome measurements take into account not only what is done to the patient, but also what subsequently happens to the patient's health status. Thus, mortality rates and complication rates (such as infections) become very important statistics in assessing individual practitioners and facilities.

Medical errors and mistakes do happen. An Institute of Medicine report indicates that as many as 44,000 to 98,000 people die in U.S. hospitals each year as the result of medical errors.[19] Clearly, we must be as proactive as possible in our health care.

what do you THINK?

Do you believe prospective patients should have access to information about practitioners' and facilities' malpractice records? ■ How about their success and failure rates or outcomes of various procedures?

Third-Party Payers

The fundamental principle of insurance underwriting is that the cost of health care can be predicted for large populations. This is how health care premiums (payments) are determined. Policyholders pay premiums into a pool, which fills as reserves until needed. When you are sick or injured, the insurance company pays out of the pool, regardless of your total amount of contribution. Depending on circumstances, you may never pay for what your medical care costs or you may pay much more for insurance than your medical bills ever total. The idea is that you pay in affordable premiums so that you never have to face catastrophic bills. In today's profit-oriented system, insurers prefer to have healthy people in their plans who put money into risk pools without taking money out.

Unfortunately, not everyone has health insurance. Forty-two million Americans (14.6 percent of the nonelderly population) are uninsured—that is, they have no private health insurance and are not eligible for Medicare, Medicaid, or other health programs.[20] The number of uninsured has grown since the late 1970s. Lack of health insurance has been associated with delayed health care and increased mortality. *Underinsurance* (that is, the inability to pay out-of-pocket expenses despite having insurance) also may result in adverse health consequences. Another 16 million Americans between the ages of 19 and 64 are estimated to be underinsured (at risk for spending more than 10 percent of their income on medical care because their insurance is inadequate).[21]

What types of things should I think about when choosing health insurance?

Contrary to the common belief that the uninsured are unemployed, 75 percent of them are either workers or the dependents of workers. One-quarter of all the uninsured are children under age 16. College students are one of the largest groups of the uninsured not in the labor force (Figure 22.4). This presents a difficult dilemma for both universities and students when they must seek care because most university insurance plans are designed as short-term, noncatastrophic plans having low upper limits of benefits. As a full-time student, you should consider purchasing a higher level catastrophic plan to protect yourself in the event of a rare, but very costly, illness or accident.

For the uninsured and many of the underinsured, health care may not be available through any source because of their inability to pay. Many either will not or cannot seek care from charitable providers, so they fail to receive the medical care they need. People without health care coverage are less likely than other Americans to have their children immunized, seek early prenatal care, obtain annual blood pressure checks, and seek attention for serious symptoms of illness. Many experts believe that this ultimately leads to higher system costs because their conditions deteriorate to a more debilitating and costly stage before they are forced to seek help.

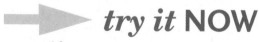

try it NOW

Be prepared for an unexpected medical emergency! Even though you may take measures to be safe and healthy, you never know when you might find yourself in an emergency medical situation, like a car accident. Right now, make sure your health insurance card is in your wallet, as well as some information on whom to contact (friend, family member) in the event of an emergency.

Private Health Insurance

Our current health system began in the past century and its growth accelerated in the post–World War II era to its current massive, complex web. Hospitals became the engines of medicine in the mid-twentieth century. Doctors became the drivers or conductors of this rapidly moving system. The system was fueled by a variety of funding sources but, chiefly, first by the growth of tax-exempt, nonprofit private insurance companies established in the 1940s and later by the growth of for-profit insurance companies.

> **Can I count on my university health care plan to cover my medical needs?**

Originally, health insurance consisted solely of coverage for hospital costs (it was called *major medical*) but gradually was extended to routine physicians' treatment and other areas such as dental services and pharmaceuticals. Payment mechanisms used until recently laid the groundwork for today's steadily rising health care costs. Hospitals were reimbursed on a cost-plus basis after services were rendered. That is, they billed for the costs of providing care plus an amount for profit. This system provided no incentive to contain costs, limit the number of procedures, or curtail capital investment in redundant equipment and facilities. Physicians were reimbursed on a fee-for-service (indemnity) basis determined by "usual, customary, and reasonable" fees. These were calculated by comparing what a doctor charged for a service with what that same doctor charged last year for the service and with what other doctors in the area charged. This system encouraged physicians to charge high fees, raise them often, and perform as many procedures as possible. At the same time, because most insurance did not cover routine or preventive services, consumers were encouraged to use hospitals whenever possible (the coverage was better) and to wait until illness developed to seek help instead of seeking preventive care. Consumers were also free to choose any provider or service they wished, including even inappropriate—and often very expensive—levels of care.

Private insurance companies have increasingly employed several mechanisms to limit potential losses and control consumers' use of insurance. These mechanisms include cost sharing (in the form of deductibles, copayments, and coinsurance), exclusions, "preexisting condition" clauses, waiting periods, and upper limits on payments. *Deductibles* are front-end payments (commonly $250 to $1,000) that you must make to your provider before your insurance company will start paying for any services you use. *Copayments* are set amounts that you pay per service received regardless of the cost of the service (for example, $20 per doctor visit or per prescription). *Coinsurance* is the percentage of the bill that you must pay throughout the course of treatment (for example, 20 percent of whatever the total is). *Preexisting condition clauses* limit the insurance company's liability for medical conditions that a consumer had before obtaining insurance coverage (for example, if a woman takes out coverage while she is pregnant, the insurance company may cover pregnancy

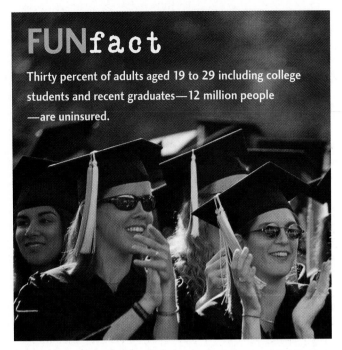

FUNfact

Thirty percent of adults aged 19 to 29 including college students and recent graduates—12 million people—are uninsured.

FIGURE 22.4 The Uninsured in America: A Closer Look at College Students and Others Aged 19–29

Source: K. Quinn et al., *Health Insurance On Their Own: Young Adults Living Without Health Insurance* (New York: The Commonwealth Fund, 2000).

complications and infant care but not charges related to "normal pregnancy"). Because many insurance companies use a combination of these mechanisms, keeping track of the costs you are responsible for can become very difficult.

Group plans of large employers (government agencies, school districts, or corporations, for example) generally do not have preexisting condition clauses in their plans. But smaller group plans (a group may be as small as two) often do. Some plans never cover services for preexisting conditions, while others specify a *waiting period* (such as six months) before they will provide coverage. All insurers set some limits on the types of services they will cover (for example, most exclude cosmetic surgery, private rooms, and experimental procedures). Some insurance plans may also include an *upper* or *lifetime limit,* after which coverage will end. Although $250,000 may seem like an enormous sum, medical bills for a sick child or chronic disease can easily run this high within a few years. Table 22.4 lists some questions you should ask yourself when considering your health care options.

Medicare and Medicaid

After years of debate about whether we should have a national health program like those of most industrialized countries, the U.S. government directed the system toward a mixed private and public approach in the 1960s. Most Americans obtained their health insurance through their employers,

TABLE 22.4 Things to Think About When Choosing Health Insurance

When deciding on a health insurance plan, you might ask yourself these questions:

- How comprehensive do I want my coverage of health care services to be?
- How do I feel about limits on my choice of doctors or hospitals?
- How convenient does my care need to be?
- How important is the cost of services?
- How much am I willing to spend on premiums and other health care costs?
- How convenient are the office hours and location?
- How long does getting an appointment with this health care provider take?
- Will the services the plan offers meet my needs?

Call the insurance plan office for details about coverage if you have questions.

but this left out two groups—the nonworking poor and the aged. In 1965, amendments to the 1935 Social Security Act established Medicare and Medicaid. Although enacted simultaneously, these programs are vastly different.

Medicare, basically federal social insurance covering 99 percent of the elderly over 65 years of age, all totally and permanently disabled people (after a waiting period), and all people with end-stage kidney failure, is a universal program that covers a broad range of services except long-term care and pharmaceuticals. It currently covers over 42 million people.[22] Medicare is widely accepted by physicians and hospitals and has relatively low administrative costs.

On the other hand, **Medicaid,** covering approximately 44 million people, is a federal–state matching funds welfare program for people who are defined as poor (blind, disabled, aged, or those receiving Aid to Families with Dependent

Medicare Federal health insurance program for the elderly and the permanently disabled.

Medicaid Federal–state health insurance program for the poor.

diagnosis-related groups (DRGs) Diagnostic categories established by the federal government to determine in advance how much hospitals will be reimbursed for the care of a particular Medicare patient.

managed care Cost-control procedures used by health insurers to coordinate treatment.

capitation Prepayment of a fixed monthly amount for each patient without regard to the type or number of services provided.

Children) and relies on matching funds provided by federal and state sources.[23] Because each state determines income eligibility levels and payments to providers, there are vast differences in the way Medicaid operates from state to state.

To control hospital costs, in 1983 the federal government set up a prospective payment system based on **diagnosis-related groups (DRGs)** for Medicare. Using a complicated formula, nearly 500 groupings of diagnoses were created to establish how much a hospital would be reimbursed for a particular patient. If a hospital can treat the patient for less than that amount, it can keep the difference. However, if a patient's care costs more than the set amount, the hospital must absorb the difference (with a few exceptions that must be reviewed by a panel). This system gives hospitals the incentive to discharge patients quickly after doing as little as possible for them, provide more ambulatory care, and admit only patients with favorable (profitable) DRGs. Many private health insurance companies have followed the federal government in adopting this type of reimbursement. In 1998, the federal HCFA expanded the prospective payment system to include payments for outpatient surgery and skilled nursing care.

In its continuing effort to control rising costs, the HCFA has encouraged the growth of prepaid HMO senior plans for Medicare-eligible persons. Under this system, commercial managed care insurance plans receive a fixed per capita premium from the HCFA and then offer more preventive services with lower out-of-pocket copayments. These managed care plans encourage providers and patients to utilize health care resources under administrative rules similar to commercial HMO plans. Similarly, states have encouraged the growth of managed Medicaid programs.

Managed Care

Managed care describes a health care delivery system comprised of the following elements:

1. A budget based on an estimate of the annual cost of delivering health care for a given population

2. A network of physicians, hospitals, and other providers and facilities linked contractually to deliver comprehensive health benefits within that predetermined budget, sharing economic risk for any budget deficit or surplus

3. An established set of administrative rules requiring patients to follow the advice of participating health care providers in order to have their health care paid for under the terms of the health plan

Many such plans pay their contracted health care providers through **capitation,** that is, prepayment of a fixed monthly amount for each patient without regard for the type or number of health services provided. Some plans pay health care providers a salary, and some are still fee-for-service plans. As with other insurance plans, enrollees are members of a risk pool, and it is expected that some persons will use no services, some will use a modest amount, and others will have high-cost utilization over a given year. Doctors have the incentive to keep their patient pool healthy and avoid catastrophic ailments that are preventable; usually such incentives come back in terms of increased salaries, bonuses, and other benefits. Thus, prevention and health education to reduce risk and intervene early to avoid major problems should be capstone components of such plans.

Managed care plans have grown steadily over the past decade with a proportionate decline of enrollment in traditional indemnity insurance plans. The reason for this shift is that indemnity insurance, which pays providers and hospitals on a fee-for-service basis with no built-in incentives to control costs, has become unaffordable or unavailable for most Americans.

With the growth of managed care organizations, concerns have arisen about the quality of care offered under this type of payment system. These concerns compelled consumer groups and public health organizations to require managed care insurers to compile quality of care "report cards," known as HEDIS (Health Employer Data Information Set) Reports, so that health outcomes could be compared across different plans. The quality measures include preventive services (childhood immunizations, Pap smears, mammograms), disease indicators (eye exams and glucose control tests for diabetics), and screening exams (routine physical exams, including gynecological exams). These reports are available from most managed care health plans on request. Still, such information is difficult for the consumer to evaluate due to inconsistent data collection and reporting techniques. This problem has given rise to skepticism and controversy over the validity of these reports.

Types of managed care plans include health maintenance organizations (HMOs), preferred provider organizations (PPOs), and point of service (POS). Approximately 166 million Americans are enrolled in HMOs, the most common type.[24]

Health Maintenance Organization (HMO)

HMOs provide a wide range of covered health benefits (such as checkups, surgery, doctor visits, lab tests) for a fixed amount prepaid by you, the employer, Medicaid, or Medicare. Usually, HMO premiums are the least expensive form of managed care (saving between 10 and 40 percent more than other plans) but also are the most restrictive (offering little or no choice in doctors and certain services). These premiums are 8 to 10 percent lower than for traditional plans; there are low or no deductibles or coinsurance payments; and copayments are $10 to $20 per office visit. HMOs contract with providers to supply health services for enrollees through various systems, such as these:[25]

- *The staff model.* You receive care from salaried staff doctors at the HMO's facility.
- *The group network model.* The HMO contracts with one or several groups of doctors, who provide care for a fixed amount per plan member. Groups often practice in one facility.
- *The independent practice association (IPA).* Doctors in private practice form an association that contracts with

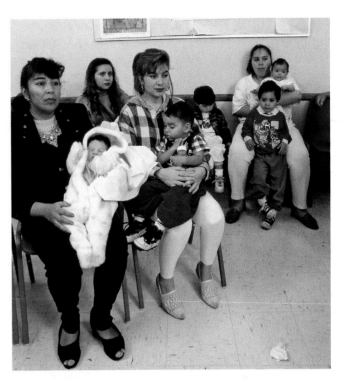

One downside to the HMO health care system is that patients often encounter crowded waiting rooms when they need to see their health care provider.

HMOs. The physicians generally work in their own offices.

The downside of HMOs is that patients are typically required to use the plan's doctors and hospitals and to get approval from a "gatekeeper" or primary care physician for treatment and referrals.[26] As more and more people enroll in HMOs, criticisms of this type of plan are mounting. Concerns about HMOs include questions such as:

- Do highly paid administrators and stockholders ration care, allocating more care to those who are better able to pay and enjoy better health?
- Does the huge administrative structure imposed by the HMO make it virtually impossible for patients to sue in the event of clear violations?
- Are patients denied costly diagnostic tests because such tests cut into bottom-line profits? Are some tests given too late because of cost concerns?
- Do HMOs really focus on prevention or intervention? Critics charge that the fee structure of many HMOs actually discourages basic preventive services, such as immunizations.
- Are doctors allowed to treat patients using their best judgment and skills, or do policies and profit-motivated concerns interfere with their roles as advocates for patients?
- Are the obstacles imposed by HMOs too daunting for patients in need of urgent care?
- Do HMO cost-saving policies force patients out of hospitals and treatment centers too early?

Preferred Provider Organization (PPO)

PPOs are networks of independent doctors and hospitals that contract to provide care at discounted rates. Although they offer greater choices in doctors than HMOs do, they are less likely to coordinate a patient's care. In addition, though members have a choice of seeing doctors who are not on the preferred list, this choice may come at considerable cost (such as having to pay 30 percent of the charges out of pocket, rather than 10 to 20 percent for PPO doctors and services).[27]

Point of Service (POS)

This option—a hybrid of the HMO and PPO types—provides a more acceptable form of managed care for those used to the traditional indemnity plan of insurance, which probably explains why it is among the fastest growing of the managed care plans. Under POS, patients can go to providers outside their HMO for care but must pay for the extra cost. Usually this is a reasonable alternative for middle-class or wealthy Americans who are willing to pay extra for choices in care.[28]

what do you THINK?

Why is it important that private insurance cover preventive or lower-level care as well as hospitalization and high-technology interventions? ■ What kinds of incentives would cause you to seek help early rather than delay care?

What Are Your Options?

The United States and South Africa are currently the only industrialized nations that do not have a national health program that guarantees all citizens access to at least a basic set of health benefits. The United States has seen four major political movements supporting national health insurance during the past century, but none has succeeded. Whether universal coverage will—or should—be achieved and through what mechanism remain hotly debated topics. Many analysts believe that health care reform has failed due to a combination of circumstances and influences: lobbying efforts by the insurance industry and the medical community, proposed plans that were too complicated, and interest groups that contended that the plans either went "too far" or "not far enough." Some people also believe that our current system serves people well.

One critical point must be made, though: we are paying for the most expensive system in the world without obtaining full coverage. We pay for people who don't have insurance through cost shifting that increases premiums and taxes, and we spend more than necessary because prevention and early treatment are not emphasized. We also pay for much duplication of services and technologies, for practitioners who practice defensive medicine and who refer patients to their own diagnostic labs for profit reasons, and for the vast bureaucracy made inevitable by over 2,000 private health insurance companies.

The Institute of Medicine, a nonpartisan organization that advises the federal government on health issues, recommends a single-payer, tax-financed scheme that severs insurance ties from employment.[29] Similar to the Canadian model, it would cover everyone—regardless of income or other factors such as health status. It would offer many different ways to tailor a plan to the needs of U.S. citizens. A single federal plan or a privately administered plan paid for by general tax funds or earmarked taxes could be created. Thus, all (or most) private insurers would be eliminated or would see their role limited to that of fiscal administrators. Benefits would be comprehensive and provide incentives for cost-effective care. Benefits would be "portable": they would remain in effect when individuals changed jobs or moved to a different area of the country. Freedom of choice in terms of providers might actually improve in a single-payer system, given how restrictive our current private health insurance system has become. Such a plan would allow far greater control over resource and personnel planning and improve access to preventive services, and it could eliminate duplicate services and technology. Claims that the Canadian system has long waiting lists have proved either entirely untrue or exaggerated: modest waits do not appear to result in any reduction of health status.

Given the delay in realizing national health care reform, several states have sought ways to contain costs and improve access for their populations. At the federal level, Congress continues to debate strategies for bolstering Social Security and Medicare.

what do you THINK?

Do you believe that the time is right for another national discussion on health care reform? ■ Do you think we are moving to a more profit-oriented health care system or to a single-payer system? ■ Which would you prefer? ■ Is health care a right or a privilege?

TAKING CHARGE

Summary

- Advertisers of health care products and services use sophisticated tactics to attract attention and get business. Advertising claims sometimes appear to be supported by spontaneous remission (symptoms disappearing without any apparent cause) or the placebo effect (symptoms disappearing because people think they should), rather than the efficacy of the product or service.
- Self-care and individual responsibility are key factors in reducing rising health care costs and improving health status. Advance planning can help a person navigate health care treatment in unfamiliar situations or emergencies. Assess health professionals by considering their qualifications, their record of treating problems like yours, and their ability to work with you.
- In theory, allopathic (conventional Western) medicine is based on scientifically validated methods and procedures. Medical doctors, specialists of various kinds, nurses, nurse practitioners, physician assistants, and other health professionals practice allopathic medicine.
- Prescription drugs are administered under medical supervision. Categories include antibiotics, sedatives, tranquilizers, antidepressants, and amphetamines. Generic drugs can often be substituted for more expensive brand-name drugs. Over-the-counter drug categories include analgesics; cold, cough, allergy, and asthma relievers; stimulants; sleeping aids and relaxants; and dieting aids. Exercise personal responsibility by reading directions for OTC drugs and asking your pharmacist or doctor if any special precautions are advised when taking these substances.
- Health care providers may provide services as solo practitioners or in group practices (which share overhead costs). Hospitals and clinics are classified by profit status, ownership, specialty, teaching status, size, and whether they are part of a chain.
- Concerns about the U.S. health care system include cost, access, choice of treatment modality, quality and malpractice, and fraud and abuse.
- Health insurance is based on the concept of spreading risk. Insurance is provided by private insurance companies (which charge premiums) and the government Medicare and Medicaid programs (funded by taxes). Managed care (in the form of HMOs, POS plans, and PPOs) attempts to control costs by streamlining administrative procedures and stressing preventive care (among other initiatives).

Chapter Review

1. When a person is suffering from an ailment and it disappears without any known cause or treatment, this is known as
   a. the placebo effect.
   b. spontaneous remission.
   c. proactive management.
   d. None of the above.

2. Which type of drug is used to fight bacterial infections in the human body?
   a. antidepressants
   b. analgesics
   c. antibiotics
   d. diuretics

3. A drug interaction characterized by the use of two or more drugs that react together to become more powerful than if taken alone is known as
   a. polydrug use.
   b. antagonism.
   c. synergism.
   d. cross-tolerance.

4. A third-party insurance company that contracts with independent physicians and hospitals to provide health care to its subscribers is known as
   a. a health maintenance organization (HMO).
   b. Medicare.
   c. a preferred provider organization (PPO).
   d. managed care.

5. Deborah, aged 28 and a single parent, is on welfare. Her medical bills are paid by a federal health insurance program for the poor. This agency is
   a. an HMO.
   b. Social Security.
   c. Medicaid.
   d. Medicare.

6. What medical practice is based on scientifically validated methods and procedures whose objective is to heal by countering the patient's symptoms?
   a. allopathic medicine
   b. nonallopathic medicine
   c. osteopathic medicine
   d. chiropractic medicine

7. Dr. Smith received training similar to that of a medical doctor's that more put emphasis on the skeletal and muscular systems. Dr. Smith is a(n):
   a. general practitioner.
   b. internist.
   c. osteopath.
   d. physical therapist.

8. Jill has diabetes, and due to a job change had to choose a new health insurance provider. The new insurance company refused to cover her diabetic care expenses under a clause in the contract which stated that Jill has
   a. a co-insurance limit.
   b. a pre-existing health condition.
   c. already exceeded lifetime upper limit.
   d. no major medical coverage on her policy.

9. An example of proactive self-care would be
   a. performing monthly breast or testicular self-examinations.
   b. taking a first aid class to learn basic procedures in case of an emergency.
   c. diagnosing cold symptoms and supplying yourself with cold remedies.
   d. All of the above.

10. One way to save money when needing to purchase a doctor-ordered prescription is to ask for the cheaper, no-name brand medicine with the same chemical formula. This is called
    a. an over-the-counter drug.
    b. a generic drug.
    c. a homeopathic drug.
    d. a no-name drug.

Answers to these questions can be found on page A-1.

Questions for Discussion and Reflection

1. What claims do marketers use to get people to try health-related products? Why are consumers susceptible to such ploys? What could be done to increase the accuracy of messages related to health care?
2. List several conditions (resulting from illness or accident) for which you don't need to seek medical help. When would you consider each condition bad enough to require medical attention? How would you decide to whom and where to go for treatment?
3. Explain the terms *synergism, antagonism,* and *inhibition.*
4. What are the advantages and disadvantages associated with generic drugs?
5. What are the pros and cons of group practices? Of non-profit and for-profit hospitals? If you had health insurance, where do you believe you would get the best care? On what do you base your answer?
6. What are the inherent benefits and risks of managed care organizations?
7. Discuss the problems of the U.S. health care system. If you were president, what would you propose as a solution? Which groups might oppose your plan? Which groups might support it?
8. Explain the differences between traditional indemnity insurance and managed health care. Which would you feel more comfortable with? Should insurance companies set rates for various medical tests and procedures in an attempt to keep prices down?

Accessing Your Health on the Internet

The following websites explore further topics and issues related to personal health. You'll also find links to each organization's website on the Companion Website for *Access to Health,* Tenth Edition, at www.aw-bc.com/donatelle.

1. *Agency for Health Care Research and Quality (AHRQ).* A gateway to consumer health information, providing links to sites that can address health care concerns and provide information on questions to ask, what to look for, and what you should know when making critical decisions about personal care. www.ahrq.gov

2. *Food and Drug Administration (FDA).* News on the latest government-approved generic drugs and investigations. www.fda.gov
3. *National Committee for Quality Assurance (NCQA).* The NCQA assesses and reports on the quality of managed care plans, including health maintenance organizations. www.ncqa.org
4. *National Institutes of Health—National Information Center on Health Services Research and Health Care Technology (NICHSR).* Collects, stores, and disseminates the latest in health services research. A good resource for consumer public health information. www.nlm.nih.gov/nichsr

Further Reading

Birenbaum, A. *Wounded Profession: American Medicine Enters the Age of Managed Care.* Westport, CT: Praeger Publishers, 2002.

Birenbaum describes the rise of HMOs in the 1990s and the increasing backlash, and he presents ideas for reform of the health care system.

Geyman, J. *Health Care in America: Can Our Ailing System Be Healed?* London: Butterworth-Heinemann, 2001.

> *Written from the perspective of a physician, this book focuses on the challenges—escalating costs, limitations of access, and a wide range of quality—facing the health care system.*

Greenburg, S. *2005 Physician's Desk Reference for Nonprescription Drugs and Dietary Supplements,* 27th ed. Montvale, NJ: Thomson, 2005.

> *Outlines proper uses, possible dangers, and effective ingredients of nonprescription medications.*

Lee, P. and C. Estes. *The Nation's Health,* 7th ed. Sudbury, MA: Jones and Bartlett, 2003.

> *Overview of factors affecting the health of Americans and the roles of public health, medical care, and the community in ensuring the nation's health. Special emphasis on health determinants, women's health, long-term care, and the uncertainties of tomorrow's health care system.*

Kawachi, I. and B. Kennedy. *The Health of Nations: Why Inequality Is Harmful to Your Health.* New York: New Press, 2006.

> *A timely summary of recent economic research that shows how extreme prosperity always comes at the expense of others' poverty.*

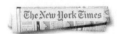

e-themes from *The New York Times*

For up-to-date articles about current health issues, visit www.aw-bc.com/donatelle, select *Access to Health,* Tenth Edition, Chapter 22, and click on "e-themes."

References

1. L. C. Baker and L. S. Baker, "Excess Cost of Emergency Department Visits for Nonurgent Care," *Health Affairs* (Winter 1994): 162–180.
2. A. B. Bernstein et al., "Introduction," *Health Care in America: Trends in Utilization* (Hyattsville, Maryland: National Center for Health Statistics, 2003), www.cdc.gov/nchs/data/misc/healthcare.pdf.
3. American Academy of Orthopaedic Surgeons, "Advisory Statement: The Importance of Good Communication in the Physician-Patient Relationship," September 2005, www.aaos.org/wordhtml/papers/advistmt/1017.htm.
4. C. Huggins, "Poll Shows Most Americans Trust Their Doctors," *Medline Plus Health Information,* 2002, www.nlm.nih.gov/medlineplus/news/fullstory_10844.html.
5. National Center for Health Statistics, "New Study Shows Critical Role for Primary Care Specialists," National Ambulatory Medical Care Survey: 2002 Summary, August 26, 2004, www.cdc.gov/nchs/pressroom/04facts/primarycare.htm.
6. H. Verdoux et al., "Is Benzodiazepine Use a Risk Factor for Cognitive Decline and Dementia?" *Psychological Medicine* 35 (2005): 307–315.
7. National Center for Health Statistics, "New Study Shows Critical Role for Primary Care Specialists."
8. J. Rowley et al., "Insomnia," June 17, 2004, www.emedicine.com/neuro/topic418.htm.
9. U.S. Food and Drug Administration, "Phenylpropanolamine (PPA) Information Page," 2002, www.fda.gov/cder/drug/infopage/ppa/default.htm.
10. U.S. Food and Drug Administration, "Sales of Supplements Containing Ephedrine Alkaloids Prohibited," April 12, 2004, www.fda.gov.
11. Institute for Global Ethics, "Malpractice Fears Are Hurting Nation's Health Care, Group Warns," *Ethics Newsline* 5, no. 16, April 22, 2002, www.globalethics.org/newsline/members/issue.tmpl?articleid=04210222410961.
12. Consumer Health, "Patient Rights: Informed Consent," 2006, www.emedicinehealth.com/articles/12033-3.asp.
13. D. E. Mittman, "Explaining Rxs with a PA or an NP Signature," *Clinician Reviews,* February 2003, www.findarticles.com/p/articles/mi_m0BUY/is_2_13/ai_98312977.
14. J. Silverman, "Consumer Report Spotlights Patient Dumping," *OB/GYN News,* September 1, 2001, www.findarticles.com/p/articles/mi_m0CYD/is_17_36/ai_78542014.
15. National Center for Health Statistics, *United States 2005 Chart Book on Trends in Health of Americans* (Hyattsville, MD: NCHS, 2005).
16. Centers for Disease Control, "Indicators for Chronic Disease Surveillance," *Morbidity and Mortality Weekly Report, Recommendations and Reports* 53, no. RR11, September 10, 2004, 1–6, www.cdc.gov/mmwr/preview/mmwrhtml/rr5311a1.htm.
17. National Center for Chronic Disease Prevention and Health Promotion, "Chronic Disease Overview," 2005, www.cdc.gov/nccdphp/overview.htm.
18. Centers for Medicare and Medicaid Services, "National Health Care Expenditures Projections: 2002–2012," 2005, www.cms.hhs.gov/statistics/nhe/projections-2005/highlights.asp.
19. Institute of Medicine, "The Chasm in Quality: Select Indicators from Recent Reports," May 2006, www.iom.edu/cms/8089/14980.aspx.
20. National Center for Health Statistics, "Health Insurance Coverage for Children Up in 2004; Number of Uninsured Adults Stable," June 29, 2005, www.cdc.gov/nchs/pressroom/05news.insur200506.htm.
21. C. Schoen et al., "Insured But Not Protected: How Many Adults are Underinsured?" *Health Affairs Web Exclusive,* June 10, 2005, http://content.healthaffairs.org.
22. Centers for Medicare and Medicaid Services, "Medicare Enrollment, July 2005," 2005, www.cms.hhs.gov/medicaiddatasourcesgeninfo/downloads/mmcpro5.pdf.
23. Ibid.
24. M. McFarlane and M. Sinnott, "Managed Care: Nursing's Friend or Foe?" *Nursing Spectrum, Education/CE Self-Study Module,* 2003, http://nsweb.nursingspectrum.com/ce/ce169.htm.
25. Tufts Health Care Institute, "Managed Care Models and Products," 2006, www.thci.org.
26. M. McFarlane and M. Sinnott, "Managed Care: Nursing's Friend or Foe?"
27. Ibid.
28. Ibid.
29. V. Kemper, "National Health Insurance Recommended," *The Miami Herald,* January 15, 2004, www.miami.com/mld/miamiherald/news/nation/7714716.htm?1c.

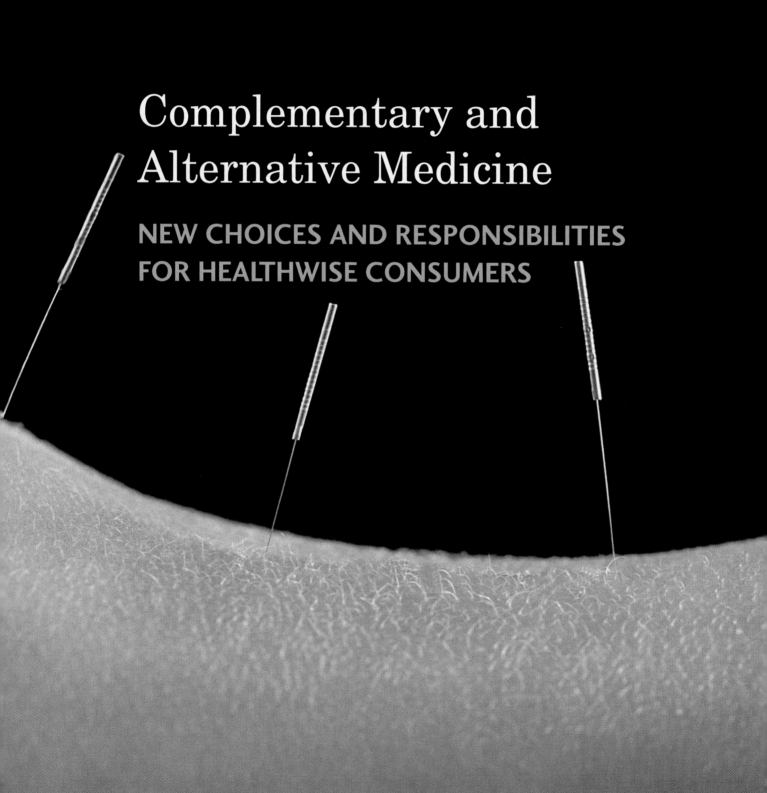

23

Complementary and Alternative Medicine

NEW CHOICES AND RESPONSIBILITIES FOR HEALTHWISE CONSUMERS

Are **chiropractors** real doctors?

What do all those little **acupuncture** needles do?

Do **herbal** remedies have any risks or side effects?

Will **echinacea** teas and cough drops cure my cold?

How do I evaluate **alternative medicine** resources for reliability?

OBJECTIVES

- Describe complementary and alternative medicine (CAM), and identify its typical domains.
- Explain the major types of complementary and alternative medicine providers, common treatments they offer, and why CAM is growing in popularity in the United States.
- Discuss the various types of complementary and alternative medicines being used in America today, their patterns of use, and their potential benefits and risks.
- Understand how to evaluate testimonials and claims related to complementary and alternative products, services, and practitioners to ensure that you are getting accurate information or safe treatment.
- Summarize the challenges and opportunities related to complementary and alternative medicine in ensuring our health and wellness.

hoosing a health care professional or health care service, or buying a health care product has never been more challenging for the average consumer. Increasingly, people are seeking *alternatives,* safer and more effective means of getting healthy and staying healthy. More and more, Americans are looking into their options outside of traditional allopathic medicine, and seek the help of alternative medical practitioners such as naturopaths or acupuncturists, or turn to various herbal and plant-based medicines. Some of these consumers may use an alternative approach in combination with the advice of their medical doctor, while others choose to use the Internet as a source for self-diagnosis and use combinations of herbal, over-the-counter, and various home remedies in search of a cure for their ailment.[1] In Chapter 22, we focused almost exclusively on your role as a consumer and making choices about allopathic medicine. In this chapter, we focus on consumer choices for complementary and alternative medicine (CAM).

Complementary and Alternative Medicine: What Is It?

Complementary and alternative medicine (CAM), as defined by the National Center for Complementary and Alternative Medicine (NCCAM), is a group of diverse medical and health care systems, practices, and products that are not presently considered part of conventional medicine.[2]

Although often used interchangeably, there is a distinction between the terms *complementary* and *alternative.* **Complementary medicine** is used *together with* conventional medicine, as part of an integrative medical approach. An aromatherapist might work with an oncologist to reduce a patient's nausea during chemotherapy, for example. **Alternative medicine** is used *in place of* conventional medicine. An example of this would be using a special diet or herbal remedy to treat cancer instead of using radiation, surgery, or other conventional treatments.

Whether one takes herbs to lift mood or reduce pain, does yoga or Pilates to reduce stress and increase strength, prac-

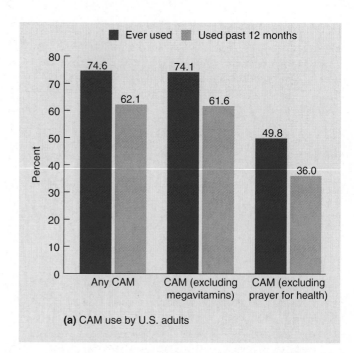

(a) CAM use by U.S. adults

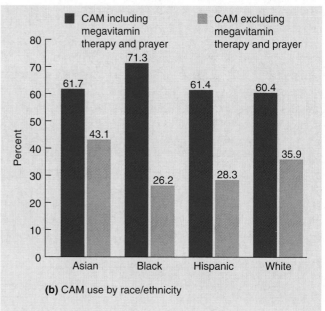

(b) CAM use by race/ethnicity

FIGURE 23.1 Use of Complementary and Alternative Medicine in the United States

Source: P. Barnes et al., "CDC Advance Data Report #343: Complementary and Alternative Medicine among Adults: United States, 2002," 2004, http://nccam.nih.gov/news/camsurvey.htm.

complementary and alternative medicine (CAM)
Forms of treatment distinct from traditional allopathic medicine that until recently were neither taught widely in U.S. medical schools nor generally available in U.S. hospitals.

complementary medicine   Treatment used in conjunction with conventional medicine.

alternative medicine   Treatment used in place of conventional medicine.

tices mind–body health techniques, receives acupuncture for low back pain, or follows naturopathic tenets for cancer treatment, over 62 percent of all Americans go outside of the conventional medicine system to prevent disease, enhance health, or treat symptoms (see Figure 23.1 for more on who uses CAM). Realizing that CAM in one form or another is here to stay and not just quackery, the National Institutes of Health (NIH) and the U.S. medical establishment now find themselves racing to evaluate many of CAM's claims and provide reliable information for consumers. In response to growing public interest, politicians and health care professionals have significantly increased the budget for CAM research; since 1999, government funding for CAM research has doubled.[3] Many argue that this is just a drop in the bucket in terms of being able to conduct the research trials necessary to study each of the CAM therapies commonly in practice. Today, someone who is interested in up-to-date information from NIH-funded research on dietary supplements, herbal medications, and any of the various CAM modalities need only click on the National Center for Complementary and Alternative Medicine (NCCAM) website for a listing of past, ongoing, and future projects. We've clearly come a long way in less than a decade.

However, in spite of the good news and apparent commitment to CAM research, progress is slow, and every minute of every day a new CAM therapy springs onto the scene. Whereas some scientific evidence exists regarding a small number of CAM therapies, for most there are still key questions that are yet to be answered through well-designed scientific studies. These questions include issues of safety and effectiveness. Differences in terminology and philosophy among practitioners, a lack of consensus on definitions, and the politics of a medical industry that emphasizes profits along with patient care often slow the availability of consumer information. How does the average consumer know what to believe? How do we separate genuinely helpful CAM therapies from those that might be risky? This chapter attempts to present a research-based perspective on modern CAM treatments. As you read, look for answers to your own questions and think about how you might access more information helpful to you and your friends in the future. Explore your own attitudes toward CAM in the Assess Yourself box on page 674.

Comparing CAM with Conventional Medicine

Various forms of CAM are increasingly being taught in U.S. medical schools and are available to patients in some clinics and hospitals. Some, such as acupuncture, are even paid for by many health insurance policies.

 However, it is important to note that complementary and alternative therapies vary widely in terms of the nature of treatment, extent of therapy, and types of problems for which they offer help. There is no national training or licensure standard and states differ in their practices (this is also true for conventional medicine). Whereas practitioners of conventional medicine have graduated from U.S.-sanctioned schools of medicine or are licensed medical practitioners recognized by the governing body for all physicians, the American Medical Association (AMA), each CAM domain has a different set of training standards, guidelines for practice, and licensure procedures. Although it is not possible to provide a detailed examination of each profession here, including the amount of training necessary, licensure, and continuing education requirements, a quick Internet search of each profession can provide you with detailed information. See the Spotlight on Your Health box on page 677 for information on finding reliable Internet resources.

It should be noted that an increasing number of conventional practitioners are partnering with or becoming involved in the actual delivery of certain CAM therapies. CAM therapies serve as alternatives to a conventional system that some regard as too invasive, too high-tech, and too toxic when it come to medications and side effects. Others continue to consult conventional medical providers, believing that there is safety in government-controlled licensing, regulation of procedures, and FDA drug testing and approval.

The History of CAM in the United States

Although the United States has been somewhat slow to accept plant remedies as standard treatment, an estimated 25 percent of all modern pharmaceutical drugs are derived from herbs, including aspirin (white willow bark), the heart medication digitalis (foxglove), and the cancer treatment Taxol (Pacific yew tree).

Although plant-based medicines were used widely in the United States until World War II, a new generation of FDA-tested pharmaceuticals took over in the later years of the twentieth century. Older treatments fell out of favor among all but a few segments of the U.S. population and became associated with the undeveloped and impoverished parts of the world. With a growing dissatisfaction of the populace with the technowizardry of early twenty-first-century U.S. medicine, many of these earlier treatments have reemerged in treatment arsenals.

To better understand why Americans behave as they do when confronted with an illness or disorder, it is necessary to understand fears, concerns, and sources of hope for a positive outcome. Many of us have a powerful distrust of traditional medical practice. Through either direct experience or media portrayals of problems with today's health care system, many people believe that when sick, the worst place to be is in a hospital or health care setting.

A number of our recent pharmacological advances have their roots in the herbal remedies used in cultures throughout the world. Ancient healing practices from China, India, and other regions may well provide reasonable alternatives to conventional Western treatments.

The Emergence of CAM in the United States

In 1997, a landmark study showed that almost half of all Americans (47 percent) were using some form of CAM.[4] Not only did this shock health care providers and public health professionals alike, but it indicated that CAM was here to stay and that we had better take a long, hard look at the implications of CAM use for American consumers. Although the

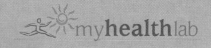
EVALUATING COMPLEMENTARY AND ALTERNATIVE MEDICINE

Fill out this assessment online at
www.aw-bc.com/MyHealthLab or
www.aw-bc.com/donatelle.

You may have a range of opinions about CAM, depending on the therapies described. Use the questions below to explore your assumptions about CAM.

1. What types of medical professionals do you think should call themselves *holistic health practitioners*?
2. What is meant by the term *mind–body medicine*?
3. What type of person do you think is most likely to seek alternative or complementary medical treatment?
4. Would you tell your doctor you were taking herbal supplements?
5. Would you tell your doctor if you were consulting an alternative-medicine practitioner?
6. Would you try hypnosis to quit smoking or lose weight? Why or why not?
7. Do you consider yoga or tai chi forms of alternative medicine?
8. If a person with severe pain claimed that wearing a magnetic bracelet worked, would you try it or recommend it to someone else?
9. Should health insurance cover complementary or alternative medical treatments?
10. Should herbal supplements be tested and regulated by the federal government?

MAKE it happen!

ASSESSMENT: The Assess Yourself activity asks you to assess your opinions about CAM. Now that you have considered your results, you may want to take steps to begin your behavior change program.

MAKING A CHANGE: In order to change your behavior, you need to develop a plan. Follow the steps below and complete your Behavior Change Contract to take action.

1. Evaluate your behavior and identify patterns and specific things you are doing. What can you change now? What can you change in the near future?

2. Select one pattern of behavior that you want to change.

3. Fill out the Behavior Change Contract found at the front of your book. It should include your long-term goal for change, your short-term goals, the rewards you'll give yourself for reaching these goals, potential obstacles along the way, and strategies for overcoming these obstacles. For each goal, list the small steps and specific actions that you will take.

4. Chart your progress in a journal. At the end of a week, consider how successful you were in following your plan. What helped you be successful? What made change more difficult? What will you do differently next week?

5. Revise your plan as needed: Are the short-term goals attainable? Are the rewards satisfying?

ONE STUDENT'S PLAN: When Melia answered the question about the type of person most likely to seek CAM treatment, she assumed that no one she knew would use anything but traditional treatment. She was surprised when she started asking her friends and family, and it turned out that several of them had tried various CAM therapies. Some had positive experiences: her uncle Louis had developed back problems after a car accident, and a chiropractor had brought him relief. Also, her friend Tony had had acupuncture for his "tennis elbow" and reported that it had helped. On the other hand, Melia's mother had taken ginkgo biloba because she felt she needed help with her memory. However, she didn't tell her regular physician that she was taking it—and, when she started taking a blood thinner he prescribed for her, the combination of the two caused dangerous bleeding. She had not experienced any memory enhancement from the ginkgo and was glad to stop it.

Melia had chronic knee pain, and her doctor had not discovered anything that could be treated with surgery or other conventional treatments. Now that she had thought more about CAM and saw how widely used some of the therapies are, Melia decided to investigate the most appropriate ones for knee pain and ask her doctor's opinion about pursuing one of them. Based on her mother's experience, she knew she would need to work together with her physician and any CAM provider to be sure that their treatments were compatible. She made an appointment with her doctor to discuss possible treatments and planned to research all of her options, including side effects and insurance coverage.

exact amount spent on CAM therapies was difficult to determine, estimates of spending in excess of $300 billion per year stunned the health care marketplace—this figure was comparable to the total out-of-pocket spending for all U.S. physician services.

Major Domains of CAM

The NCCAM has grouped the many varieties of CAM into four domains of practice (Figure 23.2 on page 676), recognizing that the domains may overlap. The domains are as follows:[5]

- **Manipulative and body-based practices** are based on manipulation or movement of one or more body parts. Examples include chiropractic or osteopathic manipulations and massage.
- **Energy medicine** involves the use of energy fields, such as magnetic fields or biofields (energy fields that some believe surround and penetrate the body).
- **Mind–body medicine** uses a variety of techniques to enhance the mind's ability to affect bodily function and symptoms. Some examples include support groups and the use of cognitive behavioral theory.
- **Biologically based practices** use substances found in nature, such as herbs, special diets, or vitamins (in doses outside those used in conventional medicine). This includes the use of natural but unproven therapies.

An additional area of study is **alternative medical systems,** which cut across all domains and are built upon complete systems of theory and practice. Often these systems evolved apart from and earlier than conventional Western medicine.

In the past decade, some specialists in nonallopathic medicine have been accepted by professional groups, and their inclusion in mainstream medicine is growing daily. Many conventional medical schools are now offering coursework in CAM, and many allopathic doctors refer patients to alternative providers, who are in turn reimbursed by the patients' health insurance plans. Modalities that have received the greatest degree of acceptance include chiropractic medicine, acupuncture, herbal and homeopathic medicine, and naturopathy, all of which we will discuss in this chapter.

Alternative Medical Systems

There are many traditional systems of medicine that have been practiced by various cultures throughout the world. Many have evolved from centuries-old Asian practices, such as traditional Chinese medicine and Ayurveda, which are at the root of much of our CAM thinking today. Other whole medical systems include homeopathy and naturopathy.

manipulative and body-based practices Treatments involving manipulation or movement of one or more body parts.

energy medicine Therapies using energy fields, such as magnetic fields or biofields.

mind–body medicine Techniques designed to enhance the mind's ability to affect bodily function and symptoms.

biologically based practices Treatments using substances found in nature, such as herbs, special diets, or vitamin megadoses.

alternative medical systems Complete systems of theory and practice that involve several CAM domains.

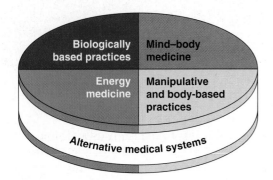

FIGURE 23.2 The Domains of Complementary and Alternative Medicine

Source: P. Barnes et al., "CDC Advance Data Report #343: Complementary and Alternative Medicine among Adults: United States, 2002," 2004, http://nccam.nih.gov/news/camsurvey.htm.

Traditional Chinese Medicine

Traditional Chinese medicine (TCM) emphasizes the proper balance or disturbances of **qi** (pronounced "chee"), or vital energy in health and disease, respectively. In TCM, diagnosis is based on history, on observation of the body (especially the tongue), on palpation, and on pulse diagnosis, an elaborate procedure requiring considerable skill and experience by the practitioner. Techniques such as acupuncture, herbal medicine, massage, and *qi gong* (a form of energy therapy described in more detail later in this chapter) are among the TCM approaches to health and healing.

Ayurveda

Ayurveda (or **Ayurvedic medicine**) refers to the "science of life," an alternative medical system that began and evolved over thousands of years in India. The goal of Ayurveda is to integrate and balance the body, mind, and spirit and restore harmony in the individual.[6] Ayurvedic practitioners use various techniques, including asking questions, observing, and touching patients before establishing a specific treatment plan. The goals of Ayurvedic treatment are to eliminate

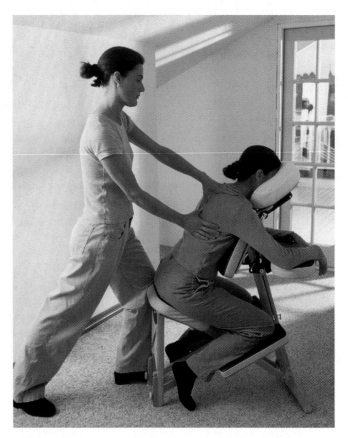

Massage therapy is a popular complementary treatment for its ability to both relax and treat pain.

impurities in the body and reduce symptoms. Dietary modification and herbal remedies drawn from the vast botanical wealth of the Indian subcontinent are common. Treatments may also include animal and mineral ingredients, powdered gemstones, yoga, stretching, meditation, massage, steam baths, exposure to the sun, and controlled breathing.[7]

Training of Ayurvedic practitioners varies. There is no national standard for certifying or training Ayurvedic practitioners, although professional groups are working toward licensure. To find out about the effectiveness of this medical system or any of its various modalities, see the NCCAM Web pages for specific topic research.[8]

Homeopathy

Homeopathic medicine, which originated in Germany during the eighteenth century, is a CAM system based on the principle that "like cures like." In other words, the same substance that in large doses produces the symptoms of an illness will, in very small doses, cure the illness.[9] Essentially, homeopathic physicians use herbal medicine, minerals, and chemicals in extremely diluted forms as natural agents to kill infectious agents or ward off illnesses that are caused by more potent forms or doses of those agents.

Homeopathic training varies considerably and is offered through diploma programs, certificate programs, short courses, and correspondence courses. Laws that detail requirements to practice vary from state to state.

traditional Chinese medicine (TCM)   Comprehensive system of diagnosis and treatment in which dietary change, touch, massage, medicinal teas, and other herbal medicines are used extensively.

qi   Element of traditional oriental medicine that refers to the vital energy force that courses through the body. When qi is in balance, health is restored.

Ayurveda (Ayurvedic medicine)   A method of treatment derived largely from ancient India, in which practitioners diagnose by observation and touch, and then assign a largely dietary treatment laced with herbal medicines.

homeopathic medicine   Unconventional Western system of medicine based on the principle that "like cures like."

SPOTLIGHT on your health

EVALUATING MEDICAL RESOURCES ON THE WEB

Planning to research health information online? The National Center for Complementary and Alternative Medicine recommends that you ask these questions about any website you visit.

How do I evaluate alternative medicine resources for reliability?

1. *Who runs this site?* Any good health-related website should be clear about who is responsible for the site and its information, with the name of the site's sponsor and a link to its home page on every major page of the site.

2. *Who pays for the site?* It costs money to run a website, so how does the site pay for its existence? The source of its funding should be clearly stated or readily apparent. For example, Web addresses ending in ".gov" denote a federal government–sponsored site. Does the site sell advertising? Is it sponsored by a drug company? The source of funding can affect the choice of content, how the information is presented, and what the site owners want to accomplish.

3. *What is the purpose of the site?* This question is related to who owns and pays for the site. An "About This Site" link appears on many sites; if it's there, use it. The purpose of the site should be clearly stated and should help you evaluate the trustworthiness of the information.

4. *Where does the information come from?* Many health and medical sites post information collected from other websites or sources. If the person or organization in charge of the site did not create the information, the original source should be clearly identified.

5. *What is the basis of the information?* In addition to identifying who wrote the material you are reading, the site should describe the evidence that the material is based on. Medical facts and figures should have references (such as to articles in medical journals). Also, opinions or advice should be clearly set apart from information that is evidence based (that is, information based on research results).

6. *How is the information selected?* Is there an editorial board listed for the site? Do people with excellent professional and scientific qualifications review the material before it is posted?

7. *How current is the information?* Websites should be reviewed and updated regularly. It is particularly important that medical information be current. The most recent update or review date should be clearly posted. Even if the information has not changed, you want to know whether the site owners have reviewed it recently to ensure that it is still valid.

8. *How does the site choose links to other sites?* Websites usually have a policy about how they establish links to other sites. Some medical sites take a conservative approach and don't link to any other sites. Some link to any site that asks—or pays—for a link. Others link only to sites that have met certain criteria.

9. *What information about you does the site collect, and why?* Websites routinely track the paths visitors take through their sites to determine which pages are being used. However, many health websites ask for you to "sub-scribe" or "become a member." In some cases, this may be so that they can collect a user fee or select information for you that is relevant to your concerns. In all cases, this will give the site personal information about you. Any credible health site asking for this kind of information should tell you exactly what will and will not be done with it. Many commercial sites sell "aggregate" (collected) data about their users to other companies—information such as what percentage of their users are women with breast cancer, for example. In some cases they may collect and reuse information that is "personally identifiable," such as your zip code, gender, and birth date. Be certain that you read and understand any privacy policy or similar language on the site, and don't sign up for anything that you do not fully understand.

10. *How does the site manage interactions with visitors?* There should always be a way for you to contact the site owner if you run across problems or have questions or feedback. If the site hosts chatrooms or other online discussion areas, it should tell visitors what the terms of using this service are. Is it moderated? If so, by whom, and why? It is always a good idea to spend time reading the discussion without joining in, so that you feel comfortable with the environment before becoming a participant.

Source: National Center for Complementary and Alternative Medicine, "Ten Things to Know about Evaluating Medical Resources on the Web," 2006, http://nccam.nih.gov/health/webresources.

TABLE 23.1	Popular Complementary Treatments
Aromatherapy	Aromatherapists use scented materials to evoke sensations through the smell centers of the body. Treatment focuses on odors regarded as pleasurable.
Food therapy	Treatment is based on the belief that many disorders are based on allergies and toxic synergism among food combinations. Naturopaths test for and treat food allergies and assign special diets designed to produce nutritional balance.
Massage	Massage involves rubbing, stroking, kneading, or lightly pounding the body with the hands or other instruments.
Megavitamins	Treatment with megavitamins promotes the consumption of large doses of common essential vitamins and minerals to prevent disease and heal illness.
Relaxation techniques	The goal is to remove stress and promote healing. Techniques include yoga, meditation, breathing exercises, posture exercises, and visualization.

Naturopathy

Naturopathic medicine, which also developed in Europe, views disease as a manifestation of an alteration in the processes by which the body naturally heals itself. Disease results from the body's effort to ward off impurities and harmful substances from the environment. Naturopathic physicians emphasize restoring health rather than curing disease. They employ an array of healing practices, including diet and clinical nutrition; homeopathy; acupuncture; herbal medicine; hydrotherapy (the use of water in a range of temperatures and methods of application); spinal and soft-tissue manipulation; physical therapies involving electric currents, ultrasound, and light therapy; therapeutic counseling; and pharmacology. Several major naturopathic schools in the United States and Canada provide training, conferring the *naturopathic doctor (ND)* degree on students who have

naturopathic medicine System of medicine that attempts to restore natural processes of the body and promote healing through natural means.

chiropractic medicine Manipulation of the spine to allow proper energy flow.

completed a four-year graduate program that emphasizes humanistically oriented family medicine.

Other Medical Systems

Though the foregoing medical philosophies and patterns of treatment have exerted great influence on populations worldwide, other, more regionally limited medical traditions are also noteworthy. American Indian, Aboriginal, African, Middle Eastern, Tibetan, and South American cultures also have their own unique medical systems. International surveys of CAM outside the United States suggest that alternative therapies are popular throughout most of the world. Public opinion polls and consumer surveys in Europe and the United Kingdom suggest high CAM use in Italy, France, Denmark, Finland, and Australia, in addition to most Asian cultures.[10]

As the number of alternative therapists grows and systems become intertwined, so do the number of health care options available to consumers (see Table 23.1 for examples). Before considering any medical systems, wise consumers will consult the most reliable resources to thoroughly evaluate risks, the scientific basis of claimed benefits, and any contraindications to using the CAM product or service. Avoid practitioners who promote their treatments as a cure-all for every health problem or who seem to promise remedies that have thus far defied the best scientific efforts of mainstream medicine. In short, apply the same strategies to researching CAM as you would to choosing allopathic care (see Chapter 22).

Manipulative and Body-Based Practices

The second domain of CAM includes methods that are based on manipulation and/or movement of the body. For example, chiropractors focus on the relationship between the body's structures (primarily the spine) and functions and on how that relationship affects the preservation and restoration of health. Chiropractors employ manipulation as a key therapy.

Chiropractic Medicine

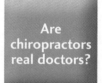

Are chiropractors real doctors?

Chiropractic medicine has been practiced for over 100 years. Allopathic medicine and chiropractic medicine were in direct competition over a century ago.[11] Today, however, many managed care organizations work closely with chiropractors, and many insurance companies will pay for chiropractic treatment, particularly if it is recommended by a medical doctor. More than 20 million Americans now visit chiropractors each year.

Chiropractic medicine is based on the idea that a life-giving energy flows through the spine via the nervous system. If the spine is subluxated (partly misaligned or dislocated), that force is disrupted. Chiropractors use a variety of techniques to manipulate the spine back into proper alignment so the life-giving energy can flow unimpeded through the nervous system. It has been established that their treatment can be effective for back pain, neck pain, and headaches.

The average chiropractic training program requires four years of intensive courses in biochemistry, anatomy, physiology, diagnostics, pathology, nutrition, and related topics, combined with hands-on clinical training. Many chiropractors continue their training to obtain specialized certification, for instance, in women's health, gerontology, or pediatrics. There are currently 16 chiropractic colleges in the United States, with a combined enrollment of over 14,000 students. Six states require a bachelor's degree in addition to the doctor of chiropractic degree for licensure. The practice of chiropractic is licensed and regulated in all 50 states.[12]

You should investigate and question a chiropractor as carefully as you would any medical doctor. As with many health professionals, you may note vast differences in technique among specialists. It is recommended that you choose a chiropractor who follows standard chiropractic regimens for treating musculoskeletal conditions. Avoid those who promote adjustment as a cure-all for all disorders or whose treatments are not based on manipulation of the spine.

Other Manipulation Therapies

There are other specialties that involve manipulation of the body. Recall from Chapter 22 that *DOs,* or *doctors of osteopathy,* place particular emphasis on the musculoskeletal system. Osteopathic practitioners believe that all of the body's systems work together and that disturbances in one system may have an impact upon function elsewhere in the body.[13] As such, they specialize in body manipulation yet also have a more traditional form of medical school training.

Energy Medicine

Energy medicine, also called energy therapy, focuses either on energy fields thought to originate within the body (biofields) or on fields from other sources (electromagnetic fields). Biofield therapies are intended to affect energy fields said to surround and penetrate the human body. The existence of these fields has not been experimentally proven. Some forms of energy therapy manipulate biofields by applying pressure and/or manipulating the body by placing the hands in, or through, these fields.[14]

Popular examples of biofield therapy include *qi gong, reiki,* and *therapeutic touch.* Qi gong, a component of traditional Chinese medicine, combines movement, meditation, and regulation of breathing to enhance the flow of vital energy (qi), improve blood circulation, and enhance immune function.[15] *Reiki,* whose name derives from the Japanese word representing "universal life energy," is based on the belief that by channeling spiritual energy through the practitioner the spirit is healed, and it in turn heals the physical body.[16] *Therapeutic touch* derives from the ancient technique

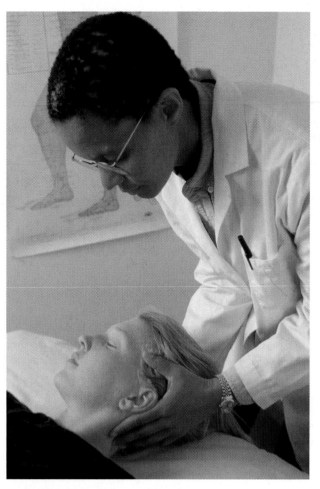

A chiropractor treats a patient using a variety of techniques to manipulate the spine into proper alignment.

of "laying on of hands" and is based on the premise that the healing force of the therapist brings about the patient's recovery and that healing is promoted when the body's energies are in balance. By passing the hands over the body, the healer identifies bodily imbalances.[17]

Bioelectromagnetic-based therapies involve the unconventional use of electromagnetic fields, such as pulsed fields, magnetic fields, or alternating current or direct current fields, to treat asthma, cancer, pain, migraines, and other conditions.

There is little scientific documentation to support claims for energy field techniques at this point. However, two derivatives of energy medicine have gained much wider acceptance in recent years: acupuncture and acupressure.

Acupuncture and Acupressure

Chinese medical treatments are growing in popularity and offer an important complement to Western biomedical care. **Acupuncture,** one of the oldest and most popular forms of

acupuncture   The insertion of long, thin needles to affect the energy flow within the body.

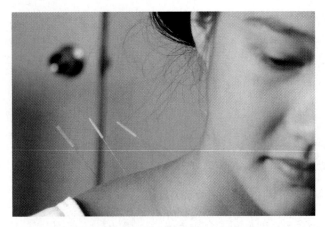

Acupuncture has been found to be effective in treating many problems but should always be performed by a licensed practitioner.

traditional Chinese medicine among Americans, is sought for a wide variety of health conditions, including musculoskeletal dysfunction, mood enhancement, and wellness promotion. It describes a family of procedures that involve stimulating anatomical points of the body with a series of needles. Following acupuncture, most respondents report high satisfaction with the treatment, improved quality of life, improvement in or cure of the condition, and reduced reliance on prescription drugs and surgery. In particular, results have been promising in the treatment of nausea associated with chemotherapy, dental pain, and knee pain.[18]

> **What do all those little acupuncture needles do?**

Acupuncturists in the United States are state licensed, and each state has specific requirements regarding training programs. Most acupuncturists have either completed a two- to three-year postgraduate program to obtain a master of traditional Oriental medicine (MTOM) degree or attended a shorter certification program in North America or Asia. They may be licensed in multiple areas—for example, the MTOM is also trained in the use of herbs. Some licensed MDs and chiropractors have trained in acupuncture and obtained certification to use this treatment.

Acupressure is similar to acupuncture but does not use needles. Instead, the practitioner applies pressure to points critical to balancing yin and yang, the two Chinese principles that interact to influence overall harmony (health) of the body. Practitioners must have the same basic understanding of energy pathways as do acupuncturists. Acupressure should

---

acupressure Application of pressure to selected body points to balance energy.

psychoneuroimmunology (PNI) Use of stress management and other techniques to enhance the function of the immune system.

---

not be applied by an untrained person to pregnant women or to anyone with a chronic health condition.

what do you THINK?

Why do you think more and more people are opting for complementary and alternative treatments? ■ What are the potential benefits of these treatments? ■ What are the potential risks? ■ What types of controls are reasonable to regulate the quality and consistency of foreign-trained health care providers?

Mind–Body Medicine

Mind–body interventions employ a variety of techniques to facilitate the mind's capacity to affect bodily functions and symptoms. Many therapies might fall into this category; but some areas, such as biofeedback, patient education, and cognitive-behavior techniques, have been so well investigated that they are no longer considered alternative. However, meditation, yoga, tai chi, certain uses of hypnosis, dance, music and art therapy, prayer and mental healing, and several others are still categorized as complementary and alternative. (See Chapter 10 for more on yoga and tai chi; see Chapters 2 and 3 for more on spirituality, and the mind–body connection).

Body Work

Body work actually consists of several different forms of exercise. *Feldenkrais* therapy work is a system of movements, floor exercises, and body work designed to retrain the central nervous system to help it find new pathways around areas of blockage or damage. It is gentle and effective in rehabilitating trauma victims. *Rolfing* is a more invasive form of body work, aimed at restructuring the musculoskeletal system by working on patterns of tension held in deep tissue. The therapist applies firm—sometimes painful—pressure to different areas of the body. Rolfing can release repressed emotions as well as dissipate muscle tension. *Shiatsu* is a traditional healing art from Japan that makes use of firm finger pressure applied to specified points on the body and is intended to increase the circulation of vital energy. The client lies on the floor, with the therapist seated alongside. *Trager therapy,* one of the least invasive forms of body work, employs gentle rocking and bouncing motions to induce states of deep, pleasant relaxation.[19]

Psychoneuroimmunology

As discussed in Chapter 3, **psychoneuroimmunology (PNI)** is a relatively new field of study. It is defined as the "interaction of consciousness (psycho), the brain and central nervous system (neuro), and the body's defense against external infection and internal aberrant cell division (immunology)."[20] A number of researchers have postulated over the years that excessive stress and maladaptive coping will ultimately serve to create dysfunction of the immune system and increase risk for a variety of infectious and chronic diseases. To counteract the negative impact on health, scientists are exploring ways in which relaxation, biofeedback, meditation, yoga, laughter, exercise, and activities that involve either conscious or unconscious mind "quieting" and harnessing of negative energy may interact to counteract negative stressors. As such, several of the above mind–body activities designed to slow heartbeat and breathing and to bring about homeostasis in the body are being studied. A classic study of PNI and mind–body health attempted to assess the effects of relaxation and coping techniques on the immune system by studying nursing home patients. Participants were divided into three groups: those who were taught relaxation techniques, those who were provided with abundant social contact, and those who received no special techniques or contact. After a one-month period, immune system function was greatly improved in those people who received stress management therapy compared with the control group.[21] Several new studies indicate positive effects of mind–body techniques that encourage relaxation and other stress-reduction strategies for those with HIV or other health problems.

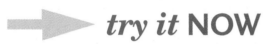

try it NOW

You don't have to take a supplement or undergo a treatment to benefit from alternative medical practices. For improved overall wellness, take a few moments to close your eyes, and think of a calm place or activity you enjoy. Perhaps you are lying on a tropical beach, or are curled up in front of a fireplace. Clear your mind of everything else, and use relaxation to improve your health.

Biologically Based Practices

Biologically based therapy is perhaps one of the most controversial domains of CAM practice, largely because of the sheer numbers of options that are available and the myriad claims that are made about their supposedly magical effects. To date, many of these claims have not been thoroughly investigated, and regulation of this aspect of CAM has been relatively slow in coming.

Biologically based practices include natural and biologically based treatments, interventions, and products, many of which overlap with conventional medicine's use of dietary supplements. Included are *herbal remedies, special dietary supplements,* and *individual* biological therapies, and foods as healing agents.

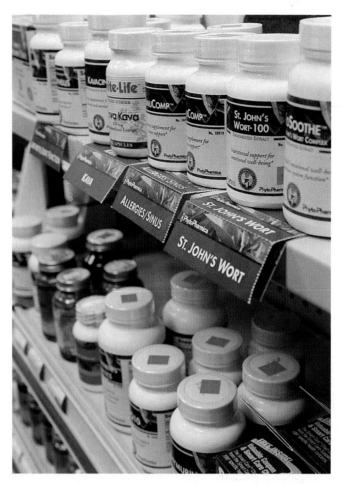

Buying herbal supplements can be confusing because so many brands exist and their manufacture is not strictly regulated for potency or quality.

Herbal Remedies

Practitioners who base their therapies primarily on the medicinal qualities of plants and herbs are referred to as *herbalists.* Derived largely from Ayurvedic or traditional Chinese medicine, herbal medications are widely available in the United States. Fueled by mass advertising and promoted as part of multiple vitamin and mineral regimens by major drug manufacturers, herbal supplements represent the hottest trend in the health market.

Herbal remedies are not to be taken lightly. Just because something is natural does not necessarily mean that it is safe. In recent years, FDA Consumer Advisories have warned that certain herbal products, kava in particular, may be associated with severe liver damage.[22] Other reports remind consumers that even rigorously tested products can be risky. Many plants are poisonous, and some can be toxic if ingested in high doses. Others may be dangerous when combined with prescription or over-the-counter drugs, or they could disrupt the normal action of the drugs.[23]

Properly trained herbalists and homeopaths have received graduate-level training in special programs such as herbal nutrition or traditional Chinese medicine. These practitioners have been trained in diagnosis; in mixing herbs, titrations, and dosages; and in the follow-up care of patients.

Herbal remedies come in several different forms. **Tinctures** (extracts of fresh or dried plants) usually contain a high percentage of grain alcohol to prevent spoilage and are among the best herbal options. Freeze-dried extracts are very stable and offer good value for your money. Standardized extracts are also among the more reliable forms of herbal preparations.

> **Do herbal remedies have any risks or side effects?**

In general, herbal medicines tend to be milder than chemical drugs and produce their effects more slowly; they also are much less likely to cause toxicity because they are diluted rather than concentrated forms of drugs.[24] But diluted or not, herbals are still drugs. They should not be taken casually, any more than you would take over-the-counter or prescription drugs without really needing them or knowing their side effects. No matter how natural they are, herbs still contain many of the same chemicals as synthetic prescription drugs. Too much of any herb can cause problems, but particularly if it is one from nonstandardized extracts. Some herbs and specific dietary supplements can pose risks to consumers by interacting with prescription drugs or causing unusual side effects.

The following discussion gives an overview of some of the most common herbal supplements on the market.

Ginkgo Biloba

Ginkgo biloba is an extract from the leaves of a deciduous tree that lives up to 1,000 years. The ginkgo was almost destroyed during the last ice age in all regions of the world except China, where it is considered a sacred tree with medicinal properties.[25] Today, ginkgo leaf extracts are widely prescribed in many countries and gaining in popularity.

Ginkgo biloba is said to have many benefits and is used to treat depression, impotence, premenstrual syndrome, diseases of the eye (such as retinopathy and macular degeneration), and general vascular disease. Although claims abound, much of this information is scientifically unsubstantiated.

What the Science Does Say Though there is no definitive verdict on the benefits of ginkgo, numerous studies have been carried out for a variety of conditions. Some promising results have been seen for Alzheimer's disease/dementia and research continues to determine the effect on its ability to enhance memory, reduce the incidence of cardiovascular disease, and decrease the rate of premature death. NCCAM is also looking at potential interactions between ginkgo and prescription drugs.[26]

Side Effects and Precautions Most nutritional experts and physicians recommend that people who are considering using ginkgo take a 40-milligram tablet three times a day for a month or so to determine whether there is any improvement. If there is none, continuing to take this supplement is largely unwarranted. It has been shown to cause gastric irritation, headache, nausea, dizziness, or allergic reactions. Also, remember that disturbing memory loss or difficulty thinking, regardless of age, should be checked by a doctor to determine underlying causes. Ginkgo should not be taken by those taking blood thinners or at risk for bleeding.

Today, much of what we know about ginkgo biloba remains controversial, even though extensive research on its effects has been conducted. Until the results of these tests are available, consumers should use caution in any use of ginkgo.[27]

St. John's Wort

The bright yellow, star-shaped flowers of St. John's wort (SJW) have a rich and varied history in Europe, Asia, and Africa. In the United States, SJW grows in abundance in northern California and southern Oregon and is also called Klamath weed.

Today, SJW enjoys global popularity. It is the favored therapy for depression in a number of countries, including Germany, actually surpassing most standard antidepressants as the first mode of treatment for clinical depression. Research into the herb has yielded mixed results: some studies have indicated it is more effective than a placebo and has fewer side effects than prescription antidepressants, while others have found no effect on depression at all.[28]

To date, several large studies of St. John's wort have been completed and NCCAM has published the following summary points about what the scientific community has discovered so far about SJW:[29]

- There is some scientific evidence that St. John's wort is useful for treating mild to moderate depression. However, two large studies, one sponsored by NCCAM, showed that the herb was no more effective than a placebo in treating major depression of moderate severity.
- Research shows that St. John's wort interacts with some drugs, including antidepressants, anticoagulants, and birth control pills.
- It is important to remember that St. John's wort is not a proven therapy for depression. If depression is not adequately treated, it can become severe. Anyone who may have depression should see a health care provider. There are effective proven therapies available.

Like other plants, SJW contains a number of different chemicals, many of which are not clearly understood. We do know that there seems to be more to SJW than myth and the simplistic explanations that many health food stores give their customers, and researchers are beginning to view the herb in a less favorable light.

The herb also has several side effects. Most are more bothersome than severe and range from slight gastrointestinal upset to fatigue, dry mouth, anxiety, sexual dysfunction,

---

tinctures Herbal extracts usually combined with grain alcohol to prevent spoilage.

dizziness, skin rashes, and itching. Some people develop extreme sensitivity to sunlight.

Due to conflicting news about SJW, consumers should proceed with caution. Because the herb is sold in the United States as a dietary supplement, not a drug, it is not regulated by the FDA and rigorous testing has not been done. Anyone suffering from clinical depression should be under a physician's and a psychologist's care.

In addition, SJW should never be taken in combination with prescription antidepressants. When combined with other serotonin-enhancing drugs, such as Prozac, SJW may result in serotonin overload, leading to tremors, agitation, or convulsions. SJW also should not be used by pregnant women or women who are nursing, by young children, or by the frail elderly, because the safety margins have not been established.[30]

Echinacea Echinacea, or the *purple coneflower,* is found primarily in the Midwest and prairie regions of the United States. Believed to be used extensively by American Indians for centuries, echinacea eventually gained widespread acceptance in the United States before being shipped to Europe, where its use grew gradually over the eighteenth and nineteenth centuries.

> Will echinacea teas and cough drops cure my cold?

Today, echinacea is the best-selling herb in health and natural food stores in the United States and is widely used throughout most of the world. It is said to stimulate the immune system and increase the effectiveness of the white blood cells that attack bacteria and viruses. Many people believe it to be helpful in preventing and treating the symptoms of a cold or flu.

However, echinacea remains controversial. Although many studies in Europe had provided preliminary evidence of its effectiveness, a recent controlled study in the United States indicates that echinacea is no more effective than a placebo in preventing or treating a cold.[31]

As with many herbal treatments, little valid research has been conducted on the benefits and risks of echinacea. Because it can affect the immune system, people with autoimmune diseases such as arthritis should not take it. Other people who should avoid echinacea include pregnant women, people with diabetes or multiple sclerosis, anyone allergic to the daisy family of plants, and anyone undergoing chemotherapy.[32] Some studies have also raised concerns about increased risks for people who take echinacea before surgery.[33]

Green Tea Although some studies have shown promising links between green and white tea consumption and cancer prevention, recent research questions the ability of tea to significantly reduce the risk of breast, lung, or prostate cancers.[34] At the same time, other research suggests that drinking two to three cups of green tea per day may reduce the risks of heart attack and hypertension, and bolster immune function.[35] Some scientists suspect that green tea may boost heart health because it contains high levels of flavonoids. These plant compounds, which are also found in fruits, vegetables, and red wine, are thought to boost health by combating oxidation, a process in which cell-damaging free radicals accumulate. Oxidative damage can be caused by outside factors, such as cigarette smoking, or by factors on the cellular level. Oxidation is suspected of increasing the risk of heart disease, stroke, and several other diseases. Although promising, more research on the role of green tea must be conducted to determine whether its perceived benefits are actually due to the tea or to some other characteristic that tea drinkers have in common.

Ephedra (Ma Huang) An herbal ingredient formerly found in many weight-loss and fitness supplements, ephedra's active ingredient is ephedrine, which is similar to amphetamine. Comprehensive research has found that ephedra has only limited effects on weight loss and athletic performance, but numerous adverse effects, including heart attack, stroke, and death. Other side effects such as heart palpitations, psychiatric problems, upper gastrointestinal effects, tremor, and insomnia were also noted.[36] In 2004, the FDA banned the sale of all supplements containing ephedra. These products are no longer legally available for sale in the United States.

See Table 23.2 on page 684 for other herbal remedies that are popular for treating common health conditions.

Special Dietary Supplements

The FDA defines dietary supplements as "products (other than tobacco) that are intended to supplement or add to the diet and contain one or more of the following ingredients: vitamins, minerals, amino acids, herbs, or other substance that increases total dietary intake, and that is intended for ingestion in the form of a capsule, powder, soft gel, or gelcap, and is not represented as a conventional food or as a sole item." Typically, people take these supplements to improve health, prevent disease, or enhance mood. In recent years, we've heard increasing reports on the health benefits of a number of vitamins and minerals.

When taken to increase work output or the potential for it, dietary supplements are labeled as **ergogenic aids.** Examples include bee pollen, caffeine, glycine, carnitine, lecithin, brewer's yeast, and gelatin. In recent years, a new generation of performance-enhancing ergogenic aids has hit the market. Many of these claim to increase muscular strength and performance, boost energy, and enhance resistance to disease.

Muscle Enhancers As described in Chapter 14, the diet supplement androstenedione, a substance that is found naturally in meat and some plants and is also produced in the human body by the adrenal glands and gonads, is a precursor

---

ergogenic aids Special dietary supplements taken to increase strength, energy, and the ability to work.

TABLE 23.2 Herbal Remedies for Common Conditions

Condition	Herbal Product	Dose	Side Effects
Constipation	Aloe	20–30 mg hydroxyanthracene derivatives/day	Electrolyte and fluid imbalance
	Buckthorn	20–30 mg glycofrangulin/day	None known
	Cascara	20–30 mg cascaroside/day	None known
	Flaxseed	1 tbs. whole flaxseed with 8 oz. water 2–3 times/day	None if taken as directed
	Manna	20–30 g/day	Nausea, flatulence
	Psyllium	12–40 g (seed) or 4–20 g (husk) daily with 8 oz. water for every 5 g drug	Allergic reaction (rare)
	Senna leaf	20–30 mg sennoside/day	Electrolyte and fluid imbalance; can produce rebound constipation if used longer than 1–2 weeks
Dysmenorrhea (menstrual cramps)	Black cohosh	40–60% extract with alcohol	Occasionally, gastric discomfort
	Potentilla	4–6 g powdered herb	Aggravates any gastric discomforts
Leg cramps and swelling	Butcher's broom	7–11 mg ruscogenin in extract	Gastric disturbance, nausea in rare cases
	Horse chestnut	250–312.5 mg extract 2 times/day	Itching, nausea in rare cases
	Sweet clover	3–30 mg coumarin/day	May cause headache
Menopausal symptoms	Black cohosh	40–60% extract with alcohol	Occasionally, gastric discomfort
	Chaste tree fruit	30–40 mg in aqueous-alcohol extracts	May cause itching, rash
Premenstrual syndrome	Black cohosh	40–60% extract with alcohol	Occasionally, gastric discomfort
	Chaste tree fruit	30–40 mg in aqueous-alcohol extracts	May cause itching, rash
	Yarrow	4.5 g powder for infusion	None known
Sleep disturbances	Hops flower	0.5 g powder for infusion	None known
	Valerian root	2–3 g powder for infusion	None known

Source: From "New Guides to Herbal Remedies: Examples of Herbs Approved by German Commission E," *Harvard Women's Health Watch,* February 1999, © 1999, President and Fellows of Harvard College. Reprinted by permission.

to the human hormone testosterone. In other words, the body converts "andro" directly into testosterone, which enables an athlete to train harder and recover more quickly. Andro is no longer available over the counter.

Research indicates that andro has a chemical structure very similar to that of anabolic steroids. When taken over time and in sufficient quantities, andro may increase the risk of serious medical conditions.

Creatine is a naturally occurring compound found primarily in skeletal muscle that helps to optimize the muscles' energy levels. In recent years, the use of creatine supplements has increased dramatically because of claims that it increases muscle energy and allows a person to work harder with less muscle fatigue and build muscle mass with less effort. Reports of creatine's benefits, however, appear exaggerated. Over one-third of those taking creatine are unable to absorb it in the muscles and thus achieve no benefit. Side effects include muscle cramping, muscle strains, and possible liver and kidney damage.[37]

Ginseng
Grown commercially throughout many regions of North America, ginseng is much prized for its reported sexual restorative value. It is believed that ginseng affects the pitu-itary gland, increasing resistance to stress, affecting metabolism, aiding skin and muscle tone, and providing the hormonal balance necessary for a healthy sex life. Other purported benefits include improved endurance, muscle strength, recovery from exercise, oxygen metabolism during exercise, auditory and visual reaction time, and mental concentration. To date, these benefits have not been scientifically validated.[38]

Studies of the effectiveness of ginseng, however, have raised questions about the appropriate dosages. Because the potency of plants varies considerably, dosage is difficult to control and side effects are fairly common. Noteworthy side effects of high doses of ginseng include nervousness, insomnia, high blood pressure, headaches, skin eruptions, chest pain, depression, and abnormal vaginal bleeding.[39]

Glucosamine
Glucosamine is a substance produced by the body that plays a key role in the growth and development of cartilage. When present in sufficient amounts, it stimulates the manufacture of substances necessary for proper joint function and joint repair. It is manufactured commercially and sold under a variety of names, usually glucosamine sulfate.

Glucosamine has been shown to be effective for treating osteoarthritis and related degenerative joint diseases and appears to relieve swelling and decrease pain. Unlike many other herbal supplements, glucosamine sulfate has a good safety record with few noteworthy side effects. However, in recent years questions have arisen as to its effectiveness. Whereas results of meta-analysis reviews and industry-sponsored research have shown it to be moderately effective, smaller independent studies have shown no significant benefits. A large study, the Glucosamine Arthritis Intervention Trial, was recently completed and the results indicate that a combination of glucosamine and chondroitin sulfate appear to alleviate moderate to severe pain associated with osteoarthritis of the knee.[40]

SAMe SAMe (pronounced "Sammy") is the nickname for S-adenosyl-L-methionine, a compound produced biochemically in all humans to help perform some 40 functions in the body, ranging from bone preservation (hence its purported osteoarthritis benefits) to DNA replication.

SAMe has long been reported to have a significant effect on mild to moderate depression without many of the typical side effects of prescription medications, such as sexual dysfunction, weight gain, and sleep disturbance. Scientists speculate that SAMe somehow affects brain levels of the neurotransmitters noradrenaline, serotonin, and, possibly, dopamine, all of which are related to the human stress response and the origins of depression in the body.[41]

Though there has been much ado about the wonders of this natural antidepressant, much of the hype has not been substantiated in large, randomized clinical trials, the type of research necessary to validate drug claims. The most recent study shows that whereas SAMe may alleviate depression and pain compared with a placebo, its benefits compared with proven medications were insignificant. Questions still remain over how much SAMe a person should take, in what form it should be administered, and whether there are long-term side effects such as liver toxicity or cancer.

Anyone considering SAMe use should consider these factors:[42]

- Though one large, randomized trial showed modest pain relief in osteoarthritis patients using SAMe, results were not significantly better than results obtained using standard treatments.
- Many question the high cost of SAMe (between $15 and $35 or higher for 20 pills).
- Clinical depression requires more than self-treatment.
- People with a family history of cardiovascular disease should not take SAMe, due to preliminary indications that it may trigger heart problems.
- Side effects such as restlessness, anxiety, insomnia, and mania occasionally occur with use and are more common in people with bipolar disorder.

Under no circumstances should SAMe be taken by anyone on prescription antidepressants. The time lag between taking the prescription medication and beginning SAMe use, and vice versa, should be carefully considered.[43]

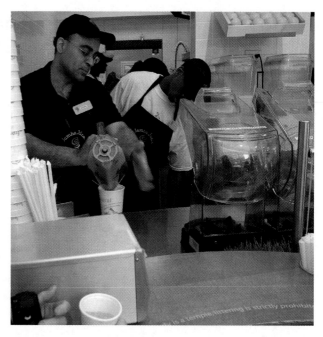

Juice drinks blended with nutraceutical ingredients ranging from protein powder to megadoses of vitamin C are popular as consumers are promised better health, more energy, and increased muscle strength by clever marketing of these products.

Antioxidants Although covered in depth in Chapter 8, it should be noted here that antioxidants are among the most sought-after supplements on the market. Primary antioxidants include beta-carotene, selenium, vitamin C, and vitamin E.

Foods as Healing Agents

Many Americans rely on *functional foods*—foods or supplements designed to improve some aspect of physical or mental functioning. Sometimes referred to as **nutraceuticals,** for their combined nutritional and pharmaceutical benefit, several are believed to actually work in much the same way as pharmaceutical drugs do in making a person well or bolstering the immune system.

Foods contain many nonnutrient active ingredients that can affect us in different ways. For example, chili peppers contain ingredients that make your eyes water and clear your sinuses. Many of these active ingredients, or constituents, can promote good health. A number of foods, such as sweet potatoes, tangerines, and red peppers, are recognized as excellent sources of antioxidants. Onion and garlic contain allium compounds that reduce blood clotting. Other foods have natural anti-inflammatory properties or aid digestion. Some are known by the term *probiotics,* foods that promote good bacteria in the body that may help fight off infection.[44]

nutraceuticals Term often used interchangeably with *functional foods;* refers to the combined nutritional and pharmaceutical benefit derived through use of foods or food supplements.

Supplement	Use	Claims of Benefits	Risks
Chaparral	Sold as teas and pills	Fights cancer and purifies blood	Linked to serious liver damage
Comfrey	Originated as a poultice to reduce swelling, but later used internally	Wound healing, infection control	Contains alkaloids toxic to the liver, and animal studies suggest it is carcinogenic
Melatonin	"Clock hormone"	Role in regulating circadian rhythms and sleep patterns	Anti-aging claims unfounded
DHEA (dehydroepiandrosterone)	Hormone that turns into estrogen and testosterone in the body	Fights aging, boosts immunity, strengthens bones, and improves brain functioning	No anti-aging benefits proven; could increase cancer risk and lead to liver damage, even when taken briefly
Dieters' teas	Herbal blends containing senna, aloe, rhubarb root, buckthorn, cascara, and castor oil	Act as laxatives	Can disrupt potassium levels and cause heart arrhythmias; linked to diarrhea, vomiting, chronic constipation, fainting, and death
Pennyroyal (member of the mint family)	—	Soothing effect in teas	Pregnancy-related complications, heart arrhythmias, coma, convulsions, death
Sassafras	Once a flavoring in root beer, used in tonics and teas	No real claims	Shown to cause liver cancer in animals
Flaxseeds	Produce linseed oil	Omega-3 fatty acid benefits	Delay absorption of medicine
Kava	Teas and pills	Relaxation	Increases the effects of alcohol and other drugs; associated with severe liver damage
High-dose vitamin E	Antioxidant	Reduces risk of heart disease; better survivability after heart attack	Causes bleeding when taking blood thinners
Vitamin C	Antioxidant, manufactures collagen, wound repair, nerve transmission	Improves blood vessel relaxation in people with CVD, diabetes, hypertension, and other problems; can relieve pain of angina pectoris	None known
L-Carnitine	Amino acid	Improves metabolism in heart muscle, purported to increase fat-burning enzymes	Heart palpitations, arrhythmias, sudden death; claims largely unsubstantiated
Licorice root	Sweetener, used in cough drops	None proven	Speeds potassium loss
Niacin (vitamin B_3)	Reduces serum lipids, vasodilation, and increases blood flow	—	Skin flushing, gastrointestinal distress, stomach pain, nausea and vomiting
Chondroitin (shark cartilage or sea cucumber)	—	Improves osteoporosis and arthritis by improving cartilage function	Fewer benefits than glucosamine; benefits still unproven

Some of the most common healthful foods and their purported benefits include (also see Chapter 8 for more information on many of these):

■ *Plant stanol.* Can lower "bad" (LDL) cholesterol.
■ *Oat fiber.* Can lower "bad" (LDL) cholesterol; serves as a natural soother of nerves; stabilizes blood sugar levels.
■ *Sunflower.* Can lower risk of heart disease; may prevent angina.

■ *Soy protein.* May lower heart disease risk; provides protective estrogen-like effect; may reduce risk from certain cancers.
■ *Garlic.* Lowers cholesterol and reduces clotting tendency of blood; lowers blood pressure; may serve as a form of antibiotic.
■ *Ginger.* Fights motion sickness, stomach pain and upset; discourages blood clots; may relieve rheumatism.
■ *Yogurt.* Yogurt that is labeled "Live Active Culture" contains active, friendly bacteria that can fight off infections.

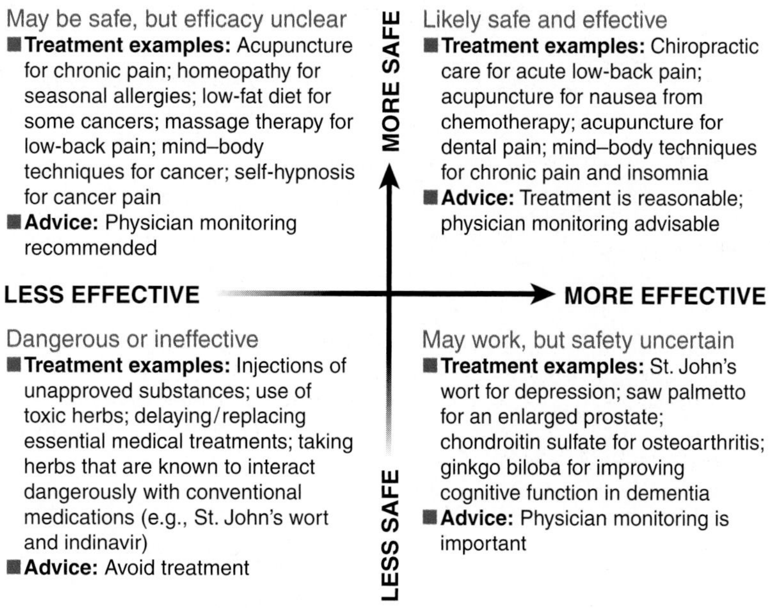

May be safe, but efficacy unclear
- **Treatment examples:** Acupuncture for chronic pain; homeopathy for seasonal allergies; low-fat diet for some cancers; massage therapy for low-back pain; mind–body techniques for cancer; self-hypnosis for cancer pain
- **Advice:** Physician monitoring recommended

Likely safe and effective
- **Treatment examples:** Chiropractic care for acute low-back pain; acupuncture for nausea from chemotherapy; acupuncture for dental pain; mind–body techniques for chronic pain and insomnia
- **Advice:** Treatment is reasonable; physician monitoring advisable

MORE SAFE

LESS EFFECTIVE ←————————————→ **MORE EFFECTIVE**

Dangerous or ineffective
- **Treatment examples:** Injections of unapproved substances; use of toxic herbs; delaying/replacing essential medical treatments; taking herbs that are known to interact dangerously with conventional medications (e.g., St. John's wort and indinavir)
- **Advice:** Avoid treatment

May work, but safety uncertain
- **Treatment examples:** St. John's wort for depression; saw palmetto for an enlarged prostate; chondroitin sulfate for osteoarthritis; ginkgo biloba for improving cognitive function in dementia
- **Advice:** Physician monitoring is important

LESS SAFE

FIGURE 23.3 Assessing the Risks and Benefits of CAM Treatments
Medical experts devised this chart to gauge the potential liability of recommending alternative treatments, but it can also help patients choose treatments based on safety and effectiveness by determining how the treatment is categorized.

Source: Figure from M. H. Cohen and D. M. Eisenberg, "Potential Physician Malpractice Liability Associated with Complementary and Integrative Medical Therapies," *Annals of Internal Medicine* 136, no. 8 (2002): 596–603.

Table 23.3 lists other foods and supplements with their risks and benefits.

Many people purchase foods labeled *organic* because they expect these products to contain only health-promoting substances. See Chapter 8 for a complete discussion of what it means for a food to be labeled organic.

Protecting Consumers and Regulating Claims

Although many CAM products appear promising, be aware that most of them are not regulated in the United States as strictly as are foods and drugs. This is in sharp contrast to nations such as Germany, where the government holds companies to strict standards for ingredients and manufacturing. In the United States, nutritional supplements have had a long history of unregulated growth, including an abundance of claims and testimonials about their supposed health-enhancing attributes. With few regulatory controls in place, many get-rich-quick charlatans have jumped into the health food and CAM market. As their profits soar, more and more companies eagerly join them. Unfortunately, this trend means that issues related to consumer safety and protection from fraudulent claims will also grow more urgent and continue to raise serious questions about our current regulatory system. It is

important to have as much information as possible to make a smart decision when evaluating CAM options (Figure 23.3).

Strategies to Protect Consumers' Health

The burgeoning popularity of nutraceuticals and functional foods concerns many scientists. According to National Institutes of Health (NIH) nutritional biochemist Dr. Terry Krakower:

> NIH does have some concerns about them, and we are looking into them, especially the potential for interaction with other medications. We advise anyone who uses them to talk to their physician. [Functional foods] are so new we don't know yet if they are good, bad, or indifferent. [Much] of the herb content in these food products is so small that it's probably ineffective, and if it were included in large amounts, it could be harmful. Anyone taking these supplements, whether in pill form or in foods, should do their homework and thoroughly research them rather than rely on health claims made by manufacturers.[45]

By legal definition, herbal remedies, dietary supplements, and functional foods are neither prescription drugs nor over-the-counter medications. Instead, classified as food supplements, they can be sold without FDA approval. As they

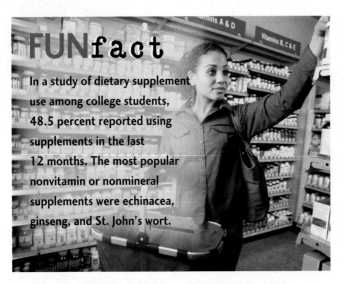

FIGURE 23.4 Do College Students Use Supplements?

Source: H. Newberry et al., "Use of Nonvitamin, Nonmineral Dietary Supplements among College Students," *Journal of American College Health* 50, no. 3 (2001): 123–129.

are not regulated by the FDA, these products are not subject to the strict guidelines that govern the research and development of medications. Many are not labeled with the precise amount of chemicals in the product, and the labels provide little guidance on how they should be used. They are not supposed to be accompanied by claims of therapeutic benefit, but they often are. Because they are available without a prescription, this poses risks for unsuspecting consumers, raising issues of consumer safety to new levels.

Even when products are dispensed by CAM practitioners, the situation can be risky. Some homeopaths and herbalists who mix their own tonics may not use standardized measures. Unfortunately, some unskilled and untrained people, who do not fully understand the potential chemical interactions of their preparations, are treating patients.

Consumer groups, members of the scientific community, and government officials are calling for action. Pressure is mounting to establish consistent standards for herbal supplements and functional foods similar to those used in Germany and other countries. Many scientists advocate a more stringent FDA approval process for virtually all supplements sold in the United States.

The German Commission E

The German Commission E has been among the most noteworthy of the international groups attempting to regulate the sale of alternative medicines and supplements. Consisting of

phytomedicines   Another name for medicinal herbs, many of which are sold over the counter in Europe.

an expert panel established in 1970, its mission was to conduct a formal evaluation of the hundreds of herbal remedies that have been part of traditional German medicine for centuries. Commission members carefully analyzed data from clinical trials, observational studies, biological experiments, and chemical analyses.

Essentially, the German Commission E analyzed a growing list of **phytomedicines,** another name for medicinal herbs, many of which are sold over the counter in Europe. Typically, phytomedicines are integrated into conventional medical practice and are prepared in several different ways, usually as tablets or powders.[46] Many are sold in much the same way as over-the-counter remedies in the United States, but research continues on many of these products.

Looking to Science for More Answers

Even as CAM treatments gain credibility, this credibility still must be tempered with good science. Although slow in coming, legislators have pushed for better science, increased funding, and an agency designed to garner information useful to consumers. One result is the National Center for Complementary and Alternative Medicine (NCCAM), which has a budget of nearly $70 million with which to fund its own projects. The NCCAM has established research centers at universities and other institutions throughout the United States, where many clinical trials are being conducted.[47] In addition, numerous studies into alternative treatments such as acupuncture, green tea, fish oil, flaxseed, shark cartilage, and others are taking place across the United States. See the New Horizons in Health box for some of the latest in research news. One of the most promising aspects of this research is the enthusiastic support of professionals who have the training and laboratory expertise to evaluate the efficacy of market-driven claims. To read about test results and new initiatives, go to the NCCAM website (http://nccam.nih.gov).

Though some alternative therapies, such as acupuncture, have been widely studied, there is little quality research to support the many claims about nutraceuticals. If you are considering the use of herbal supplements or functional foods, consult the NCCAM website or the *Cochrane Review on Complementary and Alternative Medicine* (www.cochrane.org).

Healthy Living in the New Millennium

Clearly, CAM appears to serve a very real need for consumers. But while consumers are making the adjustment to CAM in record numbers, members of the health care delivery system seem slow to act. Although progress has been noted, there is still a long way to go before CAM becomes fully accepted in mainstream medical practice.

NEWS FROM THE WORLD OF CAM RESEARCH

Research is being conducted on complementary and alternative therapies in all areas of health, with treatments for some conditions making headlines. Several new studies provide promising insight into CAM therapies. Educating yourself on the results of the most current information will help you separate fact from fiction when evaluating the benefits and risks of the many CAM therapies available today.

CANCER

Choosing CAM over conventional treatment is risky business. However, promising new research indicates that when CAM is coupled with conventional medicine, treatment may be more bearable and survival rates may improve. Interesting points include:

- High doses of vitamin E and ginkgo biloba have anticoagulant effects that could cause excessive bleeding during surgery, particularly in those already taking aspirin. Soy contains plant estrogens that have not been ruled out as having a role in causing breast or endometrial cancer.
- Although several small studies have shown that green tea prevents breast and prostate cancer, the FDA has recently reviewed several large, well-controlled studies that refute this claim.
- Mind–body therapies, acupuncture, massage, and other remedies may help comfort patients, relieve physical symptoms such as pain and insomnia, alleviate nausea, and improve recovery from treatment.

CARDIOVASCULAR DISEASE

Diet and exercise provide nearly undisputable benefits for reducing CVD risks. Research on other natural strategies is mixed. Findings include:

- The Harvard Nurses' Health Study and Health Professionals' Follow-Up Study found reduced rates of CVD in people whose diets are rich in antioxidants such as vitamin E, vitamin A, and beta-carotene. However, other studies have refuted these results.
- A large study of chelation therapy (a technique used to clear toxic metals from the bloodstream) may provide results within the next five years. Until then, the jury is out on this one.

ARTHRITIS

Traditional treatment for arthritis sufferers has focused on acetaminophen (Tylenol) or nonsteroidal anti-inflammatory drugs (NSAIDs) such as aspirin, ibuprofen (Advil), naproxen (Aleve), and celecoxib (Celebrex). However, with the safety of these drugs now in question, many people are seeking alternatives:

- *Glucosamine.* Glucosamine is a substance that occurs naturally in the body, and works to repair cartilage. Although glucosamine has been an effective anti-inflammatory in animal studies, newer research indicates that it can interfere with insulin, causing increases in blood sugar. It may also interfere with the effectiveness of certain cancer therapies and irritate asthma sufferers.
- *Chondroitin.* Often used with glucosamine, chondroitin may also elevate blood sugar levels and lead to excessive bleeding, particularly among those already on blood thinners and with other risks.

SLEEP DISORDERS

Some of the nearly 70 million Americans who have trouble sleeping turn to CAM therapies. Common CAM treatments include valerian and melatonin dietary supplements, meditation, acupuncture, and yoga. To date, most of these therapies have not been proven effective for insomnia problems.

THE COMMON COLD

Recent results of a well-controlled trial indicate that echinacea is not effective in preventing or treating the common cold. The best ways to prevent a cold are washing your hands regularly, proper nutrition, getting enough rest and exercise, and keeping stress under control.

Sources: Adapted from W. Weiger and D. Eisenberg, "Health for Life: The New Science of Alternative Medicine. Cancer: Easing the Treatment," *Newsweek,* December 2, 2002: 49; W. Haskell and D. Eisenberg, "Health for Life: The New Science of Alternative Medicine. Cardiac Disease: Ways to Heal Your Heart," *Newsweek,* December 2, 2002: 52; National Center for Complementary and Alternative Medicine, "Can't Sleep? Science Seeking New Answers," *CAM at the NIH: Focus on Complementary and Alternative Medicine* 11, no. 3 (2005): 1–2, 6–7; R. B. Turner et al., "An Evaluation of *Echinacea angustifolia* in Experimental Rhinovirus Infections," *The New England Journal of Medicine* 353, no. 4 (2005): 341–348; J. A. Tayler et al., "Efficacy and Safety of Echinacea in Treating Upper Respiratory Tract Infections in Children: A Randomized, Controlled Trial," *Journal of the American Medical Association* 290, no. 21 (2003): 2824–2930.

Enlisting Support from Insurers and Providers

More and more insurers are hiring alternative practitioners as staff or covering alternative care as a routine benefit, at least to some degree. This is especially true as criticisms of managed care increase and government agencies get involved.

The changing nature of health maintenance organizations (HMOs) and health care insurers makes it impossible to determine exactly how many insurance companies cover CAM therapies today. What is known is that the numbers are increasing despite a reimbursement system that is biased in favor of traditional treatments. For example, whereas the nation's insurers spend over $30 billion a year on bypass surgery and angioplasty for cardiovascular disease, only 40 companies cover the lifestyle-based program developed by Dr. Dean Ornish—and this despite repeated compelling research demonstrating that the program is safe, effective, and much cheaper than surgery.[48] In some cases, consumers are offered an optional "extra-cost" rider on their insurance policy, through which they may choose to consult alternative practitioners for a higher premium and copayment agreement. For many consumers, just knowing they have a choice seems to be worth the extra cost.

Support from professional organizations, such as the AMA, is also increasing, as more physician training programs require or offer electives in alternative treatment modalities. In many cases, medical schools are educating a new generation of medical doctors to be better prepared to advise patients about the pros and cons of alternative treatments and how to follow integrative practices. Studies comparing the efficacy of alternative strategies with that of conventional treatments are becoming more comprehensive. Although alternative medicine is becoming increasingly integrated into U.S. health care programs and plans, there is still a long way to go. As we learn more, we will be better able to apply both conventional and alternative care.

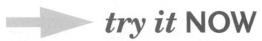

try it NOW

What kinds of CAM resources are available to you? Check with your college's health clinic and find out what types of alternative therapies it offers. Acupuncture? Massage for back injuries? Chiropractor visits? Or check with your health care insurance provider and see what is covered. Be sure to ask what expenses you'll be responsible for, and if you are limited to a certain network of practitioners.

Self-Care: Protecting Yourself

Any decision you make about your health is important, whether it be what you eat and drink, how you exercise, or other day-to-day decisions. None are more important than the decisions you make about health care treatments and whether or not you use traditional medicines or opt for some of the complementary and alternative medicine treatments discussed in this chapter.

For instance, checking on the education and training of anyone who recommends or sells herbal medications is part of intelligent consumerism as well as just plain good sense. The NCCAM website is a good place to start, because it includes summaries of recent research. In fact, it is a good resource for information on the effectiveness and risks of any CAM therapy discussed in this chapter.

To help you in making all your health care decisions, review this list of considerations from NCCAM and elsewhere:[49]

- Take charge of your health by being an informed consumer. Find out what scientific studies have been done on the safety and effectiveness of the CAM treatment in which you are interested. Don't rely on friends or testimonials.
- Remember that decisions about treatment should be made in consultation with a qualified health care provider and based on the condition and needs of each person. Discuss information on CAM with your health care provider before making any decisions.
- If you use any CAM therapy, inform your primary health care provider. This is for your safety and so your health care provider can develop a comprehensive treatment plan. It is particularly important to talk with your provider if you are thinking about replacing your prescribed treatment with one or more supplements; are currently taking a prescription drug; have a chronic medical condition; are planning to have surgery; are pregnant or nursing; or are thinking about giving supplements to children or pets.
- If you use a CAM therapy provided by a practitioner, such as acupuncture, choose the practitioner with care. Check with your insurer to see if the services will be covered. (See the Skills for Behavior Change box for more information on selecting a CAM provider.)
- Consult only reliable sources—texts, journals, periodicals, and government resources. Start with the websites listed at the end of this and every chapter.
- Remember that *natural* and *safe* are not necessarily synonyms. Many people have become seriously ill from seemingly harmless products. For example, some have suffered serious liver damage from sipping teas brewed with comfrey, an herb used in poultices and ointments to treat sprains and bruises and that should not be taken internally. Pregnant women face special risks from herbs such as echinacea, senna, comfrey, and licorice.
- Realize that in the United States, no one is closely monitoring the purity of herbal supplements. The FDA has verified industry reports that certain shipments of ginseng were contaminated with high levels of fungicides. Other problems with imported herbs have been noted.
- Recognize that dosage levels in many herbal products are not regulated. German manufacturers produce identical batches of herbal remedies as required by law. Look for reputable manufacturers.
- Always look for the word *standardized* on any herbal product you buy. This indicates that manufacturing is monitored to ensure that the dosage and content are the same in every pill or tablet.
- Be aware that herbal medications can interact with prescription and over-the-counter medications.

Also, be cautious about combining herbal medications, just as you should be cautious about combining other drugs. Always remember that just because something is natural, it doesn't mean it is safe. Remember that no herbal medicine is likely to work miracles. Monitor your health, and seek help if you notice any unusual side effects from herbal products.

SKILLS FOR *behavior change*

SELECTING A CAM PROVIDER

Selecting a CAM practitioner—indeed, any health care provider—can be difficult. Although these recommendations apply to CAM, also consider them when selecting any health care product or service. Before starting a CAM therapy or choosing a practitioner, talk with your primary health care provider(s) and others who are knowledgeable about CAM. If they dismiss the therapy, ask why. Check their explanations with other sources to see if their insights are confirmed.

FINDING A CAM PRACTITIONER

- Ask your doctor or other health professional to recommend or refer you to a CAM therapist, or consult someone you trust who has used CAM; they may have recommendations based on experience.
- If your therapy will be covered by insurance, ask your carrier for a list of approved CAM providers.
- Contact a professional organization for the type of practitioner you are seeking. Often they have standards of practice and websites or publications that list recommended providers. These resources will also answer common questions that you might have. If there is a regulatory or licensing board for this specialty, verify that your practitioner has the proper credentials.

INTERVIEWING A CAM PRACTITIONER

- Make a list of your options, and gather information about each before making your first visit. Ask basic questions about providers' credentials and experience. Where did they obtain their training? What supporting degrees, licenses, or certifications do they have?
- Write down questions to ask at your first visit. You may want to bring a friend or family member who can help you ask questions and note answers.
- Bring medical information with you, including any tests you've had, information about your health history, surgical history, allergies, and any medications (including prescription, over-the-counter, and herbal or other supplements) you are taking.
- Ask if there are diseases or health conditions in which the practitioner specializes and how frequently he or she treats patients with conditions like yours.
- Ask if there is any scientific research supporting the use of this treatment for your condition.

- Is the provider supportive of conventional as well as CAM treatments? Does he or she have a good relationship with conventional practitioners in order to give referrals to them?
- How many patients per day does the provider see, and how much time is spent with each one?
- What are the charges and payment options? What percentage of the payment might you have to pay out of pocket?

After the visit, assess the interaction and how you felt about the practitioner.

INVESTIGATING THE RECOMMENDED TREATMENT

Ask your CAM practitioner:

- What benefits can I expect from this therapy? What are the risks and side effects? Do the benefits outweigh the risks?
- Will I need to buy any special equipment or take any special supplements?
- Will this therapy interfere with any conventional medical treatments?
- If there are problems, where would I be referred for further treatment?
- What is the history of success in treating this type of condition for someone of my age and health status?

As we enter a new era of medicine, more than ever you are being called upon to take responsibility for what goes into your body. This means you must educate yourself. CAM can offer new avenues toward better health, but it is up to you to make sure that you are on the right path.

 what do you THINK?

What can you do as a consumer to obtain the greatest benefit from CAM? ■ **How can you protect yourself from possible negative risks?**

TAKING charge

Summary

- People throughout the world are choosing complementary and alternative medicine options, and these numbers are growing exponentially. Compared with other countries, the United States has been relatively slow to turn to alternative treatment and medicine.
- The National Center for Complementary and Alternative Medicine groups CAM practices into five major domains: (1) alternative medical systems (which cut across all domains); (2) manipulative and body-based methods (manipulation or movement of one or more body parts); (3) energy medicine (use of biofields or energy fields); (4) mind–body medicine (a variety of techniques designed to enhance the mind's ability to affect bodily function and symptoms); and (5) biologically based practices (including substances found in nature, such as herbs and vitamin megadoses). Acupuncture and acupressure, two derivatives of energy medicine, are among the more popular forms of traditional Chinese medicine in the United States.
- Herbal remedies, largely derived from traditional Chinese medicine, include ginkgo biloba, St. John's wort, echinacea, and green tea. Other herbal remedies have also received widespread attention as potential miracle drugs without having harmful side effects. Special supplements include muscle enhancers, ginseng, glucosamine, chromium picolinate, SAMe, and antioxidants. A number of functional foods may also serve as healing agents.
- Though many positive effects are associated with CAM, there are also many risks. The drive for profits and the lack of strict government regulation in the United States make the CAM market a free-for-all. As a consumer, you must be aware of the risks and check reputable sources to ensure that you are not being lured by false claims and promises.
- Health in the new millennium provides an interesting assortment of choices for health care consumers. By enlisting the support of health professionals and health care services and by making informed decisions, you will reap positive rewards in your quest for health enhancement in the days ahead.

Chapter Review

1. The broad range of nontraditional healing philosophies and therapies in health care are known as
   a. consumer medicine.
   b. complementary medicine.
   c. alternative medicine.
   d. Answers B and C.

2. Consumers most often turn to complementary and alternative medicines
   a. for terminal illness such as cancer.
   b. for recurring pain of the back, neck, or joints.
   c. for spiritual problems.
   d. when all else fails and this is a last resort for help.

3. Chiropractic is in which category of CAM practices?
   a. energy therapies
   b. mind–body medicine
   c. manipulative methods
   d. alternative medical systems

4. Acupuncture looks at the disturbances in the energy flows along the body and uses a series of _____ to treat the patient:
   a. needles
   b. medicines
   c. herbs
   d. hand manipulatives

5. The CAM therapy that utilizes the idea of increasing dilution and lowering the dosage of the substance to improve efficacy is
   a. ayurveda.
   b. homeopathy.
   c. naturopathy.
   d. herbal medicine.

6. Chiropractic treatment is based on the theory that diseases can be caused by
   a. misalignment of the bones.
   b. poor eating habits.
   c. taking too many drugs.
   d. muscle atrophy.

7. The use of techniques to improve the psychoneuro-immunology of the human body is called
   a. acupressure.
   b. mind–body medicine.
   c. reiki.
   d. body work.

8. The most controversial domain of the complementary and alternative medicines is
   a. mind–body medicine.
   b. manipulative medicines.
   c. energy medicines.
   d. biologically-based therapies.

9. The best-selling herbal remedy in health and natural food stores in the United States is
   a. green tea.
   b. ginkgo biloba.
   c. St. John's wort.
   d. echinacea.

10. What alternative medicine system places equal emphasis on body, mind, and spirit and strives to restore the innate harmony of the individual?
    a. ayurvedic medicine
    b. homeopathic medicine
    c. naturopathic medicine
    d. traditional Chinese medicine

Answers to these questions can be found on page A-1.

Questions for Discussion and Reflection

1. What are some of the potential benefits and risks of CAM? Why do you think these practices and products are becoming so popular?
2. What are some of the major domains of CAM treatments? Have you tried any of them? Would you feel comfortable trying any new ones? Why or why not?
3. What are the major herbal remedies? Special supplements? What are some of the risks and benefits associated with each?
4. What can you do to ensure that you are receiving accurate information regarding CAM treatments or medicines? Which federal agency oversees CAM in the United States?
5. What is being done in the United States to ensure continued growth of CAM?

Accessing Your Health on the Internet

The following websites explore further topics and issues related to personal health. You'll also find links to each organization's website on the Companion Website for *Access to Health*, Tenth Edition, at www.aw-bc.com/donatelle.

1. *Acupuncture.com.* Provides resources for consumers regarding traditional Asian therapies, geared to students and practitioners. www.acupuncture.com
2. *ClinicalTrials.gov.* Includes the latest information on CAM research and clinical trials. Search for results from NCCAM and complementary and alternative medicine. http://clinicaltrials.gov
3. *National Center for Complementary and Alternative Medicine.* A division of the National Institutes of Health dedicated to providing the latest information on complementary and alternative practices. www.nccam.nih.gov
4. *National Institutes of Health, Office of Dietary Supplements.* An excellent resource for information on dietary supplements. http://dietary-supplements.info.nih.gov
5. *CARDS (Computer Access to Research on Dietary Supplements).* This website includes a database of federally funded research projects pertaining to dietary supplements. http://dietary-supplements.info.nih.gov

Further Reading

Blumenthal, M., ed. *Complete German Commission E Monographs: Therapeutic Guide to Herbal Medicines.* Austin, TX: The American Botanical Council, 1998.

  Overview of the German Commission E findings and relevant information about supplement research for consumers. Provides an interesting perspective on international herbal research, policies, recommendations, and future directions.

Cuellar, N. *Conversations in Complementary and Alternative Medicine: Insights and Perspectives from a Leading Practitioner.* Sudbury, MA: Jones and Bartlett, 2006.

  Based on interviews with 27 leading experts in CAM, including acupuncturists, chiropractors, massage therapists, and herbalists. Includes questions about practice, education, and research.

Rakel, D. *Complementary Medicine in Practice.* Sudbury, MA: Jones and Bartlett, 2006.

  Evidence-based overview of common CAM therapies, particularly those supported by research and accepted by physicians and consumers.

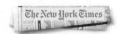

e-themes from *The New York Times*

For up-to-date articles about current health issues, visit
www.aw-bc.com/donatelle, select *Access to Health,* Tenth
Edition, Chapter 23, and click on "e-themes."

References

1. National Center for Complementary and Alternative Medicine, "The Use of Complementary and Alternative Medicine in the United States," 2006, http://nccam.nih.gov/news/camsurvey_fs1.htm.

2. National Center for Complementary and Alternative Medicine, "What Is Complementary and Alternative Medicine (CAM)?" 2006, www.nccam.nih.gov/health/whatiscam/.

3. National Center for Complementary and Alternative Medicine, "Funding Strategy: Fiscal Year 2006," 2006, http://nccam.nih.gov/research/strategy/2006.htm.

4. Eisenberg et al., "Unconventional Medicine in the United States: Prevalence, Costs, and Patterns of Use," *New England Journal of Medicine* 328, no. 4 (1993): 246–252.

5. P. Barnes et al., "CDC Advance Data Report: Complementary and Alternative Medicine among Adults: United States, 2005," 2006, http://nccam.nih.gov/news/camsurvey.htm.

6. National Center for Complementary and Alternative Medicine, "CAM at the NIH: A Closer Look at Ayurvedic Medicine," 2006, http://nccam.nih.gov/news/newsletter/2006_winter/ayurveda.htm.

7. Ibid.

8. Ibid.

9. National Center for Complementary and Alternative Medicine, "What Is Complementary and Alternative Medicine (CAM)?"

10. British Medical Association, "Complementary Medicine: New Approaches to Good Practice," 2006, www.bma.org.uk; P. DeSmet, "Herbal Medicine in Europe—Releasing Regulatory Standard," *New England Journal of Medicine,* 352 (2005): 1176–1178; D. Sibbritt et al., "A Longitudinal Analysis of Mid-Age Women's Use of CAM in Australia," *Women's Health,* 40 (2004): 41–56.

11. P. Barnes et al., "CDC Advance Data Report."

12. University of Washington School of Medicine, "Chiropractic Medicine," 2004, www.fammed.washington.edu/predoctoral/CAM/images/chiro.pdf; D. C. Cherkin et al., "A Review of the Evidence of the Effectiveness, Safety, and Cost of Acupuncture, Massage Therapy, and Spinal Manipulation for Back Pain," *Annals of Internal Medicine* 138, no. 11 (2003): 898–906.

13. National Center for Complementary and Alternative Medicine, "What Is CAM?"

14. Ibid.

15. Ibid.

16. Ibid.

17. Ibid.

18. NIH Consensus Panel, "Acupuncture: National Institutes of Health Consensus Development Panel Statement," 2006, www.odp.od.nih.gov/consensus; B. Berman et al., "Effectiveness of Acupuncture as Adjunct Therapy in Osteoarthritis of the Knee: A Randomized, Controlled Trial," *Annals of Internal Medicine* 141, no. 12 (2004): 901–910; C. Karels et al., "Treatment of Arm, Neck, and Shoulder Complaints," *Spine* 31, no. 17 (2006): E584–E589.

19. A. Weil, *Spontaneous Healing: How to Discover and Embrace Your Body's Natural Ability to Maintain and Heal Itself* (New York: Ballantine Books, 2004).

20. B. Seaward, *Managing Stress,* 5th ed. (Sudbury, MA: Jones and Bartlett, 2006); D. Tosevski et al., "Stressful Life Events and Physical Health," *Current Opinions in Psychiatry* 19, no. 2 (2006): 184–189.

21. J. Robins et al., "Research in Psychoneuroimmunology: Tai Chi as a Stress Management Approach for Individuals with HIV Disease," *Applied Nursing Research* 19, no. 1 (2006): 2–9; M. Opp et al., "Sleep and Psychoneuroimmunology," *Neurology Clinician* 24, no. 3 (2006): 493–506; A. Starkweather et al., "Immune Function, Pain, and Psychological Stress in Patients Undergoing Spinal Surgery," *Spine* 31, no. 18 (2006): E641–E647.

22. P. DeSmart, "Health Risks of Herbal Remedies: An Update," *Perspectives in Clinical Pharmacology* 76, no. 1 (2004): 1–17.

23. E. Ernst, "Herbal Remedies for Anxiety: A Systematic Review of Controlled Clinical Trials," *Phytomedicine* 13, no. 3 (2006): 205–208.

24. Ibid.

25. J. Kleignene and P. Knipschild, "Ginkgo Biloba," *The Lancet* 340 (1992): 1136–1139.

26. P. R. Solomon et al., "Ginkgo for Memory Enhancement: A Randomized, Controlled Trial," *Journal of the American Medical Association* 288, no. 7 (2002): 835–840; "Ginkgo Biloba," in *Encyclopedia of Dietary Supplements,* ed. P. Coates, M. Blackman, and G. Cragg (New York, NY: Marcel Dekker, 2005): 249–257.

27. National Center for Complementary and Alternative Medicine, "What Is CAM?"

28. National Center for Complementary and Alternative Medicine, "St. John's Wort and Depression," 2006, http://nccam.nih.gov/.

29. National Center for Complementary and Alternative Medicine, "St. John's Wort and the Treatment of Depression," 2005, http://nccam.nih.gov/; Natural Medicines Comprehensive Database, "St. John's Wort," 2005, www.naturaldatabase.com.

30. Ibid.

31. R. Turner et al., "An Evaluation of Echinacea in Experimental Rhinovirus Infections," *New England Journal of Medicine* 353, no. 4 (2005): 341–348.

32. S. M. Yu, R. M. Ghandour, and Z. J. Haung, "Herbal Supplement Use among U.S. Women, 2000" *Journal of the American Medical Women's Association,* 59, no. 1 (2004): 17–24; B. Barrett, "Efficacy and Safety of Echinacea in Treating Upper Respiratory Tract Infections in Children: A Randomized, Controlled Trial," *Journal of Pediatrics* 145, no. 1 (2004): 135–136; "Does an Echinacea Preparation Prevent Colds? The Debate Continues," *Child Health Alert,* April 22, 2004, 1–2; S. Shaber, "Echinacea for the Common Cold," *Annals of Internal Medicine* 139, no. 7 (2003): 600.

33. A. Sparreboom et al., "Herbal Remedies in the United States: Potential Adverse Interactions with Anti-Cancer Agents," *Journal of Clinical Oncology* 22, no. 12 (2004): 2489–2503.

34. Center for Food Safety and Applied Nutrition, "Green Tea and Reduced Risk of Cancer Health Claim," 2005, www.cfsan.fda.gov/~dms/ghc/gtea.html.

35. C. Cabrera et al., "Beneficial Effects of Green Tea: A Review," *Journal of American College Nutrition* 25, no. 2 (2006): 79–99.

36. U.S. Food and Drug Administration, "Sales of Supplements Containing Ephedrine Alkaloids (Ephedra) Prohibited," 2004, www.fda.gov/oc/initiatives/ephedra/february2004.

37. Mayoclinic.com, "Performance Enhancing Drugs: Dangerous, Damaging and Potentially Deadly," 2004, www.mayoclinic.com

38. T. Palisin et al., "Ginseng: Is It In the Root?" *Current Sports Medicine Report* 5, no. 4 (2006): 210–214.

39. Ibid.

40. D. Clegg et al., "Glucosamine, Chondroitin Sulfate and the Two in Combination for Painful Knee Osteoarthritis," *New England Journal of Medicine* 354 (2006): 795–808.

41. National Center for Complementary and Alternative Medicine, "What Is CAM?" 2006, www.nccam.nih.gov/health/whatiscam/.

42. Agency for Healthcare Research and Quality, "S-Adenosyl-L-Methionine for Treatment of Depression, Osteoarthritis, and Liver Disease," *Evidence Report/Technology Assessment* 64, August 2002, www.ahrq.gov/clinic/epcsums/samesum.htm.

43. Ibid.

44. Ibid.

45. S. Dixon, "Food for Thought: Prebiotics and Probiotics: What Are They and Why Should You Eat Them?" 2003, www.cancer.med.umich.edu/newspro09spr02.htm.

46. American Botanical Council, "Commission E," January 2003, www.herbalgram.org/default.asp?c=comm_e_catalog.

47. National Center for Complementary and Alternative Medicine, "What Is CAM?" 2006, http://nccam.nih.gov/health/whatiscam/.

48. National Center for Complementary and Alternative Medicine, "CAM Centers of Research: Overview of the Specialty Centers," 2004, http://nccam.nih.gov/nccam/research/centers.html.

49. "Health for Life: Inside the Science of Alternative Medicine," *Newsweek,* December 2, 2002. National Center for Complementary and Alternative Medicine, "Are You Considering Using Complementary and Alternative Medicine (CAM)?" 2002, http://nccam.nih.gov/health/decisions/index.htm.

ANSWERS TO CHAPTER REVIEW QUESTIONS

Chapter 1
1. b; 2. d; 3. c; 4. c; 5. b;
6. d; 7. b; 8. a; 9. b; 10. d

Chapter 2
1. b; 2. d; 3. d; 4. c; 5. c;
6. a; 7. b; 8. b; 9. d; 10. c

Chapter 3
1. a; 2. d; 3. d; 4. c; 5. d;
6. c; 7. b; 8. c; 9. c; 10. b

Chapter 4
1. a; 2. d; 3. d; 4. d; 5. b;
6. c; 7. a; 8. c; 9. b; 10. d

Chapter 5
1. c; 2. a; 3. b; 4. d; 5. c;
6. c; 7. c; 8. d; 9. a; 10. c

Chapter 6
1. c; 2. d; 3. c; 4. a; 5. a;
6. d; 7. b; 8. b; 9. b; 10. a

Chapter 7
1. d; 2. d; 3. d; 4. c; 5. c;
6. a; 7. b; 8. c; 9. a; 10. d

Chapter 8
1. b; 2. a; 3. d; 4. d; 5. b;
6. a; 7. c; 8. d; 9. d; 10. c

Chapter 9
1. c; 2. d; 3. b; 4. b; 5. c;
6. b; 7. d; 8. c; 9. d; 10. d

Chapter 10
1. d; 2. a; 3. b; 4. c; 5. d;
6. d; 7. a; 8. c; 9. b; 10. a

Chapter 11
1. a; 2. b; 3. b; 4. c; 5. d;
6. b; 7. d; 8. b; 9. c; 10. a

Chapter 12
1. d; 2. d; 3. d; 4. d; 5. c;
6. b; 7. b; 8. d; 9. c; 10. a

Chapter 13
1. b; 2. b; 3. c; 4. b; 5. d;
6. c; 7. d; 8. b; 9. b; 10. b

Chapter 14
1. a; 2. b; 3. d; 4. c; 5. c;
6. a; 7. d; 8. c; 9. d; 10. b

Chapter 15
1. c; 2. b; 3. a; 4. a; 5. c;
6. d; 7. b; 8. a; 9. b; 10. c

Chapter 16
1. b; 2. d; 3. d; 4. a; 5. c;
6. d; 7. c; 8. d; 9. a; 10. c

Chapter 17
1. c; 2. c; 3. c; 4. d; 5. b;
6. d; 7. c; 8. b; 9. c; 10. a

Chapter 18
1. c; 2. b; 3. b; 4. c; 5. d;
6. c; 7. b; 8. b; 9. c; 10. b

Chapter 19
1. d; 2. c; 3. d; 4. a; 5. c;
6. b; 7. d; 8. b; 9. b; 10. a

Chapter 20
1. a; 2. b; 3. c; 4. d; 5. c;
6. b; 7. d; 8. a; 9. c; 10. d

Chapter 21
1. b; 2. b; 3. c; 4. b; 5. d;
6. b; 7. d; 8. b; 9. a; 10. a

Chapter 22
1. b; 2. c; 3. c; 4. c; 5. c;
6. a; 7. c; 8. b; 9. d; 10. b

Chapter 23
1. d; 2. b; 3. c; 4. a; 5. b;
6. a; 7. b; 8. d; 9. d; 10. a

HEALTH RESOURCES

Injury Prevention and Emergency Care

Injury Prevention

Unintentional injuries are a major public health problem facing the United States today. On an average day, more than a million people will suffer a nonfatal injury; almost 100,000 people die each year as a result of unintentional injuries. Unintentional injuries are the leading cause of death for Americans under the age of 44. In the United States, unintentional injuries are the fifth leading cause of death, after heart disease, cancer, stroke, and lung disease.

Vehicle Safety

The risk of dying in an automobile crash is related to age. Young drivers (aged 16 to 24) have the highest death rate, owing to their inexperience and immaturity. Each year about 40,000 Americans die in automobile crashes and another 1.9 million are disabled, 140,000 of them permanently. Most of these car crashes were avoidable. The best way to prevent crashes is to practice risk management driving and accident-avoidance techniques and to be aware of safety technology when purchasing a car.

Risk Management Driving
Risk management driving techniques, which help reduce chances of being involved in a collision, include the following:

- *Surround your car with a bubble space.* The rear bumper of the car ahead of you should be three seconds away. To measure your safety bubble, choose a roadside landmark such as a signpost or light pole as a reference point. When the car in front of you passes this point, count "one-one-thousand, two-one-thousand." Make sure you are not passing the reference point before you've finished saying "three-one-thousand."
- *Scan the road ahead of you and to both sides.*
- *Drive with your low-beam headlights on.* Being seen is an important safety factor. Driving with your low-beam headlights on, *day and night*, makes you more visible to other drivers.

Other important techniques include anticipating other drivers' actions, driving refreshed, driving sober, obeying all traffic laws, and using safety belts.

Accident-Avoidance Techniques
Sometimes when driving, you need to react instantly to a situation. To avoid a more severe accident, you may need to steer into another, less severe, collision. The point of accident avoidance is to save lives. Here are the Automobile Association of America's (AAA) rules for avoidance:

- Generally, veer to the right.
- Steer, don't skid, off the road. (It is easy to roll a vehicle over if you swerve suddenly off the edge of the road.)
- If you have to hit a vehicle, hit one moving in the same direction as your own.
- If you have to hit a stationary object, try to hit a soft one (bushes, small trees) rather than a hard one (boulders, brick walls, giant trees).
- If you have to hit a hard object, hit it with a glancing blow.
- Avoid hitting pedestrians, motorcyclists, and bicyclists at all costs.

Safety Technology
The last line of defense against a collision is the car itself. How a car is equipped can mean the difference between life and death. When purchasing a car, the Insurance Institute for Highway Safety recommends that you look for the following features:

- Does the car have air bags? Remember, air bags do not eliminate the need for everyone to wear safety belts. Air bags inflate only in the case of frontal crashes.
- Does the car have antilock brakes? Antilock brakes rapidly pump the brakes to prevent them from locking up and, hence, prevent the car from skidding.
- Does the car have impact-absorbing crumple zones?
- Are there strengthened passenger compartment side walls?
- Is there a strong roof support? (The center door post on four-door models gives you an extra roof pillar.)

In Case of Mechanical Breakdown
- Try to get as far off the road as possible.
- Turn on your car's emergency flashers, and raise the hood. Set out flares or reflective triangles.
- Stay in the car until a law enforcement officer arrives. If others stop to help, ask them to contact the police, sheriff's office, or the state patrol.
- If you must leave your car, leave a note with the car explaining the problem (as best you can), the time and date, your name, the direction in which you are walking, and what you are wearing. This information will help anyone who needs to look for you.
- Remove all valuables from the car if you must leave it.

Safe Refueling
Gasoline is a flammable substance. Follow these guidelines from the Petroleum Equipment Institute any time you are filling up a car, truck, or motorcycle:

- Turn off the engine while refueling.
- Do not reenter your vehicle during refueling. In the unlikely event of a static-caused fire, leave the nozzle in the tank and back away from the vehicle. Notify the attendant immediately.
- Avoid prolonged breathing of gasoline vapors. Keep gasoline away from your eyes and skin; it can cause irritation. Never use it to wash your hands or as a cleaning solvent.
- If you are dispensing gasoline into a container or storing it, be sure the container is approved for such a use.
- Never siphon gasoline by mouth; it can be harmful or fatal if swallowed.

Pedestrian Safety

Each year approximately 13 percent of all motor vehicle deaths involve pedestrians, and another 82,000 pedestrians are injured each year. The highest death rates involving pedestrians occur among the very young and older populations. Pedestrian injuries occur most frequently after dark, in urban settings, and primarily in intersections where pedestrians may walk or dart into traffic. It is not uncommon for alcohol to play a role in the death or injury of a pedestrian. How can you protect yourself from being injured or becoming a fatality? AAA has the following suggestions for joggers and walkers:

- Carry or wear reflective material at night to help drivers see you.
- Cross only at crosswalks. Keep to the right in crosswalks.
- Before crossing, look both ways. Be sure the way is clear before you cross.
- Cross only on the proper signal.
- Watch for turning cars.
- Never enter the roadway from between parked cars.
- Where there is no sidewalk and it is necessary to walk in a roadway, walk on the left side, facing traffic.
- Don't wear headphones or earbuds. These may interfere with your ability to hear sounds of motor vehicles.

Cycling Safety

Currently over 63 million Americans of all ages ride bicycles for transportation, recreation, and fitness. The Consumer Product Safety Commission reports about 800 deaths per year from cycling accidents. The biggest risk factors are failure to wear a helmet, being male, and riding after dark.

Children aged 10 to 14 also are at higher risk for injury. Approximately 87 percent of fatal collisions were due to cyclists' errors, usually failure to yield at intersections. Alcohol also plays a significant role in bicycle deaths and injuries. The following are suggestions cyclists should consider to reduce risk of injury or death.

- Wear a helmet. It should be ANSI or Snell approved. This can reduce head injuries by 85 percent.
- Don't drink and ride.

- Respect traffic.
- Wear light reflective clothing that is easily seen at night and during the day.
- Avoid riding after dark.
- Ride with the flow of traffic.
- Know and use proper hand signals.
- Keep your bicycle in good working condition.
- Use bike paths whenever possible.
- Stop at stop signs and traffic lights.

Water Safety

Drowning is the third most common cause of accidental death in the United States, according to the National Safety Council. About 85 percent of drowning victims are teenage males. Many drowned swimmers are strong swimmers. Alcohol plays a significant role in many drowning cases. Most drownings occur in unorganized or unsupervised facilities, such as ponds or pools with no lifeguards present. Swimmers should take the following precautions:

- Don't drink alcohol before or while swimming.
- Don't enter the water unless you can swim at least 50 feet unassisted.
- Know your limitations; get out of the water as soon as you start to feel even slightly fatigued.
- Never swim alone, even if you are a skilled swimmer. You never know what might happen.
- Never leave a child unattended, even in extremely shallow water or wading pools.
- Before entering the water, check the depth. Most neck and back injuries result from diving into water that is too shallow.
- Never swim in muddy or dirty water that obstructs your view of the bottom.
- Never swim in a river with currents too swift for easy, relaxed swimming.

Emergency Care

In certain situations, it may be necessary to administer first aid. Ideally, first aid procedures should be performed by someone who has received formal training from the American Red Cross or some other reputable institution. If you do not have such training, contact a physician or call your local emergency medical service (EMS) by dialing 911 or your local emergency number. In life-threatening situations, however, you may not have time to call for outside assistance. In cases of serious injury or sudden illness, you may need to begin first aid immediately and continue until help arrives. This section contains basic information and general steps to follow for various emergency situations. Simply reading these directions, however, may not prepare you fully to handle these situations. For this reason, you may want to enroll in a first aid course.

Calling for Emergency Assistance

When calling for emergency assistance, be prepared to give exact details. Be clear and thorough, and do not panic. Never hang up until the dispatcher has informed you that he or she has all the information needed. Be ready to answer the following questions:

1. Where are you and the victim located? This is the most important information the EMS will need.
2. What is your phone number and name?
3. What has happened? Was there an accident, or is the victim ill?
4. How many people need help?
5. What is the nature of the emergency? What is the victim's apparent condition?
6. Are there any life-threatening situations that the EMS should know about (for example, fires, explosions, or fallen electrical lines)?
7. Is the victim wearing a medic-alert tag (a tag indicating a specific medical condition such as diabetes)?

Are You Liable?

According to the laws in most states, you are not required to administer first aid unless you have a special obligation to the victim. For example, parents must provide first aid for their children, and a lifeguard must provide aid to a swimmer.

Before administering first aid, you should obtain the victim's consent. If the victim refuses aid, you must respect that person's rights. However, you should make every reasonable effort to persuade the victim to accept your help. In emergency situations, consent is *implied* if the victim is unconscious. Once you begin to administer first aid, you are required by law to continue. You must remain with the victim until someone of equal or greater competence takes over.

Can you be held liable if you fail to provide adequate care or if the victim is further injured? To help protect people who render first aid, most states have "Good Samaritan" laws. These laws grant immunity (protection from civil liability) if you act in good faith to provide care to the best of your ability, according to your level of training. Because these laws vary from state to state, you should become familiar with the Good Samaritan laws in your state.

When Someone Stops Breathing

If someone has stopped breathing, you should perform mouth-to-mouth resuscitation. This involves the following steps:

1. Check for responsiveness by gently tapping or shaking the victim. Ask loudly, "Are you OK?"
2. Call the local EMS for help (usually 911).
3. Gently roll the victim onto his or her back.
4. Open the airway by tilting the victim's head back, placing your hand nearest the victim's head on the victim's forehead, and applying backward pressure to tilt the head back and lift the chin.

5. Check for breathing (3 to 5 seconds): look, listen, and feel for breathing.
6. Give two slow breaths.
   - Keep the victim's head tilted back.
   - Pinch the victim's nose shut.
   - Seal your lips tightly around the victim's mouth.
   - Give two slow breaths, each lasting 1½ to 2 seconds.
7. Check for pulse at side of neck; feel for pulse for 5 to 10 seconds.
8. Begin rescue breathing.
   - Keep the victim's head tilted back.
   - Pinch the victim's nose shut.
   - Give one breath every 5 to 6 seconds.
   - Look, listen, and feel for breathing between breaths.
9. Recheck pulse every minute.
   - Keep the victim's head tilted back.
   - Feel for pulse for 5 to 10 seconds.
   - If the victim has a pulse but is not breathing, continue rescue breathing. If there is no pulse, begin CPR.

There are some variations when performing this procedure on infants and children. For children aged 1 to 8, at step 8, give one slow breath every 4 seconds. For infants, you should not pinch the nose. Instead, seal your lips tightly around the infant's nose and mouth. Also for infants, at step 8, you should give one slow breath every 3 seconds.

In cases in which the victim has no pulse, cardiopulmonary resuscitation (CPR) should be performed. This technique involves a combination of artificial respiration and chest compressions. You should not perform CPR unless you have received training in it. You cannot learn CPR simply by reading directions; and, without training, you could cause further injury to the victim. The American Red Cross offers courses in mouth-to-mouth resuscitation and CPR as well as general first aid. If you have taken a CPR course in the past, you should be aware that certain changes have been made in the procedure. Consider taking a refresher course.

When Someone Is Choking

Choking occurs when an object obstructs the trachea (windpipe), thus preventing normal breathing. Failure to expel the object and restore breathing can lead to death within 6 minutes. The universal signal of distress related to choking is the clasping of the throat with one or both hands. Other signs of choking include not being able to talk and/or noisy and difficult breathing. If a victim can cough or speak, do not interfere. The most effective method for assisting choking victims is the Heimlich maneuver, which involves the application of pressure to the victim's abdominal area to expel the foreign object. The Heimlich maneuver involves the following steps:

If the Victim Is Standing or Seated

1. Recognize that the victim is choking.
2. Wrap your arms around the victim's waist from behind, making a fist with one hand.

3. Place the thumb side of the fist on the middle of the victim's abdomen, just above the navel and well below the tip of the sternum.
4. Cover your fist with your other hand.
5. Press fist into victim's abdomen, with up to five quick upward thrusts.
6. After every five abdominal thrusts, check the victim and your technique.
7. If the victim becomes unconscious, gently lower him or her to the ground.
8. Try to clear the airway by using your finger to sweep the object from the victim's mouth or throat.
9. Give two rescue breaths. If the passage is still blocked and air will not go in, proceed with the Heimlich maneuver.

If the Victim Is Lying Down
1. Facing the person, kneel with your legs astride the victim's hips. Place the heel of one hand against the abdomen, slightly above the navel and well below the tip of the sternum. Put the other hand on top of the first hand.
2. Press inward and upward using both hands with up to five quick abdominal thrusts.
3. Repeat the following steps in this sequence until the airway becomes clear or the EMS arrives:
   a. Finger sweep.
   b. Give two rescue breaths.
   c. Do up to five abdominal thrusts.

Alcohol Poisoning
Alcohol overdose is considered a medical emergency when an irregular heartbeat or coma occur. The two immediate causes of death in such cases are cardiac arrhythmia and respiratory depression. If a person is seriously uncoordinated and has possibly also taken a depressant, the risk of respiratory failure is serious enough that a physician should be contacted. When dealing with someone who is drunk, remember these points:

1. Stay calm. Assess the situation.
2. Keep the person still and comfortable.
3. Stay with the person if she or he is vomiting. When helping him or her to lie down, turn the head to the side to prevent it from falling back. This helps to prevent choking on vomit.
4. Monitor the person's breathing.
5. Keep your distance. Before approaching or touching the person, explain what you intend to do.
6. Speak in a clear, firm, reassuring manner.

When Someone Is Bleeding

External Bleeding
Control of external bleeding is an important part of emergency care. Survival is threatened by the loss of one quart of blood or more. There are three major procedures for the control of external bleeding.

1. *Direct pressure.* The best method is to apply firm pressure by covering the wound with a sterile dressing, bandage, or

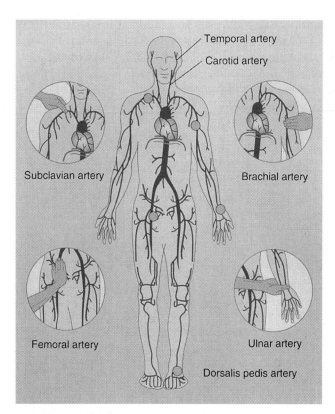

FIGURE H.1 Pressure Points
Pressure can be applied to these points to stop bleeding. However, unless absolutely necessary, avoid applying pressure to the carotid arteries, which supply blood to the brain. Never apply pressure to both carotid arteries at the same time.

clean cloth. Wearing disposable latex gloves or an equally protective barrier, apply pressure for 5 to 10 minutes to stop bleeding.
2. *Elevation.* Elevate the wounded section of the body to slow the bleeding. For example, a wounded arm or leg should be raised above the level of the victim's heart.
3. *Pressure points.* Pressure points are sites where an artery that is close to the body's surface lies directly over a bone. Pressing the artery against the bone can limit the flow of blood to the injury. This technique should be used only as a last resort when direct pressure and elevation have failed to stop bleeding.

Knowing where to apply pressure to stop bleeding is critical (see Figure H.1). For serious wounds, seek medical attention immediately.

Internal Bleeding
Although internal bleeding may not be immediately obvious, you should be aware of the following signs and symptoms:

1. Symptoms of shock (discussed on page H–6)
2. Coughing up or vomiting blood
3. Bruises or contusions of the skin
4. Bruises on chest or fractured ribs
5. Black, tarlike stools
6. Abdominal discomfort or pain (rigidity or spasms)

In some cases, a person who has suffered an injury (such as a blow to the head, chest, or abdomen) that does not cause external bleeding may experience internal bleeding. If you suspect that someone is suffering from internal bleeding, follow these steps:

1. Have the person lie on his or her back on a flat surface with knees bent.
2. Treat for shock. Keep the victim warm. Cover the person with a blanket, if possible.
3. Expect vomiting. If vomiting occurs, keep the victim on his or her side for drainage, to prevent inhalation of vomit, and to prevent expulsion of vomit from the stomach.
4. Do *not* give the victim any medications or fluids.
5. Send someone to call for emergency medical help immediately.

Nosebleeds To control a nosebleed, follow these steps:

1. Have the victim sit down and lean slightly forward to prevent blood from running into the throat. If you do not suspect a fracture, pinch the person's nose firmly closed using the thumb and forefinger. Keep the nose pinched for at least 5 minutes.
2. While the nose is pinched, apply a cold compress to the surrounding area.
3. If pinching does not work, gently pack the nostril with gauze or a clean strip of cloth. Do not use absorbent cotton, which will stick. Be sure that the ends of the gauze or cloth hang out so that it can be easily removed later. Once the nose is packed with gauze, pinch it closed again for another 5 minutes.
4. If the bleeding persists, seek medical attention.

Treatment for Burns

Minor Burns For minor burns caused by fire or scalding water, apply running cold water or cold compresses for 20 to 30 minutes. Never put butter, grease, salt water, aloe vera, or topical burn ointments or sprays on burned skin. If the burned area is dirty, gently wash it with soap and water, and blot it dry with a sterile dressing.

Major Burns For major burn injuries, call for help immediately. Wrap the victim in a clean, dry sheet. Do not clean the burns or try to remove any clothing attached to burned skin. Remove jewelry near the burned skin immediately, if possible. Keep the victim lying down and calm.

Chemical Burns Remove clothing surrounding the burn. Wash skin that has been burned by chemicals by flushing with water for at least 20 minutes. Seek medical assistance as soon as possible.

Shock

Shock is a condition in which the cardiovascular system fails to provide sufficient blood circulation to all parts of the body.

Victims of shock display the following symptoms:

- Dilated pupils
- Cool, moist skin
- Weak, rapid pulse
- Vomiting
- Delayed or unrelated responses to questions

All injuries result in some degree of shock. Therefore, treatment for shock should be given after every major injury. The following are basic steps for treating shock:

1. Have the victim lie flat with his or her feet elevated approximately 8 to 12 inches. (In the case of chest injuries, difficulty breathing, or severe pain, the victim's head should be slightly elevated if there is no sign of spinal injury.)
2. Keep the victim warm. If possible, wrap him or her in blankets or other material. Keep the victim calm and reassured.
3. Seek medical help.

Electrical Shock

Do not touch a victim of electrical shock until the power source has been turned off. Approach the scene carefully, avoiding any live wires or electrical power lines. Pay attention to the following:

1. If the victim is holding onto the live electrical wire, do not remove it unless the power has been shut off at the plug, circuit breaker, or fuse box.
2. Check the victim's breathing and pulse. Electrical current can paralyze the nerves and muscles that control breathing and heartbeat. If necessary, give mouth-to-mouth resuscitation. If there is no pulse, CPR might be necessary. (Remember that only trained people should perform CPR.)
3. Keep the victim warm and treat for shock. Once the person is breathing and stable, seek medical help or send someone else for help.

Poisoning

Of the 1 million cases of poisoning reported in the United States each year, about 75 percent occur in children under age five, and the majority are caused by household products. Most cases of poisoning involving adults are attempted suicides or attempted murders.

You should keep emergency telephone numbers for the poison control center and the local EMS close at hand. Many people keep these numbers on labels on their telephones. Check the front of your telephone book for these numbers. The National Safety Council recommends that you be prepared to give the following information when calling for help:

- What was ingested? Have the container of the product and the remaining contents ready so you can describe it. You should also bring the container to the emergency room with you.
- When was the substance taken?

- How much was taken?
- Has vomiting occurred? If the person has vomited, save a sample to take to the hospital.
- Are there any other symptoms?
- How long will it take to get to the nearest emergency room?

When caring for a person who has ingested a poison, keep these basic principles in mind:

1. Maintain an open airway. Make sure the person is breathing.
2. Call the local poison control center. Follow their advice for neutralizing the poison.
3. If the poison control center or another medical authority advises you to induce vomiting, then do so.
4. If a corrosive or caustic (that is, acid or alkali) substance was swallowed, immediately dilute it by having the victim drink at least one or two 8-ounce glasses of cold water or milk.
5. Place the victim on his or her left side. This position will delay advancement of the poison into the small intestine, where absorption into the victim's circulatory system is faster.

Injuries of Joints, Muscles, and Bones

Sprains
Sprains result when ligaments and other tissues around a joint are stretched or torn. The following steps should be taken to treat sprains:

1. Elevate the injured joint to a comfortable position.
2. Apply an ice pack or cold compress to reduce pain and swelling.
3. Wrap the joint firmly with a roller bandage.
4. Check the fingers or toes periodically to ensure that blood circulation has not been obstructed. If the bandage is too tight, loosen it.
5. Keep the injured area elevated, and continue ice treatment for 24 hours.
6. Apply heat to the injury after 48 hours if there is no further swelling.
7. If pain and swelling continue or if a fracture is suspected, seek medical attention.

Fractures
Any deformity of an injured body part usually indicates a fracture. A fracture is any break in a bone, including chips, cracks, splinters, and complete breaks. Minor fractures (such as hairline cracks) might be difficult to detect and might be confused with sprains. If there is doubt, treat the injury as a fracture until X rays have been taken.

Do not move the victim if a fracture of the neck or back is suspected because this could result in a spinal cord injury. If the victim must be moved, splints should be applied to immobilize the fracture in order to prevent further damage and to decrease pain. Following are some basic steps for treating fractures and applying splints to broken limbs:

1. If the person is bleeding, apply direct pressure above the site of the wound.
2. If a broken bone is exposed, do not try to move it back into the wound. This can cause contamination and further injury.
3. Do not try to straighten out a broken limb. Splint the limb as it lies.
4. The following materials are needed for splinting:
   - *Splint:* wooden board, pillow, or rolled up magazines and newspapers
   - *Padding:* towels, blankets, socks, or cloth
   - *Ties:* cloth, rope, or tape
5. Place splints and padding above and below the joint. Never put padding directly over the break. Padding should protect bony areas and the soft tissue of the limb.
6. Tie splints and padding into place.
7. Check the tightness of the splints periodically. Pay attention to the skin color, temperature, and pulse below the fracture to make sure the blood flow is adequate.
8. Elevate the fracture and apply ice packs to prevent swelling and reduce pain.

Head Injuries

A head injury can result from an auto accident, a fall, an assault, or a blow from a blunt object. All head injuries can potentially lead to brain damage, which may result in a cessation of breathing and pulse.

For Minor Head Injuries
1. For a minor bump on the head resulting in a bruise without bleeding, apply ice to decrease the swelling.
2. If there is bleeding, apply even, moderate pressure. Because there is always the danger that the skull may be fractured, excessive pressure should not be used.
3. Observe the victim for a change in consciousness. Observe the size of pupils, including whether both pupils are dilated to the same degree, and note signs of inability to think clearly. Check for any signs of numbness or paralysis. Allow the victim to sleep, but wake him or her periodically to check for awareness.

For Severe Head Injuries
1. If the victim is unconscious, check the airway for breathing. If necessary, perform mouth-to-mouth resuscitation.
2. If the victim is breathing, check the pulse. If it is less than 55 or more than 125 beats per minute, the victim may be in danger.
3. Check for bleeding. If fluid is flowing from the ears or nose, do not stop it.
4. Do not remove any objects embedded in the victim's skull.
5. Cover the victim with blankets to maintain body temperature, but guard against overheating.
6. Seek medical help as soon as possible.

Temperature-Related Emergencies

Frostbite Frostbite is damage to body tissues caused by intense cold. Frostbite generally occurs at temperatures below 32°F. The body parts most likely to suffer frostbite are the toes, ears, fingers, nose, and cheeks. When skin is exposed to the cold, ice crystals form beneath the skin. Avoid rubbing frostbitten tissue because the ice crystals can scrape and break blood vessels. To treat frostbite, follow these steps:

1. Bring the victim to a health facility as soon as possible.
2. Cover and protect the frostbitten area. If possible, apply a steady source of external warmth, such as a warm compress. The victim should avoid walking if the feet are frostbitten.
3. If the victim cannot be transported, you must rewarm the body part by immersing it in warm water (100°F to 105°F). Continue to rewarm until the frostbitten area is warm to the touch when removed from the bath. Do not allow the body part to touch the sides or bottom of the water container. After rewarming, dry gently and wrap the body part in bandages to protect from refreezing.

Hypothermia Hypothermia is a condition of generalized cooling of the body, resulting from exposure to cold temperatures or immersion in cold water. It can occur at any temperature below 65°F and can be made more severe by wind chill and moisture. The following are key symptoms of hypothermia:

- Shivering
- Vague, slow, slurred speech
- Poor judgment
- A cool abdomen
- Lethargy, or extreme exhaustion
- Slowed breathing and heartbeat
- Numbness and loss of feeling in extremities

After contacting the EMS, you should take the following steps to provide first aid to a victim of hypothermia:

1. Get the victim out of the cold.
2. Keep the victim in a flat position. Do not raise the legs.
3. Squeeze as much water as possible from wet clothing, and layer dry clothing over wet clothing. Removal of clothing may jostle the victim and lead to other problems.
4. Give the victim warm drinks only if he or she is able to swallow. Do not give the victim alcohol or caffeinated beverages, and do not allow the victim to smoke.
5. Do not allow the victim to exercise.

Heatstroke Heatstroke, the most serious heat-related disorder, results from the failure of the brain's heat-regulating mechanism (the hypothalamus) to cool the body. The following are signs and symptoms of heatstroke:

- Rapid pulse
- Hot, dry, flushed skin (absence of sweating)
- Disorientation leading to unconsciousness
- High body temperature

As soon as these symptoms are noticed, the body temperature should be reduced as quickly as possible. The victim should be immersed in a cool bath, lake, or stream. If there is no water nearby, loosen clothing and use a fan to help lower the victim's body temperature.

Heat Exhaustion Heat exhaustion results from excessive loss of salt and water. The onset is gradual, with the following symptoms:

- Fatigue and weakness
- Anxiety
- Nausea
- Profuse sweating
- Clammy skin
- Normal body temperature

To treat heat exhaustion, move the victim to a cool place. Have the victim lie down flat, with feet elevated 8 to 12 inches. Replace lost fluids slowly and steadily. Sponge or fan the victim.

Heat Cramps Heat cramps result from excessive sweating, resulting in an excessive loss of salt and water. Although heat cramps are the least serious heat-related emergency, they are the most painful. The symptoms include muscle cramps, usually starting in the arms and legs. To relieve symptoms, the victim should drink electrolyte-rich beverages or a light salt-water solution or eat salty foods.

First Aid Supplies

Every home, car, or boat should be supplied with a basic first aid kit. In order to respond effectively to emergences, you must have the basic equipment. This kit should be stored in a convenient place, but it should be kept out of the reach of children. Following is a list of supplies that should be included:

- Bandages, including triangular bandages (36 inches by 6 inches), butterfly bandages, a roller bandage, rolled white gauze bandages (2- and 3-inch widths), adhesive bandages
- Sterile gauze pads and absorbent pads
- Adhesive tape (2- and 3-inch widths)
- Cotton-tip applicators
- Scissors
- Thermometer
- Antibiotic ointment
- Aspirin
- Calamine lotion
- Antiseptic cream or petroleum jelly
- Safety pins
- Tweezers
- Latex gloves
- Flashlight
- Paper cups
- Blanket

You cannot be prepared for every medical emergency. Yet these essential tools and a knowledge of basic first aid will help you cope with many emergency situations.

Nutritive Value of Selected Foods and Fast Foods

This section presents nutritional information about a wide array of foods, including many fast foods. Values are given for calories, protein, carbohydrates, fiber, fat, saturated fat, and cholesterol for common foods and serving sizes. Use this information to assess your diet and make improvements. This is only a sampling of the most common foods. See the MyDietAnalysis database for a more extensive list of foods.

MDA Code	Food Name	Amt	Wt (g)	Ener (kcal)	Prot (g)	Carb (g)	Fiber (g)	Fat (g)	Sat (g)	Chol (g)
Beverages										
Alcoholic Beverages										
22831	Beer	12 fl. oz	360	157	1	13		0	0	
34053	Beer, light	12 fl. oz	353	105	1	5	0	0	0	
22606	Beer, nonalcoholic	12 fl. oz	353	73	1	14	0	0	0	
22884	Wine, red	1 fl. oz	29	24	0	1		0	0	
22861	Wine, white	1 fl. oz	29.3	24	0	1		0	0	
22514	Gin, 80 proof	1 fl. oz	27.8	64	0	0	0	0	0	
22593	Rum, 80 proof	1 fl. oz	27.8	64	0	0	0	0	0	
22515	Tequila, 80 proof	1 fl. oz	27.8	64	0	0	0	0	0	
22594	Vodka, 80 proof	1 fl. oz	27.8	64	0	0	0	0	0	
22670	Whiskey, 80 proof	1 fl. oz	27.8	64	0	0	0	0	0	
Coffee, Tea, and Dairy Drink Mixes										
20012	Coffee, brewed	1 cup	237	2	0	0	0	0	0	0
20686	Coffee, decaffeinated, brewed	1 cup	237	0	0	0	0	0	0	0
20439	Coffee, espresso	1 cup	237	5	0	0	0	0	0.2	0
20402	Coffee, from mix, French vanilla, sugar & fat free	1 ea	7	25	0	5	0	0	0.1	0
85	Chocolate milk, prepared w/syrup	1 cup	282	254	9	36	1	8	4.7	25
46	Hot cocoa, w/aspartame, sodium, vitamin A, prepared w/water	1 cup	256	74	3	14	1	1	0	0
48	Hot cocoa, prep from dry mix with water	1 cup	275	151	2	32	1	2	0.9	3
166	Hot cocoa, w/marshmallows, from dry packet	1 ea	28	112	1	24	1	1	0.4	2
39	Chocolate flavor, dry mix, prepared w/milk	1 cup	266	226	9	32	1	9	4.9	24
41	Strawberry flavor, dry mix, prepared w/milk	1 cup	266	234	8	33	0	8	5.1	32
20014	Tea, brewed	1 cup	237	2	0	1	0	0	0	0
20036	Tea, herbal (not chamomile) brewed	1 cup	237	2	0	0	0	0	0	0

Ener = energy (kilocalories); **Prot** = protein; **Carb** = carbohydrate; **Fiber** = dietary fiber; **Fat** = total fat; **Sat** = saturated fat; **Chol** = cholesterol.

*This food composition table has been prepared for Pearson Education, Inc. and is copyrighted by ESHA Research in Salem, Oregon, the developer of the MyDietAnalysis software program.

MDA Code	Food Name	Amt	Wt (g)	Ener (kcal)	Prot (g)	Carb (g)	Fiber (g)	Fat (g)	Sat (g)	Chol (g)
Fruit and Vegetable Beverages and Juices										
71080	Apple juice, canned or bottled, unsweetened	1 ea	262	123	0	31	0	0	0	0
20277	Capri Sun All Natural Juice Drink, Fruit Punch	1 ea	210	99	0	26	0	0	0	0
5226	Carrot juice, canned	1 cup	236	94	2	22	2	0	0.1	0
3042	Cranberry juice cocktail	1 cup	253	137	0	34	0	0	0	0
20024	Fruit punch, canned	1 cup	248	117	0	30	0	0	0	0
20035	Fruit punch, from frozen concentrate	1 cup	247	114	0	29	0	0	0	0
20101	Grape drink, canned	1 cup	250	153	0	39	0	0	0	0
3053	Grapefruit juice, from frozen concentrate, unsweetened	1 cup	247	101	1	24	0	0	0	0
20045	Lemonade flavor drink, from dry mix	1 cup	266	112	0	29	0	0	0	0
20047	Lemonade w/aspartame, low kcal, from dry mix	1 cup	237	5	0	1	0	0	0	0
20070	Orange drink, canned	1 cup	248	122	0	31	0	0	0	0
20004	Orange flavor drink, from dry mix	1 cup	248	122	0	31	0	0	0	0
71108	Orange juice, canned, unsweetened	1 ea	263	110	2	26	1	0	0	0
3090	Orange juice, fresh	1 cup	248	112	2	26	0	0	0.1	0
3091	Orange juice, from frozen concentrate, unsweetened	1 cup	249	112	2	27	0	0	0	0
5397	Tomato juice, canned w/o salt	1 cup	243	41	2	10	1	0	0	0
20849	Vegetable and fruit, mixed juice drink	4 oz	113	33	0	8	0	0	0	0
20080	Vegetable juice cocktail, canned	1 cup	242	46	2	11	2	0	0	0
Soft Drinks										
20006	Club soda	1 cup	237	0	0	0	0	0	0	0
20685	Low-calorie cola, with aspartame, caffeine free	12 fl. oz	355	4	0	1	0	0	0	0
20843	Cola, with higher caffeine	12 fl. oz	370	152	0	39	0	0	0	0
20008	Ginger ale	1 cup	244	83	0	21	0	0	0	0
20032	Lemon-lime soft drink	1 cup	246	98	0	25	0	0	0	0
20027	Pepper-type soft drink	1 cup	246	101	0	26	0	0	0.2	0
20009	Root beer	1 cup	246	101	0	26	0	0	0	0
Other										
20033	Soy milk	1 cup	245	127	11	12	3	5	0.6	0
20041	Water, tap	1 cup	237	0	0	0	0	0	0	0
Breakfast Cereals										
40095	All-Bran/Kellogg	0.5 cup	30	78	4	22	9	1	0.2	0
40032	Cap'n Crunch/Quaker	0.75 cup	27	108	1	23	1	2	0.4	0
40297	Cheerios/Gen Mills	1 cup	30	111	4	22	4	2	0.4	0
40126	Cinnamon Toast Crunch/ Gen Mills	0.75 cup	30	127	2	24	1	3	0.5	0
40195	Corn Flakes/Kellogg	1 cup	28	101	2	24	1	0	0.1	0
40089	Corn Grits, instant, plain, prepared/Quaker	1 pkg	137	93	2	21	1	0	0	0
40206	Corn Pops/Kellogg	1 cup	31	117	1	28	0	0	0.1	0
40179	Cream of Rice, prepared w/salt	1 cup	244	127	2	28	0	0	0	0
40182	Cream of Wheat, instant, prepared w/salt	1 cup	241	149	4	32	1	1	0.1	0
40104	Crispix/Kellogg	1 cup	29	109	2	25	0	0	0.1	0

MDA Code	Food Name	Amt	Wt (g)	Ener (kcal)	Prot (g)	Carb (g)	Fiber (g)	Fat (g)	Sat (g)	Chol (g)
40218	Froot Loops/Kellogg	1 cup	30	118	2	26	1	1	0.5	0
40217	Frosted Flakes/Kellogg	0.75 cup	31	114	1	28	1	0	0	0
11916	Frosted Mini-Wheats, bite size/Kellogg	1 cup	55	189	6	45	6	1	0.2	0
40209	Raisin Bran/Kellogg	1 cup	61	195	5	47	7	2	0.3	0
40210	Rice Krispies/Kellogg	1.25 cup	33	128	2	28	0	0	0.1	0
60887	Shredded wheat, large biscuit	2 ea	37.8	127	4	30	5	1	0.2	0
40211	Special K/Kellogg	1 cup	31	117	7	22	1	0	0.1	0

Dairy and Cheese

MDA Code	Food Name	Amt	Wt (g)	Ener (kcal)	Prot (g)	Carb (g)	Fiber (g)	Fat (g)	Sat (g)	Chol (g)
500	Cream, half & half	2 Tbs	30	39	1	1	0	3	2.1	11
11	Milk, condensed, sweetened, canned	2 Tbs	38.2	123	3	21	0	3	2.1	13
19	Milk, lowfat, 1% fat, chocolate	1 cup	250	158	8	26	1	2	1.5	8
218	Milk, 2%, w/added vitamins A & D	1 cup	245	130	8	13	0	5	3	
6	Milk, nonfat/skim, w/added vitamin A	1 cup	245	83	8	12	0	0	0.1	5
1	Milk, whole, 3.25%	1 cup	244	146	8	11	0	8	4.6	24
20	Milk, whole, chocolate	1 cup	250	208	8	26	2	8	5.3	30
72088	Yogurt, fruit variety, nonfat	1 cup	245	230	11	47	0	0	0.3	5
1287	American cheese, nonfat slices	1 pce	21.3	32	5	2	0	0	0.1	3
13349	Cheez Whiz cheese sauce/Kraft	2 Tbs	33	91	4	3	0	7	4.3	25
1014	Cottage cheese, 2% fat	0.5 cup	113	102	16	4	0	2	1.4	9
1015	Cream cheese	2 Tbs	29	101	2	1	0	10	6.4	32
1452	Cream cheese, fat free	2 Tbs	29	28	4	2	0	0	0.3	2
1016	Feta, crumbled	0.25 cup	37.5	99	5	2	0	8	5.6	33
47887	Mozzarella, whole milk, slice	1 ea	34	102	8	1	0	8	4.5	27
1075	Parmesan, grated	1 Tbs	5	22	2	0	0	1	0.9	4
1024	Ricotta, part skim	0.25 cup	62	86	7	3	0	5	3.1	19
1064	Ricotta, whole milk	0.25 cup	62	108	7	2	0	8	5.1	32

Eggs and Egg Substitutes

MDA Code	Food Name	Amt	Wt (g)	Ener (kcal)	Prot (g)	Carb (g)	Fiber (g)	Fat (g)	Sat (g)	Chol (g)
19525	Egg substitute, liquid	0.25 cup	62.8	53	8	0	0	2	0.4	1
19506	Egg, white, raw	1 ea	33.4	17	4	0	0	0	0	0
19509	Egg, whole, fried	1 ea	46	92	6	0	0	7	2	210
19515	Egg, whole, hard boiled	1 ea	37	57	5	0	0	4	1.2	157
19521	Egg, whole, poached	1 ea	37	54	5	0	0	4	1.1	156
19516	Egg, whole, scrambled	1 ea	61	101	7	1	0	7	2.2	215
19508	Egg, yolk, raw, fresh	1 ea	16.6	53	3	1	0	4	1.6	205

Fruit

MDA Code	Food Name	Amt	Wt (g)	Ener (kcal)	Prot (g)	Carb (g)	Fiber (g)	Fat (g)	Sat (g)	Chol (g)
72101	Apricots, canned, heavy syrup, drained	1 cup	182	151	1	39	5	0	0	0
3164	Fruit cocktail canned in juice	1 cup	237	109	1	28	2	0	0	0
71079	Apple w/skin, raw	1 cup	125	65	0	17	3	0	0	0
3331	w/added vitamin C	0.5 cup	128	97	0	25	2	0	0	0
3657	Apricot, raw	1 cup	165	79	2	18	3	1	0	0
3210	Avocado, California, peeled, raw	1 ea	173	289	3	15	12	27	3.7	0
71082	Banana, peeled, raw	1 ea	81	72	1	19	2	0	0.1	0
71976	Grapefruit, fresh	0.5 ea	154	60	1	16	6	0	0	
3055	Grapes, Thompson seedless, fresh	0.5 cup	80	55	1	14	1	0	0	4
3642	Melon, fresh, wedge	1 pce	69	23	1	6	1	0	0	5
3168	Mixed fruit (prune, apricot, & pear) dried	1 oz	28.4	69	1	18	2	0	0	0

MDA Code	Food Name	Amt	Wt (g)	Ener (kcal)	Prot (g)	Carb (g)	Fiber (g)	Fat (g)	Sat (g)	Chol (g)
3216	Nectarine, raw	1 cup	138	61	1	15	2	0	0	0
3726	Peach, peeled, raw	1 ea	79	31	1	8	1	0	0	0
3106	Pear, raw	1 ea	209	121	1	32	6	0	0	0
3766	Raisins, seedless	50 ea	26	78	1	21	1	0	0	0
72113	Pineapple, fresh, slice	1 pce	84	38	0	10		0		5
3085	Orange, fresh	1 ea	184	86	2	22	4	0	0	
3135	Strawberries, halves/slices, raw	1 cup	166	53	1	13	3	0	0	0

Grain Products

Breads, Rolls, and Bread Crumbs

MDA Code	Food Name	Amt	Wt (g)	Ener (kcal)	Prot (g)	Carb (g)	Fiber (g)	Fat (g)	Sat (g)	Chol (g)
71170	Bagel, cinnamon-raisin	1 ea	26	71	3	14	1	0	0.1	0
71167	Bagel, egg	1 ea	26	72	3	14	1	1	0.1	6
71152	Bagel, plain/onion/poppy/ sesame, enriched	1 ea	26	67	3	13	1	0	0.1	0
42433	Biscuit, w/butter	1 ea	82	280	5	27	0	17	4	0
71192	Biscuit, Plain or Buttermilk, refrig dough, baked, reduced fat	1 ea	21	63	2	12	0	1	0.3	0
42004	Bread crumbs, dry, plain, grated	1 Tbs	6.8	27	1	5	0	0	0.1	0
49144	Bread, crusty Italian w/garlic	1 pce	50	186	4	21	10	2.4	6	
70964	Bread, garlic, frozen/Campione	1 pce	28	101	2	12	1	5	0.8	
42069	Bread, oat bran	1 pce	30	71	3	12	1	1	0.2	0
42095	Bread, wheat, reduced kcal	1 pce	23	46	2	10	3	1	0.1	0
71247	Bread, white, commercially prepared, crumbs/cubes/slices	1 pce	9	24	1	5	0	0	0.1	0
42084	Bread, white, reduced kcal	1 pce	23	48	2	10	2	1	0.1	0
26561	Buns, hamburger, Wonder	1 ea	43	117	3	22	1	2	0.4	
42021	Hamburger/hot dog bun, plain	1 ea	43	120	4	21	1	2	0.5	0
42115	Cornbread, prepared from dry mix	1 pce	60	188	4	29	1	6	1.6	37
71227	Pita bread, white, enriched	1 ea	28	77	3	16	1	0	0	0
71228	Pita bread, whole wheat	1 ea	28	74	3	15	2	1	0.1	0
71368	Roll, dinner, plain, homemade w/reduced fat (2%) milk	1 ea	43	136	4	23	1	3	0.8	15
42161	Roll, French	1 ea	38	105	3	19	1	2	0.4	0
71056	Roll, hard/kaiser	1 ea	57	167	6	30	1	2	0.3	0
42297	Tortilla, corn, w/o salt, ready to cook	1 ea	26	58	1	12	1	1	0.1	0
90645	Taco shell, baked	1 ea	5	23	0	3	0	1	0.2	0

Crackers

MDA Code	Food Name	Amt	Wt (g)	Ener (kcal)	Prot (g)	Carb (g)	Fiber (g)	Fat (g)	Sat (g)	Chol (g)
71451	Cheez-its/Goldfish crackers, low sodium	55 pce	33	166	3	19	1	8	3.2	4
43507	Oyster/soda/soup crackers	1 cup	45	193	4	32	1	5	0.7	0
70963	Ritz crackers/Nabisco	5 ea	16	79	1	10	0	4	0.6	0
43587	Saltine crackers, original premium/Nabisco	5 ea	14	59	2	10	0	1	0.3	0
43545	Sandwich crackers, cheese filled	4 ea	28	134	3	17	1	6	1.7	1
43546	Sandwich crackers, peanut butter filled	4 ea	28	138	3	16	1	7	1.4	0
44677	Snackwell Wheat Cracker/ Nabisco	1 ea	15	62	1	12	1	2		
43581	Wheat Thins, baked/Nabisco	16 ea	29	136	2	20	1	6	0.9	0
43508	Whole wheat cracker	4 ea	32	142	3	22	3	6	1.1	0

MDA Code	Food Name	Amt	Wt (g)	Ener (kcal)	Prot (g)	Carb (g)	Fiber (g)	Fat (g)	Sat (g)	Chol (g)
Muffins and Baked Goods										
42723	English muffin, plain	1 ea	57	132	5	26		1	0.2	
62916	Muffin, blueberry, commercially prepared	1 ea	11	30	1	5	0	1	0.2	3
44521	Muffin, corn, commercially prepared	1 ea	57	174	3	29	2	5	0.8	15
44514	Muffin, oatbran	1 ea	57	154	4	28	3	4	0.6	0
44518	Toaster muffin, blueberry	1 ea	33	103	2	18	1	3	0.5	2
Noodles and Pasta										
38048	Chow mein noodles, dry	1 cup	45	237	4	26	2	14	2	0
38047	Egg noodles, enriched, cooked	0.5 cup	80	110	4	20	1	2	0.3	23
38060	Spaghetti, whole wheat, cooked	1 cup	140	174	7	37	6	1	0.1	0
38251	Egg noodles, enriched, cooked w/salt	0.5 cup	80	110	4	20	1	2	0.3	
38102	Macaroni noodles, enriched, cooked	1 cup	140	221	8	43	3	1	0.2	
38118	Spaghetti noodles, enriched, cooked	0.5 cup	70	111	4	22	1	1	0.1	4
Grains										
38076	Couscous, cooked	0.5 cup	78.5	88	3	18	1	0	0	0
38080	Oats	0.25 cup	39	152	7	26	4	3	0.5	0
38010	Rice, brown, long grain, cooked	1 cup	195	216	5	45	4	2	0.4	0
38256	Rice, white, long grain, enriched, cooked w/salt	1 cup	158	205	4	45	1	0	0.1	0
38019	Rice, white, long grain, instant, enriched, cooked	1 cup	165	193	4	41	1	1	0	0
Pancakes, French Toast, and Waffles										
42156	French toast, homemade, w/reduced fat (2%) milk	1 pce	65	149	5	16	1	7	1.8	75
45192	Pancake/waffle, buttermilk/Eggo/Kellogg	1 ea	42.5	99	3	16	0	3	0.6	5
45117	Pancakes, plain, homemade	1 ea	77	175	5	22	1	7	1.6	45
45193	Waffle, lowfat, homestyle, frozen	1 ea	35	83	2	15	0	1	0.3	9
Meat and Meat Substitutes										
Beef										
10093	Beef, average of all cuts, lean & fat (1/4" trim), cooked	3 oz	85.1	260	22	0	0	18	7.3	75
10705	Beef, average of all cuts, lean (1/4" trim), cooked	3 oz	85.1	184	25	0	0	8	3.2	73
10133	Beef, whole rib, roasted, 1/4" trim	3 oz	85.1	305	19	0	0	25	10	71
58129	Ground beef (hamburger), 25% fat, cooked, pan-browned	3 oz	85.1	236	22	0	0	15	6	76
58119	Ground beef (hamburger), 15% fat, cooked, pan-browned	3 oz	85.1	218	24	0	0	13	5	77
58109	Ground beef (hamburger), 5% fat, cooked, pan-browned	3 oz	85.1	164	25	0	0	6	2.9	76
10791	Porterhouse steak, lean & fat (1/4" trim), broiled	3 oz	85.1	280	19	0	0	22	8.7	61
58257	Rib eye steak, small end (ribs 10–12), 0" trim, broiled	3 oz	85.1	210	23	0	0	13	4.9	94

MDA Code	Food Name	Amt	Wt (g)	Ener (kcal)	Prot (g)	Carb (g)	Fiber (g)	Fat (g)	Sat (g)	Chol (g)
58094	Skirt steak, trimmed to 0" fat, broiled	3 oz	85.1	187	22	0	0	10	4	51
58328	Strip steak, top loin, 1/8" trim, broiled	3 oz	85.1	171	25	0	0	7	2.7	67
10805	T-Bone steak, lean & fat (1/4" trim), broiled	3 oz	85.1	260	20	0	0	19	7.6	55
11531	Veal, average of all cuts, cooked	3 oz	85.1	197	26	0	0	10	3.6	97
Chicken										
15057	Chicken breast, w/o skin, fried	3 oz	85.1	159	28	0	0	4	1.1	77
15080	Chicken, dark meat, w/skin, roasted	3 oz	85.1	215	22	0	0	13	3.7	77
15026	Chicken, dark meat, w/o skin, fried	3 oz	85.1	203	25	2	0	10	2.7	82
15042	Chicken drumstick, w/o skin, fried	3 oz	85.1	166	24	0	0	7	1.8	80
15048	Chicken, wing, w/o skin, fried	3 oz	85.1	180	26	0	0	8	2.1	71
15059	Chicken, wing, w/o skin, roasted	3 oz	85.1	173	26	0	0	7	1.9	72
Turkey										
51151	Turkey bacon, cooked	1 oz	28.4	108	8	1	0	8	2.4	28
51098	Turkey patty, breaded, fried	1 ea	42	119	6	7	0	8	2	26
16110	Turkey breast w/skin, roasted	3 oz	85.1	130	25	0	0	3	0.7	77
16038	Turkey breast, no skin, roasted	3 oz	85.1	115	26	0	0	1	0.2	71
16101	Turkey, dark meat w/skin, roasted	3 oz	85.1	155	24	0	0	6	1.8	100
16003	Turkey, ground, cooked	1 ea	82	193	22	0	0	11	2.8	84
Lamb										
13604	Lamb, average of all cuts (1/4" trim), cooked	3 oz	85.1	250	21	0	0	18	7.5	83
13616	Lamb, average of all cuts, lean (1/4" trim), cooked	3 oz	85.1	175	24	0	0	8	2.9	78
Pork										
12000	Bacon, broiled, pan-fried, or roasted	3 pcs	19	103	7	0	0	8	2.6	21
28143	Canadian bacon	1 pce	56	68	9	1		3	1	27
12211	Ham, cured, boneless, regular fat (11% fat), roasted	1 cup	140	249	32	0	0	13	4.4	83
12309	Pork, average of retail cuts, cooked	3 oz	85.1	232	23	0	0	15	5.3	77
12097	Pork, ribs, backribs, roasted	3 oz	85.1	315	21	0	0	25	9.4	100
12099	Pork, ground, cooked	3 oz	85.1	253	22	0	0	18	6.6	80
Lunchmeats										
13000	Beef, thin slices	1 oz	28.4	42	5	0	0	2	0.8	20
58275	Bologna, beef and pork, low fat	1 ea	14	32	2	0	0	3	1	5
13157	Chicken breast, oven roasted deluxe	1 oz	28.4	29	5	1	0	1	0.2	14
13306	Corned beef, cooked, chopped, pressed	1 ea	71	101	14	1	0	5	2	46
13264	Ham, slices, regular (11% fat)	1 cup	135	220	22	5	2	12	4	77
13101	Pastrami, beef, cured	1 oz	28.4	41	6	0	0	2	0.8	19
13215	Salami, beef, cotto	1 oz	28.4	59	4	1	0	4	1.9	24
16160	Turkey breast slice	1 pce	21	22	4	1	0	0	0.1	9
58279	Turkey ham, sliced, extra lean, prepackaged or deli-sliced	1 cup	138	163	27	2	0	5	1.8	92

MDA Code	Food Name	Amt	Wt (g)	Ener (kcal)	Prot (g)	Carb (g)	Fiber (g)	Fat (g)	Sat (g)	Chol (g)
Sausage										
13070	Chorizo, pork & beef	1 ea	60	273	14	1	0	23	8.6	53
57877	Frankfurter, beef	1 ea	45	148	5	2	0	13	5.3	24
13012	Frankfurter, turkey	1 ea	45	102	6	1	0	8	2.7	48
57890	Italian sausage, pork, cooked	1 ea	83	286	16	4	0	23	7.9	47
13021	Pepperoni sausage	1 pce	5.5	26	1	0	0	2	0.9	6
13185	Pork sausage links, cooked	2 ea	48	165	8	0	0	15	5.1	37
58227	Sausage, pork, precooked	3 oz	85	321	12	0	0	30	9.9	63
58007	Turkey sausage, breakfast links, mild	2 ea	56	132	9	1	0	10	4.4	34
Meat Substitutes										
7509	Bacon substitute, vegetarian, strips	3 ea	15	46	2	1	0	4	0.7	0
7722	Garden patties, frozen/ Worthington, Morningstar	1 ea	67	119	11	10	4	4	0.5	1
7674	Harvest burger, original flavor, vegetable protein patty	1 ea	90	138	18	7	6	4	1	0
90626	Sausage, vegetarian, meatless	1 ea	28	72	5	3	1	5	0.8	0
7726	Spicy Black Bean Burger/ Worthington, Morningstar	1 ea	78	115	12	15	5	1	0.2	1
Nuts										
4519	Cashews, dry roasted w/salt	0.25 cup	34.2	196	5	11	1	16	3.1	0
4728	Macadamia nuts, dry roasted, unsalted	1 cup	134	962	10	18	11	102	16	0
4592	Mixed nuts, w/peanuts, dry roasted, salted	0.25 cup	34.2	203	6	9	3	18	2.4	0
4626	Peanut butter, chunky w/salt	2 Tbs	32	188	8	7	3	16	2.6	0
4756	Peanuts, dry roasted w/o salt	30 ea	30	176	7	6	2	15	2.1	0
4696	Peanuts, raw	0.25 cup	36.5	207	9	6	3	18	2.5	0
4540	Pistachio nuts, dry roasted, salted	0.25 cup	32	182	7	9	3	15	1.8	0
Seafood										
17029	Bass, freshwater, cooked w/dry heat	3 oz	85.1	124	21	0	0	4	0.9	74
17037	Cod, Atlantic, baked/broiled (dry heat)	3 oz	85.1	89	19	0	0	1	0.1	47
19036	Crab, Alaskan King, boiled/ steamed	3 oz	85.1	83	16	0	0	1	0.1	45
17090	Haddock, baked or broiled (dry heat)	3 oz	85.1	95	21	0	0	1	0.1	63
17291	Halibut, Atlantic & Pacific, baked or broiled (dry heat)	3 oz	85.1	119	23	0	0	3	0.4	35
17181	Salmon, Atlantic, farmed, cooked w/dry heat	3 oz	85.1	175	19	0	0	11	2.1	54
17099	Salmon, Sockeye, baked or broiled (dry heat)	3 oz	85.1	184	23	0	0	9	1.6	74
71707	Squid, fried	3 oz	85.1	149	15	7	0	6	1.6	221
17066	Swordfish, baked or broiled (dry heat)	3 oz	85.1	132	22	0	0	4	1.2	43
56007	Tuna salad, lunchmeat spread	2 Tbs	25.6	48	4	2	0	2	0.4	3
17151	White tuna, canned in H$_2$0, drained	3 oz	85.1	109	20	0	0	3	0.7	36
17083	White tuna, canned in oil, drained	3 oz	85.1	158	23	0	0	7	1.1	26

MDA Code	Food Name	Amt	Wt (g)	Ener (kcal)	Prot (g)	Carb (g)	Fiber (g)	Fat (g)	Sat (g)	Chol (g)
Vegetables and Legumes										
Beans										
7038	Baked beans, plain or vegetarian, canned	1 cup	254	239	12	54	10	1	0.2	0
5197	Bean sprouts, mung, canned, drained	1 cup	125	15	2	3	1	0	0	0
7012	Black beans, boiled w/o salt	1 cup	172	227	15	41	15	1	0.2	0
5862	Beets, boiled w/salt, drained	0.5 cup	85	37	1	8	2	0	0	0
90018	Cowpeas, cooked w/salt	1 cup	171	198	13	35	11	1	0.2	0
7081	Hummus, garbanzo or chickpea spread, homemade	1 Tbs	15.4	27	1	3	1	1	0.2	0
7087	Kidney beans, canned	1 cup	256	210	13	37	11	2	0.2	0
7006	Lentils, boiled w/o salt	1 cup	198	230	18	40	16	1	0.1	0
7051	Pinto beans, canned	1 cup	240	206	12	37	11	2	0.4	0
6748	Snap green beans, raw	10 ea	55	17	1	4	2	0	0	0
5320	Snap yellow beans, raw	0.5 cup	55	17	1	4	2	0	0	0
90026	Split peas, boiled w/salt	0.5 cup	98	116	8	21	8	0	0.1	0
7054	White beans, canned	1 cup	262	307	19	57	13	1	0.2	0
Fresh Vegetables										
9577	Artichokes (globe or French) boiled w/salt, drained	1 ea	20	10	1	2	1	0	0	0
6033	Arugula/roquette, raw	1 cup	20	5	1	1	0	0	0	0
90406	Asparagus, raw	10 ea	35	7	1	1	1	0	0	0
5558	Broccoli stalks, raw	1 ea	114	32	3	6	4	0	0.1	0
5036	Cabbage, raw	1 cup	70	17	1	4	2	0	0	0
90605	Carrots, baby, raw	1 ea	15	5	0	1	0	0	0	0
5049	Cauliflower, raw	0.5 cup	50	12	1	3	1	0	0	0
90436	Celery, raw	1 ea	17	2	0	1	0	0	0	0
7202	Corn, white, sweet, ears, raw	1 ea	73	63	2	14	2	1	0.1	0
5900	Corn, yellow, sweet, boiled w/salt, drained	0.5 cup	82	89	3	21	2	1	0.2	0
5908	Eggplant (brinjal) boiled w/salt, drained	1 cup	99	35	1	9	2	0	0	0
5087	Lettuce, looseleaf, raw	2 pcs	20	3	0	1	0	0	0	0
51069	Mushrooms, brown, Italian, or crimini, raw	2 ea	28	6	1	1	0	0	0	0
90472	Onions, chopped, raw	1 ea	70	29	1	7	1	0	0	0
5116	Peas, green, raw	1 cup	145	117	8	21	7	1	0.1	0
7932	Peppers, jalapeno, raw	1 cup	90	27	1	5	2	1	0.1	0
90493	Peppers, sweet green, chopped/sliced, raw	10 pcs	27	5	0	1	0	0	0	0
6990	Pepper, sweet red, raw	1 ea	10	3	0	1	0	0	0	0
9251	Potatoes, red, flesh and skin, baked	1 ea	138	123	3	27	2	0	0	0
9245	Potatoes, russet, flesh and skin, baked	1 ea	138	134	4	30	3	0	0	0
5146	Spinach, raw	1 cup	30	7	1	1	1	0	0	0
90525	Squash, zucchini w/skin, slices, raw	1 ea	118	19	1	4	1	0	0	0
6924	Sweet potato, baked in skin w/salt	0.5 cup	100	90	2	21	3	0	0.1	0
5180	Tomato sauce, canned	0.5 cup	123	39	2	9	2	0	0	0
90532	Tomato, red, ripe, whole, raw	1 pce	15	3	0	1	0	0	0	0
5306	Yam, peeled, raw	0.5 cup	75	88	1	21	3	0	0	0

MDA Code	Food Name	Amt	Wt (g)	Ener (kcal)	Prot (g)	Carb (g)	Fiber (g)	Fat (g)	Sat (g)	Chol (g)
Soy and Soy Products										
7564	Tempeh	0.5 cup	83	160	15	8	9	1.8	0	
7015	Soybeans, cooked	1 cup	172	298	29	17	10	15	2.2	0
7542	Tofu, firm, silken, 1" slice	3 oz	85.1	53	6	2	0	2	0.3	0
Meals and Dishes										
92216	Tortellini with cheese filling	1 cup	108	332	15	51	2	8	3.9	45
57658	Chili con carne w/beans, canned entree	1 cup	222	269	16	25	9	12	3.9	29
57703	Chili, vegetarian chili w/beans, canned entree/Hormel	1 cup	247	205	12	38	10	1	0.1	0
57068	Macaroni and cheese, unprepared/Kraft	1 ea	70	259	11	48	1	3	1.3	10
70958	Stir fry, rice & vegetables, w/soy sauce/Hanover	1 cup	137	130	5	27	2	0		
70943	Beef & bean burrito/Las Campanas	1 ea	114	296	9	38	1	12	4.2	13
16195	Chicken & vegetables/Lean Cuisine	1 ea	297	252	19	32	5	6	1	24
70917	Hot Pockets, beef & cheddar, frozen	1 ea	142	403	16	39		20	8.8	53
70918	Hot Pockets, croissant pocket w/chicken, broccoli, & cheddar, frozen	1 ea	128	301	11	39	1	11	3.4	37
56757	Lasagna w/meat sauce/Stouffer's	1 ea	215	277	19	26	3	11	4.7	41
11029	Macaroni & beef in tomato sauce/Lean Cuisine	1 ea	283	249	14	37	3	5	1.6	23
5587	Mashed potatoes, from granules w/milk, prep w/water & margarine	0.5 cup	105	122	2	17	1	5	1.3	2
70898	Pizza, pepperoni, frozen	1 ea	146	432	16	42	3	22	7.1	22
56703	Spaghetti w/meat sauce/Lean Cuisine	1 ea	326	313	14	51	6	6	1.4	13
Snack Foods										
10051	Beef jerky	1 pce	19.8	81	7	2	0	5	2.1	10
63331	Breakfast bars, oats, sugar, raisins, coconut	1 ea	43	200	4	29	1	8	5.5	0
61251	Cheese puffs and twists, corn based, low fat	1 oz	28.4	123	2	21	3	3	0.6	0
44032	Chex snack mix	1 cup	42.5	181	5	28	2	7	2.4	0
23059	Granola bar, hard, plain	1 ea	24.5	115	2	16	1	5	0.6	0
23104	Granola bar, soft, plain	1 ea	28.4	126	2	19	1	5	2.1	0
44012	Popcorn, air-popped	1 cup	8	31	1	6	1	0	0.1	0
44076	Potato chips, plain, no salt	1 oz	28.4	152	2	15	1	10	3.1	0
5437	Potato chips, sour cream & onion	1 oz	28.4	151	2	15	1	10	2.5	2
44015	Pretzels, hard	5 pcs	30	114	3	24	1	1	0.1	0
44021	Rice cake, brown rice, plain, salted	1 ea	9	35	1	7	0	0	0.1	0
44058	Trail mix, regular	0.25 cup	37.5	173	5	17	2	11	2.1	0
Soups										
50398	Beef barley, canned/Progresso Healthy Classics	1 cup	241	142	11	20	3	2	0.7	19
50081	Chicken noodle, chunky, canned	1 cup	240	175	13	17	4	6	1.4	19

MDA Code	Food Name	Amt	Wt (g)	Ener (kcal)	Prot (g)	Carb (g)	Fiber (g)	Fat (g)	Sat (g)	Chol (g)
50085	Chicken rice, chunky, ready to eat, canned	1 cup	240	127	12	13	1	3	1	12
50088	Chicken vegetable, chunky, canned	1 cup	240	166	12	19	0	5	1.4	17
90238	Chicken, chunky, canned	1 cup	240	170	12	17	1	6	1.9	29
50697	Cup of Noodles, ramen, chicken flavor, dry/Nissin	1 ea	64	296	6	37	14	6.3		
50009	Minestrone, canned, made w/water	1 cup	241	82	4	11	1	3	0.6	2
92163	Ramen noodle, any flavor, dehydrated, dry	0.5 cup	38	172	4	25	1	6	2.9	0
50043	Tomato vegetable, from dry mix, made w/water	1 cup	253	56	2	10	1	1	0.4	0
50028	Tomato, canned, made w/water	1 cup	244	85	2	17	0	2	0.4	0
50014	Vegetable beef, canned, made w/water	1 cup	244	78	6	10	0	2	0.9	5
50013	Vegetarian vegetable, canned, made w/water	1 cup	241	72	2	12	0	2	0.3	0

Desserts

MDA Code	Food Name	Amt	Wt (g)	Ener (kcal)	Prot (g)	Carb (g)	Fiber (g)	Fat (g)	Sat (g)	Chol (g)
62904	Brownie, commercially prepared, square, lrg, 2-3/4″ × 7/8″	1 ea	56	227	3	36	1	9	2.4	10
46062	Cake, chocolate, homemade, w/o icing	1 pce	95	340	5	51	2	14	5.2	55
46091	Cake, yellow, homemade, w/o icing	1 pce	68	245	4	36	0	10	2.7	37
71337	Doughnut, cake, w/chocolate icing, lrg, 3 1/2″	1 ea	57	270	3	27	1	18	4.6	35
45525	Doughnut, cake, glazed/sugared, med, 3″	1 ea	45	192	2	23	1	10	2.7	14
47026	Animal crackers/Arrowroot/Tea Biscuits	10 ea	12.5	56	1	9	0	2	0.4	0
90636	Chocolate chip cookie, commercially prepared 3.5″ to 4″	1 ea	40	196	2	26	1	10	3.1	0
47006	Chocolate sandwich cookie, creme filled	3 ea	30	140	2	21	1	6	1.1	0
62905	Fig bar, 2 oz	1 ea	56.7	197	2	40	3	4	0.6	0
90640	Oatmeal cookie, commercially prepared, 3-1/2″ to 4″	1 ea	25	112	2	17	1	5	1.1	0
47010	Peanut butter cookie, homemade, 3″	1 ea	20	95	2	12	0	5	0.9	6
62907	Sugar cookie, refrigerated dough, baked	1 ea	23	111	1	15	0	5	1.4	7
57894	Pudding, chocolate, ready to eat	1 ea	113	158	3	26	1	5	0.8	3
2612	Pudding, vanilla, ready to eat	1 ea	113	147	3	25	0	4	1.7	8
2651	Rice pudding, ready to eat	1 ea	142	231	3	31	0	11	1.7	1
57902	Tapioca pudding, ready to eat	1 ea	113	135	2	22	0	4	1.1	1
71819	Frozen yogurts, chocolate, nonfat	1 cup	186	199	8	37	2	1	0.9	7
72124	Frozen yogurts, flavors other than chocolate	1 cup	174	221	5	38	0	6	4	23
2010	Ice cream, light, vanilla, soft serve	0.5 cup	88	111	4	19	0	2	1.4	11
90723	Ice popsicle	1 ea	59	47	0	11	0	0	0	0
42264	Cinnamon rolls w/icing, refrigerated dough/Pillsbury	1 ea	44	150	2	24	5	1.2		

MDA Code	Food Name	Amt	Wt (g)	Ener (kcal)	Prot (g)	Carb (g)	Fiber (g)	Fat (g)	Sat (g)	Chol (g)
71299	Croissant, butter	1 ea	67	272	5	31	2	14	7.8	45
45572	Danish, cheese	1 ea	71	266	6	26	1	16	4.8	11
45593	Toaster pastry, Pop Tart, apple-cinnamon/Kellogg	1 ea	52	205	2	37	1	5	0.9	0
23014	Chocolate syrup, fudge-type	2 Tbs	38	133	2	24	1	3	1.5	1
510	Whipped cream topping, pressurized	2 Tbs	7.5	19	0	1	0	2	1	6
54387	Whipped topping, frozen, low fat	2 Tbs	9.4	21	0	2	0	1	1.1	0

Fats, Oils, and Condiments

MDA Code	Food Name	Amt	Wt (g)	Ener (kcal)	Prot (g)	Carb (g)	Fiber (g)	Fat (g)	Sat (g)	Chol (g)
90210	Butter, unsalted	1 Tbs	14	100	0	0	0	11	7.2	30
8084	Oil, vegetable, canola	1 Tbs	14	124	0	0	0	14	1	0
8008	Oil, olive, salad or cooking	1 Tbs	13.5	119	0	0	0	14	1.9	0
8111	Oil, safflower, salad or cooking, greater than 70% oleic	1 Tbs	13.6	120	0	0	0	14	0.8	0
44483	Shortening, household	1 Tbs	12.8	113	0	0	0	13	2.6	0
1708	Barbecue sauce, original	2 Tbs	36	63	0	15	0			
27001	Catsup	1 ea	6	6	0	2	0	0	0	0
53523	Cheese sauce, ready to eat	0.25 cup	63	110	4	4	0	8	3.8	18
54388	Cream substitute, powdered, light	1 Tbs	5.9	25	0	4	0	1	0.2	0
50939	Gravy, brown, homestyle, canned	0.25 cup	60	25	1	3	1	0.3	2	
23003	Jelly	1 Tbs	19	51	0	13	0	0	0	0
25002	Maple syrup	1 Tbs	20	52	0	13	0	0	0	0
44476	Margarine, regular, 80% fat, with salt	1 Tbs	14.2	102	0	0	0	11	1.8	0
8145	Mayonnaise, safflower/soybean oil	1 Tbs	13.8	99	0	0	0	11	1.2	8
8502	Miracle Whip, light/Kraft	1 Tbs	16	37	0	2	0	3	0.5	4
435	Mustard, yellow	1 tsp	5	3	0	0	0	0	0	0
23042	Pancake syrup	1 Tbs	20	47	0	12	0	0	0	0
23172	Pancake syrup, reduced kcal	1 Tbs	15	25	0	7	0	0	0	0
53524	Pasta sauce, spaghetti/marinara	0.5 cup	125	92	2	14	1	3	0.4	0
53646	Salsa picante, mild	2 Tbs	30.5	8	0	1	0	0		0
504	Sour cream, cultured	2 Tbs	28.8	62	1	1	0	6	3.8	13
53063	Soy sauce	1 Tbs	18	11	2	1	0	0	0	0
53652	Taco sauce, red, mild	1 Tbs	15.7	7	0	1	0	0		0
53004	Teriyaki sauce	1 Tbs	18	15	1	3	0	0	0	0
8024	1000 Island, regular	1 Tbs	15.6	58	0	2	0	5	0.8	4
8013	Blue/Roquefort cheese, regular	2 Tbs	30.6	154	1	2	0	16	3	5
90232	French, regular	1 Tbs	12.3	56	0	2	0	6	0.7	0
44498	Italian, fat-free	1 Tbs	14	7	0	1	0	0	0	0
44696	Ranch, reduced fat	1 Tbs	15	33	0	2	0	3	0.2	3
8035	Vinegar & oil, homemade	2 Tbs	31.2	140	0	1	0	16	2.8	0

Fast Food

MDA Code	Food Name	Amt	Wt (g)	Ener (kcal)	Prot (g)	Carb (g)	Fiber (g)	Fat (g)	Sat (g)	Chol (g)
6177	Baked potato, topped w/cheese sauce	1 ea	296	474	15	47		29	10.6	18
56629	Burrito w/beans & cheese	1 ea	93	189	8	27		6	3.4	14
66023	Burrito w/beans, cheese, & beef	1 ea	102	165	7	20	2	7	3.6	62
66024	Burrito w/beef	1 ea	110	262	13	29	1	10	5.2	32
56600	Biscuit w/egg sandwich	1 ea	136	373	12	32	1	22	4.7	245
66029	Biscuit w/egg, cheese, & bacon sandwich	1 ea	144	477	16	33	0	31	11.4	261

MDA Code	Food Name	Amt	Wt (g)	Ener (kcal)	Prot (g)	Carb (g)	Fiber (g)	Fat (g)	Sat (g)	Chol (g)
66013	Cheeseburger, double, condiments & vegetables	1 ea	166	417	21	35		21	8.7	60
56649	Cheeseburger, large, one meat patty w/condiments & vegetables	1 ea	219	563	28	38		33	15	88
15063	Chicken, breaded, fried, dark meat (drumstick or thigh)	3 oz	85.1	248	17	9	1	15	4.1	95
15064	Chicken, breaded, fried, light meat (breast or wing)	3 oz	85.1	258	19	10	1	15	4.1	77
56000	Chicken filet, plain	1 ea	182	515	24	39		29	8.5	60
56635	Chimichanga w/beef & cheese	1 ea	183	443	20	39		23	11.2	51
5461	Cole slaw	0.75 cup	99	147	1	13		11	1.6	5
56606	Croissant w/egg & cheese sandwich	1 ea	127	368	13	24		25	14.1	216
56607	Croissant w/egg, cheese, & bacon sandwich	1 ea	129	413	16	24		28	15.4	215
66021	Enchilada w/cheese	1 ea	163	319	10	29		19	10.6	44
66020	Enchirito w/cheese, beef, & beans	1 ea	193	344	18	34		16	7.9	50
66031	English muffin w/cheese & sausage sandwich	1 ea	115	393	15	29	1	24	9.9	59
66010	Fish sandwich w/tartar sauce	1 ea	158	431	17	41	0	23	5.2	55
90736	French fries fried in vegetable oil, medium	1 ea	134	427	5	50	5	23	5.3	0
56638	Frijoles (beans) w/cheese	0.5 cup	83.5	113	6	14		4	2	18
56664	Ham & cheese sandwich	1 ea	146	352	21	33		15	6.4	58
56662	Hamburger, large, double, w/condiments & vegetables	1 ea	226	540	34	40		27	10.5	122
56659	Hamburger, one patty w/condiments & vegetables	1 ea	110	279	13	27		13	4.1	26
66007	Hamburger, plain	1 ea	90	274	12	31		12	4.1	35
5463	Hash browns	0.5 cup	72	151	2	16		9	4.3	9
66004	Hot dog, plain	1 ea	98	242	10	18		15	5.1	44
2032	Ice cream sundae, hot fudge	1 ea	158	284	6	48	0	9	5	21
6185	Mashed potatoes	0.5 cup	121	100	3	20		1	0.6	2
56639	Nachos w/cheese	7 pcs	113	346	9	36		19	7.8	18
6176	Onion rings, breaded, fried	8 pcs	78.1	259	3	29		15	6.5	13
6173	Potato salad	0.333 cup	95	108	1	13		6	1	57
56619	Pizza w/pepperoni 12" or 1/8	1 pce	108	275	15	30		11	3.4	22
66003	Roast beef sandwich, plain	1 ea	139	346	22	33		14	3.6	51
56671	Submarine sandwich, cold cuts	1 ea	228	456	22	51	2	19	6.8	36
57531	Taco	1 ea	171	369	21	27		21	11.4	56
71129	Shake, chocolate, 12 fl. oz	1 ea	250	317	8	51	5	9	5.8	32
71132	Shake, vanilla, 12 fl. oz	1 ea	250	369	8	49	2	16	9.9	57

Behavior Change Contract

Complete the Assess Yourself questionnaire, and read the Skills for Behavior Change box describing the stages of change. After reviewing your results and considering the various factors that influence your decisions, choose a health behavior that you would like to change, starting this quarter or semester (see other side for a sample filled-in contract). Sign the contract at the bottom to affirm your commitment to making a healthy change, and ask a friend to witness it.

My behavior change will be:

_____

My long-term goal for this behavior change is:

_____

These are three obstacles to change (things that I am currently doing or situations that contribute to this behavior or make it harder to change):

1. _____

2. _____

3. _____

The strategies I will use to overcome these obstacles are:

1. _____

2. _____

3. _____

Resources I will use to help me change this behavior include:

a friend/partner/relative: _____

a school-based resource: _____

a community-based resource: _____

a book or reputable website: _____

In order to make my goal more attainable, I have devised these short-term goals:

short-term goal _____ target date _____ reward _____

short-term goal _____ target date _____ reward _____

short-term goal _____ target date _____ reward _____

When I make the long-term behavior change described above, my reward will be:

_____ target date _____

I intend to make the behavior change described above. I will use the strategies and rewards to achieve the goals that will contribute to a healthy behavior change.

Signed: _____ Witness: _____

Sample Behavior Change Contract

Complete the Assess Yourself questionnaire, and read the Skills for Behavior Change box describing the stages of change. After reviewing your results and considering the various factors that influence your decisions, choose a health behavior that you would like to change, starting this quarter or semester (see other side for a sample filled-in contract). Sign the contract at the bottom to affirm your commitment to making a healthy change, and ask a friend to witness it.

My behavior change will be:

To snack less on junk food and more on healthy foods.

My long-term goal for this behavior change is:

Eat junk food snacks no more than once a week.

These are three obstacles to change (things that I am currently doing or situations that contribute to this behavior or make it harder to change):

1. *The grocery store is closed by the time I come home from school.*

2. *I get hungry between classes, and the vending machines only carry candy bars.*

3. *It's easier to order pizza or other snacks than to make a snack at home.*

The strategies I will use to overcome these obstacles are:

1. *I'll leave early for school once a week so I can stock up on healthy snacks in the morning.*

2. *I'll bring a piece of fruit or other healthy snack to eat between classes.*

3. *I'll learn some easy recipes for snacks to make at home.*

Resources I will use to help me change this behavior include:

a friend/partner/relative: *my roommates: I'll ask them to buy healthier snacks instead of chips when they do the shopping.*

a school-based resource: *the dining hall: I'll ask the manager to provide healthy foods we can take to eat between classes.*

a community-based resource: *the library: I'll check out some cookbooks to find easy snack ideas*

a book or reputable website: *the USDA nutrient database at www.nal.usda.gov/fnic: I'll use this site to make sure the foods I select are healthy choices*

In order to make my goal more attainable, I have devised these short-term goals:

short-term goal *Eat a healthy snack 3 times per week*   target date *September 15*   reward *new CD*

short-term goal *Learn to make a healthy snack*   target date *October 15*   reward *concert ticket*

short-term goal *Eat a healthy snack 5 times per week*   target date *November 15*   reward *new shoes*

When I make the long-term behavior change described above, my reward will be:

Ski lift tickets for winter break   target date *December 15*

I intend to make the behavior change described above. I will use the strategies and rewards to achieve the goals that will contribute to a healthy behavior change.

Signed: *Elizabeth King*   Witness: *Susan Bauer*

GLOSSARY

abortion   The medical means of terminating a pregnancy.

abstinence   Refraining from an addictive behavior.

accessory glands   The seminal vesicles, prostate gland, and Cowper's glands.

accountability   Accepting responsibility for personal decisions, choices, and actions.

acid deposition   The acidification process that occurs when pollutants are deposited in precipitation, directly on the land, or by clouds.

acquired active immunity   Immunity developed in response to a prior disease or vaccination to prevent disease.

acquired immunodeficiency syndrome (AIDS)   Extremely virulent sexually transmitted disease that renders the immune system inoperative.

active euthanasia   "Mercy killing," in which a person or organization knowingly acts to hasten the death of a terminally ill person.

activities of daily living (ADLs)   Performance of tasks of everyday living, such as bathing and walking up the stairs.

acupressure   Application of pressure to selected body points to balance energy.

acupuncture   The insertion of long, thin needles to affect the energy flow within the body.

acute bronchitis   A form of bronchitis most often caused by viruses.

acute stress   Stress that is short in duration.

adaptation energy stores   The physical and mental foundations of our ability to cope with stress.

adaptive response   Form of adjustment in which the body attempts to restore homeostasis.

adaptive thermogenesis   Theoretical mechanism by which the brain regulates metabolic activity according to caloric intake.

addiction   Continued involvement with a substance or activity despite ongoing negative consequences.

addictive exercisers   People who exercise compulsively to try to meet needs of nurturance, intimacy, self-esteem, and self-competency.

Adequate Intake (AI)   Best estimates of nutritional needs.

adrenocorticotropic hormone (ACTH)   A pituitary hormone that stimulates the adrenal glands to secrete cortisol.

aerobic capacity   The current functional status of a person's cardiovascular system; measured as VO_{2max}.

aerobic exercise   Any type of exercise that increases heart rate.

afterbirth   The expelled placenta.

ageism   Discrimination based on age.

aggravated rape   Rape that involves multiple attackers, strangers, weapons, or physical beating.

aggressive communicators   People who use hostile, loud, and blaming communication styles.

aging   The patterns of life changes that occur in members of all species as they grow older.

alcohol abuse   Use of alcohol that interferes with work, school, or personal relationships or that entails violations of the law.

alcoholic hepatitis   A condition resulting from prolonged use of alcohol in which the liver is inflamed; it can result in death.

alcoholics anonymous (AA)   An organization whose goal is to help alcoholics stop drinking; includes auxiliary branches such as Al-Anon and Alateen.

alcoholism (alcohol dependency)   A condition in which personal and health problems related to alcohol use are severe and stopping alcohol use results in withdrawal symptoms.

allergy   Hypersensitive reaction to a specific antigen or allergen in the environment in which the body produces excessive antibodies to that antigen or allergen.

allopathic medicine   Conventional, Western medical practice; in theory, based on scientifically validated methods and procedures.

allostatic load   Wear and tear on the body caused by prolonged or excessive stress responses.

alternative insemination   Fertilization accomplished by depositing a partner's or a donor's semen into a woman's vagina via a thin tube; almost always done in a doctor's office.

alternative medical systems   Complete systems of theory and practice that involve several CAM domains.

alternative medicine   Treatment used in place of conventional medicine.

alveoli   Tiny air sacs of the lungs where gas exchange occurs (oxygen enters the body and carbon dioxide is removed).

Alzheimer's disease (AD)   A chronic condition involving changes in nerve fibers of the brain that results in mental deterioration.

amino acids   The building blocks of protein.

amniocentesis   A medical test in which a small amount of fluid is drawn from the amniotic sac to test for Down's syndrome and other genetic diseases.

amniotic sac   The protective pouch surrounding the baby.

amphetamines   A large and varied group of synthetic agents, including licit and illicit drugs, that stimulate the central nervous system.

amyl nitrite   A drug that dilates blood vessels and is properly used to relieve chest pain.

anabolic steroids   Artificial forms of the hormone testosterone that promote muscle growth and strength.

analgesics   Pain relievers.

anal intercourse   The insertion of the penis into the anus.

androgyny   High levels of traditional masculine and feminine traits in a single person.

anemia   Iron-deficiency disease that results from the body's inability to produce hemoglobin.

aneurysm   A weakened blood vessel that may bulge under pressure and, in severe cases, burst.

angina pectoris   Chest pain occurring as a result of reduced oxygen flow to the heart.

angiography   A technique for examining blockages in heart arteries. A catheter is inserted into the arteries, a dye is injected, and an X ray is taken to find the blocked areas. Also called cardiac catheterization.

angioplasty   A technique in which a catheter with a balloon at the tip is inserted into a clogged artery; the balloon is inflated to flatten fatty deposits against artery walls, allowing blood to flow more freely.

anorexia nervosa   Eating disorder characterized by excessive preoccupation with food, self-starvation, and/or extreme exercising to achieve weight loss.

antagonism   A type of interaction in which two or more drugs work at the same receptor site.

antibiotics   Prescription drugs designed to fight bacterial infection.

antibodies   Substances produced by the body that are individually matched to specific antigens.

antidepressants   Prescription drugs used to treat clinically diagnosed depression.

antigen   Substance capable of triggering an immune response.

antioxidants   Substances believed to protect active people from oxidative stress and resultant tissue damage at the cellular level.

anxiety disorders   Disorders characterized by persistent feelings of threat and anxiousness in coping with everyday problems.

appetite   The desire to eat; normally accompanies hunger but is more psychological than physiological.

appraisal   The interpretation and evaluation of information provided to the brain by the senses.

arrhythmia   An irregularity in heartbeat.

arteries   Vessels that carry blood away from the heart to other regions of the body.

arterioles   Branches of the arteries.

arteriosclerosis   A general term for thickening and hardening of the arteries.

arthritis   Painful inflammatory disease of the joints.

asbestos   A substance that separates into stringy fibers and lodges in the lungs, where it can cause various diseases.

assertive communicators   People who use direct, honest communication that maintains and defends their rights in a positive manner.

assets   Internal and external resources and community supports that help a person be more resilient in difficult times and more likely to make positive choices and respond in positive, healthful ways.

asthma   A chronic respiratory disease characterized by attacks of wheezing, shortness of breath, and coughing spasms.

asymptomatic   Without symptoms, or symptom free.

atherosclerosis (coronary artery disease)   Condition characterized by deposits of fatty substances, cholesterol, cellular waste products, calcium, and fibrin in the inner lining of an artery.

atria   The two upper chambers of the heart, which receive blood.

attitude   Relatively stable set of beliefs, feelings, and behavioral tendencies in relation to something or someone.

autoerotic behaviors   Sexual self-stimulation.

autoinoculate   Transmit a pathogen from one part of your own body to another part.

autonomic nervous system (ANS)   The portion of the central nervous system that regulates bodily functions that a person does not normally consciously control.

autonomy   The ability to care for oneself emotionally, socially, and physically.

Ayurveda (Ayurvedic medicine)   A method of treatment derived largely from ancient India, in which practitioners diagnose by observation and touch, and then assign a largely dietary treatment laced with herbal medicines.

background distressors   Environmental stressors of which people are often unaware.

bacteria   Single-celled organisms that may cause disease.

barrier methods   Contraceptive methods that block the meeting of egg and sperm by means of a physical barrier (such as condom, diaphragm, or cervical cap), a chemical barrier (such as spermicide), or both.

basal metabolic rate (BMR)   The energy expenditure of the body under resting conditions at normal room temperature.

belief   Appraisal of the relationship between some object, action, or idea and some attribute of that object, action, or idea.

benign   Harmless; refers to a noncancerous tumor.

bereavement   The loss or deprivation experienced by a survivor when a loved one dies.

bidis   Hand-rolled flavored cigarettes.

binge eating disorder (BED)   Eating disorder characterized by recurrent binge eating, without excessive measures to prevent weight gain.

bioelectrical impedance analysis (BIA)   A technique of body fat assessment in which electrical currents are passed through fat and lean tissue.

biofeedback   A technique involving using a machine to self-monitor physical responses to stress.

biologically based practices   Treatments using substances found in nature, such as herbs, special diets, or vitamin megadoses.

biopsy   Microscopic examination of tissue to determine if a cancer is present.

biopsychosocial model of addiction   Theory of the relationship between an addict's biological (genetic) nature and psychological and environmental influences.

bipolar disorder   Form of depression characterized by alternating mania and depression.

bisexual   Experiencing attraction to and preference for sexual activity with people of both sexes.

black tar heroin   A dark brown, sticky form of heroin.

blood alcohol concentration (BAC)   The ratio of alcohol to total blood volume; the factor used to measure the physiological and behavioral effects of alcohol.

B lymphocytes (B cells)   Specialized white blood cells that are manufactured in the soft tissue of the hollow shafts of the long bones, and are part of the immune response system.

Bod Pod/Pea Pod   A method of body fat assessment that measures the air your body displaces in a sealed chamber.

body mass index (BMI)   A technique of weight assessment based on the relationship of weight to height.

body temperature method   A birth control method in which a woman monitors her body temperature for the rise that signals ovulation in order to abstain from intercourse around this time.

botulism   A resistant foodborne organism that is extremely virulent.

brain death   The irreversible cessation of all functions of the entire brainstem.

bronchitis   Inflammation of the lining of the bronchial tubes.

bulimia nervosa   Eating disorder characterized by binge eating followed by inappropriate measures to prevent weight gain.

burnout   Physical and mental exhaustion caused by excessive stress.

caffeine   A stimulant found in coffee, tea, chocolate, and some soft drinks.

caffeinism   Caffeine intoxication brought on by excessive use; symptoms include chronic insomnia, irritability, anxiety, muscle twitches, and headaches.

calendar method   A birth control method in which a woman's menstrual cycle is mapped on a calendar to determine presumed fertile times in order to abstain from penis–vagina contact during those times.

calorie   A unit of measure that indicates the amount of energy obtained from a particular food.

cancer   A large group of diseases characterized by the uncontrolled growth and spread of abnormal cells.

candidiasis (yeast infection, moniliasis)   Yeastlike fungal disease often triggered sexually.

capillaries   Minute blood vessels that branch out from the arterioles; their thin walls allow for the exchange of oxygen, carbon dioxide, nutrients, and waste products among body cells.

capitalization   The process by which we focus on the good things that happen to us and share those things with others.

capitation   Prepayment of a fixed monthly amount for each patient without regard to the type or number of services provided.

carbohydrates   Basic nutrients that supply the body with glucose, the energy form most commonly used to sustain normal activity.

carbon monoxide   An odorless, colorless gas that originates primarily from motor vehicle emissions. Also found in cigarette smoke.

carcinogens   Cancer-causing agents.

cardiorespiratory fitness   The ability of the heart, lungs, and blood vessels to supply oxygen to skeletal muscles during sustained physical activity.

cardiovascular disease (CVD)   Disease of the heart and blood vessels.

cardiovascular system   A complex system consisting of the heart and blood vessels that transports nutrients, oxygen, hormones, metabolic wastes, and enzymes throughout the body and regulates temperature, the water levels of cells, and the acidity levels of body components.

carotenoids   Fat-soluble compounds with antioxidant properties.

carpal tunnel syndrome   A common occupational injury in which the median nerve in the wrist becomes irritated, causing numbness, tingling, and pain in the fingers and hands.

cataracts   Clouding of the lens that interrupts the focusing of light on the retina, resulting in blurred vision or eventual blindness.

celibacy   State of not being involved in a sexual relationship.

cellulose   Fiber; a major form of complex carbohydrates.

central nervous system depressants   Sedative or hypnotic medications commonly used to treat anxiety.

cerebral cortex   The region of the brain that interprets the nature of an event.

cerebrospinal fluid   Fluid within and surrounding the brain and spinal cord tissues.

Certified Health Education Specialist (CHES)   An academically trained health educator who has passed a national competency examination for prevention and intervention programming.

cervical cap   A small cup made of latex that is designed to fit snugly over the entire cervix.

cervical mucus method   A birth control method that relies upon observation of changes in cervical mucus to determine when the woman is fertile so the couple can abstain from intercourse during those times.

cervix   Lower end of the uterus that opens into the vagina.

cesarean section (C-section)   A surgical procedure in which a baby is removed through an incision made in the mother's abdominal and uterine walls.

chancre   Sore often found at the site of syphilis infection.

chemotherapy   The use of drugs to kill cancerous cells.

chewing tobacco   A stringy type of tobacco that is placed in the mouth and then sucked or chewed.

child abuse   The systematic harming of a child by a caregiver, typically a parent.

chiropractic medicine   Manipulation of the spine to allow proper energy flow.

chlamydia   Bacterially caused STI of the urogenital tract.

chlorofluorocarbons (CFCs)   Chemicals that contribute to the depletion of the ozone layer.

cholesterol   A form of fat circulating in the blood that can accumulate on the inner walls of arteries, causing a narrowing of the channel through which blood flows.

chronic bronchitis   A serious respiratory disorder in which the bronchial tubes become so inflamed and swollen that respiratory function is impaired.

chronic fatigue syndrome (CFS)   A condition of unknown cause characterized by extreme fatigue that is not caused by other illness.

chronic lower respiratory disease   Term used to describe all conditions affecting the lower respiratory system.

chronic mood disorder   Experience of persistent sadness, despair, and hopelessness.

chronic obstructive pulmonary diseases (COPDs)   A collection of chronic lung diseases including asthma, emphysema, and chronic bronchitis.

chronic stress   Stress that is not as intense as acute stress but that exists for prolonged periods of time.

cirrhosis   The last stage of liver disease associated with chronic heavy use of alcohol during which liver cells die and damage becomes permanent.

clitoris   A pea-sized nodule of tissue located at the top of the labia minora; central to sexual arousal in women.

cocaine   A powerful stimulant drug made from the leaves of the South American coca shrub.

codeine   A drug derived from morphine; used in cough syrups and certain painkillers.

codependence   A self-defeating relationship pattern in which a person is "addicted to the addict."

cognitive restructuring   The modification of thoughts, ideas, and beliefs that contribute to stress.

cohabitation   Living together without being married.

collateral circulation   Adaptation of the heart to partial damage accomplished by rerouting needed blood through unused or underused blood vessels while the damaged heart muscle heals.

commercial preparations   Commonly used chemical substances including cosmetics, household cleaning products, and industrial by-products.

common-law marriage   Cohabitation lasting a designated period of time (usually seven years) that is considered legally binding in some states.

communication   The transmission of information and meaning from one individual to another.

comorbidity   The presence of a number of diseases at the same time.

complementary and alternative medicine (CAM)   Forms of treatment distinct from traditional allopathic medicine that until recently were neither taught widely in U.S. medical schools nor generally available in U.S. hospitals.

complementary medicine   Treatment used in conjunction with conventional medicine.

complete (high-quality) proteins   Proteins that contain all of the nine essential amino acids.

complex carbohydrates   A major type of carbohydrate, which provide sustained energy.

compulsion   Obsessive preoccupation with a behavior and an overwhelming need to perform it.

compulsive (pathological) gambler   A person addicted to gambling.

computed tomography (CT)   Use of X ray for a cross-section of the body, which can reveal intraabdominal fat.

computerized axial tomography (CAT) scan   A scan by a machine that uses radiation to view internal organs not normally visible in X rays.

concentric muscle action   Force produced while the muscle is shortening.

conception   The fertilization of an ovum by a sperm.

conflict   An emotional state that arises when the behavior of one person interferes with the behavior of another.

conflict resolution   A concerted effort by all parties to resolve points in contention in a constructive manner.

congeners   Forms of alcohol that are metabolized more slowly than ethanol and produce toxic by-products.

congenital heart disease   Heart disease that is present at birth.

congestive heart failure (CHF)   An abnormal cardiovascular condition that reflects impaired cardiac pumping and blood flow; pooling blood leads to congestion in body tissues.

conjunctivitis   Serious inflammation of the eye caused by any number of pathogens or irritants; can be caused by STIs such as chlamydia.

contraception (birth control)   Methods of preventing conception.

coping   The act of managing events or conditions to lessen the physical or psychological effects of excess stress.

coronary bypass surgery   A surgical technique whereby a blood vessel is implanted to bypass a clogged coronary artery.

coronary thrombosis   A blood clot occurring in the coronary artery.

cortisol   Hormone released by the adrenal glands that makes stored nutrients more readily available to meet energy demands.

counselor   A person with a variety of academic and experiential training who deals with the treatment of emotional problems.

Cowper's glands   Glands that secrete a fluid that lubricates the urethra and neutralizes any acid remaining in the urethra after urination.

crack   A distillate of powdered cocaine that comes in small, hard "chips" or "rocks"; not the same as rock cocaine.

cross-tolerance   Development of a tolerance to one drug that reduces the effects of another, similar drug.

cultural competency   A set of congruent attitudes and policies that come together in a system or among individuals and enables effective work in cross-cultural situations.

cunnilingus   Oral stimulation of a female's genitals.

Daily Reference Values (DRVs)   Recommended amounts for macronutrients such as total fat, saturated fat, and cholesterol.

Daily Values (DVs)   The RDIs and DRVs together make up the daily values seen on food and supplement labels.

death   The permanent ending of all vital functions.

dehydration   Abnormal depletion of body fluids; a result of lack of water.

delirium tremens (DTs)   A state of confusion brought on by withdrawal from alcohol. Symptoms include hallucinations, anxiety, and trembling.

dementias   Progressive brain impairments that interfere with memory and normal intellectual functioning.

dengue   A disease transmitted by mosquitoes; causes flulike symptoms.

dengue hemorrhagic fever   A more serious form of dengue.

denial   Inability to perceive or accurately interpret the effects of the addictive behavior.

dentist   Specialist who diagnoses and treats diseases of the teeth, gums, and oral cavity.

Depo-Provera   An injectable method of birth control that lasts for three months.

designer drugs (club drugs)   Synthetic analogs (drugs that produce similar effects) of existing illicit drugs.

detoxification   The early abstinence period during which an addict adjusts physically and cognitively to being free from the influences of the addiction.

diabetes   Disease in which the pancreas fails to produce enough insulin or to use insulin effectively.

diabetes mellitus   A disease in which the pancreas fails to produce enough insulin or the body fails to use insulin effectively.

diagnosis-related groups (DRGs)   Diagnostic categories established by the federal government to determine in advance how much hospitals will be reimbursed for the care of a particular Medicare patient.

diaphragm   A latex, cup-shaped device designed to cover the cervix and block access to the uterus; should always be used with spermicide.

diastolic pressure The lower number in the fraction that measures blood pressure, indicating pressure on the walls of the arteries during the relaxation phase of heart activity.

Dietary Reference Intakes (DRIs) A set of nutritional values; a new combined listing, including more than 26 essential vitamins and minerals, that applies to healthy people.

dietary supplements Vitamins and minerals taken by mouth that are intended to supplement existing diets.

digestive process The process by which foods are broken down and either absorbed or excreted by the body.

dilation and curettage (D&C) An abortion technique in which the cervix is dilated and the uterine walls scraped clean.

dilation and evacuation (D&E) An abortion technique that combines vacuum aspiration with dilation and curettage; fetal tissue is both sucked and scraped out of the uterus.

dioxins Highly toxic chlorinated hydrocarbons contained in herbicides and produced during certain industrial processes.

dipping Placing a small amount of chewing tobacco between the lower lip and front teeth for rapid nicotine absorption.

disaccharides Combinations of two monosaccharides.

discrimination Actions that deny equal treatment or opportunities to a group, often based on prejudice.

disease prevention Actions or behaviors designed to keep people from getting sick.

disenfranchised grief Grief concerning a loss that cannot be openly acknowledged, publicly mourned, or socially supported.

distillation The process whereby mash is subjected to high temperatures to release alcohol vapors, which are then condensed and mixed with water to make the final product.

distress Stress that can have a negative effect on health.

diuretics Drugs that increase the excretion of urine from the body.

diverticulosis A condition in which bulges form in the walls of the intestine; results in irritation and infection of the intestine.

domestic violence The use of force to control and maintain power over another person in the home environment, including both actual harm and the threat of harm.

Down's syndrome A condition characterized by mental retardation and a variety of physical abnormalities.

downshifting Conscious attempt to simplify life in an effort to reduce the stresses and strains of modern living.

drug abuse Excessive use of a drug.

drug misuse Use of a drug for a purpose for which it was not intended.

dual energy X-ray absorptiometry (DEXA) Technique using low-dose X rays that read bone and soft tissue mass at the same time.

dying The process of decline in body functions, resulting in the death of an organism.

dynamic stretching Moving parts of your body in a gradual and controlled manner, taking you to the limits of your range of motion.

dysfunctional families Families in which there is violence; physical, emotional, or sexual abuse; parental discord; or other negative family interactions that inhibit rather than enhance psychological growth.

dysmenorrhea Condition that causes pain or discomfort in the lower abdomen just before or after menstruation.

dyspareunia Pain experienced by women during intercourse.

dyspnea Shortness of breath, usually associated with disease of the heart or lungs.

dysthymia A less severe type of depression that is milder, harder to recognize, and often characterized by fatigue, pessimism, or a short temper.

eccentric muscle action Force produced while the muscle is lengthening.

eclampsia Untreated preeclampsia can develop into this potentially fatal complication that involves maternal strokes and seizures.

Ecological or Public Health Model A model in which diseases and other negative health events are viewed as a result of an individual's interaction with his or her social and physical environment.

Ecstasy A club drug that creates feelings of openness and warmth but also raises heart rate and blood pressure.

ectopic pregnancy Implantation of a fertilized egg outside the uterus, usually in a uterine tube; a medical emergency that can end in death from hemorrhage for the mother.

ejaculation The propulsion of semen from the penis.

electrocardiogram (ECG) A record of the electrical activity of the heart; may be measured during a stress test.

ELISA Blood test that detects the presence of antibodies to the HIV virus.

embryo The fertilized egg from conception until the end of two months' development.

embolus A blood clot that becomes dislodged from a blood vessel wall and moves through the circulatory system.

embryo adoption programs A procedure whereby an infertile couple is able to purchase frozen embryos donated by another couple.

embryo transfer Artificial insemination of a donor with the male partner's sperm; after a time, the embryo is transferred from the donor to the female partner's body.

emergency contraceptive pills (ECPs) Drugs taken within three days after intercourse to prevent fertilization or implantation.

emergency minipills   Contraceptive pills containing only progestin that can be taken up to three days after unprotected intercourse.

emotional health   The feeling part of psychosocial health; includes your emotional reactions to life.

emotions   Intensified feelings or complex patterns of feelings we constantly experience.

emphysema   A chronic lung disease in which the tiny air sacs in the lungs are destroyed, making breathing difficult.

enablers   People who knowingly or unknowingly protect addicts from the natural consequences of their behavior.

endemic   Describing a disease that is always present to some degree.

endometriosis   A disorder in which uterine lining tissue establishes itself outside the uterus; the leading cause of infertility in the United States.

endometrium   Soft, spongy matter that makes up the uterine lining.

endorphins   Opiate-like hormones that are manufactured in the human body and contribute to natural feelings of well-being.

energy medicine   Therapies using energy fields, such as magnetic fields or biofields.

environmental tobacco smoke (ETS)   Smoke from tobacco products, including secondhand and mainstream smoke.

enzymes   Organic substances that facilitate chemical reactions, some of which cause bodily changes and destruction of microorganisms.

epidemic   Disease outbreak that affects many people in a community or region at the same time.

epidermis   The outermost layer of the skin.

epididymis   A comma-shaped structure atop the testis where sperm mature.

epilepsy   A neurological disorder caused by abnormal electrical brain activity; can be accompanied by altered consciousness or convulsions.

epinephrine   Also called adrenaline, a hormone that stimulates body systems in response to stress.

episiotomy   A straight incision in the mother's perineum in the area between the vulva and the anus.

erectile dysfunction (ED)   Difficulty in achieving or maintaining a penile erection sufficient for intercourse.

ergogenic aids   Special dietary supplements taken to increase strength, energy, and the ability to work.

ergogenic drug   Substance believed to enhance athletic performance.

erogenous zones   Areas of the body of both males and females that, when touched, lead to sexual arousal.

essential amino acids   Nine of the basic nitrogen-containing building blocks of protein that must be obtained from foods to ensure health.

essential hypertension   Hypertension that cannot be attributed to any known cause.

Essure   A new, nonsurgical sterilization procedure in which a physician places small microcoils into the uterine tubes in order to block them.

estrogens   Hormones secreted by the ovaries; control the menstrual cycle.

ethnoviolence   Violence directed randomly at persons affiliated with a particular, usually ethnic, group.

ethyl alcohol (ethanol)   An addictive drug produced by fermentation and found in many beverages.

eustress   Stress that presents opportunities for personal growth.

exercise   Planned, structured, and repetitive bodily movement done to improve or maintain one or more components of physical fitness.

exercise metabolic rate (EMR)   The energy expenditure that occurs during exercise.

external female genitals   The mons pubis, labia majora and minora, clitoris, urethral and vaginal openings, and the vestibule of the vagina and its glands.

external male genitals   The penis and scrotum.

faith   Belief that helps each person realize a unique purpose in life.

family of origin   People present in the household during a child's first years of life—usually parents and siblings.

fats   Basic nutrients composed of carbon and hydrogen atoms; needed for the proper functioning of cells, insulation of body organs against shock, maintenance of body temperature, and healthy skin and hair.

fellatio   Oral stimulation of a male's genitals.

female condom   A single-use polyurethane sheath for internal use by women.

female orgasmic disorder   The inability to achieve orgasm.

fermentation   The process whereby yeast organisms break down plant sugars to yield ethanol.

fertility   A person's ability to reproduce.

fertility awareness methods (FAMs)   Several types of birth control that require alteration of sexual behavior rather than chemical or physical intervention in the reproductive process.

fertility drugs   Hormones that stimulate ovulation in women who are not ovulating; often responsible for multiple births.

fetal alcohol effects (FAE)   A syndrome describing children with a history of prenatal alcohol exposure but without all the physical or behavioral symptoms of FAS. Among its symptoms are low birth weight, irritability, and possible permanent mental impairment.

fetal alcohol syndrome (FAS)   A disorder that may affect the fetus when the mother consumes alcohol during pregnancy. Among its effects are mental retardation, small head, tremors, and abnormalities of the face, limbs, heart, and brain.

fetus   The term for a developing baby from the third month of pregnancy until birth.

fiber   The indigestible portion of plant foods that helps move foods through the digestive system and softens stools by absorbing water.

fibrillation   A sporadic, quivering pattern of heartbeat, resulting in extreme inefficiency in moving blood through the cardiovascular system.

fibrocystic breast condition   A common, noncancerous condition in which a woman's breasts contain fibrous or fluid-filled cysts.

fibromyalgia   A chronic, rheumatoid-like disorder that can be highly painful and difficult to diagnose.

fight-or-flight response   Physiological arousal response in which the body prepares to combat a real or perceived threat.

flexibility   The measure of the range of motion, or the amount of movement possible, at a particular joint.

flourishing   Living within an optimal range of human functioning—one that connotes goodness, productivity, growth, and resilience.

folate   A type of vitamin B that is believed to decrease levels of homocysteine, an amino acid that has been linked to vascular diseases.

follicle-stimulating hormone (FSH)   Hormone that signals the ovaries to prepare to release eggs and to begin producing estrogens.

food allergy   Overreaction by the body to normally harmless proteins, which are perceived as allergens. In response, the body produces antibodies, triggering allergic symptoms.

food intolerance   Adverse effects resulting when people who lack the digestive chemicals needed to break down certain substances eat those substances.

food irradiation   Treating foods with gamma radiation from radioactive cobalt, cesium, or some other source of X rays to kill microorganisms.

formaldehyde   A colorless, strong-smelling gas released through outgassing; causes respiratory and other health problems.

for-profit (proprietary) hospitals   Hospitals that provide a return on earnings to the investors who own them.

fourth trimester   The first six weeks of an infant's life outside the uterus.

freebase   The most powerful distillate of cocaine.

functional foods   Foods believed to be beneficial and/or to prevent disease.

fungi   A group of plants that lack chlorophyll and do not produce flowers or seeds; several microscopic varieties are pathogenic.

gallbladder disease   A disease caused by repeated irritation of the gallbladder, which leads to the formation of gallstones.

gamete intrafallopian transfer (GIFT)   Procedure in which an egg harvested from the female partner's ovary is placed with the male partner's sperm in her uterine tube, where it is fertilized and then migrates to the uterus for implantation.

gay   Sexual orientation involving primary attraction to people of the same sex; usually but not always applies to men attracted to men.

gender   The psychological condition of being feminine or masculine as defined by the society in which one lives.

genderlect   The "dialect," or individual speech pattern and conversational style, of each gender.

gender identity   Personal sense or awareness of being masculine or feminine, a male or a female.

gender-role stereotypes   Generalizations concerning how males and females should express themselves and the characteristics each possesses.

gender roles   Expression of maleness or femaleness in everyday life.

general adaptation syndrome (GAS)   The pattern followed in the physiological response to stress, consisting of the alarm, resistance, and exhaustion phases.

generalized anxiety disorder (GAD)   A constant sense of worry that may cause restlessness, difficulty in concentrating, tension, and other symptoms.

Generally Recognized as Effective (GRAE)   A list of drugs generally recognized as effective, which work for their intended purpose when used properly.

Generally Recognized as Safe (GRAS)   A list of drugs generally recognized as safe, which seldom cause side effects when used properly.

generic drugs   Drugs marketed by chemical name rather than brand name.

genital herpes   STI caused by the herpes simplex virus.

genital warts   Warts that appear in the genital area or the anus; caused by the human papillomavirus (HPV).

gerontology   The study of individual and collective aging processes.

glaucoma   Elevation of pressure within the eyeball, leading to hardening of the eyeball, impaired vision, and possible blindness.

glycogen   The polysaccharide form in which glucose is stored in the liver and, to a lesser extent, in muscles.

gonadotropin-releasing hormone (GnRH)   Hormone that signals the pituitary gland to release gonadotropins.

gonads   The reproductive organs in a male (testes) or female (ovaries).

gonorrhea   Second most common STD in the United States; if untreated, may cause sterility.

graafian follicle   Mature ovarian follicle that contains a fully developed ovum, or egg.

graded exercise test   A test of aerobic capacity administered by a physician, exercise physiologist, or other trained person; two common forms are the treadmill running test and the stationary bike test.

gratitude   A sense of thankfulness and appreciation for the good things in your life as well as for life's lessons.

greenhouse gases   Gases that contribute to global warming by trapping heat near the Earth's surface.

grief   The state of mental distress that occurs in reaction to significant loss, including one's own impending death, the death of a loved one, or a quasi-death experience.

grief work   The process of accepting the reality of a person's death and coping with memories of the deceased.

group practice   A group of physicians who combine resources, sharing offices, equipment, and staff costs, to render care to patients.

habit   A repeated behavior in which the repetition may be unconscious.

hallucinogens   Substances capable of creating auditory or visual distortions and heightened states.

hangover   The physiological reaction to excessive drinking, including symptoms such as headache, upset stomach, anxiety, depression, diarrhea, and thirst.

happiness   Feeling of contentment created when one's expectations and physical, psychological, and spiritual needs have been met and one enjoys life.

hashish   The sticky resin of the cannabis plant; it is high in THC.

hay fever   A chronic respiratory disorder that is most prevalent when ragweed and flowers bloom.

hazardous waste   Waste that, due to its toxic properties, poses a hazard to humans or to the environment.

health   The ever-changing process of achieving individual potential in the physical, social, emotional, mental, spiritual, and environmental dimensions.

Health Belief Model (HBM)   Model for explaining how beliefs may influence behaviors.

health disparities   Differences in the incidence, prevalence, mortality, and burden of diseases and other health conditions among specific population groups.

health promotion   Combined educational, organizational, policy, financial, and environmental supports to help people reduce negative health behaviors and promote positive change.

healthy life expectancy   The equivalent number of years a newborn can expect to live, based on current rates of illness and mortality.

heart attack   A blockage of normal blood supply to an area in the heart.

heat cramps   Muscle cramps that occur during or following exercise in warm or hot weather.

heat exhaustion   A heat stress illness caused by significant dehydration resulting from exercise in warm or hot conditions; frequent precursor to heatstroke.

heat stroke   A deadly heat stress illness resulting from dehydration and overexertion in warm or hot conditions; can cause body core temperature to rise from normal to 105°F to 110°F in just a few minutes.

heavy episodic (binge) drinking   Drinking for the express purpose of becoming intoxicated; five drinks or more on single occasion for men and four drinks or more for women.

hemochromatosis   Iron toxicity due to excess consumption.

hepatitis   A virally caused disease in which the liver becomes inflamed, producing symptoms such as fever, headache, and possibly jaundice.

herbal preparations   Substances of plant origin that are believed to have medicinal properties.

heroin   An illegally manufactured derivative of morphine, usually injected into the bloodstream.

heterosexual   Experiencing primary attraction to and preference for sexual activity with people of the other sex.

high-density lipoproteins (HDLs)   Compounds that facilitate the transport of cholesterol in the blood to the liver for metabolism and elimination from the body.

histamines   Chemical substances that dilate blood vessels, increase mucous secretions, and produce other symptoms of allergies.

holographic will   A will written in the testator's own handwriting and unwitnessed.

homeopathic medicine   Unconventional Western system of medicine based on the principle that "like cures like."

homeostasis   A balanced physical state in which all the body's systems function smoothly.

homicide   Death that results from intent to injure or kill.

homophobia   Irrational hatred or fear of homosexuals or homosexuality.

homosexual   Experiencing primary attraction to and preference for sexual activity with people of the same sex.

hope   Belief that allows us to look confidently and courageously to the future.

hormonal methods   Contraceptive method that introduces synthetic hormones into the woman's system to prevent ovulation, thicken cervical mucus, or prevent a fertilized egg from implanting.

hormone replacement therapies (HRTs)   Therapies that replace estrogen in postmenopausal women.

hospice   A concept of care for terminally ill patients designed to maximize quality of life.

hostility   The cognitive, affective, and behavioral tendencies toward anger and cynicism.

human chorionic gonadotropin (HCG)   Hormone detectable in blood or urine samples of a mother within the first few weeks of pregnancy; indicates fertilization has taken place.

human immunodeficiency virus (HIV)   The slow-acting virus that causes AIDS.

human papillomavirus (HPV)   A small group of viruses that cause genital warts.

hunger   An inborn physiological response to satisfy nutritional needs.

hydrocarbons   Chemical compounds that contain carbon and hydrogen.

hydrostatic weighing techniques   Method of determining body fat by measuring the amount of water displaced when a person is completely submerged.

hymen   Thin tissue covering the vaginal opening in some women.

hyperglycemia   Elevated blood sugar levels.

hyperlipidemia   Elevated levels of lipids in the blood.

hyperplasia   A condition characterized by an excessive number of fat cells.

hypertension   Sustained elevated blood pressure.

hypertrophy   Increased size (girth) of a muscle; the ability of cells to swell.

hypervitaminosis   A toxic condition caused by overuse of vitamin supplements.

hypnosis   A process that allows people to become unusually responsive to suggestion.

hyponatremia   The overconsumption of plain water, which leads to a dilution of sodium concentration in the blood and can have fatal results.

hypothalamus   An area of the brain located near the pituitary gland. The hypothalamus works in conjunction with the pituitary gland to control reproductive functions and also controls the sympathetic nervous system and directs the stress response.

hypothermia   Potentially fatal condition caused by abnormally low body core temperature.

hysterectomy   Removal of the uterus.

hysterotomy   The surgical removal of the fetus from the uterus.

"I" messages   Messages in which a person takes responsibility for communicating his or her own feelings, thoughts, and beliefs by using statements that begin with "I," not "you."

ice   A potent, inexpensive methamphetamine that has long-lasting effects.

idiopathic   Of unknown cause.

illicit drugs   Drugs that are illegal to possess, produce, or sell.

imagined rehearsal   Practicing, through mental imagery, to become better able to perform an event in actuality.

immunocompetence   The ability of the immune system to respond to assaults.

immunological competence   Ability of the immune system to defend the body from pathogens.

immunotherapy   A process that stimulates the body's own immune system to combat cancer cells.

incidence   The number of new cases.

incomplete proteins   Proteins that are lacking in one or more of the essential amino acids.

incubation period   The time between exposure to a disease and the appearance of symptoms.

induction abortion   A type of abortion in which chemicals are injected into the uterus through the uterine wall; labor begins, and the woman delivers a dead fetus.

infertility   Difficulties in conceiving.

influenza   A common viral disease of the respiratory tract.

inhalants   Products that are sniffed or inhaled in order to produce highs.

inhalation   The introduction of drugs through the nostrils.

inhibited sexual desire (ISD)   Lack of sexual appetite or simply a lack of interest and pleasure in sexual activity.

inhibition   A type of interaction in which the effects of one drug are eliminated or reduced by the presence of another drug at the receptor site.

injection   The introduction of drugs into the body via a hypodermic needle.

insomnia   Difficulty in falling asleep or staying asleep.

insulin   A hormone produced by the pancreas; required by the body for the metabolism of carbohydrates.

intentional injuries   Injuries committed on purpose with intent to harm.

intact dilation and extraction (D&X)   A late-term abortion procedure in which the body of the fetus is extracted up to the head and then the contents of the cranium are aspirated.

interconnectedness   A web of connections, including our relationship to ourselves, to others, and to a larger meaning or purpose in life.

interferon A protein substance produced by the body that aids the immune system by protecting healthy cells.

internal female genitals The vagina, uterus, uterine (fallopian) tubes, and ovaries.

internal male genitals The testes, epididymides, vasa deferentia, ejaculatory ducts, urethra, and accessory glands.

Internet addiction Compulsive use of computer activities such as fantasy games, online shopping, and chat rooms.

intersexuality Not exhibiting exclusively female or male primary and secondary sex characteristics.

interspecies transmission Transmission of disease from humans to animals or from animals to humans.

intervention A planned process of confronting an addict; carried out by significant others.

intestate Dying without a will.

intimate relationships Relationships with family members, friends, and romantic partners, characterized by closeness and understanding.

intolerance A type of interaction in which two or more drugs produce extremely uncomfortable symptoms.

intracytoplasmic sperm injection (ICSI) Fertilization accomplished by injecting a sperm cell directly into an egg.

intrauterine device (IUD) A T-shaped device that is implanted in the uterus to prevent pregnancy.

intravenous injection The introduction of drugs directly into a vein.

inunction The introduction of drugs through the skin.

in vitro fertilization Fertilization of an egg in a nutrient medium and subsequent transfer back to the mother's body.

ionizing radiation Radiation produced by photons having high enough energy to ionize atoms.

irritable bowel syndrome (IBS) Nausea, pain, gas, or diarrhea caused by certain foods or stress.

ischemia Reduced oxygen supply to a body organ or part.

isometric muscle action Force produced without any resulting joint movement.

jealousy An aversive reaction evoked by a real or imagined relationship involving a person's partner and a third person.

ketosis A condition in which the body adapts to prolonged fasting or carbohydrate deprivation by converting body fat to ketones, which can be used as fuel for some brain activity.

labia majora "Outer lips," or folds of tissue covering the female sexual organs.

labia minora "Inner lips," or folds of tissue just inside the labia majora.

lactose intolerance Inability to produce lactase, an enzyme needed to convert milk sugar into glucose.

laxatives Medications used to soften stool and relieve constipation.

leach To dissolve and filter through soil.

leachate Liquid consisting of soluble chemicals that come from garbage and industrial waste that seeps into the water supply from landfills and dumps.

lead A metal found in the exhaust of motor vehicles powered by fuel containing lead and in emissions from lead smelters and processing plants.

learned behavioral tolerance The ability of heavy drinkers to modify behavior so that they appear to be sober even when they have high BAC levels.

learned helplessness Pattern of responding to situations by giving up because of repeated failure in the past.

learned optimism Teaching oneself to think optimistically.

Lea's Shield A one-size-fits-all silicon rubber device that covers the cervix and is available by prescription.

lesbian Sexual orientation involving attraction of women to other women.

leukoplakia A condition characterized by leathery white patches inside the mouth; produced by contact with irritants in tobacco juice.

loss of control Inability to predict reliably whether a particular instance of involvement with the addictive object or behavior will be healthy or damaging.

love Acceptance, affirmation, and respect for the self and others.

low-density lipoproteins (LDLs) Compounds that facilitate the transport of cholesterol in the blood to the body's cells, and cause the cholesterol to build up on artery walls.

low sperm count A sperm count below 60 million sperm per milliliter of semen; the leading cause of infertility in men.

luteinizing hormone (LH) Hormone that signals the ovaries to release an egg and to begin producing progesterone.

lysergic acid diethylamide (LSD) Psychedelic drug causing sensory disruptions; also called acid.

macrominerals Minerals that the body needs in fairly large amounts.

macular degeneration Disease that breaks down the macula, the light-sensitive part of the retina responsible for sharp, direct vision.

magnetic resonance imaging (MRI) A device that uses magnetic fields, radio waves, and computers to generate an image of internal tissues of the body for diagnostic purposes without the use of radiation; can also be used to measure body fat.

mainstream smoke Smoke that is drawn through tobacco while inhaling.

major depressive disorder   Severe depression that entails chronic mood disorder, physical effects such as sleep disturbance and exhaustion, and mental effects such as the inability to concentrate.

male condom   A single-use sheath of thin latex or other material designed to fit over an erect penis and to catch semen upon ejaculation.

malignant   Very dangerous or harmful; refers to a cancerous tumor.

malignant melanoma   A virulent cancer of the melanocytes (pigment-producing cells) of the skin.

managed care   Cost-control procedures used by health insurers to coordinate treatment.

manipulative and body-based practices   Treatments involving manipulation or movement of one or more body parts.

marijuana   Chopped leaves and flowers of *Cannabis indica* or *Cannabis sativa* plants (hemp); a psychoactive stimulant that intensifies reactions to environmental stimuli.

masturbation   Self-stimulation of genitals.

measles   A viral disease that produces symptoms including an itchy rash and a high fever.

Medicaid   Federal–state health insurance program for the poor.

Medical Model   A model in which health status focuses primarily on the individual and a biological or diseased organ perspective.

Medicare   Federal health insurance program for the elderly and the permanently disabled.

meditation   A relaxation technique that involves deep breathing and concentration.

menarche   The first menstrual period.

meningitis   An infection of the meninges, the membranes that surround the brain and spinal cord.

menopause   The permanent cessation of menstruation, generally between the ages of 40 and 60.

menstrual phase   Final phase of the menstrual cycle in which the endometrium sloughs off, and estrogen and progesterone levels decline in response to no fertilization taking place.

mental health   The thinking part of psychosocial health; includes your values, attitudes, and beliefs.

mental illnesses   Disorders that disrupt thinking, feeling, moods, and behaviors, and impair daily functioning.

mescaline   A hallucinogenic drug derived from the peyote cactus.

metabolic syndrome   A group of three or more characteristics, including waist circumference and blood pressure, that can cause metabolic problems that raise CVD risk.

metastasis   Process by which cancer spreads from one area to different areas of the body.

methadone maintenance   A treatment for people addicted to opiates that substitutes methadone, a synthetic narcotic, for the opiate of addiction.

methamphetamine   A powerfully addictive drug that strongly activates certain areas of the brain and affects the central nervous system.

middle-old   People aged 75 to 84.

midwives   Experienced practitioners who assist with pregnancy and delivery.

mifepristone   A steroid hormone that induces abortion by blocking the action of progesterone.

migraine   A condition characterized by localized headaches that possibly result from alternating dilation and constriction of blood vessels.

mind–body medicine   Techniques designed to enhance the mind's ability to affect bodily function and symptoms.

mindfulness   Awareness and acceptance of the reality of the present moment.

minerals   Inorganic, indestructible elements that aid physiological processes.

miscarriage   Loss of the fetus before it is viable; also called spontaneous abortion.

modeling   Learning specific behaviors by watching others perform them.

monogamy   Exclusive sexual involvement with one partner.

mononucleosis   A viral disease that causes pervasive fatigue and other long-lasting symptoms.

monosaccharides   Simple sugars that contain only one molecule of sugar.

mons pubis   Fatty tissue covering the pubic bone in females; in physically mature women, the mons is covered with coarse hair.

morbidity   The relative incidence of disease.

morphine   A derivative of opium; sometimes used by medical practitioners to relieve pain.

mortality   The proportion of deaths to population.

mourning   The culturally prescribed behavior patterns for the expression of grief.

multifactorial disease   Disease caused by interactions of several factors.

multiple sclerosis (MS)   A degenerative neurological disease in which myelin, an insulator of nerves, breaks down.

municipal solid waste   Solid wastes such as durable goods, nondurable goods, containers and packaging, food waste, yard waste, and miscellaneous wastes from residential, commercial, institutional, and industrial sources.

muscle dysmorphia Sometimes referred to as "bigarexia," a pathological preoccupation with being larger and more muscular, which can lead to exercise addiction.

muscular endurance A muscle's ability to exert force repeatedly without fatiguing.

muscular strength The amount of force that a muscle is capable of exerting.

mutant cells Cells that differ in form, quality, or function from normal cells.

myocardial infarction (MI) Heart attack.

narcotic Drugs that induce sleep and relieve pain; primarily the opiates.

naturally acquired active immunity Immunity obtained by exposure to an antigen in the normal course of life.

naturopathic medicine System of medicine that attempts to restore natural processes of the body and promote healing through natural means.

near-infrared interactance (NIR) Fiber-optic measurement of tissue composition.

negative consequences Physical damage, legal trouble, financial problems, academic failure, family dissolution, and other severe problems associated with addiction.

neglect Failure to provide for a child's basic needs such as food, shelter, medical care, and clothing.

neoplasm A new growth of tissue that serves no physiological function and results from uncontrolled, abnormal cellular development.

neurotransmitters Biochemical messengers that exert influence at specific receptor sites on nerve cells.

nicotine The primary stimulant chemical in tobacco products.

nicotine poisoning Symptoms often experienced by beginning smokers, including dizziness, diarrhea, lightheadedness, rapid and erratic pulse, clammy skin, nausea, and vomiting.

nicotine withdrawal Symptoms, including nausea, headaches, irritability, and intense tobacco cravings, suffered by addicted smokers who cease using tobacco.

nitrogen dioxide An amber-colored gas found in smog; can cause eye and respiratory irritations.

nitrous oxide The chemical name for "laughing gas," a substance properly used for surgical or dental anesthesia.

nonassertive communicators Individuals who tend to be shy and inhibited in their communication with others.

nonpoint source pollutants Pollutants that run off or seep into waterways from broad areas of land.

nonprofit (voluntary) hospitals Hospitals run by religious or other humanitarian groups that reinvest their earnings in the hospital to improve health care.

nonsurgical embryo transfer In vitro fertilization of a donor egg by the male partner's (or donor's) sperm and subsequent transfer to the female partner's or another woman's uterus.

nonverbal communication All unwritten and unspoken messages, both intentional and unintentional.

nuclear meltdown An accident that results when the temperature in the core of a nuclear reactor increases enough to melt the nuclear fuel and the containment vessel housing it.

nurse Health practitioner who provides many services for patients and who may work in a variety of settings.

nurse practitioner (NP) Professional nurse with advanced training obtained through either a master's degree program or a specialized nurse practitioner program.

nurturing through avoidance Repeatedly seeking the illusion of relief to avoid unpleasant feelings or situations, a maladaptive way of taking care of emotional needs.

nutraceuticals Term often used interchangeably with *functional foods;* refers to the combined nutritional and pharmaceutical benefit derived through use of foods or food supplements.

nutrients The constituents of food that sustain humans physiologically: proteins, carbohydrates, fats, vitamins, minerals, and water.

nutrition The science that investigates the relationship between physiological function and the essential elements of foods eaten.

NuvaRing A soft, flexible ring inserted into the vagina that releases hormones, preventing pregnancy.

obesogenic The presence of several factors that make people more prone to obesity.

obesity A weight disorder generally defined as an accumulation of fat beyond that considered normal for a person based on age, sex, and body type.

obsession Excessive preoccupation with an addictive object or behavior.

old-old People aged 85 and over.

oncogenes Suspected cancer-causing genes present on chromosomes.

oncologists Physicians who specialize in the treatment of malignancies.

one repetition maximum (1 RM) The amount of weight or resistance that can be lifted or moved once, but not twice; a common measure of strength.

open relationship A relationship in which partners agree that sexual involvement can occur outside the relationship.

ophthalmologist Physician who specializes in the medical and surgical care of the eyes, including prescriptions for glasses.

opium   The parent drug of the opiates; made from the seed pod resin of the opium poppy.

optometrist   Eye specialist whose practice is limited to prescribing and fitting lenses.

oral contraceptives   Pills taken daily for three weeks of the menstrual cycle that prevent ovulation by regulating hormones.

oral ingestion   Intake of drugs through the mouth.

oral surgeon   Dentist who performs surgical procedures to correct problems of the mouth, jaw, and face.

organic   Foods that are grown without use of pesticides, chemicals, or hormones.

orthodontist   Dentist who specializes in the alignment of teeth.

Ortho Evra   A patch that releases hormones similar to those in oral contraceptives; each patch is worn for one week.

osteoarthritis (OA)   Progressive deterioration of bones and joints that has been associated with the "wear-and-tear" theory of aging.

osteopath   General practitioner who receives training similar to a medical doctor's but with an emphasis on the skeletal and muscular systems, often using spinal manipulation as part of treatment.

osteoporosis   A disease characterized by low bone mass and deterioration of bone tissue, which increase risk of fracture.

outpatient (ambulatory) care   Treatment that does not involve an overnight stay in a hospital.

ovarian follicles (egg sacs)   Areas within the ovary in which individual eggs develop.

ovaries   Almond-size organs that house developing eggs and produce hormones.

overload   A condition in which a person feels overly pressured by demands.

over-the-counter (OTC) drugs   Medications that can be purchased without a physician's prescription.

overuse injuries   Injuries that result from the cumulative effects of day-after-day stresses placed on tendons, muscles, and joints.

overweight   Increased body weight in relation to height.

ovulation   The point of the menstrual cycle at which a mature egg ruptures through the ovarian wall.

ozone   A gas formed when nitrogen dioxide interacts with hydrogen chloride.

pairings   Paired associations (such as coffee and a cigarette) that trigger cravings.

pandemic   Global epidemic of a disease.

panic attack   Severe anxiety reaction in which a particular situation, often for unknown reasons, causes terror.

Pap test   A procedure in which cells taken from the cervical region are examined for abnormal cellular activity.

parasitic worms   The largest of the pathogens, most of which are more a nuisance than a threat.

parasympathetic nervous system   Branch of the autonomic nervous system responsible for slowing systems stimulated by the stress response.

Parkinson's disease   A chronic, progressive neurological condition that causes tremors and other symptoms.

particulates   Nongaseous air pollutants.

passive euthanasia   The intentional withholding of treatment that would prolong life.

passive immunity   Antibodies formed in another person or animal, and then given to someone with a weakened immune system such as when a mother passes immunity to her fetus.

pathogens   Disease-causing agents.

pelvic inflammatory disease (PID)   An infection that scars the uterine tubes and consequently blocks sperm migration, causing infertility.

penis   Male sexual organ that releases sperm into the vagina.

peptic ulcer   Damage to the stomach or intestinal lining, usually caused by digestive juices.

perception   The process of filtering and interpreting information gathered through the senses.

perineum   Tissue that forms the "floor" of the pelvic region; it covers a kite-shaped region including the external genitalia and anus.

periodontal diseases   Diseases of the tissue around the teeth.

personal control   Belief that one's own internal resources allow one to control a situation.

pesticides   Chemicals that kill pests.

peyote   A cactus with small "buttons" that, when ingested, produce hallucinogenic effects.

phencyclidine (PCP)   A drug, commonly called "angel dust," that causes hallucinations, delusions, and delirium.

phobia   A deep and persistent fear of a specific object, activity, or situation that results in a compelling desire to avoid the source of the fear.

photochemical smog   The brownish-yellow haze resulting from the combination of hydrocarbons and nitrogen oxides.

physical activity   Any bodily movement that is produced by the contraction of skeletal muscles and that substantially increases energy expenditure.

physical fitness   The ability to perform moderate to vigorous levels of physical activity on a regular basis without excessive fatigue.

physician assistant   A midlevel practitioner trained to handle most standard cases of care.

physiological dependence   The adaptive state that occurs with regular addictive behavior and results in withdrawal syndrome.

phytomedicines   Another name for medicinal herbs, many of which are sold over the counter in Europe.

pica   Iron-deficiency disease characterized by a craving for certain foods and substances.

Pilates   Exercise programs that combine stretching with movement against resistance, aided by devices such as tension springs and heavy rubber bands.

pituitary gland   The endocrine gland located deep within the brain; controls reproductive functions.

placebo effect   An apparent cure or improved state of health brought about by a substance or product that has no medicinal value.

placenta   The network of blood vessels, connected to the umbilical cord, that carries nutrients to the developing infant and carries wastes away.

plaque   Cholesterol buildup on the inner walls of arteries; a major cause of atherosclerosis.

plateau   That point in a weight-loss program at which the dieter finds it difficult to lose more weight.

platelet adhesiveness   Stickiness of red blood cells associated with blood clots.

pneumonia   Bacterially caused disease of the lungs.

point source pollutants   Pollutants that enter waterways at a specific point.

polydrug use   Use of multiple medications or illicit drugs simultaneously.

polychlorinated biphenyls (PCBs)   Toxic chemicals that were once used as insulating materials in high-voltage electrical equipment.

polysaccharides   Complex carbohydrates formed by the combination of long chains of saccharides.

positive reinforcement   Presenting something positive following a behavior that is being reinforced.

positron emission tomography (PET) scan   Method for measuring heart activity by injecting a patient with a radioactive tracer that is scanned electronically to produce a three-dimensional image of the heart and arteries.

postpartum depression   The experience of energy depletion, anxiety, mood swings, and depression that women may feel during the postpartum period.

post-traumatic stress disorder (PTSD)   An acute stress disorder caused by experiencing an extremely traumatic event, such as rape or combat.

power   The ability to make and implement decisions.

preconception care   Medical care received prior to becoming pregnant that helps a woman assess and address potential maternal health.

preeclampsia   A complication in pregnancy characterized by high blood pressure, protein in the urine, and edema.

prejudice   A negative evaluation of an entire group of people that is typically based on unfavorable and often wrong ideas about the group.

premature ejaculation   Ejaculation that occurs prior to or almost immediately following penile penetration of the vagina.

premenstrual dysphoric disorder (PMDD)   Collective name for a group of negative symptoms similar to but more severe than PMS, including severe mood disturbances.

premenstrual syndrome (PMS)   Comprises the mood changes and physical symptoms that occur in some women during the one or two weeks prior to menstruation.

prescription drugs   Medications that can be obtained only with the written prescription of a licensed physician.

prevalence   The number of existing cases.

primary aggression   Goal-directed, hostile self-assertion that is destructive in character.

primary care practitioner   A medical practitioner who treats routine ailments, advises on preventive care, gives general medical advice, and makes appropriate referrals when necessary.

primary prevention   Actions designed to stop problems before they start.

prion   A recently identified pathogen that infects humans and animals; a self-replicating protein-based agent that systematically destroys brain cells.

probiotics   Live microorganisms found in or added to fermented foods; they optimize the bacterial environment in our intestines.

process addictions   Behaviors such as money addiction, work addiction, exercise addiction, and sex addiction that are known to be addictive because they are mood altering.

progesterone   Hormone secreted by the ovaries; helps keep the endometrium developing in order to nourish a fertilized egg; also helps maintain pregnancy.

proliferative phase   First phase of the menstrual cycle.

proof   A measure of the percentage of alcohol in a beverage.

prostaglandin inhibitors   Drugs that inhibit the production and release of prostaglandins associated with arthritis or menstrual pain.

prostate gland   Gland that secretes nutrients and neutralizing fluids into the semen.

prostate-specific antigen (PSA)   An antigen found in prostate cancer patients.

proteins The essential constituents of nearly all body cells; necessary for the development and repair of bone, muscle, skin, and blood; the key elements of antibodies, enzymes, and hormones.

protooncogenes Genes that can become oncogenes under certain conditions.

protozoa Microscopic single-celled organisms.

psilocybin The active chemical found in psilocybe mushrooms; it produces hallucinations.

psychedelics Drugs that distort the processing of sensory information in the brain.

psychiatric nurse specialist A registered nurse specializing in psychiatric practice.

psychiatrist A licensed physician who specializes in treating mental and emotional disorders.

psychoactive drugs Drugs that have the potential to alter mood or behavior.

psychoanalyst A psychiatrist or psychologist with special training in psychoanalysis.

psychoeducation The teaching of crucial psychological skills, giving people knowledge so they can help themselves.

psychological hardiness A personality trait characterized by control, commitment, and challenge.

psychological stress Stress caused by being in an environment perceived to be beyond one's control and endangering one's well-being.

psychologist A person with a PhD degree and training in psychology.

psychoneuroimmunology The science that examines the relationship between the brain and behavior and how this affects the body's immune system.

psychosocial health The mental, emotional, social, and spiritual dimensions of health.

puberty The maturation of the female or male reproduction system.

pubic lice (crabs) Parasites that can inhabit various body areas, especially the genitals.

qi Element of traditional oriental medicine that refers to the vital energy force that courses through the body. When qi is in balance, health is restored.

quasi-death experience A loss or experience that resembles death, in that it involves separation, termination, significant loss, a change of personal identity, and grief.

rabies A viral disease of the central nervous system; often transmitted through animal bites.

radiation absorbed doses (RADs) Units that measure exposure to radioactivity.

radiotherapy The use of radiation to kill cancerous cells.

radon A naturally occurring radioactive gas resulting from the decay of certain radioactive elements.

rape Sexual penetration without the victim's consent.

rational suicide The decision to kill oneself rather than endure constant pain and slow decay.

reactive aggression Emotional reaction brought about by frustrating life experiences.

rebound effects Severe withdrawal effects experienced by users of stimulants, including depression, nausea, and violent behavior.

receptor sites Specialized cells to which drugs can attach themselves.

Recommended Dietary Allowances (RDAs) The average daily intakes of energy and nutrients considered adequate to meet the needs of most healthy people in the United States under usual conditions.

recreational drugs Drugs that contain chemicals that help people relax or socialize; most, but not all, drugs in this category are legal.

Reference Daily Intakes (RDIs) Recommended amounts of 19 vitamins and minerals, also known as micronutrients.

referred pain Pain that is present at one location, although the source of pain is elsewhere.

relapse The tendency to return to the addictive behavior after a period of abstinence.

relative risk A measure of the strength of the relationship between risk factors and the condition being studied, such as a particular cancer.

repetitive stress injury (RSI) An injury to nerves, soft tissue, or joints due to the physical stress of repeated motions.

resiliency (protective factors) An individual's capacity for adapting to change and stressful events in healthy and flexible ways.

resistance exercise program A regular program of exercises designed to improve muscular strength and endurance in the major muscle groups.

respite care The care provided by substitute caregivers to relieve the principal caregiver from his or her continuous responsibility.

resting metabolic rate (RMR) The energy expenditure of the body under BMR conditions plus other daily sedentary activities.

reticular formation An area in the brain stem that is responsible for relaying messages to other areas in the brain.

Rh factor A blood protein related to the production of antibodies. If an Rh-negative mother is pregnant with an Rh-positive fetus, the mother will manufacture antibodies that can kill the fetus, causing miscarriage.

rheumatic heart disease   A heart disease caused by untreated streptococcal infection of the throat.

rheumatoid arthritis   A serious inflammatory joint disease.

RICE   Acronym for the standard first-aid treatment for virtually all traumatic and overuse injuries: rest, ice, compression, and elevation.

rickettsia   A small form of bacteria that live inside other living cells.

risk behaviors   Behaviors that increase susceptibility to negative health outcomes.

route of administration   The manner in which a drug is taken into the body.

rubella (German measles)   A milder form of measles that causes a rash and mild fever in children and may cause damage to a fetus or a newborn baby.

sarcopenia   Age-related loss of muscle mass.

satiety   The feeling of fullness or satisfaction at the end of a meal.

saturated fats   Fats that are unable to hold any more hydrogen in their chemical structure; derived mostly from animal sources; solid at room temperature.

schizophrenia   A mental illness with biological origins that is characterized by irrational behavior, severe alterations of the senses (hallucinations), and often an inability to function in society.

scrotum   Sac of tissue that encloses the testes.

seasonal affective disorder (SAD)   A type of depression that occurs in the winter months, when sunlight levels are low.

Seasonale   An extended-cycle oral contraceptive that causes a woman to menstruate only every three months.

secondary hypertension   Hypertension caused by specific factors, such as kidney disease, obesity, or tumors of the adrenal glands.

secondary prevention (intervention)   Intervention early in the development of a health problem.

secondary sex characteristics   Characteristics associated with gender but not directly related to reproduction, such as vocal pitch, degree of body hair, and location of fat deposits.

secondhand smoke (sidestream smoke)   The cigarette, pipe, or cigar smoke breathed by nonsmokers.

secretory phase   Second phase of the menstrual cycle during which the endometrium continues to prepare for a fertilized egg.

self-disclosure   The process of revealing one's inner thoughts, feelings, and beliefs to another person.

self-efficacy   Belief in one's ability to perform a task successfully.

self-esteem   Sense of self-respect or self-confidence.

self-nurturance   Developing individual potential through a balanced and realistic appreciation of self-worth and ability.

self-talk   The customary manner of thinking and talking to yourself, which can impact your self-image.

semen   Fluid containing sperm and nutrient fluids that increase sperm viability and neutralize vaginal acid.

seminal vesicles   Storage areas for sperm where nutrient fluids are added to them.

senility   A term associated with judgment and orientation problems and the loss of memory occurring in a small percentage of the elderly.

serial monogamy   A series of monogamous sexual relationships.

setpoint theory   A theory of obesity causation that suggests that fat storage is determined by a thermostatic mechanism in the body that acts to maintain a specific amount of body weight.

sexual abuse of children   Sexual interaction between a child and an adult or older child; includes, but is not limited to, sexually suggestive conversations, inappropriate kissing, touching, petting, and oral, anal, or vaginal intercourse.

sexual addiction   Compulsive involvement in sexual activity.

sexual assault   Any act in which one person is sexually intimate with another person without that person's consent.

sexual aversion disorder   Type of desire dysfunction characterized by sexual phobias and anxiety about sexual contact.

sexual dysfunction   Problems associated with achieving sexual satisfaction.

sexual fantasies   Sexually arousing thoughts and dreams.

sexual harassment   Any form of unwanted sexual attention.

sexual identity   Recognition of oneself as a sexual being; a composite of biological sex characteristics, gender identity, gender roles, and sexual orientation.

sexual orientation   A person's enduring emotional, romantic, sexual, or affectionate attraction to other persons.

sexual performance anxiety   A condition of sexual difficulties caused by anticipating some sort of problem with the sex act.

sexually transmitted infections (STIs)   Infectious diseases transmitted via some form of intimate, usually sexual, contact.

shaping   Using a series of small steps to gradually achieve a particular goal.

sick building syndrome (SBS)   Problem that exists when 80 percent of a building's occupants report maladies that tend to lessen or vanish when they leave the building.

sickle-cell anemia   Genetic disease commonly found among African Americans; results in organ damage and premature death.

simple rape Rape by one person known to the victim that does not involve physical beating or use of a weapon.

simple sugars A major type of carbohydrate, which provide short-term energy.

sinoatrial node (SA node) Cluster of electric-generating cells that serves as a form of natural pacemaker for the heart.

situational inducement Attempt to influence a behavior through situations and occasions that are structured to exert control over that behavior.

skinfold caliper technique A method of determining body fat whereby folds of skin and fat at various points on the body are grasped between thumb and forefinger and measured with calipers.

sleep apnea Disorder in which a person has numerous episodes of breathing stoppage during a normal night's sleep.

slow-acting viruses Viruses having long incubation periods and causing slowly progressive symptoms.

snuff A powdered form of tobacco that is sniffed and absorbed through the mucous membranes in the nose or placed inside the cheek and sucked.

social bonds Degree and nature of interpersonal contacts.

social death A seemingly irreversible situation in which a person is not treated like an active member of society.

social health Aspect of psychosocial health that includes interactions with others, ability to use social supports, and ability to adapt to various situations.

social learning theory Theory that people learn behaviors by watching role models—parents, caregivers, and significant others.

social phobia A phobia characterized by fear and avoidance of social situations.

social physique anxiety (SPA) A desire to look good that has a destructive effect on a person's ability to function effectively socially.

social support Network of people and services with whom you share ties and get support.

social worker A person with an MSW degree and clinical training.

socialization Process by which a society communicates behavioral expectations to its individual members.

solo practitioner Physician who renders care to patients independently of other practitioners.

spermatogenesis The development of sperm.

spermicides Substances designed to kill sperm.

spirituality A belief in a unifying force that gives meaning to life and transcends the purely physical or personal dimensions of existence.

sponge A contraceptive device, made of polyurethane foam and containing nonoxynol 9, that fits over the cervix to create a barrier against sperm.

spontaneous remission The disappearance of symptoms without any apparent cause or treatment.

stalking The willful, repeated, and malicious following, harassing, or threatening of another person.

staphylococci Round, gram-positive bacteria, usually found in clusters.

static stretching Techniques that gradually lengthen a muscle to an elongated position (to the point of discomfort) and hold that position for 10 to 30 seconds.

sterilization Permanent fertility control achieved through surgical procedures.

stillbirth The birth of a dead baby.

strain The wear and tear sustained by the body and mind in adjusting to or resisting a stressor.

streptococcus A round bacterium, usually found in chain formation.

stress Mental and physical responses to change.

stress inoculation Newer stress management technique in which a person consciously tries to prepare ahead of time for potential stressors.

stressor A physical, social, or psychological event or condition that requires our bodies to make an adjustment.

stroke A condition occurring when the brain is damaged by disrupted blood supply.

subjective well-being (SWB) That uplifting feeling of inner peace and wonder that we call happiness.

sudden cardiac death Death that occurs as a result of abrupt, profound loss of heart function.

sudden infant death syndrome (SIDS) The sudden death of an infant under one year of age for no apparent reason.

suicidal ideation A desire to die and thoughts about suicide.

sulfur dioxide A yellowish brown gaseous by-product of the burning of fossil fuels.

Superfund Fund established under the Comprehensive Environmental Response Compensation and Liability Act to be used for cleaning up toxic waste dumps.

suppositories Mixtures of drugs and a waxy medium designed to melt at body temperature that are inserted into the anus or vagina.

sympathetic nervous system Branch of the autonomic nervous system responsible for stress arousal.

sympathomimetics Food substances that can produce stresslike responses.

synergism Interaction of two or more drugs that produces more profound effects than would be expected if the drugs were taken separately.

synesthesia A drug-created effect in which sensory messages are incorrectly assigned—for example, the user hears a taste or smells a sound.

syphilis One of the most widespread STIs; characterized by distinct phases and potentially serious results.

systemic lupus erythematosus (SLE, or lupus) A disease in which the immune system attacks the body, producing antibodies that destroy or injure organs such as the kidneys, brain, and heart.

systolic pressure The upper number in the fraction that measures blood pressure, indicating pressure on the walls of the arteries when the heart contracts.

tai chi An ancient Chinese form of exercise widely practiced in the West today that promotes balance, coordination, stretching, and meditation.

tar A thick, brownish substance condensed from particulate matter in smoked tobacco.

target heart rate Calculated as a percentage of maximum heart rate (220 minus age); heart rate (pulse) is taken during aerobic exercise to check if exercise intensity is at the desired level (e.g., 60 percent of maximum heart rate).

temperature inversion A weather condition occurring when a layer of cool air is trapped under a layer of warmer air.

teratogenic Causing birth defects; may refer to drugs, environmental chemicals, X rays, or diseases.

terrorism The use of unlawful force or violence against persons or property to intimidate or coerce a government, the civilian population, or any segment thereof in furtherance of political or social objectives.

tertiary prevention Treatment and/or rehabilitation efforts.

testator A person who leaves a will or testament at death.

testes Two organs, located in the scrotum, that manufacture sperm and produce hormones.

testosterone The male sex hormone manufactured in the testes.

tetrahydrocannabinol (THC) The chemical name for the active ingredient in marijuana.

thanatology The study of death and dying.

Theory of Reasoned Action Model for explaining the importance of our intentions in determining behaviors.

thrombolysis Injection of an agent to dissolve clots and restore some blood flow, thereby reducing the amount of tissue that dies from ischemia.

thrombus Blood clot attached to the wall of a blood vessel.

tinctures Herbal extracts usually combined with grain alcohol to prevent spoilage.

T lymphocytes (T cells) Specialized white blood cells that are manufactured in the thymus, a multilobed organ that lies behind the breastbone. There are several types of T cells that aid in the immune response.

Tolerable Upper Intake Level (UL) The highest amount of a nutrient that an individual can safely consume every day without risking adverse health effects.

tolerance Phenomenon in which progressively larger doses of a drug or more intense involvement in a behavior are needed to produce the desired effects.

total body electrical conductivity (TOBEC) Technique using an electromagnetic force field to assess relative body fat.

toxic shock syndrome (TSS) A potentially life-threatening disease that occurs when specific bacterial toxins are allowed to multiply unchecked in wounds or through improper use of tampons or diaphragms.

toxins Poisonous substances produced by certain microorganisms that cause various diseases.

toxoplasmosis A disease caused by an organism found in cat feces that, when contracted by a pregnant woman, may result in stillbirth or an infant with mental retardation or birth defects.

trace minerals Minerals that the body needs in only very small amounts.

traditional Chinese medicine (TCM) Comprehensive system of diagnosis and treatment in which dietary change, touch, massage, medicinal teas, and other herbal medicines are used extensively.

***trans* fatty acids (*trans* fats)** Fatty acids that are produced when polyunsaturated oils are hydrogenated to make them more solid.

transgendered When one's gender identity does not match one's biological sex.

transient ischemic attacks (TIAs) Brief interruptions of the blood supply to the brain that cause only temporary impairment; often an indicator of impending major stroke.

transition The process during which the cervix becomes nearly fully dilated and the head of the fetus begins to move into the birth canal.

transsexuality Condition in which a person is psychologically of one sex but physically of the other.

traumatic injuries Injuries that are accidental in nature, which occur suddenly and violently (including fractured bones, ruptured tendons, and sprained ligaments).

trichomoniasis Protozoan infection characterized by foamy, yellowish discharge and unpleasant odor.

triglycerides The most common form of fat in the body; excess calories consumed are converted into triglycerides and stored as body fat.

trimester A three-month segment of pregnancy; used to describe specific developmental changes that occur in the embryo or fetus.

triple marker screen (TMS) A maternal blood test that can be used to help identify fetuses with certain birth defects and genetic abnormalities.

trust The degree of confidence felt in a relationship.

tubal ligation Sterilization of the female that involves the cutting and tying off or cauterizing of the uterine tubes.

tuberculosis (TB) A disease caused by bacterial infiltration of the respiratory system.

tumor A neoplasmic mass that grows more rapidly than surrounding tissue.

ulcerative colitis An inflammatory disorder that affects the mucous membranes of the large intestine, producing bloody diarrhea.

unintentional injuries Injuries committed without intent to harm.

unsaturated fats Fats that do have room for more hydrogen in their chemical structure; derived mostly from plants; liquid at room temperature.

urethral opening The opening through which urine is expelled.

urinary incontinence Inability to control urination.

U.S. Recommended Daily Allowances (USRDAs) Dietary guidelines developed by the Food and Drug Administration (FDA) and the U.S. Department of Agriculture.

uterine (fallopian) tubes Tubes that extend from near the ovaries to the uterus.

uterus (womb) Hollow, pear-shaped muscular organ whose function is to contain the developing fetus.

vaccination Inoculation with killed or weakened pathogens or similar, less dangerous antigens in order to prevent or lessen the effects of some disease.

vacuum aspiration The use of gentle suction to remove fetal tissue from the uterus.

vagina The passage in females leading from the vulva into the uterus.

vaginal intercourse The insertion of the penis into the vagina.

vaginismus A state in which the vaginal muscles contract so forcefully that penetration cannot be accomplished.

vaginitis Set of symptoms characterized by vaginal itching, swelling, and burning.

variant sexual behavior A sexual behavior that is not engaged in by most people.

vas deferens A tube that stores and transports sperm toward the penis.

vasectomy Sterilization of the male that involves the cutting and tying off of both ductus deferentia.

vasocongestion The engorgement of the genital organs with blood.

vegetarian A term with a variety of meanings: vegans avoid all foods of animal origin; lacto-vegetarians avoid flesh foods but eat dairy products; ovo-vegetarians avoid flesh foods but eat eggs; lacto-ovo-vegetarians avoid flesh foods but eat both dairy products and eggs; pesco-vegetarians avoid meat but eat fish, dairy products, and eggs; semivegetarians eat chicken, fish, dairy products, and eggs.

veins Vessels that carry blood back to the heart from other regions of the body.

ventricles The two lower chambers of the heart, which pump blood through the blood vessels.

venules Branches of the veins.

very low-calorie diets (VLCDs) Diets with a daily caloric value of 400 to 700 calories.

violence A set of behaviors that produce injuries, as well as the outcomes of these behaviors (the injuries themselves).

virulent Strong enough to overcome host resistance and cause disease.

viruses Minute parasitic microbes that live inside another cell.

visualization The creation of mental images to promote relaxation.

vitamins Essential organic compounds that promote growth and reproduction and help maintain life and health.

vulva Region that encloses the female's external genitalia.

waist circumference measurement Assessment of healthy weight by measurement of the circumference of the waist.

waist-to-hip ratio Ratio that indicates increased risks due to unhealthy fat distribution.

wake (viewing) Displaying of the deceased to formalize last respects and increase social support of the bereaved.

wellness The achievement of the highest level of health possible in each of several dimensions.

Western blot A more accurate test than ELISA to confirm the presence of HIV antibodies.

withdrawal A method of contraception that involves withdrawing the penis from the vagina before ejaculation. Also called *coitus interruptus*. Also, a series of temporary physical and biopsychosocial symptoms that occur when the addict abruptly abstains from an addictive chemical or behavior.

Women's Health Initiative (WHI)   National study of postmenopausal women conducted in conjunction with the NIH mandate for equal research priorities for women's health issues.

work addiction   The compulsive use of work and the work persona to fulfill needs for intimacy, power, and success.

yoga   A variety of Indian traditions geared toward self-discipline and the realization of unity; includes forms of exercise widely practiced in the West today that promote balance, coordination, flexibility, and meditation.

young-old   People aged 65 to 74.

yo-yo diets   Cycles in which people repeatedly gain weight, and then starve themselves to lose weight. This lowers their BMR, which makes regaining weight even more likely.

xanthines   The chemical family of stimulants to which caffeine belongs.

INDEX

Page references followed by *fig* indicate an illustrated figure; followed by *t* indicate a table; followed by *p* indicate a photograph.